W9-AER-334

# Med-Surg **Success**

## NCLEX®-Style Q&A Review

**FOURTH EDITION**

Q&A | Course Review | NCLEX®-Prep

# Davis's SUCCESS SERIES

- Fundamentals
- Pharmacology
- Pediatrics
- Psychiatric Mental Health Nursing
- Maternal and Newborn
- Med-Surg
- Test Prep

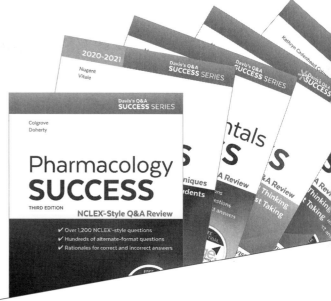

★ ★ ★ ★ ★
"My test scores definitely went up after I found these books."
—Sakin M.

★ ★ ★ ★ ★
"My #1 go-to the week before ANY exam!"
—Andrea A.

★ ★ ★ ★ ★
"The rationales are the reason I love the books in the Davis Success series."
—Lynn C.

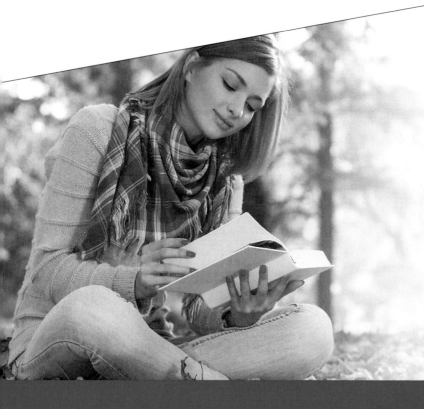

## SAVE 20% + FREE SHIPPING

Use Promo Code: DAVIS20

## Order Today!

FADavis.com

Promotion subject to change without notice.
Offer valid for individual purchases from FADavis.com in the U.S. only.

# Med-Surg **Success**

## NCLEX®-Style Q&A Review

**FOURTH EDITION**

Christi D. Doherty, DNP, MSN, RNC-OB, CNE, CHSE

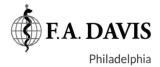

**F. A. DAVIS**

Philadelphia

F. A. Davis Company
1915 Arch Street
Philadelphia, PA 19103
www.fadavis.com

Copyright © 2021 by F.A. Davis Company

Copyright © 2021 by F.A. Davis Company. All rights reserved. This book is protected by copyright. No part of it may be reproduced, stored in a retrieval system, or transmitted in any form or by any means, electronic, mechanical, photocopying, recording, or otherwise, without written permission from the publisher.

Printed in the United States of America

Last digit indicates print number: 10 9 8 7 6 5 4 3 2 1

Acquisitions Editor, Nursing: Jacalyn Sharp
Content Project Manager: Sean P. West
Electronic Project Manager: Sandra A. Glennie
Design and Illustrations Manager: Carolyn O'Brien

As new scientific information becomes available through basic and clinical research, recommended treatments and drug therapies undergo changes. The author(s) and publisher have done everything possible to make this book accurate, up to date, and in accord with accepted standards at the time of publication. The author(s), editors, and publisher are not responsible for errors or omissions or for consequences from application of the book, and make no warranty, expressed or implied, in regard to the contents of the book. Any practice described in this book should be applied by the reader in accordance with professional standards of care used in regard to the unique circumstances that may apply in each situation. The reader is advised always to check product information (package inserts) for changes and new information regarding dose and contraindications before administering any drug. Caution is especially urged when using new or infrequently ordered drugs.

**Library of Congress Cataloging-in-Publication Data**

Names: Doherty, Christi D., author.
Title: Med-surg success: NCLEX®-style Q&A review/Christi D. Doherty.
Description: Fourth edition. | Philadelphia: F.A. Davis, [2021] | Preceded
  by Med-surg success/Kathryn Cadenhead Colgrove. Third edition. 2017. |
  Includes bibliographical references and index.
Identifiers: LCCN 2020037437 (print) | LCCN 2020037438 (ebook) | ISBN
  9781719640534 (paperback) | ISBN 9781719642972 (ebook)
Subjects: MESH: Nursing | Nursing Care | Problem Solving | Test Taking
  Skills | Examination Questions
Classification: LCC RT55 (print) | LCC RT55 (ebook) | NLM WY 18.2 | DDC
  610.73076—dc23
LC record available at https://lccn.loc.gov/2020037437
LC ebook record available at https://lccn.loc.gov/2020037438

Authorization to photocopy items for internal or personal use, or the internal or personal use of specific clients, is granted by F. A. Davis Company for users registered with the Copyright Clearance Center (CCC) Transactional Reporting Service, provided that the fee of $.25 per copy is paid directly to CCC, 222 Rosewood Drive, Danvers, MA 01923. For those organizations that have been granted a photocopy license by CCC, a separate system of payment has been arranged. The fee code for users of the Transactional Reporting Service is: 978-0-8036-4297-2/20 0 + $.25.

*Thank you to all the nursing students, nursing faculty, and nursing colleagues
I have had the privilege to work with during my career. Thank you to Jacalyn
Sharp, Acquisitions Editor at F. A. Davis, and your team for the support
and guidance on this project. Finally, thank you to Kathy Colgrove for your
mentorship and friendship.*

*This book is dedicated to my mother, Ellen Shomette, who showed me that hard
work and perseverance could make dreams come true; to my mother-in-law, Clara
June Doherty, RN, who lived her life with such kindness and generosity,
an inspiration for self-improvement every day; and to my husband and best friend,
Kevin Doherty, thank you for all the support and encouragement in all my
endeavors. You make everything worthwhile.*

—CHRISTI D. DOHERTY

# Contributor

**Kevin D. Doherty, BS, RDCS, RDMS, RVT**
Cardiovascular Sonographer
Baylor Scott and White Heart and Vascular
    Hospital
Dallas, Texas

# Table of Contents

# Test Taking

## INTRODUCTION

This book is part of a series of books published by the F.A. Davis Company designed to assist the student nurse in being successful in nursing school. This book focuses on clinical judgment and critical thinking in regard to test taking. There are the usual test questions found in review books, but the test taker will also find Test-Taking Hints in 19 of 20 chapters. Table 1-1 indicates the breakdown of the content found on the NCLEX-RN®. This book has attempted to follow this test plan. The 2019 NCLEX-RN® test plan includes additional types of alternative test questions. The end of each chapter includes these new graphic types of test questions.

The most important aspect of taking any examination is to become knowledgeable about the subject matter the test will cover. **There is no substitute for studying the material**.

Book one of this series—*Fundamentals Success: A Q&A Review Applying Critical Thinking to Test Taking*, 5th edition, by Patricia M. Nugent and Barbara A. Vitale—defines critical thinking and the RACE model for applying critical thinking to test-taking skills. The specific topics in that volume will not be repeated in this book. This book will assist the test taker to apply critical-thinking skills directly to the questions found on nursing examinations.

## GUIDELINES FOR USING THIS BOOK

This book is designed to assist the nursing student when preparing for and taking medical-surgical examinations as well as the graduate nurse who is preparing to take the national licensure examination. The book is divided into chapters according to body systems and includes chapters on pharmacology, end-of-life issues, emergency nursing, and alternative therapy, and a 100-question final examination. Chapters 2 through 18 are further divided into disease processes to more easily help the test taker identify specific content. A comprehensive final, including content areas and disease processes, is included at the end of each chapter.

In the Answers and Rationales sections of the chapters, an explanation for the correct answer and the incorrect distracters is provided. In Chapters 2 through 18, a Test-Taking Hint is provided for every question in the content area. The Test-Taking Hint provides extra advice on how to analyze each question to choose the correct answer. There are no test-taking hints provided for the comprehensive final examinations. In Chapter 19, the pharmacology chapter, the test-taking hints are discussed at the beginning of the chapter.

## PREPARING FOR CLASS

In preparation for attending class on a specific topic, the student must read the assignment and prepare notes to take to class. Any information the student does not understand should be highlighted in order to clarify the information if the instructor does not cover it in class or if, after the class, the student still does not understand the concept.

## TABLE 1–1 Client Needs Categories and Percentage of Items

| Client Needs | Percentage of Items |
|---|---|
| *SAFE AND EFFECTIVE CARE ENVIRONMENT* | |
| • Management of Care | 17–23% |
| • Safety and Infection Control | 9–15% |
| *HEALTH PROMOTION AND MAINTENANCE* | 6–12% |
| *PSYCHOSOCIAL INTEGRITY* | 6–12% |
| *PHYSIOLOGICAL INTEGRITY* | |
| • Basic Care and Comfort | 6–12% |
| • Pharmacological and Parenteral Therapies | 12–18% |
| • Reduction of Risk Potential | 9–15% |
| • Physiological Adaption | 11–17% |

The National Council of State Boards of Nursing, Inc., Chicago, IL, with permission.

A piece of paper, Word document, or study guide, divided into categories of information, should be sufficient for most disease processes. If the student is unable to limit the information to one page, the student is probably not being discriminating when reading. The idea is not to rewrite the textbook but rather to glean from the textbook the important, need-to-know information.

### Sample Study Guide

| Medical Diagnosis: | Definition: | |
|---|---|---|
| *DIAGNOSTIC TESTS:* | *SIGNS AND SYMPTOMS:* | *NURSING INTERVENTIONS:* |
| (List normal values) | | (Include teaching) |
| *PROCEDURES AND NURSING IMPLICATIONS:* | *MEDICAL INTERVENTIONS:* | |

Complete the study guide using one color pen, but take a different color pen or a pencil to class along with a highlighter and the study guide. Whatever the instructor emphasizes during the class should be highlighted in the study guide. Whatever information the instructor emphasizes that the student did not include in the study guide should be written in a different color pen or pencil. The student should reread the information in the textbook that was covered in class but not included in the study guide. When studying for the examination, the student can identify the information obtained from the textbook and the information obtained in class. The information in the study guide that is highlighted represents information that the student thought was important from reading the textbook, and the instructor emphasized during the class. This is important, need-to-know information for the examination. Please note, however, the instructor may not emphasize laboratory tests and values but still expect the student to realize the importance of this information.

The study guides can be generated on a laptop or tablet. The same highlighting and color-coding system can be used in an electronic format. The student can take the completed study guides or tablet with them to be reviewed during children's sports practices, when waiting for an appointment, or at any time the student finds a minute. This is making the most of limited time. The study guides should also be carried to clinical assignments to use when caring for clients in the hospital.

Students who prepare before attending class will find the information covered in class easier to understand, and as a result, those students will score higher on examinations. Being prepared allows the student to listen to the instructor, participate in the active learning activities, and not sit in class trying to write every word spoken.

The student should recognize the importance of the instructor's hints during the preclass preparation activities. The instructor may emphasize information in a preclass PowerPoint presentation by highlighting areas, repeating information, or emphasizing a particular fact, which usually means the instructor thinks the information is very important. *Important information usually finds its way onto tests at some point.*

## PREPARING FOR AN EXAMINATION

### Study

The student should plan to study 3 hours for every 1 hour of class. For example, a course that is 3 hours of credit requires 9 hours of study each week. Cramming immediately before the test usually indicates the student is at risk of being unsuccessful on the examination. The information acquired during cramming is not learned and will be quickly forgotten. Nursing examinations include material required by the registered nurse when caring for clients at the bedside. The knowledge required to care for clients builds on *ALL* previous knowledge as well as information newly acquired.

### Understanding What the Test Taker Does Not Know

The first time many students realize they do not understand the information is during the examination, when it is too late. Nursing examinations contain high-level application questions requiring the test taker not only to have memorized information but also to be able to interpret the data and make a judgment as to the correct course of action. Test takers must recognize their own areas of weakness before seeing an examination for the first time. This book is designed to assist test takers in identifying their areas of weakness before the examination.

Two to 3 days before the examination, the student should compose a practice test and take the examination. If a topic of study proves to be an area of strength, as evidenced by selecting the correct answer to the question, then the student should proceed to study other areas identified as weaknesses. Missing the question identifies a weakness. If the test taker does not understand the rationale for the correct answer, the test taker should read the appropriate textbook and try to understand the rationale for the correct answer. The test taker should be cautious about reading rationales for the incorrect distracters. During the examination, the test taker may remember reading the information but could become confused about whether the information applied to the correct answer or to the incorrect distracter.

### The Night Before the Exam

The night before the examination, the student should quit studying by 6:00 to 7:00 p.m. The student should do something fun or relaxing up until bedtime and get a good night's rest before taking the examination. Studying until bedtime or in an all-night cram session leaves the student tired and sleepy during the examination, which is when the mind should be at its top performance.

### The Day of the Exam

The student should eat a meal before an examination; a source of carbohydrate for energy along with a protein source makes a good meal. Skipping a meal before the examination leaves the brain without nourishment. A bagel with peanut butter and milk is an excellent meal; it provides a source of protein and sustained release of carbohydrates. Do not eat donuts or drink soft drinks. The energy from these is quickly available but will not last throughout the time required for an examination. Excessive fluid intake may cause the need to urinate during the examination and make it hard for the test taker to concentrate.

## Test-Taking Anxiety

If the student has test-taking anxiety, then it is advisable for the student to arrive at the testing site 45 minutes before the examination. Find a seat for the examination and reserve a desk. The student should walk for 15 minutes at a fast pace away from the testing site, and at the end of the 15 minutes, the student should turn and walk back. This exercise literally walks anxiety away.

If other test takers getting up and leaving the room bothers the test taker, the test taker should try to get a desk away from the group, in front of the room or facing a wall. Most schools allow students to wear earplugs during a test if noise bothers the student. Most NCLEX-RN® test sites will provide earplugs if the graduate requests them.

## TAKING THE EXAM

During the examination, if the test taker finds a question that contains totally unknown information, and the test taker is taking a pencil-and-paper test, the test taker should circle the question and skip it. Another question may help to answer the skipped question. Delaying moving on and worrying over a question will place the next few questions in jeopardy. The mind will not let go of the worry, and the test taker may miss important information in the subsequent questions.

During the NCLEX-RN® computerized test, the test taker should take some deep breaths and then select an answer. The computer examination typically does not allow the test taker to return to a question.

Test takers who become anxious during an examination should stop, put their hands in their lap, shut their eyes, and take a minimum of five deep breaths before resuming the examination. The test taker must become aware of personal body signals that indicate increasing stress levels. Some people get gastrointestinal symptoms, and others feel a tightening of muscles.

## Test-Taking Hints for the Computerized NCLEX-RN® Examination

A computer administers the NCLEX-RN® examination. Here are some test-taking hints that specifically apply to examination by computer.

- The test is composed of 75 to 265 questions. The computer determines with a 95% certainty that the test taker's ability is above the passing standard before the examination will conclude. The minimum number of questions the test taker will receive is 75 questions.
- The examination comprises multiple-choice questions and may include several types of alternate questions:
  - Fill-in-the-blank questions, which test math abilities.
  - **"Select all that apply"** questions, which require the test taker to select more than one distracter as the correct answer. In a "Select All" question, a minimum of two answers will be correct, and in some questions, all of the options may be correct. This is a new revision of the NCLEX-RN® examination. Previously, there had to be at least one incorrect option.
  - Click-and-drag questions, which require the test taker to identify a specific area of the body as the correct answer.
  - An audio component, which requires the test taker to identify body sounds.

Examples of most of these types of questions are included in this book. In an attempt to illustrate the click-and-drag questions, this book has pictures with lines to delineate A, B, C, and D. The fifth type of question, which prioritizes the answers 1, 2, 3, 4, and 5 in order of when the nurse would implement the intervention, is also included in this book.

- Test takers should not be overly concerned if they possess rudimentary computer skills. The test taker must use the mouse to select the correct answer. Every question asks for a confirmation before being submitted as the answer.
- Other than typing pertinent personal information, the test taker must be able to type numbers and use the drop-down computer calculator. The test taker can request an erase slate to calculate math problems by hand.
- The test taker should practice taking tests on the computer before taking the NCLEX-RN® examination. Many opportunities are available online to practice test taking.
- The test taker should refer to the Web site for the National Council of State Boards of Nursing (http://www.ncsbn.org) for additional information on the NCLEX-RN® examination.

## Understanding the Types of Nursing Questions

### COMPONENTS OF A MULTIPLE-CHOICE QUESTION

A multiple-choice question is called an **item**. Each item has two parts. The **stem** is the part that contains the information that identifies the topic and its parameters and then asks a question. The second part consists of one or more possible responses, which are called **options**. One of the options is the **correct answer**, and the others are the wrong answers, called **distracters**.

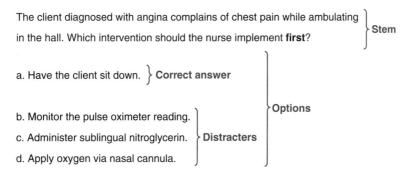

### COGNITIVE LEVELS OF NURSING QUESTIONS

Questions on nursing examinations reflect a variety of thinking processes that nurses use when caring for clients. These thinking processes are part of the cognitive domain, and they progress from the simple to the complex, from the concrete to the abstract, and from the tangible to the intangible. There are four types of thinking processes represented by nursing questions:

- Remembering Questions—The emphasis is on recalling remembered information.
- Understanding Questions—The emphasis is on understanding the meaning and intent of remembered information.
- Application Questions—The emphasis is on remembering understood information and utilizing the information in new situations.
- Analysis Questions—The emphasis is on comparing and contrasting a variety of elements of information.

## THE RACE MODEL: THE APPLICATION OF CRITICAL THINKING TO MULTIPLE-CHOICE QUESTIONS

Answering a test question is like participating in a race. Of course, the test taker wants to come in first and be the winner. However, the thing to remember about a race is that success is not based just on speed but also on strategy and tactics. The same is true about nursing examinations. Although speed may be a variable that must be considered when taking a timed test so that the amount of time spent on each question is factored into the test strategy, the emphasis on RACE is the use of critical-thinking techniques to answer multiple-choice questions. The **RACE** model presented next is a critical-thinking strategy to use when answering nursing multiple-choice questions. If the test taker follows the RACE Model every time when examining a test question, its use will become second nature. This methodical approach will improve the test taker's abilities to critically analyze a test question and improve the chances of selecting the correct answer.

The RACE model has four steps for answering a test question. The best way to remember the four steps is to refer to the acronym RACE.

**R** - **R**ecognize what information is in the stem.
  • **R**ecognize the keywords in the stem.
  • **R**ecognize who the client is in the stem.
  • **R**ecognize what the topic is about.

**A** - **A**sk what is the question asking?
  • **A**sk what keywords in the stem indicate the need for a response?
  • **A**sk what is the question asking the nurse to implement?

**C** - **C**ritically analyze the options in relation to the question asked in the stem.
  • **C**ritically scrutinize each option in relation to the information in the stem.
  • **C**ritically identify a rationale for each option.
  • **C**ritically compare and contrast the options in relation to the information in the stem and their relationships to one another.

**E** - **E**liminate as many options as possible.
  • **E**liminate one option at a time.

The text *Fundamentals Success: A Q&A Review Applying Critical Thinking to Test Taking*, 5th edition, by Patricia M. Nugent and Barbara A. Vitale, includes an in-depth discussion exploring the RACE model in relation to the thinking processes as represented in multiple-choice nursing questions.

## CONCEPT-FOCUSED QUESTIONS

A number of states and nursing programs within the states have chosen to use a *concept-based* curriculum approach to nursing education, such as Oregon, North Carolina, Texas, and many more. This is a change from the disease-based model of nursing education that followed a disease-based approach. Over the years of curriculum development in nursing, the number of topics has expanded under the disease-based curriculum to become burdensome and unwieldy for students and faculty. These schools have transitioned to teaching "concepts" of client needs, utilizing specific exemplars of commonly occurring disease processes to represent the concept to students. This is not a new idea but rather a return to a previous method of the nursing curriculum.

For example, if the curriculum being taught is **Oxygenation**, it would be taught using the exemplars of pneumonia or chronic obstructive pulmonary disease. Under the concept, there are similarities in nursing assessment guidelines and nursing interventions. Assessing the client's lung fields, elevating the head of the bed for maximum lung expansion, and administering oxygen are applicable for both exemplars and also for asthma, respiratory distress, myasthenia gravis with respiratory involvement, and other conditions that require these same interventions. The exemplars require the nurse to determine what makes this Oxygenation problem different from that of a client with myasthenia. The concept problem focus is designed to encourage critical thinking and clinical judgment. This book includes questions at the end of most chapters that focus on the larger concept with the use of exemplars.

# NEXT GENERATION NCLEX (NGN)® EXAMINATION

The goal of the NCLEX-RN® examination has always been to measure the knowledge and skills required by entry-level nurses to care for clients safely. With demographic shifts and technological advances, nurses must make increasingly complex decisions using clinical judgment and incorporate leadership, collaboration, and evidence-based practice into their nursing practice. The National Council of State Boards of Nursing (NCSBN) is currently researching and designing a better way to assess clinical judgment directly and evaluate minimal competency. The next generation NCLEX examination will include a variety of question types to address critical nursing skills such as recognizing cues, analyzing those cues, prioritizing hypotheses, generating solutions, taking action, and evaluating outcomes (NCSBN, 2018).

The new question types include unfolding case studies, enhanced hot spots, CLOZE questions, extended drag and drop, extended multiple responses, and other question formats.

- The unfolding case study includes a narrative describing a client situation. It contains assorted data, and the test taker must discern the relevant information. Then, additional data is revealed, culminating in a complete picture of the client's clinical presentation and associated interventions. The learner makes clinical judgment decisions throughout the case study, adapting the process to the evolving client information.
- Enhanced hot spots involve highlighting relevant information contained in a case study.
- CLOZE questions are fill-in-the-blank questions with drop boxes that provide four available options for the test taker to select for the blank.
- Extended drag and drop questions originate from a brief client scenario or case study. In these questions, the test taker must complete several blanks within a sentence by selecting from a list of seven to eight choices. Another format for extended drag and drop questions is the ranking or sequencing of interventions or processes.
- Extended multiple responses are select-all-that-apply questions with more than the traditional five answer options or questions requiring the learner to identify relevant or irrelevant items from a data set of no less than six options.
- Other question formats will include rich media scenarios with audio or video simulation.

# Neurological Disorders 2

*Preparation is the key to success.*

—Alexander Graham Bell

Test-taking hints are useful to discriminate information, but they cannot substitute for knowledge. The student should refer to Chapter 1 for assistance in preparing for class, studying, and taking an examination.

This chapter focuses on disorders that affect the neurological system. It provides a list of keywords, practice questions focused on disease processes, and a comprehensive examination that includes other content areas involving the neurological system and the disease processes addressed in the practice questions. Answers and reasons why the answer options provided are either correct or incorrect are also provided as test-taking hints. Subsequent chapters (Chapters 3 through 14) focus on disorders that affect other body systems and function.

## KEYWORDS

| | |
|---|---|
| Agnosia | Dysarthria |
| Akinesia | Dysphagia |
| Aphasia | Echolalia |
| Apraxia | Epilepsy |
| Areflexia | Papilledema |
| Ataxia | Paralysis |
| Autonomic dysreflexia | Paresthesia |
| Bradykinesia | Paroxysms |
| Decarboxylase | Penumbra |
| Diplopia | Postictal |

Please note: The term *health-care provider (HCP)*, as used in this text, refers to a nurse practitioner (NP), a physician (MD), an osteopath (DO), or a physician assistant (PA) having prescriptive authority. These providers are responsible for directing the care and providing orders for the clients.

# PRACTICE QUESTIONS

## Cerebrovascular Accident (Stroke)

1. A 78-year-old client is admitted to the emergency department (ED) with numbness and weakness of the left arm and slurred speech. Which nursing intervention is a **priority**?
   1. Prepare to administer recombinant tissue plasminogen activator (rtPA).
   2. Discuss the precipitating factors that caused the symptoms.
   3. Schedule for a STAT computed tomography (CT) scan of the head.
   4. Notify the speech pathologist for an emergency consult.

2. The nurse is assessing a client experiencing motor loss as a result of a left-sided cerebrovascular accident (CVA). Which clinical manifestations would the nurse document?
   1. Hemiparesis of the client's left arm and apraxia.
   2. Paralysis of the right side of the body and ataxia.
   3. Homonymous hemianopsia and diplopia.
   4. Impulsive behavior and hostility toward family.

3. Which client would the nurse identify as being **most** at risk for experiencing a CVA?
   1. A 65-year-old African American male.
   2. An 84-year-old Japanese female.
   3. A 57-year-old white male.
   4. A 25-year-old pregnant Hispanic female.

4. The client diagnosed with a right-sided CVA is admitted to the rehabilitation unit. Which interventions should be included in the nursing care plan? **Select all that apply.**
   1. Position the client to prevent shoulder adduction.
   2. Turn and reposition the client every shift.
   3. Encourage the client to move the affected side.
   4. Perform quadriceps exercises three times a day.
   5. Instruct the client to hold the fingers in a fist.

5. The nurse is planning care for a client experiencing agnosia secondary to a CVA. Which collaborative intervention will be included in the plan of care?
   1. Observe the client swallowing for possible aspiration.
   2. Position the client in a semi-Fowler's position when sleeping.
   3. Place a suction set up at the client's bedside during meals.
   4. Refer the client to an occupational therapist (OT) for an evaluation.

6. The nurse and an unlicensed assistive personnel (UAP) are caring for a client diagnosed with right-sided paralysis. Which action by the UAP **requires** the RN to **intervene**?
   1. The assistant places a gait belt around the client's waist before ambulating.
   2. The assistant places the client on the back with the client's head to the side.
   3. The assistant places a hand under the client's right axilla to move up in bed.
   4. The assistant praises the client for attempting to perform ADL independently.

7. The client diagnosed with atrial fibrillation has experienced a transient ischemic attack (TIA). Which medication would the nurse anticipate being ordered for the client on discharge?
   1. An oral anticoagulant medication.
   2. A beta blocker medication.
   3. An antihyperuricemic medication.
   4. A thrombolytic medication.

8. The client has been diagnosed with a CVA (stroke). The client's wife is concerned about her husband's generalized weakness. Which home modification should the nurse suggest to the wife **before** discharge?
   1. Obtain a rubber mat to place under the dinner plate.
   2. Purchase a long-handled bath sponge for showering.
   3. Purchase clothes with Velcro closure devices.
   4. Obtain a raised toilet seat for the client's bathroom.

9. The client is diagnosed with expressive aphasia. Which psychosocial client problem would the nurse include in the plan of care?
   1. Potential for injury.
   2. Powerlessness.
   3. Disturbed thought processes.
   4. Sexual dysfunction.

10. Which assessment data would indicate to the nurse that the client is **at risk** for a hemorrhagic stroke? **Select all that apply.**
    1. A blood glucose level of 480 mg/dL.
    2. A right-sided carotid bruit.
    3. A blood pressure (BP) of 220/120 mmHg.
    4. The presence of bronchogenic carcinoma.
    5. A lithium level of 0.8 mEq/L.

11. The 85-year-old client diagnosed with a stroke is reporting a severe headache. Which intervention should the nurse implement **first**?
    1. Administer a nonnarcotic analgesic.
    2. Prepare for STAT magnetic resonance imaging (MRI).
    3. Start an intravenous infusion with $D_5W$ at 100 mL/hr.
    4. Complete a neurological assessment.

12. A client diagnosed with a subarachnoid hemorrhage has undergone a craniotomy for the repair of a ruptured aneurysm. Which intervention will the intensive care nurse implement?
    1. Administer a stool softener bid.
    2. Encourage the client to cough hourly.
    3. Monitor neurological status every shift.
    4. Maintain the dopamine drip to keep BP at 160/90.

## Head Injury

13. The client diagnosed with a mild concussion is being discharged from the ED. Which discharge instruction should the nurse teach the client's significant other?
    1. Awaken the client every 2 hours.
    2. Monitor for increased intracranial pressure (ICP).
    3. Observe frequently for hypervigilance.
    4. Offer the client food every 3 to 4 hours.

14. The resident in a long-term care facility fell during the previous shift and has a laceration in the occipital area that has been closed with wound closure strips. Which clinical manifestations would **warrant transferring** the resident to the ED?
    1. A 4-cm area of bright red drainage on the dressing.
    2. A weak pulse, shallow respirations, and cool pale skin.
    3. Pupils that are equal, react to light, and accommodate.
    4. Reports of a headache that resolves with medication.

15. The nurse is caring for several clients. Which client would the nurse assess **first** after receiving the shift report?
    1. The 22-year-old male client diagnosed with a concussion is reporting someone is waking him up every 2 hours.
    2. The 36-year-old female client admitted with reports of left-sided weakness scheduled for an MRI scan.
    3. The 45-year-old client admitted with blunt trauma to the head after a motorcycle accident with a Glasgow Coma Scale (GCS) score of 6.
    4. The 62-year-old client diagnosed with a CVA with expressive aphasia.

16. The client has sustained a severe closed head injury and the neurosurgeon is determining if the client is "brain dead." Which data supports that the client **is** brain dead?
    1. When the client's head is turned to the right, the eyes turn to the right.
    2. The electroencephalogram (EEG) has identifiable waveforms.
    3. No eye activity is observed when the cold caloric test is performed.
    4. The client assumes decorticate posturing when painful stimuli are applied.

17. The client is admitted to the medical floor with a diagnosis of closed head injury. Which nursing intervention has **priority**?
    1. Assess neurological status.
    2. Monitor pulse, respiration, and BP.
    3. Initiate intravenous access.
    4. Maintain an adequate airway.

18. The client diagnosed with a closed head injury is admitted to the rehabilitation department. Which medication order would the nurse **question**?
    1. A subcutaneous anticoagulant.
    2. An intravenous osmotic diuretic.
    3. An oral anticonvulsant.
    4. An oral proton pump inhibitor.

19. The client diagnosed with a gunshot wound to the head assumes decorticate posturing when the nurse applies painful stimuli. Which assessment data obtained 3 hours later would indicate the client is **improving**?
    1. Purposeless movement in response to painful stimuli.
    2. Flaccid paralysis in all four extremities.
    3. Decerebrate posturing when painful stimuli are applied.
    4. Pupils that are 6 mm in size and nonreactive on painful stimuli.

20. The nurse is caring for a client diagnosed with an epidural hematoma. Which nursing interventions should the nurse implement? **Select all that apply.**
    1. Maintain the head of the bed at 60 degrees of elevation.
    2. Administer stool softeners daily.
    3. Ensure the pulse oximeter reading is higher than 93%.
    4. Perform deep nasal suction every 2 hours.
    5. Assess neurological status every 1 to 2 hours.

21. The client diagnosed with a closed head injury has clear fluid draining from the nose. Which action should the nurse implement **first**?
    1. Notify the HCP immediately.
    2. Prepare to administer an antihistamine.
    3. Test the drainage for the presence of glucose.
    4. Place a 2 × 2 gauze under the nose to collect drainage.

22. The nurse is enjoying a day at the lake and witnesses a water skier hit the boat ramp. The water skier is in the water, not responding to verbal stimuli. The nurse is the first HCP to respond to the accident. Which intervention should be implemented **first**?
    1. Assess the client's level of consciousness.
    2. Organize onlookers to remove the client from the lake.
    3. Perform a head-to-toe assessment to determine injuries.
    4. Stabilize the client's cervical spine.

23. The client is diagnosed with a closed head injury and is in a coma. The nurse writes the client problem as "**high risk** for immobility complications." Which intervention would be included in the plan of care?
    1. Position the client with the head of the bed elevated at intervals.
    2. Perform active range-of-motion (ROM) exercises every 4 hours.
    3. Turn the client every shift and massage bony prominences.
    4. Explain all procedures to the client before performing them.

24. The 29-year-old client, employed as a forklift operator, sustains a traumatic brain injury (TBI) secondary to a motor vehicle accident. The client is being discharged from the rehabilitation unit after 3 months and has cognitive deficits. Which goal would be most realistic for this client?
    1. The client will return to work within 6 months.
    2. The client is able to focus and stay on task for 10 minutes.
    3. The client will be able to dress without assistance.
    4. The client will regain bowel and bladder control.

## Spinal Cord Injury (SCI)

25. The nurse arrives at the site of a one-car motor vehicle accident and stops to render aid. The driver of the car is unconscious. After stabilizing the client's cervical spine, which action should the nurse take **next**?
    1. Carefully remove the driver from the car.
    2. Assess the client's pupils for a reaction.
    3. Assess the client's airway.
    4. Attempt to wake the client up by shaking him.

26. In assessing a client diagnosed with a thoracic SCI, which clinical manifestation would the nurse expect to find to support the diagnosis of neurogenic shock? **Select all that apply.**
    1. Warm lower extremities.
    2. Inability to move upper extremities.
    3. Reports of a pounding headache.
    4. Hypotension.
    5. Tachycardia.

27. The rehabilitation nurse caring for the client diagnosed with a lumbar SCI is developing the nursing care plan. Which intervention should the nurse implement?
    1. Keep oxygen via nasal cannula on at all times.
    2. Administer low-dose subcutaneous anticoagulants.
    3. Perform active lower extremity ROM exercises.
    4. Refer to a speech therapist for ventilator-assisted speech.

28. The nurse in the neuro-intensive care unit is caring for a client diagnosed with a new cervical (C7) SCI and breathing independently. Which nursing interventions should be implemented? **Select all that apply.**
    1. Monitor pulse oximetry reading.
    2. Provide pureed foods six times a day.
    3. Encourage coughing and deep breathing.
    4. Assess for autonomic dysreflexia.
    5. Administer intravenous corticosteroids.

29. The home health nurse is caring for a 28-year-old client diagnosed with a T10 SCI saying, "I can't do anything. Why am I so worthless?" Which statement by the nurse would be the most therapeutic?
    1. "This must be very hard for you. You're feeling worthless?"
    2. "You shouldn't feel worthless—you are still alive."
    3. "Why do you feel worthless? You still have the use of your arms."
    4. "If you attended a work rehab program, you wouldn't feel worthless."

30. The client is diagnosed with an SCI and is scheduled for an MRI scan. Which question would be **most appropriate** for the nurse to ask before taking the client to the diagnostic test?
    1. "Do you have trouble hearing?"
    2. "Are you allergic to any type of dairy products?"
    3. "Have you eaten anything in the last 8 hours?"
    4. "Are you uncomfortable in closed spaces?"

31. The client diagnosed with a C6 SCI is admitted to the ED reporting a severe pounding headache and has a BP of 180/110. Which intervention should the ED nurse implement?
    1. Keep the client flat in bed.
    2. Dim the lights in the room.
    3. Assess for bladder distention.
    4. Administer a narcotic analgesic.

32. The client diagnosed with a cervical fracture is being discharged in a halo device. Which teaching instruction should the nurse discuss with the client? **Select all that apply.**
    1. Discuss how to remove the insertion pins correctly.
    2. Instruct the client to report reddened or irritated skin areas.
    3. Inform the client that the vest liner cannot be changed.
    4. Encourage the client to remain in the recliner as much as possible.
    5. Teach the client to notify the HCP of difficulty swallowing.

33. The intensive care nurse is caring for a client diagnosed with a T1 SCI. When the nurse elevates the head of the bed 30 degrees, the client reports light-headedness and dizziness. The client's vital signs are populated in the chart below. Which action should the nurse implement?

| Vital Sign Flowsheet | Client Results | Normal Values |
|---|---|---|
| Blood pressure | 84/40 | 100–119 mmHg systolic 60–80 mmHg diastolic |
| Temperature | 99.2°F | Oral: 98°F (36.7°C) |
| Pulse | 98 | 60 to 100 beats/min |
| Respirations | 24 | 12 to 20 breaths/min |

   1. Notify the HCP as soon as possible.
   2. Calm the client down by talking therapeutically.
   3. Increase the IV rate by 50 mL/hour.
   4. Lower the head of the bed immediately.

34. The nurse is caring for clients in the rehabilitation unit. Which clients should the nurse assess **first** after receiving the change-of-shift report?
    1. The client diagnosed with a C6 SCI reporting dyspnea and has crackles in the lungs.
    2. The client diagnosed with an L4 SCI crying and very upset about being discharged home.
    3. The client diagnosed with an L2 SCI reporting a headache and feeling very hot.
    4. The client diagnosed with a T4 SCI unable to move the lower extremities.

35. Which nursing task would be **most appropriate** for the RN to delegate to the UAP?
    1. Teach Credé's maneuver to the client needing to void.
    2. Administer the tube feeding to the client diagnosed with quadriplegia.
    3. Assist with bowel training by placing the client on the bedside commode.
    4. Observe the client demonstrating the self-catheterization technique.

36. The 34-year-old male client diagnosed with an SCI is sharing with the nurse that he is worried about finding employment after being discharged from the rehabilitation unit. Which intervention should the nurse implement?
    1. Refer the client to the American Spinal Cord Injury Association (ASIA).
    2. Refer the client to the state vocational rehabilitation agency.
    3. Ask the social worker (SW) about applying for disability.
    4. Suggest the client talk with his significant other about this concern.

## Seizures

37. The male client is sitting in the chair, and his entire body is rigid with his arms and legs contracting and relaxing. The client is not aware of what is going on and is making guttural sounds. Which action should the nurse implement **first**?
    1. Push aside any furniture.
    2. Place the client on his side.
    3. Assess the client's vital signs.
    4. Ease the client to the floor.

38. The occupational health nurse is concerned about preventing occupation-related acquired seizures. Which intervention should the nurse implement?
    1. Ensure that helmets are worn in appropriate areas.
    2. Implement daily exercise programs for the staff.
    3. Provide healthy foods in the cafeteria.
    4. Encourage employees to wear safety glasses.

39. The client is scheduled for an EEG to help diagnose a seizure disorder. Which preprocedure teaching should the nurse implement? **Select all that apply.**
    1. Tell the client to take any routine antiseizure medication before the EEG.
    2. Tell the client not to eat anything for 8 hours before the procedure.
    3. Instruct the client to sleep only 4 or 5 hours before the EEG.
    4. Explain to the client that there will be some discomfort during the procedure.
    5. Tell the client to avoid hair products, such as hairspray and gels, before the EEG.

40. The nurse enters the room as the client is beginning to have a tonic-clonic seizure. What action should the nurse implement **first**?
    1. Note the first thing the client does in the seizure.
    2. Assess the size of the client's pupils.
    3. Determine if the client is incontinent of urine or stool.
    4. Provide the client with privacy during the seizure.

41. The client, after a 3-minute seizure, has no apparent injuries and is oriented to name, place, and time but is very lethargic and just wants to sleep. Which intervention should the nurse implement?
    1. Perform a complete neurological assessment.
    2. Awaken the client every 30 minutes.
    3. Turn the client to the side and allow the client to sleep.
    4. Interview the client to find out what caused the seizure.

42. The UAP is attempting to put an oral airway in the mouth of a client having a tonic-clonic seizure. Which action should the RN primary nurse take?
    1. Help the UAP to insert the oral airway in the mouth.
    2. Tell the UAP to stop trying to insert anything in the mouth.
    3. Take no action because the UAP is handling the situation.
    4. Notify the charge nurse of the situation immediately.

43. The client is prescribed phenytoin for a seizure disorder. Which statement indicates the client **understands** the discharge teaching concerning this medication?
    1. "I will brush my teeth after every meal."
    2. "I will check my phenytoin level daily."
    3. "My urine will turn orange while on phenytoin."
    4. "I won't have any seizures while on this medication."

44. The client is admitted to the intensive care unit (ICU) experiencing status epilepticus. Which collaborative intervention should the nurse anticipate?
    1. Assess the client's neurological status every hour.
    2. Monitor the client's heart rhythm via telemetry.
    3. Administer an anticonvulsant medication by intravenous push.
    4. Prepare to administer a glucocorticosteroid orally.

45. The client has been newly diagnosed with epilepsy. Which discharge instructions should be taught to the client? **Select all that apply.**
    1. Keep a record of seizure activity.
    2. Take tub baths only; do not take showers.
    3. Avoid over-the-counter medications.
    4. Have anticonvulsant medication serum levels checked regularly.
    5. Do not drive alone; have someone in the car.

46. Which statement by the female client indicates that the client **understands** factors that may precipitate seizure activity?
    1. "It is all right for me to drink coffee for breakfast."
    2. "My menstrual cycle will not affect my seizure disorder."
    3. "I am going to take a class in stress management."
    4. "I should wear dark glasses when I am out in the sun."

47. The nurse asks the male client diagnosed with epilepsy if he has auras with his seizures. The client says, "I don't know what you mean. What are auras?" Which statement by the nurse would be the **best response**?
    1. "Some people have a warning that the seizure is about to start."
    2. "Auras occur when you are physically and psychologically exhausted."
    3. "You're concerned that you do not have auras before your seizures?"
    4. "Auras usually cause you to be sleepy after you have a seizure."

48. The nurse educator is presenting an in-service on seizures. Which diseases or conditions can cause seizures in older people? **Select all that apply.**
    1. Alzheimer's disease.
    2. Cervical spondylosis.
    3. Head injuries.
    4. CVA.
    5. Brain tumors.

## Brain Tumors

49. The client is being admitted to rule out a brain tumor. Which symptoms **support** a diagnosis of a brain tumor? **Select all that apply.**
    1. Nervousness, cough, and frequent eye movements.
    2. Headache, vomiting, and papilledema.
    3. Hypotension, tachycardia, and tachypnea.
    4. Abrupt loss of motor function, diarrhea, and changes in taste.
    5. Mood changes, blurred vision, and seizures.

50. The client has been diagnosed with a brain tumor. Which presenting clinical manifestations help to localize the tumor position?
    1. Widening pulse pressure and bounding pulse.
    2. Diplopia and decreased visual acuity.
    3. Bradykinesia and scanning speech.
    4. Hemiparesis and personality changes.

51. The male client diagnosed with a brain tumor is scheduled for an MRI scan in the morning. The client tells the nurse that he is scared. Which response by the nurse indicates an appropriate therapeutic response?
    1. "MRIs are loud, but there will not be any invasive procedure done."
    2. "You're scared. Tell me about what is scaring you."
    3. "This is the last thing to be scared about—there will be worse."
    4. "I can call the MRI tech to come and talk to you about the scan."

52. The client diagnosed with breast cancer has developed metastasis to the brain. Which prophylactic measure should the nurse implement?
    1. Institute aspiration precautions.
    2. Refer the client to Reach to Recovery.
    3. Initiate seizure precautions.
    4. Teach the client about mastectomy care.

53. The significant other of a client diagnosed with a brain tumor asks the nurse for help identifying resources. Which would be the **most appropriate** referral for the nurse to make?
    1. Social worker.
    2. Chaplain.
    3. Health-care provider.
    4. Occupational therapist.

54. The nurse has written a care plan for a client diagnosed with a brain tumor. Which is an important goal regarding self-care deficit?
    1. The client will maintain body weight within 2 pounds.
    2. The client will execute an advance directive.
    3. The client will be able to perform three ADL with assistance.
    4. The client will verbalize a feeling of loss by the end of the shift.

55. The client diagnosed with a brain tumor was admitted to the ICU with decorticate posturing. Which indicates that the client's condition is becoming worse?
    1. The client has purposeful movements with painful stimuli.
    2. The client has assumed adduction of the upper extremities.
    3. The client is aimlessly thrashing in the bed.
    4. The client has become flaccid and does not respond to stimuli.

56. The client is diagnosed with a pituitary tumor and is scheduled for a transsphenoidal hypophysectomy. Which preoperative instruction is important for the nurse to teach?
    1. There will be a large turban dressing around the skull after surgery.
    2. The client will not be able to eat for 4 or 5 days postop.
    3. The client should not blow the nose for 2 weeks after surgery.
    4. The client will have to lie flat for 24 hours following the surgery.

57. The client has undergone a craniotomy for a brain tumor. Which data indicate a complication of this surgery?
    1. The client reports a headache at "3" to "4" on a 1-to-10 scale.
    2. The client has an intake of 1,000 mL and an output of 3,500 mL.
    3. The client reports a raspy, sore throat.
    4. The client experiences dizziness when trying to get up too quickly.

58. The client diagnosed with a brain tumor has a diminished gag response and weakness on the left side of the body. Which intervention should the nurse implement?
    1. Make the client NPO until seen by the HCP.
    2. Position the client in low Fowler's position for all meals.
    3. Place the client on a mechanically ground diet.
    4. Teach the client to direct food and fluid toward the right side.

59. The client is diagnosed with a metastatic brain tumor, and radiation therapy is scheduled. The client asks the nurse, "Why not try chemotherapy first? It has helped my other tumors." The nurse's response is based on which scientific rationale?
    1. Chemotherapy is only used as a last resort in caring for clients diagnosed with brain tumors.
    2. The blood-brain barrier prevents medications from reaching the brain.
    3. Radiation therapy will have fewer side effects than chemotherapy.
    4. Metastatic tumors become resistant to chemotherapy and it becomes useless.

60. The client is being discharged following a transsphenoidal hypophysectomy. Which discharge instructions should the nurse teach the client? **Select all that apply.**
    1. Sleep with the head of the bed elevated.
    2. Keep a humidifier in the room.
    3. Use caution when performing oral care.
    4. Stay on a full liquid diet until seen by the HCP.
    5. Notify the HCP if developing a cold or fever.

## Meningitis

61. The wife of the client diagnosed with septic meningitis asks the nurse, "I am so scared. What is meningitis?" Which statement would be the **most appropriate** response by the nurse?
    1. "There is bleeding into his brain, causing irritation of the meninges."
    2. "A virus has infected the brain and meninges, causing inflammation."
    3. "It is a bacterial infection of the tissues that cover the brain and spinal cord."
    4. "It is an inflammation of the brain parenchyma caused by a mosquito bite."

62. The public health nurse is giving a lecture on potential outbreaks of infectious meningitis. Which population is most at risk for an outbreak?
    1. Clients recently discharged from the hospital.
    2. Residents of a college dormitory.
    3. Individuals visiting a developing country.
    4. Employees in a high-rise office building.

63. The nurse is assessing the client diagnosed with bacterial meningitis. Which clinical manifestations would support the diagnosis of bacterial meningitis?
    1. Positive Babinski's sign and peripheral paresthesia.
    2. Negative Chvostek's sign and facial tingling.
    3. Positive Kernig's sign and nuchal rigidity.
    4. Negative Trousseau's sign and nystagmus.

64. The RN is assessing the client diagnosed with meningococcal meningitis. Which assessment data would **warrant notifying** the HCP?
    1. Purpuric lesions on the face.
    2. Reports of light hurting the eyes.
    3. Dull, aching, frontal headache.
    4. Not remembering the day of the week.

65. Which type of precautions should the nurse implement for the client diagnosed with meningococcal meningitis?
    1. Standard precautions.
    2. Airborne precautions.
    3. Contact precautions.
    4. Droplet precautions.

66. The nurse is developing a plan of care for a client diagnosed with aseptic meningitis secondary to a brain tumor. Which nursing goal would be **most appropriate** for the client problem "altered cerebral tissue perfusion"?
    1. The client will be able to complete ADL.
    2. The client will be protected from injury if seizure activity occurs.
    3. The client will be afebrile for 48 hours before discharge.
    4. The client will have elastic tissue turgor with ready recoil.

67. The nurse is preparing a client diagnosed with possible meningitis for a lumbar puncture. Which interventions should the nurse implement? **Select all that apply.**
    1. Obtain an informed consent from the client or significant other.
    2. Have the client empty the bladder before the procedure.
    3. Place the client in a side-lying position with the back arched.
    4. Instruct the client to breathe rapidly and deeply during the procedure.
    5. Explain to the client what to expect during the procedure.

68. The nurse is caring for a client diagnosed with meningitis. Which collaborative intervention should be included in the plan of care?
    1. Administer antibiotics.
    2. Obtain a sputum culture.
    3. Monitor the pulse oximeter.
    4. Assess intake and output.

69. The client is diagnosed with meningococcal meningitis. Which preventive measure would the nurse expect the HCP to order for the significant others in the home?
    1. The *Haemophilus influenzae* vaccine.
    2. Antimicrobial chemoprophylaxis.
    3. A 10-day dose pack of corticosteroids.
    4. A gamma globulin injection.

70. Which statement **best** describes the scientific rationale for alternating a nonnarcotic antipyretic and an NSAID every 2 hours to a female client diagnosed with bacterial meningitis?
    1. This regimen helps to decrease the purulent exudate surrounding the meninges.
    2. These medications will decrease ICP and brain metabolism.
    3. These medications will increase the client's memory and orientation.
    4. This will help prevent a yeast infection secondary to antibiotic therapy.

71. The client diagnosed with acute bacterial meningitis is admitted to the medical floor at noon. Which HCP's order would have the **highest priority**?
    1. Administer an intravenous antibiotic.
    2. Obtain the client's lunch tray.
    3. Provide a quiet, calm, and dark room.
    4. Weigh the client in hospital attire.

72. The 29-year-old client is admitted to the medical floor diagnosed with meningitis. Which assessment by the nurse has **priority**?
    1. Assess lung sounds.
    2. Assess the six cardinal fields of gaze.
    3. Assess the apical pulse.
    4. Assess the level of consciousness.

## Parkinson's Disease

73. The client diagnosed with Parkinson's disease is being admitted with a fever and patchy infiltrates in the lung fields on the chest x-ray. Which clinical manifestations would explain these assessment data?
    1. Masklike face and shuffling gait.
    2. Difficulty swallowing and immobility.
    3. Pill rolling of fingers and flat affect.
    4. Lack of arm swing and bradykinesia.

74. The client diagnosed with Parkinson's disease is being discharged on carbidopa and levodopa. Which statement is the scientific rationale for combining these medications?
    1. There will be fewer side effects with this combination than with carbidopa alone.
    2. Dopamine D requires the presence of both of these medications to work.
    3. Carbidopa makes more levodopa available to the brain.
    4. Carbidopa crosses the blood-brain barrier to treat Parkinson's disease.

75. The nurse caring for a client diagnosed with Parkinson's disease writes a problem of "impaired nutrition." Which nursing intervention would be included in the plan of care?

    1. Request the physical therapist to consult for equipment needed.
    2. Request a low-fat, low-sodium diet from the dietary department.
    3. Provide three meals per day that include nuts and whole-grain breads.
    4. Offer six meals per day with a soft consistency.

76. The RN and the UAP are caring for clients on a medical-surgical unit. Which task **should not** be assigned to the UAP?
    1. Feed the 69-year-old client diagnosed with Parkinson's disease having difficulty swallowing.
    2. Turn and position the 89-year-old client diagnosed with a pressure ulcer secondary to Parkinson's disease.
    3. Assist the 54-year-old client diagnosed with Parkinson's disease with toilet-training activities.
    4. Obtain vital signs on a 72-year-old client diagnosed with pneumonia secondary to Parkinson's disease.

77. The RN charge nurse is making assignments. Which client should be assigned to the new graduate nurse?
    1. The client diagnosed with aseptic meningitis reporting a headache and the light bothering his eyes.
    2. The client diagnosed with Parkinson's disease after falling during the night and is reporting difficulty walking.
    3. The client diagnosed with a CVA with vital signs P 60, R 14, and BP 198/68.
    4. The client diagnosed with a brain tumor, reporting seeing spots before the eyes.

78. The nurse is planning the care for a client diagnosed with Parkinson's disease. Which would be a therapeutic goal of treatment for the disease process?
    1. The client will experience periods of akinesia throughout the day.
    2. The client will take the prescribed medications correctly.
    3. The client will be able to enjoy a family outing with the spouse.
    4. The client will be able to carry out ADL.

79. The nurse researcher is working with clients diagnosed with Parkinson's disease. Which is an example of an experimental therapy?
    1. Stereotactic pallidotomy.
    2. Dopamine receptor agonist medication.
    3. Deep brain stimulation.
    4. Fetal tissue transplantation.

80. The client diagnosed with Parkinson's disease is being discharged. Which statement made by the significant other indicates an **understanding** of the discharge instructions?
    1. "All of my spouse's emotions will slow down now just like his body movements."
    2. "My spouse may experience hallucinations until the medication starts working."
    3. "I will schedule appointments late in the morning after his morning bath."
    4. "It is fine if we don't follow a strict medication schedule on weekends."

81. The nurse is admitting a client with the diagnosis of Parkinson's disease. Which assessment data **support** this diagnosis?
    1. Crackles in the upper lung fields and jugular vein distention.
    2. Muscle weakness in the upper extremities and ptosis.
    3. Exaggerated arm swinging and scanning speech.
    4. Masklike face and a shuffling gait.

82. Which is a common cognitive problem associated with Parkinson's disease?
    1. Emotional lability.
    2. Depression.
    3. Memory deficits.
    4. Paranoia.

83. The nurse is conducting a support group for clients diagnosed with Parkinson's disease and their significant others. Which information regarding psychosocial needs should be included in the discussion?
    1. The client should discuss feelings about being placed on a ventilator.
    2. The client may have rapid mood swings and become easily upset.
    3. Pill-rolling tremors will become worse when the medication is wearing off.
    4. The client may automatically start to repeat what another person says.

84. The nurse is caring for clients on a medical-surgical floor. Which clients should be assessed **first**?
    1. The 65-year-old client diagnosed with seizures reporting a headache that is a "2" on a 1-to-10 scale.
    2. The 24-year-old client diagnosed with a T10 SCI and cannot move his toes.
    3. The 58-year-old client diagnosed with Parkinson's disease is crying and worried about her facial appearance.
    4. The 62-year-old client diagnosed with a CVA and a resolving left hemiparesis.

## Substance Abuse

85. The friend of an 18-year-old male client brings the client to the ED. The client is unconscious, and his breathing is slow and shallow. Which action should the nurse implement **first**?
    1. Ask the friend what drugs the client has been taking.
    2. Initiate an IV infusion at a keep-open rate.
    3. Call for a ventilator to be brought to the ED.
    4. Apply oxygen at 100% via nasal cannula.

86. The chief executive officer (CEO) of a large manufacturing plant presents to the occupational health clinic with chronic rhinitis and requesting medication. On inspection, the nurse notices holes in the septum that separates the nasal passages. The nurse also notes dilated pupils and tachycardia. The facility has a "No Drug" policy. Which intervention should the nurse implement?
    1. Prepare to complete a drug screen urine test.
    2. Discuss the client's use of illegal drugs.
    3. Notify the client's supervisor about the situation.
    4. Give the client an antihistamine and say nothing.

87. The nurse is working with several clients in a substance abuse clinic. Client A tells the nurse that another client, Client B, has "started using again." Which action should the nurse implement?
    1. Tell Client A the nurse cannot discuss Client B with him.
    2. Find out how Client A got this information.
    3. Inform the HCP that Client B is using again.
    4. Get in touch with Client B and have the client come to the clinic.

88. A 20-year-old female client having tried lysergic acid diethylamide (LSD) as a teen tells the nurse that she has bad dreams that make her want to kill herself. Which is the explanation for this occurrence?
    1. These occurrences are referred to as "hold-over reactions" to the drug.
    2. These are flashbacks to a time when the client had a "bad trip."
    3. The drug is still in the client's body and causing these reactions.
    4. The client is suicidal and should be on one-to-one precautions.

89. The nurse observes a coworker acting erratically. The clients assigned to this coworker don't seem to get relief when pain medications are administered. Which action should the nurse implement?
    1. Try to help the coworker by confronting the coworker with the nurse's suspicions.
    2. Tell the coworker that the nurse will give all narcotic medications from now on.
    3. Report the nurse's suspicions to the nurse's supervisor or the facility's peer review.
    4. Do nothing until the nurse can prove the coworker has been using drugs.

90. The client is diagnosed with Wernicke-Korsakoff syndrome as a result of chronic alcoholism. Which symptoms would the nurse assess in the client?
    1. Insomnia and anxiety.
    2. Visual or auditory hallucinations.
    3. Extreme tremors and agitation.
    4. Ataxia and confabulation.

91. The client diagnosed with delirium tremens when trying to quit drinking cold turkey is admitted to the medical unit. Which medications would the nurse anticipate administering?
    1. Thiamine and chlordiazepoxide.
    2. Phenytoin and ferrous sulfate.
    3. Methadone and divalproex sodium.
    4. Mannitol and methylphenidate.

92. The client is withdrawing from a heroin addiction. Which interventions should the nurse implement? **Select all that apply.**
    1. Initiate seizure precautions.
    2. Check vital signs every 8 hours.
    3. Place the client in a quiet, calm atmosphere.
    4. Have a consent form signed for HIV testing.
    5. Administer buprenorphine.

93. The wife of the client diagnosed with chronic alcoholism tells the nurse, "I have to call his work just about every Monday to let them know he is ill or he will lose his job." Which would be the nurse's **best** response?
    1. "I am sure that this must be hard for you. Tell me about your concerns."
    2. "You are afraid he will lose his source of income."
    3. "Why would you call in for your husband? Can't he do this?"
    4. "Are you aware that when you do this, you are enabling him?"

94. The nurse caring for a client abusing amphetamines writes a problem of "cardiovascular compromise." Which nursing interventions should be implemented?
    1. Monitor the telemetry and vital signs every 4 hours.
    2. Encourage the client to verbalize the reason for using drugs.

    3. Provide a quiet, calm atmosphere for the client to rest.
    4. Place the client on bedrest and a low-sodium diet.

95. The client diagnosed with substance abuse is being discharged from a drug and alcohol rehabilitation facility. Which information should the nurse teach the client? **Select all that apply.**
    1. "Do not go anyplace where you can be tempted to use again."
    2. "It is important that you attend a 12-step meeting regularly."
    3. "Now that you are clean, your family will be willing to see you again."
    4. "You should explain to all your coworkers what has happened."
    5. "Practice breathing and relaxation techniques to manage stress."

96. The nurse is working with clients and their families regarding substance abuse. Which statement is the scientific rationale for teaching the children new coping mechanisms?
    1. The child needs to realize that the parent will be changing behaviors.
    2. The child will need to point out to the parent when the parent is not coping.
    3. Children tend to mimic the behaviors of parents when faced with similar situations.
    4. Children need to feel like they are a part of the parent's recovery.

## Amyotrophic Lateral Sclerosis (ALS or Lou Gehrig's Disease)

97. Which diagnostic tests are used to confirm the diagnosis of ALS? **Select all that apply.**
    1. Electromyogram (EMG).
    2. Nerve conduction study (NCS).
    3. Serum creatine kinase (CK).
    4. Pulmonary function test.
    5. Magnetic resonance imaging.

98. The client is diagnosed with ALS. Which client problem would be **most appropriate** for this client?
    1. Disuse syndrome.
    2. Altered body image.
    3. Fluid and electrolyte imbalance.
    4. Alteration in pain.

99. The client is being evaluated to rule out ALS. Which clinical manifestations would the nurse note to **confirm** the diagnosis?
    1. Muscle atrophy and flaccidity.
    2. Fatigue and malnutrition.
    3. Slurred speech and dysphagia.
    4. Weakness and paralysis.

100. The client diagnosed with ALS asks the nurse, "I know this disease is going to kill me. What will happen to me in the end?" Which statement by the nurse would be **most** appropriate?
    1. "You are afraid of how you will die?"
    2. "Most people with ALS die of respiratory failure."
    3. "Don't talk like that. You have to stay positive."
    4. "ALS is not a killer. You can live a long life."

101. The client diagnosed with ALS is admitted to the medical unit with shortness of breath, dyspnea, and respiratory complications. Which intervention should the nurse implement **first**?
    1. Elevate the head of the bed 30 degrees.
    2. Administer oxygen via nasal cannula.
    3. Assess the client's lung sounds.
    4. Obtain a pulse oximeter reading.

102. The client is to receive a 100-mL intravenous antibiotic over 30 minutes via an intravenous pump. At what rate should the nurse set the IV pump?

    [                    ]

103. The nurse is caring for several clients in a medical unit. Which client should the nurse assess **first**?
    1. The client diagnosed with ALS refusing to turn every 2 hours.
    2. The client diagnosed with abdominal pain reporting nausea.
    3. The client diagnosed with pneumonia and a pulse oximeter reading of 90%.
    4. The client reporting not receiving any pain medication.

104. The client is diagnosed with ALS. As the disease progresses, which intervention should the nurse implement?
    1. Discuss the need to be placed in a long-term care facility.
    2. Explain how to care for a sigmoid colostomy.
    3. Assist the client to prepare an advance directive.
    4. Teach the client how to use a motorized wheelchair.

105. The client is in the terminal stage of ALS. Which intervention should the nurse implement?
    1. Perform passive ROM every 2 hours.
    2. Maintain a negative nitrogen balance.
    3. Encourage a low-protein, soft-mechanical diet.
    4. Turn the client and have him cough and deep breathe every shift.

106. The son of a client diagnosed with ALS asks the nurse, "Is there any chance that I could get this disease?" Which statement by the nurse would be **most** appropriate?
    1. "It must be scary to think you might get this disease."
    2. "No, this disease is not genetic or contagious."
    3. "ALS does have a genetic factor and runs in families."
    4. "If you are exposed to the same virus, you may get the disease."

107. The client diagnosed with end-stage ALS requires a gastrostomy tube feeding. Which finding would require the nurse to hold a bolus tube feeding?
    1. A residual of 125 mL.
    2. The abdomen is soft.
    3. Three episodes of diarrhea.
    4. The potassium level is 3.4 mEq/L.

108. The client diagnosed with ALS is prescribed riluzole. Which instructions should the nurse discuss with the client? **Select all that apply.**
    1. Take the medication with food.
    2. Do not eat green, leafy vegetables.
    3. Use SPF 30 when going out in the sun.
    4. Report any febrile illness.
    5. Throw away unused medication after 15 days.

## Encephalitis

109. The nurse is admitting the client to rule out encephalitis. Which interventions should the nurse assess to support the diagnosis of encephalitis? **Select all that apply.**
    1. Determine if the client has recently received any immunizations.
    2. Ask if the client has had a cold in the last week.
    3. Check to see if the client has active herpes simplex 1.
    4. Find out if the client has traveled to the Great Lakes region.
    5. Assess for recent insect or mosquito bites.

110. The nurse is assessing the client admitted with encephalitis. Which data require **immediate** nursing intervention?
    1. The client has bilateral facial palsies.
    2. The client has a recurrent temperature of 100.6°F.
    3. The client has a decreased report of headaches.
    4. The client comments that the meal has no taste.

111. The client admitted to the hospital to rule out encephalitis is being prepared for a lumbar puncture. Which instructions should the nurse teach the client? **Select all that apply.**
    1. Instruct that all invasive procedures require written permission.
    2. Explain this test allows for the analysis of a sample of the cerebrospinal fluid.
    3. Tell the client to increase fluid intake for the next 48 hours.
    4. Discuss that lying supine with the head flat will prevent all hematomas.
    5. Teach the client about the spinal anesthesia used for the test.

112. The nurse is caring for a client diagnosed with encephalitis. Which is an **expected** outcome for the client?
    1. The client will regain as much neurological function as possible.
    2. The client will have no short-term memory loss.
    3. The client will have improved renal function.
    4. The client will apply hydrocortisone cream daily.

113. Which intervention should the nurse implement when caring for the client diagnosed with encephalitis? **Select all that apply**.
    1. Turn the client every 2 hours.
    2. Encourage the client to increase fluids.
    3. Keep the client in the supine position.
    4. Assess for deep vein thrombosis (DVT).
    5. Assess for any alterations in elimination.

114. The nurse is caring for the client diagnosed with encephalitis. Which intervention should the nurse implement **first** if the client is experiencing a complication?
    1. Examine pupil reactions to light.
    2. Assess level of consciousness.
    3. Observe for seizure activity.
    4. Monitor vital signs every shift.

115. The public health department nurse is preparing a lecture on the prevention of West Nile virus. Which information should the nurse include? **Select all that apply.**
    1. Change water frequently in pet dishes and birdbaths.
    2. Wear thick, dark clothing when outside to avoid bites.
    3. Apply insect repellent over face and arms only.
    4. Explain that mosquitoes are more prevalent from dusk to dawn.
    5. Get the West Nile virus vaccination yearly.

116. Which problem is the **highest priority** for the client diagnosed with West Nile virus?
    1. Alteration in body temperature.
    2. Altered tissue perfusion.
    3. Fluid volume excess.
    4. Altered skin integrity.

117. The nurse is developing a plan of care for a client diagnosed with West Nile virus. Which intervention should the nurse include in this plan?
    1. Monitor the client's respirations frequently.
    2. Refer to a dermatologist for the treatment of maculopapular rash.
    3. Treat hypothermia by using ice packs under the client's arms.
    4. Teach the client to report any swollen lymph glands.

118. Which collaborative intervention should the nurse implement when caring for the client diagnosed with West Nile virus?
    1. Complete neurovascular examinations every 8 hours.
    2. Maintain accurate intake and output at the end of each shift.
    3. Assess the client's symptoms to determine if there is an improvement.
    4. Administer intravenous fluids while assessing for overload.

119. The nurse is caring for the client diagnosed with West Nile virus. Which assessment data would require **immediate** intervention from the nurse?
    1. The vital signs are documented as T 100.2°F, P 80, R 18, and BP 136/78.
    2. The client reports generalized body aches and pains.
    3. Positive results are reported from the enzyme-linked immunosorbent assay (ELISA).
    4. The client becomes lethargic and is difficult to arouse using verbal stimuli.

120. Which rationale explains the transmission of the West Nile virus?
    1. Transmission occurs through exchange of body fluids when sneezing and coughing.
    2. Transmission occurs only through mosquito bites and not between humans.
    3. Transmission can occur from human to human in blood products and breast milk.
    4. Transmission occurs with direct contact from the maculopapular rash drainage.

# CONCEPTS

In this section of the practice questions, the focus is on a particular concept. The concepts of intracranial regulation, functional ability, and cognition, along with the exemplars (example disease processes), are directed toward the test taker recognizing the commonality that exists between one exemplar and another under the concept. There are also interrelated concepts that may be presented in a question to help the test taker understand how the concepts intertwine. The test taker must also recognize that in order to perform individualized client care, all aspects of the client's beliefs, developmental stage, and culture, as well as the disease process, must be considered.

121. The male client is admitted to the ED following a motorcycle accident. The client was not wearing a helmet and struck his head on the pavement. The nurse identifies the concept as impaired intracranial regulation. Which interventions should the ED nurse implement in the first 5 minutes? **Select all that apply.**
    1. Stabilize the client's neck and spine.
    2. Contact the organ procurement organization to speak with the family.
    3. Elevate the head of the bed to 70 degrees.
    4. Perform a Glasgow Coma Scale assessment.
    5. Ensure the client has a patent peripheral venous catheter in place.
    6. Check the client's driver's license to see if he will accept blood.

122. The client diagnosed with atrial fibrillation reports numbness and tingling of her left arm and leg. The nurse assesses facial drooping on the left side and slight slurring of speech. Which nursing interventions should the nurse implement **first**?
    1. Schedule a STAT MRI of the brain.
    2. Call a code STROKE.
    3. Notify the HCP.
    4. Have the client swallow a glass of water.

123. The nurse identifies the concept of intracranial regulation disturbance in a client diagnosed with Parkinson's disease. Which **priority** intervention should the nurse implement?
    1. Keep the bed low and call light in reach.
    2. Provide a regular diet of three meals per day.
    3. Obtain an order for home health to see the client.
    4. Perform the Braden scale skin assessment.

124. The client newly diagnosed with Parkinson's disease asks the nurse, "Why can't I control these tremors?" Which is the nurse's **best response**?
    1. "You can control the tremors when you learn to concentrate and focus on the cause."
    2. "The tremors are caused by a lack of the chemical dopamine in the brain; medication may help."

3. "You have too much acetylcholine in your brain, causing the tremors, but they will get better with time."
    4. "You are concerned about the tremors? If you want to talk, I would like to hear how you feel."

125. The concept of intracranial regulation is identified for a client diagnosed with a brain tumor. Which intervention should the nurse include in the client's plan of care?
    1. Tell the client to remain on bedrest.
    2. Maintain the intravenous rate at 150 mL/hour.
    3. Provide a soft, bland diet with three snacks per day.
    4. Place the client on seizure precautions.

126. The 80-year-old male client on an Alzheimer's unit is agitated and asking the nurse to get his father to come and see him. Which is the nurse's **best response**?
    1. Tell the client his father is dead and cannot come to see him.
    2. Give the client the phone and have him attempt to call his father.
    3. Ask the client to talk about his father with the nurse.
    4. Call the family so they can tell the client why his father cannot come to see him.

127. The 28-year-old client is on the rehabilitation unit post SCI at level T10. Which collaborative team members should participate with the RN at the case conference? **Select all that apply.**
    1. Occupational therapist (OT).
    2. Physical therapist (PT).
    3. Registered dietitian (RD).
    4. Rehabilitation physician.
    5. Social worker.
    6. Patient care tech (PCT).

128. Which diagnostic evaluation tool would the nurse use to assess the client's cognitive functioning? **Select all that apply.**
    1. The Geriatric Depression Scale (GDS).
    2. The St. Louis University Mental Status (SLUMS) scale.
    3. The Mini-Mental Status Examination (MMSE) scale.
    4. The Manic Depression vs Elderly Depression (MDED) scale.
    5. The Functional Independence Measurement Scale (FIMS).

129. Which **priority** goal would the nurse identify for a client diagnosed with Parkinson's disease?
    1. The client will be able to maintain mobility and swallow without aspiration.
    2. The client will verbalize feelings about the diagnosis of Parkinson's disease.
    3. The client will understand the purpose of medications administered for the disease.
    4. The client will have a home health agency for monitoring at home.

130. The ICU nurse is admitting a client diagnosed with a TBI. Which HCP medication order would the nurse **question**?

| Client Name: ABCD | MR# 0123456 | Diagnosis: Traumatic Brain Injury |
|---|---|---|
| Age: 29 years | Allergies: NKDA | |
| Medication | 0701–1900 | 1901–0700 |
| Dexamethasone 4 mg IVP every 6 hours | 1200<br>1800 | 2400<br>0600 |
| 0.9% saline continuous infusion at 25 mL/hour | 1600 | |
| Nicotine patch 15 mg per day<br>Apply at 0800; discontinue at 2100 | 0900 | 2100 |
| Morphine sulfate 4 mg IVP every 3 hours prn | | |
| Signature of Nurse: | Day Nurse RN/DN | Night Nurse RN/NN |

    1. Dexamethasone.
    2. 0.9% NS.
    3. Nicotine patch.
    4. Morphine sulfate.

131. The charge nurse on a medical-surgical unit is reviewing client diagnostic reports. Which report **warrants immediate** intervention?
    1. Client A—Male 64.

| Complete Blood Count | Client Values | Normal Values |
|---|---|---|
| Red blood cells (RBC) | 5 | Male: 4.21–5.81 × $10^6$ cells/microL<br>Female: 3.6–5.11 × $10^6$ cells/microL |
| Hemoglobin | 13.4 | Male: 14–17.3 g/dL<br>Female: 11.7–15.5 g/dL |
| Hematocrit | 39.5 | Male: 42%–52%<br>Female: 36%–48% |
| Platelet | 110 | 140–400 × $10^3$/microL |
| White blood cells (WBCs) | 9.2 | 4.5–11.1 × $10^3$/microL |

    2. Client B—Female 34.

| Laboratory Test | Client Values | Normal Values |
|---|---|---|
| Potassium | 3.5 | 3.5–5.3 mEq/L |
| Sodium | 142 | 135–145 mEq/L |
| Chloride | 98 | 97–107 mEq/L |
| $CO_2$ | 26 | 22–29 mEq/L |

3. Client C—Male 45.

| Laboratory Test | Client Values | Normal Values |
|---|---|---|
| Glucose | 94 | Fasting <100 mg/dL<br>Random <200 mg/dL |
| Hemoglobin A$_1$C | 13.2% | Non-diabetic 4%–5.5%<br>Prediabetes 5.7%–6.4%<br>Diabetes 6.5% or less |

4. Client D—Female 56.

| Patient | MRI Findings |
|---|---|
| MRI of brain with and without contrast | MRI brain—Finding of 5 × 4 cm mass located in the L frontal lobe; a shift in the brain tissue exerting pressure on the cerebellum and occluding the anterior portion of the L lateral ventricle. |

132. The nurse is caring for a client diagnosed with ICP and secretions pooled in the throat. Which intervention should the nurse implement **first**?
    1. Set the ventilator to hyperventilate the client in preparation for suctioning.
    2. Assess the client's lung sounds and check for peripheral cyanosis.
    3. Turn the client to the side to allow the secretions to drain from the mouth.
    4. Suction the client using the in-line suction, wait 30 seconds, and repeat.

133. The nurse is performing a GCS assessment on a client diagnosed with a problem with intracranial regulation. The client's GCS 1 hour ago was scored at 10. Which data indicate the client is improving?

**Glasgow Coma Scale**

| Best Eye Opening (E) | Best Verbal Response (V) | Best Motor Response (M) |
|---|---|---|
| 4 = Spontaneous | 5 = Normal conversation | 6 = Normal |
| 3 = To voice | 4 = Disoriented conversation | 5 = Localizes to pain |
| 2 = To pain | 3 = Words, but not coherent | 4 = Withdraws to pain |
| 1 = None | 2 = No words . . . only sounds | 3 = Flexion with pain |
| | 1 = None | 2 = Extension with pain |
| | | 1 = None |
| | | Total = E + V + M |

    1. The current GCS rating is 3.
    2. The current GCS rating is 9.
    3. The current GCS rating is 10.
    4. The current GCS rating is 12.

134. The client diagnosed with a brain abscess is experiencing a tonic-clonic seizure. Which interventions should the nurse implement? **Rank in order of performance.**
    1. Assess the client's mouth.
    2. Loosen restrictive clothing.
    3. Administer phenytoin IVP.
    4. Turn the client to the side.
    5. Protect the client's head from injury.

135. Which intervention should the nurse implement to **decrease** increased ICP for a client on a ventilator? **Select all that apply.**
    1. Position the client with the head of the bed up 30 degrees.
    2. Cluster activities of care.
    3. Suction the client every 3 hours.
    4. Administer soapsuds enemas until clear.
    5. Place the client in the Trendelenburg position.

This section provides the answers to the questions given in the previous section. The correct answers and why they are correct are provided in blue boldface. The reason why each of the other answer options is not the correct or the best answer is also given.

## Cerebrovascular Accident (Stroke)

1. 1. The drug rtPA may be administered, but a CVA must be verified by diagnostic tests before administering it. The drug rtPA helps dissolve a blood clot, and it may be administered if an ischemic CVA is verified; rtPA is not given if the client is experiencing a hemorrhagic stroke.
   2. Teaching is important to help prevent another CVA, but it is not the priority intervention on admission to the ED. Slurred speech indicates problems that may interfere with teaching.
   3. **A CT scan will determine if the client is having a stroke, has a brain tumor, or another neurological disorder. If a CVA is diagnosed, the CT scan can determine if it is a hemorrhagic or an ischemic accident and guide treatment.**
   4. The client may be referred for speech deficits and swallowing difficulty, but referrals are not the priority in the ED.

**TEST-TAKING HINT: When "priority" is used in the stem, all answer options may be appropriate for the client situation, but only one option is the priority. The client must have a documented diagnosis before treatment is started.**

2. 1. A left-sided CVA will result in right-sided motor deficits; hemiparesis is the weakness of one-half of the body, not just the upper extremity. Apraxia, the inability to perform a previously learned task, is a communication loss, not a motor loss.
   2. **The most common motor dysfunction of a CVA is paralysis of one side of the body, hemiplegia; in this case, with a left-sided CVA, the paralysis would affect the right side. Ataxia is an impaired ability to coordinate movement.**

3. Homonymous hemianopsia (loss of half of the visual field of each eye) and diplopia (double vision) are visual field deficits that a client diagnosed with a CVA may experience, but they are not motor losses.
   4. Personality disorders occur in clients diagnosed with a right-sided CVA and are cognitive deficits; hostility is an emotional deficit.

**TEST-TAKING HINT: Be sure always to notice adjectives describing something. In this case, "left-sided" describes the type of CVA. Also, be sure to identify exactly what the question is asking—in this case, about "motor loss," which will help rule out many of the possible answer options.**

3. 1. **African Americans have twice the rate of CVAs as whites and males have a higher incidence than females; African Americans are also at a higher risk of death from a stroke than people of other ethnicities. Additionally, over 75% of strokes occur in people over 65 years old (National Institute of Health, 2016).**
   2. Females are less likely to have a CVA than males, but advanced age does increase the risk for CVA. The Asian population has a lower risk.
   3. Whites have a lower risk of CVA than do African Americans, Hispanics, and American Indian/Alaska Natives.
   4. Maternal age pregnancy is a minimal risk for having a CVA, regardless of ethnicity.

**TEST-TAKING HINT: Note the age of the client if this information is given, but take this information in context with the additional information provided in the answer options. The 84-year-old may appear to be the best answer but not if the client is a female and of Asian descent, which rules out this option for the client most at risk.**

4. Correct answers are 1 and 3.
   1. **Placing a small pillow under the shoulder will prevent the shoulder from adducting toward the chest and developing a contracture.**
   2. The client should be repositioned at least every 2 hours to prevent contractures, pneumonia, skin breakdown, and other complications of immobility.

3. The client should not ignore the paralyzed side, and the nurse must encourage the client to move it as much as possible; a written schedule may assist the client in exercising.

4. These exercises are recommended, but they must be done at least five times a day for 10 minutes to help strengthen the muscles for walking.

5. The fingers are positioned so that they are barely flexed to help prevent contracture of the hand.

**TEST-TAKING HINT: Be sure to look at the intervals of time for any intervention; note that "every shift" and "three times a day" are not appropriate time intervals for this client. Because this is a "select all that apply" question, the test taker must read each answer option and decide if it is correct; one will not eliminate another.**

5. 1. Agnosia is the failure to recognize familiar objects; therefore, observing the client for possible aspiration is not appropriate.

2. A semi-Fowler's position is appropriate for sleeping, but agnosia is the failure to recognize familiar objects; therefore, this intervention is inappropriate.

3. Placing suction at the bedside will help if the client has dysphagia (difficulty swallowing), not agnosia, which is a failure to recognize familiar objects.

4. A collaborative intervention is an intervention in which another health-care discipline—in this case, occupational therapy—is used in the care of the client.

**TEST-TAKING HINT: Be sure to look at what the question is asking and see if the answer can be determined even if some terms are not understood. In this case, note that the question refers to "collaborative intervention." Only option "4" refers to collaboration with another discipline.**

6. 1. Placing a gait belt before ambulating is an appropriate action for safety and would not require the nurse to intervene.

2. Placing the client in a supine position with the head turned to the side is not a problem position, so the nurse does not need to intervene.

3. This action is inappropriate and would require intervention by the nurse because pulling on a flaccid shoulder joint could cause shoulder dislocation; the client should be pulled up by placing the arm underneath the back or using a lift sheet.

4. The client should be encouraged and praised for attempting to perform any activities independently, such as combing hair or brushing teeth.

**TEST-TAKING HINT: This type of question has three answer options that do not require a nurse to intervene to correct a subordinate. Remember to read every possible answer option before deciding on a correct one.**

7. 1. The nurse would anticipate an oral anticoagulant, warfarin (Coumadin), to be prescribed to help prevent thrombi formation in the atria secondary to atrial fibrillation. The thrombi can become embolic and may cause another TIA or a CVA (stroke).

2. Beta blockers slow the heart rate and decrease BP but would not be an anticipated medication to help prevent a TIA secondary to atrial fibrillation.

3. An antihyperuricemic medication is administered for a client experiencing gout and decreases the formation of tophi.

4. A thrombolytic medication is administered to dissolve a clot, and it may be ordered during the initial presentation for a client diagnosed with a CVA but not on discharge.

**TEST-TAKING HINT: In the stem of this question, there are two disease processes mentioned—atrial fibrillation and TIA. The reader must determine how one process affects the other before answering the question. In this question, the test taker must know atrial fibrillation predisposes the client to the formation of thrombi, and therefore, the nurse should anticipate the HCP ordering medication to prevent clot formation, an anticoagulant.**

8. 1. The rubber mat will stabilize the plate and prevent it from slipping away from the client learning to feed himself, but this does not address the generalized weakness.

2. A long-handled bath sponge will assist the client when showering hard-to-reach areas, but it is not a home modification, nor will it help with generalized weakness.

3. Clothes with Velcro closures will make dressing easier, but they do not constitute a home modification and do not address the generalized weakness.

4. Raising the toilet seat is modifying the home and addresses the client's weakness in being able to sit down and get up without straining muscles or requiring lifting assistance from the wife.

**TEST-TAKING HINT:** The test taker must read the stem of the question carefully and note that the intervention must be one in which the home is modified in some way. This would eliminate three of the options, leaving the correct answer.

9. 1. Potential for injury is a physiological, not a psychosocial, problem.
   2. **Expressive aphasia, also known as Broca's aphasia, means that the client cannot communicate thoughts but understands what is being communicated; this leads to frustration, anger, depression, and the inability to verbalize needs, which, in turn, causes the client to have a lack of control and feel powerless.**
   3. A disturbance in thought processes is a cognitive problem; with expressive aphasia, the client's thought processes are intact.
   4. Sexual dysfunction can have a psychosocial or physical component, but it is not related to expressive aphasia.

**TEST-TAKING HINT:** The test taker should always make sure that the choice selected as the correct answer matches what the question is asking. The stem has the adjective "psychosocial," so the correct answer must address psychosocial needs.

10. Correct answers are 1 and 3.
   1. **This glucose level is elevated and could predispose the client to ischemic neurological changes due to blood viscosity. However, research indicates diabetes and elevated glucose levels are risk factors for both ischemic and hemorrhagic strokes (Snarska et al., 2017).**
   2. A carotid bruit predisposes the client to an embolic or ischemic stroke but not to a hemorrhagic stroke.
   3. **Uncontrolled hypertension is a risk factor for hemorrhagic stroke, which is a ruptured blood vessel inside the cranium.**
   4. Cancer is not a precursor to developing a hemorrhagic stroke.
   5. A lithium level of 0.8 is within the therapeutic level of long-term treatment. Research indicates many mood stabilizers can increase the risk of stroke in patients with bipolar disorder, but not lithium (Chen et al., 2019).

**TEST-TAKING HINT:** Both options "1" and "2" are risk factors for an ischemic or embolic type of stroke. Knowing this, the test taker can rule out these options as incorrect.

11. 1. The nurse should not administer any medication to a client without first assessing the cause of the client's report or problem.
   2. An MRI scan may be needed, but the nurse must determine the client's neurological status before diagnostic tests.
   3. Starting an IV infusion is appropriate, but it is not the action the nurse should implement when assessing pain, and 100 mL/hr might be too high a rate for an 85-year-old client.
   4. **The nurse must complete a neurological assessment to help determine the cause of the headache before taking any further action.**

**TEST-TAKING HINT:** The test taker should always apply the nursing process when answering questions. If the test taker narrows down the choices to two possible answer options, always select the assessment option as the first intervention.

12. 1. **The client is at risk for increased ICP whenever performing the Valsalva maneuver, which will occur when straining during defecation. Therefore, stool softeners would be appropriate.**
   2. Coughing increases ICP and is discouraged for any client after a craniotomy. The client is encouraged to turn and breathe deeply but not to cough.
   3. Monitoring the neurological status is appropriate for this client, but it should be done much more frequently than every shift.
   4. Dopamine is used to increase blood pressure or to maintain renal perfusion, and a BP of 160/90 is too high for this client.

**TEST-TAKING HINT:** The test taker should always notice if an answer option has a time frame—every shift, every 4 hours, or daily. Whether or not the time frame is correct may lead the test taker to the correct answer.

## Head Injury

13. 1. **Awakening the client every 2 hours allows the identification of headache, dizziness, lethargy, irritability, and anxiety—all clinical manifestations of postconcussion syndrome—that would warrant the significant other's taking the client back to the ED.**
   2. The nurse should monitor for clinical manifestations of increased ICP, but a layperson, the significant other, would not know what these signs and medical terms mean.

3. Hypervigilance, increased alertness, and super-awareness of the surroundings is a sign of amphetamine or cocaine abuse, but it would not be expected in a client diagnosed with a head injury.

4. The client can eat food as tolerated, but feeding the client every 3 to 4 hours does not affect the development of postconcussion syndrome, the clinical manifestations of which are what should be taught to the significant other.

**TEST-TAKING HINT: Remember to pay close attention to answer options that have times (e.g., "every 2 hours," "every 3 to 4 hours"). Also, consider the likelihood of the options listed. Would a nurse teach the significant other terms such as increased ICP or hypervigilance? Probably not, so options "2" and "3" should be eliminated.**

14. 1. The scalp is a very vascular area, and a moderate amount of bleeding would be expected.

   **2. These clinical manifestations—weak pulse, shallow respirations, cool pale skin—indicate increased ICP from cerebral edema secondary to the fall, and they require immediate attention.**

   3. This is a normal pupillary response and would not warrant intervention.

   4. A headache that resolves with medication is not an emergency situation, and the nurse would expect the client to have a headache after the fall; a headache not relieved with Tylenol would warrant further investigation.

**TEST-TAKING HINT: The test taker is looking for an answer option that is not normal for the client's situation. Of the options listed, three would be expected and would not warrant a trip to the ED.**

15. 1. A client diagnosed with a head injury must be awakened every 2 hours to determine alertness; a decreasing level of consciousness is the first indicator of increased ICP.

   2. A diagnostic test, MRI, would be an expected test for a client diagnosed with left-sided weakness and would not require immediate attention.

   **3. The GCS is used to determine a client's response to stimuli (best eye-opening response, best verbal response, and best motor response) secondary to a neurological problem; scores range from 3 (deep coma) to 15 (intact neurological function). A client with a score of 6 should be assessed first by the nurse.**

4. The nurse would expect a client diagnosed with a CVA (stroke) to have some sequelae of the problem, including the inability to speak.

**TEST-TAKING HINT: This is a prioritizing question that asks the test taker to determine which client has priority when assessing all four clients. The nurse should assess the client with abnormal data for the disease process.**

16. 1. This is an oculocephalic test (doll's eye movement) that determines brain activity. If the eyes move with the head, it means the brainstem is intact, and there is no brain death.

   2. Waveforms on the EEG indicate that there is brain activity.

   **3. The cold caloric test, also called the oculovestibular test, is a test used to determine if the brain is intact or dead. No eye activity indicates brain death. If the client's eyes moved, that would indicate that the brainstem is intact.**

   4. Decorticate posturing after painful stimuli are applied indicates that the brainstem is intact; flaccid paralysis is the worse neurological response when assessing a client diagnosed with a head injury.

**TEST-TAKING HINT: The test taker needs to know what the results of the cold caloric test signify—in this case, no eye activity indicates brain death.**

17. 1. Assessing the neurological status is important, but ensuring an airway is a priority over assessment.

   2. Monitoring vital signs is important, but maintaining an adequate airway is a higher priority.

   3. Initiating an IV access is an intervention the nurse can implement, but it is not the priority intervention.

   **4. The most important nursing goal in the management of a client diagnosed with a head injury is to establish and maintain an adequate airway.**

**TEST-TAKING HINT: If the question asks for a priority intervention, it means that all of the options would be appropriate for the client, but only one intervention is the priority. Always apply Maslow's hierarchy of needs—an adequate airway is first.**

18. 1. The client in rehabilitation is at risk for the development of DVT; therefore, this is an appropriate medication.
2. An osmotic diuretic would be ordered in the acute phase to help decrease cerebral edema, but this medication would not be expected to be ordered in a rehabilitation unit.
3. Clients diagnosed with head injuries are at risk for post-traumatic seizures; thus, an oral anticonvulsant would be administered for seizure prophylaxis.
4. The client is at risk for a stress ulcer; therefore, an oral proton pump inhibitor would be an appropriate medication.

**TEST-TAKING HINT: The client is in the rehabilitation unit and, therefore, must be stable. The use of any intravenous medication should be questioned under those circumstances, even if the test taker is not sure why the medication may be considered.**

19. 1. **Purposeless movement indicates that the client's cerebral edema is decreasing. The best motor response is purposeful movement, but purposeless movement indicates an improvement over decorticate movement, which, in turn, is an improvement over decerebrate movement or flaccidity.**
2. Flaccidity would indicate a worsening of the client's condition.
3. Decerebrate posturing would indicate a worsening of the client's condition.
4. The eyes respond to light, not painful stimuli, but a 6-mm nonreactive pupil indicates a severe neurological deficit.

**TEST-TAKING HINT: The test taker must have strong assessment skills and know what specific clinical manifestations signify for each of the body systems—in this case, the significance of different stages of posturing and movement in assessing neurological status.**

20. **Correct answers are 2, 3, and 5.**
1. The head of the bed should be **elevated** no more than 30 degrees to help decrease cerebral edema by gravity.
2. **Stool softeners are initiated to prevent the Valsalva maneuver, which increases ICP.**
3. **Oxygen saturation higher than 93% ensures oxygenation of the brain tissues; decreasing oxygen levels increase cerebral edema.**
4. Noxious stimuli, such as suctioning, increase ICP and should be avoided.

5. **Frequent, serial neurological assessments, every 1 to 2 hours, should be performed**

**TEST-TAKING HINT: In "select all that apply" questions, the test taker should look at each answer option as a separate entity. In option "1" the test taker should attempt to get a mental picture of the client's position in the bed. A 60-degree angle is almost upright in the bed. Would any client diagnosed with a head injury be positioned this high? The client would be at risk of slumping over because of the inability to control the body position. Nasal suctioning, option "4," which increases ICP, should also be avoided.**

21. 1. Before notifying the HCP, the nurse should always make sure that all the needed assessment information is available to discuss with the HCP.
2. With head injuries, any clear drainage may indicate a cerebrospinal fluid leak; the nurse should not assume the drainage is secondary to allergies and administer an antihistamine.
3. **The presence of glucose in drainage from the nose or ears indicates cerebrospinal fluid, and the HCP should be notified immediately once this is determined.**
4. This would be appropriate, but it is not the first intervention. The nurse must determine where the fluid is coming from.

**TEST-TAKING HINT: The question is asking which intervention should be implemented first, and the nurse should always assess the situation before calling the HCP or taking action.**

22. 1. Assessment is important, but with clients diagnosed with a head injury, the nurse must assume SCI until it is ruled out with x-ray; therefore, stabilizing the spinal cord is the priority.
2. Removing the client from the water is an appropriate intervention, but the nurse must assume SCI until it is ruled out with an x-ray; therefore, stabilizing the spinal cord is the priority.
3. Assessing the client for further injury is appropriate, but the first intervention is to stabilize the spine because the impact was strong enough to render the client unconscious.
4. **The nurse should always assume that a client diagnosed with traumatic head injury may have sustained SCI. Moving the client could further injure the spinal**

cord and cause paralysis; therefore, the nurse should stabilize the cervical spinal cord as best as possible before removing the client from the water.

**TEST-TAKING HINT: When two possible answer options contain the same directive word—in this case, "assess"—the test taker can either rule out these two as incorrect or prioritize between the two assessment responses.**

23. 1. The head of the client's bed should be elevated to help the lungs expand and prevent stasis of secretions that could lead to pneumonia, a complication of immobility.
    2. Active ROM exercises require that the client participates in the activity. This is not possible because the client is in a coma.
    3. The client is at risk for pressure ulcers and should be turned more frequently than every shift, and research now shows that massaging bony prominences can increase the risk for tissue breakdown.
    4. The nurse should always talk to the client, even if the client is in a coma, but this will not address the problem of immobility.

**TEST-TAKING HINT: Whenever a client problem is written, interventions must address the specific problem, not the disease. Positioning the client addresses the possibility of immobility complications, whereas talking to a comatose client addresses communication deficit and psychosocial needs, not immobility issues.**

24. 1. The client is at risk for **seizures** and does not process information appropriately. Allowing him to return to his occupation as a forklift operator is a safety risk for him and other employees. Vocational training may be required.
    2. **"Cognitive" pertains to mental processes of comprehension, judgment, memory, and reasoning. Therefore, an appropriate goal would be for the client to stay on task for 10 minutes.**
    3. The client's ability to dress self addresses self-care problems, not a cognitive problem.
    4. The client's ability to regain bowel and bladder control does not address cognitive deficits.

**TEST-TAKING HINT: The test taker must note adjectives closely. The question is asking about "cognitive" deficits; therefore, the correct answer must address cognition.**

## Spinal Cord Injury

25. 1. The nurse should stabilize the client's neck and assess the airway before removal from the car.
    2. The nurse must stabilize the client's neck before doing any further assessment. Most nurses don't carry penlights, and the client's pupil reaction can be determined after stabilization.
    3. **The nurse must maintain a patent airway. The airway is the first step in resuscitation.**
    4. Shaking the patient could cause further damage, possibly leading to paralysis.

**TEST-TAKING HINT: Remember that, in a question asking about which action should be taken first, all of the answers are interventions, but only one should be implemented first. There are very few "always" situations in the healthcare profession, but in this situation, unless the client's car is on fire or underwater, stabilizing the client's neck is always the priority, followed by the airway.**

26. Correct answers are 1 and 4.
    1. **Neurogenic shock causes peripheral vasodilation below the level of the injury. Peripheral vasodilation causes heat to be carried by the blood to the skin.**
    2. Assessment of the movement of the upper extremities would be more appropriate with a higher-level injury; an injury in the cervical area might cause an inability to move the upper extremities. A lack of movement of the extremities is not a clinical manifestation of neurogenic shock.
    3. Reports of a pounding headache are not typical of neurogenic shock.
    4. **Hypotension, bradycardia, and peripheral vasodilation are clinical manifestations of neurogenic shock (Hoffman & Sullivan, 2020).**
    5. Bradycardia, not tachycardia, is a clinical manifestation of neurogenic shock.

**TEST-TAKING HINT: Neurogenic shock results from many different causes but primarily from spinal cord injuries. The test taker should be able to identify the different types of shock and clinical manifestations of each one.**

27. 1. Oxygen is administered initially to maintain a high arterial partial pressure of oxygen ($Pao_2$) because hypoxemia can worsen a neurological deficit to the spinal cord initially, but this client is in the rehabilitation

department and thus not in the initial stages of the injury.

2. DVT is a potential complication of immobility, which can occur because the client cannot move the lower extremities as a result of the L1 SCI. Low-dose anticoagulation therapy (Lovenox) helps prevent blood from coagulating, thereby preventing DVTs.
3. The client is unable to move the lower extremities. The nurse should do passive ROM exercises.
4. A client diagnosed with a spinal injury at C4 or above would be dependent on a ventilator for breathing, but a client diagnosed with an L1 SCI would not.

**TEST-TAKING HINT:** The test taker should notice any adjectives such as "rehabilitation," which should clue the test taker into ruling out oxygen, which is for the acute phase. The test taker should also be very selective if choosing an answer with a definitive word such as "all" (option "1").

28. Correct answers are 1, 3, and 5.
    1. Oxygen is administered initially to prevent hypoxemia, which can worsen the SCI; therefore, the nurse should determine how much oxygen is reaching the periphery.
    2. A C7 injury would not affect the client's ability to chew and swallow, so pureed food is not necessary.
    3. Breathing exercises are supervised by the nurse to increase the strength and endurance of inspiratory muscles, especially those of the diaphragm.
    4. Autonomic dysreflexia occurs during the rehabilitation phase, not the acute phase.
    5. Corticosteroids are administered to decrease inflammation, which will decrease edema, and help prevent edema from ascending up the spinal cord, causing breathing difficulties.

**TEST-TAKING HINT:** The test taker must notice where the client is receiving care, which may be instrumental in being able to rule out incorrect answer options and help in identifying the correct answer. Remember Maslow's hierarchy of needs—oxygen and breathing are priority nursing interventions.

29. 1. Therapeutic communication addresses the client's feelings and attempts to allow the client to verbalize feelings; the nurse should be a therapeutic listener.
    2. This is belittling the client's feelings.

3. The client does not owe the nurse an explanation of his feelings; "why" is never therapeutic.
4. This is advising the client and is not therapeutic.

**TEST-TAKING HINT:** When the question requests a therapeutic response, the test taker should select the answer option that has "feelings" in the response.

30. 1. The machine is very loud, and the technician will offer the client earplugs, but a hearing difficulty will not affect the MRI scan.
    2. Allergies to dairy products will not affect the MRI scan.
    3. The client does not need to be NPO for this procedure.
    4. MRI scans are often done in a very confined space; many people with claustrophobia must be medicated or even rescheduled for the procedure in an open MRI machine, which may be available if needed.

**TEST-TAKING HINT:** The nurse must be knowledgeable of diagnostic tests to prepare the client for the tests safely. The test taker must be realistic in determining answers—is there any test in which a hearing problem would make the diagnostic test contraindicated?

31. 1. This action will not address the client's pounding headache and hypertension.
    2. Dimming the lights will not help the client's condition.
    3. This is an acute emergency caused by exaggerated autonomic responses to stimuli and only occurs after spinal shock has resolved in the client diagnosed with a SCI above T6. The most common cause is a full bladder.
    4. The nurse should always assess the client before administering medication.

**TEST-TAKING HINT:** The test taker should apply the nursing process when answering questions, and assessing the client comes first, before administering any type of medication.

32. Correct answers are 2 and 5.
    1. The halo device is applied by inserting pins into the skull, and the client cannot remove them; the pins should be checked for signs of infection.
    2. Reddened areas, especially under the vest and brace, must be reported to the HCP because pressure ulcers can occur when wearing this appliance for an extended period.

3. The vest liner should be changed for hygiene reasons, but the halo part is not removed.
4. The client should be encouraged to ambulate to prevent complications of immobility.
5. The client should be taught to notify the HCP of difficulty swallowing. The halo may need to be adjusted.

**TEST-TAKING HINT:** The test taker would need basic knowledge about a halo device to answer this question easily, but some clues are in the stem. A cervical fracture is in the upper portion of the spine or neck area, and most people understand that a halo is something that surrounds the forehead or higher. So the test taker could get a mental image of a device that must span this area of the body and maintain alignment of the neck. If an HCP attaches pins into the head, then the test taker could assume that they were not to be removed by the client. Redness usually indicates some sort of problem with the skin.

33. 1. This is not an emergency; therefore, the nurse should not notify the HCP.
2. A physiological change in the client requires more than a therapeutic conversation.
3. Increasing the IV rate will not address the cause of the problem.
4. **Clients with SCIs are susceptible to orthostatic hypotension because BP tends to be unstable and low in the acute stage. Slight elevations of the head of the bed can cause profound hypotension; therefore, the nurse should lower the head of the bed immediately.**

**TEST-TAKING HINT:** The test taker should notice that the only answer option that addresses the "bed" is the correct answer. This does not always help identify the correct answer, but it is a hint that should be used if the test taker has no idea what the correct answer is.

34. 1. **This client has clinical manifestations of a respiratory complication and should be assessed first.**
2. This is a psychosocial need and should be addressed, but it does not have priority over a physiological problem.
3. A client diagnosed with a lower SCI would not be at risk for autonomic dysreflexia; therefore, a report of headache and feeling hot would not be a priority over an airway problem.
4. The client diagnosed with a T4 SCI would not be expected to move the lower extremities.

**TEST-TAKING HINT:** The nurse should assess the client at risk for dying or having some type of complication that requires intervention. Remember Maslow's hierarchy of needs, in which physiological problems are always priority and airway is the top physiological problem.

35. 1. The nurse cannot delegate assessment or teaching.
2. Tube feedings should be treated as if they were medications, and this task cannot be delegated.
3. **The assistant can place the client on the bedside commode as part of bowel training; the nurse is responsible for the training but can delegate this task.**
4. Evaluating the client's ability to self-catheterize must be done by the nurse.

**TEST-TAKING HINT:** Although each state has its own delegation rules, teaching, assessing, evaluating, and medication administration are nursing interventions that cannot be delegated to UAP.

36. 1. The ASIA is an appropriate referral for living with this condition, but it does not help find gainful employment after the injury.
2. **The vocational rehabilitation agency of each state will help evaluate and determine if the client can receive training or education for another occupation after injury.**
3. The client is not asking about disability; he is concerned about employment. Therefore, the nurse needs to make a referral to the appropriate agency.
4. This does not address the client's concern about gainful employment.

**TEST-TAKING HINT:** If the question mentions a specific age for a client, the nurse should consider it when attempting to answer the question. This is a young person needing to find gainful employment. Remember Erickson's stages of growth and development.

## Seizures

37. 1. The nurse needs to protect the client from injury. Moving furniture would help ensure that the client would not hit something accidentally, but this is not done first.
2. This is done to help keep the airway patent, but it is not the first intervention in this specific situation.
3. Assessment is important, but when the client is having a seizure, the nurse should provide for the client's safety before assessing vital signs.

4. The client should not remain in the chair during a seizure. He should be brought safely to the floor so that he will have room to move the extremities.

**TEST-TAKING HINT: All of the answer options are possible interventions, so the test taker should go back to the stem of the question and note that the question asks which intervention has priority. "In the chair" is the key to this question because the nurse should always think about safety, and a client having a seizure is not safe in a chair.**

38. 1. Head injury is one of the main reasons for epilepsy that can be prevented through occupational safety precautions and highway safety programs.
    2. A sedentary lifestyle is not a cause of epilepsy.
    3. Dietary concerns are not a cause of epilepsy.
    4. Safety glasses will help prevent eye injuries, but such injuries are not a cause of epilepsy.

**TEST-TAKING HINT: The nurse must be aware of risk factors that cause diseases. If the test taker does not know the correct answer, thinking about which body system the question is asking about may help rule out or rule in some of the answer options. Only options "1" and "4" have anything to do with the head, and only helmets on the head are connected with the neurological system.**

39. Correct answers are 3 and 5.
    1. Antiseizure drugs, tranquilizers, stimulants, and depressants are withheld before an EEG because they may alter the brain wave patterns.
    2. Meals are not withheld because altered blood glucose levels can cause changes in brain wave patterns.
    3. The goal is for the client to have a seizure during the EEG. Sleep deprivation, hyperventilating, or flashing lights may induce a seizure.
    4. Electrodes are placed on the client's scalp, but there are no electroshocks or any type of discomfort.
    5. The client should avoid hair products, such as conditioner, gels, and hairspray, that may interfere with electrode adherence to the scalp.

**TEST-TAKING HINT: The test taker should highlight the words "diagnose a seizure disorder" in the stem and ask which answer options are test preparation teaching for an EEG, to assist in diagnosis.**

40. 1. Noticing the first thing the client does during a seizure provides information and clues as to the location of the seizure in the brain. It is important to document whether the beginning of the seizure was observed.
    2. Assessment is important, but during the seizure, the nurse should not attempt to restrain the head to assess the eyes; muscle contractions are strong, and restraining the client could cause injury.
    3. This should be done, but it is not the first intervention when walking into a room where the client is beginning to have a seizure.
    4. The client should be protected from onlookers, but the nurse should always address the client first.

**TEST-TAKING HINT: This is a prioritizing question that asks the test taker which intervention to implement first. All four interventions would be appropriate, but only one should be implemented first. If the test taker cannot decide between two choices, always select the one that directly affects the client or the condition; privacy is important, but helping determine the origin of the seizure is a priority.**

41. 1. The client is exhausted from the seizure and should be allowed to sleep.
    2. Awakening the client every 30 minutes could possibly induce another seizure as a result of sleep deprivation.
    3. During the postictal (after-seizure) phase, the client is very tired and should be allowed to rest quietly; placing the client on the side will help prevent aspiration and maintain a patent airway.
    4. The client must rest, and asking questions about the seizure will keep the client awake, which may induce another seizure as a result of sleep deprivation.

**TEST-TAKING HINT: Options "1," "2," and "4" all have something to do with keeping the client awake. This might lead the test taker to choose the option that is different from the other three.**

42. 1. No one should attempt to put anything in the client's mouth.
    2. The nurse should tell the UAP to stop trying to insert anything in the mouth of the client experiencing a seizure. Broken teeth and injury to the lips and tongue may result from trying to place anything in the clenched jaws of a client having a tonic-clonic seizure.

3. The primary nurse is responsible for the action of the UAP and should stop the UAP from doing anything potentially dangerous to the client. No one should attempt to pry open the jaws that are clenched in a spasm to insert anything.

4. The primary nurse must correct the action of the UAP immediately, before any injury occurring to the client and before notifying the charge nurse.

**TEST-TAKING HINT:** The nurse is responsible for the actions of the UAP and must correct the behavior immediately.

43. 1. Thorough oral hygiene after each meal, gum massage, daily flossing, and regular dental care are essential to prevent or control gingival hyperplasia, which is a common occurrence in clients taking phenytoin (Dilantin), an anticonvulsant.

2. A serum (venipuncture) phenytoin (Dilantin) level is checked monthly at first and then, after a therapeutic level is attained, every 6 months.

3. Phenytoin does not turn the urine orange.

4. The use of phenytoin, an anticonvulsant, does not ensure that the client will not have any seizures, and, in some instances, the dosage may need to be adjusted, or another medication may need to be used.

**TEST-TAKING HINT:** The test taker should realize that monitoring blood glucose levels using a glucometer is about the only level that is monitored daily; therefore, option "2," which calls for daily monitoring of phenytoin (Dilantin) levels, could be eliminated. Remember, there are very few absolutes in the health-care field; therefore, option "4" could be ruled out because "won't have any" is an absolute.

44. 1. Assessment is an independent nursing action, not a collaborative one.

2. Most clients in the ICU will be placed on telemetry, which does not require an order by another HCP or collaboration with one.

3. Administering an anticonvulsant medication by intravenous push requires the nurse to have an order or confer with another member of the health-care team.

4. A glucocorticoid is a steroid and is not used to treat seizures.

**TEST-TAKING HINT:** The keyword in the stem of this question is the adjective "collaborative." The test taker would eliminate the options "1" and "2" because these do not require collaboration with another member of the health-care team and would eliminate option "4" because it is not used to treat seizures.

45. Correct answers are 1, 3, and 4.

1. Keeping a seizure and medication chart will be helpful when keeping follow-up appointments with the HCP and in identifying activities that may trigger a seizure.

2. The client should take showers, rather than tub baths, to avoid drowning if a seizure occurs. The nurse should also instruct the client never to swim alone.

3. Over-the-counter medications may contain ingredients that will interact with antiseizure medications or, in some cases, as with the use of stimulants, possibly cause a seizure.

4. Most of the anticonvulsant medications have therapeutic serum levels that should be maintained, and regular checks of the serum levels help to ensure the correct level.

5. A newly diagnosed client would have just been put on medication, which may cause drowsiness. Therefore, the client should avoid activities that require alertness and coordination and should not be driving at all until after the effects of the medication have been evaluated.

**TEST-TAKING HINT:** The test taker must select all interventions that are appropriate for the question. A keyword is the adverb "newly."

46. 1. The client diagnosed with a seizure disorder should avoid stimulants, such as caffeine.

2. The onset of menstruation can cause seizure activity in the female client.

3. Tension states, such as anxiety and frustration, induce seizures in some clients, so stress management may be helpful in preventing seizures.

4. Bright flickering lights, television viewing, and some other photic (light) stimulation may cause seizures, but sunlight does not. Wearing dark glasses or covering one eye during potential seizure-stimulating activities may help prevent seizures.

**TEST-TAKING HINT:** Caffeine is a stimulant, and its use is not recommended in many disease processes. Menstrual cycle changes are known to affect seizure disorders. Therefore, options "1" and "2" can be eliminated, as can option "4" because sunlight does not cause seizures.

47. 1. An aura is a visual, auditory, or olfactory occurrence that takes place before a seizure and warns the client a seizure is about to occur. The aura often allows time for the client to lie down on the floor or find a safe place to have a seizure.
    2. An aura is not dependent on the client being physically or psychologically exhausted.
    3. This is a therapeutic response, reflecting feelings, which is not an appropriate response when answering a client's question.
    4. Sleepiness after a seizure is very common, but the aura does not itself cause the sleepiness.

**TEST-TAKING HINT:** If the stem of the question has the client asking a question, then the nurse needs to give factual information, and option "3," a therapeutic response, would not be appropriate. Neither would option "2" or "4" because these options are worded in such a way as to imply incorrect information.

48. Correct answers are 1, 3, 4, and 5.
    1. Any disease that affects brain function, such as Alzheimer's disease, can lead to seizures.
    2. Cervical spondylosis, age-related degeneration of the bones and cartilage in the neck and spine, is not related to seizures.
    3. Head injuries from falls make the elderly client more at risk for seizures.
    4. A CVA (stroke) is the leading cause of seizures in the elderly; increased ICP associated with the stroke can lead to seizures (Centers for Disease Control and Prevention, 2019).
    5. Brain tumors are associated with seizures (CDC, 2019).

**TEST-TAKING HINT:** All answer options are associated with the brain, neurological system, and aging. However, option "2" is the only option related to the natural aging process and thus can be eliminated as a cause of seizures.

## Brain Tumors

49. Correct answers are 2 and 5.
    1. Nervousness is not a symptom of a brain tumor, and brain tumors rarely metastasize outside of the cranium. Brain tumors kill by occupying space and increasing ICP. Cough and rapid eye movements are not associated with a brain tumor.
    2. The symptoms suggesting a brain tumor include a headache that is dull, unrelenting, and worse at night; vomiting unrelated to food intake; and edema of the optic nerve (papilledema), which occurs in 70% to 75% of clients diagnosed with brain tumors. Papilledema causes visual disturbances, such as decreased visual acuity and diplopia.
    3. Hypertension and bradycardia, not hypotension and tachycardia, occur with increased ICP resulting from pressure on the cerebrum. Tachypnea does not occur with brain tumors.
    4. Abrupt loss of motor function occurs with a stroke; diarrhea does not occur with a brain tumor, and the client diagnosed with a brain tumor does not experience a change in taste.
    5. Mood changes, blurred vision, and seizures are symptoms of a brain tumor. The symptoms of a brain tumor will vary based on the location of the tumor (Hoffman & Sullivan, 2020).

**TEST-TAKING HINT:** The test taker can rule out option "4" because of the symptom of diarrhea, which is a gastrointestinal symptom, not a neurological one. Option "1" has the symptom of cough, which is a respiratory symptom and can be ruled out. Considering the other possible choices, the symptom of "headache" and "seizures" would make sense for a client diagnosed with a brain tumor.

50. 1. A widening pulse pressure and bounding pulse indicate increased ICP but do not localize the tumor.
    2. Diplopia and decreased visual pressure are symptoms indicating papilledema, a general symptom in the majority of all brain tumors.
    3. Bradykinesia is slowed movement, a symptom of Parkinson's disease, and scanning speech is symptomatic of multiple sclerosis.
    4. Hemiparesis would localize a tumor to a motor area of the brain, and personality changes localize a tumor to the frontal lobe.

**TEST-TAKING HINT:** The test taker could arrive at the correct answer if the test taker realized that specific regions of the brain control motor function and hemiparesis and that other regions are involved in personality changes.

51. 1. This is providing information and is not completely factual. MRIs are loud, but frequently the client will require an IV access

(an invasive procedure) to be started for a contrast medium to be injected.

2. This is restating and offering self. Both are therapeutic responses.

3. This statement is belittling the client's feelings.

4. This is not dealing with the client's concerns and is passing the buck. The nurse should explore the client's feelings to determine what is concerning the client. The MRI may or may not be the problem. The client may be afraid of the results of the MRI.

**TEST-TAKING HINT: When the question asks the test taker for a therapeutic response, the test taker should choose the response that directly addresses the client's feelings.**

52. 1. Nothing in the stem indicates the client has a problem with swallowing, so aspiration precautions are not needed.

2. Reach to Recovery is an American Cancer Society–sponsored program for clients diagnosed with breast cancer, but it is not prophylactic.

3. **The client diagnosed with metastatic lesions to the brain is at high risk for seizures.**

4. Teaching about mastectomy care is not prophylactic, and the stem did not indicate whether the client had a mastectomy.

**TEST-TAKING HINT: The test taker should not read into a question—for example, about mastectomy care. The test taker should be careful to read the descriptive words in the stem; in this case, "prophylactic" is the key to answering the question correctly.**

53. 1. **A SW is qualified to assist the client with referrals to any agency or personnel that is needed.**

2. The chaplain would be a referral if spiritual guidance is required, but the stem did not specify this need.

3. The HCP also can refer to the SW, but the nurse can make this referral independently.

4. The OT assists with cognitive functioning, ADL, and modification of the home, but the stem did not define these needs.

**TEST-TAKING HINT: The test taker must decide what each discipline has to offer the client; an SW has the broadest range of referral capabilities.**

54. 1. Maintaining weight is a nutritional goal.

2. Completing an advance directive is an end-of-life or psychosocial goal.

3. **Performing ADL is a goal for self-care deficit.**

4. Verbalizing feelings is a psychosocial goal.

**TEST-TAKING HINT: The test taker should read the stem of the question carefully. All of the goals could be appropriate for a client diagnosed with a brain tumor, but only one applies to self-care deficit.**

55. 1. Purposeful movement following painful stimuli would indicate an improvement in the client's condition.

2. Adducting the upper extremities while internally rotating the lower extremities is decorticate positioning and would indicate that the client's condition had not changed.

3. Aimless thrashing would indicate an improvement in the client's condition.

4. **The most severe neurological impairment result is flaccidity and no response to stimuli. This indicates that the client's condition has worsened.**

**TEST-TAKING HINT: Neurological assessment includes assessing the client for levels of consciousness; the nurse must memorize the stages of neurological progression toward a coma and death.**

56. 1. A transsphenoidal hypophysectomy is done by an incision above the gumline and through the sinuses to reach the sella turcica, where the pituitary is located.

2. The client will be given regular food when awake and able to tolerate food.

3. **Blowing the nose creates increased ICP and could result in a cerebrospinal fluid leak.**

4. The client will return from surgery with the head of the bed elevated to about 30 degrees; this allows for gravity to assist in draining the cerebrospinal fluid.

**TEST-TAKING HINT: The test taker must know the procedures for specific disease processes to answer this question, but anatomical positioning of the pituitary gland (just above the sinuses) could help to eliminate option "1," which calls for a large turban dressing.**

57. 1. A headache after this surgery would be an expected occurrence, not a complication.

2. **An output much larger than the intake could indicate the development of diabetes insipidus. Pressure on the pituitary gland can result in decreased production of vasopressin, the antidiuretic hormone (ADH).**

3. A raspy sore throat is common after surgery due to the placement of the endotracheal tube during anesthesia.
4. Dizziness when rising quickly is expected; the client should be taught to rise slowly and call for assistance for safety.

**TEST-TAKING HINT:** The test taker could eliminate options "1" and "3" as expected occurrences following the surgery and not complications. Option "4" can also be expected.

58. 1. Making the client NPO will not help the client to swallow.
2. A low Fowler's position would make it easier for the client to aspirate.
3. The consistency of the food is not an issue; the client will have difficulty swallowing this food as well as regular-consistency food.
4. To decrease the risk of aspiration, the client should direct food to the unaffected side of the throat; this helps the client to be able to use the side of the throat that is functioning.

**TEST-TAKING HINT:** The test taker should try to visualize the position of the client in the bed. A mostly recumbent position (low Fowler's) would increase the chance of aspiration; thus, option "2" should be eliminated.

59. 1. Chemotherapy is a systemic therapy that is used extensively in the care of clients diagnosed with cancer. However, most drugs have difficulty in crossing the blood-brain barrier and are not useful in treating brain tumors unless delivered by direct placement into the spinal column or directly to the ventricles of the brain by a device called an Ommaya reservoir.
2. **The blood-brain barrier is the body's defense mechanism for protecting the brain from chemical effects; in this case, it prevents chemotherapy from being able to work on the tumor in the brain.**
3. Radiation has about the same amount of side effects as chemotherapy, but the effects of radiation tend to last for a much longer time.
4. Some tumors do become resistant to the chemotherapy agents used. When this happens, the oncologist switches to different drugs.

**TEST-TAKING HINT:** The test taker can eliminate option "1" as a possible answer because it states that chemotherapy is used to treat brain tumors, but it does not tell the client why it is not being used. Option "2" is the only one that

actually informs the client of a medical reason for not administering chemotherapy for a brain tumor.

60. Correct answers are 1, 2, 3, and 5.
1. The client should sleep with the head of the bed elevated to promote drainage of the cerebrospinal fluid.
2. Humidified air will prevent drying of the nasal passages.
3. Because the incision for this surgery is just above the gum line, the client should not brush the front teeth. Oral care should be performed using a sponge until the incision has healed.
4. The client can eat a regular diet.
5. The HCP should be notified if the client develops an infection of any kind. A cold with sinus involvement and sneezing places the client at risk for opening the incision and developing a brain infection.

**TEST-TAKING HINT:** The test taker could choose option "5" because this is a standard instruction for any surgery. The test taker should look for more than one correct answer in an alternative-type question.

## Meningitis

61. 1. This is a definition of aseptic meningitis, which refers to the irritation of the meninges from viral or noninfectious sources.
2. This is another example of aseptic meningitis, which refers to the irritation of the meninges from viral or noninfectious sources.
3. Septic meningitis refers to meningitis caused by bacteria; the most common forms of bacterial meningitis are caused by the *Neisseria meningitides* and *Streptococcus pneumoniae* bacteria.
4. This is the explanation for encephalitis.

**TEST-TAKING HINT:** The nurse should explain the client's diagnosis in layperson's terms when the stem is identifying the significant other as asking the question. Be sure to notice that the adjective "septic" is the key to answering this question, ruling out options "1" and "2."

62. 1. Hospitalized clients are weakened, but they are not at risk of contracting any type of meningitis.
2. Outbreaks of infectious meningitis are most likely to occur in dense community groups such as college campuses, jails, and military installations.

3. Developing countries do not pose a risk factor for meningitis. They provide a risk for hepatitis or tuberculosis.
4. Employees in a high-rise building do not live together, and they have their own space; therefore, they are not at risk for developing meningitis.

**TEST-TAKING HINT:** The test taker must remember that the NCLEX-RN® tests all areas of nursing, so always notice the type of nurse if this is mentioned in the stem. The role of the public health nurse is to work within the community to improve health outcomes.

63. 1. Babinski's sign is used to assess brainstem activity, and paresthesia is tingling, which is not a clinical manifestation of bacterial meningitis.
2. Chvostek's sign is used to assess for hypocalcemia, and facial tingling is a sign of hypocalcemia. It is not used to assess for bacterial meningitis.
3. **A positive Kernig's sign (client unable to extend the leg when lying flat) and nuchal rigidity (stiff neck) are clinical manifestations of bacterial meningitis occurring because the meninges surrounding the brain and spinal column are irritated.**
4. Trousseau's sign is used to assess for hypocalcemia, and nystagmus is abnormal eye movement. Neither of these is a clinical manifestation of bacterial meningitis.

**TEST-TAKING HINT:** If two answer options test for the same thing (Trousseau's and Chvostek's signs), then the test taker can rule out these as possible answers because there cannot be two correct answers in the question unless the question tells the test taker that it is a "select all that apply" question.

64. 1. **In clients diagnosed with meningococcal meningitis, purpuric lesions over the face and extremity, as well as fever, are the clinical manifestations of Waterhouse-Friderichsen syndrome, which is fatal in 55% to 60% of cases (National Center for Advancing Translational Sciences, 2016).**
2. Photophobia is a common clinical manifestation of all types of meningitis and would be expected.
3. Inflammation of the meninges results in increased ICP, which causes a headache. This would be an expected occurrence and would not warrant notifying the HCP.

4. A client not being able to identify the day of the week would not in itself warrant notifying the HCP.

**TEST-TAKING HINT:** The stem is asking the nurse to identify which assessment data are abnormal for the disease process and require an immediate medical intervention to prevent the client from experiencing a complication or possible death.

65. 1. Standard precautions are mandated for all clients, but a client diagnosed with septic meningitis will require more than the standard precautions.
2. Airborne precautions are for contagious organisms that are spread on air currents and require the hospital personnel to wear an ultra-high-filtration mask; these precautions would be applied for diseases such as tuberculosis.
3. Contact precautions are for contagious organisms that are spread by blood and body fluids, such as those that occur with wounds or diarrhea.
4. **Droplet precautions are respiratory precautions used for organisms that have a limited span of transmission. Precautions include staying at least 4 feet away from the client or wearing a standard isolation mask and gloves when coming in close contact with the client. Clients are in isolation for 24 to 48 hours after the initiation of antibiotics.**

**TEST-TAKING HINT:** The test taker must know the types of isolation precautions used for different diseases and note the adjective— "septic"—in the stem of the question.

66. 1. This goal is not related to altered cerebral tissue perfusion, but it would be a goal for self-care deficit.
2. **A client diagnosed with a problem of altered cerebral tissue perfusion is at risk for seizure activity secondary to focal areas of cortical irritability; therefore, the client should be on seizure precautions.**
3. This would be an appropriate goal for the client diagnosed with an infection.
4. This would be an appropriate goal for the client diagnosed with dehydration.

**TEST-TAKING HINT:** The goal must be related to the problem—in this case, "altered cerebral tissue perfusion."

67. Correct answers are 1, 2, 3, and 5.
    1. A lumbar puncture is an invasive procedure; therefore, informed consent is required.
    2. This could be offered for client comfort during the procedure.
    3. This position increases the space between the vertebrae, which allows the HCP easier entry into the spinal column.
    4. The client is encouraged to relax and breathe normally; hyperventilation may lower elevated cerebrospinal fluid pressure.
    5. The nurse should always explain to the client what is happening before and during a procedure.

**TEST-TAKING HINT:** This is an alternative-type question, which requires the test taker to select more than one answer option.

68. 1. A nurse administering antibiotics is a collaborative intervention because the HCP must write an order for the intervention; nurses cannot prescribe medications unless they have additional education and licensure and are nurse practitioners with prescriptive authority.
    2. The nurse needs an order to send a culture to the laboratory for payment purposes, but the nurse can obtain a specimen without an order. A sputum specimen is not appropriate for meningitis.
    3. A pulse oximeter measures the amount of oxygen in the periphery and does not require an HCP to order.
    4. Intake and output are independent nursing interventions and do not require an HCP's order.

**TEST-TAKING HINT:** The test taker must note adjectives and understand that a collaborative nursing intervention is dependent on another member of the health-care team; an independent nursing intervention does not require collaboration.

69. 1. This vaccine must be administered before exposure to build up an immunity to prevent meningitis resulting from *Haemophilus influenzae*.
    2. Chemoprophylaxis includes administering a medication that will prevent infection or eradicate the bacteria and the development of symptoms in people recently in close proximity to the client. Medications include rifampin (Rifadin), ciprofloxacin (Cipro), and ceftriaxone (Rocephin).

3. Steroids are used as an adjunct therapy in the treatment of clients diagnosed with acute bacterial meningitis. They would not be given as a prophylactic measure to others in the home.
4. Gamma globulin provides passive immunity to clients exposed to hepatitis. It is not appropriate in this situation.

**TEST-TAKING HINT:** The keyword in the stem is "preventive." The test taker must pay close attention to the adjectives.

70. 1. Antibiotics would help decrease the bacterial infection in meningitis, which would cause the exudate. The drugs mentioned in the question would not.
    2. Fever increases cerebral metabolism and ICP. Therefore, measures are taken to reduce body temperature as soon as possible, and alternating Tylenol and Motrin would be appropriate.
    3. A nonnarcotic antipyretic (Tylenol) and an NSAID (Motrin) will not address the client's memory or orientation.
    4. These medications do not prevent or treat a yeast infection.

**TEST-TAKING HINT:** The test taker must have a basic knowledge of the disease process and medications that are prescribed to treat a disease. Purulent drainage would require an antibiotic. Therefore, option "1" should be eliminated as a possible answer because the question is asking about NSAIDs and a nonnarcotic antipyretic (Tylenol).

71. 1. The antibiotic has the highest priority because failure to treat a bacterial infection can result in shock, systemic sepsis, and death.
    2. The lunch tray is important and may actually arrive before the antibiotic, but the priority for the nurse must be the medication.
    3. The client's room should be kept dark because of photophobia, but photophobia is a symptom that is not life-threatening.
    4. Knowledge of the client's weight is necessary, but initial antibiotic therapy can be initiated without knowing the client's admission weight.

**TEST-TAKING HINT:** The nurse must know how to prioritize care. Which intervention has the potential to avoid a complication related to the disease process? Remember the word "priority."

**72.** 1. The client's lung sounds should be clear with meningitis, and nothing in the question stem indicates a comorbid condition. Therefore, assessing lung sounds is not a priority.
2. The client may experience photophobia and visual disturbances, but assessing the six fields of gaze will not affect the client's condition.
3. The client's cardiac status is not affected by meningitis. Therefore, the apical pulse would not be a priority.
4. **Meningitis directly affects the client's brain. Therefore, assessing the neurological status would have priority for this client.**

**TEST-TAKING HINT:** The test taker should apply a systemic approach to discerning the priority response. Maslow's hierarchy of needs would put option "1" as correct, but the disease process of meningitis does not include clinical manifestations of a respiratory component. The next highest priority would be the neurological component, and meningitis definitely is a neurological disease.

## Parkinson's Disease

**73.** 1. A masklike face is a lack of expression and is part of the motor manifestations of Parkinson's disease but is not related to the symptoms listed. Shuffling is also a motor deficit and does pose a risk for falling, but fever and patchy infiltrates on a chest x-ray do not result from a gait problem. They are manifestations of a pulmonary complication.
2. **Difficulty swallowing places the client at risk for aspiration. Immobility predisposes the client to pneumonia. Both clinical manifestations place the client at risk for pulmonary complications.**
3. Pill rolling of fingers and flat affect do not have an impact on the development of pulmonary complications.
4. Arm swing and bradykinesia are motor deficits.

**TEST-TAKING HINT:** The nurse must recognize the clinical manifestations of disease and the resulting bodily compromise. In this situation, fever and patchy infiltrates on a chest x-ray indicate a pulmonary complication. Options "1," "3," and "4" focus on motor problems and could be ruled out as too similar. Only option "2" includes dissimilar information.

**74.** 1. Carbidopa is never given alone. Carbidopa is given together with levodopa to help the levodopa cross the blood-brain barrier.
2. Levodopa is a form of dopamine given orally to clients diagnosed with Parkinson's disease.
3. **Carbidopa enhances the effects of levodopa by inhibiting decarboxylase in the periphery, thereby making more levodopa available to the central nervous system. Carbidopa and levodopa (Sinemet), an antiparkinsonian drug, are effective treatment for Parkinson's disease.**
4. Carbidopa does not cross the blood-brain barrier.

**TEST-TAKING HINT:** The nurse must be knowledgeable of the rationale for administering medication for a specific disease.

**75.** 1. PTs work on lower body assistance (gait and mobility). A PT would recommend a walker. OTs work on cognition and fine motor skills. An OT would recommend eating with adaptive appliances.
2. Clients diagnosed with Parkinson's disease are placed on high-calorie, high-protein, soft, or liquid diets. Supplemental feedings may also be ordered. If liquids are ordered because of difficulty chewing, then the liquids should be thickened to a honey or pudding consistency.
3. Nuts and whole-grain food would require extensive chewing before swallowing and would not be good for the client. Three large meals would get cold before the client can consume the meal, and one-half or more of the food would be wasted.
4. **The client's energy levels will not sustain eating for long periods. Offering frequent and easy-to-chew (soft) meals of small proportions is the preferred dietary plan.**

**TEST-TAKING HINT:** The correct answer for a nursing problem question must address the actual problem.

**76.** 1. The nurse should not delegate feeding a client at risk for complications during feeding. This requires judgment that the UAP is not expected to possess.
2. UAPs can turn and position clients diagnosed with pressure ulcers. The nurse should assist in this at least once during the shift to assess the wound area.

3. The UAP can assist the client to the bathroom every 2 hours and document the results of the attempt.
4. The UAP can obtain the vital signs on a stable client.

**TEST-TAKING HINT: When reading the answer options in a question in which the nurse is delegating to an UAP, read the stem carefully. Is the question asking what to delegate or what not to delegate? Anything requiring professional judgment should not be delegated.**

77. 1. **Headache and photophobia are expected clinical manifestations of meningitis. The new graduate could care for this client.**
    2. This client has had an unusual occurrence (fall) and now has a potential complication (a fracture). The experienced nurse should take care of this client.
    3. These vital signs indicate increased ICP. The more experienced nurse should care for this client.
    4. This could indicate a worsening of the tumor. This client is at risk for seizures and herniation of the brainstem. The more experienced nurse should care for this client.

**TEST-TAKING HINT: The test taker should determine if the clinical manifestations are expected as part of the disease process. If they are, a new graduate can care for the client; if they are not expected occurrences, a more experienced nurse should care for the client.**

78. 1. Akinesia is lack of movement. The goal in treating Parkinson's disease is to maintain mobility.
    2. This could be a goal for a problem of noncompliance with the treatment regimen but not a goal for treating the disease process.
    3. This might be a goal for a psychosocial problem of social isolation.
    4. **The major goal of treating Parkinson's disease is to maintain the ability to function. Clients diagnosed with Parkinson's disease experience slow, jerky movements and have difficulty performing routine daily tasks.**

**TEST-TAKING HINT: The test taker should match the goal to the problem. A "therapeutic goal" is the key to answering this question.**

79. 1. A stereotactic pallidotomy is a surgery that uses CT or MRI scans to localize specific areas of the brain in which to produce lesions in groups of brain cells through electrical stimulation or thermocoagulation. These procedures are done when medication has failed to control tremors.
    2. Dopamine receptor agonists are medications that activate the dopamine receptors in the striatum of the brain.
    3. Deep brain stimulation is a safe treatment, effective in controlling movement disorders but has some adverse effects such as speech and psychiatric disturbances (Stoker et al., 2018).
    4. Fetal tissue transplantation has shown some success in Parkinson's disease, but it is an experimental and highly controversial procedure (Stoker et al., 2018). Trials are being conducted with embryonic rather than fetal tissue.

**TEST-TAKING HINT: The test taker should not overlook the adjective "experimental." This would eliminate at least option "2," which refers to standard dopamine treatment, even if the test taker was not familiar with all of the procedures.**

80. 1. The emotions of a person diagnosed with Parkinson's disease are labile. The client has rapid mood swings and is easily upset.
    2. Hallucinations are a sign that the client is experiencing drug toxicity.
    3. **Scheduling appointments late in the morning gives the client a chance to complete ADL without pressure and allows the medications time to give the best benefits.**
    4. The client should take the prescribed medications at the same time each day to provide a continuous drug level.

**TEST-TAKING HINT: The test taker could eliminate option "2" because hallucinations are never an expected part of legal medication administration.**

81. 1. Crackles and jugular vein distention indicate heart failure, not Parkinson's disease.
    2. Upper extremity weakness and ptosis are clinical manifestations of myasthenia gravis.
    3. The client has very little arm swing, and scanning speech is a clinical manifestation of multiple sclerosis.
    4. **Masklike face and a shuffling gait are two clinical manifestations of Parkinson's disease.**

**TEST-TAKING HINT: Option "3" refers to arm swing and speech, both of which are affected by Parkinson's disease. The test taker needs to decide if the adjectives used to describe these**

activities—"exaggerated" and "scanning"—are appropriate. They are not, but masklike faces and shuffling gait are.

82. 1. Emotional lability is a psychosocial problem, not a cognitive one.
    2. Depression is a psychosocial problem.
    3. **Memory deficits are cognitive impairments. The client may also develop dementia.**
    4. Paranoia is a psychosocial problem.

**TEST-TAKING HINT: The test taker must know the definitions of common medical terms. "Cognitive" refers to mental capacity to function.**

83. 1. This is information that should be discussed when filling out an advance directive form. A ventilator is used to treat a physiological problem.
    2. **These are psychosocial manifestations of Parkinson's disease. These should be discussed in the support meeting.**
    3. The reduction in the unintentional pill-rolling movement of the hands is controlled at times by the medication; this is a physiological problem.
    4. Echolalia is a speech deficit in which the client automatically repeats the words or sentences of another person; this is a physiological problem.

**TEST-TAKING HINT: Psychosocial problems should address the client's feelings or interactions with another person.**

84. 1. A headache of "2" on a 1-to-10 scale is a mild headache.
    2. A SCI at T10 involves deficits at approximately the waist area. The inability to move the toes would be expected.
    3. **Body image is a concern for clients diagnosed with Parkinson's disease. This client is the one client not experiencing expected sequelae of the disease.**
    4. This client is getting better; "resolving" indicates an improvement in the client's clinical manifestations.

**TEST-TAKING HINT: At times, a psychological problem can have priority. All the physical problems are expected and are not life-threatening or life-altering.**

## Substance Abuse

85. 1. This should be done so that appropriate care can be provided, but it is not a priority action.

2. This should be done before the client ceases breathing, and a cardiac arrest follows, but it is not the first action.
3. This would be a good step to take to prepare for the worst-case scenario, but it can be done last among these answer options.
4. **Applying oxygen would be the priority action for this client. The client's breathing is slow and shallow. The greater the amount of inhaled oxygen, the better the client's prognosis.**

**TEST-TAKING HINT: When the test taker is deciding on a priority, some guidelines should be used. Maslow's hierarchy of needs places oxygen at the top of the priority list.**

86. 1. **No employee of a facility is above certain rules. In a company with a "No Drugs" policy, this includes the CEO. This client is exhibiting symptoms of cocaine abuse.**
    2. The nurse does not have definitive knowledge that the client is using drugs until a positive drug screen result is obtained. If the nurse is not a trained substance abuse counselor, this intervention would be out of the realm of the nurse's expertise.
    3. The client is the CEO of the facility; only the board of directors or the parent company is above this client in supervisory rank.
    4. Giving an antihistamine is prescribing without a license, and the nurse is obligated to intervene in this situation.

**TEST-TAKING HINT: The title of the client— CEO—eliminates option "3." The nurse has noted a potentially illegal situation.**

87. 1. **The Health Insurance Portability and Accountability Act (HIPAA) requires that a health-care professional not divulge information about one person to an unauthorized person.**
    2. This would be discussing Client B and a violation of HIPAA.
    3. The nurse does not know Client B is using drugs, so notifying the HCP is not appropriate.
    4. Client B would require an explanation for coming to the clinic, for which, if the nurse has not violated HIPAA, there is no explanation.

**TEST-TAKING HINT: Nurses are required to practice within the laws of the state and within federal laws. HIPAA is a federal law and applies to all HCPs in the United States. Legally, the nurse cannot use the information provided by**

Client A, but morally the nurse might try to identify behavior in Client B that would warrant the nurse's intervention.

88. 1. These reactions are called "flashbacks."
2. Flashback reactions occur after the use of hallucinogens in which the client relives a bad episode that occurred while using the drug.
3. The drug is gone from the body, but the mind-altering effects can occur at any time in the form of memory flashbacks.
4. The client stated that the dreams are causing her distress. She is asking for help with the dreams, not planning her suicide.

**TEST-TAKING HINT:** The client is 20 years old and took the drug in her teens; drugs do not stay in the body for extended periods. This eliminates option "3."

89. 1. The nurse is not the coworker's supervisor, and confronting the coworker about the suspicions could lead to problems if the nurse is not trained to deal with substance abusers.
2. This is circumventing the problem. The coworker will find another source of drugs if needed, and it is finding the coworker guilty without due process.
3. The coworker's supervisor or peer review committee should be aware of the nurse's suspicions so that the suspicions can be investigated. This is a client safety and care concern.
4. The nurse is obligated to report suspicious behavior to protect the clients the coworker is caring for.

**TEST-TAKING HINT:** The test taker can eliminate option "4" based on "do nothing." In this instance, direct confrontation is not recommended, but the nurse must do something—namely, report the suspicions to the supervisor or peer review.

90. 1. Insomnia and anxiety are symptoms of alcohol withdrawal, not Wernicke-Korsakoff syndrome.
2. Visual and auditory hallucinations are symptoms of delirium tremens.
3. Extreme tremors and agitation are symptoms of delirium tremens.
4. Ataxia, or lack of coordination, and confabulation, making up elaborate stories to explain lapses in memory, are both symptoms of Wernicke-Korsakoff syndrome.

**TEST-TAKING HINT:** The test taker can eliminate options "2" and "3" if the test taker knows the symptoms of delirium tremens.

91. 1. Thiamine is given in high doses to decrease the rebound effect on the nervous system as it adjusts to the absence of alcohol, and chlordiazepoxide (Librium), a benzodiazepine, is given in high doses and titrated down over several days for the tranquilizing effect of preventing delirium tremens.
2. The client may have seizures, but Valium would control this. The client does not need long-term anticonvulsant medication, phenytoin (Dilantin), and it is not known that the client needs an iron preparation, ferrous sulfate (Feosol). The vitamin deficiency associated with delirium tremens is a lack of thiamine, not iron.
3. Methadone, a synthetic narcotic, is used for withdrawing clients from heroin, and divalproex sodium (Depakote) can be used as a mood stabilizer in bipolar disorder or as an anticonvulsant.
4. The client does not need mannitol, an osmotic diuretic, and methylphenidate (Ritalin), a stimulant, would produce an effect opposite to what is desired.

**TEST-TAKING HINT:** Option "3" could be eliminated if the test taker knew the treatment for heroin withdrawal, and option "4" could be reasoned out because a stimulant would produce an undesired effect.

92. Correct answers are 3, 4, and 5.
1. Chills, sweats, and gooseflesh occur with heroin withdrawal, but seizures do not usually occur, so seizure precautions are not necessary.
2. Vital signs should be taken more frequently, every 2 to 4 hours, depending on the client's condition.
3. The client should be in an atmosphere with little stimulation. The client will be irritable and fearful.
4. Heroin is administered intravenously. Heroin addicts are at high risk for HIV as a result of shared needles and thus should be tested for HIV.
5. The client is withdrawing from heroin, so medically assisted detoxification begins with buprenorphine (Buprenex).

**TEST-TAKING HINT:** A "select all that apply" question will usually have more than one correct answer. One option cannot eliminate another.

93. 1. This is a therapeutic response. The spouse is not expressing feelings but is stating a fact. The nurse should address the problem.
    2. This is a therapeutic response. The spouse is not expressing feelings but is stating a fact. The nurse should address the problem.
    3. The spouse is not required to give an explanation to the nurse.
    4. The spouse's behavior is enabling the client to continue to drink until he cannot function.

**TEST-TAKING HINT:** The stem of the question did not ask for a therapeutic response but did ask for the nurse's best response. The best response is to address the problem.

94. 1. Telemetry and vital signs would be done to monitor cardiovascular compromise. Amphetamine use causes tachycardia, vasoconstriction, hypertension, and arrhythmias.
    2. This might be an intervention for a problem of altered coping.
    3. This would be an intervention for the problem of insomnia.
    4. These are interventions for heart failure.

**TEST-TAKING HINT:** The correct answer must address the problem of cardiovascular compromise, which eliminates options "2" and "3."

95. Correct answers are 2 and 5.
    1. This is unrealistic. Most restaurants serve some form of alcoholic beverage. It is good advice for the client to try to avoid situations that provide the temptation to use drugs or alcohol again.
    2. The client will require a follow-up program such as 12-step meetings if the client is not to relapse.
    3. The nurse does not know that this is true.
    4. The client should discuss the history with the people the client chooses.
    5. The client should use breathing and relaxation techniques to manage stress to avoid a relapse.

**TEST-TAKING HINT:** The test taker must notice descriptive words such as "all" or "do not go anywhere." These words or phrases are absolutes that should cause the test taker to eliminate the options containing them.

96. 1. The child will realize the changed behaviors when and if they happen.
    2. This could cause problems between the parent and child.
    3. Most coping behaviors are learned from parents and guardians. Children of substance abusers tend to cope with life situations by becoming substance abusers unless taught healthy coping mechanisms.
    4. Children can be a part of the parent's recovery, but this is not the rationale for teaching new coping mechanisms.

**TEST-TAKING HINT:** Most parents do not like to be corrected by their child; this could eliminate option "2." The correct answer must address a reason for teaching new coping strategies.

## Amyotrophic Lateral Sclerosis (ALS or Lou Gehrig's Disease)

97. Correct answers are 1, 2, 3, and 5.
    1. EMG is done to differentiate a neuropathy from a myopathy and can help diagnose ALS.
    2. Nerve conduction studies (NCS) can help diagnose forms of peripheral neuropathy or myopathy. If other problems are not present, this can help diagnose ALS.
    3. CK can indicate some disorders of the musculoskeletal system and can help diagnosis ALS.
    4. This is done as ALS progresses to determine respiratory involvement, but it does not diagnose ALS.
    5. An MRI is performed to reveal disorders of the brain and spinal cord and can assist in diagnosis of ALS (National Institute of Neurological Disorders and Stroke, 2019).

**TEST-TAKING HINT:** The test taker must be clear as to what the question is asking. The word "diagnose" is the key to answering this question correctly. The test taker would need to know that this disease affects the muscles to identify the answers correctly.

98. 1. Disuse syndrome is associated with complications of bedrest. Clients diagnosed with ALS cannot move and reposition themselves, and they frequently have altered nutritional and hydration status.
    2. The client does not usually have a change in body image.
    3. ALS is a disease affecting the muscles, not the kidneys or circulatory system.
    4. ALS is not painful.

**TEST-TAKING HINT:** The test taker would have to be knowledgeable about ALS to answer this question. This disease is chronic and debilitating over time and leads to wasting of the muscles.

99. 1. These clinical manifestations occur during the course of ALS, but they are not early symptoms.
    2. These clinical manifestations will occur as the disease progresses.
    3. These are late clinical manifestations of ALS.
    4. **ALS results from the degeneration and demyelination of motor neurons in the spinal cord, which results in paralysis and weakness of the muscles.**

**TEST-TAKING HINT:** This is an application question in which the test taker must know that ruling out of ALS would result in the answer being early clinical manifestations. The test taker could rule out option "1" because of atrophy, which is a long-term occurrence; rule out option "2" because these symptoms will occur as the disease progresses, and rule out option "3" because these are late clinical manifestations.

100. 1. This is a therapeutic response, but the client is asking for specific information.
    2. **About 50% of clients die within 2 to 5 years from respiratory failure, aspiration pneumonia, or another infectious process.**
    3. The nurse should allow the client to talk freely about the disease process and should provide educational and emotional support.
    4. This is incorrect information; ALS is a disease that results in death within 5 years in most cases.

**TEST-TAKING HINT:** When the client is asking for factual information, the nurse should provide accurate and truthful information. This helps foster a trusting nurse-client relationship. A therapeutic response (option "1") should be used when the client needs to express feelings and is not asking specific questions about the disease process.

101. 1. Elevating the head of the bed will enhance lung expansion, but it is not the first intervention.
    2. **Oxygen should be given immediately to help alleviate the difficulty in breathing. Remember that oxygenation is a priority.**
    3. Assessment is the first part of the nursing process and is a priority, but the

assessment will not help the client breathe easier.
    4. This is an appropriate intervention, but obtaining the pulse oximeter reading will not alleviate the client's respiratory distress.

**TEST-TAKING HINT:** The test taker should not automatically select assessment. Make sure that there is not another intervention that will directly help the client, especially if the client is experiencing a life-threatening complication.

102. **200 mL/hr.**
    This is a basic math question. The IV pump is calculated in milliliters per hour, so the nurse must double the rate to infuse the IV solution in 30 minutes.

**TEST-TAKING HINT:** This is a basic calculation that the nurse should be able to make even without a calculator.

103. 1. Refusing to turn needs to be addressed by the nurse, but it is not a priority over a life-threatening condition.
    2. Nausea needs to be assessed by the nurse, but it is not a priority over an oxygenation problem.
    3. **A pulse oximeter reading of less than 93% indicates that the client is experiencing hypoxemia, which is a life-threatening emergency. This client should be assessed first.**
    4. The nurse must address the client's reports, but it is not a priority over a physiological problem.

**TEST-TAKING HINT:** The test taker should apply Maslow's hierarchy of needs, in which oxygenation is a priority. The nurse must know normal parameters for diagnostic tools and laboratory data.

104. 1. With assistance, the client may be able to stay at home. Therefore, placement in a long-term care facility should not be discussed until the family can no longer care for the client in the home.
    2. There is no indication that a client diagnosed with ALS will need a sigmoid colostomy.
    3. **A client diagnosed with ALS usually dies within 5 years. Therefore, the nurse should offer the opportunity to determine how the client wants to die.**
    4. ALS affects both upper and lower extremities and leads to a debilitating state, so the client will not be able to transfer into and operate a wheelchair.

**TEST-TAKING HINT:** The nurse should always help the client prepare for death in disease processes that are terminal and should discuss advance directives, which include both a durable power of attorney for health care and a living will.

105. 1. Contractures can develop within a week because extensor muscles are weaker than flexor muscles. If the client cannot perform ROM exercises, then the nurse must do it for the client—passive ROM.
2. The client should maintain a positive nitrogen balance to promote optimal body functioning.
3. Adequate protein is required to maintain osmotic pressure and prevent edema.
4. The client is usually on bedrest in the last stages and should be turned and told to cough and deep breathe more often than every shift.

**TEST-TAKING HINT:** "Terminal stage" is the key term in the stem that should cause the test taker to look for an option addressing immobility issues—option "1." An intervention implemented only once in every shift should be eliminated as a possible answer when addressing immobility issues.

106. 1. The son is not sure if he may get ALS, so this is not an appropriate response.
2. This is incorrect information.
3. There is a genetic factor with ALS that is linked to mutations in the *SOD1* gene and familial ALS (National Institute of Neurological Disorders and Stroke, 2019).
4. ALS is not caused by a virus. The exact etiology is unknown, but studies indicate that some environmental factors may lead to ALS.

**TEST-TAKING HINT:** This question requires knowledge of ALS. There are some questions for which Test-taking hints are not available.

107. 1. A residual (aspirated gastric contents) of greater than 50 to 100 mL indicates that the tube feeding is not being digested and that the feeding should be held.
2. A soft abdomen is normal; a distended abdomen would be a reason to hold the feeding.
3. Diarrhea is a common complication of tube feedings, but it is not a reason to hold the feeding.

4. The potassium level is low and needs intervention, but this would not indicate a need to hold the bolus tube feeding.

**TEST-TAKING HINT:** Knowing normal assessment data would lead the test taker to eliminate option "2" as a possible correct answer. Diarrhea and hypokalemia would not cause the client not to receive a feeding. Even if the test taker did not know what "residual" means, this would be the best option.

108. Correct answers are 4 and 5.
1. The benzothiazole, riluzole (Rilutek), should be given without food at the same time each day.
2. This medication is not affected by green, leafy vegetables. (The anticoagulant warfarin [Coumadin] is a well-known medication that is affected by eating green, leafy vegetables.)
3. This medication is not affected by the sun.
4. **Riluzole, a benzothiazole, can cause blood dyscrasias. Therefore, the client is monitored for liver function, blood count, blood chemistries, and alkaline phosphatase. The client should report any febrile illness. This is the first medication developed to treat ALS.**
5. **Riluzole is an oral suspension, and 15 days after opening the bottle, the unused portion should be discarded.**

**TEST-TAKING HINT:** Blood dyscrasias occur with many medications, and this might prompt the test taker to select option "4" as the correct option. Otherwise, the test taker must be knowledgeable about medication administration.

## Encephalitis

109. Correct answers are 1, 2, 3, and 5.
1. A complication of immunizations for measles, mumps, and rubella can be encephalitis.
2. Upper respiratory tract illnesses can be a precursor to encephalitis.
3. The herpes simplex virus, specifically type 1, can lead to encephalitis.
4. Fungal encephalitis is known to occur in certain regions, and the nurse should assess for recent trips to areas where these fungal spores exist, but the common areas are the Southwest United States and central California. Some forms of mosquito-transmitted viral encephalitis are seen in the Eastern seaboard, Gulf Coast, and western and central plains states, but not the Great Lakes region.

5. Bites from some insects and mosquitoes can result in viral encephalitis (National Institute of Neurological Disorders and Stroke, 2019).

**TEST-TAKING HINT:** Encephalitis is inflammation of the brain caused by either a hypersensitivity reaction or a postinfectious state in which a virus reproduces in the brain. Encephalitis can be a life-threatening disease process. History is vital in the diagnosis.

110. 1. Bilateral facial palsies are a common initial sign and symptom of encephalitis.
2. Fever is usually one of the first clinical manifestations the client experiences.
3. A decrease in the client's headache does not indicate that the client's condition is becoming worse and thus does not warrant immediate intervention.
4. The absence of smell and taste indicates that the cranial nerves may be involved. The client's condition is becoming more serious.

**TEST-TAKING HINT:** This question requires the test taker to select an option that indicates the disease is progressing, and the client is at risk. Option "3" indicates that the client is improving, and options "1" and "2" are common early manifestations of the disease. The only option that reflects cranial nerve involvement, a sign that the client's condition is becoming worse and requires immediate intervention, is option "4."

111. Correct answers are 1, 2, and 3.
1. Written consent is needed for all invasive procedures.
2. This is information that should be shared with the client about the reason for the procedure.
3. The nurse should teach this information to decrease the possible severe, throbbing, "spinal headache" caused by the decrease in cerebrospinal fluid.
4. The client should lie with the head of the bed flat for 4 to 8 hours after the lumbar puncture, but this position would not prevent all hematomas.
5. A local anesthetic is used before a lumbar puncture, not spinal anesthesia.

**TEST-TAKING HINT:** When the test taker is trying to eliminate options, any that have absolute words, such as "all," "never," and "always," are usually wrong and can be eliminated quickly. Rarely is any activity always or never done.

112. 1. Clients diagnosed with encephalitis have neurological deficits while the inflammation is present. The therapeutic plan is to treat the disease process, decrease the edema, and return the client to an optimal level of wellness.
2. The client may have short-term memory loss from a previous condition.
3. Renal function is not affected by encephalitis. Only immobility would affect this system.
4. There is no reason to apply hydrocortisone cream for encephalitis.

**TEST-TAKING HINT:** The test taker should look at the option that reflects the body system that is involved with the disease. Refer to medical terminology; encephalon means "the brain."

113. Correct answers are 1, 2, 4, and 5.
1. Clients diagnosed with encephalitis should be treated for the disease process and also to prevent complications of immobility. Turning the client will prevent skin breakdown.
2. Increasing fluids helps prevent urinary tract infections and mobilize secretions in the lungs.
3. The client would be maintained with the head of the bed elevated 30 to 45 degrees, for gravity to assist the body in decreasing ICP.
4. Immobility causes clients to be at risk for DVT. Therefore, clients diagnosed with encephalitis should be assessed for DVT.
5. Immobility causes the gastrointestinal tract to slow, resulting in constipation. Clients can have difficulty emptying their bladders, which can cause retention and urinary tract infections and stones. Assessing these systems can identify problems early.

**TEST-TAKING HINT:** Each option should be read carefully. If the test taker does not read each one carefully, the test taker could miss important words, such as "supine" in option "3," resulting in an incorrect answer.

114. 1. This is an important area to assess for neurological deterioration, but it is not the first indication of increased ICP.
2. This is the most important assessment data. A change in level of consciousness is usually the first sign of neurological deterioration.

3. Seizures can occur with inflammation from encephalitis, but their occurrence does not indicate that the client has increased ICP resulting from a worsening condition.
4. This is important information to assess, but changes in vital signs are not the first signs and symptoms of increased ICP.

**TEST-TAKING HINT:** The word "first" asks the test taker to prioritize the interventions. Usually, all the options are interventions that the nurse should do, but the question implies that the client may be deteriorating. The level of consciousness is the most sensitive indicator of neurological deficit.

115. Correct answers are 1 and 4.
    1. **Mosquitoes breed in standing water, even pet dishes and birdbaths. All areas that collect water should be emptied, removed, covered, or turned over. Rain gutters should be cleaned.**
    2. Light-colored, long-sleeved, and loose-fitting clothing should be worn to avoid mosquito bites.
    3. Insect repellent may irritate the eyes, but it should be applied over clothing and on all exposed areas.
    4. **Mosquitoes are more prevalent at dusk, dawn, and early evening (Centers for Disease Control and Prevention, 2018).**
    5. There is no vaccine for West Nile virus licensed for human use.

**TEST-TAKING HINT:** Words such as "only" (option "3") should clue the test taker to eliminate that option. Rarely are these absolute terms correct.

116. 1. An alteration in body temperature in a client diagnosed with West Nile virus would not be the highest priority.
    2. **Altered tissue perfusion would be the highest priority because it could be life-threatening.**
    3. A problem of fluid volume excess would not apply for the client diagnosed with West Nile virus. These clients are at risk for fluid volume deficit from nausea, vomiting, and hyperthermia.
    4. A problem with skin integrity could apply to the client diagnosed with immobility caused by West Nile virus, but it would not be the highest priority problem.

**TEST-TAKING HINT:** When prioritizing client problems, oxygenation is the highest priority problem according to Maslow, and tissue perfusion is oxygenation.

117. 1. **Clients diagnosed with West Nile virus should be continuously assessed for alteration in gas exchanges or patterns.**
    2. A rash will resolve when the disease causing the rash is treated.
    3. Hypothermia is not treated with ice packs but with warming blankets.
    4. Lymph glands are edematous early in the disease process. There is no reason to teach the client to report this condition.

**TEST-TAKING HINT:** The test taker needs to read words carefully. Prefixes such as "hypo-" and "hyper-" are important in determining if an option is correct. Even if the test taker did not know if the client is hypothermic or hyperthermic, "hypo-" means "less than normal," so hypothermia would not be treated with ice packs. A client diagnosed with West Nile virus usually has a fever that should be reduced. Thus, a treatment for hypothermia is not needed.

118. 1. This intervention is independent, not collaborative.
    2. This is an independent nursing intervention.
    3. Assessment is an independent nursing intervention.
    4. **Administering an IV fluid is collaborative because it requires an order from an HCP. It does, however, require the nurse to assess the rate, fluid, and site for complications.**

**TEST-TAKING HINT:** When reading test questions, the test taker should pay attention to adjectives. In this question, the word "collaborative" makes all the options incorrect except option "4." Collaborative interventions require an order from an HCP, but the nurse uses judgment and intuition within the scope of practice.

119. 1. These vital signs are within normal ranges. The temperature is slightly elevated and may require an antipyretic but not as an immediate need.
    2. This is a common report requiring medication but not immediately.
    3. This test is used to differentiate West Nile virus from other types of encephalitis and would not require immediate intervention. Supportive care is given for West Nile virus. No definitive treatment is available.
    4. **These assessment data may indicate that the client's condition is deteriorating and require immediate intervention to prevent complications.**

**TEST-TAKING HINT:** The word "immediate" means that the nurse must recognize and intervene before complications occur. The test taker should eliminate any option that contains normal assessment data.

**120.** 1. Transmission does not occur through exposure with sneezed or coughed secretions.
2. The most common transmission of the West Nile virus to humans is through the bite of an infected mosquito.
3. The West Nile virus can be transmitted through breast milk, blood products, and organ transplants. This is a vector-borne disease. It is transmitted to mosquitoes that bite infected birds. The incubation period is 2 to 15 days.
4. Maculopapular rashes do not drain. Draining is a characteristic of a vesicle.

**TEST-TAKING HINT:** The test taker should eliminate option "2" because of the absolute word "only."

121. Correct answers are 1, 4, and 5.
  1. The first nursing action is to ensure that the client does not sustain further damage to the spinal cord. The nurse does this by placing sandbags around the client's head or by maintaining the client on a backboard with the head securely affixed to the board.
  2. This will not occur until a full assessment is made and brain death is imminent.
  3. The head of the bed has to be kept flat, with the client's head stabilized, until spinal damage has been ruled out.
  4. The GCS is a systematic tool used to assess a client's neurological status. It gives health-care workers a standard method to determine the progress of a client's condition.
  5. The client should have intravenous access to be able to administer emergency medications.
  6. In an emergency, the nurse must concentrate on the immediate care of the client. If the client requires a blood transfusion, it will take time to have the type and crossmatch completed.

**TEST-TAKING HINT:** The nurse must remember that safety is a priority when caring for clients incapable or unable to protect themselves, as in option "1." Option "3" is an appropriate assessment method for a TBI because the first step in the nursing process is assessment.

122. 1. This may be needed once the client is stable, but the first action is to get the needed personnel to intervene to prevent lasting damage for the client.
  2. A Code STROKE (for a rapid response team (RRT) related to a stroke) has been instituted in most facilities to have personnel to respond so that there is no delay in initiating interventions, thus reducing the impact of a CVA (stroke) on a client. The American Stroke Association (2020) suggests using the word FAST to help recognize the clinical manifestations of a stroke. F stands for face: ask the person to smile, and see whether one side of the face droops. A stands for arms: if both arms are raised, does one drift to the side? S stands for speech: is it slurred or strange? And T stands for

time: don't waste time before calling 911 if someone has started to show any of these signs.
  3. The first nursing intervention is to call the Code STROKE; then, the HCP would be notified next.
  4. Having the client swallow could be an assessment step, but not a glass of water and with standby suction available in case the client is unable to swallow.

**TEST-TAKING HINT:** The test taker should remember that certain physiological processes carry risks that have to be contended with. Atrial fibrillation can cause the blood to become stagnant and coat the atrial interior surfaces. If this coating of blood breaks loose, then the result can be an intracranial embolus.

123. 1. Safety is always a priority intervention when working with a client whose physical functioning is impaired or when the client's cognitive judgment is compromised.
  2. The client should receive six small meals each day. The client's swallowing ability may be impaired, and the client will be unable to consume the meal before it gets cold. The consistency should be soft so as not to require extended chewing.
  3. Home health may be needed, but the priority intervention is safety.
  4. A skin assessment is not a priority over keeping the patient safe.

**TEST-TAKING HINT:** The test taker should remember that basic nursing care is appropriate for client protection. Maslow's hierarchy of needs lists safety in the second highest priority tier. Physiological needs that involve life-threatening or life-altering complications are the only things that are more important than safety.

124. 1. Sometimes a client can temporarily overcome freezing of motion or tremor by making an intentional movement, but the issue is not enough of the neurotransmitter, dopamine, in the brain. Concentration or focusing will not increase the amount of dopamine available in the brain.
  2. This is the cause of the tremors, cogwheel motion of movement, bradykinesia, and so forth. It is also in layperson's terms that the client can

understand and provides some measure of hope that something can be done without giving false reassurance.
3. The issue is dopamine. The acetylcholine effects are caused by the dopamine not being available to counteract the acetylcholine.
4. This is a therapeutic response, and the client is asking for information.

**TEST-TAKING HINT:** The test taker should read the stem of the question carefully and determine what the client is requesting. The client is newly diagnosed and wants to know about the disease. The nurse should respond to the client's question.

125. 1. The client can be up as preferred, but the nurse should assess this and determine if the client has the functional ability to be able to accomplish this without assistance.
2. A client diagnosed with a brain tumor would be at risk for increased ICP. Fluids should be limited to decrease the amount of cerebrospinal fluid produced by the body.
3. The client can have a diet of choice. The tumor occupies space and increases the pressure on the brain, which can cause vomiting. This vomiting is not associated with the diet; it is caused by the pressure.
4. Clients diagnosed with brain issues are at risk for electrical misfiring of the neurons, a seizure. The nurse should institute measures to protect the client during a seizure.

**TEST-TAKING HINT:** The test taker should remember that basic nursing care is appropriate for client protection. Maslow's hierarchy of needs lists safety in the second highest priority tier. Physiological needs that involve life-threatening or life-altering complications are the only things that are more important than safety.

126. 1. This is presumably true, but it is not an appropriate response to someone with cognitive impairment. Rational thought processes do not apply.
2. The client would become increasingly agitated when unable to utilize the phone and be unable to reach the father.
3. The client is focused on his father. Letting the client talk about his father will allow him to focus on his father while distracting him from his impossible-to-fulfill request.

4. This is called "passing the buck." A nurse on an Alzheimer's unit should be able to assess and intervene in this type of situation.

**TEST-TAKING HINT:** Arguing with a client diagnosed with cognitive impairments only produces frustrations for the client and nurse. The nurse must remember the disease process and respond accordingly.

127. Correct answers are 1, 2, 3, 4, and 5.
1. This client is 28 years old and needs to learn how to function in the home to be able to manage ADL. The OT works with clients to help them attain the highest level of functionality.
2. The PT will work with the client to develop upper body strength.
3. The RD will make sure that nutritional needs are being met.
4. The rehabilitation physician (physiatrist) is a rehabilitation specialist and an expert in bone, muscle, and nerves and treats injuries or illnesses that affect how a client moves.
5. The SW can assist the client with financial matters and can direct the client to programs that will help the client to receive training in a skill(s) that will assist in job placement.
6. The RN represents nursing in the case conference, not the PCT.

**TEST-TAKING HINT:** The test taker can eliminate option "6" by understanding the roles of the staff members. Nurses are with the client 24 hours a day in an inpatient care facility and frequently are the coordinators of the client's care. The nurse must know which discipline should be consulted.

128. Correct answers are 2 and 3.
1. The GDS assesses the older client for depression, not cognitive functioning.
2. The SLUMS scale is a measurement tool for cognitive functioning.
3. The MMSE scale is another tool to assess cognitive functioning.
4. There is no MDED scale, and in addition, depression is not cognitive functioning.
5. The FIMS measures how well the client can perform ADL, not cognitive functioning.

**TEST-TAKING HINT:** The test taker could eliminate options "1," "4," and "5" based on the word "cognitive" in the stem of the question. The test taker should highlight any word that gives a clue as to what the question is asking. Words matter.

129. 1. The priority goal is for the client to maintain functional ability. This improves the quality and quantity of life.
2. Verbalizing feelings is a good goal, but feeling will not impact stabilizing the physiological deterioration of the client.
3. There is no way to measure the client's understanding.
4. Having a home health agency does not ensure that functional ability is maintained.

**TEST-TAKING HINT: Using Maslow's hierarchy of needs, physiological needs are higher than psychosocial needs, so the test taker can eliminate option "2." The nurse cannot determine or measure "understanding," so option "3" can be eliminated.**

130. 1. Dexamethasone is a steroid medication and is the steroid of choice to reduce cerebral edema.
2. An IV of NS at a keep-open rate (25 mL per hour is a keep-open rate) would not be questioned. It is needed for emergency access.
3. A nicotine patch could be administered if the client is a smoker and unable to smoke during hospitalization.
4. A narcotic analgesic is contraindicated until it is known that the client is neurologically stable. Narcotics, especially intravenous, can mask clinical manifestations of deterioration of the client's status.

**TEST-TAKING HINT: The test taker must know the actions of medications in order to administer them safely. Maslow's hierarchy of needs lists safety as a high priority. Many medications will be listed on the NCLEX-RN® examination using only the generic name. Dexamethasone's trade name is Decadron.**

131. 1. This complete blood count has findings that are within normal limits.
2. This chemistry report has findings that are within normal limits.
3. This glucose level and Hgb A$_1$C are within normal limits.
4. This client has abnormal findings, which could result in serious issues for the client. The nurse should first initiate seizure precautions, then notify the HCP of the results and discuss the code status of the client.

**TEST-TAKING HINT: The test taker can eliminate options "1," "2," and "3" based on the expected**

results. These values are within the ranges listed. The only option with abnormal data is option "4."

132. 1. When suctioning a client on a ventilator, it is good to hyperventilate the client before suctioning because suctioning the secretions would also suction the oxygen from the client. However, suctioning a client with ICP increases the ICP. The nurse should attempt to remove the secretions without having to suction the client.
2. The secretions pooling in the back of the throat would not be assessed by listening to lung sounds or checking for peripheral perfusion.
3. Secretions can drain if the client is turned to the side unless the secretions are too heavy. The first action is to attempt to relieve the situation without increasing the ICP even further.
4. If suctioning is absolutely needed, then a minimum of 1 minute is needed between attempts to suction.

**TEST-TAKING HINT: The test taker can eliminate options or decide between two of the options based on the fact that options "1" and "4" both involve suctioning the client. Either the nurse will perform suctioning, or it is contraindicated. Assessment is the first step of the nursing process, but the test taker must decide if the nurse is assessing the correct situation. Pooled oral secretion is not lung sounds.**

133. 1. The lowest ranking possible on the GCS is 3. The client would be considered brain dead, not improving.
2. The lower the numbers are on the GCS, the worse the client's functioning; this client is not improving.
3. This GCS rating indicates the client is the same as 1 hour ago.
4. The GCS rating is going up, which means the client is improving. (Hoffman & Sullivan, 2020).

**TEST-TAKING HINT: The test taker can eliminate options "1" and "2" because they both present a lower score; both cannot be correct in a multiple-choice question, and here, both indicate a worsening of the client's condition. Likewise, option "3" is the same score as 1 hour ago, so the test taker should be careful to note this. Therefore, because only one answer can show an improving condition, the test taker can deduce that it is option "4."**

134. Correct order is 4, 5, 2, 3, 1.
     4. The client should be turned to the side to prevent the tongue from falling back into the throat and occluding the airway. (Padded tongue blades are NOT forced into the mouth because they can break teeth and cause aspiration of the teeth.)
     5. The client's head should be protected from hitting the side rails or other objects.
     2. Clothing should be loosened to prevent airway difficulties.
     3. The medications to control the seizures should be administered to stop the seizure.
     1. Assessment, in this instance, is last because of the crisis that is occurring. The nurse should assess the mouth to determine if the client bit the tongue or buccal mucosa during the seizure or if teeth were chipped or broken.

**TEST-TAKING HINT:** Rank order questions can be difficult to answer. The test taker should remember safety. Which intervention will keep the client safe the fastest? Also important is if in stress, do not assess: Perform an intervention.

135. Correct answers are 1 and 2.
     1. Elevating the head of the bed 30 degrees will decrease ICP by using gravity to drain cerebrospinal fluid.
     2. Minimizing disturbing the client and allowing rest in between activities will decrease ICP.
     3. Suctioning increases ICP and should not be performed unless absolutely necessary.
     4. Soapsuds enemas increase intra-abdominal pressure, which, in turn, increases ICP.
     5. The Trendelenburg position is head down, feet up. This would increase ICP.

**TEST-TAKING HINT:** The test taker must be aware of interventions that increase ICP. The nursing interventions directed at facilitating drainage from the jugular venous system without inducing pressure, such as cough, suctioning, or supine positioning, are correct options.

# NEUROLOGICAL DISORDERS COMPREHENSIVE EXAMINATION

1. The client is admitted with a diagnosis of trigeminal neuralgia. Which assessment data would the nurse expect to find in this client?
   1. Joint pain of the neck and jaw.
   2. Unconscious grinding of the teeth during sleep.
   3. Sudden severe shocklike facial pain.
   4. A progressive loss of calcium in the nasal septum.

2. The client recently has been diagnosed with trigeminal neuralgia. Which intervention is the **priority** for the nurse to implement with the client?
   1. Assess the client's sense of smell and taste.
   2. Teach the client how to care for the eyes.
   3. Instruct the client to have carbamazepine levels monitored regularly.
   4. Assist the client to identify factors that trigger an attack.

3. The client comes to the clinic and reports a sudden drooping of the left side of the face and reports pain in that area. The nurse notes that the client cannot wrinkle the forehead, close the left eye, and has excessive tearing in the left eye. Which condition should the nurse **suspect**?
   1. Bell's palsy.
   2. Left-sided stroke.
   3. Tetany.
   4. Mononeuropathy.

4. The client comes to the clinic for the treatment of a dog bite. Which intervention should the clinic nurse implement **first**?
   1. Prepare the client for a series of rabies injections.
   2. Notify the local animal control department.
   3. Administer a tetanus toxoid in the deltoid.
   4. Determine if the animal has had its vaccinations.

5. The client has glossopharyngeal nerve (cranial nerve IX) paralysis secondary to a stroke. Which referral would be **most** appropriate for this client?
   1. Hospice nurse.
   2. Speech therapist.
   3. Physical therapist.
   4. Occupational therapist.

6. Which assessment data would make the nurse suspect that the client has ALS?
   1. History of a cold or gastrointestinal upset in the last month.
   2. Reports of double vision and drooping eyelids.
   3. Fatigue, progressive muscle weakness, and twitching.
   4. Loss of sensation below the level of the umbilicus.

7. The client is scheduled for an MRI of the brain to confirm a diagnosis of Creutzfeldt-Jakob disease. Which intervention should the nurse implement **before** the procedure?
   1. Determine if the client has claustrophobia.
   2. Obtain a signed informed consent form.
   3. Determine if the client is allergic to egg yolks.
   4. Start an intravenous line in both hands.

8. Which should be the nurse's **first** intervention with the client diagnosed with Bell's palsy?
   1. Explain that this disorder will resolve within a month.
   2. Tell the client to apply heat to the involved side of the face.
   3. Encourage the client to eat a soft diet.
   4. Teach the client to protect the affected eye from injury.

9. The client asks the nurse, "What causes Creutzfeldt-Jakob disease?" Which statement would be the nurse's **best** response?
   1. "The person must have been exposed to an infected prion."
   2. "It is mad cow disease, and eating contaminated meat is the cause."
   3. "This disease is caused by a virus that is in stagnant water."
   4. "A fungal spore from the lungs infects the brain tissue."

10. The client is diagnosed with Creutzfeldt-Jakob disease. Which referral would be the **most** appropriate?
    1. Alzheimer's Association.
    2. Creutzfeldt-Jakob Disease Foundation.
    3. Hospice care.
    4. A neurosurgeon.

11. The client is diagnosed with arboviral encephalitis. Which **priority** intervention should the nurse implement?
    1. Place the client in strict isolation.
    2. Administer IV antibiotics.
    3. Keep the client in the supine position.
    4. Institute seizure precautions.

12. The client is diagnosed with a brain abscess. Which clinical manifestations are present with this diagnosis? **Select all that apply.**
    1. Projectile vomiting.
    2. Disoriented behavior.
    3. Headache.
    4. Seizure activity.
    5. Fever.

13. The client diagnosed with a brain abscess has become lethargic and difficult to arouse. Which intervention should the nurse implement **first**?
    1. Implement seizure precautions.
    2. Assess the client's neurological status.
    3. Close the drapes and darken the room.
    4. Prepare to administer an IV steroid.

14. The client is diagnosed with Huntington's disease. Which interventions should the nurse implement with the family? **Select all that apply.**
    1. Refer to the Huntington's Disease Foundation.
    2. Explain the need for the client to wear safety padding.
    3. Discuss how to cope with the client's messiness.
    4. Provide three meals a day and no between-meal snacks.
    5. Teach the family how to perform chest percussion.

15. The nurse is discussing psychosocial implications of Huntington's disease with the adult child of a client diagnosed with the disease. Which psychosocial intervention should the nurse implement?
    1. Refer the adult child for genetic counseling as soon as possible.
    2. Teach the adult child to use a warming tray under the food during meals.
    3. Discuss the importance of not abandoning the parent.
    4. Allow the adult child to talk about the fear of getting the disease.

16. The client is undergoing post-thrombolytic therapy for a stroke. The HCP has ordered heparin to be infused at 1,000 units per hour. The solution comes as 25,000 units of heparin in 500 mL of D₅W. At what rate will the nurse set the pump?

    [                    ]

17. Which finding is considered to be one of the **warning signs** of developing Alzheimer's disease?
    1. Difficulty performing familiar tasks.
    2. Problems with orientation to date, time, and place.
    3. Having problems focusing on a task.
    4. Atherosclerotic changes in the vessels.

18. Which information should be shared with the client diagnosed with mild to moderate Alzheimer's disease prescribed donepezil? **Select all that apply.**
    1. The client must continue taking this medication forever to maintain function.
    2. The drug may delay the progression of the disease, but it does not cure it.
    3. A serum drug level must be obtained monthly to evaluate for toxicity.
    4. If the client develops any muscle aches, the HCP should be notified.
    5. The drug may cause bradycardia and dizziness.

19. The spouse of a recently retired man tells the nurse, "All my husband does is sit around and watch television all day long. He is so irritable and moody. I don't want to be around him." Which action should the nurse implement?
    1. Encourage the spouse to leave the client alone.
    2. Tell the spouse that he is probably developing Alzheimer's disease.
    3. Recommend that the client see an HCP for antidepressant medication.
    4. Instruct the spouse to buy him some arts and crafts supplies.

20. The nurse in a long-term care facility has noticed a change in the behavior of one of the clients. The client no longer participates in activities and prefers to stay in his room. Which intervention should the nurse implement **first**?
    1. Insist that the client go to the dining room for meals.
    2. Notify the family of the change in behavior.
    3. Determine if the client wants another roommate.
    4. Complete a Geriatric Depression Scale.

21. A family member brings the client to the ED reporting that the 78-year-old father has suddenly become very confused and thinks he is living in 1942, that he has to go to war, and that someone is trying to poison him. Which question should the nurse ask the family member?
    1. "Has your father been diagnosed with dementia?"
    2. "What medication has your father taken today?"
    3. "What have you given him that makes him think it's poison?"
    4. "Does your father like to watch old movies on television?"

22. The student nurse asks the RN, "Why do you ask the client to identify how many fingers you have up when the client hit the front of the head, not the back of the head?" The RN would base the response on which scientific rationale?
    1. This is part of the routine neurological examination.
    2. This is done to determine if the client has diplopia.
    3. This assesses the amount of brain damage.
    4. This is done to indicate if there is a rebound effect on the brain.

23. The ambulance brings the client diagnosed with a head injury to the ED. The client responds to painful stimuli by opening the eyes, muttering, and pulling away from the nurse. How would the nurse rate this client on the GCS?
    1. 3
    2. 9
    3. 10
    4. 15

### Glasgow Coma Scale

| Best Eye Opening (E) | Best Verbal Response (V) | Best Motor Response (M) |
|---|---|---|
| 4 = Spontaneous | 5 = Normal conversation | 6 = Normal |
| 3 = To voice | 4 = Disoriented conversation | 5 = Localizes to pain |
| 2 = To pain | 3 = Words, but not coherent | 4 = Withdraws to pain |
| 1 = None | 2 = No words . . . only sounds | 3 = Flexion with pain |
|  | 1 = None | 2 = Extension with pain |
|  |  | 1 = None |
|  |  | Total = E + V + M |

24. Which intervention has the **highest priority** for the client who is in the ED after a motorcycle collision with an automobile and who has a fractured left leg?
    1. Assessing the neurological status.
    2. Immobilizing the fractured leg.
    3. Monitoring the client's output.
    4. Starting an 18-gauge saline lock.

25. The nurse writes the nursing diagnosis "altered body temperature related to damaged temperature regulating mechanism" for a client diagnosed with a head injury. Which would be the **most** appropriate goal?
    1. Administer acetaminophen for elevated temperature.
    2. The client's temperature will remain less than 100°F.
    3. Maintain the hypothermia blanket at 99°F for 24 hours.
    4. The basal metabolic temperature will fluctuate no more than 2 degrees.

26. Which potential pituitary complication should the nurse assess for in the client diagnosed with a TBI?
    1. Diabetes mellitus type 2 (DM 2).
    2. Seizure activity.
    3. Syndrome of inappropriate antidiuretic hormone (SIADH).
    4. Cushing's disease.

27. The nurse is discussing seizure prevention with a female client just diagnosed with epilepsy. Which statement indicates the client **needs more** teaching?
    1. "I will take calcium supplements daily and drink milk."
    2. "I will see my HCP to have my blood levels drawn regularly."
    3. "I should not drink any type of alcohol while taking the medication."
    4. "I am glad that my periods will not affect my epilepsy."

28. The UAP is caring for a client having a seizure. Which action by the UAP would **warrant immediate** intervention by the RN?
    1. The assistant attempts to insert an oral airway.
    2. The assistant turns the client on the right side.
    3. The assistant has all the side rails padded and up.
    4. The assistant does not leave the client's bedside.

29. The nurse is preparing the male client for an electroencephalogram (EEG). Which intervention should the nurse implement?
    1. Explain that this procedure is not painful.
    2. Premedicate the client with a benzodiazepine drug.
    3. Instruct the client to shave all facial hair.
    4. Tell the client it will cause him to see "floaters."

30. Which assessment data indicate that the client diagnosed with a TBI exhibiting decorticate posturing on admission is responding **effectively** to treatment?
    1. The client has flaccid paralysis.
    2. The client has purposeful movement.
    3. The client has decerebrate posturing with painful stimuli.
    4. The client does not move the extremities.

31. The intensive care nurse is caring for the client after intracranial surgery. Which interventions should the nurse implement? **Select all that apply.**
    1. Assess for DVT.
    2. Administer IV anticoagulant.
    3. Monitor intake and output strictly.
    4. Apply warm compresses to the eyes.
    5. Perform passive ROM exercises.

32. Which client should the nurse **assess first** after receiving the shift report?
    1. The client diagnosed with a stroke and right-sided paralysis.
    2. The client diagnosed with meningitis, reporting photosensitivity.
    3. The client diagnosed with a brain tumor having projectile vomiting.
    4. The client diagnosed with epilepsy reporting tender gums.

33. The client is reporting neck pain, fever, and a headache. The nurse elicits a positive Kernig's sign. Which diagnostic test procedure should the RN anticipate the HCP ordering to **confirm** a diagnosis?
    1. A computed tomography (CT).
    2. Blood cultures times 2.
    3. Electromyogram (EMG).
    4. Lumbar puncture (LP).

34. Which behavior is a risk factor for developing and spreading bacterial meningitis?
    1. An upper respiratory infection (URI).
    2. Unprotected sexual intercourse.
    3. Chronic alcohol consumption.
    4. Use of tobacco products.

35. Which assessment data should the nurse expect to observe for the client diagnosed with Parkinson's disease?
    1. Ascending paralysis and pain.
    2. Masklike face and pill rolling.
    3. Diplopia and ptosis.
    4. Dysphagia and dysarthria.

36. The client diagnosed with Parkinson's disease is prescribed carbidopa and levodopa. Which intervention should the nurse implement **before** administering the medication?
    1. Discuss how to prevent orthostatic hypotension.
    2. Take the client's apical pulse for one (1) full minute.
    3. Inform the client that this medication is for short-term use.
    4. Tell the client to take the medication on an empty stomach.

37. The client diagnosed with ALS (Lou Gehrig's disease) is prescribed medications that require intravenous access. The HCP has ordered a primary intravenous line at a keep-vein-open (KVO) rate at 25 mL/hr. The drop factor is 10 gtts/mL. At what rate should the nurse set the IV tubing?

    [                    ]

38. Which intervention should the nurse take with the client recently diagnosed with ALS (Lou Gehrig's disease)?
    1. Discuss a percutaneous gastrostomy tube.
    2. Explain how a fistula is accessed.
    3. Provide an advance directive.
    4. Refer to a PT for leg braces.

39. The public health nurse is discussing St. Louis encephalitis with a group in the community. Which instruction should the nurse provide to help prevent an outbreak?
    1. Yearly vaccinations for the disease.
    2. Advise that the city should spray for mosquitoes.
    3. The use of gloves when gardening.
    4. Not going out at night.

40. The husband of a client with alcoholism tells the nurse, "I don't know what to do. I don't know how to deal with my wife's problem." Which response would be **most appropriate** by the nurse?
    1. "It must be difficult. Maybe you should think about leaving."
    2. "I think you should attend Alcoholics Anonymous."
    3. "I think that Alanon might be very helpful for you."
    4. "You should not enable your wife's alcoholism."

41. The client is brought to the ED by the police for public disorderliness. The client reports feeling no pain and is unconcerned that the police have arrested him. The nurse notes the client has epistaxis and nasal congestion. Which substance should the nurse suspect the client has abused?
    1. Marijuana.
    2. Heroin.
    3. Ecstasy.
    4. Cocaine.

42. The client with a history of migraine headaches comes to the clinic and reports that a migraine is coming because the client is experiencing bright spots before the eyes. Which **phase** of migraine headaches is the client experiencing?
    1. Premonitory phase.
    2. Aura phase.
    3. Headache phase.
    4. Postdromal phase.

43. The client with a history of migraine headaches comes to the ED reporting a migraine headache. Which collaborative treatment should the nurse anticipate?
    1. Administer an injection of sumatriptan.
    2. Prepare for CT of the head.
    3. Place the client in a quiet room with the lights off.
    4. Administer propranolol.

44. Which assessment data would make the nurse suspect that the client diagnosed with a C7 SCI is experiencing autonomic dysreflexia? **Select all that apply.**
    1. Abnormal diaphoresis.
    2. A severe throbbing headache.
    3. Sudden loss of motor function.
    4. Spastic skeletal muscle movement.
    5. Hypertension.

45. The nurse stops at the scene of a motor vehicle accident and provides emergency first aid at the scene. Which **law** protects the nurse as a first responder?
    1. The First Aid Act.
    2. Ombudsman Act.
    3. Good Samaritan Law.
    4. First Responder Law.

46. The nurse writes the problem "high risk for impaired skin integrity" for the client diagnosed with an L5-6 SCI. Which intervention should the nurse include in the plan of care?
    1. Perform active ROM exercise.
    2. Massage the legs and trochanters every shift.
    3. Arrange for a pressure relief cushion in the wheelchair.
    4. Apply petroleum-based lotion to the extremities.

47. The nurse is preparing to administer acetaminophen to a client diagnosed with a stroke and reporting a headache. Which intervention should the nurse implement **first**?
    1. Administer the medication in pudding.
    2. Check the client's armband.
    3. Crush the tablet and dissolve in juice.
    4. Have the client sip some water.

48. The nurse is caring for clients in a medical unit. Which client would be **most at risk** for experiencing a stroke?
    1. A 92-year-old client with alcoholism.
    2. A 54-year-old client diagnosed with hepatitis.
    3. A 60-year-old client with a Greenfield filter.
    4. A 68-year-old client diagnosed with chronic atrial fibrillation.

49. The charge nurse is making client assignments for a neuro-medical floor. Which client should be assigned to the most experienced nurse?
    1. The 80-year-old client diagnosed with a stroke in evolution.
    2. The client diagnosed with a TIA 48 hours ago.
    3. The client diagnosed with Guillain-Barré syndrome reporting leg pain.
    4. The client diagnosed with Alzheimer's disease wandering in the halls.

50. The nurse is assessing a client diagnosed with anosmia on a neurological floor. Which area should the nurse assess for cranial nerve I that is pertinent to anosmia?

    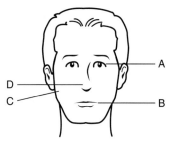

    1. A
    2. B
    3. C
    4. D

51. The nurse arrives at the scene of a motor vehicle accident, and the car is leaking gasoline. The client is in the driver's seat of the car and reports not being able to move the legs. Which actions should the nurse implement? **Rank in order of priority.**
    1. Move the client safely out of the car.
    2. Assess the client for other injuries.
    3. Stabilize the client's neck.
    4. Notify the emergency medical system.
    5. Place the client in a functional anatomical position.

52. The male client diagnosed with Parkinson's disease has undergone a minor surgical procedure and is receiving cefazolin IV piggyback every six (6) hours. Which laboratory data should the nurse **report** to the HCP?

    1.

| Complete Blood Count | Client Value | Normal Values |
|---|---|---|
| Red blood cells (RBCs) | 6 | Male: 4.21–5.81 × 10⁶ cells/microL<br>Female: 3.6–5.11 × 10⁶ cells/microL |
| Hemoglobin | 16.6 | Male: 14–17.3 g/dL<br>Female: 11.7–15.5 g/dL |
| Hematocrit | 48 | Male: 42%–52%<br>Female: 36%–48% |
| Platelet | 140 | 140–400 × 10³/microL |
| White blood cells (WBCs) | 10.3 | 4.5–11.1 × 10³/microL |

    2.

| Laboratory Test | Client Values | Normal Values |
|---|---|---|
| Potassium | 4.2 | 3.5–5.3 mEq/L |
| Sodium | 137 | 135–145 mEq/L |
| Chloride | 103 | 97–107 mEq/L |
| $CO_2$ | 30 | 22–29 mEq/L |

    3.

| Laboratory Test | Patient Results | Normal Values |
|---|---|---|
| Glucose | 115 | Fasting <100 mg/dL<br>Random <200 mg/dL |
| Hemoglobin A₁c | 6.2 | Non-diabetic 4%–5.5%<br>Prediabetes 5.7%–6.4%<br>Diabetes 6.5% or less |

    4.

| Site | Client Culture | Sensitivity | Resistant |
|---|---|---|---|
| Surgical wound | Methicillin-resistant | Vancomycin | Penicillin |
| | *Staphylococcus aureus* | | Cephalosporin |
| Intravenous line | Negative | | |

1. 1. Joint pain is usually associated with some type of arthritis.
   2. Unconscious grinding of the teeth during sleep is usually associated with temporo-mandibular joint (TMJ) disorder.
   3. **Trigeminal neuralgia affects the 5th cranial nerve and is a form of neuropathic pain characterized by sudden, extreme shocklike facial pain that lasts from a few seconds to a few minutes per episode and can have frequent episodes in quick succession. The disorder is also known as tic douloureux (National Institute of Neurological Disorders and Stroke, 2019).**
   4. The nasal structure is not made up of bone.

2. 1. The client's sense of smell and taste are not affected.
   2. The cornea is at risk for abrasions because of the twitching, which causes irritation. Therefore, the nurse must teach the client how to care for the eye, but the most important intervention is to prevent the attacks.
   3. Carbamazepine (Tegretol) is a treatment for trigeminal neuralgia, but it is not the most important intervention when the client is first diagnosed with this condition.
   4. **Stimulating specific areas of the face, called trigger zones, many initiate the onset of pain. Therefore, the nurse should help the client identify situations that exacerbate the condition, such as chewing gum, eating, brushing the teeth, or being exposed to a draft of cold air.**

3. 1. **Bell's palsy, called facial paralysis, is a disorder of the seventh cranial nerve (facial nerve) characterized by unilateral paralysis of facial muscles.**
   2. A left-sided stroke would see clinical manifestations on the right side of the body. Pain is not an immediate symptom of a stroke but can develop in the muscles and joints.
   3. Tetany is due to low calcium levels. In this disorder, the face twitches when touched; this is known as a positive Chvostek's sign.
   4. Mononeuropathy is limited to a single peripheral nerve and its branches and occurs because the trunk of the nerve is compressed, such as in carpal tunnel syndrome.

4. 1. This may be needed if it is determined the dog has not had its shots or if the dog cannot be found, but it is not the first intervention.
   2. This is an appropriate action if the client does not know the dog owner, then the dog can be found and quarantined.
   3. If the client has not had a tetanus booster in the last 10 years, one must be administered, but it is usually the last action taken before the client is discharged from the clinic.
   4. **This is a priority because if the dog has had its vaccinations, the client will not have to undergo a series of very painful injections. The nurse must obtain information about the dog, which is an assessment of the situation.**

5. 1. Clients are referred to hospice when there is a life expectancy of less than 6 months. This client has difficulty swallowing, which is not life-threatening.
   2. **Speech therapists address the needs of clients having difficulty with the innervations and musculature of the face and neck. This includes the swallowing reflex.**
   3. The PT assists the client to ambulate and transfer (e.g., from bed to chair) and with muscle strength training.
   4. The OT focuses on cognitive disability and ADL.

6. 1. A history of a cold or gastrointestinal upset in the last month would be assessment data that would make the nurse suspect Guillain-Barré syndrome.
   2. Reports of double vision and drooping eyelids would make the nurse suspect myasthenia gravis.
   3. **Fatigue, progressive muscle weakness, and twitching are clinical manifestations of ALS, a progressive neurological disease in which there is a loss of motor neurons. There is no cure, but recently a medication to slow the deterioration of the motor neurons has been found.**
   4. Loss of sensation would make the nurse suspect some type of SCI.

7. 1. **For an MRI scan, the client is placed in a very narrow tube. If claustrophobic, the client may need medication, or an open MRI machine may need to be considered.**
   2. An MRI scan is not an invasive procedure; therefore, informed consent is not needed.
   3. The nurse would need to determine allergies to shellfish or iodine, not to egg yolks.
   4. The client will need one saline lock, not two intravenous lines. Often the MRI tech is the person inserting the IV line.

8. 1. This is the correct information, but it is not a priority when discussing Bell's palsy.
   2. Heat will help promote comfort and increase blood flow to the muscles, but the safety of the client's eye is a priority.
   3. The client may have difficulty chewing on the affected side, so a soft diet should be encouraged, but it is not a priority teaching.
   4. **Teaching the client to protect the eye is a priority because the eye does not close completely, and the blink reflex is diminished, making the eye vulnerable to injury. The client should wear an eye patch at night and wraparound sunglasses or goggles during the day; the client may also need lubricating eye drops (NIH, 2019).**

9. 1. Would a layperson know what a prion is? This is using medical jargon, which is not the nurse's best response.
   2. **This is the cause of this disease and would be the best response.**
   3. A virus is not the cause of Creutzfeldt-Jakob disease.
   4. Fungal spores do not cause this disease.

10. 1. Creutzfeldt-Jakob disease is not Alzheimer's disease, although the presenting symptoms may mimic Alzheimer's disease.
    2. There is no foundation for Creutzfeldt-Jakob disease, but if there were, the significant other would not be referred to this organization because the disease progresses so rapidly that the client would not get any benefit from the organization.
    3. **This disease is usually fatal within a year, and the symptoms progress rapidly to dementia.**
    4. The nurse does not refer the client to a neurosurgeon, and the primary HCP would not refer to a neurosurgeon because there is no surgical or medical treatment for this disease.

11. 1. Arboviral encephalitis is a viral infection transmitted by mosquito bites, and isolation is not required.
    2. Antibiotics are prescribed for bacterial infections, not viral infections. There is no antiviral medication to treat this disease.
    3. Keeping the client supine would increase ICP, which is a concern when caring for clients diagnosed with brain diseases.
    4. **Seizure precautions should be instituted because any inflammation of the brain tissue will put the client at risk for seizures.**

12. **Correct answers are 2, 3, 4, and 5.**
    1. Nausea and vomiting may occur, but it is not projectile.
    2. **Disoriented behavior and confusion occur in 65% of brain abscesses.**
    3. **The most common and prevalent symptom of a brain abscess is a headache.**
    4. **The client diagnosed with a brain abscess may have seizure activity.**
    5. **Fever is present in over half of the clients diagnosed with a brain abscess.**

13. 1. This is an appropriate intervention, but it is not the first.
    2. **Remember, assessment is the first step of the nursing process and should be implemented first whenever there is a change in the client's behavior.**
    3. This helps prevent stimulation that could initiate a seizure, but it is not the first intervention.
    4. Steroids may be administered to clients diagnosed with brain abscesses to decrease inflammation, but an assessment is the first intervention.

14. **Correct answers are 1, 2, and 3.**
    1. **Foundations offer the family and client information about the disease, support groups, and up-to-date information on current research.**
    2. **The use of padding will help prevent injury from the constant movement that occurs with this disease.**
    3. **The constant movement causes the client to be messy when eating, dressing, or performing ADLs.**
    4. The constant movements expend more calories; therefore, the client should have three (3) meals plus between-meal snacks.
    5. The client is at risk for choking; therefore, teaching the Heimlich maneuver is appropriate, but teaching chest percussion is not.

15. 1. Referring the adult child is not a psycho-social intervention. The gene that determines if a client has Huntington's disease has been identified, and genetic counseling could rule out or confirm that the client's child will develop Huntington's disease.
2. This is an appropriate intervention, but it is not a psychosocial intervention. (Read the stem closely.)
3. This is placing a lot of responsibility on the child concerning the parent's debilitating, chronic, and devastating disease. The client may need to be in a long-term care facility, and the child should not feel guilty if this is necessary.
4. **The adult child would develop this disease if the gene was inherited by the adult child. It can be frightening for children to watch a parent progress through this disease and understand that they too may get it.**

16. **20 mL/hr.**
To arrive at the answer, the test taker must divide 25,000 units by 500 mL = 50 units in 1 mL.

Divide 1,000 units by 50 units = 20 mL/hr.

17. 1. The client may experience minor difficulty in work or social activities but has adequate cognitive ability to hide the loss and continue to function independently.
2. **Disorientation to time and place is a warning sign.**
3. Not being able to focus on a task is more likely a sign of attention deficit-hyperactivity disorder.
4. Atherosclerotic changes are not warning signs of Alzheimer's disease. Amyloid protein plaques do appear to have something to do with the disease, but they are not found until autopsy.

18. **Correct answers are 2 and 5.**
1. This is not a true statement. The client will no longer be prescribed this medication as the disease progresses and it becomes ineffective.
2. **Donepezil (Aricept), a cholinesterase inhibitor, does not cure Alzheimer's disease, and at some point, it will become ineffective as the disease progresses.**
3. There is no monthly drug level to be monitored. Toxicity includes jaundice and gastrointestinal distress.
4. Muscle aches are an adverse effect of the lipid-lowering medications, not of donepezil (Aricept), a cholinesterase inhibitor.

5. **Donepezil (Aricept) can cause brady-cardia and dizziness. The client should be instructed to take medication as directed and not to take higher doses because it will not increase the effects, only the side effects.**

19. 1. If the wife could leave the client alone, she would not be sharing her concerns with the nurse. The nurse needs to address the wife's concerns as well as the husband's.
2. These are not the typical clinical manifestations of stage I Alzheimer's disease.
3. **This behavior indicates the client is depressed and should be treated with antidepressants. A major life-style change has occurred, and he may need short-term medication therapy, depending on how the client adjusts to retirement.**
4. The client may not want to participate in arts and crafts.

20. 1. The nurse cannot insist that the client do anything. The nurse can encourage but, remember, this is the client's home.
2. The family may need to be notified, but the nurse should first assess what is happening that is causing this change in behavior.
3. There is nothing that indicates the client is unhappy with the roommate. In fact, the client wants to stay in the room, which does not indicate a need for a room change.
4. **A change in behavior may indicate depression. The GDS measures satisfaction with life's accomplishments. Older persons should be in Erikson's generativity versus stagnation stage of life.**

21. 1. Dementia involves behavior changes that are irreversible and occur over time. Delirium, however, occurs suddenly (as in this man's symptom onset), is caused by an acute event, and is reversible.
2. **Drug toxicity and interactions are common causes of delirium in older persons.**
3. This is blaming the family member for the client's paranoid ideation.
4. Watching old movies on television will not cause delirium.

22. 1. This is part of the neurological examination, but this is not the scientific rationale for why it is done. The nurse must understand what is being assessed to interpret the data.
2. Diplopia, double vision, is a sign of head injury, but it is not the scientific rationale.

3. The procedure does assess brain damage, but this answer does not explain why.

4. **When the client hits the front of the head, there is a rebound effect known as "coup-contrecoup," in which the brain hits the back of the skull. The occipital lobe is in the back of the head, and an injury to it may be manifested by seeing double.**

23. 1. A score of 3 is the lowest score and indicates a deep coma and impending brain death.

2. **A score of 9 indicates moderate increased ICP, but with appropriate care, the client may survive. The nurse would rate the client at an 8: 2 for opening the eyes; 3 for verbal response; and 4 for motor response.**

3. A score of 10 indicates moderately increased ICP.

4. A score of 15 is the highest score a client can receive, indicating normal function.

24. 1. **Assessment is the first step in the nursing process, and a client in a motorcycle accident must be assessed for a head injury.**

2. Neurological assessment is a priority over a fractured leg.

3. The client's urinary output is not a priority over an assessment.

4. An 18-gauge IV access should be started in case the client has to go to surgery, but it is not a priority over an assessment.

25. 1. Administering acetaminophen (Tylenol) is an intervention, which is not a goal.

2. **This is an appropriate goal. It addresses the client, addresses the problem (temperature elevation), and is measurable.**

3. Maintaining the blanket temperature is a nursing intervention, which should eliminate this as a possible answer.

4. The basal metabolic temperature is evaluated for a woman trying to get pregnant; it helps indicate ovulation.

26. 1. Diabetes mellitus type 2 is a pancreatic disease that has nothing to do with the pituitary gland or head injury.

2. Seizure activity is a possible complication of TBI, but it is not a pituitary complication.

3. **The pituitary gland produces vasopressin, the ADH, and any injury that causes increased ICP will exert pressure on the pituitary gland and can cause SIADH.**

4. Cushing's disease is caused by an excess production of glucocorticoids and mineralocorticoids from the adrenal gland.

27. 1. Because of bone loss associated with long-term use of anticonvulsants, the client should increase calcium intake to reduce the risk of osteoporosis.

2. Anticonvulsant medications have a narrow range of therapeutic value, and the levels should be checked regularly.

3. Alcohol interferes with anticonvulsant medication and should be avoided.

4. **Women with epilepsy note an increase in the frequency of seizures during menses. This is thought to be linked to the increase in sex hormones that alter the excitability of the neurons in the brain.**

28. 1. **The nurse must intervene to stop the UAP because the client's jaws are clenched. Attempting to insert anything into the mouth could cause injury to the client or to the UAP.**

2. Side-lying positions help to prevent aspiration and are an appropriate intervention.

3. The client's safety is a priority, and this will help protect the client from injury.

4. Staying with the client is appropriate behavior that would not warrant intervention by the nurse.

29. 1. **This procedure is not painful, although electrodes are attached to the scalp. The client will need to wash the hair after the procedure.**

2. An antianxiety medication would make the client drowsy and could cause a false EEG reading.

3. There is no reason for facial hair to be shaved.

4. This procedure measures the electrical conductivity in the brain and does not cause the client to see "floaters" (spots before the eyes). Flashing bright lights may be used in an attempt to evoke a seizure.

30. 1. Flaccid paralysis indicates a worsening of the increased ICP.

2. **Purposeful movement indicates the client is getting better and is responding to the treatment.**

3. Decerebrate positioning indicates a worsening of the increased ICP.

4. This is the same as flaccid paralysis and indicates a worsening of the increased ICP.

31. **Correct answers are 1, 3, and 5.**
    1. **Assessing for DVT, which is a complication of immobility, would be appropriate for this client.**
    2. Anticoagulants may cause bleeding; therefore, the client after surgery would not be prescribed this medication.
    3. **Monitoring of intake and output helps to detect possible complications of the pituitary gland, which include diabetes insipidus and SIADH.**
    4. The nurse should apply cool compresses to alleviate periocular edema.
    5. **The nurse does not want the client to be active and possibly increase ICP; therefore, the nurse should perform passive ROM for the client.**

32. 1. Paralysis is an expected occurrence with a client diagnosed with a stroke.
    2. Photosensitivity is an expected sign of meningitis.
    3. **Projectile vomiting indicates that increased ICP is exerting pressure on the vomiting center of the brain.**
    4. Tender gums could be secondary to medication given for epilepsy. The client may need to see a dentist, but this client does not need to be assessed first.

33. 1. The symptoms and a positive Kernig's sign suggest meningitis, but a CT scan is not diagnostic of meningitis.
    2. Blood cultures determine septicemia or infections of the bloodstream, not meningitis.
    3. An EMG evaluates electrical conductivity through the muscle.
    4. **The client's symptoms, along with a positive Kernig's sign, should make the nurse suspect meningitis. The definitive diagnostic test for meningitis is a LP to obtain cerebrospinal fluid for culture.**

34. 1. A URI is not a behavior. The question asked which behavior was a risk factor, so this option can be ruled out. However, a URI is a risk factor for developing and spreading bacterial meningitis because of increased droplet production.
    2. Unprotected sexual intercourse is a risk factor for sexually transmitted diseases (STIs) but not for meningitis.
    3. Chronic alcohol consumption can cause pancreatitis or hepatitis but not meningitis.
    4. **Tobacco use increases respiratory secretions and droplet production and thus is a risk factor for developing and spreading bacterial meningitis.**

35. 1. The spread of pain and paralysis are clinical manifestations of Guillain-Barré syndrome.
    2. **Masklike face and pill rolling are clinical manifestations of Parkinson's disease, along with cogwheeling, postural instability, and stooped and shuffling gait.**
    3. Diplopia and ptosis are clinical manifestations of myasthenia gravis.
    4. Dysphagia and dysarthria are clinical manifestations of myasthenia gravis.

36. 1. **Because carbidopa and levodopa (Sinemet) have been linked to hypotension, teaching a client given the medication ways to help prevent a drop in BP when standing—orthostatic hypotension—decreases the risks associated with hypotension and falling.**
    2. The medication will not cause the heart rate to change, so taking the client's apical pulse for 1 minute is not a priority.
    3. Carbidopa and levodopa (Sinemet) is prescribed for the client for life unless the medication stops working or the client experiences adverse side effects.
    4. The medication should be administered with food to help prevent gastrointestinal distress.

37. **4 gtts/min.**
    The nurse must know the formula for regulating IV drips: the amount to infuse (25 mL/hr) times the drop factor (10 gtts/mL) divided by the minutes. Thus,

    $25 \times 10 = 250 \div 60 = 4.11$ or 4 gtts/min.

38. 1. The client was diagnosed recently and at some point may need a percutaneous endoscopic gastrostomy (PEG) tube, but it is too early for this discussion.
    2. A fistula is used for hemodialysis, and ALS does not cause renal dysfunction.
    3. **It is never too early to discuss advance directives with a client diagnosed with a terminal illness.**
    4. A client diagnosed with ALS does not have leg braces as part of the therapeutic regimen.

39. 1. There is no vaccine for preventing encephalitis.
    2. **Mosquitoes are the vectors that spread the disease, and spraying to kill mosquito larvae will help prevent an outbreak in the community.**
    3. Gloves will not protect a person from being bitten by a mosquito.
    4. Mosquitoes are more prevalent at night, but this is an unrealistic intervention and will not help prevent an outbreak.

40. 1. This advice might be appropriate at some point from a professional counselor but not from the nurse.
    2. Alcoholics Anonymous is the support group that people with alcoholism—in this case, the wife, not the husband—should attend.
    3. **Alanon is the support group for significant others of individuals with alcoholism. Al-A-Teen is for teenage children of individuals with alcoholism.**
    4. This statement is making a judgment that is not given in the stem and is not applicable to all husbands of wives who have alcoholism.

41. 1. Symptoms of marijuana use are apathy, delayed time, and not wanting to eat.
    2. Heroin symptoms include pupil changes and respiratory depression.
    3. Ecstasy is a hallucinogen that is an "upper."
    4. **Disorderly behavior and the symptoms of epistaxis and nasal congestion would make the nurse suspect cocaine abuse.**

42. 1. The premonitory phase occurs hours to days before the migraine headache.
    2. **This is the aura phase, which is characterized by focal neurological symptoms.**
    3. The headache phase occurs when vasodilation occurs in the brain, along with a decline in serotonin levels, causing a throbbing headache.
    4. The postdromal phase is when the pain begins to subside gradually.

43. 1. **Sumatriptan (Imitrex), a triptan, is a medication of choice for migraine headaches. It constricts blood vessels and reduces inflammation. The nurse administering the medication is part of a collaborative effort because the nurse must act on the order or prescription of a physician or other HCP with prescriptive authority.**
    2. This is a collaborative intervention, but it is not routinely ordered because the client reports having a history of migraine headaches.
    3. This is an appropriate independent nursing intervention.
    4. Propranolol (Inderal), a beta blocker, is not used for acute migraine headaches; it is prescribed for long-term prophylaxis of migraines, so the nurse should not anticipate its use in this situation.

44. Correct answers are 1, 2, and 5.
    1. **Diaphoresis (sweating) is a sign of autonomic dysreflexia.**
    2. **A throbbing headache is the classic sign of autonomic dysreflexia, which is caused by a stimulus such as a full bladder.**
    3. Sudden loss of motor function occurs with the original injury. Autonomic dysreflexia does not occur until spinal shock has resolved; it usually occurs in the rehabilitation phase.
    4. Spastic skeletal muscle movement could be secondary to the reflex arc in lower motor neuron injuries.
    5. **Hypertension and bradycardia are signs of autonomic dysreflexia.**

45. 1. There is no such law known as the First Aid Act.
    2. The Ombudsman Act addresses many areas, such as advance directives, elderly advocacy, and several other areas.
    3. **The Good Samaritan Law protects nurses from a judgment against them when responding in an emergency situation in which the nurse is not receiving compensation for the skills and expertise rendered. The nurse must act as any reasonable and prudent nurse would in the same situation (West & Varacallo, 2019).**
    4. There is no such law known as the First Responder Law.

46. 1. A patient with an L5-6 SCI is paralyzed and cannot perform active ROM exercises.
    2. Massaging bony prominences can cause trauma to the underlying blood vessels and will increase the risk of skin breakdown.
    3. **The nurse must realize that the client is at risk for skin breakdown even when sitting in the chair. A pressure relief cushion (Roho®) is an air-filled cushion that provides reduced pressure on the ischium.**
    4. Lotion will not prevent skin breakdown and should be water based, not petroleum based.

47. 1. The medication acetaminophen (Tylenol) can be administered in pudding, but it is not the first intervention.
    2. The armband should be checked but not before determining if the client can swallow.
    3. **Acetaminophen (Tylenol) comes in liquid form, and the nurse should request this before crushing a very bitter tablet.**
    4. **Asking the client to sip some water assesses the client's ability to swallow,**

which is a priority when placing anything in the mouth of the client diagnosed with a stroke.

48. 1. An individual with alcoholism is not at risk of having a stroke any more than someone in the general population.
    2. A client diagnosed with hepatitis is not at risk of having a stroke any more than someone in the general population.
    3. A Greenfield filter is positioned in the inferior vena cava to prevent an embolism resulting from DVT; these filters prevent strokes and pulmonary emboli.
    4. A client diagnosed with atrial fibrillation is at high risk of having a stroke and is usually given oral anticoagulants to prevent a stroke.

49. 1. This client is experiencing a progressing stroke, is at risk for dying, and should be cared for by the most experienced nurse.
    2. A TIA, by definition, lasts less than 24 hours, so this client should be stable at this time.
    3. Pain is expected in clients diagnosed with Guillain-Barré syndrome, and symptoms are on the lower half of the body, which does not affect the airway. Therefore, a less experienced nurse could care for this client.
    4. The charge nurse could delegate much of the care of this client to a UAP.

50. 1. The eyes, indicated by A, would be assessed if checking cranial nerves II, III, IV, or VI.
    2. The tongue located in the mouth, indicated by B, would be assessed if checking cranial nerves IX, X, or XII.

3. The cheek, indicated by C, would be assessed if checking for cranial nerve V, the trigeminal nerve.
4. Anosmia, the loss of the sense of smell, would require the nurse to assess for cranial nerve I, the olfactory nerve, indicated by D.

51. Correct order is 3, 2, 1, 5, 4.
    3. Stabilizing the client's neck is a priority action to prevent further injury to the client, and it must be done before moving the client.
    2. The nurse should assess for any other injuries before moving the client from the vehicle.
    1. Because the vehicle is leaking fuel and there is potential for an explosion or fire, the client should be moved to an area of safety.
    5. Placing the client in a functional anatomical position is an attempt to prevent further SCI.
    4. Because the vehicle is leaking fuel, the priority is to remove the client and then obtain emergency medical assistance.

52. 1. These values are within the normal range for a male client.
    2. These values are within the normal range.
    3. These values are slightly above range for the client but not alarmingly so.
    4. The wound has methicillin-resistant *Staphylococcus aureus* (MRSA) in it, and the client is receiving cefazolin (Ancef), an antibiotic that the MRSA is resistant to; the nurse should notify the HCP for a medication change to vancomycin.

# Cardiac Disorders

3

*If you have knowledge, let others light their candles in it.*

—Margaret Fuller

The Centers for Disease Control and Prevention list heart disease as the leading cause of death in the United States. A nurse must have a thorough knowledge of the clinical manifestations of cardiac disorders and of what to expect in assessing and treating clients with heart-related problems.

## KEYWORDS

Atelectasis
Buccal
Cardiac tamponade
Crackles
Dyspnea
Dysrhythmia
Eupnea
Exacerbation
Intermittent claudication
Nocturia

Orthostatic hypotension
Paresthesia
Petechiae
Pulse oximeter
Pulsus paradoxus
Pyrosis
Splinter hemorrhages
Telemetry

## PRACTICE QUESTIONS

### Heart Failure

1. The client is admitted to the telemetry unit diagnosed with left-sided heart failure. Which clinical manifestations would the nurse expect to find when assessing this client?
   1. Apical pulse rate of 110 and crackles on auscultation.
   2. Jugular vein distention and 4+ pitting edema of feet.
   3. The client sleeping with no pillow and eupnea.
   4. Radial pulse rate of 90 and CRT less than 3 seconds.

2. The nurse is developing a nursing care plan for a client diagnosed with left-sided heart failure. A nursing diagnosis of "decreased cardiac output related to the inability of the heart to pump effectively" is written. Which short-term goal would be **best** for the client?
   1. The client will be able to ambulate in the hall by date of discharge.
   2. The client will have an audible $S_1$ and $S_2$ with no $S_3$ heard by the end of shift.
   3. The client will turn, cough, and deep breathe every 2 hours.
   4. The client will have a $Sao_2$ reading of 98% by day 2 of care.

3. The nurse is developing a discharge-teaching plan for the client diagnosed with heart failure. Which interventions should be included in the plan? **Select all that apply.**
   1. Notify the health-care provider (HCP) of a weight gain of more than 1 pound in a week.
   2. Teach the client how to count the radial pulse when taking digoxin.
   3. Instruct the client to remove the saltshaker from the dinner table.
   4. Encourage the client to monitor urine output for change to a dark color.
   5. Discuss the importance of taking furosemide at bedtime.

4. The nurse enters the room of the client diagnosed with heart failure. The client is lying in bed gasping for breath, is cool and clammy, and has buccal cyanosis. Which intervention would the nurse implement **first?**
   1. Sponge the client's forehead.
   2. Obtain a pulse oximetry reading.
   3. Take the client's vital signs.
   4. Assist the client to a sitting position.

5. The nurse is assessing the client diagnosed with heart failure. Which clinical manifestations would indicate that medical treatment has been **effective?**
   1. The client's peripheral pitting edema has gone from 3+ to 4+.
   2. The client is able to take the radial pulse accurately.
   3. The client is able to perform activities of daily living (ADLs) without dyspnea.
   4. The client has minimal jugular vein distention.

6. The nurse is assessing the client diagnosed with heart failure. Which laboratory data would indicate that the client is in heart failure?
   1. An elevated B-type natriuretic peptide (BNP).
   2. An elevated creatine kinase (CK-MB).
   3. A positive D-dimer.
   4. A positive ventilation-perfusion (VQ) scan.

7. The HCP has ordered an angiotensin-converting enzyme (ACE) inhibitor for the client diagnosed with heart failure. Which discharge instructions should the nurse include? **Select all that apply.**
   1. Instruct the client to take a cough suppressant if a cough develops.
   2. Teach the client how to prevent orthostatic hypotension.
   3. Encourage the client to eat bananas to increase potassium levels.
   4. Explain the importance of taking the medication with food.
   5. Tell the client to avoid the use of NSAIDs.

8. The nurse on the telemetry unit has just received the morning shift report. Which client should the nurse assess **first?**
   1. The client diagnosed with myocardial infarction (MI) with an audible S$_3$ heart sound.
   2. The client diagnosed with right-sided heart failure with 4+ sacral pitting edema.
   3. The client diagnosed with pneumonia with a pulse oximeter reading of 94%.
   4. The client diagnosed with chronic renal failure with an elevated creatinine level.

9. The nurse and an unlicensed assistive personnel (UAP) are caring for four clients on a telemetry unit. Which nursing task would be **best** for the RN to delegate to the UAP?
   1. Assist the client to go down to the smoking area for a cigarette.
   2. Transport the client to the intensive care unit (ICU) via a stretcher.
   3. Provide the client going home discharge-teaching instructions.
   4. Help position the client having a portable x-ray done.

10. The charge nurse is making shift assignments for the medical floor. Which client should be assigned to the **most experienced** registered nurse?
    1. The client diagnosed with chronic heart failure being discharged in the morning.
    2. The client having frequent incontinent liquid bowel movements and vomiting.
    3. The client with an apical pulse rate of 116, a respiratory rate of 26, and a blood pressure of 94/62.
    4. The client reporting chest pain on inspiration and a nonproductive cough.

11. The client diagnosed with chronic heart failure is reporting leg cramps at night. Which nursing interventions should be implemented?
    1. Check the client for peripheral edema and make sure the client takes a diuretic early in the day.
    2. Monitor the client's potassium level and assess the client's intake of bananas and orange juice.
    3. Determine if the client has gained weight and instruct the client to keep the legs elevated.
    4. Instruct the client to ambulate frequently and perform calf-muscle stretching exercises daily.

12. The nurse has written an outcome goal "demonstrates tolerance for increased activity" for a client diagnosed with heart failure. Which intervention should the nurse implement to assist the client in achieving this outcome?
    1. Measure intake and output.
    2. Provide 2 g sodium diet.
    3. Weigh the client daily.
    4. Plan for frequent rest periods.

## Angina and MI

13. Which cardiac enzyme would the nurse expect to elevate **first** in a client diagnosed with MI?
    1. Creatine kinase (CK-MB).
    2. Lactate dehydrogenase (LDH).
    3. Troponin.
    4. White blood cells (WBCs).

14. Along with persistent, crushing chest pain, which clinical manifestations would make the nurse suspect that the client is experiencing an MI?
    1. Mid-epigastric pain and eructation.
    2. Diaphoresis and cool, clammy skin.
    3. Intermittent claudication and pallor.
    4. Jugular vein distention and dependent edema.

15. The client diagnosed with possible MI is experiencing chest pain while walking to the bathroom. Which action should the nurse implement **first?**
    1. Administer sublingual nitroglycerin.
    2. Obtain a STAT electrocardiogram (ECG).
    3. Have the client sit down immediately.
    4. Assess the client's vital signs.

16. The nurse is caring for a client diagnosed with an MI experiencing chest pain. Which interventions should the nurse implement? **Select all that apply.**
    1. Administer morphine intramuscularly.
    2. Administer an acetylsalicylic acid orally.
    3. Apply oxygen via a nasal cannula.
    4. Place the client in a supine position.
    5. Administer nitroglycerin subcutaneously.

17. The client diagnosed with MI is admitted to the telemetry unit from intensive care. Which referral would be **most appropriate** for the client?
    1. Social worker.
    2. Physical therapy.
    3. Cardiac rehabilitation.
    4. Occupational therapy.

18. The client is 1 day postoperative coronary artery bypass grafting (CABG) surgery. The client reports chest pain. Which intervention should the nurse implement **first?**
    1. Medicate the client with intravenous morphine.
    2. Assess the client's chest dressing and vital signs.
    3. Encourage the client to turn from side to side.
    4. Check the client's telemetry monitor.

19. The client diagnosed with MI is 6 hours post-right femoral percutaneous coronary intervention (PCI), also known as balloon surgery. Which assessment data would **require immediate** intervention by the nurse?
    1. The client is keeping the affected extremity straight.
    2. The pressure dressing to the right femoral area is intact.
    3. The client is reporting numbness in the right foot.
    4. The client's right pedal pulse is 3+ and bounding.

20. The intensive care unit nurse is assessing the client 12 hours post-MI. The nurse assesses an $S_3$ heart sound. Which intervention should the nurse implement?
    1. Notify the HCP immediately.
    2. Elevate the head of the client's bed.
    3. Document this as a normal and expected finding.
    4. Administer morphine intravenously.

21. The nurse is administering a beta blocker to the client diagnosed with an MI. Which assessment data would cause the nurse to **question** administering this medication?
    1. The client's apical pulse is 64.
    2. The client's calcium level is elevated.
    3. The client's telemetry shows occasional premature ventricular contractions (PVCs).
    4. The client's blood pressure is 90/58.

22. The client diagnosed with an MI is on bedrest. The UAP is encouraging the client to move the legs. Which action should the RN implement?
    1. Instruct the UAP to stop encouraging the leg movements.
    2. Report this behavior to the charge nurse as soon as possible.
    3. Praise the UAP for encouraging the client to move the legs.
    4. Take no action concerning the UAP's behavior.

23. The client diagnosed with an MI asks the nurse, "What can I do to reduce my risk of another MI?" Which information should the nurse include in the teaching? **Select all that apply.**
    1. Stop smoking.
    2. Keep your blood pressure less than 140/90.
    3. Maintain a fasting glucose level of less than 120 mg/dL.
    4. Keep your weight in a normal range.
    5. Maintain total cholesterol levels less than 200 mg/dL.

24. The client has just returned from a cardiac catheterization. Which assessment data would **warrant immediate** intervention from the nurse?
    1. The client's BP is 110/70 and pulse is 90.
    2. The client's groin dressing is bloody.
    3. The client's cardiac monitor reads normal sinus rhythm.
    4. The client denies any numbness and tingling.

## Coronary Artery Disease

25. The male client is diagnosed with coronary artery disease (CAD) and is prescribed sublingual nitroglycerin. Which statement indicates the client **needs more** teaching?
    1. "I should keep the tablets in the dark-colored bottle they came in."
    2. "If the tablets do not burn under my tongue, they are not effective."
    3. "I should keep the bottle with me in my pocket at all times."
    4. "If my chest pain is not gone with one tablet, I will go to the ED."

26. The client diagnosed with CAD asks the nurse, "Why do I get chest pain?" Which statement would be the **most appropriate response** by the nurse?
    1. "Chest pain is caused by decreased oxygen to the heart muscle."
    2. "There is ischemia to the myocardium as a result of hypoxemia."
    3. "The heart muscle is unable to pump effectively to perfuse the body."
    4. "Chest pain occurs when the lungs cannot adequately oxygenate the blood."

27. The client is scheduled for a percutaneous transluminal coronary angioplasty (PCTA). Which interventions should the nurse perform **before** the procedure? **Select all that apply.**
    1. Assess the client for an allergy to seafood or contrast dye.
    2. Initiate a peripheral intravenous line.
    3. Ensure the client has been NPO for 6 to 12 hours.
    4. Teach the client about the complications of a PCTA.
    5. Confirm the client's laboratory results are available in the EHR.

28. The nurse is preparing to administer a beta blocker to the client diagnosed with CAD. Which assessment data would cause the nurse to **question** administering the medication?
    1. The client has a BP of 110/70.
    2. The client has an apical pulse of 56.
    3. The client is reporting a headache.
    4. The client's potassium level is 4.5 mEq/L.

29. Which intervention should the nurse implement when administering a loop diuretic to a client diagnosed with CAD?
    1. Assess the client's radial pulse.
    2. Assess the client's serum potassium level.
    3. Assess the client's glucometer reading.
    4. Assess the client's pulse oximeter reading.

30. Which client teaching should the nurse implement for the client diagnosed with CAD? **Select all that apply.**
    1. Encourage a low-fat, low-cholesterol diet.
    2. Instruct the client to walk 30 minutes a day.
    3. Decrease the salt intake to 2 g a day.
    4. Refer to a counselor for stress reduction techniques.
    5. Teach the client to increase fiber in the diet.

31. The older adult client has CAD. Which question should the nurse ask the client during the client's teaching?
    1. "Do you have a daily bowel movement?"
    2. "Do you get yearly chest x-rays (CXRs)?"
    3. "Are you sexually active?"
    4. "Have you had any weight change?"

32. The nurse is discussing the importance of exercise with the client diagnosed with CAD. Which intervention should the nurse implement?
    1. Perform isometric exercises daily.
    2. Walk for 15 minutes three times a week.
    3. Do not walk outside if it is less than 40°F.
    4. Wear open-toed shoes when ambulating.

33. The nurse is discussing angina with a client diagnosed with CAD. Which action should the client take **first** when experiencing angina?
    1. Put a nitroglycerin tablet under the tongue.
    2. Stop the activity immediately and rest.
    3. Document when and what activity caused angina.
    4. Notify the HCP immediately.

34. The client diagnosed with CAD is prescribed a Holter monitor. Which intervention should the nurse implement?
    1. Instruct the client to keep a diary of activity, especially when having chest pain.
    2. Discuss the need to remove the Holter monitor during morning care and showering.
    3. Explain that all medications should be withheld while wearing a Holter monitor.
    4. Teach the client the importance of decreasing activity while wearing the monitor.

35. Which statement by the client diagnosed with CAD indicates that the client **understands** the discharge teaching concerning diet?
    1. "I will not eat more than 10 eggs a week."
    2. "I should bake or grill any meats I eat."
    3. "I will drink 8 ounces of whole milk a day."
    4. "I should not eat any type of pork products."

36. The charge nurse is making assignments for clients in a cardiac unit. Which client should the charge nurse assign to a **new graduate** nurse?
    1. The 44-year-old client diagnosed with MI.
    2. The 65-year-old client admitted with unstable angina.
    3. The 75-year-old client scheduled for a cardiac catheterization.
    4. The 50-year-old client reporting chest pain.

## Valvular Heart Disease

37. A client is being seen in the clinic to rule out mitral valve stenosis. Which assessment data would be **most significant?**
    1. The client reports shortness of breath when walking.
    2. The client has jugular vein distention and 3+ pedal edema.
    3. The client reports chest pain after eating a large meal.
    4. The client's liver is enlarged and the abdomen is edematous.

38. Which assessment data would the nurse expect to auscultate in the client diagnosed with mitral valve regurgitation?
    1. A loud $S_1$, $S_2$ split, and a mitral opening snap.
    2. A holosystolic murmur heard best at the cardiac apex.
    3. A midsystolic ejection click or murmur heard at the base.
    4. A high-pitched sound heard at the third left intercostal space.

39. The client has just received a mechanical valve replacement. Which behavior by the client indicates the client **needs more** teaching?
    1. The client takes prophylactic antibiotics.
    2. The client uses a soft-bristle toothbrush.
    3. The client takes an enteric-coated acetylsalicylic acid daily.
    4. The client alternates rest with activity.

40. The nurse is teaching a class on valve replacements. Which statement identifies the disadvantage of having a biological tissue valve replacement?
    1. The client must take lifetime anticoagulant therapy.
    2. The client's infections are easier to treat.
    3. There is a low incidence of thromboembolism.
    4. The valve has to be replaced frequently.

41. The nurse is preparing to administer warfarin to a client with a mechanical valve replacement. The client's international normalized ratio (INR) is 2.7. Which action should the nurse implement?
    1. Administer the medication as ordered.
    2. Prepare to administer vitamin K.
    3. Hold the medication and notify the HCP.
    4. Assess the client for abnormal bleeding.

42. Which clinical manifestations should the nurse assess in any client diagnosed with long-term valvular heart disease? **Select all that apply.**
    1. Paroxysmal nocturnal dyspnea.
    2. Orthopnea.
    3. Cough.
    4. Pericardial friction rub.
    5. Pulsus paradoxus.

43. The client is being evaluated for valvular heart disease. Which information would be **most significant?**
    1. The client has a history of CAD.
    2. There is a family history of valvular heart disease.
    3. The client has a history of smoking for 10 years.
    4. The client has a history of rheumatic heart disease.

44. The client just had a percutaneous transluminal balloon valvuloplasty (PTBV) and is in the recovery room. Which intervention should the Post Anesthesia Care Unit nurse implement?
    1. Assess the client's chest tube output.
    2. Monitor the client's chest dressing.
    3. Evaluate the client's endotracheal (ET) lip line.
    4. Keep the client's affected leg straight.

45. The client with a mechanical valve replacement asks the nurse, "Why do I have to take antibiotics before getting my teeth cleaned?" Which response by the nurse is **most appropriate?**
    1. "You are at risk of developing an infection in your heart."
    2. "Your teeth will not bleed as much if you have antibiotics."
    3. "This procedure may cause your valve to malfunction."
    4. "Antibiotics will prevent vegetative growth on your valves."

46. The client had open-heart surgery to replace the mitral valve. Which interventions should the ICU nurse implement? **Select all that apply.**
    1. Restrict the client's fluids as ordered.
    2. Keep the client in the supine position.
    3. Maintain oxygen saturation at 90%.
    4. Administer total parenteral nutrition.
    5. Monitor the cardiac telemetry rhythm.

47. Which client would the nurse suspect of having a mitral valve prolapse?
    1. A 60-year-old female with heart failure.
    2. A 23-year-old male with Marfan's syndrome.
    3. An 80-year-old male with atrial fibrillation.
    4. A 33-year-old female with Down syndrome.

48. The RN charge nurse is making shift assignments. Which client would be **most appropriate** for the charge nurse to assign to a new graduate just having completed orientation to the medical floor?
    1. The client admitted for diagnostic tests to rule out valvular heart disease.
    2. The client 3 days post-MI being discharged tomorrow.
    3. The client exhibiting supraventricular tachycardia (SVT) on telemetry.
    4. The client diagnosed with atrial fibrillation with an INR of 5.

## Dysrhythmias and Conduction Problems

49. The telemetry nurse is unable to read the telemetry monitor at the nurse's station. Which intervention should the telemetry nurse implement **first**?
    1. Go to the client's room to check the client.
    2. Instruct the primary nurse to assess the client.
    3. Contact the client on the client call system.
    4. Request the nursing assistant to take the crash cart to the client's room.

50. The client shows ventricular fibrillation on the telemetry at the nurse's station. Which action should the telemetry nurse implement **first**?
    1. Administer epinephrine IV push (IVP).
    2. Prepare to defibrillate the client.
    3. Call a STAT code.
    4. Start cardiopulmonary resuscitation (CPR).

51. The client is experiencing multifocal PVCs. Which antidysrhythmic medication would the nurse expect the HCP to order for this client?
    1. Amiodarone.
    2. Epinephrine.
    3. Digoxin.
    4. Adenosine.

52. The client is exhibiting sinus bradycardia, is reporting syncope and weakness, and has a BP of 98/60. Which **collaborative** treatment should the nurse anticipate being implemented?
    1. Administer a thrombolytic medication.
    2. Assess the client's cardiovascular status.
    3. Prepare for the insertion of a pacemaker.
    4. Obtain a permit for synchronized cardioversion.

53. Which intervention should the nurse implement when defibrillating a client in ventricular fibrillation?
    1. Defibrillate the client at 50, 100, and 200 joules.
    2. Do not remove the oxygen source during defibrillation.
    3. Place petroleum jelly on the defibrillator pads.
    4. Shout "all clear" before defibrillating the client.

54. The client has chronic atrial fibrillation. Which discharge teaching should the nurse discuss with the client?
    1. Instruct the client to use a soft-bristle toothbrush.
    2. Discuss the importance of getting a monthly partial thromboplastin time (PTT).
    3. Teach the client about signs of pacemaker malfunction.
    4. Explain to the client the procedure for synchronized cardioversion.

55. The client is exhibiting ventricular tachycardia. Which intervention should the nurse implement **first**?
    1. Administer amiodarone IVP.
    2. Prepare to defibrillate the client.
    3. Assess the client's apical pulse and blood pressure.
    4. Start basic CPR.

56. The client is in third-degree complete heart block. Which intervention should the nurse implement **first**?
    1. Prepare to insert a pacemaker.
    2. Administer atropine.
    3. Obtain a STAT ECG.
    4. Notify the HCP.

57. The client is in ventricular fibrillation. Which interventions should the nurse implement? **Select all that apply.**
    1. Start CPR.
    2. Prepare to administer adenosine IVP.
    3. Prepare to defibrillate the client.
    4. Bring the crash cart to the bedside.
    5. Prepare to administer amiodarone IVP.

58. The client, 1 day postoperative coronary artery bypass graft surgery, is exhibiting sinus tachycardia. Which intervention should the nurse implement?
    1. Assess the apical heart rate for 1 full minute.
    2. Notify the client's cardiac surgeon.
    3. Prepare the client for synchronized cardioversion.
    4. Determine if the client is having pain.

59. The client's telemetry reading shows a P wave before each QRS complex, and the rate is 78. Which action should the nurse implement?
    1. Document this as normal sinus rhythm.
    2. Request a 12-lead electrocardiogram.
    3. Prepare to administer digoxin PO.
    4. Assess the client's cardiac enzymes.

60. Which client problem has **priority** for the client diagnosed with a cardiac dysrhythmia?
    1. Alteration in comfort.
    2. Decreased cardiac output.
    3. Impaired gas exchange.
    4. Activity intolerance.

## Inflammatory Cardiac Disorders

61. The client is diagnosed with pericarditis. Which are the **most common** clinical manifestations the nurse would expect to find when assessing the client?
    1. Pulsus paradoxus.
    2. Reports of fatigue and arthralgias.
    3. Petechiae and splinter hemorrhages.
    4. Increased chest pain with inspiration.

62. The client is diagnosed with acute pericarditis. Which clinical manifestation **warrants immediate** attention by the nurse?
    1. Muffled heart sounds.
    2. Nondistended jugular veins.
    3. Bounding peripheral pulses.
    4. Pericardial friction rub.

63. The client is admitted to the medical unit to rule out myocarditis. Which question should the nurse ask the client during the admission interview to **support** this diagnosis?
    1. "Do you have a fever or sore throat?"
    2. "Do you have atrial fibrillation?"
    3. "Do you have a family history of myocarditis?"
    4. "Do you take over-the-counter (OTC) medications?"

64. The client diagnosed with pericarditis is prescribed an NSAID. Which teaching instruction should the nurse discuss with the client?
    1. Explain the importance of tapering off the medication.
    2. Discuss that the medication will make the client drowsy.
    3. Instruct the client to take the medication with food.
    4. Tell the client to take the medication when the pain level is around "8."

65. The client diagnosed with pericarditis is reporting increased pain. Which intervention should the nurse implement **first?**
    1. Administer oxygen via nasal cannula.
    2. Evaluate the client's urinary output.
    3. Assess the client for cardiac complications.
    4. Encourage the client to use the incentive spirometer.

66. The client diagnosed with pericarditis is experiencing cardiac tamponade. Which **collaborative** intervention should the nurse anticipate for this client?
    1. Prepare for a pericardiocentesis.
    2. Request STAT cardiac enzymes.
    3. Perform a 12-lead electrocardiogram.
    4. Assess the client's heart and lung sounds.

67. The female client is diagnosed with infective endocarditis. Which statements of clinical manifestations support the diagnosis of infective endocarditis? **Select all that apply.**
    1. Osler's nodes.
    2. Chest pain.
    3. Janeway lesions.
    4. Splinter hemorrhages.
    5. Rosacea.

68. Which potential complication should the nurse assess for in the client diagnosed with infective endocarditis with embolization of vegetative lesions from the mitral valve?
    1. Pulmonary embolus (PE).
    2. Cerebrovascular accident.
    3. Hemoptysis.
    4. Deep vein thrombosis.

69. Which nursing diagnosis would be a **priority** for the client diagnosed with myocarditis?
    1. Anxiety related to possible long-term complications.
    2. High risk for injury related to antibiotic therapy.
    3. Increased cardiac output related to valve regurgitation.
    4. Activity intolerance related to impaired cardiac muscle function.

70. The client diagnosed with pericarditis is being discharged home. Which intervention should the nurse include in the discharge teaching?
    1. Be sure to allow for uninterrupted rest and sleep.
    2. Refer the client to outpatient occupational therapy.
    3. Maintain oxygen via nasal cannula at 2 L/min.
    4. Discuss upcoming valve replacement surgery.

71. The client has just had a pericardiocentesis. Which interventions should the nurse implement? **Select all that apply.**
    1. Monitor vital signs every 15 minutes for the first hour.
    2. Assess the client's heart and lung sounds.
    3. Record the amount of fluid removed as output.
    4. Evaluate the client's cardiac rhythm.
    5. Keep the client in the supine position.

72. The client diagnosed with infective endocarditis is admitted to the medical department. Which HCP's order should be implemented **first?**
    1. Administer intravenous antibiotics.
    2. Obtain blood cultures times 2.
    3. Schedule an echocardiogram.
    4. Encourage bedrest with bathroom privileges.

# CONCEPTS

The concepts covered in this chapter focus on the cardiac-related areas of nursing; perfusion-related problems of MI, dysrhythmias, heart failure, and hypertension; and the interrelated concepts of the nursing process and clinical judgment. The concept of the nursing process is displayed throughout the questions. The concept of clinical judgment is presented in any prioritizing or "first" question.

73. The nurse enters the client's room and notes an unconscious client with an absence of respirations and no pulse or blood pressure. The concept of perfusion is identified by the nurse. Which should the nurse implement **first?**
    1. Notify the HCP.
    2. Call a rapid response team (RRT).
    3. Determine the telemetry monitor reading.
    4. Activate the code blue system.

74. The 45-year-old male client diagnosed with essential hypertension has decided not to take his medications. The client's BP is 178/94, indicating a perfusion issue. Which question should the nurse ask the client **first?**
    1. "Do you have the money to buy your medication?"
    2. "Does the medication give unwanted side effects?"
    3. "Did you quit taking the medications because you don't feel bad?"
    4. "Can you tell me why you stopped taking the medication?"

75. The nurse identifies the concept of altered tissue perfusion related to a client admitted with atrial fibrillation. Which interventions should the nurse implement? **Select all that apply.**
    1. Monitor the client's blood pressure and apical rate every 4 hours.
    2. Place the client on intake and output every shift.
    3. Require the client to sleep with the head of the bed elevated.
    4. Teach the client to perform Buerger Allen exercises daily.

    5. Determine if the client is on an antiplatelet or anticoagulant medication.
    6. Assess the client's neurological status every shift and prn.

76. The nurse identifies the concept of perfusion for a client diagnosed with heart failure. Which assessment data **support** this concept?
    1. The client has a large abdomen and a positive fluid wave test.
    2. The client has paroxysmal nocturnal dyspnea.
    3. The client has 2+ glucose in the urine.
    4. The client has a comorbid condition of MI.

77. The nurse is caring for a client diagnosed with CAD. Which should the nurse teach the client before discharge? **Select all that apply.**
    1. Carry your nitroglycerin tablets in a brown bottle.
    2. Swallow a nitroglycerin tablet at the first sign of angina.
    3. If one nitroglycerin tablet does not work in 10 minutes, take another.
    4. Nitroglycerin tablets have a fruity odor if they are potent.
    5. Replace your nitroglycerin tablets after 6 months.

78. The nurse is caring for a client who suddenly reports crushing substernal chest pain while ambulating in the hall. Which nursing action should the nurse implement **first?**
    1. Call a code blue.
    2. Assess the telemetry reading.
    3. Take the client's apical pulse.
    4. Have the client sit down.

79. The client's telemetry reading is below. Which should the nurse implement?
    1. Take the client's apical pulse and blood pressure.
    2. Prepare to administer amiodarone intravenous piggyback (IVPB).
    3. Continue to monitor.
    4. Place oxygen on the client via a nasal cannula.

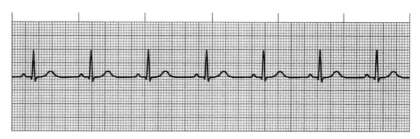

80. The nurse is functioning in the role of a medication nurse during a code. Which should the nurse implement when administering amiodarone for ventricular tachycardia?
    1. Mix the medication in 100 mL of fluid and administer over 15 minutes.
    2. Push amiodarone 300 mg directly into the nearest IV port.
    3. Question the physician's order because it is not Advanced Cardiac Life Support (ACLS) recommended.
    4. Administer via an IV pump based on mg/kg/min.

81. The client diagnosed with an ST elevation MI (STEMI) has developed 2+ edema bilaterally of the lower extremities and has crackles in all lung fields. Which should the nurse implement **first?**
    1. Notify the HCP.
    2. Assess what the client ate at the last meal.
    3. Request a STAT 12 lead electrocardiogram.
    4. Administer furosemide IVP.

82. The nurse is administering morning medications to clients on a telemetry unit. Which medication would the nurse **question?**
    1. Furosemide IVP to a client with a potassium level of 3.6 mEq/L.
    2. Digoxin orally to a client diagnosed with rapid atrial fibrillation.
    3. Enalapril orally to a client with BP 86/64 and apical pulse 65.
    4. Morphine IVP to a client who is reporting chest pain and is diaphoretic.

83. The nurse is admitting a client diagnosed with CAD and angina. Which concept is a **priority?**
    1. Sleep, rest, activity.
    2. Comfort.
    3. Oxygenation.
    4. Perfusion.

84. The home health nurse is assigned a client diagnosed with heart failure. Which should the nurse implement? **Select all that apply.**
    1. Request a dietary consult for a sodium-restricted diet.
    2. Instruct the client to elevate the feet during the day.
    3. Teach the client to weigh every morning wearing the same type of clothing.
    4. Assess for edema in the dependent areas of the body.
    5. Encourage the client to drink at least 3,000 mL of fluid per day.
    6. Have the client repeat back instructions to the nurse.

85. The telemetry monitor tech notifies the nurse of the strip shown below. Which should the RN implement **first?**
    1. Instruct the UAP to check the client.
    2. Go to the client's room and assess the client personally.
    3. Have the monitor tech check the client using a different lead.
    4. Call for the code blue team and perform CPR.

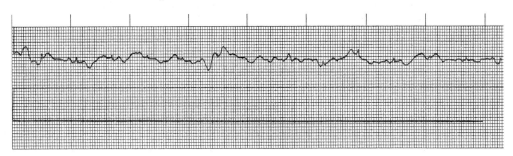

86. The nurse is working with a group of new graduates on a medical-surgical unit. Which should the RN explain about completing first morning rounds on clients?
    1. Perform a brief, focused assessment on each client soon after receiving the report.
    2. Determine which client should have a bath and inform the UAP.
    3. Give all the clients a wet wash to wash the face and a toothbrush and toothpaste.
    4. Pick up any paper on the floor and get the room ready for morning HCP rounds.

87. The nurse has received a shift report. Which client should the nurse assess **first?**
    1. The client diagnosed with CAD reporting severe indigestion.
    2. The client diagnosed with heart failure with 3+ pitting edema.
    3. The client diagnosed with atrial fibrillation with an irregular apical rate of 110.
    4. The client diagnosed with sinus bradycardia reporting being constipated.

88. The client diagnosed with MI is being discharged. Which discharge instruction(s) should the nurse teach the client?
    1. Call the HCP if any chest pain happens.
    2. Discuss when the client can resume sexual activity.
    3. Explain the pharmacology of nitroglycerin tablets.
    4. Encourage the client to sleep with the head of the bed elevated.

89. The nurse is administering morning medications. Which medication should be administered **first?**
    1. The digoxin to a client diagnosed with heart failure and with 2+ edema of the feet.
    2. The sliding scale insulin to a client with a fasting blood glucose of 345 mg/dL demanding breakfast.
    3. The furosemide to a client with a 24-hour intake of 986 mL and an output of 1,400 mL.
    4. The ARB, angiotensin receptor blocker, medication to a client with blood pressure reported by the UAP as 142/76.

90. The nurse identifies the concept of tissue perfusion as a client problem. Which is an **antecedent** of tissue perfusion?
    1. The client has a history of CAD.
    2. The client has a history of diabetes insipidus (DI).
    3. The client has a history of chronic obstructive pulmonary disease (COPD).
    4. The client has a history of multiple fractures from a motor vehicle accident.

# PRACTICE QUESTIONS ANSWERS AND RATIONALES

## Heart Failure

1. 1. The client diagnosed with left-sided heart failure would exhibit tachycardia (apical pulse rate of 110), shortness of breath, crackles on auscultation, fatigue, third heart sounds, and change in mental status.
   2. The client diagnosed with right-sided heart failure has jugular venous distention, dependent edema (4+ pitting edema of feet), and ascites.
   3. The client diagnosed with left-sided heart failure would report sleeping on at least two pillows, if not sleeping in an upright position, and labored breathing, not eupnea, which means normal breathing.
   4. In a client diagnosed with heart failure, the apical pulse, not the radial pulse, is the **best** place to assess the cardiac status.

**TEST-TAKING HINT:** In option "3," the word "no" is an absolute term and, usually, absolutes, such as "no," "never," "always," and "only," are incorrect because there is no room for any other possible answer. If the test taker is looking for abnormal data, then the test taker should exclude the options that have normal values in them, such as eupnea, pulse rate of 90, and CRT less than 3 seconds.

2. 1. Ambulating in the hall by day of discharge would be a more appropriate goal for an activity-intolerance nursing diagnosis.
   2. Audible S₁ and S₂ sounds are normal for a heart with adequate output. An audible S₃ sound might indicate left ventricular failure, which could be life-threatening.
   3. This is a nursing intervention, not a short-term goal for this client.
   4. A pulse oximeter reading would be a goal for impaired gas exchange, not for cardiac output.

**TEST-TAKING HINT:** When reading a nursing diagnosis or problem, the test taker must be sure that the answer selected addresses the problem. An answer option may be appropriate care for the disease process but may not fit with the problem or etiology. Remember, when given an etiology in a nursing diagnosis, the answer will be doing something about the problem (etiology). In this question, the test taker should look for an answer that addresses the ability of the heart to pump blood.

3. Correct answers are 2 and 3.
   1. The client should notify the HCP of weight gain of more than 2 or 3 pounds in 1 day.
   2. The client should not take digoxin, a cardiac glycoside, if the radial pulse is less than 60.
   3. The client should be on a low-sodium diet to prevent water retention.
   4. The color of the urine should not change to a dark color; if anything, it might become lighter, and the amount will increase with diuretics.
   5. Instruct the client to take the loop diuretic furosemide in the morning to prevent nocturia.

**TEST-TAKING HINT:** This is an alternative-type question—in this case, "Select all that apply." If the test taker missed this statement, it is possible to jump at the first correct answer. This is one reason that it is imperative to read all options before deciding on the correct one(s). This could be a clue to reread the question for clarity. Another hint that this is an alternative question is the number of options. The other questions have four potential answers; this one has five. Numbers in an answer option are always important. Is 1 pound enough to indicate a problem that should be brought to the attention of the HCP?

4. 1. Sponging dry the client's forehead would be appropriate, but it is not the first intervention.
   2. Obtaining a pulse oximeter reading would be appropriate, but it is not the first intervention.
   3. Taking the vital signs would be appropriate, but it is not the first intervention.
   4. The nurse must first put the client in a sitting position to decrease the workload of the heart by decreasing venous return and maximizing lung expansion. Then, the nurse could take vital signs and check the pulse oximeter and then sponge the client's forehead.

**TEST-TAKING HINT:** In a question that asks the nurse to set priorities, all the answer options can be appropriate actions by the nurse for a given situation. The test taker should apply some guidelines or principles, such as Maslow's hierarchy, to determine what will give the client the most immediate assistance.

77

5. 1. Pitting edema changing from 3+ to 4+ indicates a worsening of the right-sided heart failure.
   2. The client's ability to take the radial pulse would evaluate teaching, not medical treatment.
   3. Being able to perform ADLs without shortness of breath (dyspnea) would indicate the client's condition is improving. The client's heart is a more effective pump and can oxygenate the body better without increasing fluid in the lungs.
   4. Any jugular vein distention indicates that the right side of the heart is failing, which would not indicate effective medical treatment.

**TEST-TAKING HINT: When asked to determine whether treatment is effective, the test taker must know the clinical manifestations of the disease being treated. An improvement in the signs and symptoms indicates effective treatment.**

6. 1. BNP is a specific diagnostic test to diagnose heart failure. Levels higher than normal indicate heart failure and the need for additional assessment such as echocardiography (VanLeeuwen & Bladh, 2017).
   2. An elevated CK-MB would indicate MI, not heart failure. CK-MB is an isoenzyme.
   3. A positive D-dimer would indicate a PE, disseminated intravascular coagulation (DIC), or acute MI but not heart failure.
   4. A positive VQ scan would indicate a PE.

**TEST-TAKING HINT: This question requires the test taker to discriminate among congestive heart failure (CHF), MI, and PE. If unsure of the answer to this type of question, the test taker should eliminate any answer options that the test taker knows are wrong. For example, the test taker may not know about PE but might know that CK-MB data are used to monitor MI and be able to eliminate option "2" as a possibility. Then, there is a 1:3 chance of getting the correct answer.**

7. Correct answers are 2 and 5.
   1. If a cough develops, the client should notify the HCP because this is an adverse reaction, and the HCP will discontinue the medication.
   2. Orthostatic hypotension may occur with ACE inhibitors as a result of vasodilation. Therefore, the nurse should instruct the client to rise slowly and sit on the side of the bed until equilibrium is restored.
   3. ACE inhibitors may cause the client to retain potassium; therefore, the client should not increase potassium intake.
   4. An ACE inhibitor should be taken 1 hour before meals or 2 hours after a meal to increase absorption of the medication.
   5. ACE inhibitors taken with NSAIDs can cause an adverse effect in the kidneys and decrease the antihypertensive benefits of the ACE inhibitor.

**TEST-TAKING HINT: If the test taker knows that an ACE inhibitor is also given for hypertension, then looking at answer options referring to hypotension would be appropriate.**

8. 1. An S₃ heart sound indicates left-sided heart failure, and the nurse must assess this client first because it is an emergency situation.
   2. The nurse would expect a client diagnosed with right-sided heart failure to have sacral edema of 4+; the client diagnosed with an S₃ would be in a more life-threatening situation.
   3. A pulse oximeter reading of greater than 93% is considered normal.
   4. An elevated creatinine level is expected in a client diagnosed with chronic renal failure.

**TEST-TAKING HINT: Because the nurse will be assessing each client, the test taker must determine which client is a priority. A general guideline for this type of question is for the test taker to ask, "Is this within normal limits?" or "Is this expected for the disease process?" If the answer is yes to either question, then the test taker can eliminate these options and look for abnormal data that would make that client a priority.**

9. 1. Allowing the UAP to take a client down to smoke is not cost-effective and is not supportive of the medical treatment regimen that discourages smoking.
   2. The client going to the ICU would be unstable, and the nurse should not delegate to a UAP any nursing task that involves an unstable client.
   3. The nurse cannot delegate teaching.
   4. The UAP can assist the x-ray technician in positioning the client for the portable x-ray. This does not require judgment.

**TEST-TAKING HINT: The test taker must be knowledgeable about the individual state's Nurse Practice Act regarding what a nurse may delegate to UAPs. Generally, the answer options that require a higher level of knowledge or ability are reserved for licensed staff.**

10. 1. This client is stable because discharge is scheduled for the following day. Therefore, this client does not need to be assigned to the most experienced registered nurse.
    2. This client is more in need of custodial nursing care than care from the most experienced registered nurse. Therefore, the charge nurse could assign a less experienced nurse to this client.
    3. **This client is exhibiting clinical manifestations of shock, which makes this client the most unstable. An experienced nurse should care for this client.**
    4. These reports usually indicate muscular or pleuritic chest pain; cardiac chest pain does not fluctuate with inspiration. This client does not require the care of an experienced nurse as much as does the client diagnosed with signs of shock.

**TEST-TAKING HINT: When deciding on an answer for this type of question, the test taker should reason as to which client is stable and which has a potentially higher level of need.**

11. 1. The client diagnosed with peripheral edema will experience calf tightness but would not have leg cramping, which is the result of low potassium levels. The timing of the diuretic will not change the side effect of leg cramping resulting from low potassium levels.
    2. **The most probable cause of the leg cramping is potassium excretion as a result of diuretic medication. Bananas and orange juice are foods that are high in potassium.**
    3. Weight gain is monitored in clients with chronic heart failure, and elevating the legs would decrease peripheral edema by increasing the rate of return to the central circulation, but these interventions would not help with leg cramps.
    4. Ambulating frequently and performing leg-stretching exercises will not be effective in alleviating the leg cramps.

**TEST-TAKING HINT: The timing "at night" in this question was not important in answering the question, but it could have made the test taker jump at option "1." Be sure to read all answer options before deciding on an answer. Correctly answering this question requires knowledge of the side effects of treatments used for heart failure.**

12. 1. Measuring the intake and output is an appropriate intervention to implement for a client diagnosed with heart failure, but it does not address getting the client to tolerate activity.
    2. Dietary sodium is restricted in clients with heart failure, but this is an intervention for decreasing fluid volume, not for increasing tolerance for activity.
    3. Daily weighing monitors fluid volume status, not activity tolerance.
    4. **Scheduling activities and rest periods allows the client to participate in the care and addresses the desired outcome.**

**TEST-TAKING HINT: With questions involving nursing diagnoses or goals and outcomes, the test taker should realize that all activities referred to in the answer options may be appropriate for the disease but may not be specific for the desired outcome.**

## Angina and MI

13. 1. CK-MB elevates in 4 to 6 hours.
    2. LDH elevates in 12 to 24 hours.
    3. **Troponin is the enzyme that elevates within 2 to 6 hours (Van Leeuwen & Bladh, 2017).**
    4. WBCs elevate as a result of necrotic tissue, but this is not a cardiac enzyme.

**TEST-TAKING HINT: The test taker should be aware of the words "cardiac enzyme," which would eliminate option "4" as a possible answer. The word in the stem is "first." This question requires the test taker to have knowledge of laboratory values.**

14. 1. Midepigastric pain would support a diagnosis of peptic ulcer disease; eructation is belching.
    2. **Diaphoresis (sweating) is a systemic reaction to the MI. The blood vessels vasoconstrict to shunt blood from the periphery to the trunk of the body; this, in turn, leads to cold, clammy skin.**
    3. Intermittent claudication is leg pain secondary to decreased oxygen to the muscle, and pallor is paleness of the skin as a result of decreased blood supply. Neither is an early sign of MI.
    4. Jugular vein distension (JVD) and dependent edema are clinical manifestations of right-sided heart failure, not of MI.

**TEST-TAKING HINT: The stem already addresses chest pain; therefore, the test taker could eliminate option "1" as a possible answer. Intermittent claudication, option "3," is the classic sign of arterial occlusive disease, and JVD is very specific to right-sided heart failure. The nurse must be able to identify at least two or three clinical manifestations of disease processes.**

15. 1. The nurse must assume the chest pain is secondary to decreased oxygen to the myocardium and administer a sublingual nitroglycerin tablet, which is a coronary vasodilator, but this is not the first action.
    2. An ECG should be ordered, but it is not the first intervention.
    3. **Stopping all activity will decrease the myocardium's need for oxygen and may help decrease chest pain.**
    4. Assessment is often the first nursing intervention, but when the client has chest pain and a possible MI, the nurse must first take care of the client. Taking vital signs would not help relieve chest pain.

**TEST-TAKING HINT: Whenever the test taker wants to select an assessment intervention, be sure to think about whether that intervention will help the client, especially if the client is experiencing pain. Do not automatically select the answer option that is assessment.**

16. Correct answers are 2 and 3.
    1. Morphine should be administered intravenously, not intramuscularly.
    2. **Acetylsalicylic acid (ASA) (aspirin) is an antiplatelet medication and should be administered orally.**
    3. **Oxygen will help decrease myocardial ischemia, thereby decreasing pain.**
    4. The supine position will increase respiratory effort, which will increase myocardial oxygen consumption; the client should be in the semi-Fowler's position.
    5. Nitroglycerin, a coronary vasodilator, is administered sublingually, not subcutaneously.

**TEST-TAKING HINT: This is an alternate-type question that requires the test taker to select all options that are applicable. The test taker must identify all correct answer options to receive credit for a correct answer; no partial credit is given. Remember to read the question carefully—it is not meant to be tricky.**

17. 1. The social worker addresses financial concerns or referrals after discharge, which are not indicated for this client.
    2. Physical therapy addresses gait problems, lower extremity strength building, and assisting with a transfer, which is not required for this client.
    3. **Cardiac rehabilitation is the most appropriate referral. The client can start rehabilitation in the hospital and then attend an outpatient cardiac rehabilitation clinic, which includes progressive** exercise, diet teaching, and classes on modifying risk factors.
    4. Occupational therapy assists the client in regaining ADLs and covers mainly fine motor activities.

**TEST-TAKING HINT: The test taker must be familiar with the responsibilities of the other members of the health-care team. If the test taker had no idea which would be the most appropriate referral, the word "cardiac," which means "heart," should help the test taker in deciding that this is the most sensible option because the client had an MI, a "heart attack."**

18. 1. The nurse should medicate the client as needed, but it is not the first intervention.
    2. **The nurse must always assess the client to determine if the chest pain that is occurring is expected postoperatively or if it is a complication of the surgery.**
    3. Turning will help decrease complications from immobility, such as pneumonia, but it will not help relieve the client's pain.
    4. The nurse, not a machine, should always take care of the client.

**TEST-TAKING HINT: The stem asks the nurse to identify the first intervention that should be implemented. Therefore, the test taker should apply the nursing process and select an assessment intervention. Both options "2" and "4" involve assessment, but the nurse—not a machine or diagnostic test—should always assess the client.**

19. 1. After PCI, the client must keep the right leg straight for at least 2 to 6 hours to prevent any arterial bleeding from the insertion site in the right femoral artery.
    2. A pressure dressing is applied to the insertion site to help prevent arterial bleeding.
    3. **Any neurovascular assessment data that are abnormal require intervention by the nurse; numbness may indicate decreased blood supply to the right foot.**
    4. A bounding pedal pulse indicates that adequate circulation is getting to the right foot; therefore, this would not require immediate intervention.

**TEST-TAKING HINT: This question requires the test taker to identify abnormal, unexpected, or life-threatening data. The nurse must know that a PCI is performed by placing a catheter in the femoral artery and that internal or external bleeding is the most common complication.**

20. 1. An $S_3$ indicates left ventricular failure and should be reported to the HCP. It is a potentially life-threatening complication of MI.
  2. Elevating the head of the bed will not do anything to help a failing heart.
  3. This is not a normal finding; it indicates heart failure.
  4. Morphine is administered for chest pain, not for heart failure, which is suggested by the $S_3$ sound.

**TEST-TAKING HINT:** There are some situations in which the nurse must notify the HCP, and the test taker should not automatically eliminate this as a possible correct answer. The test taker must decide if any of the other three options will help correct a life-threatening complication. Normal assessment concepts should help identify the correct option. The normal heart sounds are $S_1$ and $S_2$ ("lubb-dupp"); $S_3$ is abnormal.

21. 1. The apical pulse is within normal limits—60 to 100 beats per minute.
  2. The serum calcium level is not monitored when beta blockers are given. Beta blockers can increase potassium, triglycerides, and blood glucose levels.
  3. Occasional PVCs would not warrant immediate intervention before administering this medication.
  4. The client's blood pressure is low, and a calcium channel blocker could cause the blood pressure to bottom out.

**TEST-TAKING HINT:** The test taker must know when to question administering medications. The test taker is trying to select an option that, if the medication is administered, would cause serious harm to the client.

22. 1. Leg movement is an appropriate action, and the UAP should not be told to stop encouraging it.
  2. This behavior is not unsafe or dangerous and should not be reported to the charge nurse.
  3. The nurse should praise and encourage UAPs to participate in the client's care. Clients on bedrest are at risk for deep vein thrombosis, and moving the legs will help prevent this from occurring.
  4. The nurse should praise subordinates for appropriate behavior, especially when it is helping to prevent life-threatening complications.

**TEST-TAKING HINT:** This is a management question. The test taker must know the chain of command and when to report the behavior. The test taker could eliminate options "1" and "2" with the knowledge that moving the legs is a safe activity for the client. When having to choose between options "3" and "4," the test taker should select doing something positive instead of taking no action. This is a management concept.

23. Correct answers are 1, 4, and 5.
  1. The American Heart Association's Life's Simple 7® (2020) defines the health behaviors that can improve cardiovascular health. Stopping smoking is the first behavior recommended.
  2. The client should keep the blood pressure less than 120/79 mm Hg.
  3. The client should maintain a fasting blood glucose level of less than 100 mg/dL.
  4. The client should maintain normal body weight, eat a healthy diet, and exercise regularly to improve cardiovascular health.
  5. The client should learn to control cholesterol levels and maintain a level of less than 200 mg/DL.

**TEST-TAKING HINT:** When attempting to answer a client's question, the nurse should provide factual information in simple, understandable terms. The test taker should be able to select the answer options that support heart-healthy living.

24. 1. These vital signs are within normal limits and would not require any immediate intervention.
  2. The groin dressing should be dry and intact; blood on the dressing indicates bleeding from the puncture site. The nurse should mark the size of the bleed, if possible, and notify the HCP.
  3. The client should be assessed for arrhythmias, and normal sinus rhythm does not require any intervention.
  4. The nurse must check the neurovascular assessment, and paresthesia would warrant immediate intervention, but no numbness and tingling is a good sign.

**TEST-TAKING HINT:** "Warrants immediate intervention" means the nurse should probably notify the HCP or do something independently because a complication may occur. Therefore, the test taker must select an answer option that is abnormal or unsafe. In the data listed, there are three normal findings and one abnormal finding.

## Coronary Artery Disease

25. 1. If the tablets are not kept in the dark bottle, they will lose their potency.
    2. The tablets should burn or sting when put under the tongue.
    3. The client should keep the tablets with him in case of chest pain.
    4. The client should take one tablet every 5 minutes and, if no relief occurs after the third tablet, have someone drive him to the emergency department or call 911.

**TEST-TAKING HINT:** This question is an "except" question, requiring the test taker to identify which statement indicates the client doesn't understand the teaching. Sometimes the test taker could restate the question and think which statement indicates the client understands the teaching.

26. 1. This is a correct statement presented in lay terms. When the coronary arteries cannot supply adequate oxygen to the heart muscle, there is chest pain.
    2. This is the explanation in medical terms that should not be used when explaining medical conditions to a client.
    3. This explains CHF but does not explain why chest pain occurs.
    4. Respiratory compromise occurs when the lungs cannot oxygenate the blood, such as occurs with an altered level of consciousness, cyanosis, and increased respiratory rate.

**TEST-TAKING HINT:** The nurse must select the option that best explains the facts in terminology a client without medical training can understand.

27. Correct answers are 1, 2, 3, and 5.
    1. The client should be assessed for an allergy to seafood or contrast dye because contrast dye is used in the percutaneous transluminal coronary angioplasty (PTCA).
    2. The nurse should initiate a peripheral intravenous line for conscious sedation and hydration during the procedure.
    3. The client should be NPO for 6 to 12 hours before the procedure.
    4. The nurse may reinforce teaching, but the HCP should thoroughly explain the procedure and its associated risks and complications to the client.

5. The nurse may ensure the appropriate laboratory tests are available for the HCP such as prothrombin time (PT), PTT, serum electrolytes, blood urea nitrogen (BUN), and creatinine.

**TEST-TAKING HINT:** The nurse should apply standard preoperative assessment to answer the question. Option "4" can be eliminated because it is the responsibility of the HCP to explain procedures to the client.

28. 1. This blood pressure is normal, and the nurse would administer the medication.
    2. A beta blocker decreases sympathetic stimulation to the heart, thereby decreasing the heart rate. An apical rate of less than 60 bpm indicates a lower-than-normal heart rate and should make the nurse question administering this medication because it will further decrease the heart rate.
    3. A headache will not affect administering the medication to the client.
    4. The potassium level is within normal limits, but it is usually not monitored before administering a beta blocker.

**TEST-TAKING HINT:** If the test taker does not know when to question the use of a certain medication, the test taker should evaluate the options to determine if any options include abnormal data based on normal parameters. This would make the test taker select option "2" because the normal apical pulse in an adult is 60 to 100.

29. 1. The nurse should always assess the apical (not radial) pulse, but the pulse is not affected by a loop diuretic.
    2. Loop diuretics cause potassium to be lost in the urine output. Therefore, the nurse should assess the client's potassium level, and if the client is hypokalemic, the nurse should question administering this medication.
    3. The glucometer provides a glucose level, which is not affected by a loop diuretic.
    4. The pulse oximeter reading evaluates peripheral oxygenation and is not affected by a loop diuretic.

**TEST-TAKING HINT:** Knowing that diuretics increase urine output would lead the test taker to eliminate glucose level and oxygenation (options "3" and "4"). In very few instances does the nurse assess the radial pulse; the apical pulse is assessed.

30. Correct answers are 1, 2, 4, and 5.
    1. A low-fat, low-cholesterol diet will help decrease the buildup of atherosclerosis in the arteries.
    2. Walking will help increase collateral circulation.
    3. Salt should be restricted in the diet of a client diagnosed with hypertension, not CAD.
    4. Stress reduction is encouraged for clients with CAD because this helps prevent excess stress on the heart muscle.
    5. Increasing fiber in the diet will help remove cholesterol via the gastrointestinal system.

**TEST-TAKING HINT: This is an alternate-type question where the test taker must select all interventions that are applicable to the situation. CAD is a common disease, and the nurse must be knowledgeable about ways to modify risk factors.**

31. 1. Bowel movements are important, but they are not pertinent to CAD.
    2. CXRs are usually done for respiratory problems, not for CAD.
    3. **Sexual activity is a risk factor for angina resulting from CAD. The fact that the client is older should not affect the nurse's assessment of the client's concerns about sexual activity.**
    4. Weight change is not significant in a client diagnosed with CAD.

**TEST-TAKING HINT: Remember, if the client is described with an adjective such as "older," this may be the key to selecting the correct answer. The nurse must not be judgmental about older clients, especially about issues concerning sexual activity.**

32. 1. Isometric exercises are weight lifting-type exercises. A client diagnosed with CAD should perform isotonic exercises, which increase muscle tone, not isometric exercises.
    2. **The client should walk at least 30 minutes a day to increase collateral circulation.**
    3. When it is cold outside, vasoconstriction occurs, and this will decrease oxygen to the heart muscle. Therefore, the client should not exercise when it is cold outside.
    4. The client should wear good, supportive tennis shoes when ambulating, not sandals or other open-toed shoes.

**TEST-TAKING HINT: The test taker should be aware of adjectives such as "isometric," which makes option "1" incorrect, and "open-toed," which makes option "4" incorrect.**

33. 1. The client should take the coronary vasodilator nitroglycerin sublingually, but it is not the first intervention.
    2. **Stopping the activity decreases the heart's need for oxygen and may help decrease angina (chest pain).**
    3. The client should keep a diary of when angina occurs, what activity causes it, and how many nitroglycerin tablets are taken before chest pain is relieved.
    4. If the chest pain (angina) is not relieved with three nitroglycerin tablets, the client should call 911 or have someone take him to the emergency department. Notifying the HCP may take too long.

**TEST-TAKING HINT: The question is asking which action the client should take first. This implies that more than one of the answer options could be appropriate for the chest pain, but that only one is done first. The test taker should select the answer that will help the client directly and quickly—and that is stopping the activity.**

34. 1. **The Holter monitor is a 24-hour electrocardiogram, and the client must keep an accurate record of activity so that the HCP can compare the ECG recordings with different levels of activity.**
    2. The Holter monitor should not be removed for any reason.
    3. All medications should be taken as prescribed.
    4. The client should perform all activity as usual while wearing the Holter monitor so the HCP can get an accurate account of heart function during a 24-hour period.

**TEST-TAKING HINT: In some instances, the test taker must be knowledgeable about diagnostic tests, and there are no test-taking hints. The test taker might eliminate option "3" by realizing that, unless the client is NPO for a test or surgery, medications are usually taken.**

35. 1. According to the American Heart Association (2020), the client should not eat more than one whole egg or two egg whites a day.
    2. **The American Heart Association recommends a low-fat, low-cholesterol diet for a client diagnosed with CAD. The client should avoid any fried foods, especially meats, and bake, broil, or grill any meat.**
    3. The client should drink low-fat milk, not whole milk.
    4. Pork products (bacon, sausage, ham) are high in sodium, which is prohibited in a low-salt diet, not a low-cholesterol, low-fat diet.

**TEST-TAKING HINT:** The test taker must be knowledgeable of prescribed diets for specific disease processes. This is mainly memorizing facts. There is no test-taking hint to help eliminate any of the options.

36. 1. This client is at high risk for complications related to necrotic myocardial tissue and will need extensive teaching, so this client should not be assigned to a new graduate.
    2. Unstable angina means this client is at risk for life-threatening complications and should not be assigned to a new graduate.
    3. **A new graduate should be able to complete a pre-procedure checklist and get this client to the catheterization laboratory.**
    4. Chest pain means this client could be having an MI and should not be assigned to a new graduate.

**TEST-TAKING HINT:** "New graduate" is the key to answering this question correctly. What type of client should be assigned to an inexperienced nurse? The test taker should not assign the new graduate an unstable client or a client at risk for a life-threatening complication.

## Valvular Heart Disease

37. 1. **Dyspnea on exertion (DOE) is typically the earliest manifestation of mitral valve stenosis.**
    2. JVD and 3+ pedal edema are clinical manifestations of right-sided heart failure and indicate worsening of the mitral valve stenosis. These signs would not be expected in a client diagnosed with early manifestations of mitral valve stenosis.
    3. Chest pain rarely occurs with mitral valve stenosis.
    4. An enlarged liver and edematous abdomen are late signs of right-sided heart failure that can occur with long-term untreated mitral valve stenosis.

**TEST-TAKING HINT:** Whenever the test taker reads "rule out," the test taker should look for data that would not indicate a severe condition of the body system that is affected. Chest pain, JVD, and pedal edema are late signs of heart problems.

38. 1. This would be expected with mitral valve stenosis.
    2. The murmur associated with mitral valve regurgitation is loud, high pitched, blowing, and holosystolic (occurring throughout systole) and is heard best at the cardiac apex.
    3. This would be expected with a mitral valve prolapse.
    4. This would be expected with aortic regurgitation.

**TEST-TAKING HINT:** This is a knowledge-based question, and there is no test-taking hint to help the test taker rule out distracters.

39. 1. Prophylactic antibiotics before invasive procedures prevent infectious endocarditis.
    2. The client is undergoing anticoagulant therapy and should use a soft-bristle toothbrush to help prevent gum trauma and bleeding.
    3. **ASA and NSAIDs interfere with clotting and may potentiate the effects of anticoagulant therapy, which the client with a mechanical valve will be prescribed. Therefore, the client should not take aspirin daily.**
    4. The client should alternate rest with activity to prevent fatigue and help decrease the workload of the heart.

**TEST-TAKING HINT:** The stem asks the test taker to identify which behavior means the client does not understand the teaching. Therefore, the test taker should select the distracter that does not agree with the condition. There is no condition for which alternating rest with activity would not be recommended.

40. 1. An advantage of having a biological valve replacement is that no anticoagulant therapy is needed. Anticoagulant therapy is needed with a mechanical valve replacement.
    2. This is an advantage of having a biological valve replacement; infections are harder to treat in clients with mechanical valve replacement.
    3. This is an advantage of having a biological valve replacement; there is a high incidence of thromboembolism in clients with mechanical valve replacement.
    4. **Biological valves deteriorate and need to be replaced frequently; this is a disadvantage of them. Mechanical valves do not deteriorate and do not have to be replaced often.**

**TEST-TAKING HINT:** This is an "except" question. The test taker might reverse the question and ask, "Which is an advantage of a biological valve?"—which might make answering the question easier.

41. 1. The therapeutic range for most clients' INR is 2 to 3, but for a client with a mechanical valve replacement, it is 2.5 to 3.5. The warfarin (Coumadin), an oral anticoagulant, should be given as ordered and not withheld.
    2. Vitamin K (AquaMephyton) is the antidote for an overdose of warfarin (Coumadin), an oral anticoagulant, but 2.7 is within the therapeutic range.
    3. This laboratory result is within the therapeutic range, INR 2 to 3, and the medication does not need to be withheld.
    4. There is no need for the nurse to assess for bleeding because 2.7 is within the therapeutic range.

**TEST-TAKING HINT:** The test taker has to know the therapeutic range for the INR to be able to answer this question correctly. The test taker should keep a list of normal and therapeutic laboratory values that must be remembered.

42. Correct answers are 1, 2, and 3.
    1. Paroxysmal nocturnal dyspnea is a sudden attack of respiratory distress, usually occurring at night because of the reclining position, and occurs in valvular disorders.
    2. This is an abnormal condition in which a client must sit or stand to breathe comfortably and occurs in valvular disorders.
    3. Coughing occurs when the client diagnosed with long-term valvular disease has difficulty breathing when walking or performing any type of activity.
    4. A pericardial friction rub is a sound auscultated in clients with pericarditis, not valvular heart disease.
    5. Pulsus paradoxus is a marked decrease in amplitude during inspiration. It is a sign of cardiac tamponade, not valvular heart disease.

**TEST-TAKING HINT:** The test taker should notice that options "1," "2," and "3" are all clinical manifestations that have something to do with the lungs. It would be a good choice to select these three as correct answers. They are similar in description.

43. 1. An acute MI can damage heart valves, causing tearing, ischemia, or damage to heart muscles that affect valve leaflet function. CAD can cause damage to the vessels, but rheumatic heart disease causes permanent damage to the heart valves.

2. Valvular heart disease does not show a genetic etiology.
3. Smoking can cause CAD, but it does not cause valvular heart disease.
4. Rheumatic heart disease is the most common cause of valvular heart disease.

**TEST-TAKING HINT:** The test taker could rule out option "1" because of knowledge of anatomy: CAD has to do with blood supply to the heart muscle, whereas the valves are a part of the anatomy of the heart.

44. 1. PTBV is not an open-heart surgery; therefore, the chest will not be open, and the client will not have a chest tube.
    2. This is not an open-heart surgery; therefore, the client will not have a chest dressing.
    3. The ET tube is inserted if the client is on a ventilator, and this surgery does not require putting the client on a ventilator.
    4. PTBV, an invasive procedure, is performed in a cardiac catheterization laboratory, and the client has a catheter inserted into the femoral artery. Therefore, the client must keep the leg straight to prevent hemorrhaging at the insertion site.

**TEST-TAKING HINT:** If the test taker knows that the word "percutaneous" means "via the skin," then options "1" and "2" could be eliminated as possible correct answers.

45. 1. The client is at risk for developing endocarditis and should take prophylactic antibiotics before any invasive procedure.
    2. Antibiotics have nothing to do with how much the teeth bleed during cleaning.
    3. Teeth cleaning will not cause the valve to malfunction.
    4. Vegetation develops on valves secondary to bacteria that cause endocarditis, but the client may not understand "vegetative growth on your valves"; therefore, this is not the most appropriate answer.

**TEST-TAKING HINT:** The test taker should select an option that answers the client's question in the easiest and most understandable terms, not in medical jargon. This would cause the test taker to eliminate option "4" as a possible correct answer. The test taker should know antibiotics do not affect bleeding and so can eliminate option "2."

46. Correct answers are 1 and 5.
    1. Fluid intake may be restricted to reduce the cardiac workload and pressures within the heart and pulmonary circuit.
    2. The head of the bed should be elevated to help improve alveolar ventilation.
    3. Oxygen saturation should be no less than 93%; 90% indicates an arterial oxygen saturation of around 60 (normal is 80 to 100).
    4. Total parenteral nutrition would not be prescribed for a client with mitral valve replacement. It is ordered for clients with malnutrition, gastrointestinal disorders, or conditions in which increased calories are needed, such as burns.
    5. The client should be on continuous cardiac monitoring to assess for any irregular heart rhythms. Atrial fibrillation is common in valvular disease.

**TEST-TAKING HINT:** A client diagnosed with a heart or lung problem should never have the head of the bed in a flat (supine) position; therefore, option "2" should be eliminated as a possible correct answer. The test taker must know normal values for monitoring techniques such as pulse oximeters and keep a list of normal values. If a client had heart surgery, monitoring of the cardiac rhythm would be expected.

47. 1. Heart failure does not predispose the female client to have a mitral valve prolapse.
    2. Clients with Marfan's syndrome have life-threatening cardiovascular problems, including mitral valve prolapse, progressive dilation of the aortic valve ring, and weakness of the arterial walls, and they usually do not live past the age of 40 because of dissection and rupture of the aorta.
    3. Atrial fibrillation does not predispose a client to a mitral valve prolapse.
    4. A client diagnosed with Down syndrome may have congenital heart anomalies but not a mitral valve prolapse.

**TEST-TAKING HINT:** The test taker could eliminate options "1" and "3" based on the knowledge that these are commonly occurring cardiovascular problems, and the nurse should know that possible complications of these problems do not include mitral valve prolapse.

48. 1. This client requires teaching and an understanding of the pre-procedure interventions for diagnostic tests; therefore, a more experienced nurse should be assigned to this client.

2. Because this client is being discharged, it would be an appropriate assignment for the new graduate.
3. Supraventricular tachycardia (SVT) is not life-threatening, but the client requires intravenous medication and close monitoring and therefore should be assigned to a more experienced nurse.
4. A client diagnosed with atrial fibrillation is usually taking the anticoagulant warfarin (Coumadin), and the therapeutic INR is 2 to 3. An INR of 5 is high, and the client is at risk for bleeding.

**TEST-TAKING HINT:** The test taker must realize that a new graduate must be assigned the least critical client. Remember, teaching is a primary responsibility of the nurse; physical care is not always the criterion that should be used when making client assignments.

## Dysrhythmias and Conduction Problems

49. 1. The telemetry nurse should not leave the monitors unattended at any time.
    2. The telemetry nurse must have someone go and assess the client, but this is not the first intervention.
    3. If the client answers the call light and is not experiencing chest pain, then there is probably a monitor artifact, which is not a life-threatening emergency. After talking with the client, send a nurse to the room to check the monitor.
    4. The crash cart should be taken to a room when the client is experiencing a code.

**TEST-TAKING HINT:** When the test taker sees the word "first," the test taker must realize that more than one answer option may be a possible intervention but that only one should be implemented first. The test taker should try to determine which intervention directly affects the client.

50. 1. There are many interventions that should be implemented before administering medication.
    2. The treatment of choice for ventricular fibrillation is defibrillation, but it is not the first action.
    3. The nurse must call a code that activates the crash cart being brought to the room and a team of HCPs that will care for the client according to an established protocol.
    4. The first person at the bedside should start CPR, but the telemetry nurse should call a code so that all necessary equipment and personnel are at the bedside.

**TEST-TAKING HINT:** The test taker must realize that ventricular fibrillation is life-threatening, and immediate action must be implemented. Remember, when the question asks "first," all options could be appropriate interventions but only one should be implemented first.

51. 1. Amiodarone suppresses ventricular ectopy and is the drug of choice for ventricular dysrhythmias.
    2. Epinephrine is a vasoconstrictor, increasing coronary and cerebral blood flow, and is administered in asystole.
    3. Digoxin slows the heart rate and increases cardiac contractility and is the drug of choice for atrial fibrillation.
    4. Adenosine is the drug of choice for supraventricular tachycardia.

**TEST-TAKING HINT:** This is a knowledge-based question, and the test taker must know the answer. The nurse must know what medications treat specific dysrhythmias.

52. 1. A thrombolytic medication is administered for a client experiencing an MI.
    2. Assessment is an independent nursing action, not a collaborative treatment.
    3. **The client is symptomatic and will require a pacemaker.**
    4. Synchronized cardioversion is used for ventricular tachycardia with a pulse or atrial fibrillation.

**TEST-TAKING HINT:** The key to answering this question is the adjective "collaborative," which means the treatment requires obtaining an HCP's order or working with another member of the health-care team. This would cause the test taker to eliminate option "2" as a possible correct answer.

53. 1. The adult client should be defibrillated at 360 joules.
    2. The oxygen source should be removed to prevent any type of spark during defibrillation.
    3. The nurse should use defibrillator pads or defibrillator gel to prevent any type of skin burns while defibrillating the client.
    4. If any member of the health-care team is touching the client or the bed during defibrillation, that person could possibly be shocked. Therefore, the nurse should shout, "all clear."

**TEST-TAKING HINT:** The test taker should always consider the safety of the client and the health-care team. Options "2" and "3" put the client at risk for injury during defibrillation.

54. 1. A client diagnosed with chronic atrial fibrillation will be taking an anticoagulant to help prevent clot formation. Therefore, the client is at risk for bleeding and should be instructed to use a soft-bristle toothbrush.
    2. The client will need a regularly scheduled INR to determine the therapeutic level for the anticoagulant warfarin (Coumadin); PTT levels are monitored for heparin.
    3. A client diagnosed with symptomatic sinus bradycardia, not a client diagnosed with atrial fibrillation, may need a pacemaker.
    4. Synchronized cardioversion may be prescribed for new-onset atrial fibrillation but not for chronic atrial fibrillation.

**TEST-TAKING HINT:** In order to choose the correct answer for this question, the test taker must recognize the disease process, then know what complications are possible, and finally, the test taker must know how the client can possibly be treated so that the complication does not occur.

55. 1. Amiodarone, an antidysrhythmic, is the drug of choice for ventricular tachycardia, but it is not the first intervention.
    2. Defibrillation may be needed, but it is not the first intervention.
    3. **The nurse must assess the apical pulse and blood pressure to determine if the client is in cardiac arrest and then treat as ventricular fibrillation. If the client's heart is beating, the nurse would then prepare for synchronized cardioversion and medication administration.**
    4. CPR is only performed on a client not breathing and without a pulse. The nurse must establish if this is occurring first before taking any other action.

**TEST-TAKING HINT:** When the stem asks the test taker to select the first intervention, all answer options could be plausible interventions, but only one is implemented first. The test taker should use the nursing process to answer the question and select the intervention that addresses assessment, which is the first step in the nursing process.

56. 1. A pacemaker will have to be inserted, but it is not the first intervention.
    2. **Atropine, an antidysrhythmic, will decrease vagal stimulation and increase the heart rate. Therefore, it is the first intervention.**
    3. A STAT ECG may be done, but the telemetry reading shows a complete heart block,

which is a life-threatening dysrhythmia and must be treated.

4. The HCP will need to be notified but not before administering a medication. The test taker must assume the nurse has the order to administer medication. Many telemetry departments have standing protocols.

**TEST-TAKING HINT:** The test taker must select the intervention that should be implemented first and will directly affect the dysrhythmia. Medication is the first intervention, and then pacemaker insertion. The test taker should not eliminate an option because the test taker thinks there is not an order by a HCP.

57. Correct answers are 1, 3, 4, and 5.
    1. Ventricular fibrillation indicates the client does not have a heartbeat. Therefore, CPR should be instituted.
    2. Adenosine, an antidysrhythmic, is the drug of choice for supraventricular tachycardia, not for ventricular fibrillation.
    3. Defibrillation is the treatment of choice for ventricular fibrillation.
    4. The crash cart has the defibrillator and is used when performing advanced CPR.
    5. Amiodarone is an antidysrhythmic that is used in ventricular dysrhythmias.

**TEST-TAKING HINT:** This is an alternate-type question that requires the test taker to select more than one option. To receive credit, the test taker must select all correct options; partial credit is not given for this type of question.

58. 1. The telemetry reading is accurate, and there is no need for the nurse to assess the client's heart rate.
    2. There is no reason to notify the surgeon for a client exhibiting sinus tachycardia.
    3. Synchronized cardioversion is prescribed for clients in acute atrial fibrillation or ventricular fibrillation with a pulse.
    4. Sinus tachycardia means the sinoatrial node is the pacemaker, but the rate is greater than 100 because of pain, anxiety, or fever. The nurse must determine the cause and treat it appropriately. There is no specific medication for sinus tachycardia.

**TEST-TAKING HINT:** The test taker must use the nursing process to determine the correct option and select an option that addresses assessment, the first step of the nursing process. Because both option "1" and option "4" address assessment, the test taker must

determine which option is more appropriate. How will taking the apical pulse help treat sinus tachycardia? Determining the cause for sinus tachycardia is the most appropriate intervention.

59. 1. The P wave represents atrial contraction, and the QRS complex represents ventricular contraction—a normal telemetry reading. A rate between 60 and 100 indicates normal sinus rhythm. Therefore, the nurse should document this as normal sinus rhythm and not take any action.
    2. A 12-lead ECG should be requested for chest pain or abnormal dysrhythmias.
    3. The cardiotonic digoxin is used to treat atrial fibrillation.
    4. Cardiac enzymes are monitored to determine if the client has had an MI. Nothing in the stem indicates the client has had an MI.

**TEST-TAKING HINT:** The test taker must know normal sinus rhythm, and there are no test-taking hints to help eliminate incorrect options. The test taker should not automatically select assessment as the correct answer, but if the test taker had no idea of the answer, remember assessment of laboratory data is not the same as assessing the client.

60. 1. Not every cardiac dysrhythmia causes an alteration in comfort; angina is caused by decreased oxygen to the myocardium.
    2. **Any abnormal electrical activity of the heart causes decreased cardiac output.**
    3. Impaired gas exchange is the result of pulmonary complications, not cardiac dysrhythmias.
    4. Not all clients with cardiac dysrhythmias have activity intolerance.

**TEST-TAKING HINT:** Option "2" has the word "cardiac," which refers to the heart. Therefore, even if the test taker had no idea what the correct answer was, this would be an appropriate option. The test taker should use medical terminology to help identify the correct option.

## Inflammatory Cardiac Disorders

61. 1. Pulsus paradoxus is the hallmark of cardiac tamponade; a paradoxical pulse is markedly decreased in amplitude during inspiration.
    2. Fatigue and arthralgias are nonspecific clinical manifestations that usually occur with myocarditis.

3. Petechiae on the trunk, conjunctiva, and mucous membranes and hemorrhagic streaks under the fingernails or toenails occur with endocarditis.
4. Chest pain is the most common symptom of pericarditis, usually has an abrupt onset, and is aggravated by respiratory movements (deep inspiration, coughing), changes in body position, and swallowing.

**TEST-TAKING HINT:** The test taker with no idea what the answer is should apply the test-taking strategy of asking which body system is affected. In this case, it is the cardiac system, specifically the outside of the heart. The test taker should select the option that has something to do with the heart, which is either option "1" or option "4."

62. 1. Acute pericardial effusion interferes with normal cardiac filling and pumping, causing venous congestion and decreased cardiac output. Muffled heart sounds, indicative of acute pericarditis, must be reported to the HCP.
2. Distended, not nondistended, jugular veins would warrant immediate intervention.
3. A decreasing quality of peripheral pulses, not bounding peripheral pulses, would warrant immediate intervention.
4. A pericardial friction rub is a classic symptom of acute pericarditis, but it would not warrant immediate intervention.

**TEST-TAKING HINT:** This is a priority setting question; the test taker should determine if the data provided is abnormal or expected for the disease process. If so, then the test taker can consider the option as being the correct answer. If the data is within normal limits or expected for the disease process, then the option is not a priority.

63. 1. Fever, chills, and a sore throat can be symptoms of Coxsackie virus in an adult and is the most common cause of myocarditis (Myocarditis Foundation, 2018).
2. Atrial fibrillation is not associated with myocarditis.
3. Myocarditis is not a genetic or congenital disease process.
4. This is an appropriate question to ask any client, but OTC medications do not cause myocarditis.

**TEST-TAKING HINT:** This is a knowledge-based question, but the test taker could eliminate option "4," realizing this is a question to ask any client, and the stem asks which question will support the diagnosis of myocarditis.

64. 1. Steroids, such as prednisone, not NSAIDs, must be tapered off to prevent adrenal insufficiency.
2. NSAIDs will not make clients drowsy.
3. NSAIDs must be taken with food, milk, or antacids to help decrease gastric distress. NSAIDs reduce fever, inflammation, and pericardial pain.
4. NSAIDs should be taken regularly around the clock to help decrease inflammation, which, in turn, will decrease pain.

**TEST-TAKING HINT:** The test taker must remember NSAIDs and steroids cause gastric distress to the point of causing peptic ulcer disease. These medications are administered for a variety of conditions and diseases.

65. 1. Oxygen may be needed, but it is not the first intervention.
2. This would be appropriate to determine if the urine output is at least 30 mL/hr, but it is not the first intervention.
3. The nurse must assess the client to determine if the pain is expected secondary to pericarditis or if the pain is indicative of a complication that requires intervention from the HCP.
4. Using the incentive spirometer will increase the client's alveolar ventilation and help prevent atelectasis, but it is not the first intervention.

**TEST-TAKING HINT:** The test taker must apply the nursing process when determining the correct answer and select the option that addresses the first step in the nursing process—assessment.

66. 1. A pericardiocentesis removes fluid from the pericardial sac and is the emergency treatment for cardiac tamponade.
2. Cardiac enzymes may be slightly elevated because of the inflammatory process, but evaluation of these would not be ordered to treat or evaluate cardiac tamponade.
3. A 12-lead ECG would not help treat the medical emergency of cardiac tamponade.
4. Assessment by the nurse is not collaborative; it is an independent nursing action.

**TEST-TAKING HINT:** "Collaborative" means another member of the health-care team must order or participate in the intervention. Therefore, option "4" could be eliminated as a possible correct answer.

67. Correct answers are 1, 3, and 4.
    1. Osler's nodes are red, painful lesions on the pads of the fingers and toes. Osler's nodes are associated with infective endocarditis.
    2. Chest pain is not present in infective endocarditis. The client will commonly experience cold and flu symptoms such as fever and fatigue.
    3. Janeway lesions are painless lesions on the palms and soles and are often indistinguishable from Osler's nodes; both are associated with infective endocarditis.
    4. Splinter hemorrhages are tiny blood spots that appear vertically under the nails of the fingers or toes and are associated with infective endocarditis.
    5. Rosacea is small, red bumps on the face with persistent redness and visible blood vessels. Rosacea is not associated with infective endocarditis.

    **TEST-TAKING HINT:** The question is asking the test taker to identify the clinical manifestations of a disease process. This is a knowledge-based question requiring memorization.

68. 1. PE would occur with embolization of vegetative lesions from the tricuspid valve on the right side of the heart.
    2. Bacteria enter the bloodstream from invasive procedures, and sterile platelet-fibrin vegetation forms on heart valves. The mitral valve is on the left side of the heart, and if the vegetation breaks off, it will go through the left ventricle into the systemic circulation and may lodge in the brain, kidneys, or peripheral tissues.
    3. Coughing up blood (hemoptysis) occurs when the vegetation breaks off the tricuspid valve in the right side of the heart and enters the pulmonary artery.
    4. Deep vein thrombosis is a complication of immobility, not of a vegetative embolus from the left side of the heart.

    **TEST-TAKING HINT:** If the test taker does not know the answer, knowledge of anatomy may help determine the answer. The mitral valve is on the left side of the heart, and any emboli would not enter the lung first, thereby eliminating options "1" and "3" as possible correct answers.

69. 1. Anxiety is a psychosocial nursing diagnosis, which is not a priority over a physiological nursing diagnosis.
    2. Antibiotic therapy does not result in injury to the client.

3. Myocarditis does not result in valve damage (endocarditis does), and there would be decreased, not increased, cardiac output.
4. Activity intolerance is the priority for the client diagnosed with myocarditis, an inflammation of the heart muscle. Nursing care is aimed at decreasing myocardial work and maintaining cardiac output.

**TEST-TAKING HINT:** If the test taker has no idea which is the correct answer, then "myo," which refers to muscle, and "card," which refers to the heart, should lead the test taker to the only option which has both muscle and heart in it, option "4."

70. 1. Uninterrupted rest and sleep help decrease the workload of the heart and help ensure the restoration of physical and emotional health.
    2. Occupational therapy addresses ADLs. The client should be referred to physical therapy to develop a realistic and progressive plan of activity.
    3. The client diagnosed with pericarditis is not usually prescribed oxygen, and 2 L/min is a low dose of oxygen that is prescribed for a client diagnosed with COPD.
    4. Endocarditis, not pericarditis, may lead to surgery for valve replacement.

**TEST-TAKING HINT:** A concept that the test taker must remember with any client being discharged from the hospital should be to alternate rest with activity to avoid problems associated with immobility. If the test taker does not know the answer to a question, using basic concepts is the best option.

71. Correct answers are 1, 2, 3, and 4.
    1. The nurse should monitor the vital signs for any client after just undergoing surgery.
    2. A pericardiocentesis involves entering the pericardial sac. Assessing heart and lung sounds allows assessment for cardiac failure.
    3. The pericardial fluid is documented as output.
    4. Evaluating the client's cardiac rhythm allows the nurse to assess for cardiac failure, which is a complication of pericardiocentesis.
    5. The client should be in the semi-Fowler's position, not in a flat position, which increases the workload of the heart.

**TEST-TAKING HINT:** This is an alternate-type question that requires the test taker to select possibly more than one option as a correct answer.

72. 1. The nurse must obtain blood cultures before administering antibiotics.
    2. Blood cultures must be done before administering antibiotics so that an adequate number of organisms can be obtained to culture and identify.
    3. An echocardiogram allows visualization of vegetations and evaluation of valve function. However, antibiotic therapy is a priority before diagnostic tests, and blood cultures must be obtained before administering medication.
    4. Bedrest should be implemented, but the first intervention should be obtaining blood cultures so that antibiotic therapy can be started as soon as possible.

**TEST-TAKING HINT:** The test taker must identify the first of the HCP's orders to be implemented. "Infective" should indicate that this is an infection, which requires antibiotics, but the nurse should always assess for allergies and obtain cultures before administering any antibiotic.

73. 1. The HCP will be notified, but the first action is to call for the code blue team and initiate CPR.
    2. A RRT is called to prevent an arrest situation from occurring. This client is in an arrest situation.
    3. The client has clinical signs of death; CPR must be initiated and the code team notified.
    4. The first action is to notify the code team and initiate CPR per protocol immediately.

**TEST-TAKING HINT:** The test taker should remember, "If in stress do not assess." The nurse has enough information given in the stem of the question to initiate an action. The question asks for a first; all of the options may be implemented but only one is first.

74. 1. Although this might be the cause of non-compliance, the actual side effects of anti-hypertensive medications may be more likely. Evidence indicates that the side effect of erectile dysfunction is a major reason for noncompliance for males.
    2. This is a mild way of introducing the subject of side effects to a client, not wishing to admit the medication causes unwanted effects. It opens the door to more probing assessment questions. The nurse should bring up the subject in order to allow the client to be forthcoming with the issues of why he is not taking his medication.
    3. This would be the second question to ask if the client denies any problems with side effects.
    4. Although, in this case, the nurse can ask "why" because it is an interview question and not therapeutic conversation being requested in the stem, a more direct question will open the conversation up better.

**TEST-TAKING HINT:** To answer this question, the test taker must remember that all medications have potential side effects. Antihypertensive medications can cause erectile dysfunction in males, frequently resulting in noncompliance with the medication regimen. The issue is a psychological as well as a physiological one.

75. Correct answers are 1, 2, 5, and 6.
    1. The client should be monitored for any cardiovascular changes.
    2. The client should be monitored for the development of heart failure as a result of increased strain on the heart from the atria not functioning as they should.
    3. There is no evidence that the client requires to sleep in the orthopneic position.
    4. Buerger Allen exercises are useful for clients with peripheral artery disease but do not have an effect on atrial fibrillation.
    5. Clients diagnosed with atrial fibrillation are at risk for developing emboli from the stasis of blood in the atria. If an embolus breaks loose from the lining of the atria, then it can travel to the lungs (right) or to the brain (left).
    6. The client diagnosed with atrial fibrillation should have their neurological status assessed frequently.

**TEST-TAKING HINT:** To answer "Select all that apply" questions, the test taker should look at each option independently of the others. Each option becomes a true or false question.

76. 1. This indicates ascites, which can happen in heart failure, but not necessarily; it can also be from liver failure or another issue.
    2. Dyspnea occurring at night when the client is in a recumbent position indicates that the cardiac muscle is not able to compensate for extra fluid returning to the heart during sleep.
    3. This could indicate diabetes but not heart failure.
    4. The client is at risk for heart failure as a result of the MI, but it does not happen with all MI clients and does not support the diagnosis.

**TEST-TAKING HINT:** The test taker should read the stem of the question carefully. It is asking for assessment data to support the client is in heart failure. Three of the answer options give assessment data; therefore, option "4" can be eliminated. Only one of the other three gives an option that only occurs with heart failure.

77. Correct answers are 1 and 5.
1. Nitroglycerin tablets are dispensed in small brown bottles to preserve the potency. The client should not change the tablets to another container.
2. The tablets are placed under the tongue to dissolve and thereby work more rapidly.
3. The client is taught to take one tablet every 5 minutes, and if the angina is not relieved after three tablets, to call 911.
4. The tablets do not have a fruity odor; they sting when placed under the tongue if they are potent.
5. The client should be taught to replace tablets 6 months after opening the bottle to maintain potency.

TEST-TAKING HINT: The test taker should be knowledgeable of common medications and what to teach the client.

78. 1. The client has not arrested. The nurse might call the RRT but not a code blue.
2. The client is in distress; the nurse should implement a procedure that will alleviate the distress.
3. The client is in distress; the nurse should implement a procedure that will alleviate the distress.
4. The client began to have a problem during physical exertion. Stopping the exertion should be the first action taken by the nurse.

TEST-TAKING HINT: The test taker should remember, "If in stress do not assess." The nurse has enough information given in the stem of the question to initiate an action. The question asks for a first. All of the options may be implemented but only one is first.

79. 1. This strip indicates normal sinus rhythm; there is no need for further action based on the strip.
2. This strip indicates normal sinus rhythm; there is no need for further action based on the strip.
3. This strip indicates normal sinus rhythm; there is no need for further action based on the strip. The nurse should continue to monitor the client.
4. This strip indicates normal sinus rhythm; there is no need for further action based on the strip.

TEST-TAKING HINT: The test taker should recognize normal values and results in order to recognize abnormal values. A normal result can rule out an answer in a "which do you assess first" question; an abnormal value

automatically elevates the need to see that client before another one.

80. 1. Amiodarone is administered during a code rapidly, not over 15 minutes.
2. Amiodarone is given 300 mg IV push according to ACLS guidelines for pulseless ventricular fibrillation or ventricular tachycardia. Amiodarone can be repeated once after 3 to 5 minutes with 150 mg IV push (maximum dose of 2.2g/24 hours) (Vallerand & Sanoski, 2019).
3. Amiodarone is ACLS recommended.
4. Dopamine is administered via mg/kg/min. The time to calculate this kind of dosage is not taken until after the code is concluded and the client is placed on a vasopressor medication such as dopamine.

TEST-TAKING HINT: The test taker should be knowledgeable about common medications and basic rules of administration.

81. 1. "Has developed" indicates a new issue; the nurse should notify the HCP of the assessment findings, which indicate that the client has developed heart failure.
2. What the client ate has no bearing on the new development of the clinical manifestations of heart failure.
3. A 12-lead ECG will not treat heart failure.
4. A diuretic may need to be administered, but notifying the HCP is first.

TEST-TAKING HINT: The test taker should read every word in the stem of the question; "has developed" indicates a newly occurring situation for the client. The nurse must notify the HCP when new issues occur in order to intervene before a failure to rescue issue occurs.

82. 1. The potassium level is within normal range; this medication would not be questioned.
2. Digoxin is given to clients with rapid atrial fibrillation to slow the heart rate; this medication would not be questioned.
3. Enalapril, an ACE inhibitor, will lower the blood pressure even more. The nurse should hold the medication and notify the HCP that the medication is being held.
4. This would be the first medication to be administered because it indicates a potential cardiac muscle perfusion issue.

TEST-TAKING HINT: The test taker should recognize normal values and results in order to recognize abnormal values. A normal result can rule out an answer in "Which do you assess first?" or "Which would the nurse question?" An abnormal value indicates a need for some action on the part of the nurse.

83. 1. Activity intolerance is a result of a lack of perfusion of the cardiac muscle, but the priority is to get the muscle perfused.
    2. Pain does not kill anyone; the reason behind the pain could. In the case of chest pain, the cardiac muscle is not being perfused, which causes pain.
    3. The problem is not having enough oxygen available to the body but that the oxygen is not being perfused to the cardiac muscle.
    4. The cardiac muscle is not perfused when there is a narrowing of the arteries caused by CAD or when an embolus or a thrombus occludes the artery. Adequate perfusion will supply oxygen to the cardiac muscle, allow for increased activity, and decrease pain.

**TEST-TAKING HINT:** The test taker should remember basic pathophysiology to answer this priority question. The other three interrelated concepts are based on the issue of tissue perfusion.

84. Correct answers are 1, 2, 3, 4, and 6.
    1. A dietitian can assist the nurse in explaining the sodium restrictions to the client as well as hidden sources of sodium.
    2. This will help the client's body to return excess fluid to the heart for removal from the body by the kidneys.
    3. The client should weigh every morning in the same type of clothing (gown, underwear, jeans, etc.) and report a weight gain of 3 pounds in a week to the HCP.
    4. The nurse should not assess for edema in the feet and lower legs, but if the client is in bed, the lowest part of the body may be in the sacral area. Whichever area is dependent is where the nurse should look for edema.
    5. The client should drink enough fluids to maintain body function, but 3,000 mL is excessive.
    6. Whenever the nurse is instructing a client, the nurse should determine if the client heard and understood the instructions. Having the client repeat the instructions is one way of determining "hearing." Having the client return instructions is a method of determining understanding.

**TEST-TAKING HINT:** The new NCLEX-RN® test plan report states that "Select all that apply" questions may have five or more answer options, and one option must be correct, but the test plan does not reveal the maximum number of answer options that must be correct. In order to answer a "Select all that apply" question, each option is considered separately as a true or false question.

85. 1. This could be nothing serious (artifact), but from the appearance of the strip, the nurse cannot tell if the client is in an arrest situation; the nurse must personally assess the situation. The nurse cannot delegate an unstable client.
    2. The nurse must determine the situation personally; this could be artifact or ventricular fibrillation.
    3. This could be nothing serious (artifact), but from the appearance of the strip, the nurse cannot tell if the client is in an arrest situation; the nurse must personally assess the situation. Telemetry monitoring is accomplished using lead II; the monitor tech does not have the ability to change the lead placement.
    4. The nurse must assess the client before making a decision as to whether to notify the code team or not.

**TEST-TAKING HINT:** The rules for delegation are the nurse cannot delegate an unstable client, teaching, assessment, evaluation, or medication administration to a UAP. This would eliminate option "1." Calling a code without assessing the client would eliminate option "4."

86. 1. A brief focused assessment of each client assigned to the nurse should be performed after receiving the shift report. This includes assessing each client for the main focus of the client's admission, any new issue that is reported from the shift report, and assessing all lines and tubes going into or coming out of the client. Once this is done, the nurse knows then that the client is stable and a full head-to-toe assessment can be done at a later time.
    2. The UAP will determine when and how to accomplish the job; the nurse may assist the UAP by informing the UAP of situations that may impact the timing of the baths, but this is not the purpose of morning rounds.
    3. This is the UAP's job.
    4. This is not the purpose of morning rounds.

**TEST-TAKING HINT:** Option "3" has the word "all," which could eliminate it from consideration because rarely does an "all" apply. Options "2" and "3" are doing the UAP's job, and option "4" is the housekeeping's job.

87. 1. A report of indigestion could be cardiac chest pain. The nurse should assess this client because of the diagnosis of CAD and the word "severe" in the option.
    2. Edema is expected for the client diagnosed with heart failure, and it is not life-threatening.
    3. An irregular heart rate is not life-threatening, and 110 is abnormal but also not life-threatening.
    4. Constipation is not life-threatening albeit uncomfortable.

**TEST-TAKING HINT:** A "first" makes the test taker determine which client has the greatest need. Expected and not life-threatening issues do not require being a priority.

88. 1. The word "any" makes this a wrong option. The nurse should teach the client what to do if chest pain occurs. Take one nitroglycerin tablet every 5 minutes times three (3), and if not relieved, call 911.
    2. **The nurse should make sure the client is aware of when sexual activity can be safely resumed.**
    3. The client needs to know how to take nitroglycerin but not the pharmacology of how the medication works.
    4. The client can sleep in any position of comfort.

**TEST-TAKING HINT:** The test taker should recognize certain words such as "any," "all," "never," or "always." These absolutes will determine if an option is incorrect or correct.

89. 1. The cardiac glycoside medication, digoxin, is a routine medication that will be administered at 0900 in most hospitals.
    2. **The client intends to eat breakfast, and this is a scheduled medication for before meals.**
    3. This client is showing that the loop diuretic, furosemide, is doing what it should do. This medication will be given at 0900.
    4. This is a slightly abnormal blood pressure but is within an acceptable range for someone prescribed an ARB. The medication can be administered at 0900.

**TEST-TAKING HINT:** The test taker should be knowledgeable of common medications and the basic rules of administration.

90. 1. CAD narrows the arteries of the heart, causing the tissues not to be perfused, especially when an embolus or a thrombus occurs.
    2. DI is a disease of the pituitary gland or the kidneys; it is not a perfusion issue.
    3. COPD is an oxygenation issue, not a perfusion one.
    4. Multiple fractures do not cause perfusion issues unless an interrelated issue occurs.

**TEST-TAKING HINT:** The test taker should remember basic pathophysiology and the resulting problems associated with different pathology.

# CARDIAC DISORDERS COMPREHENSIVE EXAMINATION

1. Which modifiable risk factors are associated with MI? **Select all that apply.**
   1. Smoking.
   2. Male sex.
   3. Postmenopausal females.
   4. Obesity.
   5. Elevated low-density lipoprotein.

2. Which **pre-procedure** information should be taught to the female client having an exercise stress test in the morning?
   1. Wear open-toed shoes to the stress test.
   2. Inform the client not to wear a bra.
   3. Do not eat anything for 4 hours.
   4. Take the beta blocker 1 hour before the test.

3. Which intervention should the nurse implement with the client diagnosed with dilated cardiomyopathy?
   1. Keep the client in the supine position with the legs elevated.
   2. Discuss a heart transplant, which is the definitive treatment.
   3. Prepare the client for coronary artery bypass graft.
   4. Teach the client to take a calcium channel blocker in the morning.

4. Which medical client problem should the nurse include in the plan of care for a client diagnosed with cardiomyopathy?
   1. Heart failure.
   2. Activity intolerance.
   3. Powerlessness.
   4. Anticipatory grieving.

5. The client has an implantable cardioverter defibrillator (ICD). Which discharge instructions should the nurse teach the client? **Select all that apply.**
   1. Do not drape MP3 headphones around your neck.
   2. Have someone drive the car for the rest of your life.
   3. Carry the cell phone on the opposite side of the ICD.
   4. Avoid using the microwave oven in the home.
   5. Walk through metal detectors at a normal pace.

6. To what area should the nurse place the stethoscope to **best** auscultate the apical pulse?

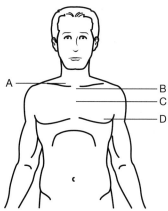

   1. A
   2. B
   3. C
   4. D

7. The telemetry nurse notes a peaked T wave for the client diagnosed with CHF. Which laboratory data should the nurse assess?
   1. CK-MB.
   2. Troponin.
   3. BNP.
   4. Potassium.

8. The client comes to the emergency department, saying, "I am having a heart attack." Which question is a **priority** when assessing the client?
   1. "Can you describe your chest pain?"
   2. "What were you doing when the pain started?"
   3. "Did you have a high-fat meal today?"
   4. "Does the pain get worse when you lie down?"

9. The client diagnosed with CAD is prescribed transdermal nitroglycerin. Which behavior indicates the client **understands** the discharge teaching concerning this medication?
   1. The client places the medication under the tongue.
   2. The client removes the old patch before placing the new.
   3. The client applies the patch to a hairy area.
   4. The client changes the patch every 36 hours.

10. Which client would **most** likely be misdiagnosed for having an MI?
    1. A 55-year-old male with crushing chest pain and diaphoresis.
    2. A 60-year-old male with an elevated troponin level.
    3. A 40-year-old female with a normal electrocardiogram.
    4. An 80-year-old female with a normal CK-MB at 12 hours.

11. Which meal would indicate the client **understands** the discharge teaching concerning the recommended diet for CAD?
    1. Baked fish, steamed broccoli, and garden salad.
    2. Enchilada dinner with fried rice and refried beans.
    3. Tuna salad sandwich on white bread and whole milk.
    4. Fried chicken, mashed potatoes, and gravy.

12. The UAP tells the primary nurse that the client diagnosed with CAD is having chest pain. Which action should the RN take **first**?
    1. Tell the UAP to go take the client's vital signs.
    2. Ask the UAP to have the telemetry nurse read the strip.
    3. Notify the client's HCP.
    4. Go to the room and assess the client's chest pain.

13. Which interventions should the nurse discuss with the client diagnosed with CAD? **Select all that apply.**
    1. Instruct the client to stop smoking.
    2. Encourage the client to exercise 3 days a week.
    3. Teach about coronary vasodilators.
    4. Prepare the client for a carotid endarterectomy.
    5. Eat foods high in monosaturated fats.

14. Which laboratory data **confirm** the diagnosis of heart failure?
    1. CXR.
    2. Liver function tests.
    3. BUN.
    4. BNP.

15. What is the **priority** problem in the client diagnosed with heart failure?
    1. Fluid volume overload.
    2. Decreased cardiac output.
    3. Activity intolerance.
    4. Knowledge deficit.

16. Which data would cause the nurse to **question** administering digoxin to a client diagnosed with CHF?
    1. The potassium level is 3.2 mEq/L.
    2. The digoxin level is 1.2 ng/mL.
    3. The client's apical pulse is 64.
    4. The client denies a yellow haze.

17. The nurse is caring for clients on a cardiac floor. Which client should the nurse assess **first**?
    1. The client diagnosed with three unifocal PVCs in 1 minute.
    2. The client diagnosed with CAD wanting to ambulate.
    3. The client diagnosed with mitral valve prolapse with an audible $S_3$.
    4. The client diagnosed with pericarditis in normal sinus rhythm.

18. The nurse is told in the report the client has aortic stenosis. Which anatomical position should the nurse auscultate to assess the murmur?
    1. Second intercostal space, right sternal notch.
    2. Erb's point.
    3. Second intercostal space, left sternal notch.
    4. Fourth intercostal space, left sternal border.

19. The nurse is caring for a client going into ventricular tachycardia. Which intervention should the nurse implement **first**?
    1. Call a code immediately.
    2. Assess the client for a pulse.
    3. Begin chest compressions.
    4. Continue to monitor the client.

20. The nurse is assisting with synchronized cardioversion on a client diagnosed with atrial fibrillation. When the machine is activated, there is a pause. What action should the nurse take?
    1. Wait until the machine discharges.
    2. Shout "all clear" and don't touch the bed.
    3. Make sure the client is all right.
    4. Increase the joules and discharge.

21. The client is diagnosed with pericarditis. When assessing the client, the nurse is unable to auscultate a friction rub. Which action should the nurse implement?
    1. Notify the HCP.
    2. Document that the pericarditis has resolved.
    3. Ask the client to lean forward and listen again.
    4. Prepare to insert a unilateral chest tube.

22. The nurse assessing the client diagnosed with pericardial effusion at 1600 notes the apical pulse is 72 and the BP is 138/94. At 1800, the client has neck vein distention, the apical pulse is 70, and the BP is 106/94. Which action would the nurse implement **first**?
    1. Stay with the client and use a calm voice.
    2. Notify the HCP immediately.
    3. Place the client left lateral recumbent.
    4. Administer morphine IVP slowly.

23. The client is admitted to the emergency department, and the nurse suspects a cardiac problem. Which assessment interventions should the nurse implement? **Select all that apply.**
    1. Obtain a midstream urine specimen.
    2. Attach the telemetry monitor to the client.
    3. Start a saline lock in the right arm.
    4. Draw a basal metabolic panel (BMP).
    5. Request an order for a STAT 12-lead ECG.

24. The client is 3 hours post-MI. Which data would **warrant immediate** intervention by the nurse?
    1. Bilateral peripheral pulses 2+.
    2. The pulse oximeter reading is 96%.
    3. The urine output is 240 mL in the last 4 hours.
    4. Cool, clammy, diaphoretic skin.

25. The nurse is transcribing the doctor's orders for a client diagnosed with heart failure. The order reads 2.5 mg of digoxin daily. Which action should the nurse implement?
    1. Discuss the order with the HCP.
    2. Take the client's apical pulse rate before administering.
    3. Check the client's potassium level before giving the medication.
    4. Determine if a digoxin level has been drawn.

26. According to the 2015 American Heart Association Guidelines, which steps of CPR for an adult suffering from a cardiac arrest should the nurse teach individuals in the community? **Rank in order of performance.**
    1. Place the hands over the lower half of the sternum.
    2. Look for obvious signs of breathing.
    3. Begin compressions at a ratio of 30:2.
    4. Call for help and an automated external defibrillator (AED) immediately.
    5. Position the victim on the back.

27. The nurse has received a report when the telemetry technician notifies the nurse of the telemetry readings. Which client should the nurse assess **first?**

1.

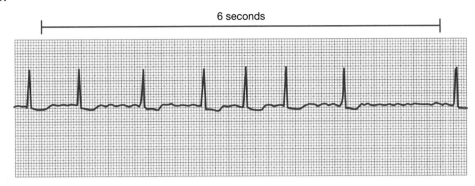

2.

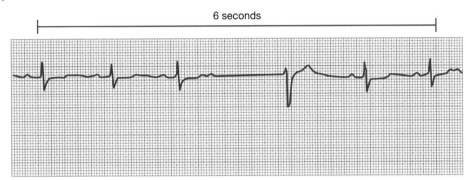

3.

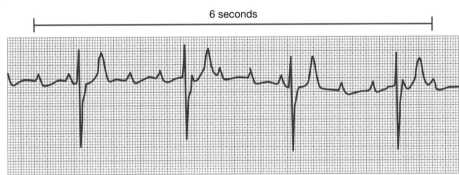

4.

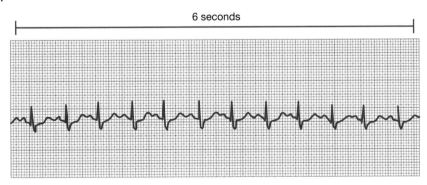

1. Correct answers are 1, 4, and 5.
   1. Smoking is a modifiable risk factor for MI and heart disease.
   2. Male sex is a nonmodifiable risk factor for MI.
   3. Postmenopausal females are at increased risk for MI, but this is not modifiable.
   4. **Obesity is a modifiable risk factor for MI and heart disease.**
   5. **An elevated low-density lipoprotein (LDL) is a modifiable risk factor for MI and heart disease.**

2. 1. The client should wear solid, well-fitting athletic shoes.
   2. The client should wear a bra to provide adequate support during the exercise.
   3. **NPO decreases the chance of aspiration in case of emergency. In addition, if the client has just had a meal, the blood supply will be shunted to the stomach for digestion and away from the heart, perhaps leading to an inaccurate test result.**
   4. A beta blocker is not taken before the stress test because it will decrease the pulse rate and blood pressure by direct parasympathetic stimulation to the heart.

3. 1. Most clients with dilated cardiomyopathy prefer to sit up with their legs in the dependent position. This position causes pooling of blood in the periphery and reduces preload.
   2. **Without a heart transplant, this client will end up in end-stage heart failure. A transplant is the only treatment for a client diagnosed with dilated cardiomyopathy.**
   3. A bypass is the treatment of choice for a client diagnosed with occluded coronary arteries.
   4. Calcium channel blockers are contraindicated in clients with dilated cardiomyopathy because they interfere with the contractility of the heart.

4. 1. **Medical client problems indicate the nurse and the physician must collaborate to care for the client; the client must have medications for heart failure.**
   2. The nurse can instruct the client to pace activities and can teach about rest versus activity without an HCP order.

3. This is a psychosocial client problem that does not require a physician's order to care for the client effectively.
4. Anticipatory grieving involves the nurse addressing issues that will occur based on the knowledge of the poor prognosis of this disease.

5. Correct answers are 1, 3, and 5.
   1. **MP3 players do not pose a risk to ICDs, but the headphones contain a magnetic material that can interfere with the ICD and pacemakers. Headphones should not be worn around the neck so they hang on the chest (American Heart Association, 2016).**
   2. There may be driving restrictions, but the client should be able to drive independently.
   3. **Cell phones may interfere with the functioning of the ICD if they are placed too close to it.**
   4. Microwave ovens should not cause problems with the ICD.
   5. **Metal detectors and electronic article surveillance or anti-theft systems will not cause problems in most client's with ICDs. The client should avoid standing near the detectors for a prolonged period of time and avoid handheld metal detector screenings if possible (American Heart Association, 2016).**

6. 1. This is the best place to auscultate the aortic valve, the second intercostal space, right sternal notch.
   2. This is the best place to auscultate the pulmonic valve, the second intercostal space, left sternal notch.
   3. This is the best place to auscultate the tricuspid valve, the third intercostal space, left sternal border.
   4. **The best place to auscultate the apical pulse is over the mitral valve area, which is the fifth intercostal space, midclavicular line.**

7. 1. CK-MB is assessed to determine if the client has had an MI. The electrical activity of the heart will not be affected by the elevation of this enzyme.
   2. Troponin is assessed to determine if the client has had an MI. The electrical activity of the heart will not be affected by the elevation of this enzyme.

3. BNP is elevated in clients with CHF, but it does not affect the electrical activity of the heart.
4. **Hyperkalemia will cause a peaked T wave; therefore, the nurse should check these laboratory data.**

8. 1. **The chest pain for an MI usually is described as an elephant sitting on the chest or a belt squeezing the substernal midchest, often radiating to the jaw or left arm.**
   2. This helps to identify if it is angina (resulting from activity) or MI (not necessarily brought on by activity).
   3. Learning about a client's intake of a high-fat meal would help the nurse to identify a gallbladder attack.
   4. This is a question the nurse might ask the client diagnosed with reflux esophagitis.

9. 1. The client does not understand how to apply this medication; it is placed on the skin, not under the tongue.
   2. **This behavior indicates the client understands the discharge teaching.**
   3. The nitroglycerin patch, a coronary vasodilator, needs to be in a nonhairy place so that it makes good contact with the skin.
   4. The patch should be worn 12 or 14 hours a day and taken off for 10 to 12 hours, but never changed every 2 hours. It takes about 1 hour for the transdermal patch to begin delivering the optimum dose of medication.

10. 1. Crushing pain and sweating are classic signs of an MI and should not be misdiagnosed.
    2. An elevated troponin level is a benchmark in diagnosing an MI and should not be misdiagnosed.
    3. **The clients misdiagnosed concerning MIs usually present with atypical symptoms. They tend to be female, be younger than 55 years old, be members of a minority group, and have normal electrocardiograms.**
    4. CK-MB may not elevate until up to 24 hours after onset of chest pain.

11. 1. **The recommended diet for CAD is low fat, low cholesterol, and high fiber. The diet described is a diet that is low in fat and cholesterol.**
    2. This is a diet very high in fat and cholesterol.
    3. The word "salad" implies something has been mixed with the tuna, usually

mayonnaise, which is high in fat, but even if the test taker did not know this, white bread is low in fiber and whole milk is high in fat.
4. Meats should be baked, broiled, or grilled—not fried. Gravy is high in fat.

12. 1. The client diagnosed with CAD having chest pain is unstable and requires further judgment to determine appropriate actions to take, and the UAP does not have that knowledge.
    2. The UAP could go ask the telemetry nurse, but this is not the first action.
    3. The client's HCP may need to be notified, but this is not the first intervention.
    4. **Assessment is the first step in the nursing process and should be implemented first; chest pain is a priority.**

13. Correct answers are 1, 2, and 3.
    1. **Smoking should be stopped in the client with CAD.**
    2. **Exercising helps develop collateral circulation and decrease anxiety; it also helps clients to lose weight.**
    3. **Clients with CAD are usually prescribed nitroglycerin, which is the treatment of choice for angina.**
    4. Carotid endarterectomy is a procedure to remove atherosclerotic plaque from the carotid arteries, not the coronary arteries.
    5. The client should eat polyunsaturated fats, not monosaturated fats, to help decrease atherosclerosis.

14. 1. The CXR will show an enlarged heart, but it is not used to confirm the diagnosis of heart failure.
    2. Liver function tests may be ordered to evaluate the effects of heart failure on the liver, but they do not confirm the diagnosis.
    3. The BUN is elevated in heart failure, dehydration, and renal failure, but it is not used to confirm heart failure.
    4. **BNP is a hormone released by the heart muscle in response to changes in blood volume and is used to diagnose and grade heart failure.**

15. 1. Fluid volume overload is a problem in clients with heart failure, but it is not the priority because, if the cardiac output is improved, then the kidneys are perfused, which leads to the elimination of excess fluid from the body.
    2. **Decreased cardiac output is responsible for all the clinical manifestations associated with heart failure and eventually**

causes death, which is why it is the priority problem.

3. Activity intolerance alters the quality of life, but it is not life-threatening.

4. Knowledge deficit is important, but it is not a priority over a physiological problem.

16. 1. **This potassium level is below normal levels; hypokalemia can potentiate digoxin toxicity and lead to cardiac dysrhythmias.**

2. This digoxin level is within the therapeutic range, 0.5 to 2 ng/mL.

3. The nurse would question the medication if the apical pulse were less than 60.

4. Yellow haze is a sign of digoxin toxicity.

17. 1. Three unifocal PVCs in 1 minute is not life-threatening.

2. The client wanting to ambulate is not a priority over a client diagnosed with a physiological problem.

3. **An audible $S_3$ indicates the client is developing left-sided heart failure and needs to be assessed immediately.**

4. A client in normal sinus rhythm will not be a priority over someone with a potentially life-threatening situation.

18. 1. **The second intercostal space, right sternal notch, is the area on the chest where the aorta can best be heard opening and closing.**

2. Erb's point allows the nurse to hear the opening and closing of the tricuspid valve.

3. The second intercostal space, left sternal notch, is the area on the chest where the pulmonic valve can best be heard opening and closing.

4. The fourth intercostal space, left sternal border, is another area on the chest that can assess the tricuspid valve.

19. 1. The nurse should call a code if the client does not have vital signs.

2. **The nurse must first determine if the client has a pulse. Pulseless ventricular tachycardia is treated as ventricular fibrillation. Stable ventricular tachycardia is treated with medications.**

3. Chest compression is only done if the client is not breathing and has no pulse.

4. Ventricular tachycardia is a potentially life-threatening dysrhythmia and needs to be treated immediately.

20. 1. Cardioversion involves the delivery of a timed electrical current. The electrical impulse discharges during ventricular

depolarization, and therefore, there might be a short delay. The nurse should wait until it discharges.

2. Calling "all clear" and not touching the bed should be done before activating the machine to discharge the electrical current.

3. A pause is an expected event, and asking if the client is all right may worry the client unnecessarily.

4. Increasing joules and discharging are implemented during defibrillation, not during synchronized cardioversion.

21. 1. These assessment data are not life-threatening and do not warrant notifying the HCP.

2. The nurse should attempt to hear the friction rub in multiple ways before documenting that it is not heard. The nurse does not determine if the pericarditis has resolved.

3. **Having the client lean forward and to the left uses gravity to force the heart nearer to the chest wall, which allows the friction rub to be heard.**

4. Chest tubes are not the treatment of choice for not hearing a friction rub.

22. 1. **This is a medical emergency; the nurse should stay with the client, keep him calm, and call the nurses' station to notify the HCP. Cardiac output declines with each contraction as the pericardial sac constricts the myocardium.**

2. The client's clinical manifestations would make the nurse suspect cardiac tamponade, a medical emergency. The pulse pressure is narrowing, and the client is experiencing severe rising central venous pressure, as evidenced by neck vein distention. Notifying the HCP is important, but the nurse should stay with the client first.

3. A left lateral recumbent position is used when administering enemas.

4. Morphine would be given to a client diagnosed with pain from MI; it is not a treatment option for cardiac tamponade.

23. Correct answers are 2, 3, and 5.

1. A midstream urine specimen is ordered for a client diagnosed with a possible urinary tract infection, not for a client diagnosed with cardiac problems.

2. **Anytime a nurse suspects cardiac problems, the electrical conductivity of the heart should be assessed.**

3. **Emergency medications for heart problems are primarily administered**

intravenously, so starting a saline lock in the right arm is appropriate.
4. This serum blood test is not specific to assess cardiac problems. A BMP evaluates potassium, sodium, glucose, and more.
5. A 12-lead ECG evaluates the electrical conductivity of the heart from all planes.

24. 1. This pulse indicates the heart is pumping adequately. Normal pulses should be 2+ to 3+.
2. A pulse oximeter reading of greater than 93% indicates the heart is perfusing the periphery.
3. An output of 30 mL/hr indicates the heart is perfusing the kidneys adequately.
4. Cold, clammy skin is an indicator of cardiogenic shock, which is a complication of MI and warrants immediate intervention.

25. 1. This digoxin (Lanoxin) dosage is 10 times the normal dose for a client diagnosed with CHF. This dose is potentially lethal.
2. No other action can be taken because of the incorrect dose.
3. No other action can be taken because of the incorrect dose.
4. No other action can be taken because of the incorrect dose.

26. Correct order is 5, 2, 4, 1, 3.
5. The victim is positioned on the back for assessment and for the rescuer to be able to begin CPR.
2. Although we now perform a quick look to determine if the victim is breathing, there is no longer a "look, listen, feel" step. The victim may not be breathing at all or may be having agonal respirations.
4. For adults, the rescuer should immediately call for an AED or 911. Research has proven the faster that defibrillation is performed the better the chance of survival for the victim.
1. Compressions are initiated immediately because the victim will have some residual oxygen in the lungs. Breathing is not initiated unless there is a barrier device available.
3. The compression rate is 30:2.

27. 1. Atrial fibrillation is not life-threatening.
2. Unifocal PVCs are common in most clients and are not life-threatening. Up to six per minute may occur before the nurse must intervene.
3. This is a complete heart block with bradycardia, a potentially life-threatening situation. The nurse should assess this client first and make interventions accordingly.
4. Sinus tachycardia may occur for different reasons, such as ambulating to the bathroom, fever, or anemia. This is not life-threatening.

# Peripheral Vascular Disorders

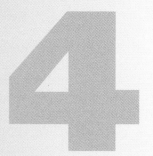

*Knowledge is a process of piling up facts; wisdom lies in their simplification.*

—Martin Fischer

Peripheral vascular disorders (PVDs) are very common disorders, affecting many people in the United States. Among the most common of these are hypertension, atherosclerosis, arterial occlusive disease, abdominal aortic aneurysms (AAA), deep vein thrombosis (DVT), and venous insufficiency. These disorders cause pain and interruption of activities and sometimes lead to life-threatening complications.

## KEYWORDS

Bruit
Dehiscence
Dependent position
Doppler device
Evisceration

Intermittent claudication
Neuropathy
Petechiae
Sequential compression device

## PRACTICE QUESTIONS

### Hypertension

1. The 66-year-old male client has his blood pressure (BP) checked at a health fair. His BP is 168/98. Which action should the nurse implement **first?**
   1. Recommend that the client have his BP checked in 1 month.
   2. Instruct the client to see his health-care provider (HCP) as soon as possible.
   3. Discuss the importance of eating a low-salt, low-fat, low-cholesterol diet.
   4. Explain that this BP is within the normal range for an older person.

2. The nurse is teaching the client recently diagnosed with essential hypertension. Which instruction should the nurse provide when discussing heart-healthy exercise? **Select all that apply.**
   1. Walk briskly for at least 30 minutes a day on flat surfaces.
   2. Perform heavy weightlifting three times a week.
   3. Recommend high-intensity aerobics every day.
   4. Encourage the client to swim laps once a week.
   5. Use resistance bands at home at least twice a week.

3. The HCP prescribes an angiotensin-converting enzyme (ACE) inhibitor for the client diagnosed with essential (or primary) hypertension. Which statement is the **most appropriate** rationale for administering this medication?
   1. ACE inhibitors prevent beta receptor stimulation in the heart.
   2. This medication blocks the alpha receptors in the vascular smooth muscle.
   3. ACE inhibitors prevent vasoconstriction and sodium and water retention.
   4. ACE inhibitors decrease BP by relaxing vascular smooth muscle.

4. The nurse is administering a beta blocker to the client diagnosed with essential hypertension. Which intervention should the nurse implement?
   1. Notify the HCP if the potassium level is 3.8 mEq.
   2. Question administering the medication if the BP is less than 90/60 mm Hg.
   3. Do not administer the medication if the client's radial pulse is greater than 100.
   4. Monitor the BP while the client is lying, standing, and sitting.

5. The male client diagnosed with essential hypertension has been prescribed an alpha-adrenergic blocker. Which intervention should the nurse discuss with the client?
   1. Eat at least one banana a day to help increase the potassium level.
   2. Explain that impotence is an expected side effect of the medication.
   3. Take the medication on an empty stomach to increase absorption.
   4. Change position slowly when going from a lying to sitting position.

6. The nurse just received the a.m. shift report. Which client should the nurse assess **first**?
   1. The client diagnosed with coronary artery disease and a BP of 170/100.
   2. The client diagnosed with DVT and reporting chest pain.
   3. The client diagnosed with pneumonia and a pulse oximeter reading of 98%.
   4. The client diagnosed with ulcerative colitis and nonbloody diarrhea.

7. The client diagnosed with essential hypertension asks the nurse, "Why do I have high blood pressure?" Which response by the nurse would be **most appropriate**?
   1. "You probably have some type of kidney disease that causes the high BP."
   2. "More than likely, you have had a diet high in salt, fat, and cholesterol."
   3. "There is no specific cause for hypertension, but there are many known risk factors."
   4. "You are concerned that you have high blood pressure. Let's sit down and talk."

8. The nurse is teaching the Dietary Approaches to Stop Hypertension (DASH) diet to a client diagnosed with essential hypertension. Which statement indicates that the client **understands** teaching concerning the DASH diet?
   1. "I should eat at least four to five servings of vegetables a day."
   2. "I should eat meat that has a lot of white streaks in it."
   3. "I should drink no more than two glasses of whole milk a day."
   4. "I should decrease my grain intake to no more than twice a week."

9. The client diagnosed with essential hypertension is taking a loop diuretic daily. Which assessment data would **require immediate** intervention by the nurse?
   1. The telemetry reads normal sinus rhythm.
   2. The client has a weight gain of 2 kg within 1 to 2 days.
   3. The client's BP is 148/92.
   4. The client's serum potassium level is 4.5 mEq.

10. The client diagnosed with essential hypertension asks the nurse, "I don't know why the doctor is worried about my blood pressure. I feel just great." Which statement by the nurse would be the **most appropriate** response?
    1. "Damage can be occurring to your heart and kidneys even if you feel great."
    2. "Unless you have a headache, your blood pressure is probably within normal limits."
    3. "When is the last time you saw your doctor? Does he know you are feeling great?"
    4. "Your blood pressure reflects how well your heart is working."

11. The intensive care unit nurse is calculating the total intake for a client diagnosed with a hypertensive crisis. What is the total intake for this client?

| | mL |
|---|---|

### Intake and Output Record

| Day One | Oral (oz) | Intravenous (mL) | Urine (mL) | Other (Specify) |
|---|---|---|---|---|
| 0701–1900 | Water: 8 oz<br>Milk: 4 oz | 680 mL (D5W)<br>100 mL (0.9% NS) | 1,000 mL | |
| 1901–0700 | Chicken broth: 6 oz | 200 mL (D5W) | 480 mL | |
| Total | | | | |

12. The nurse is teaching a class on essential hypertension. Which modifiable risk factors would the nurse include when preparing this presentation?
    1. Include information on retinopathy and nephropathy.
    2. Discuss a sedentary lifestyle and smoking cessation.
    3. Include discussions on family history and sex.
    4. Provide information on a low-fiber and high-salt diet.

## Peripheral Arterial Disease

13. The client comes to the clinic reporting muscle cramping and pain in both legs when walking for short periods of time. Which medical term would the nurse document in the client's record?
    1. Peripheral vascular disease.
    2. Intermittent claudication.
    3. Deep vein thrombosis.
    4. Dependent rubor.

14. Which instruction should the nurse include when providing discharge instructions to a client diagnosed with peripheral arterial disease?
    1. Encourage the client to use a heating pad on the lower extremities.
    2. Demonstrate to the client the correct way to apply elastic support hose.
    3. Instruct the client to walk daily for at least 30 minutes.
    4. Tell the client to check both feet for red areas at least once a week.

15. The nurse is teaching the client diagnosed with peripheral artery disease. Which interventions should the nurse include in the teaching? **Select all that apply.**
    1. Wash legs and feet daily in warm water.
    2. Apply moisturizing cream to feet.
    3. Buy shoes in the morning hours only.
    4. Avoid crossing the legs.
    5. Wear clean white cotton socks.

16. Which assessment data would **warrant immediate** intervention in the client diagnosed with peripheral arterial disease?
    1. The client has 2+ pedal pulses.
    2. The client is able to move the toes.
    3. The client has numbness and tingling.
    4. The client's feet are red when standing.

17. Which client problem would be a **priority** in a client diagnosed with peripheral arterial disease, admitted to the hospital with a foot ulcer?
    1. Impaired skin integrity.
    2. Activity intolerance.
    3. Ineffective health maintenance.
    4. Risk for peripheral neuropathy.

18. The client diagnosed with peripheral arterial disease is 1 day postoperative right femoral-popliteal bypass. Which intervention should the nurse implement?
    1. Keep the right leg in the dependent position.
    2. Apply sequential compression devices to lower extremities.
    3. Monitor the client's pedal pulses every shift.
    4. Assess the client's leg dressing every 4 hours.

19. The nurse is unable to assess a pedal pulse in the client diagnosed with peripheral arterial disease. Which intervention should the nurse implement **first**?
    1. Complete a neurovascular assessment.
    2. Use the Doppler device.
    3. Instruct the client to hang the feet off the side of the bed.
    4. Wrap the legs in a blanket.

20. The spouse of a client diagnosed with peripheral arterial disease tells the nurse, "My husband says he is having rest pain. What does that mean?" Which statement by the nurse would be **most appropriate**?
    1. "It describes the type of pain he has when he stops walking."
    2. "His legs are deprived of oxygen during periods of inactivity."
    3. "You are concerned that your husband is having rest pain."
    4. "This term is used to support that his condition is getting better."

21. The nurse is assessing the client diagnosed with long-term peripheral arterial disease. Which assessment data support the diagnosis?
    1. Hairless skin on the legs.
    2. Brittle, flaky toenails.
    3. Petechiae on the soles of feet.
    4. Nonpitting ankle edema.

22. The HCP ordered a femoral angiogram for the client diagnosed with peripheral arterial disease. Which interventions should the nurse implement? **Select all that apply.**
    1. Explain that this procedure will be done at the bedside.
    2. Discuss bedrest orders and bathroom privileges with the client.
    3. Inform the client that no intravenous access will be needed.
    4. Inform the client that fluids will be increased after the procedure.
    5. Teach the client that a local anesthetic will be used during the procedure.

23. Which medication should the nurse expect the HCP to order for a client diagnosed with peripheral arterial disease?
    1. An anticoagulant medication.
    2. An antihypertensive medication.
    3. An antiplatelet medication.
    4. A muscle relaxant.

24. The RN and an unlicensed assistive personnel (UAP) are caring for a 64-year-old client 4 hours postoperative bilateral femoral-popliteal bypass surgery. Which nursing task should be delegated to the UAP?
    1. Monitor the continuous passive motion machine.
    2. Assist the client to the bedside commode.
    3. Feed the client the evening meal.
    4. Elevate the foot of the client's bed.

## Atherosclerosis

25. The nurse is teaching a class on coronary artery disease. Which modifiable risk factor should the nurse discuss when teaching about atherosclerosis?
    1. Stress.
    2. Age.
    3. Sex.
    4. Family history.

26. The client asks the nurse, "My doctor just told me that atherosclerosis is why my legs hurt when I walk. What does that mean?" Which response by the nurse would be the **best response**?
    1. "The muscle fibers and endothelial lining of your arteries have become thickened."
    2. "The next time you see your HCP, ask what atherosclerosis means."
    3. "The valves in the veins of your legs are incompetent so your legs hurt."
    4. "You have a hardening of your arteries that decreases the oxygen to your legs."

27. The client diagnosed with peripheral vascular disease is overweight, has smoked two packs of cigarettes a day for 20 years, and sits behind a desk all day. What is the **strongest** factor in the development of atherosclerotic lesions?
    1. Being overweight.
    2. Sedentary lifestyle.
    3. High-fat, high-cholesterol diet.
    4. Smoking cigarettes.

28. The client tells the nurse that his cholesterol level is 240 mg/dL. Which action should the nurse implement?
    1. Praise the client for having a normal cholesterol level.
    2. Explain that the client needs to lower the cholesterol level.
    3. Discuss dietary changes that could help increase the level.
    4. Allow the client to verbalize feelings about the blood test result.

29. The nurse is discussing the pathophysiology of atherosclerosis with a client with a normal high-density lipoprotein cholesterol (HDLC) level. Which information should the nurse discuss with the client concerning HDLCs?
    1. A normal HDLC is good because it has a protective action in the body.
    2. The HDLC level measures the free fatty acids and glycerol in the blood.
    3. HDLC are the primary transporters of cholesterol into the cell.
    4. The client needs to decrease the amount of cholesterol and fat in the diet.

30. Which assessment data would cause the nurse to suspect the client has atherosclerosis?
    1. Change in bowel movements.
    2. Reports of a headache.
    3. Intermittent claudication.
    4. Venous stasis ulcers.

31. The nurse is teaching a class on atherosclerosis. Which statement describes the **scientific rationale** as to why diabetes is a risk factor for developing atherosclerosis?
    1. Glucose combines with carbon monoxide instead of with oxygen, and this leads to oxygen deprivation of tissues.
    2. Diabetes stimulates the sympathetic nervous system, resulting in peripheral constriction that increases the development of atherosclerosis.
    3. Diabetes speeds the atherosclerotic process by thickening the basement membrane of both large and small vessels.
    4. The increased glucose combines with the hemoglobin, which causes deposits of plaque in the lining of the vessels.

32. The nurse is discussing the importance of exercising with a client diagnosed with coronary artery disease. Which statement **best describes** the scientific rationale for encouraging 30 minutes of walking daily to help prevent complications of atherosclerosis?
    1. Exercise promotes the development of collateral circulation.
    2. Isometric exercises help develop the client's muscle mass.
    3. Daily exercise helps prevent plaque from developing in the vessel.
    4. Isotonic exercises promote the transport of glucose into the cell.

33. The HCP prescribes an HMG-CoA reductase inhibitor (statin) medication to a client diagnosed with coronary artery disease. Which should the nurse teach the client about this medication? **Select all that apply.**
    1. Take this medication on an empty stomach.
    2. This medication should be taken in the evening.
    3. Do not be concerned if muscle pain occurs.
    4. Check your cholesterol level daily.
    5. Avoid drinking grapefruit juice.

34. The nurse knows the client **understands** the teaching concerning a low-fat, low-cholesterol diet when the client selects which meal?
    1. Fried fish, garlic mashed potatoes, and iced tea.
    2. Ham and cheese on white bread and whole milk.
    3. Baked chicken, baked potato, and skim milk.
    4. A hamburger, French fries, and carbonated beverage.

35. Which interventions should the nurse include and teach the client diagnosed with atherosclerosis? **Select all that apply.**
    1. Include the significant other in the discussion.
    2. Stop smoking or using any type of tobacco products.
    3. Maintain a sedentary lifestyle as much as possible.
    4. Avoid stressful situations.
    5. Teach the client that daily exercises are important.

36. The RN is caring for clients on a telemetry floor. Which nursing task would be **most appropriate** to delegate to a UAP?
    1. Teach the client how to perform a glucometer check.
    2. Assist feeding the client diagnosed with heart failure.
    3. Check the cholesterol level for the client diagnosed with atherosclerosis.
    4. Assist the nurse to check the unit of blood at the client's bedside.

## Abdominal Aortic Aneurysm

37. Which assessment data would the nurse recognize to support the diagnosis of an AAA?
    1. Shortness of breath.
    2. Abdominal bruit.
    3. Ripping abdominal pain.
    4. Decreased urinary output.

38. Which medical treatment would be prescribed for the client diagnosed with an AAA less than 3 cm?
    1. Ultrasound every 6 months.
    2. Intravenous pyelogram yearly.
    3. Assessment of abdominal girth monthly.
    4. Repair of abdominal aortic aneurysm.

39. Which client would be **most likely** to develop an AAA?
    1. A 45-year-old female with a history of osteoporosis.
    2. An 80-year-old female with congestive heart failure.
    3. A 69-year-old male with peripheral vascular disease.
    4. A 30-year-old male with a genetic predisposition to AAA.

40. The client is diagnosed with an AAA. Which statement would the nurse expect the client to make during the admission assessment?
    1. "I have stomach pain every time I eat a big, heavy meal."
    2. "I don't have any abdominal pain or any type of problems."
    3. "I have periodic episodes of constipation and then diarrhea."
    4. "I belch a lot, especially when I lie down after eating."

41. The client is admitted for surgical repair of an 8-cm AAA. Which clinical manifestation would make the nurse suspect the client has an expanding AAA?
    1. Reports of low back pain.
    2. Weakened radial pulses.
    3. Decreased urine output.
    4. Increased abdominal girth.

42. The client is 1 day postoperative AAA repair. Which information from the UAP would **require immediate** intervention from the RN?
    1. The client refuses to turn from the back to the side.
    2. The client's urinary output is 90 mL in 6 hours.
    3. The client wants to sit on the side of the bed.
    4. The client's vital signs are T 98, P 90, R 18, and BP 130/70.

43. The client had an AAA repair 2 days ago. Which intervention should the nurse implement **first**?
    1. Assess the client's bowel sounds.
    2. Administer an IV prophylactic antibiotic.
    3. Encourage the client to splint the incision.
    4. Ambulate the client in the room with assistance.

44. Which HCP's order should the nurse **question** in a client diagnosed with an expanding AAA scheduled for surgery in the morning?
    1. Type and crossmatch for 2 units of blood.
    2. Tap water enema until clear fecal return.
    3. Bedrest with bathroom privileges.
    4. Keep nothing by mouth (NPO) after midnight.

45. The client is diagnosed with a small AAA. Which interventions should be included in the discharge teaching? **Select all that apply.**
    1. Tell the client to exercise three times a week for 30 minutes.
    2. Encourage the client to eat a low-fat, low-cholesterol diet.
    3. Instruct the client to decrease tobacco use.
    4. Discuss the importance of losing weight with the client.
    5. Teach the client to wear a truss at all times.

46. Which assessment data would **require immediate** intervention by the nurse for the client 6 hours postoperative AAA repair?
    1. Absent bilateral pedal pulses.
    2. Reports of pain at the site of the incision.
    3. Distended, tender abdomen.
    4. An elevated temperature of 100°F.

47. The nurse is discussing discharge teaching with the client 3 days postoperative AAA repair. Which discharge instructions should the nurse include when teaching the client? **Select all that apply.**
    1. Notify the HCP of any redness or irritation of the incision.
    2. Do not lift anything that weighs more than 20 pounds.
    3. Inform the client there may be pain not relieved with pain medication.
    4. Stress the importance of having daily bowel movements.
    5. Hold a pillow to the incision when you cough or sneeze.

48. On which area would the nurse place the bell of the stethoscope when assessing the client diagnosed with an AAA?

    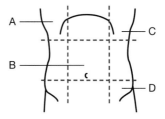

    1. A
    2. B
    3. C
    4. D

## Deep Vein Thrombosis

49. The nurse is discharging a client diagnosed with DVT from the hospital. Which discharge instructions should be provided to the client? **Select all that apply.**
    1. Have the partial thromboplastin time (PTT) levels checked weekly until the therapeutic range is achieved.
    2. Staying at home is best, but if traveling, airplanes are better than automobiles.
    3. Avoid green, leafy vegetables, such as spinach and collard greens.
    4. Wear knee stockings with an elastic band around the top.
    5. Notify the HCP of red or brown urine or emesis.

50. The nurse is caring for clients on a surgical floor. Which client should be assessed **first**?
    1. The client is 4 days postoperative abdominal surgery and is reporting left calf pain when ambulating.
    2. The client 1 day postoperative hernia repair has just been able to void 550 mL of clear amber urine.
    3. The client is 5 days postoperative open cholecystectomy, has a T-tube, and is being discharged.
    4. The client 16 hours postabdominal hysterectomy is reporting abdominal pain and is expelling flatus.

51. The male client is diagnosed with Guillain-Barré (GB) syndrome and is in the intensive care unit on a ventilator. Which cardiovascular rationale explains implementing passive range-of-motion (ROM) exercises?
    1. Passive ROM exercises will prevent contractures from developing.
    2. The client will feel better if he is able to exercise and stretch his muscles.
    3. ROM exercises will help alleviate the pain associated with GB syndrome.
    4. They help to prevent DVTs by the movement of the blood through the veins.

52. The RN and a UAP are bathing a bedfast client. Which action by the UAP **warrants immediate** intervention?
    1. The UAP closes the door and cubicle curtain before undressing the client.
    2. The UAP begins to massage and rub lotion into the client's calf.
    3. The UAP tests the temperature of the water with the wrist before starting.
    4. The UAP collects all the linens and supplies and brings them to the room.

53. The client diagnosed with a DVT is placed on a medical unit. Which nursing interventions should be implemented? **Select all that apply.**
    1. Place sequential compression devices on both legs.
    2. Instruct the client to stay in bed and not ambulate.
    3. Encourage fluids and a diet high in roughage.
    4. Monitor IV site every 4 hours and prn.
    5. Assess Homans' sign every 24 hours.

54. The nurse is caring for a client receiving heparin sodium via constant infusion. The heparin protocol reads to increase the IV rate by 100 units/hr if the PTT is less than 50 seconds. The current PTT level is 46 seconds. The heparin comes in 500 mL of D₅W with 25,000 units of heparin added. The current rate on the IV pump is 18 mL/hr. At what rate should the nurse set the pump?

    [                    ]

55. Which assessment data would **warrant immediate** intervention by the nurse?
    1. The client diagnosed with DVT reporting pain on inspiration.
    2. The immobile client refusing to turn for the last 3 hours.
    3. The client with an open cholecystectomy refuses to breathe deeply.
    4. The client with an inguinal hernia repair who must void before discharge.

56. The client diagnosed with a DVT is on a heparin drip at 1,400 units per hour, and warfarin 5 mg daily. Which intervention should the nurse implement **first**?
    1. Check the PTT and PT/INR.
    2. Check with the HCP to see which drug should be discontinued.
    3. Administer both medications.
    4. Discontinue the heparin because the client is receiving warfarin.

57. Which actions should the surgical scrub nurse take to prevent personally developing a DVT?
    1. Keep the legs in a dependent position and stand as still as possible.
    2. Flex the leg muscles and change the leg positions frequently.
    3. Wear white socks and shoes that have an elevated heel.
    4. Ask the surgeon to allow the nurse to take a break midway through each surgery.

58. The client receiving low molecular weight heparin (LMWH) subcutaneously to prevent DVT following hip replacement surgery reports to the nurse that there are small purple hemorrhagic areas on the right and left sides of the abdomen. Which action should the nurse implement?
    1. Notify the HCP immediately.
    2. Check the client's PTT level.
    3. Explain this is a result of the medication.
    4. Assess the client's vital signs.

59. The home health nurse is admitting a client diagnosed with a DVT. Which action by the client **warrants immediate** intervention by the nurse?
    1. The client takes a stool softener every day at dinnertime.
    2. The client is wearing a Medic Alert bracelet.
    3. The client takes vitamin E over-the-counter medication.
    4. The client has purchased a new recliner that will elevate the legs.

60. The client is being admitted with warfarin toxicity. Which laboratory data should the nurse monitor?
    1. Blood urea nitrogen (BUN) levels.
    2. Bilirubin levels.
    3. International normalized ratio (INR).
    4. Partial thromboplastin time (PTT).

## Peripheral Venous Disease

61. The nurse is teaching a class on venous insufficiency. The nurse would identify which condition as the **most serious** complication of chronic venous insufficiency?
    1. Arterial thrombosis.
    2. Deep vein thrombosis.
    3. Venous ulcerations.
    4. Varicose veins.

62. Which assessment data would support that the client has a venous stasis ulcer?
    1. A superficial pink open area on the medial part of the ankle.
    2. A deep pale open area over the top side of the foot.
    3. A reddened, blistered area on the heel of the foot.
    4. A necrotic gangrenous area on the dorsal side of the foot.

63. The client is employed in a job that requires extensive standing. Which intervention should the nurse include when discussing how to **prevent** varicose veins?
    1. Wear low-heeled, comfortable shoes.
    2. Wear clean white cotton socks.
    3. Move the legs back and forth often.
    4. Wear graduated compression hose.

64. The client diagnosed with varicose veins asks the nurse, "What caused me to have these?" Which statement by the nurse would be **most appropriate**?
    1. "You have incompetent valves in your legs."
    2. "Your legs have decreased oxygen to the muscle."
    3. "There is an obstruction in the saphenous vein."
    4. "Your blood is thick and can't circulate properly."

65. The nurse is caring for the client diagnosed with chronic venous insufficiency. Which statement indicates the client **understands** the discharge teaching?
    1. "I shouldn't cross my legs for more than 15 minutes."
    2. "I need to elevate the foot of my bed while sleeping."

    3. "I should take a low-dose acetylsalicylic acid every day with food."
    4. "I should increase my fluid intake to 3,000 mL a day."

66. The UAP is caring for the client diagnosed with chronic venous insufficiency. Which action would **warrant immediate** intervention from the RN?
    1. Removing compression stockings before assisting the client to bed.
    2. Taking the client's BP manually after using the machine.
    3. Assisting the client by opening the milk carton on the lunch tray.
    4. Calculating the client's shift intake and output with a pen and paper.

67. The 80-year-old client is being discharged home after having surgery to débride a chronic venous ulcer on the right ankle. Which referral would be **most appropriate** for the client?
    1. Occupational therapist.
    2. Social worker.
    3. Physical therapist.
    4. Cardiac rehabilitation.

68. Which assessment data would the nurse expect to find in the client diagnosed with chronic venous insufficiency?
    1. Decreased pedal pulses.
    2. Cool skin temperature.
    3. Intermittent claudication.
    4. Brown discolored skin.

69. Which client would be **most** at risk for developing varicose veins?
    1. A female nurse.
    2. A male bus driver.
    3. A female with no children.
    4. An elderly male with diabetes.

70. The client diagnosed with varicose veins is 6 hours postoperative vein ligation. Which nursing intervention should the nurse implement **first**?
    1. Assist the client to dangle the legs off the side of the bed.
    2. Assess and maintain pressure bandages on the affected leg.
    3. Apply a sequential compression device to the affected leg.
    4. Administer the prescribed prophylactic intravenous antibiotic.

71. The nurse has just received the morning shift report. Which client would the nurse assess **first**?
    1. The client diagnosed with a venous stasis ulcer reporting pain.
    2. The client diagnosed with varicose veins reporting dull, aching muscle cramps.
    3. The client diagnosed with peripheral arterial disease unable to move the foot.
    4. The client diagnosed with DVT and a positive Homans' sign.

72. The nurse is completing a neurovascular assessment on the client diagnosed with chronic venous insufficiency. What should be included in this assessment? **Select all that apply.**
    1. Assess for paresthesia.
    2. Assess for pedal pulses.
    3. Assess for paralysis.
    4. Assess for pallor.
    5. Assess for polar (temperature).

# CONCEPTS

The concepts covered in this chapter focus on clotting and the perfusion-related areas of nursing issues. Clotting and tissue perfusion-related problems of DVT and peripheral vascular disease, as well as the interrelated concepts of the nursing process and clinical judgment, are also covered. The concept of the nursing process is displayed throughout the questions. The concept of clinical judgment is presented in any prioritizing or "first" question.

73. The nurse is admitting a client diagnosed with peripheral vascular disease. Which data **support** a diagnosis of venous insufficiency?
    1. The client has bright red skin on the lower extremities.
    2. The client has a brownish-purple area on the lower legs.
    3. The client reports pain after ambulating for short distances.
    4. The client has nonhealing wounds on the toes and ankles.

74. The nurse identifies the concept of clotting for a client diagnosed with a DVT. Which clinical manifestations **support** the diagnosis?
    1. Brown-purple discoloration on the calf.
    2. Bright red skin on the lower legs.
    3. Swelling in the calf, warmth, and tenderness.
    4. Pain after walking for short distances that resolve with rest.

75. The client diagnosed with a DVT is prescribed heparin via continuous infusion. The client's laboratory data are listed in the table below. Based on the laboratory results, which intervention should the nurse implement?

| Laboratory Test | Client Results | Normal Values |
|---|---|---|
| PT | 12.2 Control 1.4 | 10 to 13 seconds |
| PTT | 48 Control 32 | 25 to 35 seconds |
| INR | 1 | 0.9 to 1.1 w/o anti-coagulation therapy 2 to 3 with therapy 2.5 to 3.5 if the client has a mechanical heart valve |

1. Request a change of medication to a subcutaneous anticoagulant.
2. Administer vitamin K IM.
3. Have the dietary department remove all green, leafy vegetables from the trays.
4. Administer the IV as ordered.

76. The nurse is caring for a client diagnosed with DVT. Which information reported to the RN by the UAP **requires immediate** intervention?
    1. The UAP informed the nurse the client is reporting chest pain.
    2. The UAP notified the nurse the client's BP is 100/66.
    3. The UAP reported the client is requesting to be able to take a shower.
    4. The UAP tells the nurse the client is asking for medication for a headache.

77. The client presents to the outpatient clinic reporting calf pain. The client reports returning from an airplane trip the previous day. Which should the nurse assess **first**?
    1. The nurse should auscultate the lung fields and heart sounds.
    2. The nurse should determine the length of the airplane trip.
    3. The nurse should determine if the client has had chest pain.
    4. The nurse should measure the calf and palpate the calf for warmth.

78. The client prescribed rivaroxaban is reporting dark, tarry stool. Which should the nurse implement **first**?
    1. Notify the health-care provider.
    2. Ask the client to provide a stool sample.
    3. Ask the client when the rivaroxaban was last taken.
    4. Assess the client for ecchymotic areas and bleeding.

79. The nurse is planning care for a client diagnosed with peripheral arterial disease. Which exercise instructions would the nurse teach the client?
    1. Have the client perform isometric exercises 30 minutes each day.
    2. Tell the client to start exercising on a stair stepper for 15 minutes.
    3. Inform the client that warm-up exercises are not necessary.
    4. Teach the client to walk in well-fitting shoes on level ground.

80. The nurse is teaching the client diagnosed with DVT and prescribed warfarin. Which should the nurse teach the client? **Select all that apply.**
    1. Keep a constant amount of green, leafy vegetables in the diet.
    2. Instruct the client to have regular INR laboratory work done.
    3. Tell the client to go to the hospital immediately for any bleeding.
    4. Inform the client to notify the HCP if having dark, tarry stools.
    5. Encourage the client to carry medication regimen information.
    6. Have the client take iron orally to prevent bleeding.

81. Which **complication** of anticoagulant therapy should the nurse teach the client to report to the HCP?
    1. Gastric upset.
    2. Bleeding from any site.
    3. Constipation.
    4. Myocardial infarction.

82. The nurse is teaching a class to clients diagnosed with hypertension. Which should the nurse teach the clients?
    1. The BP target range should be 120/80.
    2. Take the medication even when feeling well.
    3. Get up quickly when rising from a recumbent position.
    4. Consume a 3,000-mg sodium diet.

83. Which should the nurse include in the plan of care for a client diagnosed with venous stasis ulcers? **Select all that apply.**
    1. Elevate the legs while sitting.
    2. Wear antiembolism compression stockings.
    3. Avoid injury to the lower limbs.
    4. Trim the toenails straight across.
    5. Do not apply moisturizer to the lower legs.
    6. Allow the legs to hang over the bed in a dependent position.

84. The client on the telemetry unit is diagnosed with thromboembolism and is reporting chest pain and anxiety. Which action should the RN implement **first**?
    1. Stay with the client and call the rapid response team (RRT).
    2. Assess the client's vital signs.
    3. Have the UAP stay with the client.
    4. Check the client's telemetry reading.

85. Which arterial anticoagulant medication would the nurse anticipate being prescribed for a client diagnosed with peripheral arterial disease?
    1. Clopidogrel.
    2. Streptokinase.
    3. Protamine sulfate.
    4. Enoxaparin.

86. The nurse is caring for a male client diagnosed with essential hypertension. Which information regarding antihypertensive medication should the nurse teach?
    1. Teach the client to take his BP four times each day.
    2. Instruct the client to have regular blood levels of the medication checked.
    3. Explain the need to rise slowly from a lying or sitting position.
    4. Demonstrate how to use a blood glucose meter daily.

87. The nurse is demonstrating the use of a BP sphygmomanometer to a client newly diagnosed with hypertension. Which should the nurse teach the client? **Select all that apply.**
    1. Tell the client to make sure the cuff is placed over an artery.
    2. Teach the client to notify the HCP if the BP is >160/100.
    3. Instruct the client about orthostatic hypotension.
    4. Encourage the client to keep a record of the BP readings.
    5. Explain that even when the BP is within normal limits, the medication should still be taken.

88. The client diagnosed with a DVT is prescribed a heparin drip. The solution is 40,000 units in 500 mL of $D_5W$. The HCP ordered the client to receive 1,200 units per hour. At which rate should the nurse set the IV pump?

    ┌─────────────────────────────┐
    │                             │
    └─────────────────────────────┘

89. The client is at risk for myocardial infarction due to decreased tissue perfusion as a result of atherosclerosis. Which instructions can the nurse provide the client to **reduce** the risk?
    1. Teach the client to control the BP to less than 140/90.
    2. Instruct the client to exercise 30 minutes a day three times a week.
    3. Demonstrate how to take the BP using a battery-operated cuff.
    4. Inform the client to limit fat intake and which foods have a higher fat content.

90. The nurse is caring for a client receiving heparin therapy intravenously. Which assessment data would indicate to the nurse the client is developing heparin-induced thrombocytopenia (HIT)? **Select all that apply.**
    1. The client has spontaneous bleeding from around the IV site.
    2. The client reports chest pain on inspiration and has become restless.
    3. The client's platelet count on admission was 420 ($10^3$) and now is 200 ($10^3$).
    4. The client reports that the gums bleed when brushing the teeth.
    5. The client has developed skin lesions at the IV site.

## Hypertension

**1.** 1. This BP is elevated, and the client should have his BP checked frequently but not before seeking medical treatment.
   2. **The diastolic BP should be less than 80 mm Hg, according to the American Heart Association (2017); therefore, this client should see the HCP.**
   3. Teaching is important, but the nurse must first make sure the client sees the HCP for a thorough checkup and antihypertensive medication prescription. Diet alone should not be recommended by the nurse.
   4. This is not the normal range for an older person's BP; the diastolic should be less than 80 mm Hg.

**TEST-TAKING HINT: Remember, the question asks which action should be implemented first. Therefore, more than one answer is appropriate, but the first to be implemented should be the one that directly affects the client.**

**2.** Correct answers are 1 and 5.
   1. **Brisk walking 30 to 45 minutes a day will help to reduce BP, weight, and stress and will increase a feeling of overall well-being (American Heart Association, 2018).**
   2. Heavy weight lifting should be discouraged because performing this activity can raise systolic BP, although the research is controversial and can be addressed on an individual client basis.
   3. The client should walk, cycle, jog, or swim as moderate-intensity aerobic activity on most days, but high-level aerobic exercise is recommended at least 2 days a week.
   4. Swimming laps is recommended, but it should be daily, not once a week.
   5. **The use of resistance bands, a form of muscle-strengthening exercise, should be encouraged at least twice a week.**

**TEST-TAKING HINT: Remember to look at the frequency of interventions; it makes a difference when selecting the correct answers.**

**3.** 1. Beta-adrenergic blocking agents, not ACE inhibitors, prevent the beta receptor stimulation in the heart, which decreases heart rate and cardiac output.
   2. Alpha-adrenergic blockers, not ACE inhibitors, block alpha receptors in the vascular smooth muscle, which decreases vasomotor tone and vasoconstriction.
   3. **ACE inhibitors prevent the conversion of angiotensin I to angiotensin II, and this, in turn, prevents vasoconstriction and sodium and water retention.**
   4. Vasodilators, not ACE inhibitors, reduce BP by relaxing vascular smooth muscle, especially in the arterioles.

**TEST-TAKING HINT: The test taker needs to understand how the major classifications of medications work to answer this question.**

**4.** 1. The potassium level is within normal limits (3.5 to 5.3 mEq/L), and it is not usually checked before administering beta blockers.
   2. **The nurse should question administering the beta blocker if the BP is low because this medication will cause the BP to drop even lower, leading to hypotension.**
   3. The nurse would not administer the medication if the apical (not radial) pulse were less than 60 beats per minute.
   4. The nurse needs to assess the BP only once before administering the medication (not take all three BPs before administering the medication).

**TEST-TAKING HINT: Be sure to read the entire question and all the answer options and note the specific numbers that are identified. The test taker must know normal laboratory data and assessment findings.**

**5.** 1. The potassium level is not affected by an alpha-adrenergic blocker.
   2. Alpha-adrenergic blockers, on rare occasions, can cause sexual problems. Noncompliance with taking prescribed medications can occur in male clients who experience impotence. The noncompliance should be reported to the HCP immediately so that the medication can be changed. Impotence, however, is not an expected side effect.
   3. The medication can be taken on an empty or a full stomach, depending on whether the client becomes nauseated after taking the medication.
   4. **Orthostatic hypotension may occur when the BP is decreasing and may lead to dizziness and light-headedness, so the client should change position slowly.**

**TEST-TAKING HINT: The test taker should understand the side effects of medications. The test taker not knowing the answer may realize that**

hypertension is being treated and that hypotension is the opposite of hypertension and might be a complication of treating hypertension. Only option "4" refers to hypotension, providing advice on how to avoid orthostatic hypotension.

6. 1. This BP is elevated, but it is not life-threatening.
   2. **The chest pain could be a pulmonary embolus secondary to DVT and requires immediate intervention by the nurse.**
   3. A pulse oximeter reading of greater than 93% is within normal limits.
   4. Nonbloody diarrhea is an expected clinical manifestation of ulcerative colitis and would not require immediate intervention by the nurse.

**TEST-TAKING HINT: The nurse should assess the client with abnormal assessment data or a life-threatening condition first when determining which client is a priority.**

7. 1. Kidney disease leads to secondary hypertension; secondary hypertension is elevated BP resulting from an identifiable underlying process.
   2. A high-salt, high-fat, high-cholesterol diet is a risk factor for essential hypertension, but it is not the only cause; therefore, this would be an incorrect answer.
   3. **There is no known cause for essential hypertension, but many factors—both modifiable (obesity, smoking, diet) and nonmodifiable (family history, age, sex)—are risk factors for essential hypertension.**
   4. This is a therapeutic reply that is inappropriate because the client needs facts.

**TEST-TAKING HINT: When clients request information, the exchange should not address emotions. Just facts should be given. Therefore, option "4" can be eliminated as a correct answer.**

8. 1. **The DASH diet has proved beneficial in lowering BP. It recommends eating a diet high in vegetables, fruits, and whole grains (National Heart, Lung, and Blood Institute, n.d.).**
   2. The DASH diet recommends two or fewer servings of lean meats, which have very few white streaks; the white streaks indicate the meat is high in fat.
   3. The DASH diet recommends two to three servings of nonfat or low-fat milk, not whole milk.
   4. The DASH diet recommends six to eight servings of grain a day.

**TEST-TAKING HINT: The test taker is looking for correct information about the DASH diet. A recommended diet for hypertension would limit fatty meats and whole milk.**

9. 1. Normal sinus rhythm indicates that the client's heart is working normally.
   2. **Rapid weight gain—for example, 2 kg in 1 to 2 days—indicates that the loop diuretic is not working effectively; 2 kg equals 4.4 lb; 1 L of fluid weighs 1 kg.**
   3. This BP is not life-threateningly high and does not require immediate intervention.
   4. Loop diuretics cause an increase in potassium excretion in the urine; therefore, the potassium level should be assessed, but 4.5 mEq/L is within normal limits (3.5 to 5.3 mEq/L).

**TEST-TAKING HINT: The phrase "requires immediate intervention" should make the test taker think that the correct answer will be abnormal assessment data that require medical intervention or indicate conditions that are life-threatening.**

10. 1. **Even if the client feels great, the BP can be elevated, causing damage to the heart, kidney, and blood vessels.**
    2. A headache may indicate an elevated BP, but the client diagnosed with essential hypertension can be asymptomatic and still have a very high BP reading.
    3. This response does not answer the client's question as to why the doctor is worried about the client's BP.
    4. The BP does not necessarily reflect how well the heart is working. Many other diagnostic tests assess how well the heart is working, including an electrocardiogram (ECG), an ultrasound, and a chest x-ray.

**TEST-TAKING HINT: The test taker should select the option that provides the client with correct information in a nonthreatening, nonjudgmental approach.**

11. **1,520 mL total intake.**
    The urinary output is not used in this calculation. The nurse must add up both intravenous fluids and oral fluids to obtain the total intake for this client:

    680 + 100 + 200 = 980 IV fluids

    Oral fluids (1 ounce = 30 mL): 8 ounces × 30 mL = 240 mL, 4 ounces × 30 mL = 120 mL, 6 ounces × 30 mL = 180 mL

    240 + 120 + 180 = 540 mL oral fluids

    Total intake is 980 + 540 = 1,520 mL.

**TEST-TAKING HINT: The reader must know the conversion equivalents before performing any**

type of math problem. The key to this answer is 1 ounce = 30 mL.

12. 1. Retinopathy and nephropathy are complications of uncontrolled hypertension, not modifiable risk factors.
    2. **A sedentary lifestyle is discouraged in clients diagnosed with hypertension; daily isotonic exercises are recommended. Smoking (cigars cause problems too) increases the atherosclerotic process in and causes vasoconstriction of vessels. Carbon monoxide adheres to hemoglobin, decreasing oxygen levels.**
    3. Family history and sex are nonmodifiable risk factors. The question is asking for information on modifiable risk factors.
    4. A low-salt diet is recommended because increased salt intake causes water retention, which increases the workload of the heart. A high-fiber diet is recommended because it helps decrease cholesterol levels.

**TEST-TAKING HINT: Remember to look at the adjectives. The stem of the question is asking about "modifiable risk factors."**

## Peripheral Arterial Disease

13. 1. Peripheral vascular disease is a broad term that encompasses both venous and arterial peripheral problems of the lower extremities.
    2. **This is the classic symptom of peripheral arterial disease.**
    3. This is characterized by calf tenderness, calf edema, and a positive Homans' sign.
    4. This term is a clinical manifestation of peripheral arterial disease; the legs are pale when elevated but are dark red when in the dependent position.

**TEST-TAKING HINT: The test taker could eliminate options "1" and "3" as possible answers if the words "medical term" were noted. Both options "1" and "3" are disease processes, not medical terms.**

14. 1. External heating devices are avoided to reduce the risk of burns.
    2. Elastic support hose reduce the circulation to the skin and are avoided.
    3. **Walking promotes the development of collateral circulation to ischemic tissue and slows the process of atherosclerosis.**
    4. The feet must be checked daily, not weekly.

**TEST-TAKING HINT: The test taker must note the noun "week" in option "4," which could eliminate this distracter as a possible answer.**

15. Correct answers are 1, 2, 4, and 5.
    1. **Cold water causes vasoconstriction, and hot water may burn the client's feet; therefore, warm (tepid) water should be recommended.**
    2. **Moisturizing prevents drying of the feet.**
    3. Shoes should be purchased in the afternoon when the feet are the largest.
    4. **Crossing the legs will decrease circulation to the legs.**
    5. **Colored socks have dyes, and dirty socks may cause foot irritation that may lead to breaks in the skin.**

**TEST-TAKING HINT: The test taker must select all appropriate interventions; option "3" could be eliminated as a correct answer because of "only," which is an absolute word. There are very few absolutes in health care.**

16. 1. These are normal pedal pulses and would not require any intervention.
    2. Moving the toes is a good sign in a client diagnosed with peripheral arterial disease.
    3. **Numbness and tingling are paresthesias, which are a clinical manifestation of a severely decreased blood supply to the lower extremities.**
    4. Reddened extremities are expected secondary to increased blood supply when the legs are in the dependent position.

**TEST-TAKING HINT: "Warrants immediate intervention" indicates that the test taker must select the distracter that is abnormal, unexpected, or life-threatening for the client's disease process. Sometimes if the test taker flips the question and thinks which assessment data are normal for the disease process, it is easier to identify the correct answer.**

17. 1. **The client has a foot ulcer; therefore, the protective lining of the body—the skin—has been impaired.**
    2. This is an appropriate problem but would not take priority over impaired skin integrity.
    3. The client needs teaching, but it does not take priority over a physiological problem.
    4. The client has peripheral neuropathy, not a risk for it; this is the primary pathological change in a client diagnosed with peripheral arterial disease.

**TEST-TAKING HINT: Remember Maslow's hierarchy of needs; physiological needs are a priority.**

18. 1. The right leg should be elevated to decrease edema, not flat or hanging off the side of the bed (dependent).
    2. The left leg could have a sequential compression device to prevent DVT, but it should not be on the leg with an operative incision site.
    3. The client is 1 day postoperative, and the pedal pulses must be assessed more than once every 8 or 12 hours.
    4. The leg dressing needs to be assessed for hemorrhaging or findings of infection.

**TEST-TAKING HINT:** The test taker must be observant of time ("1 day postoperative"), and doing an intervention every "shift" should cause the test taker to eliminate this distracter. The test taker must know terms used to describe positioning, such as *dependent*, *prone*, and *supine*.

19. 1. An absent pulse is not uncommon in a client diagnosed with peripheral arterial disease, but the nurse must ensure that the feet can be moved and are warm, which indicates adequate blood supply to the feet.
    2. To identify the location of the pulse, the nurse should use a Doppler device to amplify the sound, but it is not the first intervention.
    3. This position will increase blood flow and may help the nurse palpate the pulse, but it is not the first intervention.
    4. Cold can cause vasoconstriction and decrease the ability to palpate the pulse, and warming will dilate the arteries, helping the nurse find the pedal pulse, but it is not the first intervention.

**TEST-TAKING HINT:** The stem asks the test taker to identify the first intervention, and the test taker should apply the nursing process and implement an assessment intervention.

20. 1. The pain stops when the client quits walking; therefore, it is not rest pain.
    2. Rest pain indicates a worsening of the peripheral arterial disease; the muscles of the legs are not getting enough oxygen when the client is resting to prevent muscle ischemia.
    3. This is a therapeutic response and does not answer the spouse's question.
    4. Rest pain indicates that the peripheral arterial disease is getting worse.

**TEST-TAKING HINT:** The nurse should answer questions with factual information; therefore,

option "3" could be eliminated as a possible answer. Pain usually does not indicate that a condition is getting better, which would cause the test taker to eliminate option "4."

21. 1. The decreased oxygen over time causes the loss of hair on the tops of the feet and ascending both legs.
    2. The toenails are usually thickened as a result of hypoxemia.
    3. Petechiae are tiny purple or red spots that appear on the skin as a result of minute hemorrhages within the dermal layer; this does not occur with peripheral arterial disease.
    4. There may be edema, but it is usually pitting; nonpitting edema resolves with elevation but not in clients diagnosed with peripheral arterial disease.

**TEST-TAKING HINT:** The test taker should apply the pathophysiological concept that arterial blood supplies oxygen and nutrients, and if the hair cannot get nutrients, it will not grow.

22. Correct answers are 4 and 5.
    1. This procedure will be done in a catheterization laboratory or special room, not at the bedside, because machines are used to visualize the extent of the arterial occlusion.
    2. The client will have to keep the leg straight for at least 6 hours after the procedure to prevent bleeding from the femoral artery.
    3. An intravenous contrast medium is injected, and vessels are visualized using fluoroscopy and x-rays.
    4. Fluids will help flush the contrast dye out of the body and help prevent kidney damage.
    5. A local anesthetic will be used to numb the skin at the insertion site.

**TEST-TAKING HINT:** The test taker must be knowledgeable of diagnostic tests. If not, the test taker could dissect the word "angiogram"; *angio-* means "vessel," which could help eliminate option "3" as a possible answer because some type of dye would have to be used to visualize a vessel. Adjectives should be noted—anything done in the femoral artery would require pressure at the site to prevent bleeding—this information could help the test taker to eliminate option "2" as a possible answer. Very few diagnostic tests are done at the bedside.

23. 1. Anticoagulant medication is prescribed for venous problems, such as DVT.
    2. Peripheral arterial disease is caused by atherosclerosis, which may cause hypertension as well, but antihypertensive medications are not prescribed for peripheral arterial disease.
    3. **Antiplatelet medications, such as aspirin or clopidogrel (Plavix), inhibit platelet aggregations in the arterial blood.**
    4. A muscle relaxant will not help the leg pain because the origin of the pain is decreased oxygen to the muscle.

**TEST-TAKING HINT:** The test taker should apply the knowledge learned in anatomy and physiology class. Platelets are part of the arterial blood; therefore, this would be an excellent selection if the test taker did not have any idea about the answer.

24. 1. A continuous passive motion machine is used for a client with a total knee replacement, not for this type of surgery.
    2. The client will be on bedrest at 4 hours after the surgery. Remember, the client had bilateral surgery on the legs.
    3. There is nothing in the stem that would indicate the client could not self-feed. The nurse should encourage independence as much as possible.
    4. **After the surgery, the client's legs will be elevated to help decrease edema. The surgery has corrected the decreased blood supply to the lower legs.**

**TEST-TAKING HINT:** A concept that is applicable to surgery is decreasing edema, and extremity surgeries usually include elevating the affected extremity. The test taker must apply basic concepts when answering questions.

## Atherosclerosis

25. 1. **A modifiable risk factor is a risk factor that can possibly be altered by modifying or changing behavior, such as developing new ways to deal with stress.**
    2. The client cannot do anything about getting older, so it cannot be modified.
    3. Sex is a risk factor that cannot be changed.
    4. Having a family history of coronary artery disease predisposes the client to a higher risk, but this cannot be changed by the client.

**TEST-TAKING HINT:** The test taker needs to key in on adjectives when reading the stem of a question. The word "modifiable" should cause the test taker to select "stress" because it is the only answer option referring to something that can be changed or modified.

26. 1. The nurse should assume the client is a layperson and should not explain disease processes using medical terminology.
    2. This is passing the buck; the nurse should have the knowledge to answer this question.
    3. Atherosclerosis involves the arteries, not the veins.
    4. **This response explains in plain terms why the client's legs hurt from atherosclerosis.**

**TEST-TAKING HINT:** If the test taker knows medical terminology, option "3" could be eliminated because *athero-* means "arteries," not veins. The test taker should be very cautious when choosing an option that asks the HCP to answer questions that nurses should be able to answer.

27. 1. Being overweight is not a risk factor for atherosclerotic lesions, but it does indicate that the client does not eat a healthy diet or exercise as needed.
    2. Lack of exercise is a risk factor, but it is not the strongest.
    3. Although the stem did not explicitly identify diet, the nurse should assume that an obese client would not eat a low-fat, low-cholesterol diet.
    4. **Although tobacco use has declined in the United States, tobacco use is still the strongest factor in the development of atherosclerotic lesions. Nicotine decreases blood flow to the extremities and increases heart rate and BP. It also increases the risk of clot formation by increasing the aggregation of platelets.**

**TEST-TAKING HINT:** The test taker should look at the answer options closely to determine if any are similar. This will help eliminate two options—"1" and "3"—as possible answers. An unhealthy diet will cause the client to be overweight.

28. 1. The cholesterol level should be less than 200 mg/dL.
    2. **The client needs to be taught ways to lower the cholesterol level.**
    3. The client should be taught a low-fat, low-cholesterol diet to help lower the cholesterol level.
    4. The nurse needs to discuss facts concerning the cholesterol level and teach the client. A therapeutic conversation would not be appropriate.

**TEST-TAKING HINT:** The nurse needs to know normal laboratory test findings. The test taker unaware of normal cholesterol levels could only guess the answer to the question.

29. 1. A normal HDLC level is good because HDLC transports cholesterol away from the tissues and cells of the arterial wall to the liver for excretion. This helps decrease the development of atherosclerosis.
    2. The normal HDLC level was the result of a test measuring high-density lipoproteins, not free fatty acids and glycerol in the blood, which are measured by the serum triglyceride level. Triglycerides are a source of energy.
    3. Low-density lipoproteins (LDLCs), not HDLCs, are the primary transporters of cholesterol into the cell. They have the harmful effect of depositing cholesterol into the walls of the arterial vessels.
    4. A normal HDLC level is good, and the client does not need to change the diet.

**TEST-TAKING HINT:** If the test taker has no idea what the correct answer is, the test taker should look at the specific words in the answer options. Normal laboratory data would probably be good for the client; therefore, option "1" would be a probable correct answer.

30. 1. A change in bowel movements may indicate cancer but not atherosclerosis.
    2. A headache is not a clinical manifestation of atherosclerosis.
    3. **Intermittent claudication is a clinical manifestation of generalized atherosclerosis and is a marker of atherosclerosis.**
    4. Atherosclerosis indicates arterial involvement, not venous involvement.

**TEST-TAKING HINT:** Knowledge of medical terminology—in this case, knowing that "atherosclerosis" refers to arteries—would allow the test taker to rule out all of the answer options except option "3," even if the test taker does not know what "intermittent claudication" means.

31. 1. Glucose does not combine with carbon monoxide.
    2. Vasoconstriction is not a risk factor for developing atherosclerosis.
    3. **This is the scientific rationale for why diabetes mellitus is a modifiable risk factor for atherosclerosis.**
    4. When glucose combines with the hemoglobin in a laboratory test called glycosylated hemoglobin, the result can determine the client's average glucose level over the past 3 months.

**TEST-TAKING HINT:** The nurse must understand the reason "why," or the scientific rationale, for teaching in addition to nursing interventions. This is critical thinking.

32. 1. **Collateral circulation is the development of blood supply around narrowed arteries; it helps prevent complications of atherosclerosis, including myocardial infarction, cerebrovascular accidents, and peripheral vascular disease. Exercise promotes the development of collateral circulation.**
    2. Isometric (weight-lifting) exercises help develop muscle mass, but this type of exercise does not help decrease complications of atherosclerosis.
    3. A low-fat, low-cholesterol diet may help decrease plaque formation, but exercise will not do this.
    4. Isotonic exercises, such as walking and swimming, promote the movement of glucose across the cell membrane, but this is not why such exercises are recommended for the prevention of atherosclerotic complications.

**TEST-TAKING HINT:** The test taker must understand what the stem of the question is asking and note the words "the complications of atherosclerosis." "Isometric," which refers to "muscle" (remember "m"), and "isotonic," which refers to "tone" (remember "t"), exercises do not directly help prevent the complications of atherosclerosis, so options "2" and "4" can be eliminated.

33. Correct answers are 2 and 5.
    1. Most statin medications can be taken with food or on an empty stomach. Lovastatin must be taken with food.
    2. **Most statin medications should be taken in the evening for best results because the enzyme that destroys cholesterol works best in the evening, and the medication enhances this process.**
    3. Cholesterol-reducing medications can cause serious liver problems, and if a client has muscle pain, it is an adverse effect that should be reported to the HCP.
    4. The cholesterol level is checked every few months, not on a daily basis.
    5. **Grapefruit juice should be avoided during therapy because it increases the risk of toxicity.**

**TEST-TAKING HINT:** The test taker must be aware of adverbs such as "daily." Cholesterol is not monitored daily, so option "4" can be eliminated. There are only a few medications taken on an empty stomach; most medications can and should be administered with food to help prevent gastric irritation.

34. 1. Fried foods are high in fat and cholesterol.
    2. White bread is not high in fiber; wheat bread should be recommended because it is high in fiber. Whole milk is high in fat; skim milk should be used.
    3. Baked, broiled, or grilled meats are recommended; a plain baked potato is appropriate, and skim milk is low in fat—so this meal is appropriate for a low-fat, low-cholesterol diet.
    4. Hamburger meat is high in fat, French fries are usually cooked in oil (which is high in fat), and carbonated beverages are high in calories.

**TEST-TAKING HINT:** The nurse must be aware of special diets, and a low-fat, low-cholesterol diet is often prescribed for clients diagnosed with atherosclerosis. Remember, baked, broiled, and grilled meats are lower in fat and cholesterol than fried meats.

35. Correct answers are 1, 2, and 5.
    1. Adherence to lifestyle modifications is enhanced when the client receives support from significant others.
    2. Tobacco use is the most significant modifiable risk factor that contributes to the development of atherosclerosis.
    3. A sedentary lifestyle should be discouraged; daily walking or swimming is encouraged.
    4. This is an unrealistic intervention. The nurse needs to help the client learn ways to deal with stressful situations, not avoid the situations.
    5. Daily exercise, such as walking or swimming, should be encouraged.

**TEST-TAKING HINT:** This type of alternate question requires the test taker to select all answer options that apply. Some interventions are universal to all teaching, such as including significant others. Be careful with words such as "avoid."

36. 1. Teaching cannot be delegated to a UAP.
    2. The UAP can feed a client.
    3. The UAP cannot assess the client and does not have the education to interpret laboratory data.
    4. A unit of blood must be checked by two registered nurses at the bedside.

**TEST-TAKING HINT:** Many states have rules concerning what tasks can be delegated to UAPs, but even those states that don't have delegation rules agree that teaching and assessing an unstable client cannot be delegated to UAPs.

## Abdominal Aortic Aneurysm

37. 1. Shortness of breath indicates a respiratory problem or possibly a thoracic aneurysm, not an AAA.
    2. A systolic bruit over the abdomen is a diagnostic indication of an AAA.
    3. Ripping or tearing pain indicates a dissecting aneurysm.
    4. Urine output is not diagnostic of an AAA.

**TEST-TAKING HINT:** The test taker with no idea of the answer should note that two of the options—"2" and "3"—have the word "abdominal" and choose between them, ruling out options "1" and "4," both of which refer to other systems of the body (respiratory and urinary).

38. 1. When the aneurysm is small (less than 5 cm), an abdominal sonogram will be done every 6 months until the aneurysm reaches a size at which surgery to prevent rupture is of more benefit than possible complications of an AAA repair.
    2. An intravenous pyelogram evaluates the kidney.
    3. The abdomen will not distend as the AAA enlarges.
    4. This AAA is too small to perform surgery to remove it.

**TEST-TAKING HINT:** The AAA less than 3 cm should make the test taker assume surgery is not an option; therefore, option "4" could be ruled out as a correct answer. *Pyelo-* means "kidney," so option "2" could be ruled out. The term "medical treatment" in the stem of the question should cause the test taker to rule out abdominal girth.

39. 1. AAAs affect males four to five times more often than females.
    2. AAAs affect males four to five times more often than females.
    3. The most common cause of AAA is atherosclerosis (which is the cause of peripheral vascular disease); it occurs in males four to five times more often than in females and primarily in whites.
    4. AAAs occur most often in older males, and there is no genetic predisposition.

**TEST-TAKING HINT:** If the test taker knew that AAA and peripheral vascular disease both occur with atherosclerosis, it might possibly lead to the selection of option "3" as the correct answer.

40. 1. This statement would not make the nurse suspect an AAA.
    2. **Only about two-fifths of clients diagnosed with AAA have symptoms; the remainder are asymptomatic.**
    3. Periodic episodes of constipation and diarrhea may indicate colon cancer but do not support a diagnosis of AAA.
    4. Belching does not support a diagnosis of AAA, but it could possibly indicate gastroesophageal reflux or a hiatal hernia.

**TEST-TAKING HINT:** The test taker must remember that not all disease processes or conditions have clinical manifestations. The test taker should attempt to determine what disease processes the other answer options are describing.

41. 1. **Low back pain is present because of the pressure of the aneurysm on the lumbar nerves; this is a serious symptom, usually indicating that the aneurysm is expanding rapidly and about to rupture.**
    2. If any pulses were affected, it would be the pedal pulses, not the radial pulses.
    3. Decreased urine output would not indicate an expanding AAA, but decreased urine output may occur when the AAA ruptures, causing hypovolemia.
    4. The abdominal girth would not increase for an expanding AAA, but it might increase with a ruptured AAA.

**TEST-TAKING HINT:** If the test taker knows the anatomical position of the abdominal aorta and understands the term "expanding," then it may lead the test taker to select low back pain as the correct answer.

42. 1. The nurse needs to intervene, but it does not require immediate intervention.
    2. **The client must have 30 mL of urinary output every hour. Clients post-AAA repair are at high risk for renal failure because of the anatomical location of the AAA near the renal arteries.**
    3. The client can sit on the bed the first day postoperation; this is, in fact, encouraged.
    4. These vital signs would not warrant immediate intervention by the nurse.

**TEST-TAKING HINT:** A basic concept that the test taker should remember is that any urine output less than 30 mL/hr should be cause for investigation.

43. 1. **Assessment is the first part of the nursing process and is the first intervention the nurse should implement.**
    2. Administering an antibiotic is an appropriate intervention, but it is not a priority over assessment.
    3. The client should splint the incision when coughing and deep breathing to help decrease the pain, but this intervention is not a priority over assessment.
    4. Ambulating the client as soon as possible is an appropriate intervention to help decrease complications from immobility, but it is not a priority over assessment.

**TEST-TAKING HINT:** If the test taker has difficulty in determining the first intervention, the test taker should always rely on the nursing process and select the assessment intervention if the intervention is appropriate for the disease process or condition.

44. 1. The client is at risk for bleeding; therefore, this order would not be questioned.
    2. **Increased pressure in the abdomen secondary to a tap water enema could cause the AAA to rupture.**
    3. The client should be able to ambulate to the bathroom without any problems.
    4. Clients are NPO before surgery to help prevent aspiration or problems from general anesthesia.

**TEST-TAKING HINT:** An expanding AAA should cause the test taker to realize that no additional pressure should be placed on the AAA and that, therefore, selecting option "2" would be the most appropriate answer. Options "1," "3," and "4" would be appropriate for a client scheduled for an AAA repair or most types of surgeries. Remember basic concepts.

45. **Correct answers are 1, 2, and 4.**
    1. **The most common cause of AAA is atherosclerosis, so teaching should address this area.**
    2. **A low-fat, low-cholesterol diet will help decrease the development of atherosclerosis.**
    3. The client should not decrease tobacco use—instead, the client must quit totally. Smoking is the one modifiable risk factor that is not negotiable.
    4. **Losing weight will help decrease the pressure on the AAA and will help address decreasing the cholesterol level.**
    5. A truss is worn by a client diagnosed with a hernia, not an AAA.

**TEST-TAKING HINT:** "Select all that apply" questions are an alternate-type question that requires the nurse to select all interventions that are applicable to the question. The NCLEX-RN® does not give partial credit; the test taker must select all appropriate answers to receive credit for the question.

46. 1. Any neurovascular abnormality in the client's lower extremities indicates the graft is occluded or possibly bleeding and requires immediate intervention by the nurse.
    2. The nurse would expect the client to have incisional pain 6 hours after surgery, so this is not a priority over a complication.
    3. The nurse would expect the client to have a distended, tender abdomen as a result of postoperative edema.
    4. A slightly elevated temperature would not be uncommon in a postsurgical client.

**TEST-TAKING HINT:** Any time the test taker has an answer option that has the word "absent" in it, the test taker should determine if this is normal for any client and, if not, consider it for the correct answer, especially in this case where the stem is asking which information warrants immediate intervention.

47. Correct answers are 1 and 5.
    1. Redness or irritation of the incision indicates an infection and should be reported immediately to the HCP.
    2. The client should not lift anything heavier than 5 pounds because it may cause dehiscence or evisceration of the bowel.
    3. The pain medication should keep the client comfortable; if it doesn't, the client should call the HCP.
    4. Some clients do not have daily bowel movements, but the nurse should instruct the client not to become constipated, which will increase pressure on the incision.
    5. The client should continue to splint the incision with a pillow when coughing or sneezing to protect the incision and to decrease discomfort.

**TEST-TAKING HINT:** The test taker should use basic concepts to answer questions. Clinical manifestations of incisional infection or systemic infection should always be reported to the HCP. Remember, the test taker should not eliminate an option as a possible answer just because it appears too easy an answer.

48. 1. Organs in the right upper quadrant include the liver and gallbladder.
    2. The aorta traverses the abdomen in the midline position, and that is the best location to hear an abdominal bruit.

The bell should be placed midline above the umbilicus to auscultate an abdominal bruit best.
    3. Organs in the left upper quadrant include the stomach, pancreas, and spleen.
    4. Organs in the left lower quadrant are the colon and ovaries in females.

**TEST-TAKING HINT:** There may be questions on the NCLEX-RN® that require the test taker to point to a specific area. The test taker must know correct anatomical positions for body parts and organs.

## Deep Vein Thrombosis

49. Correct answers are 3 and 5.
    1. The client will be taking an oral anticoagulant, warfarin (Coumadin). Prothrombin time (PT/INR) levels, not PTT, are monitored when this medication is taken. The client should be in the therapeutic range before discharge. The HCP will determine how often to monitor the levels, usually in 2 to 3 weeks and then at 3- to 6-month intervals.
    2. The client is not restricted to the home. The client should not take part in any activity that does not allow frequent active and passive leg exercises. In an airplane, the client should be instructed to drink plenty of fluids, move the legs up and down, and flex the muscles. If in an automobile, the client should stop to take frequent breaks to walk around.
    3. Green, leafy vegetables contain vitamin K, which is the antidote for warfarin. These foods will interfere with the action of warfarin. Red or brown urine may indicate bleeding.
    4. The client should be instructed to wear stockings that do not constrict any area of the leg.
    5. Red or brown urine, emesis, or sputum may indicate bleeding.

**TEST-TAKING HINT:** The test taker must know laboratory data for specific medications. The INR and PT are monitored for oral anticoagulants. Remember: "PT boats go to war" (warfarin). PTT monitors heparin ("tt" is like an H for heparin).

50. 1. **A complication of immobility after surgery is developing a DVT. This client diagnosed with left calf pain should be assessed for a DVT.**
    2. This is an expected finding.
    3. Clients requiring an open cholecystectomy frequently are discharged with a T-tube. This client needs to know how to care for the tube before leaving, but this is not a priority over a possible surgical complication.
    4. This is expected for this client.

**TEST-TAKING HINT: In priority-setting questions, the test taker must decide if the information in the answer option is expected or abnormal for the situation. Based on this, options "2," "3," and "4" can be eliminated.**

51. 1. Passive ROM exercises are recommended to prevent contracture formation and muscle atrophy, but this is a musculoskeletal complication, not a cardiovascular one.
    2. If the client is on a ventilator, then the paralysis associated with GB syndrome has moved up the spinal column to include the muscles of respiration. Passive ROM exercises are done by the staff; the client will not be able to do active ROM.
    3. ROM exercises will not alleviate the pain of GB syndrome.
    4. **One reason for performing ROM exercises is to assist the blood vessels in the return of blood to the heart, preventing DVT.**

**TEST-TAKING HINT: The question is asking for a cardiovascular reason for ROM exercises. Options "1," "2," and "3" do not have any cardiovascular component. Only option "4" discusses veins and blood.**

52. 1. This protects the client's privacy.
    2. **The UAP could dislodge a blood clot in the leg when massaging the calf. The UAP can apply lotion gently, being sure not to massage the leg.**
    3. Testing the temperature of the water prevents scalding the client with water that is too hot or making the client uncomfortable with water that is too cold.
    4. Collecting supplies needed before beginning the bath is using time wisely and avoids interrupting the bath to go and get items needed.

**TEST-TAKING HINT: This is an "except" question, so all options except one will be actions that should be encouraged. The test taker should not jump to the first option and choose it as the correct answer.**

53. Correct answers are 2, 3, and 4.
    1. Sequential compression devices provide gentle compression of the legs to prevent DVT, but they are not used to treat DVT because the compressions could cause the clot to break loose.
    2. **Clients should be on bedrest for 5 to 7 days after diagnosis to allow time for the clot to adhere to the vein wall, thereby preventing embolization.**
    3. **Bedrest and limited activity predispose the client to constipation. Fluids and diets high in fiber will help prevent constipation. Fluids will also help provide adequate fluid volume in the vasculature.**
    4. **The client will be administered a heparin IV drip, which should be monitored.**
    5. Homans' sign is assessed to determine if a DVT is present. This client has already been diagnosed with a DVT. Manipulating the leg to determine the presence of Homans' sign could dislodge the clot.

**TEST-TAKING HINT: Two of the answer options are used to determine if a DVT is present or to prevent one. The test taker should not become confused about treatment and prevention or early diagnosis.**

54. 20 mL/hr.
    To determine the rate, the test taker must first determine how many units are in each milliliter of fluid; 25,000 divided by 500 = 50 units of heparin in each milliliter of fluid, and 50 divided into 100 = 2, and 2 + 18 = 20.

**TEST-TAKING HINT: This math question is worked in several steps, but every step is a simple addition or division.**

55. 1. **A potentially life-threatening complication of DVT is a pulmonary embolus, which causes chest pain. The nurse should determine if the client has "thrown" a pulmonary embolus.**
    2. An immobile client should be turned at least every 2 hours, but a pressure area is not life-threatening.
    3. This is expected in a client with a large upper abdominal incision. It hurts to breathe deeply. The nurse should address this but has some time. The life-threatening complication is a priority.
    4. Clients with inguinal hernia repair often have difficulty voiding afterward. This is expected.

**TEST-TAKING HINT: The test taker should determine which option contains information that**

indicates a potentially life-threatening situation. This is the priority client.

56. 1. The nurse should check the laboratory values pertaining to the medications before administering the heparin and warfarin (Coumadin), both anticoagulant medications.
    2. The client will be administered an oral medication while still receiving a heparin drip to allow time for the client to achieve a therapeutic level of the oral medication before discontinuing the heparin. The effects of oral medications take 3 to 5 days to become therapeutic.
    3. The laboratory values should be noted before administering the heparin and warfarin (Coumadin), both anticoagulant medications.
    4. The heparin will be continued for 3 to 5 days before being discontinued.

**TEST-TAKING HINT:** Knowing the actions of each medication, as well as the laboratory tests that monitor the safe range of dosing, is important. Remember, assessment is first. Assess blood levels and then administer the medication.

57. 1. Keeping the legs dependent and standing still will promote the development of a DVT.
    2. Flexing the leg muscles and changing positions assist the blood in returning to the heart and move out of the peripheral vessels.
    3. The nurse should wear support stockings, not socks, and change the types of shoes worn from day to day, varying the type of heels.
    4. This is not in the client's best interest.

**TEST-TAKING HINT:** The test taker can eliminate option "4" by imagining the reaction of the HCP if this were done. The words "dependent" and "still" make option "1" wrong.

58. 1. This occurs from the administration of the LMWH and is not a reason to notify the HCP.
    2. A therapeutic range will not be achieved with LMWH, and PTT levels are usually not done.
    3. This is not hemorrhaging, and the client should be reassured that this is a side effect of the medication.
    4. Assessing the vital signs will not provide any pertinent information to help answer the client's question.

**TEST-TAKING HINT:** Before selecting "Notify the HCP," the test taker should ask, "What will the HCP do with this information? What can the HCP order or do to help the purple hemorrhaged areas?" This would cause the test taker to eliminate option "1" as a possible answer.

59. 1. There is nothing that contraindicates the use of a stool softener, and the use of one may be recommended if the client is prone to constipation and hard stool that could cause some bleeding from hemorrhoids.
    2. A Medic Alert bracelet notifies any emergency HCP of the client's condition and medications.
    3. **Vitamin E can affect the action of warfarin. The nurse should explain to the client that these and other medications could potentiate the action of warfarin.**
    4. This will be recommended for the client if the footrest does not restrict blood flow in the calves.

**TEST-TAKING HINT:** The test taker can eliminate option "1" by realizing that a stool softener would not cause a problem and could help with an unrelated problem. Medic Alert bracelets are frequently recommended for many clients diagnosed with certain diseases and conditions.

60. 1. BUN laboratory tests are measurements of renal functioning.
    2. Bilirubin is a liver function test.
    3. **PT/INR is a test to monitor warfarin (Coumadin), an anticoagulant, action in the body.**
    4. PTT levels monitor heparin activity.

**TEST-TAKING HINT:** The test taker should devise some sort of memory-jogging mnemonic or aid to remember which laboratory test monitors for which condition. Try "PT boats go to war," to recall that PT monitors warfarin.

## Peripheral Venous Disease

61. 1. Venous insufficiency is a venous problem, not an arterial problem.
    2. DVT is not a complication of chronic venous insufficiency, but it may be a cause.
    3. **Venous ulcerations are the most serious complication of chronic venous insufficiency. It is very difficult for these ulcerations to heal, and often clients must be seen in wound care clinics for treatment.**
    4. Varicose veins may lead to chronic venous insufficiency, but they are not a complication.

**TEST-TAKING HINT:** The test taker must use knowledge of anatomy, which would eliminate option "1" because "venous" and "arterial" refer to different parts of the vascular system. The test taker must key in on the most serious complication to select the correct answer.

62. 1. The medial part of the ankle usually ulcerates because of edema that leads to stasis, which, in turn, causes the skin to break down.
    2. A deep, pale, open area over the top side of the foot describes an arterial ulcer.
    3. A reddened, blistered area on the heel describes a blister that may result from wearing shoes that are too tight or that rub on the heel.
    4. Gangrene does not usually occur with venous problems; it occurs with arterial ulcers.

**TEST-TAKING HINT:** There are some questions that require the test taker to be knowledgeable of the disease process.

63. 1. Low-heeled, comfortable shoes should be recommended to help decrease foot pain, but they will not help prevent varicose veins.
    2. Wearing clean white socks will help prevent irritation to the feet, but they will not help prevent varicose veins.
    3. Moving the legs back and forth often may help prevent DVT, but it will not prevent varicose veins.
    4. Graduated compression hose help decrease edema and increase the circulation back to the heart; this helps prevent varicose veins.

**TEST-TAKING HINT:** Options "1" and "2" could be eliminated as possible answers if the test taker knows that the varicose veins are in the leg because options "1" and "2" are addressing the feet.

64. 1. Varicose veins are irregular, tortuous veins with incompetent valves that do not allow the venous blood to ascend the saphenous vein.
    2. Decreased oxygen to the muscle occurs with arterial occlusive disease.
    3. This is the explanation for a DVT.
    4. Thick, poorly circulating blood could be an explanation for diabetic neuropathy.

**TEST-TAKING HINT:** Knowing that veins have valves and arteries do not might help the test taker select the correct answer. The test taker should use knowledge of anatomy and physiology to determine the answer.

65. 1. The client should not cross the legs at all because this further **impedes** the blood from ascending the saphenous vein.
    2. Elevating the foot of the bed while sleeping helps the venous blood return to the heart and decreases pressure in the lower extremity.
    3. Antiplatelet therapy, low-dose acetylsalicylic acid (baby aspirin), is for arterial blood, not venous blood.
    4. Fluid intake will not help prevent or improve chronic venous insufficiency.

**TEST-TAKING HINT:** Knowing about the venous and arterial blood systems will help the test taker eliminate or identify the correct answer. Venous blood goes back to the heart, so elevating the feet will help return it. Options "3" and "4" do not have anything to do with the extremities.

66. 1. Research shows that removing the compression stockings while the client is in bed promotes perfusion of the subcutaneous tissue. The foot of the bed should be elevated.
    2. The UAP can take the BP with a machine or manually; therefore, the nurse would not need to intervene.
    3. The UAP can help the client with meals as long as the client is stable.
    4. The UAP can calculate the intake and output, but the nurse must evaluate the data to determine if they are normal for the client.

**TEST-TAKING HINT:** This is a backward "except" question. Flipping the question and asking which actions would be appropriate for the UAP to implement might make it easier for the test taker to answer the question.

67. 1. The occupational therapist assists the client with activities of daily living skills, such as eating, bathing, or brushing teeth.
    2. The social worker would assess the client to determine if home health-care services or financial interventions were appropriate for the client. The client is older, immobility is a concern, and wound care must be a concern when the client is discharged home.
    3. The physical therapist addresses gait training and transferring.
    4. Cardiac rehabilitation helps clients after myocardial infarctions, cardiac bypass surgery, or congestive heart failure recover.

**TEST-TAKING HINT:** The test taker must be aware of the responsibilities of other members of the health-care team. "Discharge" is the keyword in the stem. The test taker should select an answer that will help the client in the home.

68. 1. Pedal pulses are normal in venous insufficiency, but pulses are decreased or absent in arterial insufficiency.
    2. The skin is warm in venous insufficiency; the skin is cool in arterial insufficiency.
    3. Intermittent claudication, pain that occurs when walking, is a symptom of arterial insufficiency.
    4. Chronic venous insufficiency leads to chronic edema that, in turn, causes a brownish pigmentation to the skin.

**TEST-TAKING HINT:** The test taker could apply anatomical concepts to eliminate both options "1" and "2" because it is the arteries that have pulses and control the temperature of the skin.

69. 1. Varicose veins are more common in females, Hispanic ethnicity, increasing age, obesity, and in occupations that involve prolonged standing or sitting.
    2. Driving a bus requires prolonged sitting, which is a risk factor for developing varicose veins, but women are more prone to developing varicose veins.
    3. Studies suggest that the increased risk for varicose veins is common during pregnancy and may be the result of venous stasis.
    4. Diabetes may lead to diabetic neuropathy and arterial occlusive disease, but it does not lead to varicose veins.

**TEST-TAKING HINT:** The test taker must know that prolonged standing or sitting, occupations that have people on their feet for long periods of time, female sex, Hispanic ethnicity, increasing age, and obesity are risk factors for varicose veins.

70. 1. Because the saphenous vein is removed during vein ligation, standing and sitting are prohibited during the initial recovery period to prevent increased pressure in the lower extremities.
    2. Pressure bandages are applied for up to 6 weeks after vein ligation to help prevent bleeding and to help venous return from the lower extremities when in the standing or sitting position.
    3. Sequential compression devices are used to help prevent DVT.
    4. Antibiotics would be ordered prophylactically for surgery, but it is not the first intervention.

**TEST-TAKING HINT:** When the question asks the test taker to implement the first intervention, two or more of the answer options could be possible interventions, but only one is implemented first. Apply the nursing process and select the intervention that addresses assessment, which is the first part of the nursing process.

71. 1. The client diagnosed with a venous stasis ulcer should have pain, so this would be expected.
    2. Dull, aching muscle cramps are expected with varicose veins.
    3. The inability to move the foot means that a severe neurovascular compromise has occurred, and the nurse should assess this client first.
    4. A positive Homans' sign is expected in a client diagnosed with DVT.

**TEST-TAKING HINT:** The nurse should first assess the client experiencing an abnormal, unexpected, or life-threatening complication of the disease process. Do not automatically select the client diagnosed with pain; pain in many instances is not life-threatening or unexpected.

72. Correct answers are 1, 2, 3, 4, and 5.
    1. The nurse should determine if the client has any numbness or tingling.
    2. The nurse should determine if the client has pulses, the presence of which indicates there is no circulatory compromise.
    3. The nurse should determine if the client can move the feet and legs.
    4. The nurse should determine if the client's feet are pink or pale.
    5. The nurse should assess the feet to determine if they are cold or warm.

**TEST-TAKING HINT:** These five assessment interventions, along with assessing for pain, are known as the 6 Ps, which is the neurovascular assessment.

73. 1. Bright red tissue indicates an arterial problem.
    2. **Purplish-brown areas on the skin indicate venous stasis of the blood in the legs.**
    3. This indicates arterial occlusive disease.
    4. This could indicate diabetic foot ulcers but does not mean venous problems.

**TEST-TAKING HINT: The test taker should apply pathophysiology knowledge to answer this question. Venous blood is darker than arterial blood, which is a brighter red.**

74. 1. Brown-purple discoloration on the calf indicates a venous insufficiency issue, not a clot.
    2. Bright red skin on the lower legs indicates an arterial issue, not a clot.
    3. **A clot disrupts the blood flow; swelling and warmth, along with pain, indicate a potential blood clot.**
    4. Pain after walking for short distances that resolves with rest indicates peripheral arterial disease, usually caused by the narrowing of the arteries as a result of atherosclerosis.

**TEST-TAKING HINT: The test taker should apply pathophysiology knowledge to answer this question. Venous blood is returning to the heart to pick up oxygen from the lungs and be redistributed to the body, making it a bright red color; oxygen in the blood makes the blood bright red. This could eliminate both options "1" and "2."**

75. 1. The client is in the therapeutic range for intravenous heparin; the nurse has no reason to ask for a change of medication.
    2. Heparin is administered based on the activated PTT results; phytonadione (Aqua-Mephyton or vitamin K) is the antidote for warfarin (Coumadin).
    3. Limiting green, leafy vegetables applies to warfarin, not heparin, and all green, leafy vegetables are not prohibited. The client should consume a consistent amount of green, leafy vegetables in order for the INR levels to maintain a therapeutic range.
    4. **The client is in the therapeutic range for intravenous heparin; the nurse should administer the heparin as ordered.**

**TEST-TAKING HINT: The test taker should be aware of therapeutic levels as they apply to commonly administered medications. This will allow the test taker to make decisions as to the appropriate nursing actions to implement.**

76. 1. **The UAP has informed the nurse that a client is having chest pain. A DVT can break loose and become an embolism, which can cause life-threatening problems for the client.**
    2. The BP is within normal limits (WNL).
    3. This is not an unusual request, and the nurse should discuss the need for limited activity, but it does not require immediate intervention.
    4. A headache is not life-threatening. It does not require immediate intervention.

**TEST-TAKING HINT: The test taker should consider which could be the most serious of the situations listed for the client. This is the one that requires immediate intervention.**

77. 1. Auscultation of heart and lung sounds is part of a full assessment, but the first action is to focus on the client's chief concern; the results of this assessment will guide the remainder of the nurse's actions.
    2. The length of the trip is implicated in the client developing a blood clot because of the lower moisture content in the air being breathed and the lack of movement of the lower extremities during the flight; however, if the client has developed a clot, then that is the issue now.
    3. If the client had experienced chest pain, that would have been the chief concern; the nurse needs to assess the client for a DVT.
    4. **Measuring the client's calf and assessing for warmth are part of a focused assessment for DVT, for which the flight placed the client at risk.**

**TEST-TAKING HINT: The test taker should apply decision-making questions when determining which to do first. One such question is, Which option will give the nurse the most needed information the fastest? The nurse should acquire information that will eliminate or support the suspected diagnosis.**

78. 1. The nurse must complete the assessment before notifying the HCP.
    2. This can be done, but most clients cannot provide a stool sample immediately.
    3. The timing is not important at this time; the client has been taking the rivaroxaban (Xarelto), an anticoagulant.
    4. Ecchymotic areas (bruising) indicate bleeding; the nurse should determine the extent of the client's bleeding before notifying the HCP.

**TEST-TAKING HINT:** When answering a question and the test taker wishes to choose "notify the HCP," the test taker should read all the options carefully; if any option has needed information to report to the HCP, then that option comes before notifying the HCP.

79. 1. Isometric exercises are "pumping iron" or body-building exercises. Isotonic exercises are what the nurse teaches the client to perform.
    2. A stair stepper places considerable requirements for lower body strength on the client. The client diagnosed with peripheral arterial disease may not have the ability to use this machine.
    3. Warm-up exercises are needed to prevent injury to the client.
    4. The client should walk as the preferred form of exercise; the shoes should fit the client without causing blisters, and walking on level ground decreases the risk of injury or excessive stress on the muscles.

**TEST-TAKING HINT:** The test taker could eliminate option "1" if aware of the definition of isometric; the test taker must be knowledgeable regarding medical terminology.

80. Correct answers are 1, 2, 4, and 5.
    1. Green, leafy vegetables contain vitamin K, which is the antidote for warfarin; when achieving a therapeutic range for the INR, a change in the consumption of green, leafy vegetables will change the anticoagulant effects on the body.
    2. The INR is the level that the HCP will use to gauge the anticoagulant effects occurring in the body and should be monitored regularly.
    3. The nurse should teach the client to apply pressure on any bleeding for 5 minutes to see if a minor cut will stop bleeding on its own. The client should not go to the hospital unless bleeding cannot be stopped.
    4. Dark, tarry stools indicate upper GI bleeding, and the HCP should be informed.

    5. The client should carry information describing the client's medication regimen and inform any HCPs before lab tests, procedures, or surgery.
    6. Iron does not prevent bleeding.

**TEST-TAKING HINT:** When answering a "Select all that apply" question, the test taker should read each option as a true or false option. If the option is true, then the test taker should choose it. All of the options may be correct or only one may be.

81. 1. Gastric upset is not an issue for a client receiving anticoagulant therapy.
    2. Anticoagulant therapy reduces the client's ability to form clots; bleeding is the most important issue to discuss with the client.
    3. Constipation is not caused by anticoagulant therapy.
    4. Myocardial infarction is not caused by anticoagulant therapy, but it could be prevented by it.

**TEST-TAKING HINT:** When answering questions about medications, the nurse must be aware of common instructions. In the case of any medication that involves changing the body's ability to form a clot, bleeding must always be an issue.

82. 1. Clients diagnosed with hypertension must have had a BP of 140/90 on three separate occasions unless the client has diabetes, and the BP reading is 135/85. The numbers may reach much higher levels. Over 160 systolic and 90 to 95 diastolic places the client at risk for cardiovascular events. The client's BP should be controlled according to the HCP instructions but 120/80 is not a realistic goal.
    2. Many clients decide that because they do not feel ill, medication is not needed. Hypertension is called the silent killer because damage to the body can occur without the client realizing it.
    3. The client should be taught to rise slowly from a recumbent position to prevent dizziness and falls.
    4. The client should limit sodium in the diet to less than 2,300 mg/day (American Heart Association, 2018).

**TEST-TAKING HINT:** The test taker should be aware of commonly administered medications and which instructions apply. This will allow the test taker to make decisions as to the appropriate nursing actions to implement.

**83.** Correct answers are 1, 2, 3, and 4.
   1. Elevating the legs will assist the blood in returning to the heart.
   2. Antiembolism stockings compress the veins and prevent stasis in the legs.
   3. The circulation in the legs is compromised. Injuries will take longer to heal.
   4. Trimming the toenails straight across prevents ingrown toenails.
   5. The client may apply moisturizer to the legs.
   6. The legs being in a dependent position applies to clients diagnosed with peripheral arterial disease. This assists the arterial flow to the feet. The problem with venous stasis is getting the blood back to the heart; the feet should be elevated.

**TEST-TAKING HINT:** When answering a "Select all that apply" question, the test taker should read each option as a true or false option. If the option is true, then the test taker should choose it. All of the options may be correct or only one may be. By knowing the pathophysiology of blood circulation, the test taker can choose option "1" because venous circulation is returning blood to the heart. The test taker could eliminate option "6" because it is the opposite of option "1."

**84.** 1. These clinical manifestations could indicate a pulmonary embolus. The nurse should not leave the client but should get help as soon as possible. The rules of the RRT are that anyone can call an RRT if a concern is noted, and no one will suffer consequences if one was called and it was determined that the client was not in serious danger.
   2. The nurse's first action is to stay with the client and call for help.
   3. The UAP cannot be assigned an unstable client.
   4. The telemetry reading is not important in regard to the current clinical manifestations.

**TEST-TAKING HINT:** Remember, "if in distress, do not assess"; the nurse must implement an intervention that will directly affect the client outcome.

**85.** 1. Clopidogrel (Plavix) is an arterial antiplatelet that prevents clots from occurring in the lower extremity arteries.
   2. Streptokinase is an enzyme that breaks down existing clots, a "clot buster."
   3. Protamine sulfate is the antidote for heparin.

   4. Enoxaparin (Lovenox) is a subcutaneous LMWH and not usually administered for peripheral arterial disease.

**TEST-TAKING HINT:** The test taker should be aware of commonly administered medications and which instructions apply. This will allow the test taker to make decisions as to the appropriate nursing actions to implement.

**86.** 1. The client should occasionally monitor his BP but not four times a day.
   2. Antihypertensive medications do not have established therapeutic blood levels.
   3. Antihypertensive medications can cause a drop in the BP when the client changes positions from a sitting or lying position to an upright position because of gravity and relaxed blood vessels. This is orthostatic hypotension; the blood vessels will adjust if the client rises slowly or sits on the side of the bed for a short time.
   4. Blood glucose meters measure glucose levels, which is not what should be monitored for hypertension.

**TEST-TAKING HINT:** The test taker should be aware of commonly administered medications and which instructions apply. This will allow the test taker to make decisions as to the appropriate nursing actions to implement.

**87.** Correct answers are 1, 2, 3, 4, and 5.
   1. BP readings measure arterial pressures; the cuff should be placed so the pressure in an artery can be read.
   2. The client should be instructed as to when to notify the HCP. BP readings over 160 systolic or 100 diastolic indicate the BP is not controlled, and the medication regimen might need to be adjusted.
   3. Antihypertensive medications can cause a drop in the BP when the client changes from a sitting or lying position to an upright position because of gravity and relaxed blood vessels. This is orthostatic hypotension; the blood vessels will adjust if the client rises slowly or sits on the side of the bed for a short time.
   4. A record of the BP reading obtained by the client can assist the HCP in planning the suggested regimen.
   5. Many clients decide that if they are WNL, the medication is no longer needed. The client should understand if the readings are WNL, it is because of the medication, and stopping the medication will stop the desired effect.

**TEST-TAKING HINT:** The test taker should be aware of commonly administered medications and which instructions apply. This will allow the test taker to make decisions as to the appropriate nursing actions to implement.

88. **15 mL per hour.** The nurse must first determine how many units are in each milliliter of fluid. $40,000 \div 500$ mL = 80 units per milliliter. Next, the nurse must determine how many milliliter should be administered each hour: $1200 \div 80 = 15$ mL per hour.

**TEST-TAKING HINT:** The test taker should be aware of common mathematical equations in order to administer the correct dose of medication.

89. 1. The usual guideline is to keep the BP to less than 160/100; 140/90 is the low number to diagnose hypertension.
    2. This will improve cardiovascular fitness but will not directly cause an increase in atherosclerosis.
    3. This will allow the client to monitor the BP but does not reduce the risk of an MI.
    4. Atherosclerosis is caused by plaque buildup in the arteries. Plaque is primarily caused by fat in the diet compounded by clotting mechanisms.

**TEST-TAKING HINT:** The test taker must be aware of the recommended treatment for the prevention of the problems associated with disease processes in order to teach the client about the disease.

90. **Correct answers are 2, 3, and 5.**
    1. Type 2 HIT is an immune-mediated disorder that typically occurs after exposure to heparin for 4 to 10 days and has life-threatening and limb-threatening thrombotic complications. The client clots rather than bleeds. Spontaneous bleeding is not associated with HIT.
    2. HIT is not manifested by bleeding but by the development of clots, either deep venous or pulmonary, and sometimes arterially, which can cause a myocardial infarction. These are symptoms of a pulmonary embolus.
    3. HIT is a decrease in baseline platelet count by 50% of baseline.
    4. Bleeding is not associated with HIT.
    5. Clinically, HIT may manifest itself as skin lesions at the site of heparin injections or chills, fever, dyspnea, or chest pain.

**TEST-TAKING HINT:** The test taker must remember diseases and syndromes that do not match with the general picture of what is occurring. In HIT, the thrombocytopenia is not associated with bleeding but rather with clotting. This could eliminate options "1" and "4" because both are options indicating the client is bleeding.

# PERIPHERAL VASCULAR DISORDERS COMPREHENSIVE EXAMINATION

1. Which client behavior would be a **causative factor** for developing thromboangiitis obliterans (Buerger's disease)?
   1. Drinking alcohol daily.
   2. Eating a high-fat diet.
   3. Chewing tobacco.
   4. Inhaling gasoline fumes.

2. Which clinical manifestation would the nurse expect to find when assessing a client diagnosed with subclavian steal syndrome?
   1. Reports of arm tiredness with exertion.
   2. Reports of shortness of breath while resting.
   3. Jugular vein distention when sitting at a 35-degree angle.
   4. Dilated blood vessels above the nipple line.

3. Which question should the nurse ask the male client diagnosed with aortoiliac disease during the admission interview?
   1. "Do you have trouble sitting for long periods of time?"
   2. "How often do you have a bowel movement and urinate?"
   3. "When you lie down, do you feel throbbing in your abdomen?"
   4. "Have you experienced any problems having sexual intercourse?"

4. The client is 4 hours postoperative AAA repair. Which nursing intervention should be implemented for this client?
   1. Assist the client to ambulate.
   2. Assess the client's bilateral pedal pulses.
   3. Maintain a continuous IV heparin drip.
   4. Provide a clear liquid diet to the client.

5. Which referral would be **most appropriate** for the client newly diagnosed with thoracic outlet syndrome?
   1. The physical therapist.
   2. The thoracic surgeon.
   3. The occupational therapist.
   4. The social worker.

6. Which instructions should the nurse discuss with the client diagnosed with Raynaud's phenomenon? **Select all that apply.**
   1. Explain exacerbations will not occur in the summer.
   2. Use nicotine gum to help quit smoking.

   3. Wear extra-warm clothing during cold exposure.
   4. Avoid prolonged exposure to direct sunlight.
   5. Practice relaxation techniques to reduce stress.

7. The client diagnosed with diabetes mellitus type 2 is admitted to the hospital with cellulitis of the right foot secondary to an insect bite. Which intervention should the nurse implement **first?**
   1. Administer intravenous antibiotics.
   2. Apply warm moist packs every 2 hours.
   3. Elevate the right foot on two pillows.
   4. Teach the client about skin and foot care.

8. Which discharge instructions should the nurse discuss with the client to **prevent** recurrent episodes of cellulitis? **Select all that apply.**
   1. Soak your feet daily in Epsom salts for 20 minutes.
   2. Wear thick white socks when working in the yard.
   3. Use a mosquito repellent when going outside.
   4. Inspect the feet between the toes for cracks in the skin.
   5. Apply moisturizers to skin daily.

9. Which discharge instruction should the nurse teach the client diagnosed with varicose veins receiving sclerotherapy?
   1. Walk 15 to 20 minutes three times a day.
   2. Keep the legs in the dependent position when sitting.
   3. Remove compression bandages before going to bed.
   4. Perform Buerger-Allen exercises four times a day.

10. The nurse is teaching the client diagnosed with peripheral vascular disease. Which interventions should the nurse discuss with the client? **Select all that apply.**
    1. Wash your feet in antimicrobial soap.
    2. Wear comfortable, well-fitting shoes.
    3. Cut your toenails in an arch.
    4. Keep the area between the toes dry.
    5. Use a heating pad when feet are cold.

11. The UAP is applying elastic compression stockings to the client. Which action by the UAP would **warrant immediate** intervention by the RN?
    1. The UAP is putting the stockings on while the client is in the chair.
    2. The UAP inserted two fingers under the proximal end of the stocking.
    3. The UAP elevated the feet while lying down before putting on the stockings.
    4. The UAP made sure the toes were warm after putting the stockings on.

12. The nurse is administering a beta blocker to the client diagnosed with essential hypertension. Which data would cause the nurse to **question** administering the medication?
    1. The client's BP is 110/70.
    2. The client's potassium level is 3.4 mEq/L.
    3. The client has a barky cough.
    4. The client's apical pulse is 56.

13. The client diagnosed with acute DVT is receiving a continuous heparin drip. The HCP orders warfarin. Which action should the nurse take?
    1. Discontinue the heparin drip before initiating the warfarin.
    2. Check the client's INR before beginning warfarin.
    3. Clarify the order with the HCP as soon as possible.
    4. Administer the warfarin along with the heparin drip as ordered.

14. The nurse is caring for the client on strict bedrest. Which intervention is a **priority** when caring for this client?
    1. Encourage the client to drink liquids.
    2. Perform active ROM exercises.
    3. Elevate the head of the bed to 45 degrees.
    4. Provide a high-fiber diet to the client.

15. The nurse is caring for clients on the medical floor. Which client will the nurse assess **first**?
    1. The client diagnosed with an AAA and is constipated.
    2. The client on bedrest and ambulated to the bathroom.
    3. The client diagnosed with essential hypertension having epistaxis and a headache.
    4. The client diagnosed with peripheral arterial disease and a decreased pedal pulse.

16. The client diagnosed with peripheral venous disease is scheduled to go to the whirlpool for a dressing change. Which is the nurse's **priority** intervention?
    1. Escort the client to the physical therapy department.
    2. Medicate the client 30 minutes before going to the whirlpool.

3. Obtain sterile dressing supplies for the client.
4. Assist the client to the bathroom before the treatment.

17. The client is receiving prophylactic LMWH. There are no PT/PTT or INR results in the client's electronic health record since admission 3 days ago. Which action should the nurse implement?
    1. Administer the medication as ordered.
    2. Notify the health-care provider immediately.
    3. Obtain the PT/PTT and INR before administering the medication.
    4. Hold the medication until the HCP makes rounds.

18. The client diagnosed with atherosclerosis asks the nurse, "I have heard of atherosclerosis for many years, but I never really knew what it meant. Am I going to die?" Which statement would be the nurse's **best response**?
    1. "This disease process will not kill you, so don't worry."
    2. "The blood supply to your brain is being cut off."
    3. "It is what caused you to have your high BP."
    4. "Atherosclerosis is a buildup of plaque in your arteries."

19. Which clinical manifestations would the nurse expect to find in the female client diagnosed with Marfan's syndrome?
    1. Xerostomia, dry eyes, and reports of a dry vagina.
    2. A triad of arthritis, conjunctivitis, and urethritis.
    3. Very tall stature and long bones in the hands and feet.
    4. Spinal deformities of the vertebral column and malaise.

20. The nurse is preparing to administer 7.5 mg of an oral anticoagulant. The medication available is 5 mg per tablet. How many tablets should the nurse administer?

    _____

21. Which dietary selection indicates the client diagnosed with essential hypertension **understands** the discharge teaching?
    1. Fried pork chops, a loaded baked potato, and coffee.
    2. Spaghetti and meatballs, garlic bread, and iced tea.
    3. Baked ham, macaroni and cheese, and milk.
    4. Broiled fish, steamed broccoli, and garden salad.

22. The client diagnosed with thromboangiitis obliterans (Buerger's disease) asks the nurse, "What is the worst thing that could happen if I don't quit smoking? I love my cigarettes." Which statement is the nurse's **best response**?
    1. "You are concerned about quitting smoking. Let's sit down and talk about it."
    2. "Many clients end up having to have an amputation, especially a leg."
    3. "You should consider attending a smoking cessation program."
    4. "Your coronary arteries could block and cause a heart attack."

23. The client diagnosed with subclavian steal syndrome has undergone surgery. Which assessment data would **warrant immediate** intervention by the nurse?
    1. The client's pedal pulse on the left leg is absent.
    2. The client reports numbness in the right hand.
    3. The client's brachial pulse is strong and bounding.
    4. The client's capillary refill time (CRT) is less than 3 seconds.

24. The client with a left-sided mastectomy is diagnosed with elephantiasis of the left arm. Which clinical manifestations should the nurse expect to assess? **Select all that apply.**
    1. Edematous arm from the axillary area to the fingertips.
    2. Painful, edematous, reddened lower forearm.
    3. Tented skin turgor over the entire left arm.
    4. Nipple retraction and *peau d'orange* skin.
    5. Dry, thickened left arm with pebbly appearance.

25. The client is 4 hours postoperative femoral-popliteal bypass surgery. Which pulse would be **best** for the nurse to assess for complications related to an occluded vessel?

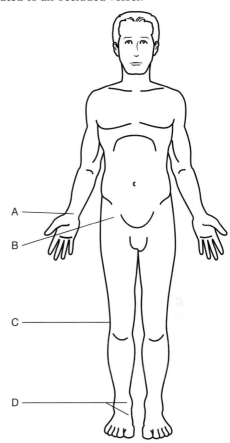

    1. A
    2. B
    3. C
    4. D

26. The client admitted with a diagnosis of pneumonia reports tenderness and pain in the left calf, and the nurse assesses a positive Homans' sign. Which interventions should the nurse implement? **Rank in order of priority.**
    1. Notify the health-care provider.
    2. Initiate an intravenous line.
    3. Monitor the client's PTT.
    4. Administer a continuous heparin infusion.
    5. Instruct the client not to get out of the bed.

27. The nurse is caring for clients on a medical-surgical floor. Which information **warrants immediate** investigation?

1.

### Intake and Output Record

| Day 1 | Oral (oz) | Intravenous (mL) | Urine (mL) | Nasogastric Tube (mL) | Other (Specify) (mL) |
|---|---|---|---|---|---|
| 0701–1900 | 3,600 | 2,575 | 3,000 | | |
| 1901–0700 | 1,380 | 3,500 | 1,270 | | |
| Total | 4,980 | 6,075 | 4,270 | | |

2.

### Intake and Output Record

| Day 1 | Oral (oz) | Intravenous (mL) | Urine (mL) | Nasogastric Tube (mL) | Other (Specify) (mL) |
|---|---|---|---|---|---|
| 0701–1900 | 700 | 1,650 | 2,700 | 200 | |
| 1901–0700 | 700 | 1000 | 1,800 | 0 | |
| Total | 1,400 | 2,650 | 4,500 | 200 | |

3.

### Intake and Output Record

| Day 1 | Oral (oz) | Intravenous (mL) | Urine (mL) | Nasogastric Tube (mL) | Other (Specify) (mL) |
|---|---|---|---|---|---|
| 0701–1900 | 1,000 | 1,500 | 2,350 | | JP drain 64 |
| 1901–0700 | 750 | 1,500 | 1600 | | 44 |
| Total | 1,750 | 3,000 | 3,950 | | 108 |

4.

### Intake and Output Record

| Day 1 | Oral (oz) | Intravenous (mL) | Urine (mL) | Nasogastric Tube (mL) | Other (Specify) (mL) |
|---|---|---|---|---|---|
| 0701–1900 | 1,320 | 150 | 1,600 | | |
| 1901–0700 | 697 | 100 | 785 | | |
| Total | 2,017 | 250 | 2,385 | | |

1. 1. Drinking alcohol on a daily basis is not a cause of thromboangiitis obliterans (Buerger's disease).
   2. Eating a high-fat diet is not a cause of thromboangiitis obliterans (Buerger's disease).
   3. **Heavy smoking or chewing tobacco is a causative or an aggravating factor for thromboangiitis obliterans (Buerger's disease). Cessation of tobacco use may cause cessation of the disease process in some clients.**
   4. Inhaling gasoline fumes is not a cause of thromboangiitis obliterans (Buerger's disease); however, this can cause neurological damage.

2. 1. **Subclavian steal syndrome occurs in the upper extremities from a subclavian artery occlusion or stenosis, which causes arm tiredness, paresthesia, and exercise-induced pain in the forearm when the arms are elevated. This is also known as upper extremity arterial occlusive disease (Shaikh, O'Leary, & Bajwa, 2015).**
   2. Shortness of breath could be a clinical manifestation of a variety of diseases, including heart failure, pneumonia, or chronic obstructive pulmonary disease.
   3. Jugular vein distention could indicate heart failure.
   4. Dilated vessels above the nipple line are a clinical manifestation of superior vena cava syndrome, an oncologic emergency.

3. 1. The client would not experience problems sitting; walking causes the pain.
   2. The client does not have elimination dysfunction.
   3. This would indicate an AAA but not an aortoiliac problem.
   4. **Aortoiliac disease, also known as aortoiliac occlusive disease, is caused by atherosclerosis of the aortoiliac arch, which causes fatigue, cramping, or pain in the lower back and buttocks, and impotence in men (Vallabhaneni, n.d.).**

4. 1. At 4 hours postoperative, the client would not be able to ambulate and would be in the intensive care department. The client usually ambulates the first day postoperatively.
   2. **A neurovascular assessment is a priority to make sure the graft is perfusing the lower extremities.**
   3. Intravenous anticoagulant therapy would cause the client to bleed postoperatively. Prophylactic anticoagulant therapy may be ordered to help prevent DVT.
   4. The client will be NPO and have a nasogastric tube for at least 24 hours.

5. 1. **Thoracic outlet syndrome is a compression of the subclavian artery at the thoracic outlet by an anatomical structure such as a rib or muscle. Physical therapy, exercises, and avoiding aggravating positions are recommended treatments.**
   2. The nurse does not refer to a surgeon when newly diagnosed. Surgery is rare.
   3. The occupational therapist helps with activities of daily living and cognitive disorders that do not occur with this syndrome.
   4. The social worker would not need to be consulted for a client diagnosed with this syndrome.

6. Correct answers are 3 and 5.
   1. During the summer, a sweater **should** be available when entering an air-conditioned room.
   2. Nicotine of any type causes vasoconstriction and may induce attacks.
   3. **Raynaud's phenomenon is a form of intermittent arteriolar vasoconstriction that results in coldness, pain, and pallor of fingertips or toes; therefore, the client should keep warm to prevent vasoconstriction of the extremities.**
   4. Sunlight does not cause an exacerbation of this disease.
   5. **Stress can cause an exacerbation of Raynaud's phenomenon, and the client should be encouraged to use relaxation techniques to reduce stress.**

7. 1. This would be an appropriate intervention but not before elevating the foot.
   2. Warm, moist packs cause necessary dilation, but it is not the first intervention.
   3. **Elevating the foot above the heart will decrease edema and thereby help decrease the pain. It is the easiest and first intervention for the nurse to implement.**
   4. Educating the client is important, but it is not the first intervention. The client will be hospitalized for several days.

8. **Correct answers are 4 and 5.**
   1. Soaking the feet will not help prevent cellulitis; salt would be drying to the tissue, causing cracks that may lead to cellulitis.
   2. Thick white socks do not prevent cellulitis.
   3. Mosquito repellent would help to prevent encephalitis but not cellulitis.
   4. **The key to preventing cellulitis is by identifying the sites of bacterial entry. The most commonly overlooked areas are the cracks and fissures that occur between the toes.**
   5. **Moisturizers applied to the skin daily is one of the best nonantibiotic interventions for the prevention of cellulitis (Teasdale et al., 2019).**

9. 1. After sclerotherapy, clients are taught to perform walking activities to maintain blood flow in the leg and enhance the dilution of the sclerosing agent.
   2. The legs should be elevated to decrease edema. The legs should not be below the level of the heart, which is the dependent position.
   3. The compression bandages should be kept on at all times for at least 5 days or until the HCP removes them for the first time.
   4. These exercises are recommended for clients diagnosed with peripheral arterial disease, not a venous disease.

10. **Correct answers are 2 and 4.**
    1. Antimicrobial soap is harsh and can dry the skin; the client should use mild soap and room-temperature water.
    2. **Shoes must be comfortable to prevent blisters or ulcerations of the feet.**
    3. The toenails should be cut straight across; cutting in an arch increases the risk for ingrown toenails.
    4. **Moisture between the toes increases fungal growth, leading to skin breakdown.**

5. The client diagnosed with PVD has decreased sensation in the feet and should not use a heating pad.

11. 1. **Stockings should be applied after the legs have been elevated for a period of time when the amount of blood in the leg veins is at its lowest; therefore, the nurse should intervene when the UAP is putting them on while the client is in the chair.**
    2. The top of the stocking should not be tight; being able to insert two fingers indicates it is not too tight.
    3. This is the correct way to apply stockings.
    4. Warm toes mean the stockings are not too tight and that there is adequate circulation.

12. 1. This BP indicates the medication is effective and in the desired range, and the nurse should not question administering the medication.
    2. This potassium level is low, but a beta blocker does not affect the potassium level.
    3. A barky cough is associated with an ACE inhibitor, not a beta blocker.
    4. **The beta blocker decreases sympathetic stimulation to the beta cells of the heart. Therefore, the nurse should question administering the medication if the apical pulse is less than 60 beats per minute.**

13. 1. This is an inappropriate intervention.
    2. The INR is checked to determine if the medication is within the therapeutic range, not before administering the first dose.
    3. The order does not need to be clarified.
    4. **It will require several days for the oral anticoagulant, warfarin (Coumadin), to reach therapeutic levels; the client will continue receiving the intravenous anticoagulant, heparin drip until the therapeutic range can be attained.**

14. 1. Fluids will help prevent dehydration and renal calculi, but this is not the priority nursing intervention.
    2. **Preventing DVT is the priority nursing intervention because the client is on strict bedrest; ROM exercises should be done every 4 hours.**
    3. Elevating the head of the bed will not help prevent immobility complications.
    4. High-fiber diets will help prevent constipation, but this is not a priority.

15. 1. This is not a priority unless the client is actively having a bowel movement and is performing the Valsalva maneuver.
    2. This client needs to be addressed, and orders need to be clarified, but this is not a priority.
    3. **A bloody nose and a headache indicate the client is experiencing very high BP and should be assessed first because of a possible myocardial infarction or stroke.**
    4. A decreased pedal pulse is expected in this client.

16. 1. The physical therapy department comes and gets the client; if not, the UAP should escort the client to physical therapy.
    2. **The client's pain is a priority, and the nurse should premedicate before treatment.**
    3. The physical therapy department will have the supplies for dressing the wound.
    4. This could be done, but it is not a priority for the nurse.

17. 1. **Subcutaneous LMWH will not achieve a therapeutic level because of the short half-life of the medication; therefore, the nurse should administer the medication.**
    2. There is no need to notify the HCP.
    3. There is no need to monitor these laboratory tests.
    4. There is no need to notify the HCP.

18. 1. This is not a true statement. Atherosclerosis causes strokes, heart attacks, and hypertension, which are all possibly lethal diseases.
    2. This may occur, but it does not answer the client's question.
    3. This may occur, but it does not answer the client's question.
    4. **A buildup of plaque in the arteries is occurring in the body when the client has atherosclerosis. The nurse cannot tell the client atherosclerosis will lead to death because there are many other things that could cause the client's death. The statement does inform the client what atherosclerosis is.**

19. 1. Xerostomia, dry eyes, and dry vagina are symptoms of Sjögren's syndrome.
    2. A triad of arthritis, conjunctivitis, and urethritis are symptoms of Reiter's syndrome.
    3. Clients diagnosed with Marfan's syndrome are very tall and have long bones in the hands and feet. They also have abnormalities of the cardiovascular system, resulting in valvular problems and aneurysms, which are the leading cause of death during the late 20s.
    4. Spinal deformities and malaise are symptoms of ankylosing spondylitis.

20. **1.5 tablets.**
    The nurse must score and divide one tablet and administer one and a half tablets to ensure that the correct dose is administered.

21. 1. Fried foods have a lot of grease, a loaded baked potato is high in fat, and coffee has caffeine. This is a high-calorie, high-sodium diet that is not recommended.
    2. Spaghetti is high in carbohydrates, meat is high in fat, garlic bread is high in carbohydrates, and iced tea has caffeine.
    3. Ham is cured meat and is high in sodium, but many clients do not realize this; cheese and milk are high in sodium.
    4. **The client should be eating a low-fat, low-cholesterol, low-sodium diet. This meal reflects this diet.**

22. 1. This is a therapeutic response and does not answer the client's question.
    2. **Smoking aggravates Buerger's disease. Aggravated or severe Buerger's disease can lead to arterial occlusion caused by superficial thrombophlebitis, resulting in poor wound healing and poor circulation. This can lead to the need for amputation.**
    3. This is an appropriate referral, but it does not answer the question.
    4. Buerger's disease affects the arteries and veins of the upper and lower extremities, but it does not affect the coronary arteries.

23. 1. Subclavian steal syndrome affects the upper extremities only.
    2. **Subclavian steal syndrome occurs in the upper extremities from a subclavian artery occlusion or stenosis; therefore, any abnormal neurovascular assessment would warrant intervention.**
    3. This is a normal finding and would not warrant immediate intervention.
    4. This is a normal finding and would not warrant immediate intervention.

24. Correct answers are 1 and 5.
    1. **Elephantiasis is obstruction of the lymphatic vessels that causes chronic fibrosis, thickening of the subcutaneous tissue, and hypertrophy of the skin; this**

condition causes chronic edema of the extremity that recedes only slightly with elevation.

2. This may be cellulitis.
3. This may indicate dehydration of the tissue.
4. Nipple retraction and *peau d'orange* skin would be an indication of late-stage breast cancer.
5. Elephantiasis causes the skin of the affected area to be dry, thickened, and have a pebbly appearance. The skin may become ulcerated, pitted, and darkened (hyperkeratosis) (National Organization for Rare Disorders, 2019).

25. 1. An absent radial pulse would not indicate a complication of a lower extremity surgery.
2. The femoral pulse would be an appropriate pulse to assess, but it is not the best because the nurse needs to determine if the blood is getting to the most distal area of the leg.
3. The popliteal pulse would be an appropriate pulse to assess, but it is not the best because the nurse needs to determine if the blood is getting to the most distal area of the leg.
4. **The pedal pulse is the best pulse to assess because it indicates if there is adequate circulation to the most distal site of the extremity. The bypass extends from the midthigh to the mid-calf area.**

26. Correct order is 5, 1, 2, 4, 3.
5. The nurse should suspect a DVT and should not allow the client to get out of the bed.
1. This is a medical emergency, and the HCP should be notified as soon as possible.
2. The client needs an intravenous line so that IV heparin can be administered.
4. The treatment for DVT is to prevent further coagulation until the clot dissolves.
3. The client's PTT is monitored when receiving heparin therapy.

27. 1. **This client has had 11,055 mL of intake compared to 4,270 mL of output; even with an insensible loss, the nurse should assess the client to determine if the client is becoming fluid volume overloaded.**
2. This client has had 4,050 mL of intake compared to 4,700 mL of output. This client has a deficit but not one to be concerned with at this time.
3. This client has had 4,750 mL of intake compared to 4,058 mL of output. The insensible loss would account for the difference and make this client's intake and output basically even.
4. This client has had 2,267 mL of intake compared to 2,385 mL of output, basically even.

# Hematological Disorders

**5**

*Believe you can and you're halfway there.*

—Theodore Roosevelt

Hematological disorders include a broad range of blood dyscrasias, which may be hereditary or have an unknown etiology; some may be fatal, and some clients may live a normal life. Among the most serious blood disorders—types of cancer—are leukemia and lymphoma. Others include bleeding disorders, both hereditary (hemophilia and von Willebrand's disease) and nonhereditary (thrombocytopenic purpura); clotting disorders (disseminated intravascular coagulation); and anemias characterized by abnormal red blood cells (sickle cell disease, thalassemia). The nurse must know the clinical manifestations of these disorders, what is expected with the disorder, and when immediate intervention is necessary. The questions and answers that follow cover these topics.

## KEYWORDS

| | |
|---|---|
| Angiogram | Leukocytosis |
| Apoptosis | Leukopenia |
| Autologous | Melena |
| Epistaxis | Menorrhagia |
| Hemarthrosis | Neutropenia |
| Hematemesis | Pancytopenia |
| Hematoma | Placenta previa |
| Hematuria | Purpura |

## PRACTICE QUESTIONS

### Leukemia

1. The nurse is caring for clients on an oncology unit. Which **neutropenia** precautions should be implemented? **Select all that apply.**
   1. Hold all venipuncture sites for at least 5 minutes.
   2. Limit fresh fruits and flowers.
   3. Place all clients in reverse isolation.
   4. Have the clients use a soft-bristle toothbrush.
   5. Screen visitors for infectious diseases.

2. The nurse is assessing a client diagnosed with acute myelogenous leukemia (AML). Which assessment data support this diagnosis?
   1. Fever and infections.
   2. Nausea and vomiting.
   3. Excessive energy and high platelet counts.
   4. Cervical lymph node enlargement and positive acid-fast bacillus.

3. The client diagnosed with leukemia has central nervous system involvement. Which instruction should the nurse teach?
   1. Sleep with the HOB elevated to prevent increased intracranial pressure.
   2. Take an analgesic medication for pain only when the pain becomes severe.
   3. Explain that radiation therapy to the head may result in permanent hair loss.
   4. Discuss end-of-life decisions before cognitive deterioration.

4. The client diagnosed with leukemia is scheduled for a peripheral stem cell transplantation (PSCT). Which interventions should be implemented to prepare the client for this procedure? **Select all that apply.**
   1. Administer high-dose chemotherapy.
   2. Teach the client about autologous transfusions.
   3. Have the family members' HLA typed.
   4. Monitor the complete blood cell count daily.
   5. Provide central line care per protocol.

5. The client is diagnosed with chronic lymphocytic leukemia (CLL) after routine laboratory tests during a yearly physical. Which is the **scientific rationale** for the random nature of discovering the illness?
   1. CLL is not serious, and clients die from other causes first.
   2. There are no symptoms with this form of leukemia.
   3. This is a childhood illness and is self-limiting.
   4. In the early stages of CLL, the client may be asymptomatic.

6. The client diagnosed with leukemia is being admitted for an induction course of chemotherapy. Which laboratory values indicate a **diagnosis** of leukemia?
   1. A left shift in the white blood cell (WBC) count differential.
   2. A large number of WBCs that decreases after the administration of antibiotics.
   3. An abnormally low hemoglobin (Hgb) and hematocrit (Hct) level.
   4. Red blood cells (RBCs) that are larger than normal.

7. Which medication is **contraindicated** for a client diagnosed with leukemia?
   1. Sulfamethoxazole and trimethoprim.
   2. Morphine.
   3. Epoetin alpha.
   4. Imatinib mesylate.

8. The laboratory results for a male client diagnosed with leukemia are listed in the chart below. Based on these results, which intervention should the nurse teach the client?

| Complete Blood Count | Client Value | Normal Values |
|---|---|---|
| Red blood cells | 2.1 | Male: 4.21–5.81 ($10^6$ cells/microL) Female: 3.61–5.11 ($10^6$ cells/microL) |
| Sodium (Na$^+$) | 139 | 135–145 mEq/L or mmol/L |
| Potassium (K$^+$) | 3.8 | 3.5–5.3 mEq/L or mmol/L |
| Platelet | 22 | 140–400 × ($10^3$/microL) |
| WBCs | 4.3 | 4.5–11.1 × ($10^3$/cells/microL) |

   1. Encourage the client to eat foods high in iron.
   2. Instruct the client to use an electric razor when shaving.
   3. Discuss the importance of limiting sodium in the diet.
   4. Instruct the family to limit visits to once a week.

9. The nurse writes a nursing problem of "altered nutrition" for a client diagnosed with leukemia following a treatment regimen of chemotherapy and radiation. Which nursing intervention should be implemented?
   1. Administer an antidiarrheal medication before meals.
   2. Monitor the client's serum albumin levels.
   3. Assess for clinical manifestations of infection.
   4. Provide skincare to irradiated areas.

10. The nurse and the licensed practical nurse (LPN) are caring for clients on an oncology floor. Which clients could be assigned to the LPN? **Select all that apply.**
    1. The client newly diagnosed with chronic lymphocytic leukemia.
    2. The client 4 hours postprocedure bone marrow biopsy.
    3. The client who received 2 units of PRBCs on the previous shift.
    4. The client receiving multiple intravenous piggyback medications.
    5. The client diagnosed with neutropenia with a fever.

11. The nurse is completing a care plan for a client diagnosed with leukemia. Which **independent** problem should be addressed?
    1. Infection.
    2. Anemia.
    3. Nutrition.
    4. Grieving.

12. The nurse is caring for a client diagnosed with AML. Which assessment data **warrant immediate** intervention?
    1. T 99, P 102, R 22, and BP 132/68.
    2. Hyperplasia of the gums.
    3. Weakness and fatigue.
    4. Pain in the left upper quadrant.

## Lymphoma

13. The client diagnosed with non-Hodgkin's lymphoma is scheduled for a lymphangiogram. Which information should the nurse teach?
    1. The scan will identify any malignancy in the vascular system.
    2. A radiopaque dye will be injected between the toes.
    3. The test will be done similar to a cardiac angiogram.
    4. The test will be completed in about 5 minutes.

14. The client asks the nurse, "They say I have cancer. How can they tell if I have Hodgkin's disease from a biopsy?" The nurse's answer is based on which **scientific rationale**?
    1. Biopsies are nuclear medicine scans that can detect cancer.
    2. A biopsy is a laboratory test that detects cancer cells.
    3. It determines which kind of cancer the client has.
    4. The health care provider (HCP) takes a small piece out of the tumor and looks at the cells.

15. The nurse is admitting a client with a diagnosis of rule out Hodgkin's lymphoma. Which assessment data **support** this diagnosis? **Select all that apply.**
    1. Drenching night sweats and fever.
    2. Edematous lymph nodes in the groin.
    3. Malaise and reports of an upset stomach.
    4. Rapid onset of pain after alcohol consumption.
    5. Anemia and occult gastrointestinal bleeding.

16. Which client is at the **highest risk** for developing non-Hodgkin's lymphoma?
    1. The client diagnosed with chronic lung disease taking a steroid.
    2. The client diagnosed with breast cancer and extensive lymph involvement.
    3. The client with a kidney transplant several years ago.
    4. The client diagnosed with a neurogenic bladder and ureteral stent placements.

17. The female client recently diagnosed with Hodgkin's lymphoma asks the nurse about the prognosis. Which is the nurse's **best response**?
    1. Survival for Hodgkin's disease is relatively good with standard therapy.
    2. Survival depends on becoming involved in an investigational therapy program.
    3. Survival is poor, with more than 50% of clients dying within 6 months.
    4. Survival is fine for primary Hodgkin's, but secondary cancers occur within a year.

18. The nurse writes the problem of "grieving" for a client diagnosed with non-Hodgkin's lymphoma. Which collaborative intervention should be included in the plan of care?
    1. Encourage the client to talk about feelings of loss.
    2. Arrange for the family to plan a memorable outing.
    3. Refer the client to the American Cancer Society's Dialogue group.
    4. Have the chaplain visit with the client.

19. Which test is considered **diagnostic** for Hodgkin's lymphoma?
    1. A magnetic resonance image (MRI) of the chest.
    2. A computed tomography (CT) scan of the cervical area.
    3. An erythrocyte sedimentation rate (ESR).
    4. A biopsy of the cervical lymph nodes.

20. Which client should be assigned to the **experienced** medical-surgical nurse during the first week of orientation to the oncology floor?
    1. The client diagnosed with non-Hodgkin's lymphoma having daily radiation treatments.
    2. The client diagnosed with Hodgkin's disease receiving combination chemotherapy.
    3. The client diagnosed with leukemia and petechiae covering both anterior and posterior body surfaces.
    4. The client diagnosed with diffuse histolytic lymphoma to receive 2 units of packed red blood cells (PRBCs).

21. Which information about reproduction should be taught to the 27-year-old female client diagnosed with Hodgkin's disease?
    1. The client's reproductive ability will be the same after the treatment is completed.
    2. The client should practice birth control for at least 2 years following therapy.
    3. All clients become sterile from the therapy and should plan to adopt.
    4. The therapy will temporarily interfere with the client's menstrual cycle.

22. Which clinical manifestation of stage I non-Hodgkin's lymphoma would the nurse expect to find when assessing the client?
    1. Enlarged lymph tissue anywhere in the body.
    2. Tender left upper quadrant.
    3. No symptom in this stage.
    4. Elevated B-cell lymphocytes on the complete blood count (CBC).

23. The nurse and an unlicensed assistive personnel (UAP) are caring for clients in a bone marrow transplantation unit. Which nursing task should the RN delegate?
    1. Take the hourly vital signs on a client receiving blood transfusions.
    2. Monitor the infusion of antineoplastic medications.
    3. Transcribe the HCP's laboratory orders into the EHR.
    4. Determine the client's response to the therapy.

24. The 33-year-old client diagnosed with stage IV Hodgkin's lymphoma is at the 5-year remission mark. Which information should the nurse teach the client?
    1. Instruct the client to continue scheduled screenings for cancer.
    2. Discuss the need for follow-up appointments every 5 years.
    3. Teach the client that the cancer risk is the same as for the general population.
    4. Have the client talk with the family about funeral arrangements.

## Anemia

25. The nurse is admitting a client with a history of gastric bypass surgery for obesity 4 years ago presenting now with pale mucous membranes, dyspnea on exertion, and vitals populated in the flowsheet below. Which **type** of anemia would the nurse suspect the client has developed?

| Client: African American Female | | Diagnosis: Rule Out Anemia |
|---|---|---|
| Age: 24 | Height: 5'5" | Weight: 75 kg |
| Vital Sign Flowsheet | Client Results | Normal Values |
| Blood pressure | 104/66 | 100–119 mm Hg systolic 60–80 mm Hg diastolic |
| Pulse | 110 | 60–100 beats/min |
| Respirations | 27 | 12–20 breaths/min |

    1. Vitamin $B_{12}$ deficiency.
    2. Folic acid deficiency.
    3. Iron deficiency.
    4. Sickle cell disease.

26. The client diagnosed with menorrhagia reports to the nurse of feeling listless and tired all the time. Which scientific rationale would explain why these symptoms occur?
    1. The pain associated with the menorrhagia does not allow the client to rest.
    2. The client's symptoms are unrelated to the diagnosis of menorrhagia.
    3. The client probably has been exposed to a virus that causes chronic fatigue.
    4. Menorrhagia has caused the client to have decreased levels of hemoglobin.

27. The nurse writes a diagnosis of altered tissue perfusion for a client diagnosed with anemia. Which interventions should be included in the plan of care? **Select all that apply.**
    1. Monitor the client's Hgb and hematocrit.
    2. Move the client to a room near the nurse's desk.
    3. Limit the client's dietary intake of green vegetables.
    4. Assess the client for numbness and tingling.
    5. Allow for rest periods during the day for the client.

28. The client diagnosed with iron-deficiency anemia is prescribed ferrous gluconate orally. Which should the nurse teach the client?
    1. Take loperamide, over-the-counter, daily.
    2. Limit exercise for several weeks until tolerance is achieved.
    3. The stools may be very dark, and this can mask blood.
    4. Eat only red meats and organ meats for protein.

29. The nurse and a UAP are caring for clients in a medical unit. Which task should the RN delegate to the UAP?
    1. Check on the bowel movements of a client diagnosed with melena.
    2. Take the vital signs of a client who received blood the day before.
    3. Evaluate the dietary intake of a client non-compliant with eating.
    4. Shave the client diagnosed with severe hemolytic anemia.

30. The client is diagnosed with heart failure and anemia. The HCP ordered a transfusion of 2 units of PRBCs. The unit has 250 mL of RBCs plus 45 mL of additive. At what rate should the nurse set the IV pump to infuse each unit of PRBCs?

31. The client is being admitted with folic acid deficiency anemia. Which would be the **most appropriate** referral?
    1. Alcoholics Anonymous.
    2. Leukemia Society of America.
    3. A hematologist.
    4. A social worker.

32. The charge nurse is making assignments on a medical floor. Which client should be assigned to the **most** experienced nurse?
    1. The client diagnosed with iron-deficiency anemia prescribed iron supplements.
    2. The client diagnosed with pernicious anemia receiving vitamin B$_{12}$ intramuscularly.
    3. The client diagnosed with aplastic anemia and has pancytopenia.
    4. The client diagnosed with renal disease and deficiency of erythropoietin.

33. The client diagnosed with anemia reports dyspnea when ambulating in the hall. Which intervention should the nurse implement **first**?
    1. Apply oxygen via nasal cannula.
    2. Get a wheelchair for the client.
    3. Assess the client's lung fields.
    4. Assist the client when ambulating in the hall.

34. The nurse is transcribing the HCP's order for an iron supplement on the MAR. At which time should the nurse schedule the daily dose?
    1. 0900.
    2. 1000.
    3. 1200.
    4. 1630.

35. The nurse is discharging a client diagnosed with anemia. Which discharge instructions should the nurse teach? **Select all that apply.**
    1. Take the prescribed iron until it is completely gone.
    2. Monitor pulse and blood pressure at a local pharmacy weekly.
    3. Have a CBC checked at the HCP's office.
    4. Perform isometric exercise three times a week.
    5. Increase the amount of iron-rich foods in the diet.

36. The nurse writes a client problem of "activity intolerance" for a client diagnosed with anemia. Which interventions should the nurse implement? **Select all that apply.**
    1. Pace activities according to tolerance.
    2. Provide supplements high in iron and vitamins.
    3. Administer packed red blood cells.
    4. Monitor vital signs every 4 hours.
    5. Assist with personal care as needed.

## Bleeding Disorders

37. The charge nurse in the intensive care unit is making client assignments. Which client should the charge nurse assign to the graduate nurse after 3 months of orientation?
    1. The client with an abdominal peritoneal resection and a colostomy.
    2. The client diagnosed with pneumonia and acute respiratory distress syndrome.
    3. The client diagnosed with a head injury developing disseminated intravascular coagulation.
    4. The client admitted with a gunshot wound and an H&H of 7 and 22.

38. Which client would be **most at risk** for developing disseminated intravascular coagulation (DIC)?
    1. A 35-year-old pregnant client diagnosed with placenta previa.
    2. A 42-year-old client diagnosed with a pulmonary embolus.
    3. A 60-year-old client receiving hemodialysis 3 days a week.
    4. A 78-year-old client diagnosed with septicemia.

39. The client admitted with full-thickness burns may be developing DIC. Which clinical manifestations would support the diagnosis of DIC?
    1. Oozing blood from the IV catheter site.
    2. Sudden onset of chest pain and frothy sputum.
    3. Foul-smelling, concentrated urine.
    4. A reddened, inflamed central line catheter site.

40. Which laboratory results would the nurse expect in the client diagnosed with DIC? **Select all that apply.**
    1. A decreased prothrombin time.
    2. A low fibrinogen level.
    3. An increased platelet count.
    4. An increased WBC count.
    5. Elevated fibrin split products.

41. Which **collaborative** treatment would the nurse anticipate for the client diagnosed with DIC?
    1. Administer oral anticoagulants.
    2. Prepare for plasmapheresis.
    3. Administer frozen plasma.
    4. Calculate the intake and output.

42. The UAP asks the primary nurse, "How does someone get hemophilia A?" Which statement would be the RN's **best response**?
    1. "It is an inherited X-linked recessive disorder."
    2. "There is a deficiency of the clotting factor VIII."
    3. "The person is born with hemophilia A."
    4. "The mother carries the gene and gives it to the son."

43. Which clinical manifestation should the nurse expect to assess in the client diagnosed with hemophilia A?
    1. Epistaxis.
    2. Petechiae.
    3. Subcutaneous emphysema.
    4. Intermittent claudication.

44. Which situation might cause the nurse to think that the client has von Willebrand's disease?
    1. The client has had unexplained episodes of hematemesis.
    2. The client has microscopic blood in the urine.
    3. The client has prolonged bleeding following surgery.
    4. The female client developed abruptio placentae.

45. The client diagnosed with hemophilia A is experiencing hemarthrosis. Which intervention should the nurse recommend to the client?
    1. Alternate acetylsalicylic acid and acetaminophen to help with the pain.
    2. Apply cold packs for 24 to 48 hours to the affected area.
    3. Perform active range-of-motion exercise on the extremity.
    4. Put the affected extremity in the dependent position.

46. Which clinical manifestation would the nurse expect to assess in the client diagnosed with idiopathic thrombocytopenic purpura (ITP)?
    1. Petechiae on the anterior chest or lower legs.
    2. Capillary refill of less than 3 seconds.
    3. An enlarged spleen.
    4. Pulse oximeter reading of 95%.

47. The nurse is caring for the following clients. Which client should the nurse assess **first**?
    1. The client with partial thromboplastin time (aPTT) of 38 seconds.
    2. The client with Hgb 14 g/dL and Hct 45%.
    3. The client with platelet count 75,000 per cubic millimeter of blood.
    4. The client with a red blood cell count of $4.8 \times 10^6$/microL.

48. Which nursing interventions should the nurse implement when caring for a client diagnosed with hemophilia A? **Select all that apply.**
    1. Instruct the client to use a razor blade to shave.
    2. Avoid administering enemas to the client.
    3. Encourage participation in contact sports.
    4. Teach the client how to apply direct pressure if bleeding occurs.
    5. Explain the importance of not flossing the gums.

## Blood Transfusions

49. The client has laboratory values populated in the chart below. The HCP has ordered 2 units of PRBCs to be transfused. Which interventions should the nurse implement? **Select all that apply.**

| Complete Blood Count | Client Value | Normal Values |
|---|---|---|
| Hgb | 7.7 | Male: 14–17.3 g/dL Female: 11.7–15.5 g/dL |
| Hct | 22.3 | Male: 42%–52% Female: 36%–48% |

    1. Obtain a signed consent.
    2. Initiate a 22-gauge IV.
    3. Assess the client's lungs.
    4. Check for allergies.
    5. Hang a keep-open IV of $D_5W$.

50. The client is admitted to the emergency department after a motor vehicle accident. The nurse notes profuse bleeding from a right-sided abdominal injury. Which intervention should the nurse implement **first**?
    1. Type and crossmatch for RBCs immediately (STAT).
    2. Initiate an IV with an 18-gauge needle and hang normal saline.
    3. Have the client sign a consent for an exploratory laparotomy.
    4. Notify the significant other of the client's admission.

51. The nurse is working in a blood bank facility procuring units of blood from donors. Which clients would be candidates to donate blood? **Select all that apply.**
    1. The client with wisdom teeth removed a week ago.
    2. The nursing student after receiving a rubella immunization 2 weeks ago.
    3. The mother with a 6-week-old newborn.
    4. The client diagnosed with an allergy to acetylsalicylic acid in childhood.
    5. The client who got a tattoo 18 months ago.

52. The client with O+ blood is in need of an emergency transfusion, but the laboratory does not have any O+ blood available. Which potential unit of blood could be given to the client?
    1. The O− unit.
    2. The A+ unit.
    3. The B+ unit.
    4. Any Rh+ unit.

53. The client is scheduled to have a total hip replacement in 2 months and has chosen to prepare for autologous transfusions. Which medication would the nurse administer to prepare the client?
    1. Prednisone.
    2. Azithromycin.
    3. Lorazepam.
    4. Epoetin alpha.

54. The client undergoing knee replacement surgery has an autologous blood recovery apparatus attached to the knee when he arrives in the postanesthesia care unit (PACU). Which intervention should the nurse implement to care for this drainage system?
    1. Infuse the drainage into the client when a prescribed amount fills the chamber.
    2. Attach an hourly drainage collection bag to the unit and discard the drainage.
    3. Replace the unit with a continuous passive motion (CPM) unit and start it on low.
    4. Have another nurse verify the unit number before reinfusing the blood.

55. Which statement is the scientific rationale for infusing a unit of blood in less than 4 hours?
    1. The blood will coagulate if left out of the refrigerator for more than 4 hours.
    2. The blood has the potential for bacterial growth if allowed to infuse longer.
    3. The blood components begin to break down after 4 hours.
    4. The blood will not be affected; this is a laboratory procedure.

56. The HCP orders 2 units of blood to be administered over 8 hours each for a client diagnosed with heart failure. Which intervention(s) should the nurse implement?
    1. Call the HCP to question the order because blood must infuse within 4 hours.
    2. Retrieve the blood from the laboratory and run each unit at an 8-hour rate.
    3. Notify the laboratory to split each unit into half-units and infuse each half for 4 hours.
    4. Infuse each unit for 4 hours, the maximum rate for a unit of blood.

57. The client receiving a unit of PRBCs begins to chill and develop hives. Which action should be the nurse's **first** response?
    1. Notify the laboratory and health-care provider.
    2. Administer diphenhydramine, IV.
    3. Assess the client for further complications.
    4. Stop the transfusion and change the tubing at the hub.

58. The RN and a UAP are caring for clients on an oncology floor. Which nursing task would be delegated to the UAP?
    1. Assess the urine output on a client diagnosed with a blood transfusion reaction.
    2. Take the first 15 minutes of vital signs on a client receiving a unit of PRBCs.
    3. Auscultate the lung sounds of a client before a transfusion.
    4. Assist a client with brushing teeth after receiving 10 units of platelets.

59. The nurse is caring for clients on the medical floor. After the shift report, which client should be assessed **first**?
    1. The client two-thirds of the way through a blood transfusion reporting no dyspnea or hives.
    2. The client diagnosed with leukemia, Hct of 18%, and petechiae covering the body.
    3. The client diagnosed with peptic ulcer disease calling over the intercom to report vomiting blood.
    4. The client diagnosed with Crohn's disease reporting perineal discomfort.

60. The client received 2 units of PRBCs of 250 mL with 63 mL of preservative each during the shift. There was 240 mL of saline remaining in the 500-mL bag when the nurse discarded the blood tubing. How many milliliters of fluid should be documented on the intake and output (I&O) record?

    | |
    |---|

## Sickle Cell Disease

61. The student nurse asks the nurse, "What is sickle cell disease?" Which statement by the nurse would be the **best answer** to the student's question?
    1. "There is some written material at the desk that will explain the disease."
    2. "It is a congenital disease of the blood in which the blood does not clot."
    3. "The client has decreased synovial fluid that causes joint pain."
    4. "The blood becomes thick when the client is deprived of oxygen."

62. The client's nephew has just been diagnosed with sickle cell disease (SCD). The client asks the nurse, "How did my nephew get this disease?" Which statement would be the **best response** by the nurse?
    1. "Sickle cell disease is an inherited autosomal recessive disease."
    2. "He was born with it, and both his parents were carriers of the disease."
    3. "At this time, the cause of sickle cell disease is unknown."
    4. "Your sister was exposed to a virus while she was pregnant."

63. The client diagnosed with SCD comes to the emergency department reporting joint pain throughout the body. The oral temperature is 102.4°F, and the pulse oximeter reading is 91%. Which action should the emergency department nurse implement **first**?
    1. Request arterial blood gases (ABGs) STAT.
    2. Administer oxygen via nasal cannula.
    3. Start an IV with an 18-gauge angiocath.
    4. Prepare to administer analgesics as ordered.

64. The client diagnosed with SCD is experiencing a vaso-occlusive sickle cell crisis secondary to an infection. Which medical treatments should the nurse anticipate the HCP ordering for the client? **Select all that apply.**
    1. Administer meperidine intravenously.
    2. Admit the client to a private room and keep in reverse isolation.
    3. Infuse D$_5$W 0.33% NS at 150 mL/hr via pump.
    4. Insert a 22-French Foley catheter with a urinometer.
    5. Give oxygen therapy via nasal cannula.

65. The nurse is assessing an African American client diagnosed with sickle cell crisis. Which assessment datum is **most** pertinent when assessing for cyanosis in clients with dark skin?
    1. Assess the client's oral mucosa.
    2. Assess the client's metatarsals.
    3. Assess the client's capillary refill time (CRT).
    4. Assess the sclera of the client's eyes.

66. The client is diagnosed with sickle cell crisis. The nurse is calculating the client's I&O for the shift. What is the client's total intake for this shift?

    | mL |
    | --- |

### Intake and Output Record

| Day 1 | Oral (ounces) | Intravenous (mL) | Urine (mL) | Other (Specify) |
| --- | --- | --- | --- | --- |
| 0701–1900 | Water: 10 oz<br>Milk: 8 oz<br>Apple juice: 8 oz | 1200 mL (0.9% NS) | 800 mL | |
| 1901–0700 | Milk: 4 oz<br>Water: 10 oz | 600 mL (0.9% NS) | 400 mL | |
| Total | | | | |

67. The nurse is caring for the female client recovering from a sickle cell crisis. The client tells the nurse about a planned family trip to Yellowstone National Park. Which response would be **best** for the nurse?
    1. "That sounds like a wonderful trip to take this summer."
    2. "Have you talked to your doctor about taking the trip?"
    3. "You really should not take a trip to areas with high altitudes."
    4. "Why do you want to go to Yellowstone National Park?"

68. Which is a potential complication that occurs specifically to a male client diagnosed with SCD during a sickle cell crisis?
    1. Chest syndrome.
    2. Compartment syndrome.
    3. Priapism.
    4. Hypertensive crisis.

69. The nurse is completing discharge teaching for the client diagnosed with a sickle cell crisis. The nurse recommends the client getting the flu and pneumonia vaccines. The client asks, "Why should I take those shots? I hate shots." Which statement by the nurse is the **best response**?
    1. "These vaccines promote health in clients diagnosed with chronic illnesses."
    2. "You are susceptible to infections. These shots may help prevent a crisis."
    3. "The vaccines will help your blood from sickling secondary to viruses."
    4. "The doctor wanted to make sure that I discussed the vaccines with you."

70. The client diagnosed with SCD asks the nurse, "Should I join the Sickle Cell Foundation? I received some information from the Sickle Cell Foundation. What kind of group is it?" Which statement is the **best response** by the nurse?
    1. "It is a foundation that deals primarily with research for a cure for SCD."
    2. "It provides information on the disease and on support groups in this area."
    3. "I recommend joining any organization that will help deal with your disease."
    4. "The foundation arranges for families that have children with sickle cell to meet."

71. Which clinical manifestation will the nurse expect to assess in the client diagnosed with a vaso-occlusive sickle cell crisis?
    1. Lordosis.
    2. Epistaxis.
    3. Hematuria.
    4. Petechiae.

72. The male client diagnosed with SCD comes to the emergency department with a temperature of 101.4°F and tells the nurse that he is having a sickle cell crisis. Which diagnostic test should the nurse anticipate the emergency department doctor ordering for the client?
    1. Spinal tap.
    2. Hemoglobin electrophoresis.
    3. Sickle cell screen.
    4. Blood cultures.

## CONCEPTS

The concepts covered in this chapter focus on hematological regulation problems such as leukemia, lymphoma, and clotting issues such as SCD and bleeding. Interrelated concepts of the nursing process and clinical judgment are covered throughout the questions. The test taker will be challenged to apply clinical judgment, particularly in the questions about priority interventions or "first" choices.

73. The nurse has identified the concept of cellular deviation for a client diagnosed with chronic myelogenous leukemia. Which intervention should the nurse implement? **Select all that apply.**
    1. Screen visitors for infection before allowing them to enter the room.
    2. Assess the client's vital signs every 4 hours.
    3. Do not allow fresh fruits and vegetables on diet trays.
    4. Monitor the client's WBC count.
    5. Place the client on droplet isolation.
    6. Check the client's bone marrow results daily.

74. The client is diagnosed with non-Hodgkin's lymphoma. Which nursing concept should the nurse identify as the **priority**?
    1. Immunity.
    2. Grieving.
    3. Perfusion.
    4. Clotting.

75. The nurse is caring for a client diagnosed with SCD. Which should the nurse include in the client's plan of care? **Select all that apply.**
    1. Teach the client to limit fluids.
    2. Discuss interventions to maintain hydration.
    3. Measure the client's calf for swelling.

    4. Have the client take narcotic pain medication every 8 hours.
    5. Administer hydroxyurea by mouth.

76. The nurse identified clotting as a concept related to SCD. Which intervention should the nurse implement?
    1. Assess for cerebrovascular symptoms.
    2. Keep the HOB elevated.
    3. Order a 2,000-mg sodium diet.
    4. Apply antiembolism stockings.

77. The client is diagnosed with Hodgkin's disease. Which data are **diagnostic** for Hodgkin's disease?
    1. Night sweats and low-grade fever.
    2. Cavitation noted on the chest x-ray.
    3. Reed-Sternberg cells found on biopsy.
    4. Weight loss and palpable inguinal lymph nodes.

78. Which interrelated psychological concept is a **priority** for the nurse caring for a client diagnosed with leukemia?
    1. Comfort.
    2. Stress.
    3. Grieving.
    4. Coping.

79. The client diagnosed with SCD is experiencing a vaso-occlusive crisis. Which **priority** interventions should the nurse implement?
    1. Maintain IV fluids and administer pain medications.
    2. Encourage frequent ambulation in the hallways.
    3. Administer oxygen via nasal cannula at 10 liters per minute (LPM).
    4. Monitor the client's RBC count every 4 hours.

80. The nurse is assessing a client diagnosed with a vaso-occlusive crisis. Which indicates the client is **not meeting** an appropriate stage of growth and development, according to Erikson?
    1. The 32-year-old client does not have a significant other and is on disability.
    2. The 28-year-old client is actively involved in the care of a 6-year-old child.
    3. The 40-year-old client has a full-time job and cares for an aged parent.
    4. The 19-year-old client is a full-time college student and has many friends.

81. The nurse identifies the concept of hematologic regulation for a client diagnosed with leukemia. Which clinical manifestations support the concept?
    1. The client has petechiae on the trunk and extremities.
    2. The client reports pain and swelling in the joints.
    3. The client has Hgb of 9.7 and Hct of 32%.
    4. The client reports a headache and slurred speech.

82. Which concepts could the nurse identify for a client diagnosed with lymphoma? **Select all that apply.**
    1. Coping.
    2. Hematologic regulation.
    3. Tissue perfusion.
    4. Clotting.
    5. Clinical judgment.

# PRACTICE QUESTIONS ANSWERS AND RATIONALES

## Leukemia

1. **Correct answers are 2 and 5.**
   1. This would be done for thrombocytopenia (low platelets), not neutropenia (low WBCs).
   2. **Fresh fruits and flowers may carry bacteria or insects on the skin of the fruit or dirt on the flowers and leaves, so they are restricted around clients diagnosed with low WBC counts.**
   3. Clients with severe neutropenia may be placed in reverse isolation, but not all clients diagnosed with neutropenia will be placed in reverse isolation. Clients are at a greater risk for infecting themselves from endogenous fungi and bacteria than from being exposed to noninfectious individuals.
   4. This is an intervention for thrombocytopenia.
   5. **All visitors should be screened for infectious diseases that could be transmitted to the client.**

**TEST-TAKING HINT: The test taker must match the problem with the answer options. Options "1" and "4" would be implemented for the client diagnosed with a bleeding disorder. Option "3" has the word "all" in it, which would make the test taker not select this option. Option "5" is appropriate for any client in the hospital.**

2. 1. **Fever and infection are hallmark symptoms of leukemia. They occur because the bone marrow is unable to produce WBCs of the number and maturity needed to fight infection.**
   2. Nausea and vomiting are symptoms related to the treatment of cancer but not to the diagnosis of leukemia.
   3. The clients are frequently fatigued and have low platelet counts. The platelet count is as a result of the inability of the bone marrow to produce the needed cells. In some forms of leukemia, the bone marrow is not producing cells at all, and in others, the bone marrow is producing tens of thousands of immature cells.
   4. Cervical lymph node enlargement is associated with Hodgkin's lymphoma, and positive acid-fast bacillus is diagnostic for tuberculosis.

**TEST-TAKING HINT: Option "3" could be eliminated because of the excessive energy. Illness normally drains energy reserves; it does not increase them.**

3. 1. Sleeping with the HOB elevated might relieve some intracranial pressure, but it will not prevent increased intracranial pressure from occurring.
   2. Analgesic medications for clients diagnosed with cancer are given on a scheduled basis with a fast-acting analgesic administered prn for breakthrough pain.
   3. **Radiation therapy to the head and scalp area is the treatment of choice for central nervous system involvement of any cancer. Radiation therapy has longer lasting side effects than chemotherapy. If radiation therapy destroys the hair follicles, the hair will not grow back.**
   4. Cognitive deterioration does not usually occur.

**TEST-TAKING HINT: The test taker must be aware of the treatments used for the disease processes to answer this question but might eliminate option "2" because it violates the basic principles of pain management.**

4. **Correct answers are 1, 3, 4, and 5.**
   1. The client will receive high-dose chemotherapy and radiation therapy to destroy the cancer cells before transfusing the donor stem cells via blood transfusion. The PSCT procedure is more commonly utilized for donor comfort. The donor only needs to give blood rather than have bone marrow harvested from the iliac bone.
   2. Autologous transfusions are infusions from the client's own blood. Since this client has cancer involving blood tissue, the client does not have healthy cells to infuse.
   3. **The best stem cell or bone marrow donor comes from an identical twin; the next best comes from a matching sibling. The most complications occur from a matched unrelated donor (MUD). The client's body recognizes the marrow as foreign and tries to reject it, resulting in graft-versus-host disease (GVHD).**
   4. **The CBC must be monitored daily to assess for infections, anemia, and thrombocytopenia.**
   5. **Clients will have at least one multiple-line central venous access. These clients are seriously ill and require multiple transfusions and antibiotics.**

**TEST-TAKING HINT: If the test taker knows the definition of "autologous," then option "2" could be eliminated.**

5. 1. All types of leukemia are serious and can cause death. The chronic types of leukemia are more insidious in the onset of symptoms and can have a slower progression of the disease. Chronic types of leukemia are more common in the adult population.
   2. The symptoms may have a slower onset, but anemia causing fatigue and weakness and thrombocytopenia causing bleeding can be present (usually in the later stages of the disease). Organ enlargement from infiltration may be present. Secondary symptoms of fever, night sweats, and weight loss may also be present.
   3. This disease is usually found in adults.
   4. In this form of leukemia, the cells seem to escape apoptosis (programmed cell death), which results in many thousands of mature cells clogging the body. Because the cells are mature, the client may be asymptomatic in the early stages.

**TEST-TAKING HINT: The test taker can eliminate option "1" based on the words "not serious"; common sense lets the test taker know this is not true.**

6. 1. A left shift indicates immature WBCs are being produced and released into the circulating blood volume. This should be investigated for the malignant process of leukemia.
   2. Leukocytosis (elevated WBCs) is normal in the presence of an infection, but it should decrease as the infection clears.
   3. Low Hgb and Hct levels indicate anemia and can be caused by a number of factors. Anemia does occur in leukemia, but it is not diagnostic for leukemia.
   4. RBCs larger than normal occur in macrocytic anemias (vitamin $B_{12}$ and folic acid deficiency). They are not characteristic of leukemia.

**TEST-TAKING HINT: The test taker should recognize that elevated WBCs resolve with antibiotics as an infection. Option "3" is not specific enough to be the correct answer.**

7. 1. Because of the ineffective or nonexistent WBCs (segmented neutrophils) characteristic of leukemia, the body cannot fight infections, and sulfamethoxazole and trimethoprim (Bactrim), a sulfa antibiotic, is given to treat infections.
   2. Leukemic infiltrations into the organs or the central nervous system cause pain. Morphine, a narcotic analgesic, is the drug of choice for most clients diagnosed with cancer.
   3. **Epoetin alpha (Epogen) is a biologic response modifier that stimulates the bone marrow to produce RBCs. The bone marrow is the area of malignancy in leukemia. Stimulating the bone marrow would be generally ineffective for the desired results and would have the potential to stimulate malignant growth.**
   4. Imatinib mesylate (Gleevec), a genetic blocking agent, is a drug that specifically works in leukemic cells to block the expression of the BCR-ABL protein, preventing the cells from growing and dividing.

**TEST-TAKING HINT: If the test taker were not familiar with the drug mentioned in option "4," then this option would not be a good choice. Options "1" and "2" are common drugs and should not be chosen as the answer unless the test taker knows for sure they are contraindicated.**

8. 1. The anemia that occurs in leukemia is not related to iron deficiency, and eating foods high in iron will not help.
   2. **The platelet count of $22 \times 10^3$/microL indicates a platelet count of 22,000. The definition of thrombocytopenia is a count of less than 100,000. This client is at risk for bleeding. Bleeding precautions include decreasing the risk by using soft-bristle toothbrushes and electric razors and holding all venipuncture sites for a minimum of 5 minutes.**
   3. The sodium level is within normal limits. The client is encouraged to eat whatever is desired unless some other disease process limits food choices.
   4. The client is at risk for infection, but unless the family or significant others are ill, they should be encouraged to visit whenever possible.

**TEST-TAKING HINT: The test taker could eliminate option "3" based on a normal laboratory value. The RBC, WBC, and platelet values are all not in the normal range. The correct answer option must address one of these values.**

9. 1. The nurse should administer an anti-emetic before meals, not an antidiarrheal medication.
   2. **Serum albumin is a measure of the protein content in the blood that is derived from the foods eaten; albumin monitors nutritional status.**
   3. Assessment of the nutritional status is indicated for this problem, not an assessment of the clinical manifestations of infections.
   4. This addresses an altered skin integrity problem.

**TEST-TAKING HINT: The stem of the question asks for interventions for "altered nutrition." Assessment is the first step of the nursing process, but option "3" is not assessing nutrition.**

10. Correct answers are 2, 3, and 4.
   1. The newly diagnosed client will need to be taught about the disease and about treatment options. The RN cannot delegate teaching to an LPN.
   2. **This client is postprocedure and could be cared for by the LPN.**
   3. **This client has already received the blood products; this client requires routine monitoring, which the LPN could perform.**
   4. **The LPN can administer antibiotic medications.**
   5. The client with neutropenia and fever is unstable. The client could have an infection that could become a medical emergency. The RN should care for this client.

**TEST-TAKING HINT: The nurse cannot assign assessment, teaching, or evaluation. The clients in options "2," "3," and "4" are stable or have expected situations.**

11. 1. Treating infections, which require HCP orders for cultures and antibiotics, is a collaborative problem.
   2. The treatment of anemia is a collaborative problem.
   3. The provision of adequate nutrition requires collaboration among the nurse, HCP, and dietitian.
   4. **Grieving is an independent problem, and the nurse can assess and treat this problem with or without collaboration.**

**TEST-TAKING HINT: The stem of the question asks for an independent intervention. If the test taker understands the problem and the treatment needs, options "1," "2," and "3" can be eliminated.**

12. 1. These vital signs are not alarming. The vital signs are slightly elevated and indicate monitoring at intervals, but they do not indicate an immediate need.
   2. Hyperplasia of the gums is a symptom of myelogenous leukemia, but it is not an emergency.
   3. Weakness and fatigue are symptoms of the disease and are expected.
   4. **Pain is expected, but it is a priority, and pain control measures should be implemented.**

**TEST-TAKING HINT: If all the answer options contain expected events, the test taker must decide which is a priority—and pain is a priority need.**

## Lymphoma

13. 1. The scan detects abnormalities in the lymphatic system, not the vascular system.
   2. **A dye is injected between the toes of both feet and then scans are performed in a few hours, at 24 hours, and then possibly once a day for several days.**
   3. Cardiac angiograms are performed through the femoral or brachial arteries and are completed in one session.
   4. The test takes 30 minutes to 1 hour and then is repeated at intervals.

**TEST-TAKING HINT: The test taker must be aware of diagnostic tests used to diagnose specific diseases. Options "1" and "3" could be eliminated because of the words "vascular" and "cardiac"; these words pertain to the cardiovascular system, not the lymphatic system.**

14. 1. Biopsies are surgical procedures requiring needle aspiration or excision of the area; they are not nuclear medicine scans.
   2. The biopsy specimen is sent to the pathology laboratory for the pathologist to determine the type of cell. "Laboratory test" refers to tests of body fluids performed by a laboratory technician.
   3. A biopsy is used to determine if the client has cancer and, if so, what kind. However, this response does not answer the client's question.
   4. **A biopsy is the removal of cells from a mass and examination of the tissue under a microscope to determine if the cells are cancerous. Reed-Sternberg cells are diagnostic for Hodgkin's disease. If these cells are not found in the biopsy, the HCP can rebiopsy to make sure the specimen provided the**

needed sample or, depending on the involvement of the tissue, diagnose a non-Hodgkin's lymphoma.

**TEST-TAKING HINT:** Option "1" can be eliminated if the test taker knows what the word "biopsy" means. Option "3" does not answer the question and can be eliminated for this reason.

15. Correct answers are 1 and 4.
    1. Clients with Hodgkin's disease experience drenching diaphoresis, especially at night, fever, and unintentional weight loss. Early-stage disease is indicated by painless enlargement of a lymph node on one side of the neck (cervical area). Pruritus is also a common symptom.
    2. Lymph node enlargement with Hodgkin's disease is in the neck area.
    3. Malaise and stomach issues are not associated with Hodgkin's disease.
    4. Rapid onset of pain after the ingestion of small amounts of alcohol is a clinical manifestation of Hodgkin's disease. The cause of this is unknown.
    5. Anemia and occult gastrointestinal bleeding are not associated with Hodgkin's disease.

**TEST-TAKING HINT:** The test taker must notice the descriptive words, such as "groin" and "fatty," to decide if these options could be correct.

16. 1. Long-term steroid use suppresses the immune system and has many side effects, but it is not the highest risk for the development of non-Hodgkin's lymphoma.
    2. This client would be considered to be in late-stage breast cancer. Cancers are described by the original cancerous tissue. This client has breast cancer that has metastasized to the lymph system.
    3. Clients after a transplant must take immunosuppressive medications to prevent rejection of the organ. This immunosuppression blocks the immune system from protecting the body against cancers and other diseases. There is a high incidence of non-Hodgkin's lymphoma among transplant recipients.
    4. A neurogenic bladder is a benign disease; stent placement would not put a client at risk for cancer.

**TEST-TAKING HINT:** To answer this question, the test taker must be aware of the function of the immune system in the body and of the treatments of the disease processes.

17. 1. Up to 90% of clients respond well to standard treatment with chemotherapy and radiation therapy. Relapse clients usually respond to a change in chemotherapy medications. Survival depends on the individual client and the stage of disease at diagnosis.
    2. Investigational therapy regimens would not be recommended for clients initially diagnosed with Hodgkin's disease because of the expected prognosis with standard therapy.
    3. Clients usually achieve a significantly longer survival rate than 6 months. Many clients survive to develop long-term secondary complications.
    4. Secondary cancers can occur as long as 20 years after remission of Hodgkin's disease has occurred.

**TEST-TAKING HINT:** The test taker must have a basic knowledge of the disease process but could rule out option "2" based on the word "investigational."

18. 1. Encouraging clients to verbalize feelings is an independent nursing intervention.
    2. Discussing activities that will make pleasant memories and planning a family outing improve the client's quality of life and assist the family in the grieving process after the client dies, but this is an independent nursing intervention.
    3. Nurses can and do refer clients diagnosed with cancer to the American Cancer Society–sponsored groups independently. Dialogue is a group support meeting that focuses on dealing with the feelings associated with a cancer diagnosis.
    4. Collaborative interventions involve other departments of the health-care facility. A chaplain is a referral that can be made, and the two disciplines should work together to provide the needed interventions.

**TEST-TAKING HINT:** The stem of the question asks for a collaborative intervention, which means that another health-care discipline must be involved. Options "1," "2," and "3" are all interventions the nurse can do without another discipline being involved.

19. 1. An MRI of the chest area will determine numerous disease entities, but it cannot determine the specific morphology of Reed-Sternberg cells, which are diagnostic for Hodgkin's disease.
    2. A CT scan will show tumor masses in the area, but it is not capable of pathological diagnosis.

3. ESR laboratory tests are sometimes used to monitor the progress of the treatment of Hodgkin's disease, but ESR levels can be elevated in several disease processes.

4. Cancers of all types are definitively diagnosed through biopsy procedures. The pathologist must identify Reed-Sternberg cells for a diagnosis of Hodgkin's disease.

**TEST-TAKING HINT:** The test taker can eliminate the first three answer options based on these tests giving general information on multiple diseases. A biopsy procedure of the involved tissues is the only procedure that provides a definitive diagnosis.

20. 1. This client is receiving treatments that can have life-threatening side effects; the nurse is not experienced with this type of client.

2. Chemotherapy is administered only by nurses after receiving training in chemotherapy medications and their effects on the body and are aware of necessary safety precautions; this nurse is in the first week of orientation.

3. This is expected in a client diagnosed with leukemia, but it indicates a severely low platelet count; a nurse with more experience should care for this client.

4. **This client is receiving blood. The nurse with experience on a medical-surgical floor should be able to administer blood and blood products.**

**TEST-TAKING HINT:** The key to this question is the fact, although the nurse is an experienced medical-surgical nurse, the nurse is not experienced in oncology. The client subject to treatment on a medical-surgical floor should be assigned to the nurse.

21. 1. This is a false promise. Many clients undergo premature menopause as a result of cancer therapy.

2. **The client should be taught to practice birth control during treatment and for at least 2 years after treatment has ceased. The therapies used to treat cancer can cause cancer. Antineoplastic medications are carcinogenic, and radiation therapy has proved to be a precursor to leukemia. A developing fetus would be subjected to the internal conditions of the mother.**

3. Some clients—but not all—do become sterile. The client must understand the risks of therapy, but the nurse should give a realistic picture of what the client can

expect. It is correct procedure to tell the client the nurse does not know the absolute outcome of therapy. This is the ethical principle of veracity.

4. The therapy may interfere with the client's menses, but it may be temporary.

**TEST-TAKING HINT:** Option "3" can be eliminated on the basis that it says "all" clients; if the test taker can think of one case where "all" does not apply, then the option is incorrect.

22. 1. Enlarged lymph tissue would occur in stage III or IV Hodgkin's lymphoma.

2. A tender left upper quadrant would indicate spleen infiltration and occurs at a later stage.

3. **Stage I lymphoma presents with no symptoms; for this reason, clients are usually not diagnosed until the later stages of lymphoma (National Cancer Institute, 2019).**

4. B-cell lymphocytes are the usual lymphocytes involved in the development of lymphoma, but a serum blood test must be done specifically to detect B cells. They are not tested on a CBC.

**TEST-TAKING HINT:** Most cancers are staged from 0 to IV. Stage 0 is microinvasive and stage I is minimally invasive, progressing to stage IV, which is a large tumor load or distant disease. If the test taker noted the "stage I," then choosing the option that presented with the least amount of known disease—option "3"—would be a good choice.

23. 1. **After the first 15 minutes during which the client tolerates the blood transfusion, it is appropriate to ask the UAP to take the vital signs as long as the UAP has been given specific parameters for the vital signs. Any vital signs outside the normal parameters must have an intervention by the nurse.**

2. Antineoplastic medication infusions must be monitored by a chemotherapy-certified, competent nurse.

3. This is the responsibility of the unit secretary or the nurse, not the UAP.

4. This represents the evaluation portion of the nursing process and cannot be delegated.

**TEST-TAKING HINT:** The test taker must decide what is within the realm of duties of a UAP. Three of the options have the UAP doing some action with medications. This could eliminate all of these. Option "1" did not say monitor or evaluate or decide on a nursing action; this option only says the UAP can take vital signs on a presumably stable client because the infusion has been going long enough to reach the hourly time span.

24. 1. The 5-year mark is a time for celebration for clients diagnosed with cancer, but the therapies can cause secondary malignancies and there may be a genetic predisposition for the client to develop cancer. The client should continue to be tested regularly.
   2. Follow-up appointments should be at least yearly.
   3. The client's risk for developing cancer has increased as a result of the therapies undergone for the lymphoma.
   4. This client is in remission, and death is not imminent.

**TEST-TAKING HINT:** The test taker should look at the time frames in the answer options. It would be unusual for a client to be told to have a checkup every 5 years. Option "4" can be eliminated by the stem, which clearly indicates the client is progressing well at the 5-year remission mark.

## Anemia

25. 1. The rugae in the stomach produce intrinsic factor, which allows the body to use vitamin $B_{12}$ from the foods eaten. Gastric bypass surgery reduces the amount of rugae drastically. Clients develop pernicious anemia (vitamin $B_{12}$ deficiency). Other symptoms of anemia include dizziness and the tachycardia and dyspnea listed in the stem.
   2. Folic acid deficiency is usually associated with chronic alcohol intake.
   3. Iron deficiency is the result of chronic blood loss or inadequate dietary intake of iron.
   4. SCD is associated with African Americans, but the symptoms and history indicate a different anemia.

**TEST-TAKING HINT:** The question did not give a lifetime history of anemia, which would be associated with SCD. The stem related to a history of obesity and surgery. The test taker should look for an answer related to the intake of vitamins and minerals. A review of the anatomy of the stomach is the key to the question.

26. 1. Menorrhagia (excessive blood loss during menses) does not cause pain. Fibroids or other factors that cause the menorrhagia may cause pain, but lack of rest or sleep is not responsible for the listlessness or fatigue.
   2. The symptoms are the direct result of excessive blood loss.
   3. Some viruses do cause chronic fatigue syndrome, but there is a direct cause and effect from the menorrhagia.
   4. Menorrhagia is excessive blood loss during menses. If the blood loss is severe, then the client will not have the blood's oxygen-carrying capacity needed for daily activities. The most frequent symptom and complication of anemia is fatigue. It frequently has the greatest impact on the client's ability to function and quality of life.

**TEST-TAKING HINT:** Three of the answer options have the word "menorrhagia" in them, but option "3" detours from the subject to talk about viruses; this could eliminate it as a consideration. This question requires the test taker to understand medical terminology—in this case, what menorrhagia means—and then decide what results from that process in the body.

27. Correct answers are 1, 2, 4, and 5.
   1. The nurse should monitor the Hgb and Hct in all clients diagnosed with anemia.
   2. Because decreased oxygenation levels to the brain can cause the client to become confused, a room where the client can be observed frequently—near the nurse's desk—is a safety issue.
   3. The client should include leafy, green vegetables in the diet. These are high in iron.
   4. Numbness and tingling may occur in anemia as a result of neurological involvement.
   5. Fatigue is the number-one presenting symptom of anemia.

**TEST-TAKING HINT:** This is an alternative-type question requiring the test taker to select multiple correct answers. The test taker could eliminate option "3" because the only clients told to limit green, leafy vegetables are those receiving Coumadin, an oral anticoagulant.

28. 1. Iron is constipating; loperamide (Imodium), an antidiarrheal, for diarrhea is contraindicated for this drug.
    2. Iron can cause gastrointestinal distress, and tolerance to it is built up gradually; exercise has nothing to do with tolerating iron.
    3. **The stool will be a dark green-black, which can mask the appearance of blood in the stool.**
    4. The client should eat a well-balanced diet high in iron, vitamins, and protein. Fowl and fish are encouraged.

**TEST-TAKING HINT:** **The test taker could eliminate option "4" as a possible answer because of the absolute word "only." Health-care professionals usually encourage the client to limit red and organ meats.**

29. 1. **The RN should evaluate the stools of a client diagnosed with melena (dark, tarry stools indicate blood) as part of the ongoing assessment.**
    2. The UAP can take the vital signs of a stable client; this client received the blood the day before.
    3. Evaluation is the nurse's responsibility; the nurse should know what the client is eating.
    4. A client diagnosed with severe hemolytic anemia would have pancytopenia and is at risk for bleeding.

**TEST-TAKING HINT:** **Melena indicates a problem with the bowel movements and would indicate a need for nursing judgment. A nurse cannot delegate judgment decisions.**

30. **74 mL/hr.**
    Pumps are set at an hourly rate. The client in heart failure should receive blood at the slowest possible rate to prevent the client from further complications of fluid volume overload. Each unit of blood must be infused within 4 hours of initiation of the infusion.

    250 mL + 45 mL = 295 mL
    295 mL ÷ 4 = 73¾ mL/hr, which rounded is 74 mL/hr.

**TEST-TAKING HINT:** **The test taker must think about the disease process and the normal requirement for administering blood to arrive at the correct answer.**

31. 1. **Most clients diagnosed with folic acid deficiency anemia have developed anemia from chronic alcohol abuse. Alcohol consumption increases the use of folates, and the alcoholic diet is usually deficient in folic acid. A referral to Alcoholics Anonymous would be appropriate.**
    2. There is no connection between folic acid deficiency and leukemia; therefore, this referral would not be appropriate.
    3. A hematologist may see the client, but nurses usually don't make this kind of referral; the HCP would make this referral if the HCP felt incapable of caring for the client.
    4. The social worker is not the most appropriate referral.

**TEST-TAKING HINT:** **The stem asks the test taker to decide which referral is most appropriate. Option "4" might be appropriate for a number of different clients, but nothing in the stem indicates a specific need for social services. The test taker must decide which could be a possible cause of folic acid deficiency anemia.**

32. 1. Any nurse should be able to administer iron supplements, which are oral iron preparations.
    2. Any nurse should be able to give intramuscular medication.
    3. **Pancytopenia is a situation that develops in clients diagnosed with aplastic anemia because the bone marrow is not able to produce cells of any kind. The client has anemia, thrombocytopenia, and leukopenia. This client could develop an infection or hemorrhage, go into congestive heart failure, or have a number of other complications develop. This client needs the most experienced nurse.**
    4. A deficiency of erythropoietin is common in clients diagnosed with renal disease. The current treatment for this is to administer erythropoietin, a biologic response modifier, subcutaneously, or, if the anemia is severe enough, a blood transfusion.

**TEST-TAKING HINT:** **The test taker could eliminate options "1" and "2" because of the words "most experienced nurse" in the stem.**

33. 1. The client may need oxygen, but getting the client a wheelchair and getting the client back to bed is the priority.
    2. **The client is experiencing dyspnea on exertion, which is common for clients diagnosed with anemia. The client needs a wheelchair to limit exertion.**
    3. The problem with this client is not a pulmonary one; it is a lack of Hgb.
    4. Even if the nurse helps the client ambulate, the client still will not have the needed oxygen for the tissues.

**TEST-TAKING HINT:** The test taker should ask, "What is causing the distress, and what will alleviate the distress the fastest?" The distress is caused by exertion and it is occurring in the hallway. The most expedient intervention is to have the client stop the activity that is causing the distress; a chair will accomplish this, but the client should be returned to the room, so it needs to be a wheelchair.

34. 1. The usual medication dosing time for daily medications is 0900, but this is only an hour after the breakfast meal. Iron absorption is reduced when taken with food.
    2. This is approximately 2 hours after breakfast and is the correct dosing time for iron to achieve the best effects. Iron preparations should be administered 1 hour before a meal or 2 hours after a meal. Iron can cause gastrointestinal upset, but if administered with a meal, absorption can be diminished by as much as 50%.
    3. This is the usual time health-care facilities serve lunch.
    4. This time would be very close to the evening meal and would decrease the absorption of the iron.

**TEST-TAKING HINT:** The test taker could eliminate options "3" and "4" if the test taker realized both of these times are very close to mealtimes, so, with this in common, food must pose a problem for the medication.

35. Correct answers are 3 and 5.
    1. This is an instruction for antibiotics, not iron. The client will take iron for an indefinite period.
    2. Pulse is indirectly affected by anemia when the body attempts to compensate for the lack of oxygen supply, but this is an indirect measure, and blood pressure is not monitored for anemia.
    3. The client should have a CBC regularly to determine the status of the anemia.
    4. Isometric exercises are bodybuilding exercises, and the client should not exert in this manner.
    5. The client should be encouraged to eat foods high in iron such as red meat, organ meats, legumes, spinach, and pumpkin seeds.

**TEST-TAKING HINT:** The test taker could eliminate option "1" because this applies to antibiotics and option "4" because it is an isometric exercise.

36. Correct answers are 1 and 5.
    1. The client's problem is activity intolerance, and the pacing of activities directly affects the diagnosis.
    2. This is an appropriate intervention for iron or vitamin deficiency, but it is not for activity intolerance.
    3. This may be done but not specifically for the diagnosis.
    4. This would not help activity intolerance.
    5. Assisting the client with personal care and ambulation will address activity intolerance

**TEST-TAKING HINT:** The test taker should read the stem closely and choose only interventions that directly affect an activity. The word "activity" is in the diagnosis and in the correct answer. When answer options match the stem, they are good choices.

## Bleeding Disorders

37. 1. This is a major surgery but has a predictable course with no complications identified in the stem, and a colostomy is expected with this type of surgery. The graduate nurse could be assigned to this client.
    2. Acute respiratory distress syndrome (ARDS) is a potentially life-threatening complication and should be assigned to a more experienced nurse.
    3. DIC is life-threatening. The client is unstable and should be assigned to a more experienced nurse.
    4. This client is experiencing hypovolemia, which means hemorrhaging and potential emergency surgery; therefore, this client should be assigned to a more experienced nurse.

**TEST-TAKING HINT:** The test taker must think about what type of client a new graduate should be assigned. The least critical client is the correct choice.

38. 1. DIC is a complication in many obstetric problems, including septic abortion, abruptio placentae, amniotic fluid embolus, and retained dead fetus, but it is not a complication of placenta previa.
    2. A client diagnosed with a fat embolus is at risk for DIC, but a client diagnosed with a pulmonary embolus is not.
    3. Hemodialysis is not a risk factor for developing DIC.

4. DIC is a clinical syndrome that develops as a complication of a wide variety of other disorders, with sepsis being the most common cause of DIC.

**TEST-TAKING HINT:** The test taker could eliminate option "3" if the test taker knew that DIC is a complication of another disorder. Age is not a risk factor for developing DIC.

39. 1. The clinical manifestations of DIC result from clotting and bleeding, ranging from oozing blood to bleeding from every body orifice and into the tissues.
    2. Chest pain and frothy sputum may indicate a pulmonary embolus.
    3. Foul-smelling, concentrated urine may indicate dehydration or urinary tract infection.
    4. A reddened, inflamed central line catheter site indicates a possible infection.

**TEST-TAKING HINT:** If the test taker realized that coagulation deals with blood, then the only answer option that addresses any type of bleeding is option "1."

40. Correct answers are 2 and 5.
    1. The prothrombin time (PT), along with the partial thromboplastin time (PTT) and thrombin time, are prolonged or increased in a client diagnosed with DIC.
    2. **The fibrinogen level helps predict bleeding in DIC. As it becomes lower, the risk of bleeding increases.**
    3. The platelet count is decreased in DIC. The platelets are used up because clotting and bleeding are occurring simultaneously.
    4. WBC counts increase as a result of infection, not from DIC.
    5. Fibrin split products are elevated.

**TEST-TAKING HINT:** An understanding of bleeding may help the test taker rule out options "3" and "4" because platelets are needed for clotting, so an increased platelet count would not cause bleeding, and WBCs are associated with infection. If the test taker thinks about oral anticoagulant therapy and remembers that PT is prolonged with bleeding, it might lead to eliminating option "1" as a possible correct answer. Option "5" is the breakdown of fibrin (also fibrinogen degradation products) and this could be associated with option "2."

41. 1. Heparin, a parenteral anticoagulant, is administered to interfere with the clotting cascade and may prevent further clotting factor consumption as a result of uncontrolled bleeding, but its use is controversial. Oral anticoagulants are not administered.

2. Plasmapheresis involves the removal of plasma from withdrawn blood by centrifugation, reconstituting it in an isotonic solution, and then reinfusing the solution back into the body, but it is not a treatment for DIC.
3. Fresh frozen plasma, cryoprecipitate, and platelet concentrates are administered to restore clotting factors and platelets.
4. Calculating the I&O is adding up how much oral and intravenous fluids went into the client and how much fluid came out of the client. It does not require an HCP's order and thus is not a collaborative treatment.

**TEST-TAKING HINT:** "Collaborative" means another health-care discipline must order or perform the intervention. A test-taking hint that may help with unit examinations, but not with the NCLEX-RN®, is that if the test taker has studied the assigned content and has never heard of one of the words in the answer options, the test taker should not select that answer—in this case, perhaps the word "plasmapheresis."

42. 1. This is a true statement, but it is medical jargon explaining how someone gets hemophilia A and thus is not the best response.
    2. This is a true statement, but it refers to the pathophysiology of hemophilia A and does not explain how someone gets the disease.
    3. This is a true statement, but it does not answer the question of how someone gets it.
    4. **This is a true statement and explains exactly how someone gets hemophilia A: The mother passes it to the son.**

**TEST-TAKING HINT:** When the stem has the word "best" in it, then all four answer options could be correct and, in this case, statements that the RN could reply, but only one answer option is best. The test taker needs to evaluate the stem and identify terms that may help select the best option; in this case, a UAP is asking the question, and a direct answer without using medical jargon should be given.

43. 1. Nosebleeds, along with hemarthrosis, cutaneous hematoma formation, bleeding gums, hematemesis, occult blood, and hematuria, are all clinical manifestations of hemophilia.
    2. Petechiae are tiny purple or red spots that appear on the skin as a result of minute hemorrhages within the dermal or

submucosal layers, but they are not clinical manifestations of hemophilia.

3. Subcutaneous emphysema is air under the skin, which may occur with a chest tube or tracheostomy insertion.

4. Intermittent claudication is severe leg pain that occurs from decreased oxygenation to the leg muscles.

**TEST-TAKING HINT: If the test taker knows that hemophilia is a bleeding disorder, the test taker should eliminate any answer options that don't address bleeding—in this case, options "3" and "4."**

44. 1. Vomiting blood is not a situation that would indicate the client has von Willebrand's disease.

2. Microscopic blood in the urine is not a clinical manifestation of von Willebrand's disease.

3. von Willebrand's disease is a type of hemophilia. The most common hereditary bleeding disorder, it is caused by a deficiency in von Willebrand's factor (vWF) and is often diagnosed after prolonged bleeding following surgery or dental extraction (National Hemophilia Foundation, 2020).

4. Abruptio placentae is not a situation that might cause von Willebrand's disease.

**TEST-TAKING HINT: The test taker must be knowledgeable about vWF to be able to answer this question. Risk factors or situations are facts that need to be memorized.**

45. 1. The client should avoid prescription and OTC drugs containing acetylsalicylic acid (aspirin) because these drugs may have an antiplatelet effect, leading to bleeding.

2. Hemarthrosis is bleeding into the joint. Applying ice to the area can cause vasoconstriction, which can help decrease bleeding.

3. The joint should be immobilized for 24 to 48 hours after the bleeding starts.

4. The dependent position is putting the extremity below the level of the heart; the extremity should be elevated if possible.

**TEST-TAKING HINT: If the test taker does not know the answer, the test taker could apply medical terminology; in this case, the terminology contains _hem-_, which refers to "blood." A basic concept with bleeding is that cold causes vasoconstriction; therefore, option "2" would be a good choice to select.**

46. 1. ITP is caused by bleeding from small vessels and mucous membranes. Petechiae, tiny purple or red spots that appear on the skin as a result of minute hemorrhages within the dermal or submucosal layers, and purpura, hemorrhaging into the tissue beneath the skin and mucous membranes, are the first clinical manifestations of ITP.

2. A CRT less than 3 seconds is a normal assessment finding and would not indicate ITP.

3. A splenectomy is the treatment of choice if glucocorticosteroid therapy does not treat the ITP, but the spleen is not enlarged.

4. ITP causes bleeding, but it does not affect the oxygen that gets to the periphery.

**TEST-TAKING HINT: Knowing medical terminology—in this case, that _thrombo-_ refers to "platelets"—the test taker could conclude that an answer option that includes something about bleeding would be the most appropriate selection for the correct answer. Options "2" and "4" could be eliminated as possible answers based on the knowledge that these are normal values.**

47. 1. A range for the normal activated PTT is 25 to 35 seconds.

2. These are normal Hgb and Hct levels for either a male or a female client.

3. A platelet count of less than 100,000 per cubic millimeter of blood indicates thrombocytopenia.

4. This is a normal red blood cell count.

**TEST-TAKING HINT: The test taker must be knowledgeable of normal laboratory values. The test taker should write these normal values on a 3 × 5 card, carry it, and memorize the values.**

48. Correct answers are 2, 3, and 4.

1. The client should use an electric razor, which minimizes the opportunity to develop superficial cuts that may result in bleeding.

2. Enemas, rectal thermometers, and intramuscular injections can pose a risk of tissue and vascular trauma that can precipitate bleeding.

3. Even minor trauma can lead to serious bleeding episodes; safer activities such as swimming or golf should be recommended.

4. Direct pressure occludes bleeding vessels.

5. There is no reason why the client can't floss the teeth.

**TEST-TAKING HINT:** This type of question requires the test taker to select all interventions that apply. Bleeding is the priority concern with hemophilia A, so all interventions should be based around activities that can potentially cause bleeding and ways to treat bleeding.

## Blood Transfusions

49. Correct answers are 1, 3, and 4.
    1. The client must give permission to receive blood or blood products because of the nature of potential complications.
    2. Most blood products require at least a 20-gauge IV because of the size of the cells. RBCs are best infused through an 18-gauge IV. If unable to achieve cannulation with an 18-gauge, a 20-gauge is the smallest acceptable IV. Smaller IVs damage the cell walls of the RBCs and reduce the life expectancy of the RBCs.
    3. Because infusing IV fluids can cause fluid volume overload, the nurse must assess for heart failure. Assessing the lungs includes auscultating for crackles and other clinical manifestations of left-sided heart failure. Additional assessment findings of jugular vein distention, peripheral edema, and liver engorgement indicate right-sided failure.
    4. Checking for allergies is important before administering any medication. Some medications are administered before blood administration.
    5. A keep-open IV of 0.9% saline would be hung. $D_5W$ causes RBCs to hemolyze in the tubing.

**TEST-TAKING HINT:** This is an alternative-type question. This type of question can appear anywhere on the NCLEX-RN® examination. Each answer option must be evaluated on its own merit. One will not rule out another. Assessing is the first step of the nursing process. Unless the test taker is absolutely sure that an option is wrong, the test taker could select an option based on "assessing," such as options "3" and "4." Ethically speaking, informed consent should always be given for any procedure unless a life-or-death emergency situation exists. The other options require knowledge of blood and blood product administration.

50. 1. This should be done, but the client requires the IV first. This client is at risk for shock.
    2. The first action in a situation in which the nurse suspects the client has a fluid volume loss is to replace the volume as quickly as possible.
    3. The client will probably need to have surgery to correct the source of the bleeding, but stabilizing the client with fluid resuscitation is the first priority.
    4. This is the last thing on this list in order of priority.

**TEST-TAKING HINT:** The question requires the test taker to decide which of the actions comes first. Only one of the options actually has the nurse treating the client. The test taker must not read into a question—for example, that consent is needed to send a client to surgery to correct the problem, so that could be first. Only one answer option has the potential to stabilize the client.

51. Correct answers are 1, 3, 4, and 5.
    1. Oral surgeries are associated with transient bacteremia, and the client cannot donate for 72 hours after oral surgery. This client had oral surgery a week ago so is eligible to donate
    2. The client cannot donate blood for 1 month following rubella immunization. This client had a rubella vaccination 2 weeks ago.
    3. The client cannot donate blood for 6 weeks after pregnancy. This client may donate blood.
    4. Recent allergic reactions prevent donation because the passive transference of hypersensitivity can occur. This client has an allergy to acetylsalicylic acid (aspirin) developed during childhood.
    5. The client with a tattoo must wait 12 months to donate blood if the state where the tattoo was applied is not regulated. Currently District of Columbia, Georgia, Idaho, Maryland, Massachusetts, New Hampshire, New York, Pennsylvania, Utah, and Wyoming do not regulate tattoos. This client can donate because the tattoo was applied over 1 year ago (American Red Cross, 2020).

**TEST-TAKING HINT:** All of the answer options have a given time period, and these time frames make each option correct or incorrect. The test taker must pay particular attention whenever an option contains time frames. Is it long enough or not frequent enough?

52. 1. O– (O-negative) blood is considered the universal donor because it does not contain the antigens A, B, or Rh. (AB+ is considered the universal recipient because a person with this blood type has all the antigens on the blood.)
2. A+ blood contains the antigen A that the client will react to, causing the development of antibodies. The unit being Rh+ is compatible with the client.
3. B+ blood contains the antigen B that the client will react to, causing the development of antibodies. The unit being Rh+ is compatible with the client.
4. This client does not have antigens A or B in the blood. Administration of these types would cause an antigen-antibody reaction within the client's body, resulting in massive hemolysis of the client's blood and death.

**TEST-TAKING HINT: This is a knowledge-based question that requires memorization of the particular facts regarding blood typing. Three of the possible answer options have a positive (+) Rh factor; only one has a negative (−) Rh factor.**

53. 1. Prednisone, a glucocorticoid, is a steroid that could delay healing time after the surgery and has no effect on the production of RBCs.
2. Azithromycin (Zithromax), an antibiotic, does not increase the production of RBCs. Orthopedic surgeries frequently involve blood loss. The client wishes to donate blood for the surgery (autologous).
3. Lorazepam (Ativan) is a tranquilizer. Tranquilizers do not affect the production of RBCs.
4. **Epoetin alpha (Epogen) and (Procrit), biologic response modifiers, are forms of erythropoietin, the substance in the body that stimulates the bone marrow to produce RBCs. A client may be prescribed iron preparations to prevent the depletion of iron stores and erythropoietin to increase RBC production. A unit of blood can be withdrawn once a week beginning at 6 weeks before surgery. No phlebotomy will be done within 72 hours of surgery.**

**TEST-TAKING HINT: The test taker should examine the keywords "autologous" and "transfusion." If the test taker did not know the meaning of the word "autologous," "auto-" as a prefix refers to "self," such as an autobiography, one's own story. Pairing "self" with** "transfusion" then should make the test taker look for an option that would directly affect the production of blood cells.

54. 1. **An autologous blood recovery apparatus, or cell saver, is a device to catch the blood lost during orthopedic surgeries to reinfuse into the client, rather than giving the client donor blood products. The cells are washed with saline and reinfused through a filter into the client. The salvaged cells cannot be stored and must be used within 4 hours or discarded because of bacterial growth.**
2. The cell saver has a measuring device; an hourly drainage bag is part of a urinary drainage system. A cell saver is a sterile system that should not be broken until ready to disconnect for reinfusion.
3. The PACU nurse would not replace the cell saver; it is inserted into the surgical wound. A CPM machine can be attached on the outside of the bandage and started if the surgeon so orders, but this has nothing to do with the blood.
4. The blood has not been crossmatched, so there is no a crossmatch number.

**TEST-TAKING HINT: The test taker could discard option "4" if the test taker realized that the laboratory is not involved with this blood at all. The test taker must have basic knowledge of surgical care.**

55. 1. Blood will coagulate if left out for an extended period, but blood is stored with a preservative that prevents this and prolongs the life of the blood.
2. **Blood is a medium for bacterial growth, and any bacteria contaminating the unit will begin to grow if left outside of a controlled refrigerated temperature for longer than 4 hours, placing the client at risk for septicemia.**
3. Blood components are stable and do not break down after 4 hours.
4. These are standard nursing and laboratory procedures to prevent the complication of septicemia.

**TEST-TAKING HINT: The test taker must know the rationale behind nursing interventions to be able to answer this question.**

56. 1. The HCP has written an appropriate order for this client diagnosed with heart failure and does not need to be called to verify the order before the nurse implements it.
2. Blood or blood components have a specified amount of infusion time, and this is

not 8 hours. The time constraints are for the protection of the client.
3. The correct procedure for administering a unit of blood over 8 hours is to have the unit split into halves. Each half-unit is treated as a new unit and checked accordingly. This slower administration allows the compromised client, such as one with heart failure, to assimilate the extra fluid volume.
4. This rate has already been determined by the HCP to be unsafe for this client.

**TEST-TAKING HINT:** The key to this question is the time frame of 8 hours and the client's diagnosis of heart failure. Basic knowledge of heart failure allows the test taker to realize that fluid volume is the problem. Only one option addresses administering a smaller volume at a time.

57. 1. This should be done, but after preventing any more of the PRBCs from infusing.
2. Diphenhydramine (Benadryl), a histamine-1 blocker, may be administered to reduce the severity of the transfusion reaction, but it is not the first priority.
3. The nurse should assess the client, but in this case, the nurse has all the assessment data needed to stop the transfusion.
4. **The priority in this situation is to prevent a further reaction if possible. Stopping the transfusion and changing the fluid out at the hub will prevent any more of the transfusion from entering the client's bloodstream.**

**TEST-TAKING HINT:** In a question that requires the test taker to determine a priority action, the test taker must decide what will have the most impact on the client. Option "4" does this. All the options are interventions that should be taken, but only one will be first.

58. 1. UAPs cannot assess. The RN cannot delegate the assessment.
2. The likelihood of a reaction is the greatest during the first 15 minutes of a transfusion. The nurse should never leave the client until after this time. The nurse should take and assess the vital signs during this time.
3. Auscultation of the lung sounds and administering blood based on this information are the nurse's responsibility. Any action requiring nursing judgment cannot be delegated.

4. **The UAP can assist a client in brushing the teeth. Instructions about using soft-bristle toothbrushes and the need to report to the nurse any pink or bleeding gums should be given before delegating the procedure.**

**TEST-TAKING HINT:** The test taker must be aware of delegation guidelines. The RN cannot delegate assessment or any intervention requiring nursing judgment. Options "1," "2," and "3" require judgment and cannot be delegated to a UAP.

59. 1. The likelihood of a client having a transfusion reaction after receiving more than half of the blood product is slim. The first 15 minutes have passed, and to this point, the client is tolerating the blood.
2. Clients diagnosed with leukemia have cancer involving blood cell production. These are expected findings in a client diagnosed with leukemia.
3. **This client has a potential for hemorrhage and is reporting blood in the vomitus. This client should be assessed first.**
4. Crohn's disease involves frequent diarrhea stools, leading to perineal irritation and skin excoriation. This is expected and not life-threatening. Clients "1," "2," and "3" should be seen before this client.

**TEST-TAKING HINT:** In a prioritizing question, the test taker should be able to rank in order which client to see first, second, third, and fourth. Expected, but not immediately life-threatening, situations are seen after a situation in which the client has a life-threatening problem.

60. **886 mL of fluid has infused.**
   250 mL + 63 mL = 313 mL per unit
   313 + 313 = 626 mL
   500 mL of saline – 240 mL remaining = 260 mL infused.
   626 mL + 260 mL = 886 mL of fluid infused.

**TEST-TAKING HINT:** This problem has several steps but only requires basic addition and subtraction. The test taker should use the drop-down calculator on the computer to check or double-check the answer to make sure that simple mistakes are not made.

## Sickle Cell Disease

61. 1. Offering the nursing student written material is appropriate, but the nurse's best statement would be to answer the student's question.
    2. The problem in SCD is that the blood clots inappropriately when there is a decrease in oxygenation.
    3. This is a true statement, but it is not the best response because it is not answering the nursing student's question.
    4. SCD is a disorder of the RBCs characterized by abnormally shaped red cells that sickle or clump together, leading to oxygen deprivation and resulting in crisis and severe pain.

**TEST-TAKING HINT:** When answering a question, the test taker should close the eyes and answer the question exactly as if in the clinical setting. Most nurses would answer the student's question and not offer written material.

62. 1. This is the etiology for SCD, but a layperson would not understand this explanation.
    2. This explains the etiology in terms that a layperson could understand. When both parents are carriers of the disease, each pregnancy has a 25% chance of producing a child with SCD.
    3. The cause of SCD is known, and genetic counseling can explain it to the prospective parent.
    4. A virus does not cause SCD.

**TEST-TAKING HINT:** When discussing disease processes with laypersons, the nurse should explain the facts in terms that the person can understand. Would a layperson know what "autosomal recessive" means? The test taker should consider terminology when selecting an answer.

63. 1. The HCP could order STAT ABGs, but caring directly for the client is always the first priority.
    2. A pulse oximeter reading of less than 93% indicates hypoxia, which warrants oxygen administration.
    3. The nurse should start an 18-gauge IV catheter because the client may need blood, but this is not the nurse's first intervention.
    4. The medication will be administered intravenously, so the IV will have to be started before administering the medication.

**TEST-TAKING HINT:** If the test taker can eliminate two options and cannot decide between the other two, the test taker should apply a rule such as Maslow's hierarchy of needs and select the intervention that addresses oxygenation or airway.

64. **Correct answers are 3 and 5.**
    1. Meperidine (Demerol) is not given in sickle cell crisis to control pain or recommended for long-term pain management because the accumulative effect of normeperidine can cause seizures. Morphine is the drug of choice.
    2. The client does not need to be in reverse isolation because other people will not affect the crisis.
    3. The increased intravenous fluid reduces the viscosity of blood, thereby preventing further sickling as a result of dehydration.
    4. The client needs to be receiving I&O monitoring, but there is no reason to insert a Foley catheter.
    5. Oxygen therapy is given to the client in sickle cell crisis or vaso-occlusive crisis.

**TEST-TAKING HINT:** The test taker would have to know that sickling is caused by decreased oxygen or dehydration to know this answer. Possibly looking at the word "infection" and increasing fluids may help the test taker select this option.

65. 1. The oral mucosa and conjunctiva should be assessed for cyanosis (blueness) in individuals with dark skin because cyanosis cannot be assessed in the lips or fingertips.
    2. Metacarpals are the fingers, which should not be assessed for cyanosis.
    3. CRT is not a reliable indicator of cyanosis in individuals with dark skin.
    4. The nurse should assess the conjunctiva for paleness, indicating hypoxemia; the sclera is assessed for jaundice.

**TEST-TAKING HINT:** The test taker must realize that assessing different skin colors requires different assessment techniques and data.

66. **3,000 mL.**
    The key is knowing that 1 ounce is equal to 30 mL. Then, 20 ounces (20 × 30) = 600 mL, 8 ounces (8 × 30) = 240 mL, and 4 ounces (4 × 30) = 120 × 3 cartons = 360 mL for a total of 600 + 240 + 360 = 1,200 mL of oral fluids. That, plus 1,800 mL of IV fluids, makes the total intake for this shift 3,000 mL.

**TEST-TAKING HINT:** The test taker must memorize equivalents, such as how many milliliters are in an ounce. This is the only way that the test taker can convert the client's intake to be able to assess the balance between intake and output.

67. 1. Whenever an opportunity presents itself, the nurse should teach the client about the medical condition. This client should not go to areas that have decreased oxygen, such as Yellowstone National Park, which is at high altitude.
    2. This is passing the buck. The nurse can respond to this comment.
    3. **High altitudes have decreased oxygen, which could lead to a sickle cell crisis.**
    4. It is none of the nurse's business why the client wants to go to Yellowstone National Park. The client's safety comes first, and the nurse needs to teach the client.

**TEST-TAKING HINT: Even if the test taker did not know the answer to this question, the only answer option that does any teaching is option "3," which would be the best choice. Yellowstone National Park, because of its altitude, has something to do with the answer.**

68. 1. Chest syndrome refers to chest pain, fever, and a dry, hacking cough with or without pre-existing pneumonia and is not a fatal complication. It can occur in males and females.
    2. Compartment syndrome is a complication of a cast that has been applied too tightly or a fracture in which there is edema in a muscle compartment.
    3. **This is a term that means painful and constant penile erection that can occur in male clients diagnosed with SCD during a sickle cell crisis.**
    4. A hypertensive crisis is potentially fatal, but it is not a complication of SCD. The client diagnosed with SCD usually has cardiomegaly or systolic murmurs; all sexes have this.

**TEST-TAKING HINT: This is a knowledge-based question, but if the test taker realized that priapism could only occur in males, this might help the test taker select option "3" as a correct answer. Whenever there is an indicated sex for the client, it usually has something to do with the correct answer.**

69. 1. Health promotion is important in clients diagnosed with chronic illnesses, but the best answer should address the client's specific disease process, not chronic illnesses in general.

2. An individual with SCD has a reduction in splenic activity from infarcts occurring during crises. This situation progresses to the spleen no longer being able to function, and this increases the client's susceptibility to infection.
    3. These vaccines do nothing to prevent the sickling of the blood cells.
    4. Teaching the client is an independent nursing intervention, and the nurse does not need to rely on the HCP to designate what should be taught to the client.

**TEST-TAKING HINT: Vaccines are recommended to clients diagnosed with chronic problems to help prevent the flu and pneumonia. The test taker should see if a widely accepted concept could help answer the question and not get caught up in the client's disease process.**

70. 1. Research and a search for a cure are not the missions of the Sickle Cell Foundation.
    2. **The foundation's mission is to provide information about the disease and about support groups in the area. This information helps decrease the client's and significant others' feelings of frustration and helplessness.**
    3. The nurse should not force personal thoughts on the client. The nurse should provide information and let the client make decisions. This empowers the client.
    4. The nurse can arrange for families to meet, but this is not the mission of the foundation.

**TEST-TAKING HINT: The nurse should know about organizations for specific disease processes in the geographic area, but most organizations provide information on the disease process and support groups.**

71. 1. Skeletal deformities, such as lordosis or kyphosis, are common. They are secondary to chronic vaso-occlusive crisis, not an acute crisis.
    2. A bloody nose is not an expected finding in a client diagnosed with an acute vaso-occlusive crisis.
    3. **Vaso-occlusive crisis, the most frequent crisis, is characterized by organ infarction, which will result in bloody urine secondary to kidney infarction.**
    4. Petechiae are small pinpoint blood spots on the skin, but they are not clinical manifestations of a vaso-occlusive crisis.

**TEST-TAKING HINT:** Understanding medical terminology of assessment data is an important part of being able to answer NCLEX-RN® questions. These terms can help eliminate or select an answer option.

72. 1. A spinal tap is a test used to diagnose meningitis.
    2. Hemoglobin electrophoresis is a test used to help diagnose SCD; it is the "fingerprinting" of the protein, which detects homozygous and heterozygous forms of the disease.
    3. The sickle cell screen is only used to screen for SCD.
    4. The elevated temperature is the first clinical manifestation of bacteremia. Bacteremia leads to a sickle cell crisis. Therefore, the bacteria must be identified so that the appropriate antibiotics can be prescribed to treat the infection. Blood cultures assist in determining the type and source of infection so that it can be treated appropriately.

**TEST-TAKING HINT:** The client's temperature in the stem is the key to selecting blood cultures as the correct answer.

**73.** Correct answers are 1, 2, 3, and 4.

1. The client is at risk of infection because of the lack of mature WBCs in the circulating blood. Leukemia is a disease process involving the hematological system. WBCs are produced in the bone marrow. The nurse screens visitors for infection because there are insufficient functioning WBCs to protect the client from developing an infection if exposed to a virus or bacteria.
2. The client should be monitored for infection; one way to do this is to monitor the temperature.
3. Fresh fruits and vegetables may have bacteria on the skins, which could expose the client to infection.
4. The WBC count indicates the presence or absence of granulocytes, also called neutrophils or segmented neutrophils.
5. The client might be placed on reverse isolation or neutropenic precautions because the client is at risk from anyone entering the room; however, there is no reason to suspect the client is a risk to others, which droplet precautions are initiated to prevent.
6. Bone marrow biopsies are not performed daily.

**TEST-TAKING HINT:** The test taker must answer "Select all that apply" questions by viewing each option as true or false.

**74.** 1. Immunity is compromised when the hematopoietic system is impaired. The bone marrow is part of the initial response by the immune system to prevent disease.
2. Grieving is a possible interrelated concept because the client must adjust to the diagnosis but is not a priority over a physiological problem.
3. Perfusion is not a concept normally associated with lymphoma.
4. Clotting is not a concept normally associated with lymphoma.

**TEST-TAKING HINT:** The test taker must match the problem with the answer option. Options "3" and "4" would probably be implemented for the client diagnosed with a bleeding disorder. Option "2" is a psychological problem; physiological issues are priority over psychological problems.

**75.** Correct answers are 2 and 5.

1. The client should be encouraged to push fluids to maintain hydration. When the client becomes dehydrated, then the sickling of the abnormal RBCs will occur.
2. The client should maintain hydration status to prevent the sickling of the RBCs.
3. Swelling from sickling cells usually occurs in the joints and into the organs. Measuring the calf would be assessing for deep vein thrombosis.
4. The client should receive pain medication on a prn basis, not routinely around the clock, unless experiencing a sickle cell crisis.
5. Hydroxyurea, an FDA-approved medication, has been proven to reduce the frequency of painful sickling episodes (American Society of Hematology, 2019).

**TEST-TAKING HINT:** The test taker must be aware of the cause of physiological changes in the body. The sickling of cells occurs when the client experiences a lack of oxygen to the cells or becomes dehydrated.

**76.** 1. The client is at risk of forming clots, which can lead to cerebrovascular accidents [CVAs] (stroke).
2. There is no reason to keep the HOB elevated.
3. A low-sodium diet is for fluid volume overload, not dehydration.
4. Antiembolism hose are not needed for sickle cell crisis.

**TEST-TAKING HINT:** The test taker must be aware of the cause of physiological changes in the body. The sickling of cells occurs when the client experiences a lack of oxygen to the cells or becomes dehydrated. The results of clot formation can lead to strokes and other CVAs.

**77.** 1. Night sweats and low-grade fever do occur in Hodgkin's disease but also occur in diseases associated with an HIV infection.
2. Cavitation occurs with tuberculosis.
3. Reed-Sternberg cells found on biopsy are diagnostic for Hodgkin's disease.
4. Weight loss and palpable lymph nodes should be investigated but are not definitive in the diagnosis of Hodgkin's disease.

**TEST-TAKING HINT:** The test taker must be aware of the cause of physiological changes in the body. The test taker should read every word; "diagnostic" means not just clinical manifestations, which could be attributed to several different diseases, but something that is only attributed to the disease in question.

78. 1. Comfort is appropriate for the disease but is not the priority concept. Pain alerts the client that a problem is occurring but is not life-threatening.
    2. Stress could be a concept, but coping problems are the priority.
    3. Grieving is an interrelated concept but is limited in the scope of the client's needs.
    4. Coping includes dealing with stress, anxiety, and grief. The nurse can help the client most by assisting in identifying the client's coping mechanisms.

**TEST-TAKING HINT:** The test taker must be aware of concepts that are interrelated. Coping encompasses stress and grieving. The word "psychological" can rule out option "1" because comfort is related to pain.

79. 1. The nurse's priority is to treat the cause of the crisis and pain.
    2. During a crisis and the administration of narcotic medication, frequent ambulation is not encouraged.
    3. The client has the ability to oxygenate the cells; if used, then the rate would not be at 10 LPM.
    4. The client's RBCs would be monitored but not every 4 hours.

**TEST-TAKING HINT:** The test taker must be aware of the cause of physiological changes in the body. The nurse must treat a client's discomfort if the cause of the pain is known, and no other complications are occurring.

80. 1. According to Erikson's growth and development stages, the 32-year-old should be in the intimacy versus isolation stage. In this stage, the client should have developed a close relationship with another human being, have a job, and become self-supporting. This client is not meeting Erikson's expected stage of development for his age.
    2. This client is caring for a child; based on this statement, the client is meeting Erikson's growth and development stages.

3. This client is caring for a parent and working. Based on this statement, the client is meeting Erikson's growth and development stages.
4. This client is actively involved in preparing for a career and has friends. Based on this statement, this client is meeting Erikson's growth and development stages.

**TEST-TAKING HINT:** The test taker must be aware of the cause of psychological changes as growth across the life span occurs. Basic psychology principles are frequently used by nurses to assess the client's status. The test taker has to memorize the stages of development.

81. 1. Petechiae indicate a lack of clotting ability caused by decreased production of platelets.
    2. Pain and joint swelling could indicate several different disease processes.
    3. The H&H are low but not indicative of leukemia.
    4. A headache and slurred speech could indicate a CVA or other disease processes.

**TEST-TAKING HINT:** The test taker must be aware of the cause of physiological changes in the body in order to answer this option. Platelets are produced by the bone marrow, and a deficient number results in bleeding (small pinpoint areas of bleeding appear on the body).

82. Correct answers are 1 and 2.
    1. Coping could be applied to any diagnosis of cancer.
    2. Hematologic regulation is the top priority identified for a client diagnosed with lymphoma because the client has a problem with the cells produced by the bone marrow.
    3. Tissue perfusion is not associated with lymphoma.
    4. Clotting is not associated with lymphoma.
    5. Clinical judgment is a concept for the nurse, not the client.

**TEST-TAKING HINT:** The test taker must consider each option in a "Select all that apply" question as a true or false option. The lymphocytes are produced on the bone marrow; the test taker has to remember the pathophysiology of the disease process.

# HEMATOLOGICAL DISORDERS COMPREHENSIVE EXAMINATION

1. The client is diagnosed with severe iron-deficiency anemia. Which statement is the scientific rationale regarding oral replacement therapy?
   1. Iron supplements are well tolerated without side effects.
   2. There is no benefit from oral preparations; the best route is IV.
   3. Oral iron preparations cause diarrhea if not taken with food.
   4. Very little of the iron supplement will be absorbed by the body.

2. The client's laboratory values are populated in the chart below. Which intervention should the nurse implement?

   | Complete Blood Count | Client Value | Normal Values |
   | --- | --- | --- |
   | RBCs | 5.5 | Male: 4.21–5.81 ($10^6$ cells/microL) Female: 3.61–5.11 ($10^6$ cells/microL) |
   | Platelet | 189 | 140–400 × ($10^3$/microL) |
   | WBCs | 8.9 | 4.5–11.1 × ($10^3$/cells/microL) |

   1. Prepare to administer PRBCs.
   2. Continue to monitor the client.
   3. Request an order for filgrastim.
   4. Institute bleeding precautions.

3. The client diagnosed with anemia is admitted to the emergency department with dyspnea, cool pale skin, and diaphoresis. Which assessment data **warrant immediate** intervention?
   1. The vital signs are T 98.6° F, P 116, R 28, and BP 88/62.
   2. The client is allergic to multiple antibiotic medications.
   3. The client has a history of receiving chemotherapy.
   4. ABGs are pH 7.35, $Pco_2$ 44, $Hco_3$ 22, $Pao_2$ 92.

4. The client diagnosed with anemia has an Hgb of 6.1 g/dL. Which **complication** should the nurse assess for?
   1. Decreased pulmonary functioning.
   2. Impaired muscle functioning.
   3. Congestive heart failure.
   4. Altered gastric secretions.

5. The nurse writes a diagnosis of "activity intolerance" for a client diagnosed with anemia. Which intervention should the nurse implement?
   1. Encourage isometric exercises.
   2. Assist the client with activities of daily living (ADLs).
   3. Provide a high-protein diet.
   4. Refer to the physical therapist.

6. The client diagnosed with cancer has been undergoing systemic treatments and has RBC deficiency. Which clinical manifestations should the nurse teach the client to manage?
   1. Nausea associated with cancer treatment.
   2. Shortness of breath and fatigue.
   3. Controlling mucositis and diarrhea.
   4. The emotional aspects of having cancer.

7. The nurse is assisting the HCP with a bone marrow biopsy. Which intervention postprocedure has **priority?**
   1. Apply pressure to site for 5 to 10 minutes.
   2. Medicate for pain with morphine slow IVP.
   3. Maintain head of the bed in high Fowler's position.
   4. Apply oxygen via nasal cannula at 5 L/min.

8. The client diagnosed with end-stage renal disease has developed anemia. Which would the nurse anticipate the HCP prescribing for this client?
   1. Place the client in reverse isolation.
   2. Discontinue treatments until blood count improves.
   3. Monitor CBC daily to assess for bleeding.
   4. Give the client erythropoietin.

9. The nurse is planning the care of a client diagnosed with aplastic anemia. Which interventions should be taught to the client? **Select all that apply.**
   1. Avoid alcohol.
   2. Pace activities.
   3. Stop smoking.
   4. Eat a balanced diet.
   5. Use a safety razor.

10. The nurse is caring for a client in a sickle cell crisis. Which is the pain **regimen of choice** to relieve pain?
    1. Frequent acetylsalicylic acid.
    2. Ibuprofen prn.
    3. Meperidine every 4 hours.
    4. Morphine every 3 hours.

11. The client is diagnosed with hereditary spherocytosis. Which treatment or procedure would the nurse prepare the client to receive?
    1. Bone marrow transplant.
    2. Splenectomy.
    3. Frequent blood transfusions.
    4. Liver biopsy.

12. Which is the **primary** goal of care for a client diagnosed with SCD?
    1. The client will call the HCP if feeling ill.
    2. The client will be compliant with the medical regimen.
    3. The client will live as normal a life as possible.
    4. The client will verbalize an understanding of treatments.

13. The client diagnosed with thalassemia, a hereditary anemia, is to receive a transfusion of PRBCs. The crossmatch reveals the presence of antibodies that cannot be crossmatched. Which **precaution** should the nurse implement when initiating the transfusion?
    1. Start the transfusion at 10 to 15 mL/hr for 15 to 30 minutes.
    2. Recrossmatch the blood until the antibodies are identified.
    3. Have the client sign a permit to receive uncrossmatched blood.
    4. Have the unlicensed assistive personnel stay with the client.

14. The client is diagnosed with polycythemia vera. The nurse would prepare to perform which intervention?
    1. Type and crossmatch for a transfusion.
    2. Assess for petechiae and purpura.
    3. Perform phlebotomy of 500 mL of blood.
    4. Monitor for low Hgb and Hct.

15. The client diagnosed with leukemia has received a bone marrow transplant. The nurse monitors the client's absolute neutrophil count (ANC). What is the client's neutrophil count if the WBCs are $2.2 \times 10^3$/microL, neutrophils are 25%, and bands are 5%?

16. The client is diagnosed with leukemia and has leukocytosis. Which laboratory value would the nurse expect to assess?
    1. An elevated Hgb.
    2. A decreased sedimentation rate.
    3. A decreased red cell distribution width.
    4. An elevated WBC count.

17. The client is placed on neutropenia precautions. Which information should the nurse teach the client?
    1. Shave with an electric razor and use a soft toothbrush.
    2. Eat plenty of fresh fruits and vegetables.
    3. Perform perineal care after every bowel movement.
    4. Some blood in the urine is not unusual.

18. The client is diagnosed with chronic myelogenous leukemia and leukocytosis. Which clinical manifestations would the nurse expect to find when assessing this client?
    1. Frothy sputum and jugular vein distention.
    2. Dyspnea and slight confusion.
    3. Right upper quadrant tenderness and nausea.
    4. Increased appetite and weight gain.

19. The client's CBC laboratory results are populated in the chart below. Which intervention should the nurse implement?

| Complete Blood Count | Client Value | Normal Values |
|---|---|---|
| RBCs | 6 | Male: 4.21–5.81 ($10^6$ cells/microL) Female: 3.61–5.11 ($10^6$ cells/microL) |
| Hgb | 14.2 | Male: 14–17.3 g/dL Female: 11.7–15.5 g/dL |
| Hct | 42 | Male: 42%–52% Female: 36%–48% |
| Platelet | 69 | 140–400 × ($10^3$/microL) |

    1. Teach the client to use a soft-bristle toothbrush.
    2. Monitor the client for elevated temperature.
    3. Check the client's blood pressure.
    4. Hold venipuncture sites for 1 minute.

20. The 24-year-old female client is diagnosed with ITP. Which question would be **important** for the nurse to ask during the admission interview?
    1. "Do you become short of breath during an activity?"
    2. "How heavy are your menstrual periods?"
    3. "Do you have a history of deep vein thrombosis?"
    4. "How often do you have migraine headaches?"

21. The client is diagnosed with hemophilia. Which **safety** precaution should the nurse encourage?
    1. Wear helmets and pads during contact sports.
    2. Take antibiotics before any dental work.
    3. Keep clotting factor VIII on hand at all times.
    4. Use ibuprofen for mild pain.

22. The nurse writes a diagnosis of "potential for fluid volume deficit related to bleeding" for a client diagnosed with DIC. Which would be an **appropriate goal** for this client?
    1. The client's clot formations will resolve in 2 days.
    2. The saturation of the client's dressings will be documented.
    3. The client will use lemon-glycerin swabs for oral care.
    4. The client's urine output will be greater than 30 mL per hour.

23. The client diagnosed with atrial fibrillation is admitted with warfarin toxicity. Which HCP order would the nurse anticipate?
    1. Protamine sulfate.
    2. Heparin sodium.
    3. Enoxaparin sodium.
    4. Vitamin K.

24. Fifteen minutes after the nurse has initiated a transfusion of PRBCs, the client becomes restless and reports itching on the trunk and arms. Which intervention should the nurse implement **first?**
    1. Collect urine for analysis.
    2. Notify the laboratory of the reaction.
    3. Administer diphenhydramine.
    4. Stop the transfusion at the hub.

25. The HCP has ordered 1 unit of packed red blood cells (PRBCs) for the right-handed client. Which area would be the **best place** to insert the intravenous catheter?

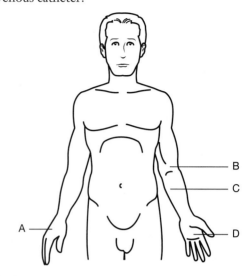

    1. A
    2. B
    3. C
    4. D

26. The nurse is administering a transfusion of PRBCs to a client. Which interventions should the nurse implement? **Rank in order of performance.**
    1. Start the transfusion slowly.
    2. Have the client sign a permit.
    3. Assess the IV site for size and patency.
    4. Check the blood with another nurse at the bedside.
    5. Obtain the blood from the laboratory.

27. The charge nurse is reviewing the laboratory values on clients on a medical floor. Which laboratory data should be **reported** to the HCP **immediately?**

1.

| Complete Blood Count | Client Value | Normal Values |
|---|---|---|
| Red blood cells | 4.7 | Male: 4.21–5.81 ($10^6$ cells/microL)<br>Female: 3.61–5.11 ($10^6$ cells/microL) |
| Hemoglobin | 12.8 | Male: 14–17.3 g/dL<br>Female: 11.7–15.5 g/dL |
| Hematocrit | 35 | Male: 42%–52%<br>Female: 36%–48% |
| Platelet | 39 | 140–400 $\times$ ($10^3$/microL) |
| White blood cells | 10.8 | 4.5–11.1 $\times$ ($10^3$/cells/microL) |

2.

| Complete Blood Count | Client Value | Normal Values |
|---|---|---|
| Red blood cells | 4.2 | Male: 4.21–5.81 ($10^6$ cells/microL)<br>Female: 3.61–5.11 ($10^6$ cells/microL) |
| Hemoglobin | 10.6 | Male: 14–17.3 g/dL<br>Female: 11.7–15.5 g/dL |
| Hematocrit | 30.4 | Male: 42%–52%<br>Female: 36%–48% |
| Platelet | 148 | 140–400 $\times$ ($10^3$/microL) |
| White blood cells | 4.3 | 4.5–11.1 $\times$ ($10^3$/cells/microL) |

3.

| Complete Blood Count | Client Value | Normal Values |
|---|---|---|
| Red blood cells | 7.2 | Male: 4.21–5.81 ($10^6$ cells/microL)<br>Female: 3.61–5.11 ($10^6$ cells/microL) |
| Hemoglobin | 18.9 | Male: 14–17.3 g/dL<br>Female: 11.7–15.5 g/dL |
| Hematocrit | 56 | Male: 42%–52%<br>Female: 36%–48% |
| Platelet | 125 | 140–400 $\times$ ($10^3$/microL) |
| White blood cells | 4.3 | 4.5–11.1 $\times$ ($10^3$/cells/microL) |

4.

| Complete Blood Count | Client Value | Normal Values |
|---|---|---|
| Red blood cells | 5.5 | Male: 4.21–5.81 ($10^6$ cells/microL)<br>Female: 3.61–5.11 ($10^6$ cells/microL) |
| Hemoglobin | 15 | Male: 14–17.3 g/dL<br>Female: 11.7–15.5 g/dL |
| Hematocrit | 45 | Male: 42%–52%<br>Female: 36%–48% |
| Platelet | 200 | 140–400 $\times$ ($10^3$/microL) |
| White blood cells | 6.3 | 4.5–11.1 $\times$ ($10^3$/cells/microL) |

1. 1. Iron supplements can be poorly tolerated. The supplements can cause nausea, abdominal discomfort, and constipation.
   2. There is benefit from oral preparations, but in severe cases of iron deficiency, the client may need parenteral replacement.
   3. Iron supplements cause constipation and should be taken 1 hour before a meal or 2 hours after a meal for the best absorption of the medication. As much as 50% of the iron is not absorbed when taken with food.
   4. **At best, only about 20% to 35% of the medication is absorbed through the gastrointestinal tract.**

2. 1. The normal RBC is 4.21 to 5.81 ($\times 10^6$ cells/microL) for males and 4.21 to 5.814 ($\times 10^6$ cells/microL) for females. The RBC is within normal limits.
   2. **All the laboratory values are within normal limits. The nurse should continue to monitor the client.**
   3. The normal WBC is 4.5 to 11.1 ($\times 10^3$/microL), so filgrastim (Neupogen), a biologic response modifier, to increase the numbers of WBCs is not needed.
   4. Thrombocytopenia does not occur until the client's platelet count is less than 100 ($\times 10^3$); there is no reason to institute bleeding precautions.

3. 1. **The pulse of 116 and BP of 88/62, in addition to the other symptoms, indicate the client is in shock. This is an emergency situation.**
   2. The client is in shock; allergies to medications are not the most important thing.
   3. This may be the cause of the anemia, and complications from the chemotherapy may be causing the shock, but the priority intervention is to treat the shock, regardless of the cause.
   4. These are normal blood gases, so no immediate intervention regarding arterial blood gases is needed.

4. 1. A low Hgb level will not decrease pulmonary functioning. In fact, the lungs will try to compensate for the anemia by speeding up respirations to oxygenate the RBCs and provide oxygen to the tissues.
   2. The client may have difficulty with activity intolerance, but this will be from lack of oxygen, not lack of ability of the muscles to function.
   3. **General complications of severe anemia include heart failure, paresthesias, and confusion. The heart tries to compensate for the lack of oxygen in the tissues by becoming tachycardic. The heart will be able to maintain this compensatory mechanism for only so long and then will show evidence of failure.**
   4. The gastric secretions will not be altered. The blood supply to the stomach may be shunted to the more vital organs, leaving the acidic stomach to deal with the production of acid, and this could cause the client to develop a gastric ulcer.

5. 1. Isometric exercises are bodybuilding exercises; these types of exercises would deplete the client's energy stores.
   2. **The client with activity intolerance will need assistance to perform ADLs.**
   3. A high-protein diet may be needed, but this does not address activity intolerance.
   4. Activity intolerance is not a problem for a physical therapist. The client's blood counts must increase to increase the ability to perform activities.

6. 1. RBC deficiency is anemia. The client should be taught to deal with the effects of anemia, not nausea.
   2. **Anemia causes the client to experience dyspnea and fatigue. Teaching the client to pace activities and rest often, to eat a balanced diet, and to cope with changes in lifestyle is needed.**
   3. Mucositis and diarrhea may occur with chemotherapy administration, but this client's problem is anemia.
   4. All clients diagnosed with cancer should be assisted to discuss the impact of cancer on their lives, but this client's problem is anemia.

7.  1. After a bone marrow biopsy, it is important that the client form a clot to prevent bleeding. The nurse should hold direct pressure on the site for 5 to 10 minutes.
    2. The nurse might premedicate for pain, but once the procedure is completed, a mild oral medication is usually sufficient to relieve any residual discomfort.
    3. The head of the bed can be in any position of comfort for the client.
    4. The procedure is performed on the iliac crest or the sternum and does not cause respiratory distress.

8.  1. The client is anemic, not neutropenic, so reverse isolation is not needed.
    2. This client will be receiving a form of dialysis to maintain life. Discontinuing treatments until the counts improve would be resigning the client to death.
    3. The RBC count would not appreciably improve from one day to the next unless a transfusion had been given.
    4. **Erythropoietin is a biologic response modifier produced by the kidneys in response to a low RBC count in the body. It stimulates the body to produce more RBCs.**

9.  Correct answers are 1, 2, and 4.
    1. **Alcohol consumption interferes with the absorption of nutrients.**
    2. **The client will be short of breath with activity and therefore should pace activities.**
    3. Although all clients should be told to stop smoking, smoking will not directly affect the client's diagnosis.
    4. **The client should eat a well-balanced diet to be able to manufacture blood cells.**
    5. The client should use an electric razor to diminish the risk of cuts and bleeding.

10. 1. Acetylsalicylic acid (aspirin), a nonnarcotic analgesic, is an option for mild pain, but it would not be strong enough during a crisis.
    2. Ibuprofen (Motrin) is an NSAID. NSAIDs are helpful because they relieve pain and decrease inflammation, but they are not used during a crisis because they are not strong enough.
    3. Meperidine (Demerol), a narcotic analgesic, breaks down in the body into normeperidine, which can cause seizures in large doses.

    4. **Morphine, a narcotic analgesic, is the drug of choice for a crisis; it does not have a ceiling effect and can be given in large amounts and frequent doses.**

11. 1. A bone marrow transplant is a treatment option for aplastic anemia and some clients diagnosed with thalassemia, but not for spherocytosis.
    2. **Hereditary spherocytosis is a hemolytic anemia that affects 1 in 2,000 people in the United States. It is characterized by an abnormal permeability of the RBC, which permits it to become spherical in shape. The spheres are then destroyed by the spleen. A splenectomy is the treatment of choice (National Organization for Rare Disorders, 2019).**
    3. The client may require blood transfusions, but preventing the destruction of RBCs by the spleen is the better option.
    4. A liver biopsy will not affect the client's condition.

12. 1. All clients should know when to notify the HCP. This is not the primary goal of living with a chronic illness.
    2. The client should be compliant with recommendations, but this is a lifestyle choice and not the primary goal.
    3. **The primary goal for any client coping with a chronic illness is that the client will be able to maintain as normal a life as possible.**
    4. This is a goal for a client diagnosed with knowledge-deficit problems.

13. 1. **It can be difficult to crossmatch blood when antibodies are present. If imperfectly crossmatched blood must be transfused, the nurse must start the blood very slowly and stay with the client, frequently monitoring for clinical manifestations of a hemolytic reaction.**
    2. The antibodies have been identified. The donor blood does not crossmatch perfectly to the blood of the client.
    3. The blood has been crossmatched. Client permits regarding uncrossmatched blood are used for emergency transfusions when time does not allow any attempt to crossmatch. In such a case, O− blood, the universal donor, will be used.
    4. The nurse cannot delegate an unstable client to an unlicensed assistive personnel. The nurse must stay with the client.

14. 1. The client has too many RBCs and does not need more.
   2. Petechiae and purpura occur when a client does not have adequate platelets.
   3. **The client has too many RBCs, which can cause as much damage as too few. The treatment for this disease is to remove the excess blood; 500 mL at a time is removed.**
   4. The client's hemoglobin and hematocrit are high, not low.

15. **660 ANC.**
   To determine the ANC, first, the WBC count must be determined: 2.2 multiplied by 1,000 ($10^3$) = 2,200. Multiply that by 30 (25% neutrophils + 5% bands) to obtain 66,000 and divide that by 100 to determine the ANC of 660. The ANC is used to determine a client's risk of developing an infection.

16. 1. Clients with leukemia are usually anemic because of the bone marrow's inability to produce cells or, in this case, the bone marrow, stuck in high gear, producing immature WBCs that are unable to function normally.
   2. Sedimentation rates increase in some diseases, such as rheumatoid arthritis, but there will be no change in leukemia.
   3. The red cell distribution width (RDW), shown in the CBC report, reports on the size of the RBCs.
   4. **An elevated WBC count is what is being described in the term "leukocytosis"— *leuko-* means "white" and *cyto-* refers to "cell." Leukocytosis is the opposite of leukopenia.**

17. 1. Shaving with an electric razor and using a soft toothbrush are interventions for thrombocytopenia.
   2. Fresh fruits and vegetables are limited because they may harbor microbes.
   3. **Perineal care after each bowel movement, preferably with antimicrobial soap, is performed to reduce bacteria on the skin.**
   4. Blood in the urine would indicate a complication and is not expected.

18. 1. Frothy sputum and jugular vein distention are symptoms of heart failure, which could occur as a complication of anemia.
   2. **Clients with leukocytosis may be short of breath and somewhat confused as a result of decreased capillary perfusion to the lung and brain from excessive**

numbers of WBCs inhibiting blood flow through the capillaries.
   3. The client may have left upper quadrant pain and tenderness from WBC infiltration of the spleen, but the client will not have right upper quadrant tenderness.
   4. The client may be anorexic and lose weight.

19. 1. **The client has a low platelet count (thrombocytopenia) and should be on bleeding precautions, such as using a soft-bristle toothbrush.**
   2. Monitoring for a fever, a clinical manifestation of infection, would be an intervention for low WBCs.
   3. Assessing blood pressure is not indicated for any of the blood cell count abnormalities.
   4. Holding the venipuncture site would be done for a minimum of 5 minutes.

20. 1. Thrombocytopenia is low platelets and would not cause shortness of breath.
   2. **Because thrombocytopenia causes bleeding, the nurse should assess for any type of bleeding that may be occurring. A young female client would present with excessive menstrual bleeding.**
   3. The problems associated with ITP are bleeding, not clotting.
   4. ITP does not cause migraine headaches.

21. 1. The client should not participate in contact sports because even minimal injury can cause massive bleeding.
   2. The client should have factor VIII on hand for any dental procedure to ensure clotting, but antibiotics are not needed.
   3. **The client must have the clotting factor on hand in case of injury to prevent massive bleeding.**
   4. Ibuprofen is an NSAID. NSAIDs prolong bleeding and should be avoided.

22. 1. The body dissolves clots over a period of several days to a week or more. The problem in DIC is that the body is bleeding and clotting simultaneously.
   2. This is a nursing goal, not a client goal.
   3. Lemon-glycerin swabs are drying to the mucosa and should be avoided because they will increase bleeding from the mucosa.
   4. **The problem is addressing the potential for hemorrhage; a urine output of greater than 30 mL/hr indicates the kidneys are being adequately perfused, and the body is not in shock.**

23. 1. Protamine sulfate, an anticoagulant anti-
       dote, is the antidote for a heparin overdose,
       not for warfarin toxicity.
    2. Administering heparin sodium, an antico-
       agulant, would increase the client's risk of
       bleeding.
    3. Enoxaparin sodium (Lovenox), a low
       molecular weight heparin, would increase
       the client's risk of bleeding.
    4. **The antidote for warfarin (Coumadin)
       is vitamin K, an anticoagulant agonist.**

24. 1. The question asks for a first action; urine
       will be collected for analysis, but this is not
       the first intervention.
    2. The question asks for the first action. The
       laboratory should be notified, but this is
       not the first action to take.
    3. Administering diphenhydramine, an anti-
       histamine, may be done, but it is more
       important to stop the transfusion causing
       the reaction.
    4. **Anytime the nurse suspects the client
       is having a reaction to blood or blood
       products, the nurse should stop the
       infusion at the spot closest to the client
       and not allow any more of the blood to
       enter the client's body.**

25. 1. The client is right-handed; therefore, the
       nurse should attempt to place the IV cathe-
       ter in the nondominant arm.
    2. The antecubital area should not be used
       as an IV site because the movement of
       the elbow will crimp the cannula, and it is
       uncomfortable for the client to keep the
       arm straight all the time.
    3. **The left forearm is the best site to start
       the IV because it has larger veins that
       will accommodate an 18-gauge catheter,
       which should be used when adminis-
       tering blood. This area is less likely to
       have extravasation because there is no
       joint movement, and this site is on the
       client's nondominant side.**

    4. The hand area usually has smaller veins
       that do not accommodate a larger gauge
       catheter, and hand movement can cause
       extravasation more readily than forearm
       movement.

26. Correct order is 2, 3, 5, 4, 1.
    2. The client must give consent before
       receiving blood; therefore, this is the
       first intervention.
    3. Blood products should be administered
       within 30 minutes of obtaining the
       blood from the laboratory; therefore,
       the nurse should determine that the
       IV is patent and the catheter is large
       enough to administer blood, preferably
       an 18-gauge catheter, before obtaining
       the blood.
    5. The nurse must then obtain the blood
       from the laboratory.
    4. Blood must be checked by two RNs at
       the bedside to check the client's cross-
       match bracelet with the unit of blood.
    1. After all of the previous steps are com-
       pleted, then the nurse should start the
       infusion of the blood slowly for the first
       15 minutes to determine if the client is
       going to have a reaction.

27. 1. **This client has a critically low platelet
       count, even though the other labora-
       tory values are in a normal or near-
       normal range. This client is at risk of
       hemorrhaging.**
    2. This client has low values but not dan-
       gerously so. The HCP can be shown the
       results on rounds.
    3. This client's laboratory values are high, but
       not dangerously so; these can be shown to
       the HCP on rounds.
    4. This client has normal laboratory values.

# Respiratory Disorders

*Any piece of knowledge I acquire today has a value at this moment exactly proportional to my skill to deal with it. Tomorrow when I know more, I recall that piece of knowledge and use it better.*

—Mark Van Doren

Respiratory disorders include some of the most common disorders that nurses and other health-care providers (HCPs) encounter. They range from the simple cold to chronic conditions such as asthma to life-threatening diseases such as lung cancer. Whether it is teaching a client the correct way to blow the nose; administering oxygen, antibiotics, or pain-relieving medications; or checking ventilators, chest tubes, and other equipment used in the treatment of clients diagnosed with respiratory disorders, the nurse must know the correct procedures, medications, and interventions to use. One of the most important interventions—and perhaps, the most important—is assessment and monitoring of the client's breathing status and oxygenation level. Oxygenation is the first priority in Maslow's hierarchy—and in terms of saving lives.

## KEYWORDS

Adenoidectomy
Ambu
Antral
Aphonia
Bronchoscopy
Caldwell-Luc antrostomy
Dorsiflexion
Enteral
Eupnea
Exacerbation
Extrinsic
Hypoxemia
Iatrogenic

Intrinsic
Laryngectomy
Laryngoscopy
Lobectomy
Pleurodesis
Pneumonectomy
Polysomnography
Rhinitis
Rhinorrhea
Rhonchi
Thoracentesis
Thoracotomy

# PRACTICE QUESTIONS

## Upper Respiratory Infection (URI)

1. The home health-care nurse is talking on the telephone to a male client diagnosed with hypertension and hears the client sneezing. The client tells the nurse he has been blowing his nose frequently. Which question should the nurse ask the client?
   1. "Have you had the flu shot in the last 2 weeks?"
   2. "Are there any small children in the home?"
   3. "Are you taking over-the-counter medicine for these symptoms?"
   4. "Do you have any cold sores associated with your sneezing?"

2. The school nurse is presenting a class to students at a primary school on how to prevent the transmission of the common cold virus. Which information should the nurse discuss?
   1. Instruct the children to always keep a tissue or handkerchief with them.
   2. Explain that children current with immunizations will not get a cold.
   3. Tell the children they should go to the doctor if they get a cold.
   4. Demonstrate to the students how to wash hands correctly.

3. Which information should the nurse teach the client diagnosed with acute rhinosinusitis? **Select all that apply.**
   1. Instruct the client to complete all the ordered antibiotics.
   2. Teach the client how to irrigate the nasal passages.
   3. Have the client demonstrate how to blow the nose.
   4. Give the client samples of a narcotic analgesic for the headache.
   5. Educate the client on limiting decongestant nasal sprays.

4. The client has been diagnosed with chronic rhinosinusitis. Which clinical manifestation alerts the nurse to a potentially **life-threatening** complication?
   1. Muscle weakness.
   2. Purulent sputum.
   3. Nuchal rigidity.
   4. Intermittent loss of muscle control.

5. The client diagnosed with tonsillitis is scheduled to have surgery in the morning. Which assessment data should the nurse **notify** the health-care provider (HCP) about **before** surgery?
   1. The client has a hemoglobin of 14.2 g/dL and hematocrit of 42.5%.
   2. The client has an oral temperature of 100.2°F and a dry cough.
   3. There are one to two white blood cells (WBCs) in the urinalysis.
   4. The client's current international normalized ratio (INR) is 1.

6. The influenza vaccine is in short supply. Which group of clients would the public health nurse consider **priority** when administering the vaccine?
   1. Elderly and chronically ill clients.
   2. Child-care workers and elementary school children.
   3. Pregnant women and infants.
   4. Schoolteachers and students living in a dormitory.

7. The client diagnosed with chronic rhinosinusitis has undergone a Caldwell-Luc antrostomy and is reporting pain. Which intervention should the nurse implement **first**?
   1. Administer the narcotic analgesic intravenous push (IVP).
   2. Perform gentle oral hygiene.
   3. Place the client in semi-Fowler's position.
   4. Assess the client's pain.

8. The charge nurse on a surgical floor is making assignments. Which client should be assigned to the **most experienced** registered nurse (RN)?
   1. The 36-year-old client diagnosed with glottic cancer after laser microsurgery yesterday with moderate pain.
   2. The 6-year-old client scheduled for a tonsillectomy and adenoidectomy this morning refusing to swallow medication.
   3. The 18-year-old client after a Caldwell-Luc procedure 3 days ago with purulent drainage on the drip pad.
   4. The 45-year-old client diagnosed with a peritonsillar abscess requiring IVPB antibiotic therapy four times a day.

9. The client diagnosed with influenza A is being discharged from the emergency department with a prescription for antibiotics. Which statement by the client indicates an **understanding** of this prescription?
   1. "These pills will make me feel better fast, and I can return to work."
   2. "The antibiotics will help prevent me from developing bacterial pneumonia."
   3. "If I had gotten this prescription sooner, I could have prevented this illness."
   4. "I need to take these pills until I feel better; then I can stop taking the rest."

10. The nurse is developing a plan of care for a client diagnosed with laryngitis and identifies the client's problem "altered communication." Which intervention should the nurse implement?
    1. Instruct the client to drink a mixture of brandy and honey several times a day.
    2. Encourage the client to whisper instead of trying to speak at a normal level.
    3. Provide the client with a blank note pad for writing any communication.
    4. Explain that the client's aphonia may become a permanent condition.

11. Which task is **most appropriate** for the RN to delegate to an unlicensed assistive personnel (UAP)?
    1. Feed the postoperative tonsillectomy client the first meal of clear liquids.
    2. Encourage the client diagnosed with a cold to drink a glass of orange juice.
    3. Obtain a throat culture on a client diagnosed with bacterial pharyngitis.
    4. Escort the client diagnosed with laryngitis outside to smoke a cigarette.

12. The nurse is caring for a client diagnosed with a cold. Which is an example of **alternative** therapy?
    1. Vitamin C, 2,000 mg daily.
    2. Strict bedrest.
    3. Humidification of the air.
    4. Decongestant therapy.

## Lower Respiratory Infection

13. The nurse is assessing a 79-year-old client diagnosed with pneumonia. Which clinical manifestations should the nurse expect to assess in the client? **Select all that apply.**
    1. Confusion and lethargy.
    2. High fever and chills.
    3. Frothy sputum and edema.
    4. Bradypnea and jugular vein distention.
    5. Low body temperature and cough.

14. The nurse is planning the care of a client diagnosed with pneumonia and writes a problem of "impaired gas exchange." Which is an **expected** outcome for this problem?
    1. Performs chest physiotherapy three times a day.
    2. Able to complete activities of daily living.
    3. Ambulates in the hall several times during each shift.
    4. Alert and oriented to person, place, time, and events.

15. The nurse in a long-term care facility is planning the care for a client with a percutaneous endoscopic gastrostomy (PEG) feeding tube used for bolus feedings. Which intervention should the nurse include in the plan of care?
    1. Inspect the insertion line at the naris before instilling formula.
    2. Elevate the head of the bed (HOB) while feeding the client.
    3. Place the client in the Sims position following each feeding.
    4. Change the dressing on the feeding tube every 3 days.

16. The client diagnosed with community-acquired pneumonia is being admitted to the medical unit. Which nursing intervention has the **highest priority**?
    1. Administer the ordered oral antibiotic immediately (STAT).
    2. Order the meal tray to be delivered as soon as possible.
    3. Obtain a sputum specimen for culture and sensitivity.
    4. Have the unlicensed assistive personnel weigh the client.

17. The 56-year-old client diagnosed with tuberculosis (Tb) is being discharged. Which statement made by the client indicates an **understanding of** the discharge instructions?
    1. "I will take my medication for the full 3 weeks prescribed."
    2. "I must stay on the medication for months if I am to get well."
    3. "I can be around my friends because I have started taking antibiotics."
    4. "I should get a Tb skin test every 3 months to determine if I am well."

18. The employee health nurse is administering tuberculin skin testing to employees exposed to a client diagnosed with active tuberculosis (Tb). Which statement indicates the **need** for radiological evaluation instead of skin testing?
    1. The client's first skin test indicates a flat purple area at the site of injection.
    2. The client's second skin test indicates a red area measuring 4 mm.
    3. The client's previous skin test was read as positive.
    4. The client has never shown a reaction to the tuberculin medication.

19. The nurse is caring for the client diagnosed with pneumonia. Which information should the nurse include in the teaching plan? **Select all that apply.**
    1. Place the client on oxygen delivered by nasal cannula.
    2. Plan for periods of rest during activities of daily living.
    3. Place the client on a fluid restriction of 1,000 mL/day.
    4. Restrict the client's smoking to two to three cigarettes per day.
    5. Monitor the client's pulse oximetry readings every 4 hours.

20. The nurse is feeding a client diagnosed with aspiration pneumonia. The client becomes dyspneic, begins to cough, and is turning blue. Which nursing intervention should the nurse implement **first?**
    1. Suction the client's nares.
    2. Turn the client to the side.
    3. Place the client in the Trendelenburg position.
    4. Notify the health-care provider.

21. The day shift charge nurse on a medical unit is making rounds after the report. Which client should be seen **first?**
    1. The 65-year-old client diagnosed with tuberculosis has a sputum specimen to be sent to the laboratory.
    2. The 76-year-old client diagnosed with aspiration pneumonia has a clogged feeding tube.
    3. The 45-year-old client diagnosed with pneumonia has a pulse oximetry reading of 92%.
    4. The 39-year-old client diagnosed with bronchitis has an arterial oxygenation level of 89%.

22. The client is admitted with a diagnosis of rule out tuberculosis. Which type of isolation procedures should the nurse implement?
    1. Standard precautions.
    2. Contact precautions.
    3. Droplet precautions.
    4. Airborne precautions.

23. The nurse observes the UAP entering an airborne isolation room and leaving the door open. Which action is the RN's **best response?**
    1. Close the door and discuss the UAP's action after coming out of the room.
    2. Make the UAP come back outside the room and then reenter, closing the door.
    3. Say nothing to the UAP but report the incident to the nursing supervisor.
    4. Enter the client's room and discuss the matter with the UAP immediately.

24. The client is admitted to a medical unit with a diagnosis of pneumonia. Which clinical manifestations should the nurse assess in the client?
    1. Pleuritic chest discomfort and anxiety.
    2. Asymmetrical chest expansion and pallor.
    3. Leukopenia and CRT less than 3 seconds.
    4. Substernal chest pain and diaphoresis.

## Chronic Obstructive Pulmonary Disease (COPD)

25. The nurse is assessing the client diagnosed with COPD. Which health-promotion information is **most important** for the nurse to obtain?
    1. The number of years the client has smoked.
    2. Risk factors for complications.
    3. Ability to administer inhaled medication.
    4. Willingness to modify lifestyle.

26. The client diagnosed with an exacerbation of COPD is in respiratory distress. Which intervention should the nurse implement **first?**
    1. Assist the client to a sitting position at 90 degrees.
    2. Administer oxygen at 6 LPM via nasal cannula.
    3. Monitor vital signs with the client sitting upright.
    4. Notify the health-care provider about the client's status.

27. The nurse is assessing the client diagnosed with COPD. Which data require **immediate intervention** by the nurse?
    1. Large amounts of thick white sputum.
    2. Oxygen flowmeter set on 8 liters.
    3. Use of accessory muscles during inspiration.
    4. Presence of a barrel chest and dyspnea.

28. The nurse is caring for the client diagnosed with COPD. Which outcome requires a revision in the plan of care?
    1. The client has no signs of respiratory distress.
    2. The client shows an improved respiratory pattern.
    3. The client demonstrates intolerance to activity.
    4. The client participates in establishing goals.

29. The nurse is caring for the client diagnosed with end-stage COPD. Which data **warrant immediate intervention** by the nurse?
    1. The client's pulse oximeter reading is 92%.
    2. The client's arterial blood gas level is 74.
    3. The client has SOB when walking to the bathroom.
    4. The client's sputum is rusty colored.

30. Which statement made by the client diagnosed with chronic bronchitis indicates to the nurse **more teaching** is required?
    1. "I should contact my health-care provider if my sputum changes color or amount."
    2. "I will take my bronchodilator regularly to prevent having bronchospasms."
    3. "This metered-dose inhaler gives a precise amount of medication with each dose."
    4. "I need to return to the HCP to have my blood drawn with my annual physical."

31. Which client problems are appropriate for the nurse to include in the plan of care for the client diagnosed with COPD? **Select all that apply.**
    1. Impaired gas exchange.
    2. Inability to tolerate temperature extremes.
    3. Activity intolerance.
    4. Inability to cope with changes in roles.
    5. Alteration in nutrition.

32. Which outcome is appropriate for the client problem "ineffective gas exchange" for the client recently diagnosed with COPD?
    1. The client demonstrates the correct way to perform pursed-lip breathing.
    2. The client lists three clinical manifestations to report to the HCP.
    3. The client will drink at least 2,500 mL of water daily.
    4. The client will be able to ambulate 100 feet with dyspnea.

33. The nurse observes the UAP removing the nasal cannula from the client diagnosed with COPD while ambulating the client to the bathroom. Which action should the RN implement?
    1. Praise the UAP because this prevents the client from tripping on the oxygen tubing.
    2. Place the oxygen back on the client while sitting in the bathroom and say nothing.
    3. Explain to the UAP in front of the client oxygen must be left in place at all times.
    4. Discuss the UAP's action with the charge nurse so appropriate action can be taken.

34. Which clinical manifestations should the nurse expect to assess in the client recently diagnosed with COPD? **Select all that apply.**
    1. Clubbing of the client's fingers.
    2. Infrequent respiratory infections.
    3. Chronic sputum production.
    4. Nonproductive hacking cough.
    5. Shortness of breath.

35. Which statement made by the client indicates the nurse's discharge teaching is **effective** for the client diagnosed with COPD?
    1. "I need to get an influenza vaccine each year, even when there is a shortage."
    2. "I need to get a vaccine for pneumonia each year with my influenza shot."
    3. "If I reduce my cigarettes to six a day, I won't have difficulty breathing."
    4. "I need to restrict my drinking liquids to keep from having so much phlegm."

36. Which referral is **most appropriate** for a client diagnosed with end-stage COPD?
    1. The Asthma Foundation of America.
    2. The American Cancer Society.
    3. The American Lung Association.
    4. The American Heart Association.

## Reactive Airway Disease (Asthma)

37. The nurse is completing the admission assessment on a 13-year-old client diagnosed with an acute exacerbation of asthma. Which clinical manifestations would the nurse expect to find?
    1. Fever and crepitus.
    2. Rales and hives.
    3. Dyspnea and wheezing.
    4. Normal chest shape and eupnea.

38. The nurse is planning the care of a client diagnosed with asthma and has written a problem of "anxiety." Which nursing intervention should be implemented?
    1. Remain with the client.
    2. Notify the health-care provider.
    3. Administer an anxiolytic medication.
    4. Encourage the client to drink fluids.

39. The case manager is arranging a care planning meeting regarding the care of a 65-year-old client diagnosed with adult-onset asthma. Which health-care disciplines should participate in the meeting? **Select all that apply.**
    1. Nursing.
    2. Pharmacy.
    3. Social work.
    4. Occupational therapy.
    5. Speech therapy.

40. The client is diagnosed with mild intermittent asthma. Which medication should the nurse discuss with the client?
    1. Daily inhaled corticosteroids.
    2. Use of a "rescue inhaler."
    3. Use of systemic steroids.
    4. Leukotriene agonists.

41. Which statements indicate to the nurse the client diagnosed with asthma **understands** the teaching regarding inhaled corticosteroid medications? **Select all that apply.**
    1. "I should call my doctor if I have a sore throat or mouth."
    2. "I must taper off the medications and not stop taking them abruptly."
    3. "These drugs will be most effective if taken at bedtime."
    4. "These drugs are not good at the time of an attack."
    5. "If I need both inhalers, I should take my bronchodilator first."

42. The client diagnosed with asthma is admitted to the emergency department with difficulty breathing and a blue color around the mouth. Which diagnostic test will be ordered to determine the status of the client?
    1. Complete blood count.
    2. Pulmonary function test.
    3. Allergy skin testing.
    4. Drug cortisol level.

43. The nurse and a licensed practical nurse (LPN) are caring for five clients in a medical unit. Which clients would the RN assign to the LPN? **Select all that apply.**
    1. The 32-year-old female diagnosed with exercise-induced asthma and a forced vital capacity of 3,000 mL.
    2. The 45-year-old male with adult-onset asthma reporting difficulty completing all of the ADLs at one time.
    3. The 92-year-old client diagnosed with respiratory difficulty, beginning to be confused, and keeps climbing out of bed.
    4. The 6-year-old client diagnosed with intrinsic asthma, scheduled for discharge, and the mother needs teaching about the medications.
    5. The 20-year-old client diagnosed with asthma has a pulse oximetry reading of 95%, and wants to sleep all the time.

44. The charge nurse is making rounds. Which client should the nurse assess **first**?
    1. The 29-year-old client diagnosed with reactive airway disease reporting the nurse caring for him was rude.
    2. The 76-year-old client diagnosed with heart failure and has 2+ edema of the lower extremities.

3. The 15-year-old client diagnosed with diabetic ketoacidosis after a bout with the flu and a blood glucose reading of 189 mg/dL.
4. The 62-year-old client diagnosed with COPD and pneumonia receiving $O_2$ by nasal cannula at 2 liters per minute.

45. The client diagnosed with exercise-induced asthma (EIA) is being discharged. Which information should the nurse include in the discharge teaching?
    1. Take two puffs on the rescue inhaler and wait 5 minutes before exercise.
    2. Warm-up exercises will increase the potential for developing asthma attacks.
    3. Use the bronchodilator inhaler immediately before beginning exercise.
    4. Increase dietary intake of food high in monosodium glutamate (MSG).

46. The client diagnosed with restrictive airway disease (asthma) has been prescribed a glucocorticoid inhaled medication. Which information should the nurse teach regarding this medication? **Select all that apply.**
    1. Do not abruptly stop taking this medication; it must be tapered off.
    2. Immediately rinse the mouth following the administration of the drug.
    3. Hold the medication in the mouth for 15 seconds before swallowing.
    4. Take the medication immediately when an attack starts.
    5. Clean the mouthpiece of the inhaler with soapy water monthly.

47. The nurse is discussing the care of a child diagnosed with asthma with the parent. Which referral is **important** to include in the teaching?
    1. Referral to a dietitian.
    2. Referral for allergy testing.
    3. Referral to the developmental psychologist.
    4. Referral to a home health nurse.

48. The nurse is discharging a client newly diagnosed with restrictive airway disease (asthma). Which statement indicates the client **understands** the discharge instructions?
    1. "I will call 911 if my medications don't control an attack."
    2. "I should wash my bedding in warm water."
    3. "I can still eat at the Chinese restaurant when I want."
    4. "If I get a headache, I should take a nonsteroidal anti-inflammatory drug."

## Lung Cancer

49. The nurse is taking the social history from a client diagnosed with small cell carcinoma of the lung. Which information is **significant** for this disease?
    1. The client worked with asbestos for a short time many years ago.
    2. The client has no family history for this type of lung cancer.
    3. The client has numerous tattoos covering both upper and lower arms.
    4. The client has smoked two packs of cigarettes a day for 20 years.

50. The nurse writes a problem of "impaired gas exchange" for a client diagnosed with cancer of the lung. Which interventions should be included in the plan of care? **Select all that apply.**
    1. Apply $O_2$ via nasal cannula.
    2. Have the dietitian plan for six small meals per day.
    3. Place the client in respiratory isolation.
    4. Assess vital signs for fever.
    5. Listen to lung sounds every shift.

51. The nurse is discussing cancer statistics with a group from the community. Which information about death rates from lung cancer is **accurate?**

**Trends in Age-Adjusted Cancer Death Rates\* by Site, Males U.S., 1930–2017**

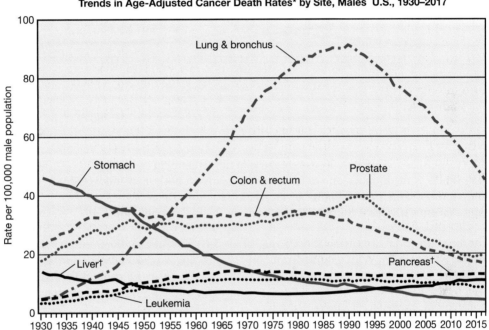

\*Per 100,000 age-adjusted to the 2000 U.S. standard population. †Mortality rates for pancreatic and liver cancer are increasing.

**Note:** Due to changes in ICD coding, numerator information has changed over time. Rates for cancers of the liver, lung & bronchus, and colon & rectum are affected by these coding changes.

**Source:** U.S. Mortality Volumes 1930 to 1959 and U.S. Mortality Data 1960 to 2017, National Center for Health Statistics, Centers for Disease Control and Prevention.

©2020, American Cancer Society Inc., Surveillance Research.

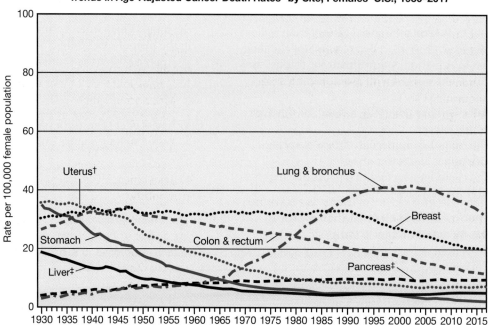

**Trends in Age-Adjusted Cancer Death Rates\* by Site, Females  U.S., 1930–2017**

\*Per 100,000 age-adjusted to the 2000 U.S. standard population. †Uterus refers to uterine cervix and uterine corpus combined.
‡Mortality rates for pancreatic and liver cancers are increasing.

**Note:** Due to changes in ICD coding, numerator information has changed over time. Rates for cancers of the liver, lung & bronchus, and colon & rectum are affected by these coding changes.

**Source:** U.S. Mortality Volumes 1930 to 1959, National Center for Health Statistics, Centers for Disease Control and Prevention. ©2020, American Cancer Society Inc., Surveillance Research.

1. Lung cancer has a low mortality rate because of new treatment options.
2. Lung cancer is the number-one cause of cancer deaths in both men and women.
3. Lung cancer deaths are not significant in relation to other cancers.
4. Lung cancer deaths have continued to increase in the male population.

52. The nurse and a UAP are caring for a group of clients in a medical unit. Which information provided by the UAP **warrants immediate intervention** by the RN?
    1. The client diagnosed with cancer of the lung has a small amount of blood in the sputum collection cup.
    2. The client diagnosed with chronic emphysema is sitting on the side of the bed and leaning over the bedside table.
    3. The client receiving epoetin alfa has a T 99.2°F, P 68, R 24, and BP of 198/102.
    4. The client receiving prednisone is reporting an upset stomach after eating breakfast.

53. The client diagnosed with lung cancer has been told the cancer has metastasized to the brain. Which intervention should the nurse implement?
    1. Discuss implementing an advance directive.
    2. Explain the use of chemotherapy for brain involvement.
    3. Teach the client to discontinue driving.
    4. Have the significant other make decisions for the client.

54. The client diagnosed with lung cancer is in an investigational program and receiving a vaccine to treat the cancer. Which information regarding investigational regimens should the nurse teach?
    1. Investigational regimens provide a better chance of survival for the client.
    2. Investigational treatments have not been proven to be helpful to clients.
    3. Clients will be paid to participate in an investigational program.
    4. Only dying clients qualify for investigational treatments.

55. The nursing staff on an oncology unit is interviewing applicants for the unit manager position. Which type of organizational structure does this represent?
    1. Centralized decision making.
    2. Decentralized decision making.
    3. Shared governance.
    4. Pyramid with filtered-down decisions.

56. The client diagnosed with lung cancer is being discharged. Which statement made by the client indicates **more teaching** is required?
    1. "It doesn't matter if I smoke now. I already have cancer."
    2. "I should see the oncologist at my scheduled appointment."
    3. "If I begin to run a fever, I should notify the HCP."
    4. "I should plan for periods of rest throughout the day."

57. The clinic nurse is interviewing clients. Which information provided by a client **warrants further** investigation? **Select all that apply.**
    1. The client uses a topical analgesic chest rub every night before bed.
    2. The client has had an appendectomy.
    3. The client takes a multiple vitamin pill daily.
    4. The client has been coughing up blood in the mornings.
    5. The client practices meditation every day.

58. The client is 4 hours postlobectomy for cancer of the lung. Which assessment data **warrant immediate** intervention by the nurse?
    1. The client has an intake of 1,500 mL IV and an output of 1,000 mL.
    2. The client has 450 mL of bright-red drainage in the chest tube.
    3. The client is reporting pain at a "10" on a 1-to-10 scale.
    4. The client has absent lung sounds on the side of the surgery.

59. The client is admitted to the outpatient surgery center for a bronchoscopy to rule out cancer of the lung. Which information should the nurse teach? **Select all that apply.**
    1. The test will confirm the results of the MRI.
    2. The client can eat and drink immediately after the test.
    3. The HCP can do a biopsy of the tumor through the scope.
    4. There is no discomfort associated with this procedure.
    5. Continuous cardiac monitoring is performed during the procedure.

60. The client diagnosed with small cell carcinoma of the lung tells the nurse, "I am so tired of all this. I might as well just end it all." Which statement should be the nurse's **first** response?
    1. Say, "This must be hard for you. Would you like to talk?"
    2. Tell the HCP of the client's statement.
    3. Refer the client to a social worker or spiritual advisor.
    4. Find out if the client has a plan to carry out suicide.

## Cancer of the Larynx

61. The nurse is admitting a client with a diagnosis of rule out cancer of the larynx. Which information should the nurse teach?
    1. Demonstrate the proper method of gargling with normal saline.
    2. Perform voice exercises for 30 minutes three times a day.
    3. Explain that a lighted instrument will be placed in the throat to biopsy the area.
    4. Teach the client to self-examine the larynx monthly.

62. The client is diagnosed with cancer of the larynx and is to have radiation therapy to the area. Which prophylactic procedure should the nurse prepare the client for?
    1. Have a dental examination with frequent check-ups.
    2. Take antiemetic medications every 4 hours.
    3. Wear sunscreen on the area at all times.
    4. Placement of a nasogastric feeding tube.

63. The client is 3 days post-partial laryngectomy. Which type of nutrition should the nurse offer the client?
    1. Total parenteral nutrition.
    2. Soft, regular diet.
    3. Partial parenteral nutrition.
    4. Clear liquid diet.

64. The nurse is preparing the client diagnosed with laryngeal cancer for a laryngectomy in the morning. Which intervention is the nurse's **priority?**
    1. Take the client to the intensive care unit for a visit.
    2. Explain that the client will need to ask for pain medication.
    3. Demonstrate the use of an antiembolism hose.
    4. Find out if the client can read and write.

65. The client has had a total laryngectomy. Which referral is **specific** for this surgery?
    1. CanSurmount.
    2. Dialogue.
    3. Lost Chord Club.
    4. SmokEnders.

66. The nurse and a UAP are caring for a group of clients on a surgical floor. Which information provided by the UAP requires **immediate intervention** by the nurse?
    1. The client, after modified radical neck dissection, has a small, continuous amount of bright-red drainage coming out from under the dressing.
    2. The client, after right upper lobectomy, is reporting the patient-controlled analgesia (PCA) pump is not providing any relief.

3. The client diagnosed with cancer of the lung is reporting being tired and short of breath.
4. The client admitted with chronic obstructive pulmonary disease is making a whistling sound with every breath.

67. The RN charge nurse is assigning clients for the shift. Which client should be assigned to the **new graduate** nurse?
    1. The client diagnosed with cancer of the lung, chest tubes in place.
    2. The client diagnosed with laryngeal spasms exhibiting stridor.
    3. The client diagnosed with laryngeal cancer and multiple fistulas.
    4. The client 2 hours post-partial laryngectomy.

68. The nurse is writing a care plan for a client newly diagnosed with cancer of the larynx. Which problem is the **highest priority**?
    1. Wound infection.
    2. Hemorrhage.
    3. Respiratory distress.
    4. Knowledge deficit.

69. The male client has had a radical neck dissection for cancer of the larynx. Which action by the client indicates a disturbance in body image?
    1. The client requests a consultation by the speech therapist.
    2. The client has a towel placed over the mirror.
    3. The client is attempting to shave his face.
    4. The client practices neck and shoulder exercises.

70. The HCP has recommended a total laryngectomy for a male client diagnosed with cancer of the larynx, but the client refuses. Which intervention by the nurse illustrates the ethical principle of **nonmaleficence**?
    1. The nurse listens to the client explaining why he is refusing surgery.
    2. The nurse and significant other insist that the client have the surgery.
    3. The nurse refers the client to a counselor for help with the decision.
    4. The nurse asks a cancer survivor to come and discuss the surgery with the client.

71. The client diagnosed with cancer of the larynx has had 4 weeks of radiation therapy to the neck. The client is reporting severe pain when swallowing. Which **scientific rationale** explains the pain?
    1. The cancer has grown to obstruct the esophagus.
    2. The treatments are working on the cancer, and the throat is edematous.
    3. Cancers are painful, and this is expected.
    4. The treatments are also affecting the esophagus, causing ulcerations.

72. The client, after radical neck dissection and tracheostomy for cancer of the larynx, is being discharged. Which discharge instructions should the nurse teach? **Select all that apply.**
    1. The client will be able to speak again after the surgery area has healed.
    2. The client should wear a protective covering over the stoma when showering.
    3. The client should clean the stoma and then apply a petroleum-based ointment.
    4. The client should use a humidifier in the room.
    5. The client can get a special telephone for communication.

## Pulmonary Embolus

73. The client is diagnosed with a pulmonary embolus (PE) and is receiving a heparin drip. The bag hanging is 20,000 units/500 mL of $D_5W$ infusing at 22 mL/hr. How many units of heparin is the client receiving each hour?

    _____

74. The client is suspected of having a PE. Which diagnostic test suggests the presence of a pulmonary embolus and requires further investigation?
    1. Plasma D-dimer test.
    2. Arterial blood gases.
    3. Chest x-ray (CXR).
    4. Magnetic resonance imaging (MRI).

75. Which nursing assessment data **support** that the client has experienced a pulmonary embolism?
    1. Calf pain with dorsiflexion of the foot.
    2. Sudden onset of chest pain and dyspnea.
    3. Left-sided chest pain and diaphoresis.
    4. Bilateral crackles and low-grade fever.

76. The client diagnosed with a pulmonary embolus is in the intensive care department. Which assessment data **warrant immediate intervention** from the nurse?
    1. The client's ABGs are pH 7.36, $Po_2$ 95, $Pco_2$ 38, $Hco_3$ 24.
    2. The client's telemetry exhibits occasional premature ventricular contractions (PVCs).
    3. The client's pulse oximeter reading is 90%.
    4. The client's urinary output for the 12-hour shift is 800 mL.

77. The client is admitted to the medical unit diagnosed with a pulmonary embolus. Which intervention should the nurse implement? **Select all that apply.**
    1. Administer oral anticoagulants.
    2. Assess the client's bowel sounds.
    3. Prepare the client for a thoracentesis.
    4. Institute and maintain bedrest.
    5. Provide oxygen therapy.

78. The nurse is preparing to administer warfarin to a client with the laboratory results populated in the chart below. What action should the nurse implement?

| Laboratory Test | Client Results | Normal Values |
|---|---|---|
| PT | 22 | 10–13 sec |
| aPTT | 35 | 25–35 seco |
| INR | 2.8 | 0.9–1.1 w/o anti-coagulation therapy 2–3 with therapy 2.5–3.5 if the client has a mechanical heart valve |

   1. Assess the client for abnormal bleeding.
   2. Prepare to administer vitamin K.
   3. Administer the medication as ordered.
   4. Notify the HCP to obtain an order to increase the dose.

79. The nurse identified the client problem "decreased cardiac output" for the client diagnosed with a pulmonary embolus. Which intervention should be included in the plan of care?
   1. Monitor the client's arterial blood gases
   2. Assess skin color and temperature.
   3. Check the client for signs of bleeding.
   4. Keep the client in the Trendelenburg position.

80. Which nursing interventions should the nurse implement for the client diagnosed with a pulmonary embolus undergoing thrombolytic therapy? **Select all that apply.**
   1. Keep protamine sulfate readily available.
   2. Avoid applying pressure to venipuncture sites.
   3. Assess for overt and covert signs of bleeding.
   4. Avoid invasive procedures and injections.
   5. Administer stool softeners as ordered.

81. Which statement by the client diagnosed with a pulmonary embolus indicates the discharge teaching is **effective**?
   1. "I am going to use a hard-bristle toothbrush."
   2. "I will take antibiotics before having my teeth cleaned."
   3. "I can take enteric-coated acetylsalicylic acid for my headache."
   4. "I will wear a medical alert bracelet at all times."

82. The client diagnosed with a pulmonary embolus is being discharged. Which intervention should the nurse discuss with the client? **Select all that apply.**
   1. Increase fluid intake to 2 to 3 L/day.
   2. Eat a low-sodium, low-fat diet.

   3. Avoid being around large crowds.
   4. Receive pneumonia and flu vaccines.
   5. Stop smoking.

83. The nurse is preparing to administer medications to the following clients. Which medication should the nurse **question** administering?
   1. Warfarin to the client with an INR of 1.9.
   2. Regular insulin to a client with a blood glucose level of 218 mg/dL.
   3. Hang the heparin bag on a client with a PT/aPTT of 12.9/98.
   4. A calcium channel blocker to the client with a BP of 112/82.

84. The client is getting out of bed and becomes very anxious and has a feeling of impending doom. The nurse thinks the client may be experiencing a pulmonary embolism. Which action should the nurse implement **first**?
   1. Administer oxygen 10 L via nasal cannula.
   2. Place the client in high Fowler's position.
   3. Obtain a STAT pulse oximeter reading.
   4. Auscultate the client's lung sounds.

## Chest Trauma

85. The client is admitted to the emergency department with chest trauma. Which clinical manifestations indicate to the nurse the diagnosis of a pneumothorax?
   1. Bronchovesicular lung sounds and bradypnea.
   2. Unequal lung expansion and dyspnea.
   3. Frothy, bloody sputum, and consolidation.
   4. Barrel chest and polycythemia.

86. The client had a right-sided chest tube inserted 2 hours ago for a pneumothorax. Which action should the nurse implement if there is no fluctuation (tidaling) in the water-seal compartment?
   1. Obtain an order for a STAT CXR.
   2. Increase the amount of wall suction.
   3. Check the tubing for kinks or clots.
   4. Monitor the client's pulse oximeter reading.

87. Which intervention should the nurse implement for a male client with a left-sided chest tube in place for 6 hours refusing to take deep breaths because of pain?
   1. Medicate the client and have the client take deep breaths.
   2. Encourage the client to take shallow breaths to help with the pain.
   3. Explain that deep breaths do not have to be taken at this time.
   4. Tell the client if he doesn't take deep breaths, he could die.

88. The UAP assists the client with a chest tube to ambulate to the bathroom. Which situation **warrants immediate intervention** from the RN?
    1. The UAP keeps the chest tube below the chest level.
    2. The UAP has the chest tube attached to suction.
    3. The UAP allowed the client out of bed.
    4. The UAP uses a bedside commode for the client.

89. The nurse is caring for a client with a right-sided chest tube that is accidentally pulled out of the pleural space. Which action should the nurse implement **first**?
    1. Notify the HCP to have chest tubes reinserted STAT.
    2. Instruct the client to take slow, shallow breaths until the tube is reinserted.
    3. Take no action and assess the client's respiratory status every 15 minutes.
    4. Tape a petroleum jelly or dry sterile dressing to the insertion site.

90. The nurse is presenting a class on chest tubes. Which statement best describes a tension pneumothorax?
    1. A tension pneumothorax develops when an air-filled bleb on the surface of the lung ruptures.
    2. When a tension pneumothorax occurs, the air moves freely between the pleural space and the atmosphere.
    3. The injury allows air into the pleural space but prevents it from escaping from the pleural space.
    4. A tension pneumothorax results from a puncture of the pleura during central line placement.

91. Which action should the nurse implement for the client diagnosed with a hemothorax complicated by a right-sided chest tube with excessive bubbling in the water-seal compartment?
    1. Check the amount of wall suction being applied.
    2. Assess the tubing for any blood clots.
    3. Milk the tubing proximal to distal.
    4. Encourage the client to cough forcefully.

92. Which assessment data indicate to the nurse the chest tubes inserted 3 days ago have been **effective** in treating the client diagnosed with a hemothorax?
    1. Gentle bubbling in the suction compartment.
    2. No fluctuation (tidaling) in the water-seal compartment.
    3. The drainage compartment has 250 mL of blood.
    4. The client is able to deep breathe without any pain.

93. The nurse is caring for a client with a right-sided chest tube secondary to a pneumothorax. Which interventions should the nurse implement when caring for this client? **Select all that apply.**
    1. Place the client in the low Fowler's position.
    2. Assess the chest tube drainage system frequently.
    3. Maintain strict bedrest for the client.
    4. Secure a loop of drainage tubing to the sheet.
    5. Observe the site for subcutaneous emphysema.

94. The charge nurse is making client assignments on a medical floor. Which client should the RN charge nurse assign to the LPN?
    1. The client diagnosed with pneumonia, pulse oximeter reading of 91%.
    2. The client diagnosed with a hemothorax, Hb of 9 g/dL, and Hct of 20%.
    3. The client with chest tubes, jugular vein distention, and BP of 96/60.
    4. The client 2 hours postbronchoscopy procedure.

95. The alert and oriented client is diagnosed with a spontaneous pneumothorax, and the HCP is preparing to insert a left-sided chest tube. Which intervention should the nurse implement **first**?
    1. Gather the needed supplies for the procedure.
    2. Obtain a signed informed consent form.
    3. Assist the client to a side-lying position.
    4. Discuss the procedure with the client.

96. Which intervention should the nurse implement **first** for the client diagnosed with a hemothorax, having a right-sided chest tube for 3 days, and has no fluctuation (tidaling) in the water compartment?
    1. Assess the client's bilateral lung sounds.
    2. Obtain an order for a STAT CXR.
    3. Notify the HCP as soon as possible.
    4. Document the findings in the client's EHR.

## Acute Respiratory Distress Syndrome

97. The UAP is bathing the client diagnosed with acute respiratory distress syndrome (ARDS). The bed is in a high position with the opposite side rail in the low position. Which action should the RN implement?
    1. Demonstrate the correct technique for giving a bed bath.
    2. Encourage the UAP to put the bed in the lowest position.
    3. Instruct the UAP to get another person to help with the bath.
    4. Provide praise for performing the bath safely for the client and the UAP.

98. The client diagnosed with ARDS is transferred to the intensive care department and placed on a ventilator. Which intervention should the nurse implement **first?**
    1. Confirm that the ventilator settings are correct.
    2. Verify that the ventilator alarms are functioning properly.
    3. Assess the respiratory status and pulse oximeter reading.
    4. Monitor the client's arterial blood gas results.

99. The nurse suspects the client may be developing ARDS. Which assessment data **confirm** the diagnosis of ARDS?
    1. Low arterial oxygen when administering a high concentration of oxygen.
    2. The client has dyspnea and tachycardia and is feeling anxious.
    3. Bilateral breath sounds clear, and pulse oximeter reading is 95%.
    4. The client has jugular vein distention and frothy sputum.

100. The two-pack-a-day cigarette smoker develops ARDS after a near-drowning. The client asks the nurse, "What is happening to me? Why did I get this?" Which statement by the nurse is **most appropriate?**
    1. "Most people develop ARDS after a near-drowning."
    2. "Platelets and fluid enter the alveoli due to permeability instability."
    3. "Your lungs are filling up with fluid, causing breathing problems."
    4. "Smoking has caused your lungs to become weakened, so you got ARDS."

101. Which assessment data indicate to the nurse the client diagnosed with ARDS has experienced a complication secondary to the ventilator?
    1. The client's urine output is 100 mL in 4 hours.
    2. The pulse oximeter reading is greater than 95%.
    3. The client has asymmetrical chest expansion.
    4. The telemetry reading shows sinus tachycardia.

102. The HCP ordered STAT ABGs for the client diagnosed with ARDS. The results are populated in the chart below. Which action should the nurse implement?

| Arterial Blood Gas | Client Values | Normal Values |
|---|---|---|
| pH | 7.38 | 7.35–7.45 |
| Pco$_2$ | 38 | 35–45 mmHg |
| Hco$_3$ | 24 | 22–26 mEq/L |
| Pao$_2$ | 92 | 80–95 mmHg |

   1. Continue to monitor the client without taking any action.
   2. Encourage the client to take deep breaths and cough.
   3. Administer one ampule of sodium bicarbonate IVP.
   4. Notify the respiratory therapist of the ABG results.

103. The client diagnosed with ARDS is on a mechanical ventilator. Which interventions should be included in the nursing care plan addressing the endotracheal tube (ET) care? **Select all that apply.**
   1. Do not move or touch the ET tube.
   2. Obtain a chest x-ray daily.
   3. Determine if the ET cuff is deflated.
   4. Ensure that the ET tube is secure.
   5. Assess lung sounds every 2 hours.

104. Which procedure or test should the nurse anticipate the HCP ordering to diagnose ARDS?
   1. Chest x-ray.
   2. Complete blood count.
   3. Airway pressure-release ventilation test.
   4. Sputum culture.

105. The client diagnosed with ARDS is in respiratory distress, and the ventilator is malfunctioning. Which intervention should the nurse implement **first?**
   1. Notify the respiratory therapist immediately.
   2. Ventilate with a manual resuscitation bag.
   3. Request STAT arterial blood gases.
   4. Auscultate the client's lung sounds.

106. The nurse is caring for the client diagnosed with ARDS. Which interventions should the nurse implement? **Select all that apply.**
   1. Assess the client's level of consciousness.
   2. Monitor urine output every shift.
   3. Turn the client every 2 hours.
   4. Maintain intravenous fluids as ordered.
   5. Place the client in the prone position.

107. Which instruction is a **priority** for the nurse to discuss with the client diagnosed with ARDS being discharged from the hospital?
    1. Avoid smoking and exposure to smoke.
    2. Do not receive flu or pneumonia vaccines.
    3. Avoid any type of alcohol intake.
    4. It will take about 1 month to recuperate.

108. The client diagnosed with ARDS is on a ventilator, and the high alarm indicates an increase in the peak airway pressure. Which intervention should the nurse implement **first**?
    1. Check the tubing for any kinks.
    2. Suction the airway for secretions.
    3. Assess the lip line of the ET tube.
    4. Sedate the client with a muscle relaxant.

# CONCEPTS

The concepts covered in this chapter focus on oxygenation and acid-base problems. Exemplars that are covered are COPD, pneumonia, lung cancer, and respiratory distress. Interrelated concepts of the nursing process and clinical judgment are covered throughout the questions. The concept of clinical judgment is presented in prioritizing or "first" questions.

109. The client is admitted to the emergency department reporting shortness of breath and fever. The vital signs are populated in the chart below. Which concept should the nurse identify as a concern for the client? **Select all that apply.**

| Vital Sign Flowsheet | Client Results | Normal Values |
|---|---|---|
| Blood Pressure | 134/86 | 100–119 mmHg systolic 60–80 mmHg diastolic |
| Temperature | 100.4°F | Oral: 98°F (36.7°C) |
| Pulse | 94 | 60–100 beats/min |
| Respirations | 26 | 12–20 breaths/min |

    1. Clotting.
    2. Oxygenation.
    3. Infection.
    4. Perfusion.
    5. Coping.

110. The nurse observes the client sitting on the side of the bed with the arms propped on the over-bed table. The chest is barrel-shaped and the client is breathing through lips spaced close together and is exhaling slowly. Which concept is the **priority** for this client?
    1. Mobility.
    2. Nutrition.
    3. Activity intolerance.
    4. Oxygenation.

111. The client diagnosed with community-acquired pneumonia is admitted to the medical unit. Which HCP order should the nurse implement **first**?
    1. Start IV with 1,000 mL 0.9% saline.
    2. Ceftriaxone 1 gm IVPB every 12 hours.
    3. Obtain sputum and blood cultures.
    4. CBC and basic metabolic panel.

112. The client diagnosed with COPD is admitted to the medical unit. The client has thin extremities, truncal obesity, and multiple ecchymotic areas on the arms. Based on the assessment data, which question should the nurse ask the client?
    1. "Do you take prednisone?"
    2. "Can you tell me who hurts you?"
    3. "May I check your coccyx for pressure areas?"
    4. "Do you sleep with the head of the bed elevated?"

113. The client is diagnosed with COPD and pneumonia. Which medication should the day nurse **question** administering?

| Client Name: A. B. | MR# 1258637 | Diagnosis: COPD and Pneumonia |
|---|---|---|
| Age: 56 years | Allergies: Cephalosporins | |
| Medication | 0701–1900 | 1901–0700 |
| Methylprednisolone 100 mg IVP every 8 hours | 0800, 1600 | 2400 |
| Ceftriaxone 1 g IVPB every 12 hours | 0900 | 2100 |
| Benzonatate orally every 12 hours | 0900 | 2100 |
| Morphine 30 mg orally every day | 0900 | |
| Signature of Nurse: | Day Nurse RN/DN | Night Nurse RN/NN |

1. Methylprednisolone.
2. Ceftriaxone.
3. Benzonatate.
4. Morphine.

114. The nurse is reviewing the EHRs of the clients. Which data should the nurse report to the HCP?
A. Client A—Diagnosis: Pneumonia

| Complete Blood Count | Client Value | Normal Values |
|---|---|---|
| Red blood cells | 5.2 | Male: 4.21– 5.81 $\times$ 10$^6$ cells/microL<br>Female: 3.61–5.11 $\times$ 10$^6$ cells/microL |
| Hemoglobin | 12.1 | Male: 14 to 17.3 g/dL<br>Female: 11.7–15.5 g/dL |
| Hematocrit | 38 | Male: 42%–52%<br>Female: 36%–48% |
| White blood cells | 18.3 | 4.5–11.1 $\times$ 10$^3$ cells/microL |
| Platelets | 582 | 140– 400 $\times$ 10$^3$/microL |

B. Client B—Diagnosis: Respiratory Distress

| Arterial Blood Gas | Client | Normal Values |
|---|---|---|
| pH | 7.35 | 7.35–7.45 |
| $Pco_2$ | 45 | 35–45 mmHg |
| $Hco_3$ | 28 | 22–26 mEq/L |
| $Pao_2$ | 82 | 80–95 mmHg |

C. Client C—Diagnosis: Acute Exacerbation of COPD

| Laboratory Test | Client Results | Normal Values |
|---|---|---|
| Glucose | 132 | Fasting < 100 mg/dL<br>Random < 200 mg/dL |
| Hemoglobin A$_{1c}$ | 6.9 | Non-diabetic 4%–5.5%<br>Prediabetes 5.7%–6.4%<br>Diabetes 6.5% or less |

D. Client D—Diagnosis: Sepsis

| Site | Client Culture | Sensitivity |
|------|----------------|-------------|
| Sputum culture | Positive for gram-negative Streptococcus | Keflex Ceftriaxone |
| Gram stain | Gram-negative organism | |

1. Client A.
2. Client B.
3. Client C.
4. Client D.

115. Which intervention should the nurse institute for the client diagnosed with COPD and cor pulmonale based on the intake and output record?

### Intake and Output Record

| Day 1 | Oral (in mL) | Intravenous (in mL) | Urine (in mL) | Nasogastric Tube (in mL) | Other (Specify) (in mL) |
|-------|--------------|---------------------|---------------|--------------------------|-------------------------|
| 0701–1900 | 1,475 | 1,850 | 1,600 | | |
| 1901–0700 | 740 | 1,400 | 1,200 | | |
| Total | 2,215 | 3,250 | 2,800 | | |

1. Administer methylprednisolone IVP.
2. Administer guaifenesin orally.
3. Request an order to reduce the IV rate.
4. Continue to monitor the client.

116. The client diagnosed with respiratory distress has the following ABG laboratory results. Which should the nurse implement? **Select all that apply.**

| Arterial Blood Gas | Client | Normal Values |
|--------------------|--------|---------------|
| pH | 7.45 | 7.35–7.45 |
| $Pco_2$ | 54 | 35–45 mmHg |
| $Hco_3$ | 25 | 22–26 mEq/L |
| $Pao_2$ | 52 | 80–95 mmHg |

1. Apply oxygen via nonrebreather mask.
2. Call the rapid response team (RRT).
3. Elevate the head of the bed.
4. Stay with the client.
5. Notify the health-care provider (HCP).

117. The nurse is applying oxygen via nasal cannula to a client diagnosed with COPD. The client reports extreme shortness of breath. At which rate should the nurse set the flowmeter?
    1. 2 LPM.
    2. 4 LPM.
    3. 6 LPM.
    4. 10 LPM.

118. The charge nurse receives morning laboratory and respiratory data on the clients. Which data **requires immediate** intervention?
    1. ABG results of pH 7.35, $Pco_2$ 56, $Hco_3$ 29, $Po_2$ 78 for a client diagnosed with COPD.
    2. Pulse oximetry reading of 89% on a 2-day postsurgical total knee replacement client.
    3. Hgb of 9 g/dL and Hct of 28% on a client receiving the second unit of blood.
    4. B-type natriuretic peptide (BNP) of 100 on a client diagnosed with stage 4 congestive heart failure.

119. The nurse is caring for clients in the medical unit. Which assessment data indicate a **critical** oxygenation problem for the client?
    1. The client with an anterior upper left chest tube is splinting the dressing with a pillow.
    2. The male client on oxygen is coughing forcefully, making it hard to catch his breath.
    3. The client diagnosed with circumoral cyanosis at rest and is difficult to arouse.
    4. The female client reports shortness of breath while ambulating in the hallway.

120. The 75-year-old male nursing home resident is found wandering in the hall and has a new onset of confusion. Which should the RN implement **first**?
    1. Assess the resident's lung fields and temperature.
    2. Have the resident return to his room.
    3. Notify the resident's family to come and sit with him.
    4. Ask the UAP to push fluids.

## Upper Respiratory Infection

1. 1. Influenza is a viral illness that might cause these symptoms; however, immunization would not give the client the illness.
   2. Coming into contact with small children increases the risk of contracting colds and the flu, but the client has a problem—not just a potential one.
   3. A client diagnosed with hypertension should not take many of the over-the-counter medications because they work by causing vasoconstriction, which will increase hypertension.
   4. Cold sores are actually an infection by the herpes simplex virus. Colds and coldlike symptoms are caused by the rhinovirus or influenza virus. The term "cold sore" is a common term that still persists in the populace.

   **TEST-TAKING HINT:** The keys to answering this question are the words "hypertension" and "cold." Any time a client has a chronic illness, the client should discuss over-the-counter medications with the HCP or a pharmacist. Many of the routine medications for chronic illnesses interact with over-the-counter medications.

2. 1. It is not feasible for a child to always have a tissue or handkerchief available.
   2. There is no immunization for the common cold. Colds are actually caused by at least 200 separate viruses, and the viruses mutate frequently.
   3. Colds are caused by a virus, and antibiotics do not treat a virus; therefore, there is no need to go to an HCP.
   4. Hand washing is the single most useful technique for the prevention of disease.

   **TEST-TAKING HINT:** Option "1" contains the word "always," an absolute word, and in most questions, absolutes such as "always," "never," and "only" make that answer option incorrect.

3. Correct answers are 1, 2, 3, and 5.
   1. The client should be taught to take all antibiotics as ordered. Discontinuing antibiotics before the full dose results in the development of antibiotic-resistant bacteria. Sinus infections are difficult to treat and may become chronic and will then require several weeks of therapy or possibly surgery to control.
   2. The client should be taught how to perform a normal saline nasal irrigation to remove debris, allergens, and bacteria. The client pours or squeezes NS in one nostril, and it flows through the nasal cavity to the other nostril and drains out into the sink.
   3. Forcefully blowing the nose will increase pressure in the sinus cavities and cause the client increased pain; therefore, the client should be taught to blow the nose gently, one nostril at a time.
   4. The nurse is not licensed to prescribe medications, so this is not in the nurse's scope of practice. Also, narcotic analgesic medications are controlled substances and require written documentation of being prescribed by the HCP; samples are not available.
   5. The client should be taught to limit the use of decongestant nasal sprays to fewer than 4 days to avoid rebound rhinitis.

   **TEST-TAKING HINT:** Note in this situation an "all" is one of the correct answers. There are very few cases in which absolute adjectives will describe the correct answer. The test taker must be aware that general rules will not always apply.

4. 1. Muscle weakness is a clinical manifestation of myalgia, but it is not a life-threatening complication of rhinosinusitis.
   2. Purulent sputum would be a clinical manifestation of a lung infection, but it is not a life-threatening complication of rhinosinusitis.
   3. Nuchal rigidity is a clinical manifestation of meningitis, which is a potentially life-threatening complication of rhinosinusitis resulting from the close proximity of the sinus cavities to the meninges.
   4. Intermittent loss of muscle control can be a symptom of multiple sclerosis, but it would not be a life-threatening complication of rhinosinusitis.

   **TEST-TAKING HINT:** A basic knowledge of anatomy and physiology would help to answer this question. The sinuses lie in the head and surround the orbital cavity. Options "1" and "4" refer to muscle problems, so both could be ruled out as wrong.

5. 1. The hemoglobin and hematocrit (H&H) given are within the normal range. This would not warrant notifying the HCP.
   2. **A low-grade temperature and a cough could indicate the presence of an infection, in which case the HCP would not want to subject the client to anesthesia and the possibility of further complications. The surgery would be postponed.**
   3. One to two WBCs in a urinalysis is not uncommon because of the normal flora in the bladder.
   4. The INR indicates that the client's bleeding time is within the normal range.

**TEST-TAKING HINT: In this question, all the answer options contain normal data except for one. The nurse would not call the HCP to notify them of normal values.**

6. 1. Clients who are older and chronically ill are at risk for developing serious complications if they contract the influenza virus, but in a national shortage, pregnant women and infants are to receive the vaccination first (tier one) before older clients who are chronically ill (tier 4).
   2. It is recommended people in contact with children receive the flu vaccine whenever possible, but these clients should be able to withstand the flu if their immune systems are functioning normally.
   3. **According to the Centers for Disease Control and Prevention (2018) guidelines for influenza vaccination during a period of vaccine shortage, the first tier of the general population to be vaccinated are pregnant women, infants, and toddlers 6 to 35 months. Pregnant women and infants are at high risk of severe complications or death. National security personnel, health-care and community support services, and other critical infrastructure are vaccinated before the general population.**
   4. During flu season, the more people the individual comes into contact with, the greater the risk the client will be exposed to the influenza virus, but this group of people would not receive the vaccine before the pregnant women and infants or older people who are chronically ill.

**TEST-TAKING HINT: The test taker may think the answer is too easy and obvious, but the test taker should not try to second-guess the question. Item writers are not trying to trick the test taker; they are trying to evaluate knowledge.**

7. 1. The client has reported pain, and the nurse should first determine the severity of the pain, then, barring any complications in the client, administer pain medication after completion of the assessment.
   2. Oral hygiene helps to prevent the development of infections and promotes comfort, but it will not relieve the pain.
   3. Placing the client in the semi-Fowler's position will reduce edema of inflamed sinus tissue, but it will not immediately affect the client's perception of pain.
   4. **Before intervening, the nurse must assess to determine the amount of pain and possible complications occurring that could be masked if narcotic medication is administered.**

**TEST-TAKING HINT: Whenever there is an assessment answer among the answer options, the test taker should look carefully at what is being assessed. If the option says to assess the problem identified in the question, it will usually be the correct answer. Remember, the first step in the nursing process is assessment.**

8. 1. This client is 1 day postoperative and has moderate pain, which is to be expected after surgery. A less experienced nurse can care for this client.
   2. A child about to go to surgery involving the throat area can be expected to have painful swallowing. This does not require the most experienced nurse.
   3. **The postoperative client with purulent drainage could be developing an infection. The experienced nurse would be needed to assess and monitor the client's condition.**
   4. Any nurse capable of administering IVPB medications can care for this client.

**TEST-TAKING HINT: In this type of question, the test taker must determine if the situation described is expected or within normal limits. The option that gives unexpected data or data not within normal limits requires a nurse with more knowledge and experience.**

9. 1. A person with a viral infection should not return to work until the virus has run its course because the antibiotics help prevent complications of the virus, but they do not make the client feel better faster.
   2. **Secondary bacterial infections often accompany influenza, and antibiotics are often prescribed to help prevent the development of a bacterial infection resulting from a weakened client immune system.**

3. Antibiotics will not prevent the flu. Only the flu vaccine will prevent the flu.

4. When people take portions of the antibiotic prescription and stop taking the remainder, an antibiotic-resistant strain of bacteria may develop, and the client may experience a return of symptoms—but this time, the antibiotics will not be effective.

**TEST-TAKING HINT: Knowing drug classifications and how the drugs within the classification work would assist the test taker in determining the correct answer. Antibiotics work to destroy bacterial invasions of the body.**

10. 1. The client diagnosed with laryngitis is instructed to avoid all alcohol. Alcohol causes increased irritation of the throat.
2. Whispering places added strain on the larynx.
3. Voice rest is encouraged for the client experiencing laryngitis.
4. Aphonia, or inability to speak, is a temporary condition associated with laryngitis.

**TEST-TAKING HINT: Encouraging the use of alcohol, with the exception of a glass of red wine, is not accepted medical practice; therefore, option "1" could be eliminated. Option "4" has an absolute—"permanent"—in it and, therefore, could be eliminated from consideration.**

11. 1. Tonsillectomies cause throat edema and difficulty swallowing; the nurse must observe the client's ability to swallow before this task can be delegated.
2. Clients diagnosed with colds are encouraged to drink 2,000 mL of liquids a day. The UAP could do this.
3. Throat swabs for culture must be done correctly, or false-negative results can occur. The nurse should obtain the swab.
4. Clients diagnosed with laryngitis are instructed not to smoke. Smoking is discouraged in all health-care facilities. Sending nursing personnel outside encourages an unhealthy practice, which is not the best use of the personnel.

**TEST-TAKING HINT: Interventions requiring assessment, teaching, and evaluation cannot be delegated. Levels of activities being delegated should be appropriate for the level of training of the staff member carrying out the task. Tasks delegated must conform to safe health-care practice.**

12. 1. Alternative therapies are therapies not accepted as standard medical practice. These may be encouraged as long as they do not interfere with the medical regimen. Vitamin C in large doses is thought to improve the immune system's functions.
2. Bedrest is accepted standard advice for a client diagnosed with a cold.
3. Humidifying the air helps to relieve congestion and is standard practice.
4. Decongestant therapy is a standard therapy for a cold.

**TEST-TAKING HINT: Only one of the answer options is not common advice for a client diagnosed with a cold. When all options but one match each other, then the odd option should be selected as the correct answer.**

## Lower Respiratory Infection

13. Correct answers are 1, 2, and 5.
1. The older client diagnosed with pneumonia may present with weakness, fatigue, lethargy, confusion, and poor appetite but not have any of the classic clinical manifestations of pneumonia.
2. Fever and chills are classic symptoms of pneumonia and can be present in the older client.
3. Frothy sputum and edema are clinical manifestations of heart failure, not pneumonia.
4. The client has tachypnea (fast respirations), not bradypnea (slow respirations), and jugular vein distention accompanies heart failure.
5. Low body temperature is an atypical sign of pneumonia in older clients. Cough is a common symptom of pneumonia.

**TEST-TAKING HINT: The question provides the client's age, so age can be expected to affect the disease process—in this case, causing atypical symptoms. The prefix *brady-* means "slow" when attached to a word. Knowing the definition of medical prefixes can assist the test taker in determining the correct answers. Often the test taker would not select opposite symptoms such as high fever and low body temperature, but the older client could have typical or atypical symptoms.**

14. 1. Clients do not perform chest physiotherapy; this is normally done by the respiratory therapist. This is a staff goal, not a client goal.
    2. This would be a goal for self-care deficit but not for impaired gas exchange.
    3. This would be a goal for the problem of activity intolerance.
    4. Impaired gas exchange results in hypoxia, the earliest clinical manifestation of which is a change in the level of consciousness.

**TEST-TAKING HINT:** The test taker should match the answer option to the listed nursing problem. Option "1" is a staff goal to accomplish. When writing goals for the client, it is important to remember they are written in terms of what is expected of the client. Options "2" and "3" are appropriately written client goals, but they do not evaluate gas exchange.

15. 1. A gastrostomy tube is placed directly into the stomach through the abdominal wall; the naris is the opening of the nostril.
    2. **Elevating the head of the bed uses gravity to keep the formula in the gastric cavity and help prevent it from refluxing into the esophagus, which predisposes the client to aspiration.**
    3. The Sims position is the left lateral side-lying flat position. This position is used for administering enemas and can be used to prevent aspiration in clients sedated by anesthesia. The sedated client would not have a full stomach.
    4. Dressings on PEG tubes should be changed at least daily. If there is no dressing, the insertion site is still assessed daily.

**TEST-TAKING HINT:** The test taker should try to picture the positioning of the client to determine the correct answer. In option "4," the test taker should question if the time given, 3 days, is the correct time interval for performing this intervention.

16. 1. Broad-spectrum IV antibiotics are a priority, but before antibiotics are administered, it is important to obtain culture specimens to determine the correct antibiotic for the client's infection. Clients are placed on oral medications only after several days of IVPB therapy.
    2. Meal trays are not a priority over cultures.
    3. **Specimens for culture are taken before beginning the medication to determine the antibiotic that will effectively treat an infection. Administering antibiotics**

before cultures may make it impossible to determine the actual agent causing the pneumonia.
    4. Admission weights are important to determine the appropriate dosing of medication, but they are not a priority over sputum collection.

**TEST-TAKING HINT:** Option "1" has a medication classification and a route, and the test taker should question if the route is appropriate for the client being admitted. Clients will not die from a delayed meal, but a client could die from delayed IV antibiotic therapy.

17. 1. Clients diagnosed with Tb will need to take the medications for 6 months to a year.
    2. **Compliance with treatment plans for Tb includes multidrug therapy for 6 months to 1 year for the client to be free of the Tb bacteria.**
    3. Clients are no longer contagious when three morning sputum specimens are cultured negative, but this will not occur until after several weeks of therapy.
    4. The Tb skin test only determines possible exposure to the bacteria, not the active disease.

**TEST-TAKING HINT:** The test taker should determine if the time of 3 weeks in option "1," months in option "2," or immediately in option "3" is the correct time interval.

18. 1. A flat purple area indicates that the client became bruised when the intradermal injection was given, but it has no bearing on whether the test is positive.
    2. **A positive skin test is 15 mm or greater with induration in clients with no known risk factors; 10 mm or greater in recent immigrants, IV drug users, or clients residing in prisons or institutions; and 5 mm or greater in clients diagnosed with HIV, recent Tb, organ transplant clients, and immunosuppressed clients (Centers for Disease Control and Prevention, 2019).**
    3. If the client has ever reacted positively, then the client should have a CXR to look for causation and inflammation.
    4. These are negative findings and do not indicate the need to have x-ray determination of disease.

**TEST-TAKING HINT:** The test taker should note descriptive terms such as "purple," "flat," or "4 mm" before determining the correct answer. Option "4" has the absolute word "never," and absolutes usually indicate incorrect answers.

19. Correct answers are 1, 2, and 5.
    1. The client diagnosed with pneumonia will have some degree of gas-exchange deficit. Administering oxygen would help the client.
    2. Activities of daily living require energy and therefore oxygen consumption. Spacing the activities allows the client to rebuild oxygen reserves between activities.
    3. Clients are encouraged to drink at least 2,000 mL daily to thin secretions.
    4. Cigarette smoking depresses the action of the cilia in the lungs. Any smoking should be prohibited.
    5. Pulse oximetry readings provide the nurse with an estimate of oxygenation in the periphery.

**TEST-TAKING HINT:** Maslow's hierarchy of needs lists oxygenation as the top priority. Therefore, the test taker should select interventions addressing oxygenation.

20. 1. The nares are the openings of the nostrils. Suctioning, if done, would be of the posterior pharynx.
    2. Turning the client to the side allows for the food to be coughed up and come out of the mouth, rather than be aspirated into the lungs.
    3. Placing the client in the Trendelenburg position increases the risk of aspiration.
    4. An immediate action is needed to protect the client.

**TEST-TAKING HINT:** In a question requiring the test taker to determine the first action, all the answer options may be correct for the situation. The test taker must determine which has the greatest potential for improving the client's condition.

21. 1. The specimen needs to be taken to the laboratory within a reasonable time frame, but a UAP can take specimens to the laboratory.
    2. Clogged feeding tubes occur with some regularity. Delay in feeding a client will not result in permanent damage.
    3. A pulse oximetry reading of 92% means that the arterial blood oxygen saturation is somewhere around 60% to 70%.
    4. Arterial oxygenation normal values are 80% to 100%.

**TEST-TAKING HINT:** Be sure to read all the answer options. Pulse oximetry readings do not give the same information as ABG readings.

22. 1. Standard precautions are used to prevent exposure to blood and body secretions on all clients. Tuberculosis is caused by airborne bacteria.
    2. Contact precautions are used for wounds.
    3. Droplet precautions are used for infections spread by sneezing or coughing but not transmitted over distances of more than 3 to 4 feet.
    4. Tuberculosis bacteria are capable of disseminating over long distances on air currents. Clients diagnosed with tuberculosis are placed in negative air pressure rooms where the air in the room is not allowed to cross-contaminate the air in the hallway.

**TEST-TAKING HINT:** Standard precautions and contact precautions can be ruled out as the correct answer if the test taker is aware that Tb is usually a respiratory illness. This, at least, gives the reader a 1:2 chance of selecting the correct answer if the answer is not known.

23. 1. Closing the door reestablishes the negative air pressure, which prevents the air from entering the hall and contaminating the hospital environment. When correcting an individual, it is always best to do so in a private manner.
    2. The employee is an adult and, as such, should be treated with respect and corrected accordingly.
    3. Problems should be taken care of at the lowest level possible. The nurse is responsible for any task delegated, including the appropriate handling of isolation.
    4. Correcting staff should never be done in the presence of the client. This undermines the UAP and creates doubt of the staff's competency in the client's mind.

**TEST-TAKING HINT:** An action must be taken; the test taker must determine which action would have the desired results with the least amount of disruption to client care. Correcting the UAP in this manner has the greatest chance of creating a win-win situation.

24. 1. Pleuritic chest pain and anxiety from diminished oxygenation occur along with fever, chills, dyspnea, and cough.
    2. Asymmetrical chest expansion occurs if the client has a collapsed lung from a pneumothorax or hemothorax, and the client would be cyanotic from decreased oxygenation.

3. The client would have leukocytosis, not leukopenia, and a capillary refill time (CRT) of less than 3 seconds is normal.
4. Substernal chest pain and diaphoresis are symptoms of myocardial infarction.

**TEST-TAKING HINT:** Options "1" and "4" have chest pain as part of the answer. The adjectives describing the chest pain determine the correct answer.

## Chronic Obstructive Pulmonary Disease (COPD)

25. 1. The number of years of smoking is information needed to treat the client but not the most important in health promotion.
2. The risk factors for complications are important in planning care.
3. Assessing the ability to deliver medications is an important consideration when teaching the client.
4. The client's attitude toward lifestyle changes is the most important consideration in health promotion, in this case, smoking cessation. The nurse should assess if the client is willing to consider cessation of smoking and carry out the plan.

**TEST-TAKING HINT:** The test taker should read the stem for words such as "health promotion." These words make all the other answer options incorrect because they do not promote health.

26. 1. The client should be assisted to a sitting position either on the side of the bed or in the bed. This position decreases the work of breathing. Some clients find it easier sitting on the side of the bed leaning over the bed table. The nurse needs to maintain the client's safety.
2. Oxygen will be applied as soon as possible, but the least amount possible. If levels of oxygen are too high, the client may stop breathing.
3. Vital signs need to be monitored, but this is not the first priority. If the equipment is not in the room, another member of the health-care team should bring it to the nurse. The nurse should stay with the client.
4. The HCP needs to be notified, but the client must be treated first. The nurse should get assistance if possible, so the nurse can treat this client quickly.

**TEST-TAKING HINT:** When a question asks for the test taker to choose the intervention to implement first, the test taker should select an intervention directly caring for the client. Remember: in distress, do not assess.

27. 1. A large amount of thick sputum is a common symptom of COPD. There is no cause for immediate intervention.
2. The nurse should decrease the oxygen rate to 2 to 3 L. Hypoxemia is the stimulus for breathing in the client diagnosed with COPD. If the hypoxemia improves and the oxygen level increases, the drive to breathe may be eliminated.
3. It is common for clients diagnosed with COPD to use accessory muscles when inhaling. These clients tend to lean forward.
4. In clients diagnosed with COPD, there is a characteristic barrel chest from chronic hyperinflation, and dyspnea is common.

**TEST-TAKING HINT:** This question requires interpreting the data to determine which are abnormal or unexpected and require intervention. Options "1," "3," and "4" are expected for the client's disease process.

28. 1. The expected outcome showing no signs of respiratory distress indicates the plan of care is effective and should be continued.
2. An improved respiratory pattern indicates the plan should be continued.
3. The expected outcome should be that the client has tolerance for activity; because the client is not meeting the expected outcome, the plan of care needs revision.
4. The client should participate in planning the course of care. The client is meeting the expected outcome.

**TEST-TAKING HINT:** This question is an "except" question. Three of the options indicate desired outcomes, and only one option indicates the need for improvement.

29. 1. The client diagnosed with end-stage COPD has decreased peripheral oxygen levels; therefore, this would not warrant immediate intervention.
2. The client's ABGs would normally indicate a low oxygen level; therefore, this would not warrant immediate intervention.
3. The client diagnosed with dyspnea on exertion should stop the exertion but does

not require intervention by the nurse if the dyspnea resolves.

4. Rusty-colored sputum indicates blood in the sputum and requires further assessment by the nurse.

**TEST-TAKING HINT:** The test taker could rule out options "1" and "2" as correct answers because both describe the same data of decreased oxygen, which is characteristic of COPD.

30. 1. When sputum changes in color or amount, or both, this indicates infection, and the client should report this information to the HCPs. This statement indicates the client understands the teaching.
    2. Bronchodilators should be taken routinely to prevent bronchospasms. This statement indicates the client understands the teaching.
    3. Clients use metered-dose inhalers because they deliver a precise amount of medication with correct use. This statement indicates the client understands the teaching.
    4. Clients should have blood levels drawn every 6 months when taking bronchodilators, not yearly. This indicates the client needs more teaching.

**TEST-TAKING HINT:** When evaluating whether the client has learned the information presented, the test taker is observing for incorrect information. The test taker should pay close attention to time frames such as "every 12 months."

31. Correct answers are 1, 2, 3, 4, and 5.
    1. The client diagnosed with COPD has difficulty exchanging oxygen with carbon dioxide, which is manifested by physical signs such as fingernail clubbing and respiratory acidosis, as seen on ABGs.
    2. The client should avoid extremes in temperatures. Warm temperatures cause an increase in metabolism and increase the need for oxygen. Cold temperatures cause bronchospasms.
    3. The client has increased respiratory effort during activities and can be fatigued. Activities should be timed, so rest periods are scheduled to prevent fatigue.
    4. The client may have difficulty adapting to the role changes brought about because of the disease process. Many cannot maintain the activities involved in meeting responsibilities at home and

at work. Clients should be assessed for these issues.
    5. Clients often lose weight because of the effort expended to breathe.

**TEST-TAKING HINT:** This is an example of an alternate-type question. There may be more than one correct answer. The test taker should consider all options independently and understand that the question is not a trick.

32. 1. Pursed-lip breathing helps keep the alveoli open to allow for better oxygen and carbon dioxide exchange.
    2. This would be an appropriate outcome for a knowledge-deficit problem.
    3. This outcome does not ensure the client has an effective airway; increasing fluid does not ensure an effective airway.
    4. This is not an appropriate outcome for any client problem because the client should be able to ambulate without dyspnea for 100 feet.

**TEST-TAKING HINT:** The test taker needs to identify the outcome for the client problem cited—namely, "ineffective gas exchange." The only answer option addressing the airway is option "1," pursed-lip breathing.

33. 1. The client diagnosed with COPD needs oxygen at all times, especially when exerting energy, such as ambulating to the bathroom.
    2. The client needs the oxygen, and the nurse should not correct the UAP in front of the client; it is embarrassing for the UAP, and the client loses confidence in the staff.
    3. The nurse should not verbally correct a UAP in front of the client; the nurse should correct the behavior and then talk to the UAP in private.
    4. The primary nurse should confront the UAP and take care of the situation. Continued unsafe client care would warrant notifying the charge nurse.

**TEST-TAKING HINT:** The test taker must know management concepts, and the nurse should first address the behavior with the person directly, then follow the chain of command.

34. Correct answers are 3 and 5.
    1. Clubbing of the fingers is the result of chronic hypoxemia, which is expected with chronic COPD but not recently diagnosed COPD.
    2. These clients have frequent respiratory infections.

3. Sputum production, along with cough and dyspnea on exertion, are the early clinical manifestations of COPD.

4. These clients have a productive cough, not a nonproductive cough.

5. Shortness of breath is the classic symptom of COPD due to the increased work to breathe.

**TEST-TAKING HINT:** The test taker must be observant of terms such as "recently diagnosed," which help to rule out incorrect answers such as option "1." Option "2" has the word "infrequent." The test taker must notice these words.

35. 1. Clients diagnosed with COPD should receive the influenza vaccine each year. If there is a shortage, these clients have tier 4 priority (CDC, 2018).

2. The pneumococcal vaccine should be administered every 5 years.

3. Reducing the number of cigarettes smoked does not stop the progression of COPD, and the client will continue to experience clinical manifestations such as shortness of breath or dyspnea on exertion.

4. Clients diagnosed with COPD should increase their fluid intake unless contraindicated for another health condition. The increased fluid assists the client in expectorating the thick sputum.

**TEST-TAKING HINT:** Nurses are expected to serve as community resources. The nurse should be knowledgeable about health-promotion activities such as immunizations. One option describes a desired goal, but the other three do not.

36. 1. The Asthma Foundation of America is not appropriate for a client diagnosed with this stage of COPD.

2. The American Cancer Society is helpful for a client diagnosed with lung cancer but not for a client diagnosed with COPD.

3. The American Lung Association has information helpful for a client diagnosed with COPD.

4. Many clients diagnosed with COPD end up with heart problems, but the American Heart Association does not have information for clients diagnosed with COPD.

**TEST-TAKING HINT:** The test taker should be familiar with organizations, but if the test taker had no idea what the answer was, the only option containing a word referring to respiration—"lung"—is option "3."

## Reactive Airway Disease (Asthma)

37. 1. Fever is a sign of infection, and crepitus is air trapped in the layers of the skin.

2. Rales indicate fluid in the lung, and hives are a skin reaction to a stimulus such as occurs with an allergy to a specific substance.

3. During an asthma attack, the muscles surrounding the bronchioles constrict, causing a narrowing of the bronchioles. The lungs then respond with the production of secretions that further narrow the lumen. The resulting symptoms include wheezing from air passing through the narrow, clogged spaces and dyspnea.

4. During an attack, the chest will be expanded from air being trapped and not being exhaled. A CXR will reveal a lowered diaphragm and hyperinflated lungs.

**TEST-TAKING HINT:** The test taker must have a basic knowledge of common medical terms to answer this question. *Dyspnea*, *wheezing*, and *rales* are common terms used when describing respiratory function and lung sounds. *Crepitus* and *eupnea* are not as commonly used, but they are also terms that describe respiratory processes and problems.

38. 1. Anxiety is an expected sequela of being unable to meet the oxygen needs of the body. Staying with the client lets the client know the nurse will intervene, and the client is not alone.

2. Because anxiety is an expected occurrence with asthma, it is not necessary to notify the HCP.

3. An anxiolytic medication could decrease respiratory drive and increase respiratory distress. Also, the medication will require a delayed time period to begin to work.

4. Drinking fluids will not treat an asthma attack or anxiety.

**TEST-TAKING HINT:** Before choosing an answer option that directs the test taker to notify an HCP, the test taker should determine if the option is describing an expected event or data for the disease process being discussed. If it is expected, then notifying the HCP would not be the correct answer.

39. Correct answers are 1, 2, and 3.

1. Nursing is the one discipline remaining with the client around the clock. Therefore, nurses have knowledge of the client that other disciplines might not have.

2. The pharmacist will be able to discuss the medication regimen the client is receiving and make suggestions regarding other medications or medication interactions.
3. The social worker may be able to assist with financial information or home care arrangements.
4. Occupational therapists help clients with activities of daily living and modifications to home environments; nothing in the stem indicates a need for these services.
5. Speech therapists assist clients diagnosed with speech and swallowing problems; nothing in the stem indicates a need for these services.

**TEST-TAKING HINT:** Cost containment issues are always a concern the nurse must address. The use of limited resources (health-care personnel) should be on an as-needed basis only. Cost containment must be considered when using other disciplines or supplies.

40. 1. Daily inhaled steroids are used for mild, moderate, or severe persistent asthma, not for intermittent asthma.
    2. Clients diagnosed with intermittent asthma will have exacerbations treated with rescue inhalers. Therefore, the nurse should teach the client about rescue inhalers.
    3. Systemic steroids are frequently used by clients diagnosed with severe persistent asthma, not with mild intermittent asthma.
    4. Leukotriene agonists are prescribed for clients diagnosed with mild persistent asthma.

**TEST-TAKING HINT:** In the stem, there are two words giving the test taker a clue about the correct answer. "Mild" and "intermittent" are words that indicate the client is not experiencing frequent or escalating symptoms. Steroid medications can have multiple side effects.

41. 1. Inhaled corticosteroids, such as fluticasone (Flovent HFA), can cause sore throat or mouth. The client should notify the HCP if this symptom occurs.
    2. Tapering of medications is done for inhaled and systemic steroids because of adrenal functioning.
    3. The drugs are taken daily, not necessarily at bedtime.
    4. Inhaled corticosteroids are routine maintenance medications and do not treat an attack.
    5. The client should be taught to use the inhaled bronchodilator first in the event of an acute attack. The corticosteroid is not used in acute asthma attacks. The client should wait 5 minutes after the bronchodilator to use the inhaled corticosteroid (Vallerand & Sanoski, 2019).

**TEST-TAKING HINT:** The test taker must be knowledgeable about medications. There are not many test-taking hints. If the test taker knows that a specific option applies to a medication other than the one mentioned in the stem, the test taker can eliminate that option.

42. 1. A complete blood count determines the oxygen-carrying capacity of the hemoglobin in the body, but it will not identify the immediate problem.
    2. Pulmonary function tests are completed to determine the forced vital capacity (FVC), the forced expiratory volume in the first second ($FEV_1$), and $FEV_1$/FVC ratio. A decline in the FVC, $FEV_1$, and $FEV_1$/FVC ratio indicates respiratory compromise.
    3. Allergy skin testing will be done to determine triggers for allergic asthma, but it is not done during an attack.
    4. Drug cortisol levels do not relate to asthma.

**TEST-TAKING HINT:** If the test taker is unsure about the correct response, it is helpful to choose the option that directly relates to the topic. Asthma is a pulmonary problem, and only one option has the word "pulmonary" in it.

43. Correct answers are 1, 2, and 5.
    1. An FVC of 3,000 mL is considered normal for most females; therefore, the LPN could care for this client. The FVC averages 3,000 to 5,000 mL (approximate) (Van Leeuwen & Bladh, 2017).
    2. The client should be encouraged to pace the activities of daily living; this is expected for a client diagnosed with asthma, so the LPN could care for this client.
    3. Confusion could be a sign of decreased oxygen to the brain and requires the RN's expertise. This client should not be assigned to the LPN.
    4. The client's mother requires teaching, which is the nurse's responsibility and cannot be assigned to an LPN.
    5. A pulse oximetry level of 95% is normal, so this client could be assigned to an LPN.

**TEST-TAKING HINT:** The nurse cannot assign an LPN assessment, teaching, evaluation, or an unstable client.

44. 1. The charge nurse is responsible for all clients. At times it is necessary to see clients diagnosed with a psychosocial need before clients with expected and non–life-threatening situations.
2. Two (2)+ edema of the lower extremities is expected in a client diagnosed with heart failure.
3. A blood glucose reading of 189 mg/dL is not within the normal range, but it is not in a range indicating the client is catabolizing the fats and proteins in the body. No ketones will be produced at this blood glucose level, so the ketoacidosis has resolved itself.
4. Most clients diagnosed with COPD are receiving oxygen at a low level.

**TEST-TAKING HINT:** All the options with physiological data are expected and not life-threatening, so the nurse should address the client diagnosed with a psychosocial problem.

45. 1. Rescue inhalers are used to treat attacks, not prevent them, so this should not be administered before exercising.
2. Warm-up exercises decrease the risk of developing an asthma attack.
3. Using a bronchodilator immediately before exercising will help reduce bronchospasms.
4. Monosodium glutamate, a food preservative, has been shown to initiate asthma attacks.

**TEST-TAKING HINT:** Option "1" has two words that are opposed—"rescue" and "wait"—which might lead the test taker to eliminate this option. Remember basic concepts, which are contradicted in option "2." There are a few disease processes that encourage intake of sodium, but asthma is not one of them, which would cause option "4" to be eliminated.

46. Correct answers are 1 and 2.
1. This applies to both inhaled and systemically administered steroids.
2. The steroids must pass through the oral cavity before reaching the lungs. Allowing the medication to stay within the oral cavity will suppress the normal flora found there, and the client could develop a yeast infection of the mouth (oral candidiasis).
3. Holding the medication in the mouth increases the risk of an oral yeast infection, and the medication is inhaled, not swallowed.

4. Inhaled steroids are not used first; the bronchodilators are used for an acute attack.
5. The plastic inhaler cover can be cleaned with warm water weekly or more frequently. The metal canister should not be placed in water.

**TEST-TAKING HINT:** Option "3" suggests that an inhaled medication is swallowed; the two terms do not match.

47. 1. A child with asthma can eat a regular diet if the child is not allergic to the components of the diet.
2. Because asthma can be a reaction to an allergen, it is important to determine which substances may trigger an attack.
3. The stem did not indicate the child is developmentally delayed.
4. The child does not require a home health nurse solely on the basis of asthma; the school nurse or any child-care provider should be informed of the child's diagnosis, and the parents must know the individual caring for the child is prepared to intervene during an attack.

**TEST-TAKING HINT:** The test taker must be aware of the disease process, determine causes, and then make a decision based on interventions required.

48. 1. The client must be able to recognize a life-threatening situation and initiate the correct procedure.
2. Bedding is washed in hot water to kill dust mites.
3. Many Chinese dishes are prepared with monosodium glutamate, an ingredient that can initiate an asthma attack.
4. Nonsteroidal anti-inflammatory medications, aspirin, and beta blockers have been known to initiate asthma attacks.

**TEST-TAKING HINT:** Dietary questions or answer options should be analyzed for the content. The test taker should decide, "What about Chinese foods could be a problem for a client diagnosed with asthma?" or "What might be good for the client about this diet?"

## Lung Cancer

49. 1. Working with asbestos is significant for mesothelioma of the lung, cancer with a very poor prognosis, but not for small cell carcinoma.

2. Family history is not a significant risk factor for small cell carcinoma. Smoking is the number-one risk factor.

3. Tattoos may be implicated in the development of blood-borne pathogen disease (if sterile needles were not used), but they do not have any association with cancer.

4. Smoking is the number-one risk factor for developing cancer of the lung. More than 85% of lung cancers are attributable to the inhalation of chemicals. There are more than 400 chemicals in each puff of cigarette smoke, 17 of which are known to cause cancer.

**TEST-TAKING HINT: If the test taker did not know this information, option "3" has no anatomical connection to the lungs and could be eliminated. This information has been widely disseminated in the media for more than 40 years since the Surgeon General's office first warned about the dangers of smoking in the early 1960s.**

50. Correct answers are 1, 2, 4, and 5.
    1. Respiratory distress is a common finding in clients diagnosed with lung cancer. As the tumor grows and takes up more space or blocks air movement, the client may need to be taught positioning for lung expansion. The administration of oxygen will help the client to use the lung capacity that is available to get oxygen to the tissues.
    2. Clients diagnosed with lung cancer frequently become fatigued, trying to eat. Providing six small meals spaces the amount of food the client eats throughout the day.
    3. Cancer is not communicable, so the client does not need to be in isolation.
    4. Clients diagnosed with cancer of the lung are at risk for developing an infection from lowered resistance as a result of treatments or from the tumor blocking secretions in the lung. Therefore, monitoring for the presence of fever, a possible indication of infection, is important.
    5. Assessment of the lungs should be completed on a routine and prn basis.

**TEST-TAKING HINT: This alternative-type question is an all-or-nothing situation. The NCLEX-RN® examination requires the test taker to answer each option correctly to receive credit for the question. Each option has the potential to be right or wrong.**

51. 1. Lung cancer is the number-one cause of cancer deaths in the United States.
    2. **Lung cancers are responsible for almost twice as many deaths among males as any other cancer and more deaths than breast cancer in females.**
    3. Lung cancers are the most deadly cancers among the U.S. population.
    4. Lung cancer deaths have remained relatively stable among the male population but have continued to increase among females steadily.

**TEST-TAKING HINT: The nurse must be able to interpret data to the public. The nurse will be asked about the incidence and severity of diseases.**

52. 1. This is expected from this client and does not warrant immediate attention.
    2. This is called a 3-point stance. It is a position many clients diagnosed with lung disease will assume because it assists in the expansion of the lung.
    3. Epoetin alfa (Procrit), a biologic response modifier, stimulates the bone marrow and can increase the client's blood pressure to dangerous levels. This BP is high and warrants immediate attention.
    4. This client can be seen after taking care of the client in "3." The nurse should intervene, but it is not a life-threatening situation.

**TEST-TAKING HINT: Even if the test taker did not know the side effects of Procrit, a BP of 198/102 warrants immediate attention.**

53. 1. This situation indicates a terminal process, and the client should make decisions for the end of life.
    2. Radiation therapy is used for tumors in the brain. Chemotherapy, as a whole, will not cross the blood-brain barrier.
    3. There is no indication the client cannot drive at this time. Clients may develop seizures from the tumors at some point.
    4. The client should make personal decisions for as long as possible. However, the client should discuss personal wishes with the person named in an advance directive to make decisions.

**TEST-TAKING HINT: The ethical principle of autonomy could help the test taker to discard option "4" as a correct answer.**

**54.** 1. If the investigational regimen proves to be effective, then this statement is true. However, many investigational treatments have not proved to be efficacious.

2. **Investigational treatments are just that—treatments being investigated to determine if they are effective in the care of clients diagnosed with cancer. There is no guarantee the treatments will help the client. Investigational treatments and medicines are sometimes called compassionate medicine use.**

3. Clients receive medical care and associated treatments and laboratory tests at no cost, but the client is not paid. Paying the client is unethical.

4. Frequently clients failing standard treatments and without hope for further treatment become involved in investigational protocols. The protocols can be used by other qualified volunteers for investigational treatment.

**TEST-TAKING HINT: The test taker should think about the word "investigational" and understand its meaning. Investigational means looking into something. This should lead the test taker to choose option "2."**

**55.** 1. A centralized system of organization means decisions are made at the top and given to the staff underneath to accept and implement.

2. A decentralized decision-making pattern means there is a fairly flat accountability chart. The unit manager has more autonomy in managing the unit, but this does not mean the staff has input into decisions.

3. **Shared governance is a system where the staff is empowered to make decisions such as scheduling and hiring of certain staff. Staff members are encouraged to participate in developing policies and procedures to reach set goals.**

4. A pyramid decision-making tree is an example of a centralized system.

**TEST-TAKING HINT: Answer options "1" and "4" basically say the same thing and could be eliminated for this reason.**

**56.** 1. **Research indicates smoking will still interfere with the client's response to treatment, so more teaching is needed.**

2. It is expected for the client to follow up with a specialist regarding subsequent treatment; therefore, the client does not need more teaching.

3. Clients diagnosed with cancer and undergoing treatment are at risk for developing infections, so more teaching is not needed.

4. Lung cancers produce fatigue as a result of physiological drains on the body in the areas of lack of adequate oxygen to the tissues, the tumor burden on the body, and the toll taken by the effects of the treatments. Cancer-related fatigue syndrome is a very real occurrence, so the client understands the teaching.

**TEST-TAKING HINT: Two options—"2" and "3"—are instructions given to all clients regardless of the disease process.**

**57.** Correct answers are 1 and 4.

1. **The use of a topical analgesic chest rub, such as Vicks VapoRub, could be an individual, cultural, or familial routine. It can be encouraged unless it interferes with the medical treatment plan. However, the nurse should assess the client to determine if this is an individual routine or an indicator of a health-care issue.**

2. An appendectomy in the past should be documented, but no further information is required.

3. Many clients take a multivitamin, so this would not warrant intervention.

4. **Coughing up blood is not normal and is cause for investigation. It could indicate lung cancer.**

5. Many clients use meditation for stress relief and self-awareness; no intervention would be warranted.

**TEST-TAKING HINT: The test taker should read all distracters carefully. "Further investigation" means something abnormal is occurring. Coughing up blood is always abnormal.**

**58.** 1. This is an adequate output. After a major surgery, clients will frequently have an intake greater than the output because of the fluid shift occurring as a result of trauma to the body.

2. **This is about a pint of blood loss and could indicate the client is hemorrhaging.**

3. The nurse should intervene and medicate the client, but pain, although a client comfort issue, is not life-threatening.

4. The client will have a chest tube to assist in reinflation of the lung, and absent lung sounds are expected at this point in the client's recovery.

**TEST-TAKING HINT: Blood is always a priority.**

59. Correct answers are 3 and 5.
   1. A bronchoscopy is not performed to confirm another test; it is performed to confirm diagnoses, such as cancer, *Pneumocystis* pneumonia, tuberculosis, fungal infections, and other lung diseases.
   2. The client's throat will be numbed with a local anesthetic to prevent gagging during the procedure. The client will not be able to eat or drink until this medication has worn off.
   3. **The HCP can take biopsies and perform washing of the lung tissue for pathological diagnosis during the procedure.**
   4. Most HCPs use an anesthetic procedure called twilight sleep to perform endoscopies, but there is no guarantee the client will not experience some discomfort.
   5. **Continuous cardiac monitoring, pulse oximetry, and blood pressure will be monitored throughout the procedure.**

**TEST-TAKING HINT:** The test taker must read each stem and answer option carefully. When in medicine does one test confirm another? Tests are done to confirm diagnoses. Option "4" has a false promise. Option "5" is standard during procedures.

60. 1. The nurse might enter into a therapeutic conversation, but client safety is the priority.
   2. The nurse must first assess the seriousness of the client's statement and any plans to carry out suicide. Depending on the client's responses, the nurse will notify the HCP.
   3. The client can be referred for assistance in dealing with the disease and its ramifications, but this is not the priority.
   4. **The priority action anytime a client makes a statement regarding suicide is to determine if the client has thought it through and has a plan. A plan indicates an emergency situation.**

**TEST-TAKING HINT:** In a question that asks for a first response, all answer options may be actions the nurse would take. Ranking the options in order of action—"4," "1," "2," "3"— may help the test taker to make a decision. Applying Maslow's hierarchy of needs, safety comes first.

## Cancer of the Larynx

61. 1. Gargling with salt water is good for sore throats, but it does not diagnose cancer of the larynx.
   2. Clients thought to have a vocal cord problem are encouraged to practice voice rest. Vocal cord exercises would not assist in the diagnosis of cancer.
   3. **A laryngoscopy will be performed to allow for visualization of the vocal cords and to obtain a biopsy for pathological diagnosis.**
   4. There is no monthly self-examination of the larynx. To visualize the vocal cords, the HCP must numb the throat and pass a fiberoptic instrument through the throat and into the trachea.

**TEST-TAKING HINT:** The test taker must understand that, if the question states the client is admitted to "rule out" a disease, then diagnostic tests and procedures will be done to determine if, in fact, the client has the diagnosis that the HCP suspects.

62. 1. **The teeth will be in the area of radiation, and the roots of teeth are highly sensitive to radiation, which results in root abscesses. The client should have a dental examination before radiation treatments and frequently throughout treatments (American Cancer Society, 2017).**
   2. An antiemetic on a routine scheduled basis is prophylactic for nausea, and the schedule is 30 minutes before a meal. Radiation to the throat does not encompass nausea-producing areas.
   3. Sunscreen is used to prevent the penetration of ultraviolet (UV) rays into the dermis. Radiation is gamma rays.
   4. The client may receive a PEG tube for severe esophagitis from the irradiation of the esophagus. The client does not have a nasogastric tube.

**TEST-TAKING HINT:** The test taker could eliminate option "4" as a form of nutritional treatment, not prophylaxis. The test taker must recognize which anatomical structures would lie within the radiation beam. The teeth of the lower jaw definitely are within the port, and the upper teeth possibly would be in range.

63. 1. The client is 3 days postoperative partial removal of the larynx and should be eating by this time.
    2. The client should be eating normal foods at this time. The consistency should be soft to allow for less chewing of the food and easier swallowing because a portion of the throat musculature has been removed. The client should be taught to turn the head toward the affected side when swallowing to help prevent aspiration.
    3. The client should be capable of enteral nutrition at this time.
    4. The client should have progressed to a diet with a more normal consistency and amount.

**TEST-TAKING HINT:** The keys to this question are "3 days" and "partial." Clients are progressed rapidly after surgery to as normal a life as possible.

64. 1. This is an appropriate preoperative intervention, but it is not the priority.
    2. The client should be taught about pain medication administration, but this is not the highest priority.
    3. The client should be told about an anti-embolism hose, but it is not necessary to demonstrate the hose because the nurse will apply and remove the hose initially.
    4. The client is having the vocal cords removed and will be unable to speak. Communication is a high priority for this client. If the client is able to read and write, a Magic Slate, a pad of paper, or a programmable speech-generating device should be provided. If the client is illiterate, the nurse and the client should develop a method of communication using pictures or hand signals.

**TEST-TAKING HINT:** Questions addressing the highest priority include all of the options being possible interventions, but only one is the priority. Use Maslow's hierarchy of needs to answer the question—safety is a priority.

65. 1. CanSurmount is a program of volunteer cancer survivors. The volunteers talk to clients about having cancer or what the treatments involve. This group is based on the success of Reach to Recovery for breast cancer, but it is not specific to a particular cancer.
    2. Dialogue is a cancer support group that brings together clients diagnosed with cancer to discuss the feelings associated with having cancer.

3. The Lost Chord Club is an American Cancer Society–sponsored group of survivors of larynx cancer. These clients are able to discuss feelings and needs with survivors of laryngectomies because they have all had this particular surgery.
    4. SmokEnders is a group of clients working together to stop smoking. It is a group to which any smoker can be referred.

**TEST-TAKING HINT:** The larynx is commonly referred to as the "vocal cords." If the test taker were not aware of the various support groups, option "3" has "lost" and "cords" in it and is the best choice.

66. 1. The most serious complication resulting from a radical neck dissection is the rupture of the carotid artery. Continuous bright-red drainage indicates bleeding, and this client should be assessed immediately (Thyroid, Head & Neck Cancer Foundation, n.d.).
    2. Pain is a priority but not over hemorrhaging.
    3. Clients diagnosed with cancer of the lung have fatigue and are short of breath; these are expected findings.
    4. Clients diagnosed with chronic lung problems are taught pursed-lip breathing to assist in expelling air. This type of breathing often produces a whistling sound.

**TEST-TAKING HINT:** If the test taker is not sure of the answer and airway compromise is not one of the answer options, then an option dealing with bleeding is the best choice.

67. 1. Chest tubes are part of the nursing education curriculum. The new graduate should be capable of caring for this client or at least knowing when to get assistance.
    2. This client is in respiratory compromise, and an experienced nurse should care for the client.
    3. A client diagnosed with multiple fistulas in the neck area is at high risk for airway compromise and should be assigned to a more experienced nurse.
    4. This client is at risk for developing edema of the neck area and should be cared for by a more experienced nurse.

**TEST-TAKING HINT:** The question is asking for the least compromised or most stable client. The client in option "1" already has chest tubes in place and is presumably stable.

**68.** 1. Wound infection is a concern, but in the list of the answer options, it is not the highest priority. A wound infection can be treated, but a client not breathing is in a life-threatening situation, and the problem must be addressed immediately.
2. Hemorrhage is normally a priority, but bleeding is not a priority over not breathing.
3. Respiratory distress is the highest priority. Hemorrhaging and infection are serious problems, but the airway is the priority.
4. Knowledge deficit is the lowest on this priority list. It is a psychosocial problem, and these problems rank lower in priority than physiological ones.

**TEST-TAKING HINT: This option concurs with Maslow's hierarchy of needs, which places oxygenation at the top of the hierarchy.**

**69.** 1. This request indicates the client is accepting the situation and trying to deal with it.
2. Placing a towel over the mirror indicates the client is having difficulty looking at his reflection, a body-image problem.
3. In attempting to shave his face, the client is participating in self-care activities and also must look at his neck in the mirror, both good steps toward adjustment.
4. Neck and shoulder exercises are done to strengthen the remaining musculature, but they have nothing to do with body image.

**TEST-TAKING HINT: The test taker must try to match the problem with the answer choices. This would eliminate options "1" and "4." Shaving his face is a positive action, and the question asks for an action indicating a disturbance in body image.**

**70.** 1. This is an example of nonmaleficence, where the nurse "does no harm." In attempting to discuss the client's refusal, the nurse is not trying to influence the client; the nurse is merely attempting to listen therapeutically.
2. This is an example of paternalism, telling the client what he should do, and it is also coercion, an unethical action.
3. This is an example of beneficence, "to do good"; it is a positive action and a step up from nonmaleficence.
4. This is an example of beneficence.

**TEST-TAKING HINT: If the test taker were not aware of the terms of ethical principles, then**

dissecting the word "nonmaleficence" into its portions might help. *Non-* means "nothing" or "none," and *mal-* means "bad," so "no bad action" could be inferred. This would eliminate option "2."

**71.** 1. The cancer may have grown, but this would not be indicated by the type of pain described.
2. Painful swallowing is caused by esophageal irritation.
3. Most cancers are not painful unless obstructing an organ or pressing on a nerve. This is not what is being described.
4. The esophagus is extremely radiosensitive, and esophageal ulcerations are common. The pain can become so severe the client cannot swallow saliva. This is a situation in which the client will be admitted to the hospital for IV narcotic pain medication and possibly total parenteral nutrition.

**TEST-TAKING HINT: The test taker must remember not to jump to conclusions and to realize what a word is actually saying. Swallowing is an action involving the esophagus, so the best choice would be either option "1" or option "4," both of which contain the word "esophagus."**

**72.** Correct answers are 2, 4, and 5.
1. This surgery removed the vocal cords, so the client will not be able to speak again unless the client learns esophageal speech, uses an electric larynx, or has a surgically created transesophageal puncture.
2. The client breathes through a stoma in the neck. Care should be taken not to allow water to enter the stoma.
3. The stoma should be cleaned, but petroleum-based products should not be allowed near the stoma. A petroleum-based product is contraindicated because it is not water-soluble, could contribute to an occlusion, and is flammable.
4. The client has lost the use of the nasal passages to humidify the inhaled air, and artificial humidification is useful until the client's body adapts to the change.
5. Special equipment is available for clients unable to hear or speak.

**TEST-TAKING HINT: Option "1" can be eliminated as a false promise that would undermine the nurse-client relationship.**

# Pulmonary Embolus

**73.** 880 units.

If there are 20,000 units of heparin in 500 mL of $D_5W$, there are 40 units in each milliliter:

$20,000 \div 500 = 40$ units

If 22 mL are infused per hour, then 880 units of heparin are infused each hour:

$40 \times 22 = 880$

**TEST-TAKING HINT:** The test taker must know how to calculate heparin drips from two aspects: the question may give the mL/hr, and the test taker has to determine units/hr, or the question may give units/hr, and the test taker has to determine mL/hr. Remember to learn how to use the drop-down calculator on the computer or request an erase slate during the NCLEX-RN®.

**74.** 1. The plasma D-dimer test is highly specific for the presence of a thrombus; an elevated D-dimer indicates a thrombus formation and lysis. This result would require a computed tomography (CT) or ventilation and perfusion VQ scan to confirm the diagnosis.
2. An ABG evaluates the oxygenation level, but it does not diagnose a PE.
3. A CXR shows pulmonary infiltration and pleural effusions, but it does not diagnose a PE.
4. An MRI is a noninvasive test that detects a deep vein thrombosis (DVT), but it does not diagnose a PE. A CT scan or VQ scan would be used to confirm the diagnosis.

**TEST-TAKING HINT:** The key to answering this question is the phrase, "confirms the diagnosis." The test taker should eliminate options "2" and "3" based on the fact these are diagnostic tests used for many disease processes and conditions.

**75.** 1. This is a sign of a DVT, which is a precursor to a PE, but it is not a sign of a pulmonary embolism.
2. The most common signs of a PE are sudden onset of chest pain when taking a deep breath and shortness of breath.
3. These are signs of myocardial infarction.
4. These could be signs of pneumonia or other pulmonary complications but not specifically a PE.

**TEST-TAKING HINT:** The key to selecting option "2" as the correct answer is sudden onset. The test taker would need to note "left-sided" in option "3" to eliminate this as a possible

correct answer, and option "4" is nonspecific for a PE.

**76.** 1. The ABGs are within normal limits and would not warrant immediate intervention.
2. Occasional PVCs are not unusual for any client and would not warrant immediate intervention.
3. The normal pulse oximeter reading is 93% to 100%. A reading of 90% indicates the client has an arterial oxygen level of around 60.
4. Urinary output of 800 mL over 12 hours indicates an output of greater than 30 mL/ hour and would not warrant immediate intervention by the nurse.

**TEST-TAKING HINT:** This question is asking the test taker to select abnormal, unexpected, or life-threatening assessment data in relation to the client's disease process. A pulse oximeter reading of less than 93% indicates severe hypoxia and requires immediate intervention.

**77.** Correct answers are 4 and 5.
1. The intravenous anticoagulant heparin will be administered immediately after the diagnosis of a PE, not oral anticoagulants.
2. The client's respiratory system will be assessed, not the gastrointestinal system.
3. Thoracentesis is used to aspirate fluid from the pleural space; it is not a treatment for a PE.
4. Bedrest reduces the risk of another clot becoming an embolus leading to a PE. Bedrest reduces metabolic demands and tissue needs for oxygen in the lungs.
5. The nurse should administer oxygen therapy to the client as ordered by the HCP.

**TEST-TAKING HINT:** The test taker must be aware of adjectives such as "oral" in option "1," which makes this option incorrect. The test taker should apply the body system of the disease process to eliminate option "2" as a correct answer.

**78.** 1. The client would not be experiencing abnormal bleeding with this INR.
2. Vitamin K (AquaMephyton) is the antidote for an overdose of anticoagulant, and the INR does not indicate this.
3. A therapeutic INR is 2 to 3; therefore, the nurse should administer the oral anticoagulant warfarin (Coumadin).
4. There is no need to increase the dose; this result is within the therapeutic range.

**TEST-TAKING HINT:** The test taker must know normal laboratory values; this is the only way the test taker will be able to answer this question. The test taker should make a list of laboratory values that must be memorized for successful test taking.

79. 1. Arterial blood gases would be included in the client problem "impaired gas exchange."
    2. These assessment data monitor tissue perfusion, which evaluates for decreased cardiac output.
    3. This would be appropriate for the client problem "high risk for bleeding."
    4. The client should not be put in a position with the head lower than the legs because this would increase difficulty breathing.

**TEST-TAKING HINT:** The test taker must think about which answer option addresses the problem of the heart's inability to pump blood. Decreased blood to the extremities results in cyanosis and cold extremities.

80. Correct answers are 1, 3, 4, and 5.
    1. Heparin is administered during thrombolytic therapy, and the antidote is protamine sulfate and should be available to reverse the effects of the anticoagulant.
    2. Firm pressure reduces the risk of bleeding into the tissues.
    3. Obvious (overt) as well as hidden (covert) signs of bleeding should be assessed for.
    4. Invasive procedures increase the risk of tissue trauma and bleeding.
    5. Stool softeners help prevent constipation and straining, which may precipitate bleeding from hemorrhoids.

**TEST-TAKING HINT:** Thrombolytic therapy is ordered to help dissolve the clot resulting in the PE. Therefore, all nursing interventions should address bleeding tendencies. The test taker must select all interventions applicable to these alternative questions.

81. 1. The client should use a soft-bristle toothbrush to reduce the risk of bleeding, so teaching is not effective.
    2. This is appropriate for a client with a mechanical valve replacement, not a client receiving anticoagulant therapy, so the teaching is not effective.
    3. Acetylsalicylic acid [ASA] (aspirin), enteric-coated or not, is an antiplatelet, which may increase bleeding tendencies and should be avoided, so the teaching is not effective.
    4. The client should wear a medical alert bracelet (Medic Alert band) at all times so that, if any accident or situation

occurs, the HCPs will know the client is receiving anticoagulant therapy. The client understands the teaching.

**TEST-TAKING HINT:** This is a higher-level question in which the test taker must know clients diagnosed with a PE are prescribed anticoagulant therapy on discharge from the hospital. If the test taker had no idea of the answer, the option stating "wear a Medic Alert band" is a good choice because many disease processes require the client to take long-term medication, and an HCP should be aware of this.

82. Correct answers are 1, 2, and 5.
    1. Increasing fluids will help increase fluid volume, which will, in turn, help prevent the development of DVT, the most common cause of PE.
    2. Pulmonary emboli are not caused by atherosclerosis, but a diet low in fat and sodium is an appropriate discharge instruction for a client diagnosed with a PE because a heart-healthy diet can reduce damage to the vasculature. A clot forms in response to damage to blood vessels.
    3. Infection does not cause a PE; this is not an appropriate teaching instruction.
    4. Pneumonia and flu do not cause a pulmonary embolism.
    5. Smoking causes damage to the vascular system and vasoconstriction, which increases the risk of clot formation.

**TEST-TAKING HINT:** The test taker must know DVT is the most common cause of PE, and preventing dehydration is an important intervention. Measures to avoid damage to the vascular system and prevent clots should be included in the teaching. The test taker can attempt to eliminate answers by trying to determine which disease process is appropriate for the intervention.

83. 1. An INR of 2 to 3 is therapeutic; therefore, the nurse would administer the oral coagulant warfarin (Coumadin).
    2. This is an elevated blood glucose level; therefore, the nurse should administer the insulin.
    3. A normal aPTT is 25 to 35 seconds, and for heparin to be therapeutic, it should be 1.5 to 2 times the normal value or 37.5 to 70. A PTT of 98 indicates the client is not clotting, and the medication should be held.
    4. This is normal blood pressure, and the nurse should administer the medication.

**TEST-TAKING HINT:** This question is asking the test taker to select a distracter with assessment data that are unsafe for administering the medication. The test taker must know normal laboratory values to administer medication safely.

84. 1. The client needs oxygen, but the nurse can intervene to help the client before applying oxygen.
    2. Placing the client in this position facilitates maximal lung expansion and reduces venous return to the right side of the heart, thus lowering pressures in the pulmonary vascular system.
    3. A pulse oximeter reading is needed, but it is not the first intervention.
    4. Assessing the client is indicated, but it is not the first intervention in this situation.

**TEST-TAKING HINT:** The test taker must select the option that will directly help the client breathe easier. Therefore, assessment is not the first intervention, and option "4" can be eliminated as the correct answer. When the client is in distress, do not assess.

## Chest Trauma

85. 1. The client diagnosed with pneumothorax has absent breath sounds and tachypnea.
    2. Unequal lung expansion and dyspnea indicate a pneumothorax.
    3. Consolidation occurs when there is no air moving through the alveoli, as in pneumonia; frothy sputum occurs with heart failure.
    4. Barrel chest and polycythemia are signs of chronic obstructive pulmonary disease.

**TEST-TAKING HINT:** The test taker can use "chest trauma" or "pneumothorax" to help select the correct answer. Both of these terms should cause the test taker to select option "2" because unequal chest expansion would result from trauma.

86. 1. A STAT CXR would not be needed to determine why there is no fluctuation in the water-seal compartment.
    2. Increasing the amount of wall suction does not address why there is no fluctuation in the water-seal compartment.
    3. The key to the answer is "2 hours." The air from the pleural space is not able to get to the water-seal compartment, and the nurse should try to determine why. Usually, the client is lying on the tube, it is kinked, or there is a dependent loop.

4. The stem does not state the client is in respiratory distress, and a pulse oximeter reading detects hypoxemia but does not address any fluctuation in the water-seal compartment.

**TEST-TAKING HINT:** The test taker should apply the nursing process to answer the question correctly. The first step in the nursing process is assessment, and "check" (option "3") is a word that can be used synonymously for "assess." Monitoring (option "4") is also assessing, but the test taker should not check a diagnostic test result before caring for the client.

87. 1. The client must take deep breaths to help push the air out of the pleural space into the water-seal drainage, and deep breaths will help prevent the client from developing pneumonia or atelectasis.
    2. The client must take deep breaths; shallow breaths could lead to complications.
    3. Deep breaths must be taken to prevent complications.
    4. This is a cruel intervention; the nurse can medicate the client and then encourage deep breathing.

**TEST-TAKING HINT:** If the test taker reads options "2" and "3" and notices that both reflect the same idea—namely, that deep breaths are not necessary—then both can either be eliminated as incorrect answers or kept as possible correct answers. Option "4" should be eliminated based on being a very rude and threatening comment.

88. 1. Keeping the drainage system lower than the chest promotes drainage and prevents reflux.
    2. The chest tube system can function as a result of gravity and does not have to be attached to suction. Keeping it attached to suction could cause the client to trip and fall. Therefore, this is a safety issue, and the nurse should intervene and explain this to the UAP.
    3. Ambulation facilitates lung ventilation and expansion; drainage systems are portable to allow ambulation while chest tubes are in place.
    4. The client should ambulate, but getting up and using the bedside commode is better than staying in bed, so no action would be needed.

**TEST-TAKING HINT:** "Warrants immediate intervention" means the test taker must identify the situation in which the nurse should correct the action, demonstrate a skill, or somehow intervene with the UAP's behavior.

89. 1. The HCP will have to be notified, but this is not the first intervention. Air must be prevented from entering the pleural space from the outside atmosphere.
   2. The client should breathe regularly or take deep breaths until the tubes are reinserted.
   3. The nurse must take action and prevent air from entering the pleural space.
   4. The nurse should immediately apply pressure to the insertion site, have the client perform the Valsalva maneuver, and cover the site with petroleum gauze or dry sterile dressing (per hospital policy).

**TEST-TAKING HINT:** The words "implement first" in the stem of the question indicate to the test taker that possibly more than one intervention could be warranted in the situation, but only one is implemented first. Remember, do not select an assessment first without reading the question. If the client is in any type of crisis, then the nurse should first do something to help the client's situation.

90. 1. This statement describes a spontaneous pneumothorax.
   2. This statement describes an open pneumothorax.
   3. This describes a tension pneumothorax. It is a medical emergency requiring immediate intervention to preserve life.
   4. This is called an iatrogenic pneumothorax, which also may be caused by thoracentesis or lung biopsy. A tension pneumothorax could occur from this procedure, but the statement does not describe a tension pneumothorax.

**TEST-TAKING HINT:** The test taker must always be clear about what the question is asking before answering the question. If the test taker can eliminate options "1" and "2" and can't decide between options "3" and "4," the test taker must go back to the stem and clarify what the question is asking.

91. 1. Checking to see if someone has increased the suction rate is the simplest and a noninvasive action for the nurse to implement; if it is not on high, then the nurse must check to see if the problem is with the client or the system.
   2. No fluctuation (tidaling) would cause the nurse to assess the tubing for a blood clot.

3. The tube is milked to help dislodge a blood clot that may be blocking the chest tube, causing no fluctuation (tidaling) in the water-seal compartment. The chest tube is never stripped, which creates negative air pressure and could suck lung tissue into the chest tube.
   4. Encouraging the client to cough forcefully will help dislodge a blood clot blocking the chest tube, causing no fluctuation (tidaling) in the water-seal compartment.

**TEST-TAKING HINT:** The test taker should always think about assessing the client if there is a problem, and the client is not in immediate danger. This would cause the test taker to eliminate options "3" and "4." The test taker should know bubbling has to do with suctioning.

92. 1. This is an expected finding in the suction compartment of the drainage system, indicating adequate suctioning is being applied.
   2. At 3 days postinsertion, no fluctuation (tidaling) indicates the lung has re-expanded, which indicates the treatment has been effective.
   3. Blood in the drainage bottle is expected for a hemothorax but does not indicate the chest tubes have re-expanded the lung.
   4. Taking a deep breath without pain is good, but it does not mean the lungs have re-expanded.

**TEST-TAKING HINT:** The test taker must be knowledgeable about chest tubes to be able to answer this question. The test taker must know the normal time frame and what is expected for each compartment of the chest tube drainage system.

93. Correct answers are 2, 4, and 5.
   1. The client should be in the high Fowler's position to facilitate lung expansion.
   2. The system must be patent and intact to function properly.
   3. The client can have bathroom privileges, and ambulation facilitates lung ventilation and expansion.
   4. Looping the tubing prevents direct pressure on the chest tube itself and keeps tubing off the floor, addressing both a safety and a potential clogging of the tube.
   5. Subcutaneous emphysema is air under the skin, which is a common occurrence at the chest tube insertion site.

**TEST-TAKING HINT:** The test taker should be careful with adjectives. In option "1," the word "low" makes it incorrect; in option "3," the word "strict" makes this option incorrect.

94. 1. This pulse oximeter reading indicates the client is hypoxic and therefore is not stable and should be assigned to an RN.
    2. These H&H levels are very low; therefore, the client is not stable and should be assigned to an RN.
    3. Jugular vein distention and hypotension are signs of a tension pneumothorax, which is a medical emergency, and the client should be assigned to an RN.
    4. A client 2 hours post-bronchoscopy procedure could safely be assigned to an LPN.

**TEST-TAKING HINT: The test taker must understand that the LPN should be assigned the least critical client or the stable client not exhibiting any complications secondary to the admitting disease or condition.**

95. 1. The nurse should gather a thoracotomy tray and the chest tube drainage system and take it to the client's bedside, but it is not the first intervention.
    2. **The insertion of a chest tube is an invasive procedure and requires informed consent. Without a consent form, this procedure should not be done on an alert and oriented client.**
    3. This is a correct position to place the client in for a chest tube insertion, but it is not the first intervention.
    4. The HCP will discuss the procedure with the client, then informed consent must be obtained, and the nurse can do further teaching.

**TEST-TAKING HINT: The test taker must know invasive procedures require informed consent, and legally it must be obtained first before anyone can touch the client.**

96. 1. Assessment of the lung sounds could indicate the client's lung has re-expanded because it has been 3 days since the chest tube has been inserted.
    2. This should be done to ensure the lung has re-expanded, but it is not the first intervention.
    3. The HCP will need to be notified so the chest tube can be removed, but it is not the first intervention.
    4. This situation needs to be documented, but it is not the first intervention.

**TEST-TAKING HINT: When the stem asks the test taker to identify the first intervention, all four answer options could be interventions appropriate for the situation, but only one is the first intervention. Remember to apply the nursing process: the first step is assessment.**

## Acute Respiratory Distress Syndrome

97. 1. The opposite side rail should be elevated so the client will not fall out of the bed. Safety is the priority, and the nurse should demonstrate the proper way to bathe a client in the bed.
    2. The bed should be at a comfortable height for the UAP to bathe the client, not in the lowest position.
    3. The UAP can bathe a client without assistance if the client's safety can be ensured.
    4. The UAP is not ensuring the client's safety because the opposite side rail is not elevated to prevent the client from falling out of the bed.

**TEST-TAKING HINT: Although the test taker should always be concerned with the disease process of the client, many times the answer may be selected based on basic nursing skills, and not require an understanding of the client's disease process.**

98. 1. Maintaining ventilator settings and checking to ensure they are specifically set as prescribed is appropriate, but it is not the first intervention.
    2. Making sure alarms are functioning properly is appropriate, but checking a machine is not the priority.
    3. **Assessment is the first part of the nursing process and is the first intervention the nurse should implement when caring for a client on a ventilator.**
    4. Monitoring laboratory results is an appropriate intervention for the client on a ventilator, but monitoring laboratory data is not the priority intervention.

**TEST-TAKING HINT: The test taker should apply the nursing process, which identifies assessment as the first step. Therefore, if the test taker is not sure of the answer, the best-educated choice is to select an option addressing assessment data.**

99. 1. **The classic sign of ARDS is decreased arterial oxygen level ($Pao_2$) while administering high levels of oxygen; the oxygen is unable to cross the alveolar membrane.**
    2. These are early signs of ARDS, but they could also indicate pneumonia, atelectasis, and other pulmonary complications, so they do not confirm the diagnosis of ARDS.
    3. Clear breath sounds and the oxygen saturation indicate the client is not experiencing any respiratory difficulty or compromise.

4. These are signs of congestive heart failure; ARDS is noncardiogenic (without signs of cardiac involvement) pulmonary edema.

**TEST-TAKING HINT:** If the test taker does not know the clinical manifestations of ARDS, the test taker should eliminate option "2" because this could be any respiratory disorder, option "3" because these are normal data, and option "4" because jugular vein distention usually occurs with heart problems.

100. 1. This is an incorrect statement. ARDS has multiple etiologies, such as hemorrhagic shock, septic shock, drug overdose, burns, and near-drowning. Many people with near-drowning do not develop ARDS.
2. The layperson may not know what the term *alveoli* means, and the near-drowning is the initial insult that caused the ARDS.
3. This is a basic layperson's terms explanation of ARDS and explains why the client is having trouble breathing.
4. Smoking increases the risk of developing ARDS, but the etiology is unknown; however, an initial insult occurs less than 7 days before the development of ARDS.

**TEST-TAKING HINT:** The test taker should select the answer option presenting facts and easiest for the client to understand. The test taker should not select the distracter with medical jargon the client may not understand. The test taker, as a rule, can eliminate any distracter using medical jargon in the answer.

101. 1. A urine output of 30 mL/hr or 120 mL in 4 hours indicates the kidneys are functioning properly.
2. This indicates the client is being adequately oxygenated.
3. Asymmetrical chest expansion indicates the client has had a pneumothorax, which is a complication of mechanical ventilation.
4. An increased heart rate does not indicate a complication; this could result from numerous reasons, not specifically because of the ventilator.

**TEST-TAKING HINT:** The test taker should be looking for an answer option describing abnormal, unexpected, or life-threatening data because of the word "complication" in the stem. Understanding medical suffixes and prefixes could help the test taker select the correct answer. Any time there is an "a" before the word, it means "without," as in "asymmetrical," which means "without symmetry."

102. 1. These arterial blood gases are within normal limits, and therefore, the nurse should not take any action except to continue to monitor the client.
2. The nurse would recommend deep breaths and coughing if the client's ABGs revealed respiratory acidosis.
3. Sodium bicarbonate is administered when the client is in metabolic acidosis.
4. This is a normal ABG, and the respiratory therapist does not need to be notified.

**TEST-TAKING HINT:** This question requires the test taker to know normal ABG results: pH 7.35 to 7.45, $Pao_2$ 80 to 100, $Paco_2$ 35 to 45, $Hco_3$ 22 to 26. The test taker must know how to evaluate the results.

103. Correct answers are 4 and 5.
1. Alternating the ET tube position will help prevent a pressure ulcer on the client's tongue and mouth.
2. A CXR is performed immediately after the insertion of the ET tube but not daily.
3. The cuff should be inflated but no more than 25 cm $H_2O$ to ensure no air leakage and must be checked every 4 to 8 hours, not daily.
4. The ET tube should be secure to ensure it does not enter the right main bronchus. The ET tube should be 1 inch above the bifurcation of the bronchi.
5. The lung sounds should be assessed every 2 hours to determine if suctioning is needed and to confirm ET tube placement.

**TEST-TAKING HINT:** The test taker must be knowledgeable about ventilator care. Radiation is dangerous; therefore, a daily CXR (option "2") may be eliminated as the correct answer.

104. 1. The CRX will identify bilateral infiltrates in the lungs, the classic sign of ARDS.
2. A complete blood count can determine if the cause of ARDS is an infection but is not diagnostic of ARDS.
3. Airway pressure-release ventilation is a ventilator mode with a longer inspiration-to-expiration ratio that facilitates oxygenation and gas exchange.
4. A sputum culture is not diagnostic of ARDS.

**TEST-TAKING HINT:** ARDS would indicate a problem with the lungs; if the test taker identifies a CRX as direct visualization of the lungs, this would be an appropriate selection as the correct answer.

105. 1. The nurse must first address the client's acute respiratory distress and then notify other members of the multidisciplinary team.
     2. **If the ventilator system malfunctions, the nurse must ventilate the client with a manual resuscitation (Ambu) bag until the problem is resolved.**
     3. The nurse must first address the client's respiratory distress before requesting any laboratory data.
     4. Assessment is not always a priority. In this situation, the client is in obvious acute respiratory distress; therefore, the nurse needs to intervene to help the client breathe.

**TEST-TAKING HINT: When the question asks the test taker to select the first intervention, and the client is in a life-threatening situation, the nurse should select an intervention that directly helps the client.**

106. Correct answers are 1, 3, 4, and 5.
     1. Altered level of consciousness is the earliest sign of hypoxemia.
     2. Urine output of less than 30 mL/hr indicates decreased cardiac output, which requires immediate intervention; it should be assessed every 1 or 2 hours, not once during a shift.
     3. The client is at risk for complications of immobility; therefore, the nurse should turn the client at least every 2 hours to prevent pressure ulcers.
     4. The client is at risk for fluid volume overload, so the nurse should monitor and maintain fluid intake.
     5. The prone position has been demonstrated to facilitate lung expansion and improve oxygenation by opening more alveoli (Hoffman & Sullivan, 2020).

**TEST-TAKING HINT: The client diagnosed with ARDS is critically ill, and interventions should address complications of immobility, decreased cardiac output, and respiratory distress. Remember, how often an intervention is implemented is important when selecting the correct answer to the question. More than one answer is possible in these alternate-type questions.**

107. 1. Not smoking is vital to prevent further lung damage.
     2. The client should get vaccines to help prevent further episodes of serious respiratory distress.
     3. Avoiding alcohol intake is appropriate for many serious illnesses, but it is not the most important when discussing ARDS.
     4. It usually takes about 6 months to recover maximal respiratory function after ARDS.

**TEST-TAKING HINT: ARDS means something is wrong with the respiratory system. Therefore, the test taker should select an answer option addressing the lungs and possible lung damage.**

108. 1. **When peak airway pressure is increased, the nurse should implement the intervention least invasive for the client. This alarm goes off with a plugged airway, "bucking" in the ventilator, decreasing lung compliance, kinked tubing, or pneumothorax.**
     2. The alarm may indicate the client needs suctioning, but the nurse should always do the least invasive procedure when troubleshooting a ventilator alarm.
     3. The lip line on the ET tube determines how far the ET tube is in the trachea. It should always stay at the same number, but it would not have anything to do with the ventilator alarms.
     4. This may be needed, but the nurse should not sedate the client unless absolutely necessary.

**TEST-TAKING HINT: If the test taker has no idea what peak airway pressure is, the test taker should not give up on being able to figure out the correct answer. When something is going wrong with a machine, the nurse should either assess or do something for the client. Always select the easiest and least invasive intervention to help the client.**

109. Correct answers are 2 and 3.
    1. These symptoms indicate a respiratory and an infection problem, not clotting.
    2. Shortness of breath and a low-grade fever indicate pneumonia; the oxygenation concept applies to this client.
    3. Shortness of breath and a low-grade fever indicate pneumonia; the infection concept applies to this client.
    4. Perfusion does not apply for this client based on the presenting symptoms.
    5. Coping does not apply for this client based on the presenting symptoms.

**TEST-TAKING HINT: The keys to answering this question are the client's presenting symptoms and the vital signs.**

110. 1. The symptoms are seen in clients diagnosed with COPD. Oxygenation is the highest priority. Mobility can be an issue but is not the priority.
    2. The symptoms are seen in clients diagnosed with COPD. Oxygenation is the highest priority. Nutrition can be an issue but is not the priority.
    3. The symptoms are seen in clients diagnosed with COPD. Oxygenation is the highest priority. Activity intolerance can be an issue but is not the priority.
    4. **The symptoms are seen in clients diagnosed with COPD. Oxygenation is the highest priority.**

**TEST-TAKING HINT: The test taker should use Maslow's hierarchy of needs to answer this question. The lowest level of the hierarchy pyramid is physiological needs; the client will die quickly if tissues do not receive oxygen.**

111. 1. This is the second order to implement; an IVPB cannot be administered without IV access.
    2. This is the third order to implement; the goal is to initiate the IV antibiotic 1 to 2 hours from when the order was written by the HCP.
    3. Culture specimens should be obtained before the initiation of antibiotic medication to prevent skewing of results.
    4. This is the fourth order for the nurse to initiate.

**TEST-TAKING HINT: The test taker must be aware of the basic steps in medication delivery.**

In the case of an antibiotic, any or all cultures must be obtained before initiating the antibiotic, or the culture results will be skewed.

112. 1. The symptoms described indicate Cushing's syndrome, developed as a result of long-term steroid use. The steroid of choice for home administration is prednisone. The client must continue to receive a form of glucocorticoid medication, or the client may develop symptoms of cortisol insufficiency.
    2. The symptoms indicate steroid-induced Cushing's syndrome, not a potential abuse situation.
    3. Nothing indicates the client is immobile or has an issue with the coccyx.
    4. Whether or not the client sleeps with the HOB elevated does not address the described symptoms.

**TEST-TAKING HINT: The keys to answering this question are the client's presenting symptoms; the test taker must be knowledgeable of treatments for certain diseases and the side effects of those treatments.**

113. 1. The client should be on a form of glucocorticosteroid medication. The nurse would not question administering this medication.
    2. **A client diagnosed with COPD and pneumonia would be placed on an antibiotic, but the client lists an allergy to cephalosporin antibiotics; ceftriaxone is a third-generation cephalosporin. The nurse should investigate further before administering the medication.**
    3. Benzonatate (Tessalon Perles) is an antitussive cough suppressant; the nurse would not question this medication.
    4. Continuous release morphine is prescribed for the mild bronchodilating effect of morphine over a sustained period of time. The nurse would not question administering this medication.

**TEST-TAKING HINT: The key to answering this question is for the test taker to read all the portions of the graph (MAR) carefully. Noting the allergy to a "ceph" medication would have provided a clue as to choosing a "ceph" answer.**

114. 1. This client has an elevated platelet count, which is not an expected result for a client diagnosed with pneumonia. The nurse should notify the HCP so that the client can be evaluated for a comorbid problem. The WBC count is high, but it is expected in a client diagnosed with pneumonia.
2. The only value that is abnormal is the $Hco_3$ level, which indicates that complete compensation has occurred by the client's body. This is a good ABG report. There is no reason to notify the HCP.
3. A client diagnosed with an exacerbation of COPD would be on steroid medication, which can cause an increase in blood glucose.
4. Cultures take 24 to 48 hours to obtain results. The client should already be on antibiotic medication. The information provided did not mention which antibiotics the client is on.

**TEST-TAKING HINT:** The test taker should not read into a question, such as option "4," based on the knowledge that cultures take 24 to 48 hours. Then the nurse would be aware that the client has been receiving antibiotic therapy currently.

115. 1. This EHR graphic indicates the client is not processing the amount of fluid being taken in. A steroid medication will not affect this situation.
2. Guaifenesin is an antitussive medication. This medication will not affect fluid balance.
3. The client is not processing the amount of fluid received via the oral or parenteral route. The nurse should request the HCP to change the fluid to a saline lock. Cor pulmonale is heart failure resulting from increased pressure in the lungs from COPD.
4. The nurse should take action to prevent further fluid overload.

**TEST-TAKING HINT:** The test taker should recognize an imbalance between the intake and output numbers and make a decision based on this fact.

116. Correct answers are 1, 2, 3, 4, and 5.
1. The $Pao_2$ level is very low; this client should be placed on a ventilator. The nurse should provide as much oxygen as possible until this can be done.
2. The RRT is called when an individual identifies a situation that requires

immediate intervention to prevent the client from going into an arrest situation.
3. Elevating the HOB allows for better lung expansion.
4. The nurse should not leave the client but should direct care from the bedside.
5. The HCP should be notified of the client's status.

**TEST-TAKING HINT:** The keys to answering this question are knowledge of normal values. The nurse makes decisions based on deviations from normal.

117. 1. The nurse should set the flow rate for 2 LPM (20%) because of the diagnosis of COPD. The client diagnosed with COPD develops carbon dioxide narcosis, which does not allow the brain to recognize high levels of carbon dioxide as a stimulus to breathe. The only remaining stimulus for breathing is oxygen hunger. Giving high levels of oxygen removes the client's stimulus to breathe.
2. The client should receive 2 LPM only.
3. The client should receive 2 LPM only.
4. The client should receive 2 LPM only.

**TEST-TAKING HINT:** The test taker must recognize safety precautions in relation to therapies that are being administered. Knowledge of basic pathophysiology of the brain's respiratory center will help the test taker choose the correct option.

118. 1. The body has compensated for the abnormally high level of carbon dioxide (acid) in the blood by holding on to the base ($Hco_3$), and the pH is within the normal range. This is an expected blood gas for the client diagnosed with COPD.
2. This pulse oximetry reading indicates arterial blood oxygen of less than 60. The client should be seen immediately to prevent respiratory failure.
3. This client is receiving blood to correct the lower levels of H&H.
4. A BNP of less than 100 is considered within normal limits. A BNP of 100 would not be a concern to report for a client diagnosed with stage 4 heart failure.

**TEST-TAKING HINT:** The test taker must be aware of critical laboratory and respiratory results to determine the correct answer to this question.

119. 1. Chest tubes are painful; splinting the insertion site can help to lessen the pain.
     2. Coughing indicates the ability to move air in and out of the lungs. This is not a critical issue.
     3. This client, lacking oxygenation at rest, blueness around the mouth, and difficulty in arousing, indicates a decrease in neurological functioning.
     4. Dyspnea on exertion is not a critical issue.

**TEST-TAKING HINT:** The key to answering this question is reading every word in the stem. "Critical" should indicate that a non-life-threatening issue cannot be the correct answer.

120. 1. The only clinical manifestation of pneumonia in older clients may be confusion caused by a lack of oxygen to the brain. The nurse should assess the client for a respiratory cause for the new onset of confusion and wandering.
     2. The nurse should assist the resident in returning to the room so an assessment can be performed but should not tell him to return to the room without the nurse.
     3. This may be done, but the assessment is the first priority.
     4. Pushing fluids may help to liquefy secretions, but the assessment is first.

**TEST-TAKING HINT:** The test taker should use the nursing process to answer this first question. Assess is the first step of the nursing process.

# RESPIRATORY DISORDERS COMPREHENSIVE EXAMINATION

1. Which diagnostic test should the nurse anticipate the HCP ordering to **rule out** the diagnosis of asthma in clients diagnosed with COPD?
   1. A bronchoscopy.
   2. An immunoglobulin E.
   3. An arterial blood gas.
   4. A bronchodilator reversibility test.

2. Which statement indicates the client diagnosed with asthma **needs more teaching** concerning the medication regimen?
   1. "I will take montelukast every day to prevent allergic asthma attacks."
   2. "I need to use my cromolyn inhaler 15 minutes before I begin my exercise."
   3. "I need to take oral glucocorticoids every day to prevent my asthma attacks."
   4. "If I have an asthma attack, I need to use my albuterol inhaler."

3. Which intervention should the emergency department nurse implement **first** for the client admitted for an acute asthma attack?
   1. Administer glucocorticoids intravenously.
   2. Administer oxygen 5 L per nasal cannula.
   3. Establish and maintain a 20-gauge saline lock.
   4. Assess breath sounds every 15 minutes.

4. Which isolation procedure should be instituted for the client admitted for possible novel coronavirus (COVID-19)?
   1. Airborne isolation.
   2. Droplet isolation.
   3. Reverse isolation.
   4. Strict isolation.

5. The client is admitted with a diagnosis of possible COVID-19. Which information is **most important** for the nurse to ask related to this diagnosis?
   1. Current prescription and over-the-counter medication use.
   2. Dates of and any complications associated with recent immunizations.
   3. Any problems with recent or past use of blood or blood products.
   4. Recent travel to an area with a high rate of COVID-19 transmission.

6. The nurse suspects the client admitted with a near-drowning is developing ARDS. Which data **support** the nurse's suspicion?
   1. The client's arterial blood gases are within normal limits.
   2. The client appears anxious, has dyspnea, and is tachypneic.

3. The client has intercostal retractions and is using accessory muscles.
4. The client's bilateral lung sounds have crackles and rhonchi.

7. Which client's ABG results support the diagnosis of ARDS after the client has received $O_2$ at 10 LPM?

   1.

   | Arterial Blood Gas | Client Values | Normal Values |
   |---|---|---|
   | pH | 7.38 | 7.35–7.45 |
   | $Pco_2$ | 44 | 35–45 mmHg |
   | $Hco_3$ | 24 | 22–26 mEq/L |
   | $Pao_2$ | 94 | 80–95 mmHg |

   2.

   | Arterial Blood Gas | Client Values | Normal Values |
   |---|---|---|
   | pH | 7.46 | 7.35–7.45 |
   | $Pco_2$ | 34 | 35–45 mmHg |
   | $Hco_3$ | 22 | 22–26 mEq/L |
   | $Pao_2$ | 82 | 80–95 mmHg |

   3.

   | Arterial Blood Gas | Client Values | Normal Values |
   |---|---|---|
   | pH | 7.48 | 7.35–7.45 |
   | $Pco_2$ | 30 | 35–45 mmHg |
   | $Hco_3$ | 26 | 22–26 mEq/L |
   | $Pao_2$ | 59 | 80–95 mmHg |

   4.

   | Arterial Blood Gas | Client Values | Normal Values |
   |---|---|---|
   | pH | 7.33 | 7.35–7.45 |
   | $Pco_2$ | 44 | 35–45 mmHg |
   | $Hco_3$ | 20 | 22–26 mEq/L |
   | $Pao_2$ | 94 | 80–95 mmHg |

8. The nurse is planning the activities for the client diagnosed with asbestosis. Which activity should the nurse schedule at 0900 if breakfast is served at 0800?
   1. Assist with the client's bath and linen change.
   2. Administer an inhalation bronchodilator treatment.
   3. Provide the client with a 1-hour rest period.
   4. Have respiratory therapy perform chest physiotherapy.

9. Which datum requires **immediate intervention** by the nurse for the client diagnosed with asbestosis?
   1. The client develops an $S_3$ heart sound.
   2. The client has clubbing of the fingers.
   3. The client is fatigued in the afternoon.
   4. The client has basilar crackles in all lobes.

10. Which clinical manifestation would the nurse assess in the client newly diagnosed with lung cancer? **Select all that apply.**
    1. Dysphagia.
    2. Foul-smelling breath.
    3. Hoarseness.
    4. Weight loss.
    5. Hemoptysis.

11. Which **priority** intervention should the nurse implement for the client diagnosed with coal workers' pneumoconiosis?
    1. Monitor the client's intake and output.
    2. Assess for black-streaked sputum.
    3. Monitor the white blood cell count daily.
    4. Assess the client's activity level every shift.

12. Which statement indicates the client with a total laryngectomy **requires more teaching** concerning the care of the tracheostomy?
    1. "I must avoid hair spray and powders."
    2. "I should take a shower instead of a tub bath."
    3. "I will need to cleanse around the stoma daily."
    4. "I can use an electric larynx to speak."

13. The occupational nurse for a mining company is planning a class on the risks of working with toxic substances to comply with the "Right to Know" law. Which information should the nurse include in the presentation? **Select all that apply.**
    1. Cigarette smokers have a drastically increased risk of lung cancer.
    2. Floors need to be clean, and dust needs to be wet to prevent the transfer of dust.
    3. The air needs to be monitored at specific times to evaluate for exposure.
    4. Surface areas need to be painted every year to prevent the accumulation of dust.
    5. Employees should wear the appropriate personal protective equipment.

14. Which data are significant when assessing a client diagnosed for possible Legionnaires' disease?
    1. The number of cigarettes smoked a day and the age when they started smoking.
    2. Symptoms of aching muscles, high fever, malaise, and coughing.
    3. Exposure to a saprophytic water bacterium transmitted into the air.
    4. Decreased bilateral lung sounds in the lower lobes.

15. Which assessment data indicate to the nurse the client diagnosed with Legionnaires' disease is experiencing a complication?
    1. The client has an elevated body temperature.
    2. The client has less than 30 mL urine output an hour.
    3. The client has a decrease in body aches.
    4. The client has an elevated white blood cell count.

16. Which statement indicates to the nurse the client diagnosed with sleep apnea **needs further** teaching?
    1. "If I lose weight I may not need treatment for sleep apnea."
    2. "The CPAP machine holds my airway open with pressure."
    3. "The CPAP will help me stay awake during the day while I am at work."
    4. "It is all right to have a couple of beers because I have this CPAP machine."

17. The nurse is preparing to administer influenza vaccines to a group of clients in a long-term care facility. Which client should the nurse **question** receiving the vaccine?
    1. The client diagnosed with congestive heart failure.
    2. The client diagnosed with a documented allergy to eggs.
    3. The client previously diagnosed with an anaphylactic reaction to penicillin.
    4. The client with elevated blood pressure and pulse.

18. The nurse is preparing the client for a polysomnography to confirm sleep apnea. Which preprocedure instruction should the nurse include?
    1. The client should not eat or drink past midnight.
    2. The client will receive a sedative for relaxation.
    3. The client will sleep in a laboratory for evaluation.
    4. The client will wear a monitor at home for this test.

19. The client in the intensive care unit diagnosed with end-stage COPD has a Swan-Ganz mean pulmonary artery pressure of 35 mmHg. Which HCP order would the nurse **question?**
    1. Administer intravenous fluids of normal saline at 125 mL/hr.
    2. Provide supplemental oxygen per nasal cannula at 2 L/min.
    3. Continuous telemetry monitoring with strips every 4 hours.
    4. Administer a loop diuretic intravenously every 6 hours.

20. The RN and a UAP are caring for a client diagnosed with emphysema. Which nursing tasks could be delegated to the UAP to improve gas exchange? **Select all that apply.**
    1. Keep the head of the bed elevated.
    2. Encourage deep breathing exercises.
    3. Record pulse oximeter reading.
    4. Assess the level of consciousness.
    5. Auscultate breath sounds.

21. The nurse is preparing the plan of care for the client after a talc pleurodesis. Which **collaborative** intervention should the nurse include?
    1. Monitor the amount and color of drainage from the chest tube.
    2. Perform a complete respiratory assessment every 2 hours.
    3. Administer morphine sulfate intravenously.
    4. Keep a sterile dressing and bottle of sterile normal saline at the bedside.

22. Which problem is **appropriate** for the nurse to identify for the client 1 day postoperative thoracotomy?
    1. Alteration in comfort.
    2. Altered level of consciousness.
    3. Alteration in elimination pattern.
    4. Knowledge deficit.

23. The nurse is caring for the client diagnosed with bacterial pneumonia. Which **priority** intervention should the nurse implement?
    1. Assess respiratory rate and depth.
    2. Provide for an adequate rest period.
    3. Administer oxygen as prescribed.
    4. Teach slow abdominal breathing.

24. The nurse is caring for a client diagnosed with pneumonia, having shortness of breath, and difficulty breathing. Which intervention should the nurse implement **first?**
    1. Take the client's vital signs.
    2. Check the client's pulse oximeter reading.
    3. Administer oxygen via a nasal cannula.
    4. Notify the respiratory therapist STAT.

25. The postanesthesia care nurse is caring for the client diagnosed with lung cancer, experiencing frequent PVCs after a thoracotomy. Which intervention should the nurse implement **first?**
    1. Request STAT arterial blood gases.
    2. Administer lidocaine intravenous push.
    3. Assess for possible causes.
    4. Request a STAT electrocardiogram.

26. The nurse is caring for the postoperative client diagnosed with lung cancer recovering from a thoracotomy. Which data require **immediate intervention** by the nurse?
    1. The client refuses to perform shoulder exercises.
    2. The client reports a sore throat and is hoarse.
    3. The client has crackles that clear with a cough.
    4. The client is coughing up frothy pink sputum.

27. Which information should the nurse include in the teaching plan for the mother of a child diagnosed with cystic fibrosis (CF)? **Select all that apply.**
    1. Perform postural drainage and percussion every 4 hours.
    2. Modify activities to accommodate daily physiotherapy.
    3. Increase fluid intake to 1 L daily to thin secretions.
    4. Recognize and report clinical manifestations of respiratory infections.
    5. Avoid anyone suspected of having an upper respiratory infection.

28. Which clinical manifestation indicates to the nurse the child has cystic fibrosis?
    1. Wheezing with a productive cough.
    2. Excessive salty sweat secretions.
    3. Multiple vitamin deficiencies.
    4. Clubbing of all fingers.

29. The client is diagnosed with bronchiolitis obliterans. Which data indicate the glucocorticoid therapy is **effective?**
    1. The client has an elevation in the blood glucose.
    2. The client has a decrease in sputum production.
    3. The client has an increase in the temperature.
    4. The client has a decrease in wheezing.

30. The nurse is discharging the client diagnosed with bronchiolitis obliterans. Which **priority** intervention should the nurse include?
    1. Refer the client to the American Lung Association.
    2. Notify the physical therapy department to arrange for activity training.
    3. Arrange for oxygen therapy to be used at home.
    4. Discuss advance directives with the client.

31. The client admitted for recurrent aspiration pneumonia is at risk for bronchiectasis. Which intervention should the nurse anticipate the HCP to order?
    1. Administer intravenous antibiotics for 7 days.
    2. Insert a subclavian line and initiate total parenteral nutrition.
    3. Provide a low-calorie and low-sodium restricted diet.
    4. Encourage the client to turn, cough, and deep breathe frequently.

32. Which **collaborative** intervention should the nurse implement when caring for the client diagnosed with bronchiectasis?
    1. Prepare the client for an emergency tracheostomy.
    2. Discuss postoperative teaching for a lobectomy.
    3. Administer bronchodilators with postural drainage.
    4. Obtain informed consent form for chest tube insertion.

33. The nurse is discussing the results of a tuberculosis skin test. Which explanation should the nurse provide the client?
    1. A red area is a positive reading that means the client has tuberculosis.
    2. The skin test is the only procedure needed to diagnose tuberculosis.
    3. A positive reading means exposure to the tuberculosis bacilli.
    4. Do not get another skin test for 1 year if the skin test is positive.

34. The client diagnosed with tuberculosis has been treated with antitubercular medications for 6 weeks. Which data would indicate the medications have been **effective**?
    1. A decrease in the WBCs in the sputum.
    2. The client's symptoms are improving.
    3. No change in the chest x-ray.
    4. The skin test is now negative.

35. The nurse is caring for a client on a ventilator and the alarm goes off. Which action should the nurse implement **first**?
    1. Notify the respiratory therapist immediately.
    2. Check the ventilator to determine the cause.
    3. Elevate the head of the client's bed.
    4. Assess the client's oxygen saturation.

36. The client diagnosed with DVT suddenly reports severe chest pain and a feeling of impending doom. Which **complication** should the nurse suspect the client has experienced?
    1. Myocardial infarction.
    2. Pneumonia.
    3. Pulmonary embolus.
    4. Pneumothorax.

37. The nurse is preparing to administer warfarin to a client diagnosed with a PE. Which laboratory data would cause the nurse to **question** administering the medication?

| Laboratory Test | Client Results | Normal Values |
|---|---|---|
| PT | 22 | 10–13 sec |
| aPTT | 38 | 25–35 sec |
| INR | 5 | 0.9–1.1 w/o anti-coagulation therapy 2–3 with therapy 2.5–3.5 if the client has a mechanical heart valve |
| ESR | 10 | Adult < 50 yr: Male: 0–15 mm/hr Female: 0–25 mm/hr Adult ≥ 50 yr: Male: 0–20 mm/hr Female: 0–30 mm/hr |

1. The client's activated partial thromboplastin time (aPTT).
2. The client's international normalized ratio (INR).
3. The client's prothrombin time (PT).
4. The client's erythrocyte sedimentation rate (ESR).

38. The nurse is caring for a client diagnosed with a pneumothorax and chest tubes inserted 4 hours ago. There is no fluctuating (tidaling) in the water-seal compartment of the closed chest drainage system. Which action should the nurse implement **first**?
    1. Milk the chest tube.
    2. Check the tubing for kinks.
    3. Instruct the client to cough.
    4. Assess the insertion site.

39. The HCP has ordered a continuous intravenous infusion of aminophylline. The client weighs 165 pounds. The infusion order is 0.3 mg/kg/hr. The bag is mixed with 500 mg of aminophylline in 250 mL of $D_5W$. At which rate should the nurse set the pump?

    [                    ]

40. The client diagnosed with a cold is taking an antihistamine. Which statement indicates to the nurse the client **needs more teaching** concerning the medication?
    1. "If my mouth gets dry I will suck on hard candy."
    2. "I will not drink beer or any type of alcohol."
    3. "I need to be careful when I drive my car."
    4. "This medication will make me sleepy."

41. The client diagnosed with a cold asks the nurse, "Is it all right to take echinacea for my cold?" Which statement is the nurse's **best response**?
    1. "You should discuss that with your health-care provider."
    2. "No, you should not take any type of herbal medicine."
    3. "Yes, but do not take it for more than 3 days."
    4. "Echinacea may help with the symptoms of your cold."

42. Which intervention should the nurse implement for the client experiencing bronchospasms?
    1. Administer intravenous epinephrine.
    2. Administer albuterol via nebulizer.
    3. Request a STAT portable CXR at the bedside.
    4. Insert a small nasal trumpet in the right nostril.

43. The nurse is caring for an anxious female client with a respiratory rate of 40, and who is reporting her fingers tingling and her lips feeling numb. Which intervention should the nurse implement **first**?
    1. Have the client take slow, deep breaths.
    2. Instruct her to put her head between her legs.
    3. Determine why she is feeling so anxious.
    4. Administer alprazolam.

44. The client diagnosed with pneumonia has the following ABGs. Which intervention should the nurse implement?

    | Arterial Blood Gas | Client | Normal Values |
    | --- | --- | --- |
    | pH | 7.33 | 7.35–7.45 |
    | Pco$_2$ | 47 | 35–45 mmHg |
    | Hco$_3$ | 25 | 22–26 mEq/L |
    | Pao$_2$ | 94 | 80–95 mmHg |

    1. Administer sodium bicarbonate.
    2. Administer oxygen via nasal cannula.
    3. Have the client cough and deep breathe.
    4. Instruct the client to breathe into a paper bag.

45. The nurse is assessing the client diagnosed with a lung abscess. Which information **supports** the diagnosis of lung abscess?
    1. Tympanic sounds elicited by percussion over the site.
    2. Inspiratory and expiratory wheezes heard over the upper lobes.
    3. Decreased breath sounds with a pleural friction rub.
    4. Asymmetric movement of the chest wall with inspiration.

46. The public health department nurse is caring for the client diagnosed with active tuberculosis placed on directly observed therapy (DOT). Which statement **best describes** this therapy?
    1. The nurse accounts for all medications administered to the client.
    2. The nurse must complete federal, state, and local forms for this client.
    3. The nurse must report the client to the Centers for Disease Control.
    4. The nurse must watch the client take the medication daily.

47. Which intervention should the nurse implement **first** when caring for a client diagnosed with a respiratory disorder?
    1. Administer a respiratory treatment.
    2. Check the client's radial pulses daily.
    3. Monitor the client's vital signs daily.
    4. Assess the client's capillary refill time.

48. The nurse is preparing to hang the next bag of aminophylline for the client diagnosed with asthma. The current theophylline level is 18 mcg/mL. Which intervention should the nurse implement?
    1. Hang the next bag and continue the infusion.
    2. Do not hang the next bag and decrease the rate.
    3. Notify the HCP of the level.
    4. Confirm the current serum theophylline level.

49. Which intervention should the nurse implement **first** when administering the first dose of intravenous antibiotic to the client diagnosed with a respiratory infection?
    1. Monitor the client's current temperature.
    2. Monitor the client's white blood cells.
    3. Determine if a culture has been collected.
    4. Determine the compatibility of fluids.

50. Which nursing interventions should the nurse implement for the client diagnosed with a respiratory disorder? **Select all that apply.**
    1. Administer oxygen via a nasal cannula.
    2. Assess the client's lung sounds.
    3. Encourage the client to cough and deep breathe.
    4. Monitor the client's pulse oximeter reading.
    5. Increase the client's fluid intake.

51. The client in the intensive care unit (ICU) on a mechanical ventilator is bucking the ventilator, causing the alarms to sound, and is in respiratory distress. Which assessment data should the nurse obtain? **Rank in order of priority.**
    1. Assess the ventilator alarms.
    2. Assess the client's pulse oximetry reading.
    3. Assess the client's lung sounds.
    4. Assess for symmetry of the client's chest expansion.
    5. Assess the client's endotracheal tube for secretions.

**52.** The nurse is checking the vital signs flowsheet in the EHR at 0800 on a client diagnosed with pneumonia secondary to COPD who has received prednisone therapy for several years. Which flowsheet should the nurse expect to see?

1.

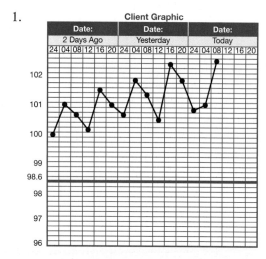

2.

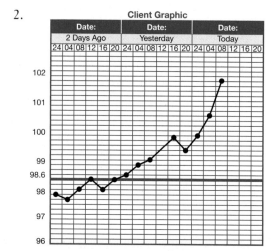

3.

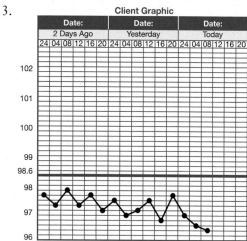

4.

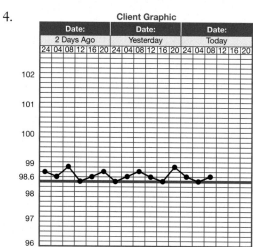

# RESPIRATORY DISORDERS COMPREHENSIVE EXAMINATION ANSWERS AND RATIONALES

1. 1. A bronchoscope visualizes the bronchial tree under sedation, but it does not confirm the diagnosis of asthma.
   2. An immunoglobulin E is a blood test for the presence of an antibody protein indicating allergic reactions.
   3. Arterial blood gases analyze levels providing information about the exchange of oxygen and carbon dioxide, but they are not diagnostic of asthma.
   4. **During a bronchodilator reversibility test, the client's positive response to a bronchodilator confirms the diagnosis of asthma. It is useful in clients diagnosed with COPD because airway reversibility is characteristic of asthma but not emphysema or bronchitis.**

2. 1. Leukotrienes, such as montelukast (Singulair), should be taken daily to prevent an asthma attack triggered by an allergen response.
   2. Cromolyn inhalers, such as Intal, are used to prevent exercise-induced asthma attacks.
   3. **Glucocorticoids are administered orally or intravenously during acute exacerbations of asthma, not on a daily basis because of the long-term complications of steroid therapy.**
   4. Albuterol inhaler, a beta$_2$ agonist, is used during attacks because of the fast action.

3. 1. Glucocorticoids are a treatment of choice, but they are not the first intervention.
   2. **The client is in distress, so the nurse must do something for the client's airway.**
   3. A saline lock is needed for intravenous fluids, but it is not the first intervention.
   4. Assessment is the first step of the nursing process, but in distress, do not assess.

4. 1. **The CDC recommends clients known or suspected of having COVID-19 be placed in airborne isolation when the infectious agent can remain in the air and be transported greater than 3 feet and recommends wearing specially fitted masks to prevent transmission (Centers for Disease Control and Prevention, 2020).**
   2. The client suspected of having COVID-19 should be placed in standard, contact, and airborne precautions.
   3. "Reverse isolation" is a term for using equipment to prevent the client from being exposed to organisms from other people.
   4. "Strict isolation" is an old term used to describe isolation to prevent transmission of organisms to other people. It is vague and not used today in infection control standards.

5. 1. This information is important during an admission interview but is not specific to COVID-19.
   2. The information would not be specific to the diagnosis of COVID-19.
   3. This would be important to ask before the administration of any blood products, but it is not specific for COVID-19.
   4. **Recent travel to an area with a high rate of COVID-19 transmission is a risk factor for contracting Novel coronavirus (CDC, 2020).**

6. 1. The client would have low arterial oxygen when developing ARDS.
   2. **Initial clinical manifestations of ARDS usually develop 24 to 48 hours after the initial insult leading to hypoxia and include anxiety, dyspnea, and tachypnea.**
   3. As ARDS progresses, the client has more difficulty breathing, resulting in intercostal retractions and the use of accessory muscles.
   4. Lungs are initially clear; crackles and rhonchi develop in later stages of ARDS.

7. 1. This ABG is within normal limits and would not be expected in a client diagnosed with ARDS.
   2. These ABG levels indicate respiratory alkalosis, but the oxygen level is within normal limits and would not be expected in a client diagnosed with ARDS.
   3. **ABGs initially show hypoxemia with a Pao$_2$ of less than 60 mmHg and respiratory alkalosis resulting from tachypnea in a client diagnosed with ARDS.**
   4. This ABG is metabolic acidosis and would not be expected in a client diagnosed with ARDS.

8. 1. Bathing is too strenuous an activity immediately after eating.
2. Inhalation bronchodilators should be administered 1 hour after meals. The nurse should realize the client will require 20 to 30 minutes to eat, and scheduling these activities at 0900 would not give the client sufficient time to digest the food or rest before the activity.
3. **Periods of rest should be alternated with periods of activity (American Lung Association, 2019).**
4. Chest physiotherapy should be performed at least 1 hour after meals. The nurse should realize the client will require 20 to 30 minutes to eat, and scheduling these activities at 0900 would not give the client sufficient time to digest the food or rest before the activity.

9. 1. The appearance of $S_3$ heart sounds indicates the client is developing heart failure, which is a medical emergency.
2. Clubbing of the fingers indicates the client has a chronic respiratory condition, but this would not require immediate intervention.
3. Fatigue is a common occurrence in clients diagnosed with respiratory conditions, such as asbestosis, as a result of the effort required to breathe.
4. Bibasilar crackles are common symptoms experienced by clients diagnosed with asbestosis and do not require immediate intervention. Bibasilar means basilar on both sides.

10. Correct answers are 3, 4, and 5.
1. Dysphagia is a late sign of lung cancer.
2. Foul-smelling breath is a late sign of lung cancer.
3. **Hoarseness is an early clinical manifestation of lung cancer.**
4. **Weight loss is a common sign of most types of cancers, including lung cancer.**
5. **Hemoptysis is coughing up blood and is an early sign of lung cancer.**

11. 1. Fluids should be encouraged to help to liquefy sputum; therefore, intake and output should be monitored, but this is not the priority intervention.
2. **Black-streaked sputum is a classic sign of coal workers' pneumoconiosis (black lung), and the sputum should be assessed for color and amount. Remember Maslow's hierarchy of needs when answering priority questions.**
3. The client's WBCs should be monitored to assess for infection, but it is not the priority and is not done daily.

4. Activity tolerance is important to assess for clients diagnosed with all respiratory diseases, but it is not the priority intervention.

12. 1. The client should not let any spray or powder enter the stoma because it goes directly into the lung.
2. **The client should not allow water to enter the stoma; therefore, the client should take a tub bath, not a shower.**
3. The stoma site should be cleaned to help prevent infection.
4. The client's vocal cords were removed; therefore, the client must use an alternate form of communication.

13. Correct answers are 1, 2, 3, and 5.
1. **Cigarette smokers working with toxic substances have an increased risk of lung cancer because many of the substances are carcinogenic.**
2. **When floors and surfaces are kept clean, toxic dust particles, such as asbestos and silica, are controlled, and this decreases exposure. Covering areas with water controls dust.**
3. **The quality of air is monitored to determine what toxic substances are present and in what amount. The information is then used in efforts to minimize the amount of exposure.**
4. Applying paint to a surface does not eliminate or minimize exposure and can trap more dust.
5. **Employees must wear protective coverings, goggles, and other equipment needed to eliminate exposure to toxic substances.**

14. 1. Smoking cigarettes is important to assess in any respiratory disease. Legionnaires' disease is contracted with a bacterium, not by smoking.
2. Aching muscles, high fever, malaise, and coughing are symptoms of most respiratory illnesses, including influenza and pneumonia, but these symptoms are not specific to Legionnaires' disease.
3. **Legionnaires' disease is caused by a saprophytic water bacterium that is transmitted through the air from places where these bacteria are found: rivers, lakes, evaporative condensers, respiratory apparatuses, or water distribution centers.**
4. Abnormal breath sounds can be heard in many respiratory illnesses.

**15.** 1. The temperature is elevated and does not indicate a complication.
2. **Multiple organ failure is a common complication of Legionnaires' disease. Renal failure should be suspected as a complication if the client does not have a urine output of 30 mL/hr.**
3. A decrease in body aches does not indicate a complication.
4. An elevation of WBCs is expected in a client diagnosed with Legionnaires' disease and is not a complication.

**16.** 1. The contributing factors to developing sleep apnea are obesity, smoking, drinking alcohol, and a short neck. In some situations, modifying lifestyle will improve sleep apnea.
2. Many clients need a continuous positive airway pressure (CPAP) machine, which continuously administers positive pressure to assist sleep during the night.
3. When clients have sleep apnea, the buildup of carbon dioxide causes the client to arouse constantly from sleep to breathe. This, in turn, causes the client to be sleepy during the day.
4. **Drinking alcohol before sleep sedates the client, causing the muscles to relax, which, in turn, causes an obstruction of the client's airway. Drinking alcohol should be avoided even if the client uses a CPAP machine.**

**17.** 1. There would be no reason to question administering a vaccine to a client diagnosed with heart failure.
2. **Clients allergic to egg protein may experience a significant hypersensitivity response after receiving the influenza vaccine.**
3. There would be no reason to question administering a vaccine to a client previously diagnosed with a reaction to penicillin.
4. There would be no reason to question administering a vaccine to a client with elevated blood pressure and pulse.

**18.** 1. Preparation for the polysomnography does not require the client to avoid having anything by mouth (NPO) after midnight.
2. The examination is a recording of the natural sleep of the client. No sedative is administered.
3. **The polysomnography is completed in a sleep laboratory to observe all the stages of sleep. Equipment is attached to the client to monitor the depth and stage of sleep and movement, respiratory effort, and oxygen saturation level during sleep.**
4. The client could perform this test at home, but the evaluation is not as reliable, and the visual observation is not included; therefore, this is not recommended.

**19.** 1. **Normal mean pulmonary artery pressure is about 15 mmHg, and an elevation indicates right ventricular heart failure or cor pulmonale, which is a comorbid condition of COPD. The nurse should question this order because the rate is too high.**
2. Supplemental oxygen should be administered at the lowest amount; therefore, this order should not be questioned.
3. Clients diagnosed with hypoxia and cor pulmonale are at risk for dysrhythmias, so monitoring the electrocardiogram (ECG) is an appropriate intervention.
4. Loop diuretics are administered to decrease the fluid and decrease the circulatory load on the right side of the heart; therefore, this order would not be questioned.

**20.** Correct answers are 1, 2, and 3.
1. **Keeping the head of the bed elevated maximizes lung excursion and improves gas exchange and can be delegated.**
2. **Encouraging breathing exercises can be delegated.**
3. **Recording pulse oximeter readings can be delegated. Evaluating is the responsibility of the nurse.**
4. Assessment cannot be delegated. Confusion is one of the first symptoms of hypoxia.
5. Auscultation is a technique of assessment and cannot be delegated.

**21.** 1. Monitoring the amount and color of drainage from the chest tube is an independent nursing intervention.
2. Respiratory assessment is an independent intervention.
3. **Administering morphine sulfate, an opioid analgesic, is a collaborative intervention because it requires an HCP's order.**
4. Keeping supplies at the bedside is an independent intervention the nurse may take in case the chest tube becomes dislodged.

**22.** 1. Pain and discomfort are major problems for clients after a thoracotomy because the chest wall has been opened and closed.
2. The client would be on a mechanical ventilator and have an adequate airway;

therefore, altered consciousness would not be an appropriate client problem.
3. Altered elimination problem is not specific for the client with a thoracotomy.
4. A knowledge-deficit problem is not an appropriate problem for the client 1 day postoperative thoracotomy because the client is on a ventilator.

23. 1. **The assessment of respiratory rate and depth is the priority intervention because tachypnea and dyspnea may be early indicators of respiratory compromise.**
2. Rest reduces metabolic demands, fatigue, and the work of breathing, which promotes a more effective breathing pattern, but it is not a priority over assessment.
3. Oxygen therapy increases the alveolar oxygen concentration, reducing hypoxia and anxiety, but it is not a priority over assessment in this situation.
4. This breathing pattern promotes lung expansion, but it is not a priority over assessment.

24. 1. Taking the client's vital signs will not help the client's shortness of breath and difficulty in breathing.
2. Checking the pulse oximeter reading will not help the client's shortness of breath and difficulty breathing.
3. **After elevating the head of the bed, the nurse should administer oxygen to the client in respiratory difficulty.**
4. Notifying the respiratory therapist will not help the client's shortness of breath and difficulty breathing.

25. 1. ABGs may show hypoxia, which is a cause of PVCs, but it is not the first intervention the nurse should implement.
2. Beta blockers are used to treat frequent PVCs, but it is not the first intervention. Other treatments include calcium channel blockers and ablation.
3. **The nurse should assess for possible causes of the PVCs; these causes may include hypoxia or hypokalemia.**
4. An ECG further evaluates the heart function, but it is not the first intervention.

26. 1. The client refusing to perform shoulder exercises is pertinent, but it does not require immediate intervention.
2. Sore throats and hoarseness are common postintubation and would not require immediate intervention.

3. Crackles that clear with coughing would not require immediate intervention.
4. **Pink frothy sputum indicates pulmonary edema and would require immediate intervention.**

27. **Correct answers are 1, 2, 4, and 5.**
1. **Clients and family members should be taught chest physiotherapy, including postural drainage, chest percussion, and vibration and breathing techniques to keep the lungs clear of the copious secretions.**
2. **Daily activities should be modified to accommodate the client's treatments.**
3. Clients should increase fluids up to 3,000 mL each day to thin secretions and ease expectoration.
4. **Clients should be taught the clinical manifestations of infections to report to the HCP.**
5. **Clients diagnosed with CF are susceptible to respiratory infections and should avoid anyone suspected of having an infection.**

28. 1. Wheezing and productive coughs are symptoms experienced by clients diagnosed with respiratory diseases, but they are not specific to CF.
2. **The excessive excretion of salt from the sweat glands is specific to CF. Repeated values greater than 60 mEq/L of sweat chloride is diagnostic for CF.**
3. Multiple vitamin deficiencies are experienced with some pulmonary diseases, but they are not specific to CF.
4. Clubbing of the fingers is an indicator of chronic hypoxia, but it is not specific to the diagnosis of CF.

29. 1. An elevation in the blood glucose level is a common side effect of corticosteroids and does not indicate the effectiveness of the treatment for bronchiolitis obliterans.
2. Bronchiolitis obliterans causes a dry cough, no sputum is produced.
3. An elevated temperature indicates the client is becoming worse; therefore, the medication is not effective.
4. **Treatment with corticosteroids decreases the shortness of breath, fatigue, and wheezing noted with bronchiolitis obliterans, which would indicate the medication is effective (National Center for Advancing Translational Sciences, n.d.).**

30. 1. The American Lung Association is an excellent resource for educational material, but it is not a priority intervention for the client.
    2. Physical therapy is an appropriate intervention, but it is not the priority intervention.
    3. **The client diagnosed with bronchiolitis obliterans will need long-term use of oxygen.**
    4. Advance directives are an important intervention but are not the priority intervention.

31. 1. **Antibiotics should be administered intravenously for 7 to 10 days. Bronchiectasis is an irreversible condition caused by repeated damage to the bronchial walls secondary to repeated aspiration of gastric contents and release of inflammatory mediators by the body to combat the foreign substances.**
    2. Total parenteral nutrition is not an expected treatment for a client diagnosed with bronchiectasis.
    3. Clients should have a high-calorie and high-protein diet as a result of the high expenditure of energy used to breathe and tissue healing.
    4. Turning, coughing, and deep breathing are appropriate independent nursing interventions but do not require an HCP's order.

32. 1. Medical treatment for bronchiectasis does not include a tracheostomy.
    2. Removing a lobe of the lung is not the expected medical treatment for a client diagnosed with bronchiectasis.
    3. **Administering bronchodilators is a collaborative intervention (requiring an order from an HCP) appropriate for this client.**
    4. The insertion of chest tubes is not an expected treatment for bronchiectasis.

33. 1. A red and raised area at the injection site indicates that the client has been exposed to tuberculosis bacilli, but it does not indicate active disease.
    2. The skin test indicates the client has been exposed to the tuberculosis bacilli, but further tests must be performed to confirm the diagnosis of tuberculosis.
    3. **A positive reading indicates the client has been exposed to the bacilli.**
    4. Once a positive reading occurs, then the client should never receive a Tb skin test again.

34. 1. Antitubercular medications target the tubercular bacilli, not WBCs.
    2. **As the bacilli are being destroyed, the client should begin to feel better and have fewer symptoms.**
    3. At 6 weeks, the chest x-ray may not have changed.
    4. The skin test will always be positive.

35. 1. The nurse needs to notify the respiratory therapist to check the ventilator, but it is not the first intervention.
    2. **The nurse must determine what is causing the alarm; a high or low alarm will make a difference in the nurse's next assessment or action.**
    3. Elevating the head of the bed will help lung expansion, but it is not the first intervention.
    4. The ventilator alarm indicates something is wrong, and the nurse must first determine if the problem is with the ventilator or the client.

36. 1. The nurse would not suspect a myocardial infarction for a client diagnosed with a DVT and sudden chest pain.
    2. These clinical manifestations should not make the nurse think the client has pneumonia.
    3. **Part of the clot in the deep veins of the legs dislodges and travels up the inferior vena cava, lodges in the pulmonary arterial system, and causes the chest pain; the client often has feelings of impending doom or death.**
    4. Chest pain is a sign of pneumothorax, but it is not a complication of DVT.

37. 1. The aPTT is not monitored to determine a therapeutic serum level for warfarin (Coumadin), an oral anticoagulant; normal aPTT is 25 to 35.
    2. **The INR therapeutic range is 2 to 3 for a client receiving warfarin (Coumadin), an oral anticoagulant. The INR may be allowed to go to 3.5 if the client has a mechanical cardiac valve, but nothing in the stem of the question indicates this.**
    3. The PT is monitored for oral anticoagulant therapy and should be 1.5 to 2 times the normal of 12; therefore, 22 is within therapeutic range and would not warrant the nurse questioning administering this medication.
    4. The ESR is not monitored for oral anticoagulant therapy.

38. 1. No fluctuation in the water-seal chamber 4 hours postinsertion indicates the tubing is blocked; the nurse should not milk the chest tube.
    2. **The nurse should implement the least invasive intervention first. The nurse should check to see if the tubing is kinked, causing a blockage between the pleural space and the water-seal bottle.**
    3. Coughing may help push a clot in the tubing into the drainage bottle, but the first intervention is to check and see if the client is lying on the tubing or the tube is kinked somewhere.
    4. The insertion site can be assessed, but it will not help determine why there is no fluctuation in the water-seal drainage compartment.

39. **11 mL/hr.**
    First, convert pounds to kilograms:

    165 pounds ÷ 2.2 = 75 kg

    Then, determine how many milligrams of aminophylline per hour should be administered:

    0.3 mg × 75 kg = 22.5 mg/hr

    Then, determine how much aminophylline is delivered per milliliter:

    500 mg ÷ 250 mL = 2 mg/1 mL

    If 2 mg/1 mL is delivered, then to deliver the prescribed 22.5 mg/hr, the rate must be set at:

    22.5 ÷ 2 = 11.25 mL/hr

    Less than 0.5 should be rounded down, 0.5 and above is rounded up.

40. 1. Antihistamines dry respiratory secretions through an anticholinergic effect; therefore, the client will have a dry mouth.
    2. Antihistamines cause drowsiness; therefore, the client should not drink any type of alcohol.
    3. **Antihistamines cause drowsiness, so the client should not drive or operate any type of machinery.**
    4. Antihistamines cause drowsiness; therefore, the client understands the teaching.

41. 1. The nurse can answer the client's questions concerning herbal medication. Passing the buck should be eliminated as a possible correct answer.
    2. The nurse should not be judgmental. If the client does not have comorbid conditions, is not taking other medications, or is not pregnant, herbal medications may be helpful in treating the common cold.
    3. Echinacea should not be taken for more than 2 weeks, not 3 days. Nothing cures the common cold; the cold must run its course.
    4. **Echinacea is an herb that may reduce the duration and symptoms of the common cold, but nothing cures the common cold. If the client does not have comorbid conditions, is not taking other medications, and is not pregnant, herbal medications may be helpful in treating the common cold.**

42. 1. Epinephrine, a bronchodilator, is administered intravenously during an arrest in a code situation, but it is not a treatment of choice for bronchospasms.
    2. **Albuterol, a bronchodilator, given via nebulizer, is administered to stop the bronchospasms. If the client continues to have the bronchospasms, intubation may be needed.**
    3. A STAT portable x-ray will be ordered, but the goal is to prevent respiratory arrest.
    4. Nasal trumpet airways would not be helpful in stopping the bronchospasm and respiratory arrest.

43. 1. **The client is hyperventilating and blowing off too much $CO_2$, which is why her fingers are tingling and her mouth is numb; she needs to retain $CO_2$ by taking slow, deep breaths.**
    2. Putting the head between the legs sometimes helps a client about to faint, but it is not the first intervention.
    3. The client is hyperventilating; determining why is not appropriate at this time.
    4. Medications such as alprazolam (Xanax), an antianxiety agent, take up to 30 minutes to 1 hour to work and are not the first intervention for the hyperventilating client.

44. 1. Sodium bicarbonate is administered for metabolic acidosis.
    2. The arterial oxygen level is within normal limits (80 to 100); therefore, the client does not need oxygen.
    3. **The client is retaining $CO_2$, which causes respiratory acidosis, and the nurse should help the client remove the $CO_2$ by instructing the client to cough and deep breathe.**
    4. Breathing into a paper bag is not recommended for clients diagnosed with respiratory acidosis.

45. 1. Dull sounds would be heard over the site of a lung abscess as a result of the solid mass.
    2. Crackles may be heard, but wheezes indicate a narrowing of airways, not exudates-filled airways.
    3. **Diminished or absent sounds are heard with intermittent pleural friction rubs. A lung abscess is the accumulation of pus in an area where pneumonia was present that becomes encapsulated and can extend to the bronchus or pleural space.**
    4. Even with a lung abscess, the chest should move symmetrically.

46. 1. Nurses are responsible for accounting for medications, but it is not the rationale for DOT.
    2. Nurses complete forms as required by all governmental agencies, but this is not the rationale for DOT.
    3. Documentation of events concerning the client's treatment is completed, but this is not the rationale for DOT.
    4. **To ensure compliance with all medications regimens, the health department has adapted a DOT where the nurse actually observes the client taking the medication every day.**

47. 1. The nurse should gather data before implementing an intervention.
    2. The radial pulse would indicate the cardiovascular status of the client, not the respiratory status, and the nurse should assess the apical pulse.
    3. Daily vital signs would not indicate the respiratory status of the client.
    4. **Assessing the client's capillary refill time has the highest priority for the nurse because it indicates the oxygenation of the client.**

48. 1. **The therapeutic level is 10 to 20 mcg/mL; therefore, the nurse should hang the bag of aminophylline, a bronchodilator, and continue the infusion to maintain the aminophylline level.**
    2. There is no reason not to hang the next bag of aminophylline.
    3. There is no need to notify the HCP for a level of 18 mcg/mL.
    4. There is no need for the nurse to confirm the laboratory results.

49. 1. The client's current temperature would not affect the administration of the antibiotic.
    2. The client's WBCs may be elevated because of the infection, but this would not affect administering the medication.
    3. **A culture needs to be collected before the first dose of antibiotics, or the culture and sensitivity will be skewed and the appropriate antibiotic needed to treat the respiratory infection may not be identified.**
    4. Compatibility of fluids should be assessed before administering each intravenous antibiotic, but when administering the first dose of an antibiotic, the nurse must check to make sure the sputum culture was obtained.

50. Correct answers are 1, 2, 3, 4, and 5.
    1. **A client diagnosed with a respiratory disorder may have decreased oxygen saturation; therefore, administering oxygen via a nasal cannula is appropriate.**
    2. **The client's lung sounds should be assessed to determine how much air is being exchanged in the lungs.**
    3. **Coughing and deep breathing will help the client expectorate sputum, thus clearing the bronchial tree.**
    4. **The pulse oximeter evaluates how much oxygen is reaching the periphery.**
    5. **Increasing fluids will help thin secretions, making them easier to expectorate.**

51. Correct order is 5, 2, 3, 4, 1.
    5. **The most common cause of bucking the ventilator is obstructed airway, which could be secondary to secretions in the airway, so assessing the client would be most appropriate.**
    2. **Clients in the ICU are constantly monitored by pulse oximetry; therefore, the nurse should determine if the client has decreased oxygen saturation, and if so, the nurse should start to "bag" the client. The client is in respiratory distress.**
    3. **The nurse should assess the client's lung fields to determine if any air movement is occurring because the client is in respiratory distress.**
    4. **A complication of mechanical ventilation is a pneumothorax, and the nurse should assess for this because the client is in respiratory distress.**
    1. **The machine is alerting the nurse there is a problem with the client; because the client is in respiratory distress, the client should be assessed first. If the client were not in distress, then the nurse should assess the machine first to determine which alarm is sounding.**

**52.** 1. This client has an immune system that is responding to an infection, not one suppressed by steroids.
2. This client's graphic indicates that the client was admitted without an infection and now has developed one, and the immune system is responding.
3. This client's pattern of temperatures does not indicate an infection exists.
4. **The client diagnosed with COPD on long-term prednisone therapy, a** glucocorticoid steroid, has a suppressed immune system. Temperatures are in the normal range because steroids mask the symptoms of infection by suppressing the immune system. The only common symptoms would be rusty-colored sputum or a change in sputum color and confusion.

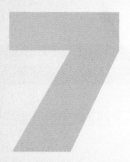

# Gastrointestinal Disorders

*Science is knowledge; wisdom is organized life.*

—Immanuel Kant

The many organs making up the gastrointestinal system—the mouth, esophagus, stomach, upper and lower intestine, and related organs—are subject to many disorders and diseases. Some are relatively minor, such as temporary constipation or a short bout of diarrhea and gastroenteritis. Others, such as diverticulosis and inflammatory bowel disease, may be chronic, requiring the client to follow a specific diet and other lifestyle modifications. Some chronic diseases, including gastroesophageal reflux, may eventually lead to life-threatening problems such as esophageal cancer. Still, other diseases affect the gastrointestinal tract. One—colon cancer—is one of the most common cancers in the United States. In addition, eating disorders rooted in psychological problems can be serious if not addressed promptly and effectively. Because gastrointestinal diseases and disorders are so common, the nurse must be aware of the clinical manifestations of each, what is considered normal or abnormal for the disease process, and how the specific problem is treated.

## KEYWORDS

Asterixis
Borborygmus
Caput medusae
Cathartic
Cruciferous
Dyspepsia
Dysphagia
Eructation
Esophagogastroduodenoscopy
Evisceration
Exacerbation
Feces
Hematemesis
Hypoalbuminemia

Jaundice
Lower esophageal sphincter
Melena
Nosocomial
Odynophagia
Oligomenorrhea
Peritonitis
Pruritus
Pyrosis
Sedentary
Steatorrhea
Tenesmus
Water brash

# PRACTICE QUESTIONS

## Gastroesophageal Reflux (GERD)

1. The male client tells the nurse he has been experiencing "heartburn" at night that awakens him. Which assessment question should the nurse ask?
   1. "How much weight have you gained recently?"
   2. "What have you done to alleviate the heartburn?"
   3. "Do you consume many milk and dairy products?"
   4. "Have you been around anyone with a stomach virus?"

2. The nurse caring for a client diagnosed with GERD writes the client problem of "behavior modification." Which intervention should be included for this problem?
   1. Teach the client to sleep with a wedge pillow under the head.
   2. Encourage the client to decrease the amount of smoking.
   3. Instruct the client to take over-the-counter medication for relief of pain.
   4. Discuss the need to attend Alcoholics Anonymous to quit drinking.

3. The nurse is preparing a client diagnosed with GERD for discharge following an esophagogastroduodenoscopy (EGD). Which statement indicates the client **understands** the discharge instructions?
   1. "I should not eat for at least 1 day following this procedure."
   2. "I can lie down whenever I want after a meal. It won't make a difference."
   3. "The stomach contents won't bother my esophagus but will make me nauseous."
   4. "I should avoid orange juice and eating tomatoes after this procedure."

4. The nurse is planning the care of a client diagnosed with lower esophageal sphincter dysfunction. Which dietary modifications should be included in the plan of care? **Select all that apply.**
   1. Allow any of the client's favorite foods as long as the amount is limited.
   2. Have the client perform eructation exercises several times a day.
   3. Eat four to six small meals a day and limit fluids during mealtimes.
   4. Encourage the client to consume a glass of red wine with one meal a day.
   5. Maintain an ideal body weight with a healthy diet and exercise.

5. The nurse is caring for a client diagnosed with GERD. Which nursing interventions should be implemented?
   1. Place the client prone in bed and administer nonsteroidal anti-inflammatory medications.
   2. Have the client remain upright at all times and walk for 30 minutes three times a week.
   3. Instruct the client to maintain a supine position and take antacids before meals.
   4. Elevate the head of the bed (HOB) 30 degrees and discuss lifestyle modifications with the client.

6. The nurse is caring for an adult client diagnosed with GERD. Which condition is the **most** common comorbid disease associated with GERD?
   1. Adult-onset asthma.
   2. Pancreatitis.
   3. Peptic ulcer disease.
   4. Increased gastric emptying.

7. The nurse is administering morning medications at 0730. Which medication should have **priority**?
   1. A proton pump inhibitor.
   2. A nonnarcotic analgesic.
   3. A histamine receptor antagonist.
   4. A mucosal barrier agent.

8. The nurse is preparing a client diagnosed with GERD for surgery. Which information **warrants notifying** the health-care provider (HCP)?
   1. The client's esophageal pH test was positive.
   2. The client's abdominal x-ray shows a hiatal hernia.
   3. The client's WBC count is 14,000/mm³.
   4. The client's hemoglobin is 13.8 g/dL.

9. The RN charge nurse is making assignments. Staffing includes a registered nurse with 5 years of medical-surgical experience, a newly graduated registered nurse, and two unlicensed assistive personnel (UAPs). Which client should be assigned to the **most experienced nurse**?
   1. The 39-year-old client diagnosed with lower esophageal dysfunction reporting pyrosis.
   2. The 54-year-old client diagnosed with Barrett's esophagus scheduled to have an endoscopy this morning.
   3. The 46-year-old client diagnosed with gastroesophageal reflux disease wheezing in all five lobes.
   4. The 68-year-old client 3 days postoperative for hiatal hernia needs to be ambulated four times today.

10. Which statement made by the client indicates to the nurse the client may be experiencing GERD?
    1. "My chest hurts when I walk up the stairs in my home."
    2. "I take antacid tablets with me wherever I go."
    3. "My spouse tells me I snore very loudly at night."
    4. "I drink six to seven soft drinks every day."

11. The nurse is performing an admission assessment on a client diagnosed with GERD. Which clinical manifestations would indicate GERD?
    1. Pyrosis, water brash, and eructation.
    2. Weight loss, dysarthria, and diarrhea.
    3. Decreased abdominal fat, proteinuria, and constipation.
    4. Mid-epigastric pain, positive *Helicobacter pylori* test, and melena.

12. Which disease is the client diagnosed with GERD at **greater risk** for developing?
    1. Hiatal hernia.
    2. Gastroenteritis.
    3. Esophageal cancer.
    4. Gastric cancer.

## Inflammatory Bowel Disease (IBD)

13. Which clinical manifestation should the nurse expect to find in a client diagnosed with ulcerative colitis?
    1. Twenty bloody stools a day.
    2. Oral temperature of 102°F.
    3. Hard, rigid abdomen.
    4. Urinary stress incontinence.

14. The client diagnosed with type 2 diabetes is prescribed prednisone for an acute exacerbation of IBD. Which intervention should the nurse discuss with the client?
    1. Take this medication on an empty stomach.
    2. Notify the HCP if experiencing a moon face.
    3. Take the steroid medication as prescribed.
    4. Notify the HCP if the blood glucose is over 160.

15. The client diagnosed with IBD has a serum potassium level of 3.4 mEq/L. Which action should the nurse implement **first?**
    1. Notify the health-care provider.
    2. Assess the client for muscle weakness.
    3. Request telemetry for the client.
    4. Prepare to administer potassium IV.

16. The client is diagnosed with an acute exacerbation of ulcerative colitis. Which intervention should the nurse implement?
    1. Provide a low-residue diet.
    2. Rest the client's bowel.
    3. Assess vital signs daily.
    4. Administer antacids orally.

17. The client diagnosed with IBD is prescribed total parenteral nutrition (TPN). Which intervention should the nurse implement?
    1. Check the client's glucose level.
    2. Administer an oral hypoglycemic.
    3. Assess the peripheral intravenous site.
    4. Monitor the client's oral food intake.

18. The client is diagnosed with an acute exacerbation of IBD. Which **priority** intervention should the nurse implement?
    1. Weigh the client daily and document in the client's EHR.
    2. Teach coping strategies such as dietary modifications.
    3. Record the frequency, amount, and color of stools.
    4. Monitor the client's oral fluid intake every shift.

19. The client diagnosed with Crohn's disease is crying and tells the nurse, "I can't take it anymore. I never know when I will get sick and end up here in the hospital." Which statement is the nurse's **best response**?
    1. "I understand how frustrating this must be for you."
    2. "You must keep thinking about the good things in your life."
    3. "I can see you are very upset. I'll sit down, and we can talk."
    4. "Are you contemplating committing suicide?"

20. The client diagnosed with ulcerative colitis has an ileostomy. Which statement indicates the client **needs more** teaching concerning the ileostomy?
    1. "My stoma should be pink and moist."
    2. "I will irrigate my ileostomy every morning."
    3. "If I get a red, bumpy, itchy rash, I will call my HCP."
    4. "I will change my pouch if it starts leaking."

21. The client diagnosed with IBD is prescribed sulfasalazine. Which statement **best** describes the rationale for administering this medication?
    1. It is administered rectally to help decrease colon inflammation.
    2. This medication slows gastrointestinal (GI) motility and reduces diarrhea.
    3. This medication kills the bacteria causing the exacerbation.
    4. It acts topically on the colon mucosa to decrease inflammation.

22. The client is diagnosed with Crohn's disease. Which statement by the client **supports** this diagnosis?
    1. "My pain is on the right lower side of my abdomen."
    2. "I have bright red blood in my stool all the time."
    3. "I have episodes of diarrhea and constipation."
    4. "My abdomen is hard and rigid, and I have a fever."

23. The client diagnosed with ulcerative colitis is prescribed a low-residue diet during exacerbations. Which meal selection indicates the client **understands** the diet teaching?
    1. Grilled hamburger on a wheat bun and fried potatoes.
    2. A chicken salad sandwich and lettuce and tomato salad.
    3. Roast pork, white rice, and plain custard.
    4. Fried fish, whole grain pasta, and fruit salad.

24. The client diagnosed with ulcerative colitis is scheduled for a continent ileostomy. The nurse is aware the client's stoma will be located in which area of the abdomen?

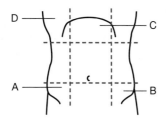

    1. A
    2. B
    3. C
    4. D

## Peptic Ulcer Disease

25. Which assessment data support the client's diagnosis of gastric ulcer to the nurse?
    1. Presence of blood in the client's stool for the past month.
    2. Reports of a burning sensation moving like a wave.
    3. Sharp pain in the upper abdomen after eating a heavy meal.
    4. Reports of epigastric pain shortly after ingesting food.

26. The nurse is caring for a client diagnosed with rule out peptic ulcer disease. Which test **confirms** this diagnosis?
    1. Esophagogastroduodenoscopy (EGD).
    2. Magnetic resonance imaging (MRI).
    3. Occult blood test.
    4. Gastric acid stimulation test.

27. Which specific data should the nurse obtain from the client suspected of having peptic ulcer disease?
    1. History of side effects experienced from all medications.
    2. Use of NSAIDs.
    3. Any known allergies to drugs and environmental factors.
    4. Medical histories of at least three generations.

28. Which physical examination should the nurse implement **first** when assessing the client diagnosed with peptic ulcer disease?
    1. Auscultate bowel sounds in all four quadrants.
    2. Palpate the abdominal area for tenderness.
    3. Percuss the abdominal borders to identify organs.
    4. Assess the tender area progressing to nontender.

29. Which problems should the nurse include in the plan of care for the client diagnosed with peptic ulcer disease to observe for physiological complications?
    1. Alteration in bowel elimination patterns.
    2. Knowledge deficit in the causes of ulcers.
    3. Inability to cope with changing family roles.
    4. Potential for alteration in gastric emptying.

30. The nurse is caring for a client diagnosed with hemorrhaging duodenal ulcer. Which collaborative interventions should the nurse implement? **Select all that apply.**
    1. Perform a complete pain assessment.
    2. Assess the client's vital signs frequently.
    3. Administer a proton pump inhibitor intravenously.
    4. Obtain permission and administer blood products.
    5. Monitor the intake of a soft, bland diet.

31. Which expected outcome should the nurse include for a client diagnosed with peptic ulcer disease?
    1. The client's pain is controlled with the use of NSAIDs.
    2. The client maintains lifestyle modifications.
    3. The client has no clinical manifestations of hemoptysis.
    4. The client takes antacids with each meal.

32. The nurse has been assigned to care for a client diagnosed with peptic ulcer disease. Which assessment data **require further** intervention?
    1. Bowel sounds auscultated 15 times in 1 minute.
    2. Belching after eating a heavy and fatty meal late at night.
    3. A decrease in systolic blood pressure (BP) of 20 mmHg from lying to sitting.
    4. A decreased frequency of distress located in the epigastric region.

33. Which oral medication should the nurse **question** before administering to the client diagnosed with peptic ulcer disease?
    1. Celecoxib.
    2. Omeprazole.
    3. Metronidazole.
    4. Acetaminophen.

34. The nurse has administered an antibiotic, a proton pump inhibitor, and bismuth subsalicylate for peptic ulcer disease secondary to *H. pylori*. Which data would indicate to the nurse the medications are **effective**?
    1. A decrease in alcohol intake.
    2. Maintaining a bland diet.
    3. A return to previous activities.
    4. A decrease in gastric distress.

35. Which assessment data indicate to the nurse the client's gastric ulcer has perforated?
    1. Reports of sudden, sharp pain in the back.
    2. Rigid, boardlike abdomen with rebound tenderness.
    3. Frequent, clay-colored, liquid stool.
    4. Reports of vague abdominal pain in the right upper quadrant.

36. The client with a history of peptic ulcer disease is admitted into the intensive care department with frank gastric bleeding. Which **priority** intervention should the nurse implement?
    1. Maintain a strict record of intake and output.
    2. Insert a nasogastric (NG) tube and begin saline lavage.
    3. Assist the client with keeping a detailed calorie count.
    4. Provide a quiet environment to promote rest.

## Colorectal Disease

37. The occupational health nurse is preparing a presentation to a group of factory workers about preventing colon cancer. Which information should be included in the presentation? **Select all that apply.**

1. Wear a high-filtration mask when around chemicals.
2. Eat several servings of cruciferous vegetables daily.
3. Take a multivitamin every day.
4. Do not engage in high-risk sexual behaviors.
5. Avoid smoking and tobacco use.

38. The nurse is admitting a client to a medical floor with a diagnosis of adenocarcinoma of the rectosigmoid colon. Which assessment data support this diagnosis?
    1. The client reports up to 20 bloody stools per day.
    2. The client has a feeling of fullness after a heavy meal.
    3. The client has diarrhea alternating with constipation.
    4. The client reports right lower quadrant pain.

39. The 85-year-old male client diagnosed with cancer of the colon asks the nurse, "Why did I get this cancer?" Which statement is the nurse's **best response**?
    1. "Research shows a lack of fiber in the diet can cause colon cancer."
    2. "It is not common to get colon cancer at your age; it is usually in young people."
    3. "No one knows why anyone gets cancer; it just happens to certain people."
    4. "Women usually get colon cancer more often than men but not always."

40. The nurse is planning the care of a client with an abdominal–perineal resection for cancer of the colon. Which interventions should the nurse implement? **Select all that apply.**
    1. Provide meticulous skincare to the stoma.
    2. Assess the flank incision.
    3. Maintain the indwelling catheter.
    4. Irrigate the (JP) drains every shift.
    5. Position the client semirecumbent.

41. The client had an abdominal perineal resection and is being discharged. Which discharge information should the nurse teach?
    1. The stoma should be a white, blue, or purple color.
    2. Limit ambulation to prevent the pouch from coming off.
    3. Take pain medication when the pain level is at an "8."
    4. Empty the pouch when it is one-third to one-half full.

42. The nurse caring for a client 1 day postoperative sigmoid resection notes a moderate amount of dark reddish-brown drainage on the midline abdominal incision. Which intervention should the nurse implement **first**?
    1. Mark the drainage on the dressing with the time and date.
    2. Change the dressing immediately using sterile technique.
    3. Notify the health-care provider immediately.
    4. Reinforce the dressing with a sterile gauze pad.

43. The client reports unhappiness with the HCP to the nurse. Which intervention should the nurse implement **next**?
    1. Call the HCP and suggest a talk with the client.
    2. Determine what about the HCP is bothering the client.
    3. Notify the nursing supervisor to arrange a new HCP to take over.
    4. Explain the client cannot request another HCP until after discharge.

44. The client with a new colostomy is being discharged. Which statement made by the client indicates the **need for further** teaching?
    1. "If I notice any skin breakdown, I will call the HCP."
    2. "I should drink only liquids until the colostomy starts to work."
    3. "I should not take a tub bath until the HCP okays it."
    4. "I should not drive or lift more than 5 pounds."

45. The nurse is preparing to hang a new bag of total parenteral nutrition for a client with an abdominal perineal resection. The bag has 1,500 mL of 50% dextrose, 10 mL of trace elements, 20 mL of multivitamins, 20 mL of potassium chloride, and 500 mL of lipids. The bag is to infuse over the next 24 hours. At what rate should the nurse set the pump?

    _____

46. The nurse is caring for clients in an outpatient clinic. Which information should the nurse teach regarding the American Cancer Society's recommendations for the early detection of colon cancer in persons of average risk?
    1. A digital rectal examination should be done yearly beginning at age 60.
    2. At middle age, a fecal occult blood test should be done every 3 years.
    3. Have a colonoscopy at age 45 and then once every 10 years.
    4. A stool-based DNA test should be done yearly after age 40.

47. The nurse writes a psychosocial problem of "risk for altered sexual functioning related to new colostomy." Which intervention should the nurse implement?
    1. Tell the client there should be no intimacy for at least 3 months.
    2. Ensure the client and significant other are able to change the ostomy pouch.
    3. Demonstrate with charts possible sexual positions for the client to assume.
    4. Teach the client to protect the pouch from becoming dislodged during sex.

48. The client presents with a complete blockage of the large intestine from a tumor. Which HCP's order would the nurse **question**?
    1. Obtain consent for a colonoscopy and biopsy.
    2. Start an IV of 0.9% saline at 125 mL/hr.
    3. Administer 3 L of polyethylene glycol.
    4. Give tap water enemas until it is clear.

## Diverticulosis and Diverticulitis

49. The client diagnosed with diverticulitis is reporting severe pain in the left lower quadrant and has an oral temperature of 100.6°F. Which intervention should the nurse implement **first**?
    1. Notify the health-care provider.
    2. Document the findings in the EHR.
    3. Administer an oral antipyretic.
    4. Assess the client's abdomen.

50. The nurse is teaching the client diagnosed with diverticulosis. Which instruction should the nurse include in the teaching session?
    1. Discuss the importance of drinking 1,000 mL of water daily.
    2. Instruct the client to exercise at least three times a week.
    3. Teach the client about eating a low-residue diet.
    4. Explain the need to have regular bowel movements.

51. The client is admitted to the medical unit with a diagnosis of acute diverticulitis. Which HCP's order should the nurse **question**?
    1. Insert a nasogastric tube.
    2. Start an IV with $D_5W$ at 125 mL/hr.
    3. Put the client on a clear liquid diet.
    4. Place the client on bedrest with bathroom privileges.

52. The nurse is discussing the therapeutic diet for the client diagnosed with diverticulosis. Which meal indicates the client **understands** the discharge teaching?
    1. Fried fish, mashed potatoes, and iced tea.
    2. Ham sandwich, applesauce, and whole milk.

3. Chicken salad on whole-wheat bread and water.
4. Lettuce, tomato, and cucumber salad and coffee.

53. The client is 2 hours postcolonoscopy. Which assessment data **warrant immediate** intervention by the nurse?
    1. The client has a soft, nontender abdomen.
    2. The client has a loose, watery stool.
    3. The client has hyperactive bowel sounds.
    4. The client's pulse is 104 and BP is 98/60.

54. The nurse is preparing to administer the initial dose of an aminoglycoside antibiotic to the client diagnosed with acute diverticulitis. Which intervention should the nurse implement?
    1. Obtain a serum trough level.
    2. Ask about drug allergies.
    3. Monitor the peak level.
    4. Assess the vital signs.

55. The client diagnosed with acute diverticulitis is reporting severe abdominal pain. On assessment, the nurse finds a hard, rigid abdomen and T 102°F. Which intervention should the nurse implement?
    1. Notify the health-care provider.
    2. Prepare to administer a sodium phosphate enema.
    3. Administer an antipyretic suppository.
    4. Continue to monitor the client closely.

56. The nurse is preparing to administer a 250 mL intravenous antibiotic to the client. The medication must infuse in 1 hour. An intravenous pump is not available, and the nurse must administer the medication via gravity with IV tubing at 10 gtts/min. At what rate should the nurse infuse the medication?

    _____

57. The client diagnosed with acute diverticulitis has a nasogastric tube draining green liquid bile. Which intervention should the nurse implement?
    1. Document the findings as normal.
    2. Assess the client's bowel sounds.
    3. Determine the client's last bowel movement.
    4. Insert the NG tube at least 2 more inches.

58. The nurse is teaching a class on diverticulosis. Which interventions should the nurse discuss when teaching ways to prevent an acute exacerbation of diverticulosis? **Select all that apply.**
    1. Eat a high-fiber diet.
    2. Increase fluid intake.
    3. Elevate the HOB after eating.
    4. Walk 30 minutes a day.
    5. Take an antacid every 2 hours.

59. The nurse is working in an outpatient clinic. Which client is **most likely** to have a diagnosis of diverticulosis?
    1. A 60-year-old male with a sedentary lifestyle.
    2. A 72-year-old female with multiple childbirths.
    3. A 63-year-old female with hemorrhoids.
    4. A 40-year-old male with a family history of diverticulosis.

60. The client is admitted to the medical floor with acute diverticulitis. Which **collaborative** intervention should the nurse anticipate the HCP ordering?
    1. Administer total parenteral nutrition.
    2. Maintain NPO and nasogastric tube.
    3. Maintain on a high-fiber diet and increase fluids.
    4. Obtain consent for abdominal surgery.

## Gallbladder Disorders

61. The morbidly obese client is 4 hours postoperative open cholecystectomy. Which data **warrant immediate** intervention by the nurse?
    1. Absent bowel sounds in all four quadrants.
    2. The T-tube has 60 mL of green drainage.
    3. Urine output of 100 mL in the past 3 hours.
    4. Refusal to turn, cough, and deep breathe.

62. The client 2 hours postoperative laparoscopic cholecystectomy is reporting severe pain in the right shoulder. Which nursing intervention should the nurse implement?
    1. Apply a heating pad to the abdomen for 15 to 20 minutes.
    2. Administer morphine sulfate intravenously after diluting with saline.
    3. Contact the surgeon for an order to x-ray the right shoulder.
    4. Apply a sling to the right arm, which was injured during surgery.

63. The nurse is teaching a client recovering from a laparoscopic cholecystectomy. Which statement indicates the discharge teaching is **effective**?
    1. "I will take my lipid-lowering medicine at the same time each night."
    2. "I may experience some discomfort when I eat a high-fat meal."
    3. "I need someone to stay with me for about a week after surgery."
    4. "I should not splint my incision when I deep breathe and cough."

64. Which clinical manifestations should the nurse report to the HCP for the client recovering from a laparoscopic cholecystectomy? **Select all that apply.**
    1. Clay-colored stools.
    2. Yellow-tinted sclera.
    3. Dark-colored urine.
    4. Incision approximated.
    5. Abdominal pain.

65. The nurse is caring for the immediate postoperative laparoscopic cholecystectomy client. Which task could the RN delegate to the UAP?
    1. Check the abdominal dressings for bleeding.
    2. Increase the IV fluid if the blood pressure is low.
    3. Ambulate the client to the bathroom.
    4. Auscultate the breath sounds in all lobes.

66. Which data should the nurse expect to assess in the client after an upper gastrointestinal (UGI) series?
    1. Chalky white stools.
    2. Increased heart rate.
    3. A firm, hard abdomen.
    4. Hyperactive bowel sounds.

67. The client is 1 hour post-endoscopic retrograde cholangiopancreatography (ERCP). Which intervention should the nurse include in the plan of care?
    1. Instruct the client to cough forcefully.
    2. Encourage early ambulation.
    3. Assess for return of a gag reflex.
    4. Administer held medications.

68. Which outcome should the nurse identify for the client scheduled to have a cholecystectomy?
    1. Decreased pain management.
    2. Ambulate the first day postoperatively.
    3. No breaks in skin integrity.
    4. Knowledge of postoperative care.

69. Which assessment data indicate to the nurse the client recovering from an open cholecystectomy may require pain medication?
    1. The client's pulse is 65 beats per minute.
    2. The client has shallow respirations.
    3. The client's bowel sounds are 20 per minute.
    4. The client uses a pillow to splint when coughing.

70. The charge nurse is monitoring client laboratory values. Which value is expected in the client diagnosed with cholecystitis and chronic inflammation?
    1. An elevated white blood cell (WBC) count.
    2. A decreased lactate dehydrogenase (LDH).
    3. An elevated alkaline phosphatase.
    4. A decreased direct bilirubin level.

71. Which problem is the **highest priority** for the nurse to identify in the client after cholecystectomy surgery?
    1. Alteration in nutrition.
    2. Alteration in skin integrity.
    3. Alteration in urinary pattern.
    4. Alteration in comfort.

72. The nurse assesses a large amount of red drainage on the dressing of a client 6 hours postoperative open cholecystectomy. Which intervention should the nurse implement?
    1. Measure the abdominal girth.
    2. Palpate the lower abdomen for a mass.
    3. Turn client onto side to assess for further drainage.
    4. Remove the dressing to determine the source.

## Liver Disease

73. The client diagnosed with end-stage liver disease is admitted with esophageal bleeding. The HCP recommends endoscopic treatment. Which nursing interventions should the nurse implement before this treatment? **Select all that apply.**
    1. Position the client in a lateral position.
    2. Stay with the client at all times.
    3. Have a suction catheter at the bedside.
    4. Administer lactulose.
    5. Monitor the client's oxygen saturation.

74. The client has had a liver biopsy. Which **post-procedure** interventions should the nurse implement? **Select all that apply.**
    1. Instruct the client to void immediately.
    2. Keep the client NPO for 8 hours.
    3. Place the client on the right side.
    4. Monitor blood urea nitrogen (BUN) and creatinine level.
    5. Assess the client's level of consciousness every 15 minutes.

75. The client diagnosed with end-stage liver disease is admitted with hepatic encephalopathy. Which dietary restriction should be implemented by the nurse to address this complication?
    1. Restrict sodium intake to 2 g/day.
    2. Limit oral fluids to 1,500 mL/day.
    3. Decrease daily fat intake.
    4. Reduce protein intake to 60 to 80 g/day.

76. The client diagnosed with end-stage liver disease and ascites is scheduled for a paracentesis. Which client teaching should the nurse discuss with the client?
    1. Explain the procedure will be done in the operating room.
    2. Instruct the client a Foley catheter will have to be inserted.

3. Tell the client vital signs will be taken frequently after the procedure.
4. Provide instructions on holding the breath when the HCP inserts the catheter.

77. The client diagnosed with liver disease is experiencing pruritus secondary to severe jaundice. Which action by the UAP **warrants intervention** by the RN?
    1. The UAP is assisting the client in taking a hot, soapy shower.
    2. The UAP applies an emollient to the client's legs and back.
    3. The UAP puts mittens on both hands of the client.
    4. The UAP pats the client's skin dry with a clean towel.

78. The nurse identifies the client problem "excess fluid volume" for the client diagnosed with liver failure. Which short-term goal would be **most appropriate** for this problem?
    1. The client will not gain more than 2 kg a day.
    2. The client will have no increase in abdominal girth.
    3. The client's vital signs will remain within normal limits.
    4. The client will receive a low-sodium diet.

79. The client diagnosed with end-stage liver disease has vitamin K deficiency. Which interventions should the nurse implement? **Select all that apply.**
    1. Avoid rectal temperatures.
    2. Use only a soft toothbrush.
    3. Monitor the platelet count.
    4. Use small-gauge needles.
    5. Assess for asterixis.

80. Which GI assessment data should the nurse expect to find when assessing the client diagnosed with end-stage liver disease?
    1. Hypoalbuminemia and muscle wasting.
    2. Oligomenorrhea and decreased body hair.
    3. Clay-colored stools and hemorrhoids.
    4. Dyspnea and caput medusae.

81. Which assessment question is a **priority** for the nurse to ask the client diagnosed with end-stage liver disease secondary to alcoholic cirrhosis?
    1. "How many years have you been drinking alcohol?"
    2. "Have you completed an advance directive?"
    3. "When did you have your last alcoholic drink?"
    4. "What foods did you eat at your last meal?"

82. The client has end-stage liver disease secondary to alcoholic cirrhosis. Which complication indicates the client is **at risk** for developing hepatic encephalopathy?
    1. Gastrointestinal bleeding.
    2. Hypoalbuminemia.
    3. Splenomegaly.
    4. Hyperaldosteronism.

83. The client is diagnosed with end-stage liver disease. The client asks the nurse, "Why is my doctor decreasing the doses of my medications?" Which statement is the nurse's **best response**?
    1. "You are worried because your doctor has decreased the dosage."
    2. "You really should ask your doctor. I am sure there is a good reason."
    3. "You may have an overdose of the medications because your liver is damaged."
    4. "The half-life of the medications is altered because the liver is damaged."

84. The client is admitted with end-stage liver disease and is prescribed lactulose. Which statement indicates the client **needs more** teaching concerning this medication?
    1. "I should have two to three soft stools a day."
    2. "I must check my ammonia level daily."
    3. "If I have diarrhea, I will call my doctor."
    4. "I should check my stool for any blood."

## Hepatitis

85. The client is in the **prodromal** or **preicteric** phase of hepatitis. Which clinical manifestations should the nurse expect the client to exhibit during this phase?
    1. Clay-colored stools and jaundice.
    2. Normal appetite and pruritus.
    3. Being afebrile and left upper quadrant pain.
    4. Reports of fatigue and diarrhea.

86. The public health nurse is teaching day-care workers. Which type of hepatitis is transmitted by the fecal-oral route via contaminated food, water, or direct contact with an infected person?
    1. Hepatitis A.
    2. Hepatitis B.
    3. Hepatitis C.
    4. Hepatitis D.

87. Which type of precaution should the nurse implement to protect from being exposed to any of the hepatitis viruses?
    1. Airborne precautions.
    2. Standard precautions.
    3. Droplet precautions.
    4. Exposure precautions.

88. The school nurse is discussing methods to prevent an outbreak of hepatitis A with a group of high school teachers. Which action is the **most important** to teach the high school teachers?
    1. Do not allow students to eat or drink after each other.
    2. Drink bottled water as much as possible.
    3. Encourage protected sexual activity.
    4. Sing the "Happy Birthday" song while washing hands.

89. Which instruction should the nurse discuss with the client in the **icteric** phase of hepatitis C?
    1. Decrease alcohol intake.
    2. Encourage rest periods.
    3. Eat a large evening meal.
    4. Drink diet drinks and juices.

90. The public health nurse is discussing hepatitis B with a group in the community. Which health promotion activities should the nurse discuss with the group? **Select all that apply.**
    1. Do not share needles or equipment.
    2. Use barrier protection during sex.
    3. Get the hepatitis B vaccine.
    4. Obtain immune globulin injections.
    5. Avoid any type of hepatotoxic medications.

91. The client diagnosed with hepatitis asks the nurse, "I went to an herbalist, who recommended I take milk thistle. What do you think about the herb?" Which statement is the nurse's **best response**?
    1. "You are concerned about taking an herb."
    2. "The herb has been used to treat liver disease."
    3. "I would not take anything that is not prescribed."
    4. "Why would you want to take any herbs?"

92. The nurse writes the problem "imbalanced nutrition: less than body requirements" for the client diagnosed with hepatitis. Which intervention should the nurse include in the plan of care?
    1. Provide a high-calorie intake diet.
    2. Discuss total parenteral nutrition (TPN).
    3. Instruct the client to decrease salt intake.
    4. Encourage the client to increase water intake.

93. The female nurse sticks herself with a contaminated needle. Which action should the nurse implement **first**?
    1. Notify the infection control nurse.
    2. Cleanse the area with soap and water.
    3. Request postexposure prophylaxis.
    4. Check the hepatitis status of the client.

94. The client diagnosed with liver problems asks the nurse, "Why are my stools clay-colored?" On which scientific rationale should the nurse base the response?
    1. There is an increase in the serum ammonia level.
    2. The liver is unable to excrete bilirubin.
    3. The liver is unable to metabolize fatty foods.
    4. A damaged liver cannot detoxify vitamins.

95. Which statement by the client diagnosed with hepatitis **warrants immediate** intervention by the clinic nurse?
    1. "I will not drink any type of beer or mixed drink."
    2. "I will get adequate rest, so I don't get exhausted."
    3. "I had a big hearty breakfast this morning."
    4. "I took some cough syrup for this nasty head cold."

96. Which task is **most appropriate** for the RN to delegate to the UAP?
    1. Draw the serum liver function test.
    2. Evaluate the client's intake and output.
    3. Perform the bedside glucometer check.
    4. Help the unit clerk transcribe orders.

## Gastroenteritis

97. The female client came to the clinic reporting abdominal cramping and at least 10 episodes of diarrhea every day for the last 2 days. The client just returned from a trip to Mexico. Which intervention should the nurse implement?
    1. Instruct the client to take a cathartic laxative daily.
    2. Tell the client to take an oral glucose electrolyte solution.
    3. Discuss the need to increase protein in the diet.
    4. Explain the client should weigh herself daily.

98. Which intervention should the nurse include when discussing ways to help **prevent** potential episodes of gastroenteritis from *Clostridium botulism*?
    1. Make sure all hamburger meat is well cooked.
    2. Ensure all dairy products are refrigerated.
    3. Discuss why campers should drink only bottled water.
    4. Discard damaged canned goods.

99. The client is diagnosed with a Salmonella infection secondary to eating some slightly cooked hamburger meat. Which clinical manifestations should the nurse expect the client to report?
    1. Abdominal cramping, nausea, and vomiting.
    2. Neuromuscular paralysis and dysphagia.
    3. Gross amounts of explosive bloody diarrhea.
    4. Frequent "rice-water stool" with no fecal odor.

100. The client is diagnosed with gastroenteritis. Which laboratory data warrant immediate intervention by the nurse?
    1. A serum sodium level of 137 mEq/L.
    2. Arterial blood gases of pH 7.37, Po$_2$ 95, Pco$_2$ 43, HCO$_3$ 24.
    3. A serum potassium level of 3.3 mEq/L.
    4. A stool sample positive for fecal leukocytes.

101. The client diagnosed with gastroenteritis is being discharged from the emergency department. Which interventions should the nurse include in the discharge teaching? Select all that apply.
    1. If diarrhea persists for more than 96 hours, contact the health-care provider.
    2. Instruct the client to wash hands thoroughly before handling any type of food.
    3. Explain the importance of decreasing steroids gradually as instructed.
    4. Discuss how to collect all stool samples for the next 24 hours.
    5. Tell the client to drink clear liquids or electrolyte solutions.

102. Which medication should the nurse expect the HCP to order to treat the client diagnosed with botulism secondary to eating contaminated canned goods?
    1. An antidiarrheal medication.
    2. An aminoglycoside antibiotic.
    3. An antitoxin medication.
    4. An ACE inhibitor medication.

103. Which nursing problem is a priority for the 76-year-old client diagnosed with gastroenteritis from staphylococcal food poisoning?
    1. Fluid volume deficit.
    2. Nausea.
    3. Acute pain.
    4. Impaired urinary elimination.

104. Which data should the nurse expect to assess in the client diagnosed with acute gastroenteritis?
    1. Decreased gurgling sounds on auscultation of the abdominal wall.
    2. A hard, firm, edematous abdomen on palpation.
    3. Frequent, small melena-type liquid bowel movements.
    4. Bowel assessment reveals loud, rushing bowel sounds.

105. The 79-year-old client diagnosed with acute gastroenteritis is admitted to the medical unit. Which task would be most appropriate for the RN to delegate to the UAP?
    1. Evaluate the client's intake and output.
    2. Take the client's vital signs.
    3. Change the client's intravenous solution.
    4. Assess the client's perianal area.

106. Which statement indicates to the emergency department nurse the client diagnosed with acute gastroenteritis understands the discharge teaching?
    1. "I will probably have some leg cramps while I have gastroenteritis."
    2. "I should decrease my fluid intake until the diarrhea subsides."
    3. "I should reintroduce solid foods very slowly back into my diet."
    4. "I should only drink bottled water until the abdominal cramping stops."

107. Which nursing interventions should be included in the care plan for the 84-year-old client diagnosed with acute gastroenteritis? Select all that apply.
    1. Assess the skin turgor on the back of the client's hands.
    2. Monitor the client for orthostatic hypotension.
    3. Record the frequency and characteristics of sputum.
    4. Use standard precautions when caring for the client.
    5. Institute safety precautions when ambulating the client.

108. The nurse has received the a.m. shift report. Which client should the nurse assess first?
    1. The 44-year-old client diagnosed with peptic ulcer disease reporting acute epigastric pain.
    2. The 74-year-old client diagnosed with acute gastroenteritis and four diarrhea stools during the night.
    3. The 65-year-old client diagnosed with IBD, tented skin turgor, and dry mucous membranes.

4. The 15-year-old client diagnosed with food poisoning, who vomited several times during the night shift.

## Abdominal Surgery

109. The male client had abdominal surgery, and the nurse suspects the client has peritonitis. Which assessment data support the diagnosis of peritonitis?
    1. Absent bowel sounds and potassium level of 3.9 mEq/L.
    2. Abdominal cramping and hemoglobin of 14 g/dL.
    3. Profuse diarrhea and stool specimens show *Campylobacter*.
    4. Hard, rigid abdomen and WBC count 22 ($10^3$ cells/microL).

110. The client, after abdominal surgery, tells the nurse, "I felt something give way in my stomach." Which intervention should the nurse implement **first**?
    1. Notify the surgeon immediately.
    2. Instruct the client to splint the incision.
    3. Assess the abdominal wound incision.
    4. Administer pain medication intravenously.

111. The client is 1 day postoperative major abdominal surgery. Which client problem is the **priority**?
    1. Impaired skin integrity.
    2. Fluid and electrolyte imbalance.
    3. Altered bowel elimination.
    4. Altered body image.

112. The client has an eviscerated abdominal wound. Which intervention should the nurse implement?
    1. Apply sterile normal saline dressing.
    2. Use sterile gloves to replace protruding parts.
    3. Place the client in a reverse Trendelenburg position.
    4. Administer intravenous antibiotics immediately (STAT).

113. The client is diagnosed with peritonitis. Which assessment data indicate to the nurse the client's condition is **improving**?
    1. The client is using more pain medication on a daily basis.
    2. The client's nasogastric tube is draining coffee-ground material.
    3. The client has a decrease in temperature and a soft abdomen.
    4. The client has had two soft-formed bowel movements.

114. The client developed a paralytic ileus after abdominal surgery. Which intervention should the nurse include in the plan of care?
    1. Administer a laxative of choice.
    2. Encourage the client to increase oral fluids.
    3. Instruct the client to take deep breaths.
    4. Maintain a patent nasogastric tube.

115. The client following abdominal surgery has a Jackson Pratt (JP) drainage device. Which assessment data **warrant immediate** intervention by the nurse?
    1. The bulb is round and has 40 mL of fluid.
    2. The drainage tube is taped to the dressing.
    3. The JP insertion site is pink and has no drainage.
    4. The JP bulb has suction and is sunken in.

116. The postanesthisia care nurse is caring for a client after abdominal surgery with gastric decompression in place and reporting nausea. Which intervention should the nurse implement **first**?
    1. Medicate the client with a narcotic analgesic (IVP).
    2. Assess the nasogastric tube for patency.
    3. Check the temperature for elevation.
    4. Hyperextend the neck to prevent stridor.

117. The nurse is assessing the client recovering from abdominal surgery. The client is using a patient-controlled analgesia (PCA) pump, has shallow respirations, and refuses to deep breathe. Which intervention should the nurse implement?
    1. Insist the client take deep breaths.
    2. Notify the surgeon to request a chest x-ray.
    3. Determine the last time the client used the PCA pump.
    4. Administer oxygen at 2 L/min via nasal cannula.

118. The client has a nasogastric tube. The HCP orders IV fluid replacement based on the previous hour's output plus the baseline IV fluid ordered of 125 mL/hr. From 0800 to 0900, the client's NG tube drained 45 mL. At 0900, what rate should the nurse set for the IV pump?

    

119. The nurse is caring for clients in a surgical unit. Which client should the nurse assess **first**?
    1. The client 4 hours after an inguinal hernia repair with an absence of voiding.
    2. The client admitted with abdominal pain who suddenly has no pain.
    3. The client 4 hours postoperative abdominal surgery with no bowel sounds.
    4. The client 1 day post-appendectomy who is being discharged.

120. The 84-year-old client comes to the clinic reporting right lower abdominal pain. Which question is **most appropriate** for the nurse to ask the client?
1. "When was your last bowel movement?"
2. "Did you have a high-fat meal last night?"
3. "Can you describe the type of pain?"
4. "Have you been experiencing any gas?"

## Eating Disorders

121. The female client presents to the clinic for an examination because she has not had a menstrual cycle for several months and wonders if she could be pregnant. The client is 5'10" tall and weighs 45 kg. Which assessment data should the nurse obtain **first**?
1. Ask the client to recall what she ate for the last 24 hours.
2. Determine what type of birth control the client has been using.
3. Reweigh the client to confirm the data.
4. Take the client's pulse and blood pressure.

122. The occupational health nurse observes the chief financial officer eat large lunch meals then disappear into the restroom for about 20 minutes. Which observation by the nurse would indicate the client has bulimia?
1. The client jogs 2 miles a day.
2. The client has not gained weight.
3. The client's teeth are a green color.
4. The client has smooth knuckles.

123. The nurse is caring for a client diagnosed with bulimia nervosa. Which nursing intervention should the nurse implement **after** the client's evening meal?
1. Praise the client for eating all the food on the tray.
2. Stay with the client for 45 minutes to an hour.
3. Allow the client to work out on the treadmill.
4. Place the client on bedrest until morning.

124. The nurse writes the problem "low self-esteem" for a 16-year-old client diagnosed with anorexia. Which client goal should be included in the plan of care?
1. The client will spend 1 hour a day with the parents.
2. The client eats 50% of the meals provided.
3. Dietary will provide high-protein milkshakes (tid).
4. The client will verbalize one positive attribute.

125. The female client diagnosed with anorexia nervosa is admitted to the hospital. The client is 67 inches tall and weighs 40 kg. Which client problem has the **highest priority**?
1. Altered nutrition.
2. Low self-esteem.
3. Disturbed body image.
4. Altered sexuality.

126. Which diagnostic test should the nurse monitor for the client diagnosed with severe anorexia nervosa?
1. Liver function tests.
2. Kidney function tests.
3. Cardiac function tests.
4. Bone density scan.

127. The female client is more than 10% over ideal body weight. Which nursing intervention should the nurse implement **first?**
1. Ask the client why she is eating too much.
2. Refer the client to a gymnasium for exercise.
3. Have the client set a realistic weight loss goal.
4. Determine the client's eating patterns.

128. The morbidly obese client has undergone gastric bypass surgery. Which **immediate** postoperative intervention has the **greatest priority**?
1. Monitor respiratory status.
2. Weigh the client daily.
3. Teach a healthy diet.
4. Assist in behavior modification.

129. The obese client presents to the clinic before beginning a weight loss program. Which interventions should the nurse teach? **Select all that apply.**
1. Walk for 30 minutes three times a day.
2. Determine situations that initiate eating behavior.
3. Weigh at the same time every day.
4. Limit sodium in the diet.
5. Refer to a weight support group.

130. The 22-year-old obese female is discussing weight loss programs with the nurse. Which information should the nurse teach? **Select all that apply.**
1. Jog for 2 to 3 hours every day.
2. Lifestyle behaviors must be modified.
3. Eat one large meal every day in the evening.
4. Eat 1,000 calories a day, and don't take vitamins.
5. Drink water a half hour before each meal.

131. The 36-year-old female client diagnosed with anorexia nervosa tells the nurse "I am so fat. I won't be able to eat today." Which response by the nurse is **most appropriate**?
    1. "Can you tell me why you think you are fat?"
    2. "You are skinny. Many women wish they had your problem."
    3. "If you don't eat, we will have to restrain you and feed you."
    4. "Not eating might cause physical problems."

132. The client is being admitted to the outpatient psychiatric clinic diagnosed with bulimia. Which question should the nurse ask to identify behaviors suggesting bulimia?
    1. "When was the last time you exercised?"
    2. "What over-the-counter medications do you take?"
    3. "How long have you had a positive self-image?"
    4. "Do you eat a lot of high-fiber foods for bowel movements?"

## Constipation and Diarrhea Disorders

133. The client admitted from the emergency department is diagnosed with a fecal impaction. Which nursing intervention should be implemented?
    1. Administer an antidiarrheal medication every day and prn.
    2. Perform bowel training every 2 hours.
    3. Administer an oil retention enema.
    4. Prepare for a upper gastrointestinal (UGI) series x-ray.

134. The nurse is caring for a client using cathartics frequently. Which statement made by the client indicates an **understanding** of the discharge teaching?
    1. "In the future, I will eat a banana every time I take the medication."
    2. "I don't have to have a bowel movement every day."
    3. "I should limit the fluids I drink with my meals."
    4. "If I feel sluggish, I will eat a lot of cheese and dairy products."

135. The client has been experiencing difficulty and straining when expelling feces. Which intervention should the nurse discuss with the client?
    1. Explain some blood in the stool will be normal for the client.
    2. Instruct the client in manual removal of feces.
    3. Encourage the client to use a cathartic laxative on a daily basis.
    4. Place the client on a high-fiber diet.

136. The client has dark, watery, and shiny-appearing stool. Which intervention should the nurse implement **first**?
    1. Check for a fecal impaction.
    2. Encourage the client to drink fluids.
    3. Check the EHR for sodium and potassium levels.
    4. Apply a protective barrier cream to the perianal area.

137. The charge nurse has just received the shift report. Which client should the nurse see **first**?
    1. The client diagnosed with Crohn's disease who, on the previous shift, had two semi-formed stools.
    2. The elderly client admitted from another facility, reporting constipation.
    3. The client diagnosed with AIDS had a 200-mL diarrhea stool and has elastic skin tissue turgor.
    4. The client diagnosed with hemorrhoids having spots of bright red blood on the toilet tissue.

138. The dietitian and the nurse in a long-term care facility are planning the menu for the day. Which foods should be recommended for the immobile clients with no swallowing issues?
    1. Cheeseburger and milk shake.
    2. Canned peaches and a sandwich on whole-wheat bread.
    3. Mashed potatoes and mechanically ground red meat.
    4. Biscuits and gravy with bacon.

139. The client diagnosed with AIDS is experiencing voluminous diarrhea. Which interventions should the nurse implement? **Select all that apply.**
    1. Monitor diarrhea, documenting amount, character, and consistency.
    2. Assess the client's tissue turgor every day.
    3. Encourage the client to drink carbonated soft drinks.
    4. Weigh the client daily in the same clothes and at the same time.
    5. Assist the client with a warm sitz bath prn.

140. The RN, a licensed practical nurse (LPN), and a UAP are caring for clients on a medical floor. Which nursing task would be **most appropriate** to assign to the LPN?
    1. Assist the UAP to learn to perform blood glucose checks.
    2. Monitor the potassium levels of a client diagnosed with diarrhea.
    3. Administer a bulk laxative to a client diagnosed with constipation.
    4. Assess the abdomen of a client reporting abdominal pain.

141. The client is placed on percutaneous endoscopic gastrostomy (PEG) tube feedings. Which occurrence **warrants immediate** intervention by the nurse?
    1. The client tolerates the feedings being infused at 50 mL/hr.
    2. The client pulls the nasogastric feeding tube out.
    3. The client reports being thirsty.
    4. The client is incontinent of green, watery stool.

142. The client presents to the emergency department experiencing frequent watery, bloody stools after eating some undercooked meat at a fast-food restaurant. Which intervention should be implemented **first**?
    1. Obtain a stool sample from the client.
    2. Initiate antibiotic therapy intravenously.
    3. Have the laboratory draw a complete blood count.
    4. Administer diphenoxylate and atropine.

143. The clinic nurse is talking on the phone to a client with diarrhea. Which intervention should the nurse discuss with the client?
    1. Tell the client to measure the amount of stool.
    2. Recommend the client come to the clinic immediately.
    3. Explain the client should follow the BRAT diet.
    4. Discuss taking an over-the-counter histamine-2 blocker.

144. The nurse is caring for clients on a medical unit. Which client information should be brought to the attention of the HCP **immediately**?
    1. A serum sodium of 128 mEq/L in a client diagnosed with obstipation.
    2. The client diagnosed with fecal impaction after two hard formed stools.
    3. A serum potassium level of 3.8 mEq/L in a client diagnosed with diarrhea.
    4. The client diagnosed with diarrhea after two semiliquid stools totaling 300 mL.

# CONCEPTS

The concepts covered in this chapter focus on nutrition and acid-base problems. Exemplars that are covered are eating disorders and dietary recommendations and gastrointestinal disorders. Interrelated concepts of the nursing process and clinical judgment are covered throughout the questions. The concept of clinical judgment is presented in prioritizing or "first" questions.

145. The nurse is caring for a postoperative client with a nasogastric tube set to low intermittent suction. Which intervention should the nurse implement **first** based on the blood gas results?

| Arterial Blood Gas | Client | Normal Values |
|---|---|---|
| pH | 7.48 | 7.35–7.45 |
| $Pco_2$ | 46 | 35–45 mmHg |
| $Hco_3$ | 20 | 22–26 mEq/L |
| $O_2$ saturation | 96 | 95%–99% |

    1. Assess the output in the suction canister.
    2. Apply oxygen by nasal cannula.
    3. Have the client take slow, deep breaths.
    4. Place the client on stool specimen collection.

146. The 70-year-old client is admitted to the medical unit diagnosed with acute diverticulitis. Which interventions should the nurse implement? **Select all that apply.**
    1. Tell the client not to eat or drink.
    2. Start an intravenous line.
    3. Assess the client for abdominal tenderness.
    4. Have the dietitian consult for a low-residue diet.
    5. Place the client on bedrest with bathroom privileges.

147. The nurse is admitting a client diagnosed with protein calorie malnutrition. Which interventions should the RN implement? **Select all that apply.**
    1. Place the client on a 72-hour calorie count.
    2. Ask the client to describe the stools.
    3. Have the UAP weigh the client.
    4. Obtain a list of current medications.
    5. Make a referral to the dietitian.

148. The client at the eating disorder clinic weighs 35 kg and is 5 ft 7 inches tall. What would the nurse document as the body mass index (BMI)?

[        ]

149. The client presents to the outpatient clinic reporting diarrhea for 2 days. Which laboratory data should the nurse monitor?
    1. The sodium level.
    2. The albumin level.
    3. The potassium level.
    4. The glucose level.

150. The clinic nurse is returning client calls. Which client should the nurse call **first**?
    1. The 39-year-old client reporting headache pain with a 3 on the pain scale.
    2. The 45-year-old client needing a prescription refill for warfarin.
    3. The 54-year-old client diagnosed with diabetes type 1 who is vomiting.
    4. The 60-year-old client needing financial aid to buy food.

151. The occupational health nurse has had five clients come to the clinic reporting abdominal cramping, nausea, and vomiting. Which information should the nurse teach the employees to **decrease** the spread of this condition?
    1. Teach the employees to cough into the sleeve.
    2. Teach the housekeepers to use an antibacterial soap.
    3. Teach the coworkers to get a hepatitis vaccine.
    4. Teach the employees to wash their hands frequently.

152. Which diagnostic data should be reported to the HCP **immediately?**
    1.

| Client: A.C. | | Diagnosis: Type 1 Diabetes |
| --- | --- | --- |
| Arterial Blood Gas | Client Results | Normal Values |
| pH | 7.11 | 7.35–7.45 |
| $Pco_2$ | 45 | 35–45 mmHg |
| $Hco_3$ | 20 | 22–26 mEq/L |
| $Pao_2$ | 98 | 80–95 mmHg |

2.

| Client: U.T. | | Diagnosis: Gastroenteritis |
| --- | --- | --- |
| Laboratory Test | Client Results | Normal Values |
| Glucose | 120 | Fasting < 100 mg/dL<br>Random < 200 mg/dL |
| Sodium ($Na^+$) | 137 | 135–145 mEq/L or mmol/L |
| Potassium ($K^+$) | 4 | 3.5–5.3 mEq/L or mmol/L |

3.

| Client: G.B. | | Diagnosis: 12 Hours Post–Blood Transfusion |
| --- | --- | --- |
| Complete Blood Count (CBC) | Client Value | Normal Values |
| Hemoglobin (Hgb) | 9.4 | Male: 14–17.3 g/dL<br>Female: 11.7–15.5 g/dL |
| Hematocrit (Hct) | 29 | Male: 42%–52%<br>Female: 36%–48% |

4.

| Client: B.D. | | Diagnosis: COPD |
| --- | --- | --- |
| Arterial Blood Gas | Client Results | Normal Values |
| Pulse oximetry ($O_2$ saturation) | 93 | 95%–99% |

153. The parents of a female toddler bring the child to the pediatrician's office with nausea, vomiting, and diarrhea. Which intervention should the nurse implement **first?**
    1. Ask the parent about the child's diet.
    2. Assess the child's tissue turgor.
    3. Give the child a sucker if she is "good."
    4. Notify the HCP the child is waiting to be seen.

154. The weight loss clinic nurse identifies the concept of nutrition for a client diagnosed with obesity. Which interventions should the nurse implement? **Select all that apply.**
    1. Ask the client about previous diet attempts.
    2. Refer the client to the dietitian.
    3. Discuss maintaining a sedentary lifestyle.
    4. Weigh the client.
    5. Assist the client to set a realistic weight loss goal.

155. The client diagnosed with bulimia has a BMI of 20. Which scientific rationale explains this finding?

**Body Mass Index**

| Category | BMI Lower Range | BMI Upper Range |
|---|---|---|
| Underweight | Less than 18.5 | — |
| Ideal weight | 18.5 | 24.9 |
| Overweight | 25 | 29.9 |
| Obese | 30 or greater | — |

1. The BMI is low because the client does not eat and exercises frequently.
    2. The BMI is within the normal range because the client's therapy is effective.
    3. The BMI is WNL because the client vomits or uses laxatives to prevent weight gain.
    4. The BMI is high, and the client needs to try new methods of weight control.

156. The nurse is teaching the American Diabetes Association diet to a client diagnosed with diabetes mellitus type 2. Which should the nurse teach the client?
    1. Instruct the client to weigh all food before cooking it.
    2. Teach the client to eat only carbohydrates if the blood glucose is low.
    3. Demonstrate how to determine the number of carbohydrates being eaten.
    4. Explain that proteins should be 75% of the recommended diet.

### Gastroesophageal Reflux (GERD)

1. 1. Clients having heartburn are frequently diagnosed as having GERD. GERD can occasionally cause weight loss but not weight gain.
   2. **Most clients diagnosed with GERD have been self-medicating with over-the-counter medications before seeking advice from an HCP. It is important to know what the client has been using to treat the problem.**
   3. Milk and dairy products contain lactose, which is important if considering lactose intolerance but is not important for "heartburn."
   4. Heartburn is not a symptom of a viral illness.

**TEST-TAKING HINT: Clients will use common terms such as "heartburn" to describe symptoms. The nurse must be able to interpret or clarify the meaning of terms used with the client. Part of the assessment of a symptom requires determining what aggravates and alleviates the symptom.**

2. 1. **The client should elevate the HOB on blocks or use a foam wedge to use gravity to help keep the gastric acid in the stomach and prevent reflux into the esophagus. Behavior modification is changing one's behavior.**
   2. The client should be encouraged to quit smoking altogether. Referral to support groups for smoking cessation should be made.
   3. The nurse should be careful when recommending over-the-counter (OTC) medications. This is not the most appropriate intervention for a client diagnosed with GERD.
   4. The client should be instructed to discontinue using alcohol, but the stem does not indicate the client is an alcoholic.

**TEST-TAKING HINT: Clients are encouraged to quit, not decrease, smoking. Current research indicates smoking is damaging to many body systems, including the gastrointestinal system. The test taker should not assume anything not in the stem of a question.**

3. 1. The client is allowed to eat as soon as the gag reflex has returned.
   2. An esophagogastroduodenoscopy is a diagnostic procedure, not a cure. Therefore, the client still has GERD and should be instructed to stay in an upright position for 2 to 3 hours after eating.
   3. Stomach contents are acidic and will erode the esophageal lining.
   4. **Orange juice and tomatoes are acidic and prone to trigger acid reflux. The client diagnosed with GERD should avoid acidic foods to allow the esophagus to heal and to reduce heartburn.**

**TEST-TAKING HINT: This question assumes the test taker has knowledge of diagnostic procedures for specific disease processes.**

4. **Correct answers are 3 and 5.**
   1. The client is instructed to avoid spicy and acidic foods and any food that produces symptoms.
   2. Eructation means belching, which is a symptom of GERD.
   3. **Clients should eat small, frequent meals and limit fluids with the meals to prevent reflux into the esophagus from a distended stomach.**
   4. Clients are encouraged to forgo all alcoholic beverages because alcohol relaxes the lower esophageal sphincter and increases the risk of reflux.
   5. **Clients should maintain an ideal body weight because obesity increases intraabdominal pressure, causing GERD.**

**TEST-TAKING HINT: The word "any" in option "1" should give the test taker a clue that, unless there are absolutely no dietary restrictions, this is an incorrect answer. Option "2" requires knowledge of medical terminology.**

5. 1. The client is encouraged to lie with the HOB elevated, but this is difficult to achieve when on the stomach. NSAIDs inhibit prostaglandin synthesis in the stomach, which places the client at risk for developing gastric ulcers. The client is already experiencing gastric acid difficulty.
   2. The client will need to lie down at some time, and walking will not help with GERD.

3. The client should not lie supine flat on the back. The bed should be elevated. Antacids are taken 1 and 3 hours after a meal.
4. **The HOB should be elevated to allow gravity to help in preventing reflux. Lifestyle modifications of losing weight, making dietary modifications, attempting smoking cessation, discontinuing the use of alcohol, and not stooping or bending at the waist all help to decrease reflux.**

**TEST-TAKING HINT: Option "2" has an "all," which should alert the test taker to eliminate this option. If the test taker has no idea of the answer, lifestyle modifications are an educated guess for most chronic problems.**

6. 1. **In adult-onset asthma, a large number of cases are caused by GERD. Additionally, GERD can make existing asthma symptoms difficult to control (Banki, 2020).**
   2. Pancreatitis is not related to GERD.
   3. Peptic ulcer disease, gastritis, and gastric cancer are related to *H. pylori* bacterial infections and can lead to changes in the levels of gastric acid, but it is not related to reflux (Waldum, Kleveland, & Sordal, 2016).
   4. GERD is related to gastric emptying because increased gastric emptying would be a benefit to a client diagnosed with decreased functioning of the lower esophageal sphincter. However, increased gastric emptying is not a disease.

**TEST-TAKING HINT: Option "4" is not a disease, only a gastrointestinal process, which should alert the test taker to eliminate this option.**

7. 1. Proton pump inhibitors can be administered at routine dosing times, usually 0900 or after breakfast.
   2. Pain medication is important, but a non-narcotic medication, such as Tylenol, can be administered after a medication, which must be timed.
   3. A histamine receptor antagonist can be administered at routine dosing times.
   4. **A mucosal barrier agent must be administered on an empty stomach for the medication to coat the stomach.**

**TEST-TAKING HINT: Basic knowledge of how medications work is required to administer medications for peak effectiveness. There are very few medications requiring a specific time. The test taker should memorize these specific medications.**

8. 1. In esophageal pH monitoring, gastric pH is monitored for 24 hours for esophageal symptoms. A positive result would be expected for a client diagnosed with GERD. This would not warrant notifying the HCP.
   2. Hiatal hernias are frequently the cause of GERD; therefore, this finding would not warrant notifying the HCP.
   3. **The client's WBC count is elevated, indicating a possible infection, which warrants notifying the HCP.**
   4. This is a normal hemoglobin result and would not warrant notifying the HCP.

**TEST-TAKING HINT: When the test taker is deciding when to notify a HCP, the answer should be data not normal for the disease process or signaling a potential or life-threatening complication.**

9. 1. Pyrosis is heartburn and is expected in a client diagnosed with GERD. The new graduate can care for this client.
   2. Barrett's esophagus is a complication of GERD; new graduates can prepare a client for a diagnostic procedure.
   3. **This client is exhibiting symptoms of asthma, a complication of GERD. This client should be assigned to the most experienced nurse.**
   4. This client can be cared for by the new graduate, and ambulating can be delegated to the UAP.

**TEST-TAKING HINT: The most experienced nurse should be assigned to the client requiring more experience and knowledge about the disease process, potential complications, and medications for assessment and care. The term "most experienced" in the stem is the key to answering this question.**

10. 1. Pain in the chest when walking up stairs indicates angina.
    2. **Frequent use of antacids indicates an acid reflux problem.**
    3. Loud snoring could indicate sleep apnea but not GERD.
    4. Carbonated beverages increase stomach pressure. Six to seven soft drinks a day would not be tolerated by a client diagnosed with GERD.

**TEST-TAKING HINT: The stem of the question indicates an acid problem. The drug classification of antacid, or "against acid," provides the test taker a hint as to the correct answer.**

11. 1. Pyrosis is heartburn, water brash is the feeling of saliva secretion as a result of reflux, and eructation is burping or belching—all symptoms of GERD.
   2. Gastroesophageal reflux disease does not cause weight loss.
   3. There is no change in abdominal fat, no proteinuria (the result of a filtration problem in the kidney), and no alteration in bowel elimination for the client diagnosed with GERD.
   4. Midepigastric pain, a positive *H. pylori* test, and melena are associated with gastric ulcer disease.

**TEST-TAKING HINT:** Frequently, incorrect answer options will contain the symptoms of a disease of the same organ system.

12. 1. A hiatal hernia places the client at risk for GERD; GERD does not predispose the client for developing a hiatal hernia.
   2. Gastroenteritis is an inflammation of the stomach and intestine, usually caused by a virus.
   3. Barrett's esophagus results from long-term erosion of the esophagus as a result of the reflux of stomach contents secondary to GERD. This is a precursor to esophageal cancer.
   4. The problems associated with GERD result from the reflux of acidic stomach contents into the esophagus, which is not a precursor to gastric cancer.

**TEST-TAKING HINT:** The test taker may associate hiatal hernia with GERD. One can be a result of the other, and this can confuse the test taker. If the test taker did not have any idea of the correct answer, option "3" has the word "esophageal" in it, as does the stem of the question, and, therefore, the test taker should select this as the correct answer.

## Inflammatory Bowel Disease (IBD)

13. 1. The colon is ulcerated and unable to absorb water, resulting in bloody diarrhea. Ten to 20 bloody diarrhea stools are the most common symptom of ulcerative colitis.
   2. Inflammation and dehydration can cause a low-grade temperature elevation but this is not an expected finding in the client diagnosed with ulcerative colitis.
   3. A hard, rigid abdomen indicates peritonitis, which is a complication of ulcerative colitis but not an expected symptom.
   4. Stress incontinence is not a symptom of colitis.

**TEST-TAKING HINT:** If the test taker is not sure of the answer, the test taker should use knowledge of anatomy and physiology to help identify the correct answer. The colon is responsible for absorbing water, and if the colon can't do its job, then water will not be absorbed, causing diarrhea (option "1"). Colitis is inflammation of the colon; therefore, option "4" referring to the urinary system can be eliminated.

14. 1. Steroids can cause erosion of the stomach and should be taken with food.
   2. A moon face is an expected side effect of steroids.
   3. Prednisone, a steroid, must be tapered off to prevent adrenal insufficiency; therefore, the client must take this medication as prescribed.
   4. Steroids may increase the client's blood glucose, but diabetic medication regimens are usually not altered for the short period of time the client, diagnosed with an acute exacerbation, is prescribed steroids.

**TEST-TAKING HINT:** The test taker should know few medications must be taken on an empty stomach, which would cause option "1" to be eliminated. All medications should be taken as prescribed—don't think the answer is too easy.

15. 1. The HCP should be notified so potassium supplements can be ordered, but this is not the first intervention.
   2. Muscle weakness may be a clinical manifestation of hypokalemia; hypokalemia can lead to cardiac dysrhythmias and can be life-threatening. Assessment is a priority for a potassium level just below the normal level, which is 3.5 to 5.3 mEq/L.
   3. Hypokalemia can lead to cardiac dysrhythmias; therefore, requesting telemetry is appropriate, but it is not the first intervention.
   4. The client will need potassium to correct the hypokalemia, but it is not the first intervention.

**TEST-TAKING HINT:** When the question asks which action should be implemented first, remember assessment is the first step in the nursing process. If the answer option addressing assessment is appropriate for the situation in the question, then the test taker should select it as the correct answer.

16. 1. The client's bowel should be placed on rest, and no foods or fluids should be introduced into the bowel.
   2. Whenever a client has an acute exacerbation of a gastrointestinal disorder,

the first intervention is to place the bowel on rest. The client should be NPO with intravenous fluids to prevent dehydration.

3. The vital signs must be taken more often than daily in a client having an acute exacerbation of ulcerative colitis.

4. The client will receive anti-inflammatory and antidiarrheal medications, not antacids, which are used for gastroenteritis.

**TEST-TAKING HINT:** "Acute exacerbation" is the key phrase in the stem of the question. The word "acute" should cause the test taker to eliminate any daily intervention.

17. 1. TPN is high in dextrose, which is glucose; therefore, the client's blood glucose level must be monitored closely.

2. The client may be on sliding-scale regular insulin coverage for the high glucose level.

3. The TPN must be administered via a central line in the subclavian vein because of the high glucose level.

4. The client is NPO to put the bowel at rest, which is the rationale for administering the TPN.

**TEST-TAKING HINT:** The test taker may want to select option "3" because it has the word "assess," but the test taker should remember to note the adjective "peripheral," which makes this option incorrect. Remember, the words "check" and "monitor" are words meaning "assess."

18. 1. Weighing the client each day will help identify if the client is experiencing malnutrition, but it is not the priority intervention during an acute exacerbation.

2. Coping strategies help develop healthy ways to deal with this chronic disease, which has remissions and exacerbations, but it is not the priority intervention.

3. **The severity of diarrhea helps determine the need for fluid replacement. The liquid stool should be measured as part of the total output.**

4. The client will be NPO when there is an acute exacerbation of IBD to allow the bowel to rest.

**TEST-TAKING HINT:** The test taker can apply Maslow's hierarchy of needs and select the option addressing a physiological need.

19. 1. The nurse should never state an understanding of what the client is going through.

2. Telling the client to think about the good things is not addressing the client's feelings.

3. **The client is crying and is expressing feelings of powerlessness; therefore, the nurse should allow the client to talk.**

4. The client is crying and states, "I can't take it anymore," but this is not a suicidal comment or situation.

**TEST-TAKING HINT:** There are rules applied to therapeutic responses. Do not say "understand" and do not ask "why." The test taker should select an option where some type of feeling is being reflected in the statement.

20. 1. A pink and moist stoma indicates viable tissue and adequate circulation. A purple stoma indicates necrosis.

2. **An ileostomy will drain liquid all the time and should not routinely be irrigated. A sigmoid colostomy may need daily irrigation to evacuate feces.**

3. A red, bumpy, itchy rash indicates infection with the yeast *Candida albicans*, which should be treated with medication.

4. The ileostomy drainage has enzymes and bile salts, which are irritating and harsh to the skin; therefore, the pouch should be changed if any leakage occurs.

**TEST-TAKING HINT:** This is an "except" question, and the test taker must identify which option is not a correct action for the nurse to implement. Sometimes flipping the question—"Which interventions indicate the client understands the teaching?"—can assist in identifying the correct answer.

21. 1. Sulfasalazine (Azulfidine), a disease-modifying antirheumatic drug (DMARD), cannot be administered rectally. Mesalamine, a similar gastrointestinal anti-inflammatory, can be given by mouth, enema, or rectally. Corticosteroids may be administered by enema for the local effect of decreasing inflammation while minimizing the systemic effects.

2. Antidiarrheal agents slow the gastrointestinal motility and reduce diarrhea.

3. IBD is not caused by bacteria.

4. **Sulfasalazine (Azulfidine), a DMARD, acts topically on the colonic mucosa to inhibit the inflammatory process.**

**TEST-TAKING HINT:** If the test taker doesn't know the answer, then the test taker could eliminate options "2" and "3" because they do not contain the word "inflammation"; IBD is inflammatory bowel disease.

22. 1. The terminal ileum is the most common site for Crohn's disease (previously called regional enteritis), which causes right lower quadrant pain.
2. Stools are liquid or semiformed and usually do not contain blood.
3. Episodes of diarrhea and constipation may be a clinical manifestation of colon cancer, not Crohn's disease.
4. A fever and hard, rigid abdomen are clinical manifestations of peritonitis, a complication of Crohn's disease.

**TEST-TAKING HINT:** The test taker should eliminate option "2" because of the word "all," which is an absolute. There are very few absolutes in the health-care arena.

23. 1. Fried potatoes, along with pastries and pies, should be avoided.
2. Raw vegetables should be avoided because they are hard to digest.
3. A low-residue diet is a low-fiber diet. Products made of refined flour or finely milled grains, along with roasted, baked, or broiled meats, are recommended.
4. Fried foods should be avoided, and whole grains are high in fiber. Nuts and fruits with peels should be avoided.

**TEST-TAKING HINT:** The test taker must know about therapeutic diets prescribed by HCPs. Remember, a low-residue diet is the same as low fiber.

24. 1. The cure for ulcerative colitis is a proctocolectomy, which is removing the entire large colon and rectum and bringing the terminal end of the ileum up to the abdomen in the right lower quadrant. A continent ileostomy (Koch or Kock pouch) has a reservoir that is emptied by inserting a catheter into the stoma.
2. This site is the left lower quadrant.
3. This site is the transverse colon.
4. This site is the right upper quadrant.

**TEST-TAKING HINT:** The test taker must identify the area by using the computer mouse. These are called "hot spots" on the NCLEX-RN®.

## Peptic Ulcer Disease

25. 1. The presence of blood does not specifically indicate the diagnosis of an ulcer. The client could have hemorrhoids or cancer, resulting in the presence of blood.
2. A wavelike burning sensation is a symptom of gastroesophageal reflux.

3. Sharp pain in the upper abdomen after eating a heavy meal is a symptom of gallbladder disease.
4. In a client diagnosed with a gastric ulcer, the pain usually occurs shortly after eating a meal. In contrast, a client diagnosed with a duodenal ulcer has pain beginning 2 to 3 hours after meals that is often relieved by eating. A duodenal ulcer often causes pain during the night due to nocturnal gastric acid secretion.

**TEST-TAKING HINT:** This question asks the test taker to identify assessment data specific to the disease process. Many diseases have similar symptoms, but the timing of symptoms or their location may help rule out some diseases and provide the HCP with a key to diagnose a specific disease—in this case, peptic ulcer disease. Nurses are usually the major source of information for the health-care team.

26. 1. The EGD, or upper GI endoscopy, is an invasive diagnostic test that visualizes the esophagus, stomach, and duodenum to diagnose an ulcer accurately and evaluate the effectiveness of the client's treatment.
2. An MRI shows cross-sectional images of tissue or blood flow.
3. An occult blood test shows the presence of blood but not the source.
4. A gastric acid stimulation test is used to understand the pathophysiology of ulcer disease and evaluate gastric fluid, but it is not a definitive diagnosis for ulcers (Van Leeuwen & Bladh, 2017).

**TEST-TAKING HINT:** If the test taker has no idea what the correct answer is, knowledge of anatomy can help identify the answer. A peptic ulcer is an ulcer in the stomach, and in option "1" the word "esophagogastroduodenoscopy" has "gastro," which refers to the stomach. Therefore, this would be the best option to select as the correct answer.

27. 1. A history of problems the client has experienced with medications is taken during the admission interview. This information does not specifically address peptic ulcer disease.
2. The use of NSAIDs places the client at risk for peptic ulcer disease and hemorrhage. NSAIDs suppress the production of prostaglandin in the stomach, which is a protective mechanism to prevent damage from hydrochloric acid.
3. Allergies are included for safety, but this is not specific for peptic ulcer disease.

4. Information needs to be obtained about past generations so the nurse can analyze any potential health problems, but this is not specific for peptic ulcer disease.

**TEST-TAKING HINT: The words "specific data" indicate there will be appropriate data in one or more of the answer options, but only one is specific to peptic ulcer disease.**

28. 1. **Auscultation should be used before palpation or percussion when assessing the abdomen. Manipulation of the abdomen can alter bowel sounds and give false information.**
    2. Palpation gives appropriate information the nurse needs to collect, but if done before auscultation, the sounds will be altered.
    3. Percussion of the abdomen does not give specific information about peptic ulcer disease.
    4. Tender areas should be assessed last to prevent guarding and altering the assessment. This includes palpation, which should be done after auscultation.

**TEST-TAKING HINT: The word "first" requires the test taker to rank in order the interventions needing to be performed. The test taker should visualize caring for the client. This will assist the test taker in making the correct choice.**

29. 1. There is no indication from the question there is a problem or potential problem with bowel elimination.
    2. Knowledge deficit does not address physiological complications.
    3. This client may have problems from changing roles within the family, but the question asks for potential physiological complications, not psychosocial problems.
    4. **Potential for alteration in gastric emptying is caused by edema or scarring associated with an ulcer, which may cause a feeling of "fullness," vomiting of undigested food, or abdominal distention.**

**TEST-TAKING HINT: This question asks the test taker to identify a physiological problem identifying a complication of the disease process. Therefore, options "2" and "3" could be eliminated because they do not address physiological problems.**

30. Correct answers are 3 and 4.
    1. A pain assessment is an independent intervention the nurse should implement frequently.
    2. Evaluating vital signs is an independent intervention the nurse should implement.

If the client is able, BPs should be taken lying, sitting, and standing to assess for orthostatic hypotension.
3. **This is a collaborative intervention the nurse should implement. It requires an order from the HCP.**
4. **Administering blood products is collaborative, requiring an order from the HCP.**
5. The diet requires an order by the HCP, but a diet will not be ordered because the client is NPO.

**TEST-TAKING HINT: Descriptive words such as "collaborative" or "independent" can be the deciding factor when determining if an answer option is correct or incorrect. These are key-words the test taker should identify.**

31. 1. Use of NSAIDs increases and causes problems associated with peptic ulcer disease.
    2. **Maintaining lifestyle changes such as following an appropriate diet and reducing stress indicates the client is complying with the medical regimen. Compliance is the goal of treatment to prevent complications.**
    3. Hemoptysis is coughing up blood, which is not a clinical manifestation of peptic ulcer disease. This would not be an expected outcome.
    4. Antacids should be taken 1 to 3 hours after meals, not with each meal.

**TEST-TAKING HINT: Expected outcomes are positive completion of goals; maintaining lifestyle modifications would be an appropriate goal for any client diagnosed with any chronic illness.**

32. 1. The range for normoactive bowel sounds is from 5 to 35 times per minute. This would require no intervention.
    2. Belching after a heavy, fatty meal is a symptom of gallbladder disease. Eating late at night may cause symptoms of esophageal disorders.
    3. **A decrease of 20 mmHg in BP after changing position from lying to sitting to standing is orthostatic hypotension. This could indicate the client is bleeding.**
    4. A decrease in the quality and quantity of discomfort shows an improvement in the client's condition. This would not require further intervention.

**TEST-TAKING HINT: When the question asks about further intervention, the test taker should examine the answer options for an unexpected outcome requiring further assessment.**

33. 1. Celecoxib (Celebrex) is an NSAID used to treat arthritis. NSAIDs can cause irritation to the stomach, and the use by a client diagnosed with peptic ulcer disease should be questioned.
    2. Prilosec, a proton pump inhibitor, decreases gastric acid production, and its use should not be questioned by the nurse.
    3. Metronidazole (Flagyl), an antimicrobial, is administered to treat peptic ulcer disease secondary to *H. pylori* bacteria.
    4. Acetaminophen (Tylenol), a nonnarcotic analgesic, can be safely administered to a client diagnosed with peptic ulcer disease.

**TEST-TAKING HINT:** The test taker needs to understand how medications work, adverse effects of medications, when to question administering a specific medication, and how to administer the medication safely. By learning classifications, the test taker should be able to make a knowledgeable selection in most cases.

34. 1. Decreasing alcohol intake indicates the client is making some lifestyle changes.
    2. The client diagnosed with PUD is prescribed a regular diet, but the type of diet does not determine if the medication is effective.
    3. The return to previous activities indicates the client has not adapted to the lifestyle changes and has returned to the previous behaviors, which precipitated the peptic ulcer disease.
    4. Antibiotics, proton pump inhibitors, and bismuth subsalicylate (Pepto-Bismol) are administered to decrease the irritation of the ulcerative area and cure the ulcer. A decrease in gastric distress indicates the medication is effective.

**TEST-TAKING HINT:** To determine the effectiveness of a medication, the test taker must know the scientific rationale for administering the medication. Peptic ulcer disease causes gastric distress. If gastric distress is relieved, then the medication is effective.

35. 1. Sudden sharp pain felt in the back, chest, and upper body indicates angina or myocardial infarction.
    2. A rigid, boardlike abdomen with rebound tenderness is the classic clinical manifestation of peritonitis, which is a complication of a perforated gastric ulcer.
    3. Clay-colored stools indicate liver disorders, such as hepatitis.
    4. Clients diagnosed with gallbladder disease report vague to sharp abdominal pain in the right upper quadrant.

**TEST-TAKING HINT:** The only two answer options that refer to the abdomen are options "2" and "4." Therefore, the test taker should select one of these two because a gastric ulcer involves the stomach.

36. 1. Maintaining a strict record of intake and output is important to evaluate the progression of the client's condition, but it is not the most important intervention.
    2. Inserting a nasogastric tube and lavaging the stomach with saline is the most important intervention because this removes blood and may slow the bleeding (Hoffman & Sullivan, 2020).
    3. A calorie count is important information assisting in the prevention and treatment of a nutritional deficit, but this intervention does not address the client's immediate and life-threatening problem.
    4. Promoting a quiet environment aids in the reduction of stress, which can cause further bleeding, but this will not stop the bleeding.

**TEST-TAKING HINT:** The test taker is required to rank the importance of interventions in the question. Using Maslow's hierarchy of needs to rank physiological needs first, the test taker should realize inserting a nasogastric tube and beginning lavage is solving a circulation or fluid deficit problem.

## Colorectal Disease

37. Correct answers are 2 and 5.
    1. Some cancers have a higher risk of development when the client is occupationally exposed to chemicals, but cancer of the colon is not one of them.
    2. Cruciferous vegetables, such as broccoli, cauliflower, and cabbage, are high in fiber. One of the risks for cancer of the colon is a high-fat, low-fiber, and high-protein diet. The longer the transit time (the time from ingestion of the food to the elimination of the waste products), the greater the chance of developing cancer of the colon.
    3. A multivitamin may improve immune system function, but it does not prevent colon cancer.
    4. High-risk sexual behavior places the client at risk for sexually transmitted diseases.

A history of multiple sexual partners and initial sexual experience at an early age does increase the risk for the development of cancer of the cervix in females.

5. Smoking and tobacco use are risk factors for many disease processes, including the development of colorectal cancer.

**TEST-TAKING HINT:** The colon processes waste products from eating foods, and option "2" is the only option to mention food. Therefore, option "2" would be an option to select. Option "5" discusses smoking and tobacco use, which is a common risk factor for many diseases.

38. 1. Frequent bloody stools are a symptom of IBD. IBD is a risk factor for cancer of the colon, but the symptoms are different when the colon becomes cancerous.
    2. Most people have a feeling of fullness after a heavy meal; this does not indicate cancer.
    3. **The most common symptom of colon cancer is a change in bowel habits, specifically, diarrhea alternating with constipation.**
    4. Lower right quadrant pain with rebound tenderness would indicate appendicitis.

**TEST-TAKING HINT:** The test taker could eliminate option "4" based on anatomical position. The rectosigmoid colon is in the left lower quadrant.

39. 1. **A long history of low-fiber, high-fat, and high-protein diets results in prolonged transit time. This allows the carcinogenic agents in the waste products to have greater exposure to the lumen of the colon.**
    2. The older the client, the greater the risk of developing cancer of the colon.
    3. Risk factors for cancer of the colon include increasing age, family history of colon cancer or polyps, a history of IBD, obesity, cigarette and alcohol use, and eating a high-fat, high-protein, low-fiber diet.
    4. Males have a slightly higher incidence of colon cancers than do females.

**TEST-TAKING HINT:** The test taker should realize cancers, in general, have an increasing incidence with age. Cancer etiologies are not an exact science, but most cancers have some risk factor if only advancing age.

40. **Correct answers are 1, 3, and 5.**
    1. **Colostomy stomas are openings through the abdominal wall into the colon, through which feces exit the body. Feces can be irritating to**
    the abdominal skin, so careful and thorough skin care is needed.
    2. There are midline and perineal incisions, not flank incisions.
    3. **The client will have an indwelling catheter to monitor the urine output after surgery, assessing renal perfusion.**
    4. Jackson Pratt drains are emptied every shift, but they are not irrigated.
    5. **The client should not sit upright because this causes pressure on the perineum.**

**TEST-TAKING HINT:** The test taker could eliminate option "2" because flank and abdominal perineal are not in the same areas. This is an alternative-type question requiring the test taker to choose more than one option.

41. 1. **The stoma should be light to a medium pink, the color of the intestines. A blue or purple color indicates a lack of circulation to the stoma and is a medical emergency.**
    2. The stoma should be pouched securely for the client to be able to participate in normal daily activities. The client should be encouraged to ambulate to aid in recovery.
    3. Pain medication should be taken before the pain level reaches a "5." Delaying taking medication will delay the onset of pain relief, and the client will not receive full benefit from the medication.
    4. The pouch should be emptied when it is one-third to one-half full to prevent the contents from becoming too heavy for the seal to hold and to prevent leakage from occurring.

**TEST-TAKING HINT:** Normal mucosa is pink, not white, and clients are always encouraged to ambulate after surgery to prevent the complications related to immobility. Remember basic concepts when answering questions, especially about postoperative nursing care.

42. 1. **The nurse should mark the drainage on the dressing to determine if active bleeding is occurring because dark reddish-brown drainage indicates old blood. This allows the nurse to assess what is actually happening.**
    2. Surgical dressings are initially changed by the surgeon; the nurse should not remove the dressing until the surgeon orders the dressing change to be done by the nurse.
    3. The nurse should assess the situation before notifying the HCP.
    4. The nurse may need to reinforce the dressing if the dressing becomes saturated, but this would be after a thorough assessment is completed.

**TEST-TAKING HINT:** The question is asking the test taker to determine which intervention must be implemented first, and assessment is the first step of the nursing process. Options "2," "3," and "4" would not be implemented before assessing. Marking the dressing allows the nurse to assess the dressing and determine if active bleeding is occurring.

43. 1. The nurse should first assess the situation before informing the HCP of the client's concerns and then allow the HCP and client to discuss the situation.
    2. The nurse should determine what is concerning the client. It could be a misunderstanding or a real situation where the client's care is unsafe or inadequate.
    3. If a new HCP is to be arranged, it is the HCP's responsibility to arrange for another HCP to assume responsibility for the care of the client.
    4. The choice of HCP is ultimately the client's. If the HCP cannot arrange for another HCP, the client may be discharged and obtain a new HCP.

**TEST-TAKING HINT:** The nurse should assess the situation; the first step in the nursing process is assessment.

44. 1. If the tissue around the stoma becomes excoriated, the client will be unable to pouch the stoma adequately, resulting in discomfort and leakage. The client understands the teaching.
    2. **The client should be on a regular diet, and the colostomy will have been working for several days before discharge. The client's statement indicates the need for further teaching.**
    3. Until the incision is completely healed, the client should not sit in bathwater because of the potential contamination of the wound by the bathwater. The client understands the teaching.
    4. The client has had major surgery and should limit lifting to minimal weight. The client understands the teaching.

**TEST-TAKING HINT:** This is an abdominal surgery, and all instructions for major surgery apply. This is an "except" question; therefore, three options would indicate the client understands the teaching.

45. 85 mL/hr.
    First, determine the total amount to be infused over 24 hours:

$$1500 + 500 + 20 + 20 = 2,040 \text{ mL over } 24 \text{ hours}$$

Then, determine the rate per hour:

$$2,040 \div 24 = 85 \text{ mL/hr}$$

**TEST-TAKING HINT:** Check and recheck calculations. The division should be carried out to the second or third decimal place before rounding.

46. 1. A digital rectal examination is done to detect prostate cancer and should be started at age 40 years.
    2. "Middle age" is a relative term; specific ages are used for recommendations. At the age of 45 years, the American Cancer Society (2018) recommends a fecal occult blood test every year.
    3. **The American Cancer Society recommends a colonoscopy at age 45 and every 10 years thereafter for people at average risk of colorectal cancer. Screening can be performed with a stool-based test at more frequent intervals (American Cancer Society, 2018).**
    4. A stool-based test is an option for persons at low risk of colon cancer, beginning at 45 years old. A fecal immunochemical test is done yearly, and a multitargeted stool DNA test (MT-sDNA) is done every 3 years.

**TEST-TAKING HINT:** A digital examination is an examination performed by the examiner's finger and does not examine the entire colon.

47. 1. Intimacy involves more than sexual intercourse. The client can be sexually active whenever the wounds are healed sufficiently not to cause pain.
    2. This is an appropriate nursing intervention for home care, but it has nothing to do with sexual activity.
    3. The nurse is not a sexual counselor and would not have these types of charts. The nurse should address sexuality with the client but would not be considered an expert capable of explaining the advantages and disadvantages of sexual positioning.
    4. **A pouch that becomes dislodged during the sexual act would cause embarrassment for the client with body image issues already.**

**TEST-TAKING HINT:** Option "2" does not address the issue, and option "3" is outside of the nurse's professional expertise. Option "1" could be eliminated because of the word "no," which is an absolute word.

48. 1. The client will need to have diagnostic tests, so this is an appropriate intervention.
    2. The client with an intestinal blockage will need to be hydrated.

3. This client has an intestinal blockage from a solid tumor blocking the colon. Although the client needs to be cleaned out for the colonoscopy, polyethylene glycol (GoLYTELY) could cause severe cramping without a reasonable benefit to the client and could cause a medical emergency.

4. Tap water enemas until clear would be instilling water from below the tumor to try to rid the colon of any feces. The client can expel this water.

**TEST-TAKING HINT:** The stem states a "complete blockage," which indicates the client needs surgery. Therefore, options "1" and "2" are appropriate for surgery. The stem asks the test taker which order would be questioned, so this is an "except" question.

## Diverticulosis and Diverticulitis

49. 1. These are classic clinical manifestations of diverticulitis; therefore, the HCP does not need to be notified.

2. These are normal findings for a client diagnosed with diverticulitis, but on admission, the nurse should assess the client and document the findings in the client's EHR.

3. The nurse should not administer any food or medications.

4. The nurse should assess the client to determine if the abdomen is soft and nontender. A rigid tender abdomen may indicate peritonitis.

**TEST-TAKING HINT:** The test taker must remember to apply the nursing process when answering test questions. Assessment is the first step in the nursing process. Although the clinical manifestations are normal and could be documented, the nurse should always assess.

50. 1. The client should drink at least 3,000 mL of water daily to help prevent constipation.

2. The client should exercise daily to help prevent constipation.

3. The client should eat a high-fiber diet to help prevent constipation.

4. The client should have regular bowel movements. Frequency of bowel movements varies by individual, but daily or every 2 days is common. Constipation may cause diverticulitis, which is a potentially life-threatening complication of diverticulosis.

**TEST-TAKING HINT:** The test taker must be careful to distinguish between -*osis* and -*itis*. Diverticulosis is the condition of having small pouches in the colon, and preventing constipation is the most important action the client can take to prevent diverticulitis (inflammation of the diverticulum).

51. 1. The client will have a nasogastric tube because the client will be NPO, which will decompress the bowel and remove hydrochloric acid.

2. Preventing dehydration is a priority with the NPO client.

3. The nurse should question a clear liquid diet because the bowel must be put on total rest, which means NPO.

4. The client is in severe pain and should be on bedrest, which will help rest the bowel.

**TEST-TAKING HINT:** This is an "except" question. Therefore, the test taker must identify which answer option is incorrect for the stem. Sometimes flipping the question helps in selecting the correct answer. In this question, the test taker could ask, "Which HCP orders would be expected for a client diagnosed with diverticulitis?" The unexpected option would be the correct answer.

52. 1. Fried foods increase cholesterol. Mashed potatoes do not have the peel, which is needed for increased fiber.

2. Applesauce does not have the peel, which is needed for increased fiber, and the option does not identify which type of bread; whole milk is high in fat.

3. Chicken salad, which has vegetables such as celery, grapes, and apples, and whole-wheat bread are high in fiber, which is the therapeutic diet prescribed for clients diagnosed with diverticulosis. An adequate intake of water helps prevent constipation.

4. Tomatoes and cucumbers have seeds, and many HCPs recommend clients diagnosed with diverticulosis avoid seeds because of the possibility of the seeds entering the diverticulum and becoming trapped, leading to peritonitis.

**TEST-TAKING HINT:** The test taker must know a high-fiber diet is prescribed for diverticulosis, and at least five to six foods are encouraged or discouraged for the different types of diets. High-fiber foods are foods with peels (potato, apple) and whole-wheat products.

53. 1. The client's abdomen should be soft and nontender; therefore, this finding would not require immediate intervention.
2. The client had to clean the bowel before the colonoscopy; therefore, the watery stool is expected.
3. The client was NPO and received bowel preparation before the colonoscopy; therefore, hyperactive bowel sounds might occur and do not warrant immediate intervention.
4. Bowel perforation is a potential complication of a colonoscopy. Therefore, clinical manifestations of hypotension—decreased BP and increased pulse—warrant immediate intervention from the nurse.

**TEST-TAKING HINT:** This is an "except" question. The test taker is being asked to select which data are abnormal for a procedure. The test taker should remember any invasive procedure could possibly lead to hemorrhaging, and signs of shock should always be considered a possible correct answer.

54. 1. Peak and trough levels are drawn after the client has received at least three to four doses of medication, not after the initial dose because the client has just been admitted.
2. The nurse should always ask about allergies to any medication when administering medications, but especially when administering antibiotics, which are notorious for allergic reactions.
3. The peak and trough levels are not drawn before the first dose; they are ordered after multiple doses.
4. The nurse should question when to administer the medication, but there is no vital sign preventing the nurse from administering an antibiotic.

**TEST-TAKING HINT:** The test taker must read the stem closely to realize the client is receiving the initial dose, causing the test taker to eliminate options "1" and "3" as possible correct answers. Both options "2" and "4" are assessment data, but the test taker should ask which one will directly affect the administration of the medication.

55. 1. These are signs of peritonitis, which is life-threatening. The HCP should be notified immediately.
2. A sodium phosphate (Fleet's) enema will not help a life-threatening complication of diverticulitis.

3. A medication administered to help decrease the client's temperature will not help a life-threatening complication.
4. These are clinical manifestations indicating a possible life-threatening situation and require immediate intervention.

**TEST-TAKING HINT:** In most instances, the test taker should not select the option stating to notify the HCP immediately, but in some situations, it is the correct answer. The test taker should look at all the other options and determine if the option is information the HCP requires or if it is an independent intervention that will help the client.

56. 42 gtts/min.
The nurse must use the formula:

$$\frac{\text{amount to be infused} \times \text{drops per minute}}{\text{minutes for infusion}}$$

$$\frac{250 \text{ mL} \times 10 \text{ gtts}}{60 \text{ minutes}}$$

or, 2,500 ÷ 60 minutes = 41.66 gtts/min, which should be rounded up to 42 gtts/min.

**TEST-TAKING HINT:** The test taker must know how to calculate dosage and understand calculation questions. Remember to use the drop-down calculator if needed; the test taker can ask for an erase slate during state board examinations.

57. 1. Green bile contains hydrochloric acid and should be draining from the NG tube; therefore, the nurse should take no action and document the findings.
2. There is no reason for the nurse to assess the client's bowel sounds because the drainage is normal.
3. The client's last bowel movement would not affect the NG tube drainage.
4. Bile draining from the NG tube indicates the tube is in the stomach, and there is no need to advance the tube farther.

**TEST-TAKING HINT:** The test taker must know what drainage is normal for tubes inserted into the body. Any type of blood or coffee-ground drainage would be abnormal and require intervention by the nurse.

58. Correct answers are 1, 2, and 4.
1. A high-fiber diet will help to prevent constipation, which is the primary reason for diverticulitis.
2. Increased fluids will help keep the stool soft and prevent constipation.
3. This will not do anything to help prevent diverticulitis.
4. Exercise will help prevent constipation.

5. No medications are prescribed to prevent an acute exacerbation of diverticulitis. Antacids are used to neutralize hydrochloric acid in the stomach.

**TEST-TAKING HINT: This is an alternate-type question where the test taker must select more than one option. To correctly identify the answers, the test taker should think about what part of the GI system is affected. Knowing diverticulosis occurs in the sigmoid colon would help eliminate options "3" and "5" because these would be secondary to stomach disorders.**

59. 1. A sedentary lifestyle may lead to obesity and contribute to hypertension or heart disease but usually not to diverticulosis.
    2. Multiple childbirths are not a risk factor for developing diverticulosis.
    3. Hemorrhoids would indicate the client has chronic constipation, which is a strong risk factor for diverticulosis. Constipation increases the intraluminal pressure in the sigmoid colon, leading to weakness in the intestinal lining, which, in turn, causes outpouchings, or diverticula.
    4. Family history is not a risk factor. Having daily bowel movements and preventing constipation will decrease the chance of developing diverticulosis.

**TEST-TAKING HINT: The test taker must know constipation is the leading risk factor for diverticulosis, and if the test taker knows hemorrhoids are caused by constipation, it would lead the test taker to select option "3" as the correct answer.**

60. 1. Total parenteral nutrition is not an expected order for this client.
    2. The bowel must be put at rest. Therefore, the nurse should anticipate orders for maintaining the client NPO and a nasogastric tube.
    3. These orders would be instituted when the client is getting better, and the bowel is not inflamed.
    4. Surgery is not the first consideration when the client is admitted to the hospital.

**TEST-TAKING HINT: "Collaborative" means the nurse must care for the client with another discipline, and the HCP would have to order all of the distracters. The test taker should remember food and fluid probably should be stopped in the client diagnosed with lower gastrointestinal problems.**

## Gallbladder Disorders

61. 1. After abdominal surgery, it is not uncommon for bowel sounds to be absent.
    2. This is a normal amount and color of drainage.
    3. The minimum urine output is 30 mL/hr.
    4. Refusing to turn, cough, and deep breathe places the client at risk for pneumonia, and the client is already at increased risk for complications due to morbid obesity. This client needs immediate intervention to prevent complications.

**TEST-TAKING HINT: The test taker should recognize normal data such as the normal urine output and normal data for postoperative clients. The test taker should apply basic concepts when answering questions. Normal or expected outcomes do not require action.**

62. 1. A heating pad should be applied for 15 to 20 minutes to assist the migration of the $CO_2$ used to insufflate the abdomen. Shoulder pain is an expected occurrence.
    2. Morphine sulfate does not affect the etiology of the pain.
    3. The surgeon would not order an x-ray for this condition.
    4. There is no indication an injury occurred during surgery. A sling would not benefit the migration of the $CO_2$. Shoulder pain is expected.

**TEST-TAKING HINT: The test taker must understand laparoscopic surgery to be able to answer this question. Option "4" could be eliminated because of the phrase "injured during surgery."**

63. 1 This surgery does not require lipid-lowering medications, but eating high-fat meals may cause discomfort.
    2. After the removal of the gallbladder, some clients experience abdominal discomfort when eating fatty foods.
    3. Laparoscopic cholecystectomy surgeries are performed in day surgery, and clients usually do not need assistance for a week.
    4. Using a pillow to splint the abdomen provides support for the incision and should be continued after discharge.

**TEST-TAKING HINT: When answering questions stating, "teaching is effective," the test taker should look for the correct information. Basic concepts should help the test taker answer questions, and because pain often occurs after surgeries, option "2" would probably be a correct answer.**

64. Correct answers are 1, 2, 3, and 5.
    1. Clay-colored stools are caused by recurring stricture of the common bile duct, which is a clinical manifestation of postcholecystectomy syndrome.
    2. Yellow-tinted sclera and skin indicate residual effects of a stricture of the common bile duct, which is a clinical manifestation of postcholecystectomy syndrome.
    3. Dark-colored urine could indicate a bile duct block in postcholecystectomy syndrome.
    4. An approximated incision is intact and does not warrant intervention by the nurse.
    5. Abdominal pain indicates a residual effect of a stricture of the common bile duct, inflammation, or calculi, which is a clinical manifestation of postcholecystectomy syndrome.

**TEST-TAKING HINT:** The test taker must use knowledge of anatomy to answer this question. All answer options have something to do with the abdominal area, and the common bile duct is anatomically near the hepatic duct, which causes liver clinical manifestations.

65. 1. This is an assessment and cannot be delegated.
    2. This intervention would require nursing judgment, and increasing IV fluid is medication administration; neither task can be delegated.
    3. A day surgery client can be ambulated to the bathroom, so this task can be delegated to the UAP.
    4. This would require assessment and cannot be delegated.

**TEST-TAKING HINT:** The RN cannot delegate teaching, assessing, medication administration, and evaluating or any task for an unstable client to a UAP.

66. 1. A UGI series requires the client to swallow barium, which passes through the intestines, making the stools a chalky white color.
    2. Increased heart rate is abnormal data and would be cause for further assessment.
    3. A firm, hard abdomen is not expected from the UGI series.
    4. Hyperactive bowel sounds are not an expected sequela of a UGI series.

**TEST-TAKING HINT:** Option "2" could be eliminated because it does not have anything to do with the gastrointestinal system. A firm, hard abdomen is seldom ever expected, so option "3" could be eliminated.

67. 1. Asking the client to cough forcefully may irritate the client's throat.
    2. Early ambulation does not enhance safety because the client will be sedated.
    3. The ERCP requires an anesthetic spray be used before insertion of the endoscope. If medications, food, or fluid are given orally before the return of the gag reflex, the client may aspirate.
    4. Medications are not administered until the gag reflex has returned.

**TEST-TAKING HINT:** The test taker must notice adjectives such as "endoscopic," which means the procedure includes going down the mouth; option "3" is the only option that has anything to do with the mouth. Selecting a distracter addressing assessment would be appropriate because assessment is the first step of the nursing process.

68. 1. The expected outcome is pain control for both preoperative and postoperative care.
    2. Postoperative care includes ambulation.
    3. Prevention of additional impaired skin integrity is a desired postoperative outcome. The incision would be a break in skin integrity.
    4. This would be an expected outcome for the client scheduled for surgery. This indicates preoperative teaching has been effective.

**TEST-TAKING HINT:** The time element is important in this question. The expected outcome is required for the preoperative period. Option "1" is incorrect because of the adjective "decreased." Adjectives commonly determine the accuracy of the options.

69. 1. An increased pulse is expected for the client in acute pain.
    2. An open cholecystectomy requires a large incision under the diaphragm. Deep breathing places pressure on the diaphragm and the incision, causing pain. Shallow respirations indicate inadequate pain control, and the nurse should intervene.
    3. Twenty bowel sounds a minute is normal data and does not require further action.
    4. Splinting the abdomen allows the client to increase the strength of the cough by increasing comfort and does not indicate a need for pain medication.

**TEST-TAKING HINT:** The stem asks which data would warrant pain medication. Therefore, the test taker should select an answer not expected or not normal for clients postoperative abdominal surgery.

70. 1. The WBC should be elevated in clients diagnosed with chronic inflammation.
    2. A decreased LDH indicates liver abnormalities.
    3. An elevated alkaline phosphatase indicates liver abnormalities.
    4. A decreased bilirubin indicates an obstructive process.

**TEST-TAKING HINT: If the test taker does not know what the values mean, the test taker should look to the disease process. The -*itis* means inflammation, and an educated guess would be elevated WBCs in an inflammatory process.**

71. 1. Alteration in nutrition may be an appropriate client problem, but it is not the priority.
    2. Alteration in skin integrity may be an appropriate client problem but is not the priority.
    3. Alteration in urinary elimination may be an appropriate client problem but is not the priority.
    4. Acute pain management is the highest priority client problem after surgery because pain may indicate a life-threatening problem.

**TEST-TAKING HINT: When a question asks for the highest priority problem, the test taker should look for a life-threatening complication. Pain may be expected, but it may indicate a complication.**

72. 1. Measuring the abdominal girth helps further assess internal bleeding, not external bleeding.
    2. Palpating the lower abdomen assesses the bladder, not bleeding.
    3. **Turning the client to the side to assess the amount of drainage and possible bleeding is important before contacting the surgeon.**
    4. The first dressing change is usually done by the surgeon; the nurse can reinforce the dressing.

**TEST-TAKING HINT: The adjectives "large" and "red" indicate the client is bleeding, and assessment is always a priority when the client is having a possible complication of surgery. Remember, assessment is the first step in the nursing process.**

## Liver Disease

73. Correct answers are 1, 2, 3, and 5.
    1. The client should be placed in a lateral position, and the HOB elevated to protect the client's airway.
    2. The client must not be left unattended in case the bleeding becomes active. This is a safety issue as esophageal bleeding can be life-threatening.
    3. A Yankauer suction catheter should be kept at the bedside in case it is needed to prevent aspiration.
    4. Lactulose (Chronulac), a laxative, is administered to decrease the ammonia level, but the question does not say the client's ammonia level is elevated.
    5. Clients with esophageal bleeding should have frequent vital signs, including oxygen saturation and cardiac monitoring.

**TEST-TAKING HINT: The test taker should select the options directly related to client safety. Option "4" is the only action not expected in an emergent situation; therefore, this option could be eliminated, containing the word "all," but in some instances, it may be the correct answer.**

74. Correct answers are 3 and 5.
    1. The client should empty the bladder immediately before the liver biopsy, not after the procedure.
    2. Foods and fluids are usually withheld 2 hours after the biopsy, after which the client can resume the usual diet.
    3. **Direct pressure is applied to the site, and then the client is placed on the right side to maintain site pressure.**
    4. BUN and creatinine levels are monitored for kidney function, not liver function, and the renal system is not affected by a liver biopsy.
    5. **The client's level of consciousness and vital signs should be assessed every 15 minutes for the first hour after the liver biopsy. Changes in the level of consciousness and a decrease in BP can indicate bleeding.**

**TEST-TAKING HINT: The adjective "postprocedure" should help the test taker rule out option "1." Knowing the anatomical position of the liver should help the test taker select option "3" as a correct answer. The test taker must know laboratory data for each organ, which helps rule out option "4" as a possible correct answer. Option "5" is standard postprocedure care.**

75. 1. Sodium is restricted to reduce ascites and generalized edema, not for hepatic encephalopathy.
    2. Fluids are calculated based on diuretic therapy, urine output, and serum electrolyte values; fluids do not affect hepatic encephalopathy.
    3. A diet high in calories and moderate in fat intake is recommended to promote healing.
    4. Ammonia is a by-product of protein metabolism and contributes to hepatic encephalopathy. Reducing protein intake should decrease ammonia levels. Research indicates that a diet higher in vegetable protein than animal protein is preferred (Nguyen & Morgan, 2014).

**TEST-TAKING HINT:** The test taker could eliminate options "1" and "2" based on the knowledge sodium and water work together and address edema, not encephalopathy. The test taker's knowledge of biochemistry—protein breaks down to ammonia, carbohydrates break down to glucose, and fat breaks down to ketones—may be helpful in selecting the correct answer.

76. 1. The procedure is done in the client's room, with the client seated either on the side of the bed or in a chair.
    2. The client should empty the bladder before the procedure to avoid bladder puncture, but there is no need for an indwelling catheter to be inserted.
    3. The client is at risk for hypovolemia; therefore, vital signs will be assessed frequently to monitor for clinical manifestations of hemorrhaging.
    4. The client does not have to hold the breath when the catheter is inserted into the peritoneum; this is done when obtaining a liver biopsy.

**TEST-TAKING HINT:** If the test taker had no idea what the answer is, knowing vital signs are assessed after all procedures should make the test taker select this option.

77. 1. Hot water increases pruritus, and soap will cause dry skin, which increases pruritus; therefore, the RN should discuss this with the UAP.
    2. Applying emollient lotion will help prevent dry skin, which will help decrease pruritus; therefore, this would not require any intervention by the nurse.
    3. Mittens will help prevent the client from scratching the skin and causing skin breakdown. This would not require intervention by the nurse.

4. The skin should be patted dry, not rubbed, because rubbing the skin will cause increased irritation. This action does not require intervention by the nurse.

**TEST-TAKING HINT:** A concept accepted for most clients during morning care is not to use hot water because it causes dilation of vessels, which may cause orthostatic hypotension. This is not the rationale for avoiding the use of hot water for a client with pruritus, but sometimes the test taker can apply broad concepts when answering questions.

78. 1. Two kilograms is more than 4 pounds, which indicates severe fluid retention and is not an appropriate goal.
    2. Excess fluid volume could be secondary to portal hypertension. Therefore, no increase in abdominal girth would be an appropriate short-term goal, indicating no excess of fluid volume.
    3. Vital signs are appropriate to monitor, but they do not yield specific information about fluid volume status.
    4. Having the client receive a low-sodium diet does not ensure the client will comply with the diet. The short-term goal must evaluate if the fluid volume is within normal limits.

**TEST-TAKING HINT:** Remember, goals evaluate the interventions; therefore, option "4" could be eliminated as the correct answer because it is an intervention, not a goal. Short-term weight fluctuations tend to reflect fluid balance, and any weight gain in 24 hours indicates retention of fluid, which is not an appropriate goal.

79. Correct answers are 1, 2, 3, and 4.
    1. Vitamin K deficiency causes impaired coagulation; therefore, rectal thermometers should be avoided to prevent bleeding.
    2. Soft-bristle toothbrushes will help prevent bleeding of the gums.
    3. Platelet count, partial thromboplastin time/prothrombin time (PTT/PT), and INR should be monitored to assess coagulation status.
    4. Injections should be avoided, if at all possible, because the client is unable to clot, but if they are absolutely necessary, the nurse should use small-gauge needles.
    5. Asterixis is a flapping tremor of the hands when the arms are extended and indicates an elevated ammonia level not associated with vitamin K deficiency.

**TEST-TAKING HINT: The test taker must know the function of specific vitamins. Vitamin K is responsible for blood clotting. This is an alternate-type question, which requires the test taker to select all applicable interventions; the test taker should select interventions addressing bleeding.**

80. 1. Hypoalbuminemia (decreased albumin) and muscle wasting are metabolic effects, not gastrointestinal effects.
    2. Oligomenorrhea is no menses, which is a reproductive effect, and decreased body hair is an integumentary effect.
    3. **Clay-colored stools and hemorrhoids are gastrointestinal effects of liver failure.**
    4. Dyspnea is a respiratory effect, and caput medusae (dilated veins around the umbilicus) is an integumentary effect, although it is on the abdomen.

**TEST-TAKING HINT: The adjective "gastrointestinal" is the keyword guiding the test taker to select the correct answer. The test taker must rule out options not addressing gastrointestinal symptoms. Although liver failure affects every body system, the question asks for a gastrointestinal effect.**

81. 1. It really doesn't matter how long the client has been drinking alcohol. The diagnosis of alcoholic cirrhosis indicates the client has probably been drinking for many years.
    2. An advance directive is important for the client diagnosed with a terminal illness, but it is not the priority question.
    3. **The nurse must know when the client had the last alcoholic drink to be able to determine when and if the client will experience delirium tremens, the physical withdrawal from alcohol.**
    4. This is not a typical question asked by the nurse unless the client is malnourished, which is not information provided in the stem.

**TEST-TAKING HINT: Because the word "alcohol" is in the stem of the question, if the test taker has no idea what the correct answer is, the test taker should select an option with the word "alcohol" in it and look closely at options "1" and "3."**

82. 1. **Blood in the intestinal tract is digested as a protein, which increases serum ammonia levels and increases the risk of developing hepatic encephalopathy.**
    2. Decreased albumin causes the client to develop ascites.

3. An enlarged spleen increases the rate at which red blood cells (RBCs), WBCs, and platelets are destroyed, causing the client to develop anemia, leukopenia, and thrombocytopenia, but not hepatic encephalopathy.
4. An increase in aldosterone causes sodium and water retention, resulting in the development of ascites and generalized edema.

**TEST-TAKING HINT: Some questions require the test taker to have specific knowledge to be able to identify the correct answer. This is one of those questions.**

83. 1. This is a therapeutic response and is used to encourage the client to verbalize feelings but does not provide factual information.
    2. This is passing the buck; the nurse should be able to answer this question.
    3. **This is the main reason the HCP decreases the client's medication dose and is an explanation appropriate for the client.**
    4. This is the medical explanation as to why the medication dose is decreased, but it should not be used to explain to a layperson.

**TEST-TAKING HINT: The test taker should provide factual information when the client asks "why." Therefore, options "1" and "2" could be eliminated as possible correct answers. Both options "3" and "4" explain the rationale for decreasing the medication dose, but the nurse should answer in terms the client can understand. Would a layperson know what "half-life" means?**

84. 1. Two to three soft stools a day indicates the laxative lactulose (Chronulac) is effective.
    2. There is no instrument used at home to test daily ammonia levels. A new ammonia in the breath measurement device is currently in development and is not FDA approved. At this time, the ammonia level is a serum level requiring venipuncture and laboratory diagnostic equipment.
    3. Diarrhea indicates an overdosage of the laxative lactulose (Chronulac), possibly requiring the dosage to be decreased. The HCP needs to make this change in dosage, so the client understands the teaching.
    4. The client should check the stool for bright red blood as well as a dark, tarry stool.

**TEST-TAKING HINT: This is an "except" question. The test taker must realize three options indicate an understanding of the teaching. If**

the test taker does not know the answer, notice that all the options except "2" have something to do with stool, and laxative affects the stool.

## Hepatitis

85. 1. Clay-colored stools and jaundice occur in the icteric phase of hepatitis.
    2. Normal appetite and itching occur in the icteric phase of hepatitis.
    3. Fever subsides in the icteric phase, and the pain is in the right upper quadrant.
    4. "Flu-like" symptoms are the first reports of the client diagnosed with the preicteric phase of hepatitis, which is the initial phase and may begin abruptly or insidiously.

**TEST-TAKING HINT:** The test taker must use anatomy knowledge in ruling out incorrect answers; option "3" could be ruled out because the liver is in the right upper quadrant.

86. 1. The hepatitis A virus is in the stool of infected people and takes up to 2 weeks before symptoms develop.
    2. Hepatitis B virus is spread through contact with infected blood and body fluids.
    3. Hepatitis C virus is transmitted through infected blood and body fluids.
    4. Hepatitis D virus only causes infection in people also infected with hepatitis B.

**TEST-TAKING HINT:** This is a knowledge question; the nurse must be aware of how the various types of hepatitis viruses are transmitted.

87. 1. Airborne precautions are required for transmission occurring by the dissemination of either airborne droplet nuclei or dust particles containing the infectious agent.
    2. Standard precautions apply to blood, all body fluids, secretions, and excretions, except sweat, regardless of whether they contain visible blood.
    3. Droplet transmission involves contact of the conjunctivae of the eyes or mucous membranes of the nose or mouth with large-particle droplets generated during coughing, sneezing, talking, or suctioning.
    4. Exposure precautions is not a designated isolation category.

**TEST-TAKING HINT:** The test taker must know standard precautions are used by all health-care workers having direct contact with clients or with their body fluids or have indirect contact with objects used by infected clients, such as would be involved in emptying trash, changing linens, or cleaning the room.

88. 1. Eating after each other should be discouraged, but it is not the most important intervention.
    2. Only bottled water should be consumed in developing countries, but this precaution is not necessary for American high schools.
    3. Hepatitis B and C, not hepatitis A, are transmitted by sexual activity.
    4. **Hepatitis A is transmitted via the fecal-oral route. Good handwashing helps to prevent its spread. Singing the "happy birthday" song takes approximately 20 seconds, which is how long an individual should wash hands (Centers for Disease Control and Prevention, 2019).**

**TEST-TAKING HINT:** The test taker must realize good hand washing is the most important action in preventing transmission of the hepatitis A virus. Often, the test taker will not select the answer option that seems too easy—but remember, do not overlook the obvious.

89. 1. The client must avoid alcohol altogether, not decrease intake, to prevent further liver damage and promote healing.
    2. **Adequate rest is needed for maintaining optimal immune function.**
    3. Clients are more often anorexic and nauseated in the afternoon and evening; therefore, the main meal should be in the morning.
    4. Diet drinks and juices provide few calories, and the client needs an increased-calorie diet for healing.

**TEST-TAKING HINT:** The test taker must be aware of keywords in both the stem and answer options. The "icteric" phase means the acute phase. The word "decrease" should cause the test taker to eliminate option "1" as a possible correct answer, and "large" should cause the test taker to eliminate "3" as a possible correct answer.

90. Correct answers are 1, 2, and 3.
    1. **Hepatitis B can be transmitted by sharing any type of needles, especially those used by drug abusers.**
    2. **Hepatitis B can be transmitted through sexual activity; therefore, the nurse should recommend abstinence, mutual monogamy, or barrier protection.**
    3. **Three doses of hepatitis B vaccine provide immunity in 90% of healthy adults.**
    4. Immune globulin injections are administered as postexposure prophylaxis (after

being exposed to hepatitis B), but encouraging these injections is not a health promotion activity.

5. Hepatotoxic medications should be avoided in clients diagnosed with hepatitis or who have had hepatitis. The HCP prescribes medications, and the layperson does not know which medications are hepatotoxic.

**TEST-TAKING HINT: In this "Select all that apply" type of question, there may be only one correct answer, there may be several, or all five options may be correct answers.**

91. 1. This is a therapeutic response, and the nurse should provide factual information.
    2. Milk thistle has an active ingredient, silymarin, which has been commonly used to treat liver disease. The efficacy of milk thistle in the treatment of hepatitis B is controversial (Hepatitis B Foundation, 2019).
    3. The nurse should not discourage complementary therapies.
    4. This is a judgmental statement, and the nurse should encourage the client to ask questions.

**TEST-TAKING HINT: The test taker may not have any idea what milk thistle is but should apply test-taking strategies, including not selecting options with "why" unless interviewing the client. Only use therapeutic responses when unable to provide factual information. At times, the test taker may not like any answer option but should always apply the rules to help determine the correct answer.**

92. 1. Sufficient energy is required for healing. Adequate carbohydrate intake can spare protein. An energy content of 35 to 40 kcal/kg/day will help restore and maintain nutritional status and enhance liver regeneration.
    2. TPN is not routinely prescribed for the client diagnosed with hepatitis; the client must lose a large amount of weight and be unable to eat anything for TPN to be ordered.
    3. Salt intake does not affect the healing of the liver.
    4. Water intake does not affect the healing of the liver, and the client should not drink so much water as to decrease caloric food intake.

**TEST-TAKING HINT: The test taker should key in on "less than body requirements" in the stem and select the answer option addressing increasing calories, which eliminates options "3" and "4."**

93. 1. The nurse must notify the infection control nurse as soon as possible, so treatment can start if needed, but this is not the first intervention.
    2. **The nurse should first clean the needle stick site with soap and water and attempt to "milk" the area to encourage bleeding to help remove any virus injected into the skin.**
    3. Postexposure prophylaxis may be needed, but this is not the first action.
    4. The infection control and employee health nurse will determine the client needle recipient status before the nurse contaminated needle stick incident.

**TEST-TAKING HINT: The question requires the test taker to identify the first intervention. The test taker should think about which intervention will directly help the nurse—and that is to clean the area.**

94. 1. The serum ammonia level is increased in liver failure, but it is not the cause of clay-colored stools.
    2. **Bilirubin, the by-product of red blood cell destruction, is metabolized in the liver and excreted via the feces, which causes the feces to be brown in color. If the liver is damaged, the bilirubin is excreted via the urine and skin.**
    3. The liver excretes bile into the gallbladder, and the body uses the bile to digest fat, but it does not affect the feces.
    4. Vitamin deficiency, resulting from the liver's inability to detoxify vitamins, may cause steatorrhea, but it does not cause clay-colored stool.

**TEST-TAKING HINT: The test taker should have a grasp of physiology to help answer this question. Clay-colored stool indicates no color in the feces. Because the color in the feces is caused by bilirubin, lack of color would be the result of the liver's inability to excrete bilirubin.**

95. 1. The client should avoid alcohol to prevent further liver damage and promote healing.
    2. Rest is needed for the healing of the liver and to promote optimum immune function.
    3. Clients diagnosed with hepatitis need increased caloric intake, so this is a good statement.
    4. **The client needs to understand some types of cough syrup have alcohol, and all alcohol must be avoided to prevent further injury to the liver; therefore, this statement requires intervention.**

**TEST-TAKING HINT:** If the test taker did not know the answer, the test taker could apply the rule of avoiding any OTC medications unless approved by an HCP.

96. 1. The laboratory technician draws serum blood studies, not the UAP.
    2. The UAP can obtain the intake and output, but the RN must evaluate the data to determine if the results are normal for the client's disease process or condition.
    3. The UAP can perform a bedside glucometer check, but the RN must evaluate the result and determine any action needed.
    4. The unit clerk has specific training that allows the transcribing of HCP orders.

**TEST-TAKING HINT:** The test taker must be knowledgeable of delegation rules; the nurse cannot delegate assessing, teaching, medication administration, evaluating, and any task for an unstable client.

## Gastroenteritis

97. 1. The client would be taking antidiarrheal medication, not medications to stimulate bowel movements.
    2. The client probably has traveler's diarrhea, and oral rehydration is the preferred choice for replacing fluids lost as a result of diarrhea. An oral glucose electrolyte solution, such as Gatorade, All-Sport, or Pedialyte, is recommended.
    3. The client should be encouraged to stay on liquids and eat bland foods of all three food groups—carbohydrates, proteins, and fats.
    4. There is no need for the client to weigh daily. Symptoms usually resolve within 2 to 3 days without complications.

**TEST-TAKING HINT:** Be sure to note the adjectives and adverbs in the stem and the answer options, such as "cathartic" laxative and weigh "daily." These words are very often important in ruling out answers and identifying the correct answer.

98. 1. Well-cooked meat will help prevent gastroenteritis secondary to staphylococcal food poisoning.
    2. Refrigerating dairy products will help prevent gastroenteritis secondary to eating foods kept at room temperature, causing staphylococcal food poisoning.
    3. Drinking bottled water will help prevent gastroenteritis secondary to *Escherichia coli* found in contaminated water.
    4. Any discolored food, food from a damaged can or jar, or food from a can or jar not having a tight seal should be destroyed without tasting or touching it.

**TEST-TAKING HINT:** The test taker should be careful with words such as "all," "only," and "never"; few absolutes exist in the health-care field.

99. 1. Symptoms develop 6 hours to 6 days after ingesting the *Salmonella* bacteria and include diarrhea, abdominal cramping, nausea, and vomiting, along with a low-grade fever (CDC, 2019).
    2. Neuromuscular paralysis and dysphagia occur with botulism, a severe life-threatening form of food poisoning caused by *C. botulinum*.
    3. Gross explosive bloody diarrhea is a clinical manifestation of hemorrhagic colitis caused by *E. coli*.
    4. Gray cloudy diarrhea with no fecal odor, blood, or pus is caused by cholera, which is endemic in parts of Asia, the Middle East, and Africa.

**TEST-TAKING HINT:** Often when two options have the same clinical manifestation, such as diarrhea and stool, this should make the test taker realize either one of these two options is correct, so the other two options can be eliminated, or both are incorrect.

100. 1. The normal serum sodium level is 135 to 145 mEq/L; therefore, an intervention by the nurse is not needed.
    2. These are normal arterial blood gas results; therefore, the nurse would not need to intervene.
    3. In gastroenteritis, diarrhea often results in metabolic acidosis and loss of potassium. The normal serum potassium level is 3.5 to 5.3 mEq/L; therefore, a level of 3.3 mEq/L would require immediate intervention. Hypokalemia can lead to life-threatening cardiac dysrhythmias.
    4. A stool specimen showing fecal leukocytes supports the diagnosis of gastroenteritis and does not warrant immediate intervention by the nurse.

**TEST-TAKING HINT:** The test taker should read the stem and be certain what the question is asking—in this case, which data require "immediate intervention"? Therefore, the test taker is identifying an answer not normal for the disease process.

**101.** Correct answers are 2 and 5.
  1. If diarrhea persists more than 48 hours, the client should notify the HCP. Diarrhea for more than 96 hours could lead to metabolic acidosis, hypokalemia, and possible death.
  2. **Washing hands should be done by the client at all times, but especially when the client has gastroenteritis. The bacteria in feces may be transferred to other people via food if hands are not washed properly.**
  3. Steroids are not used in the treatment of gastroenteritis; antidiarrheal medication is usually prescribed.
  4. The client may be asked to provide a stool specimen for culture, ova, parasites, and fecal leukocytes, but the client is not asked for a 24-hour stool collection.
  5. **The client should be instructed to drink clear fluids or electrolyte solutions to replace lost fluids and prevent dehydration.**

**TEST-TAKING HINT: If the test taker did not know any of the answers to this question, hand washing should be selected because it is the number-one intervention for preventing any type of contamination or nosocomial infection.**

**102.**
  1. Antidiarrheal medications are contraindicated with botulism because the toxin needs to be expelled from the body.
  2. Aminoglycoside antibiotics will not be ordered because there is no bacterium with botulism; it is caused by a neurotoxin.
  3. A botulism antitoxin neutralizes the circulating toxin and is prescribed for a client diagnosed with botulism.
  4. An angiotensin-converting enzyme (ACE) inhibitor is prescribed for a client diagnosed with cardiovascular disease.

**TEST-TAKING HINT: The keyword in this question is "treat." Because botulism does not end in -*itis*, and thus is not an infection, the use of an antibiotic can be eliminated.**

**103.**
  1. Fluid volume deficit secondary to diarrhea is the priority because of the potential for metabolic acidosis and hypokalemia, which are both life-threatening, especially in older clients.
  2. Nausea may occur, but it is not the priority. However, excessive vomiting could lead to potential complications.

  3. Acute pain secondary to abdominal cramping may occur, but it is not the priority.
  4. Impaired urinary elimination is not a priority. The client has diarrhea, not urine output problems.

**TEST-TAKING HINT: Always notice the client's age because it is usually a significant clue as to the correct answer. Prioritizing questions may have more than one potential appropriate nursing problem, but only one has priority. Remember Maslow's hierarchy of needs.**

**104.**
  1. The client would have increased gurgling sounds, revealing hyperactive bowel movements.
  2. A hard, firm, edematous abdomen is not expected in a client diagnosed with gastroenteritis; this would indicate a possible complication and require further assessment.
  3. The client has increased liquid bowel movements (diarrhea) but should not have blood in the stool, which is the definition of melena.
  4. **Borborygmi, or loud, rushing bowel sounds, indicates increased peristalsis, which occurs in clients diagnosed with diarrhea and is the primary clinical manifestation in a client diagnosed with acute gastroenteritis.**

**TEST-TAKING HINT: The test taker should realize that, in an acute condition, the assessment data would be abnormal, which may help select the correct answer for some questions.**

**105.**
  1. The UAP can calculate the client's intake and output, but the nurse must evaluate the data to determine if it is normal for the elderly client diagnosed with acute gastroenteritis.
  2. The UAP can take the vital signs for a stable client; the nurse must interpret and evaluate the vital signs.
  3. The UAP cannot administer medications, and IV solutions are considered to be medications.
  4. **The nurse cannot delegate assessment. The client may have an excoriated perianal area secondary to diarrhea; therefore, the nurse should assess the client.**

**TEST-TAKING HINT: The nurse should not delegate any nursing task requiring judgment or assessment and cannot delegate the administration of medications. Words such as "evaluate" mean the same thing as "assess"; therefore, options "1," "3," and "4" can be eliminated.**

106. 1. Leg cramps could indicate hypokalemia, which is a potential complication of excessive diarrhea and should be reported to the HCP.
    2. The client should increase fluid intake because oral rehydration is the primary treatment for gastroenteritis to replace lost fluid as a result of diarrhea and to prevent dehydration.
    3. Reintroducing solid foods slowly, in small amounts, will allow the bowel to rest and the mucosa to return to normal functioning after acute gastroenteritis.
    4. Bottled water should be consumed when contaminated water is suspected, and an oral glucose electrolyte solution, such as Gatorade or Pedialyte, should be recommended.

**TEST-TAKING HINT:** Both options "2" and "4" refer to fluids, which should make the test taker either eliminate both of these or select from one of these two as the right answer.

107. Correct answers are 2, 4, and 5.
    1. The nurse should assess skin turgor over the sternum in the older client because the loss of subcutaneous fat associated with aging makes skin turgor assessment on the arms less reliable.
    2. Orthostatic hypotension indicates fluid volume deficit, which can occur in an older client having many episodes of diarrhea.
    3. The nurse should record the frequency and characteristics of stool, not sputum, in the client diagnosed with gastroenteritis.
    4. Standard precautions, including wearing gloves and hand washing, help prevent the spread of the infection to others.
    5. The older client is at risk for orthostatic hypotension; therefore, safety precautions should be instituted to ensure the client doesn't fall as a result of a decrease in BP.

**TEST-TAKING HINT:** This is an alternate-type question requiring the test taker to choose all interventions that apply. The test taker should look at each option and consider if this is an intervention for an "older" client. Older people are a special population, usually requiring specific interventions addressing the aging process no matter what the disease process.

108. 1. Epigastric pain is expected in a client diagnosed with peptic ulcer disease.
    2. Four diarrheal stools are not unusual in a client diagnosed with gastroenteritis.

3. Tented skin turgor and dry mucous membranes indicate dehydration, which warrants the nurse assessing this client first.
4. Vomiting is expected in a client diagnosed with food poisoning.

**TEST-TAKING HINT:** When managing clients, the nurse must be able to prioritize care. Therefore, the test taker must be able to determine which client's reports or clinical manifestations are not expected of the disease process. The test taker should always look at the client's age because it may help determine the best answer.

## Abdominal Surgery

109. 1. Absent bowel sounds indicate a paralytic ileus, not peritonitis, and the potassium level is within normal limits (3.5 to 5.3 mEq/L).
    2. Abdominal cramping would not make the nurse suspect peritonitis, and the hemoglobin is normal (male 14 to 17 g/dL, female 11.7 to 15.5 g/dL).
    3. *Campylobacter* is a cause of profuse diarrhea, but it does not support a diagnosis of peritonitis.
    4. A hard, rigid abdomen indicates an inflamed peritoneum (abdominal wall cavity) resulting from an infection, which results in an elevated WBC level.

**TEST-TAKING HINT:** The -*itis* of peritonitis means inflammation, and if the test taker has no idea what the answer is, an elevated WBC count should provide the key to selecting option "4" as the correct answer.

110. 1. The nurse may notify the surgeon if warranted, but it is not the first intervention.
    2. The nurse should instruct the client to splint the incision when coughing, then take further action.
    3. Assessing the surgical incision is the first intervention because this may indicate the client has wound dehiscence.
    4. The nurse should never administer pain medication without assessing for potential complications.

**TEST-TAKING HINT:** The stem is asking which intervention is first. This means all four answer options could be possible actions, but only one is first. The test taker should use the nursing process and select the option addressing assessment because it is the first step in the nursing process.

111. 1. The client has a surgical incision, which impairs the skin integrity, but it is not the priority because it is sutured under sterile conditions.
2. After abdominal surgery, the body distributes fluids to the affected area as part of the healing process. These fluids are shifted from the intravascular compartment to the interstitial space, which causes potential fluid and electrolyte imbalance.
3. Bowel elimination is a problem, but after general anesthesia wears off, the bowel sounds will return, and this is not a life-threatening problem.
4. Psychosocial problems are not a priority over actual physiological problems.

**TEST-TAKING HINT:** When identifying priority problems, the test taker can eliminate any psychosocial problem as a potentially correct answer if there are applicable physiological problems.

112. 1. Evisceration is a life-threatening condition in which the abdominal contents protrude through the ruptured incision. The nurse must protect the bowel from the environment by placing a sterile normal saline gauze on it, which prevents the intestines from drying out and necrosing.
2. The nurse should not attempt to replace the protruding bowel.
3. This position places the client with the HOB elevated, which will make the situation worse.
4. Antibiotics will not protect the protruding bowels, which must be the priority. Antibiotics will be administered at a later time to prevent infection, but this is not urgent.

**TEST-TAKING HINT:** The test taker must understand the word "evisceration" to answer this question.

113. 1. The client needing more pain medication indicates the client's condition is getting worse.
2. Coffee-ground material indicates old blood from the gastrointestinal system.
3. Because the clinical manifestations of peritonitis are elevated temperature and rigid abdomen, a reversal of these clinical manifestations indicates the client is getting better.
4. Two soft-formed bowel movements are normal, but this does not have anything to do with peritonitis.

**TEST-TAKING HINT:** The -*itis* of peritonitis means inflammation, which is associated with an elevated temperature. A decrease in temperature would be a sign the client is improving.

114. 1. The client is NPO; therefore, no medication would be administered.
2. The client is NPO, so no food or fluids are allowed.
3. Deep breathing will help prevent pulmonary complications but does not address the client's paralytic ileus.
4. A paralytic ileus is the absence of peristalsis; therefore, the bowel will be unable to process any oral intake. A nasogastric tube is inserted to decompress the bowel until surgical intervention or until bowel sounds return spontaneously.

**TEST-TAKING HINT:** If the test taker realizes the stem of the question says part of the gastrointestinal system, the ileus, is paralyzed, the test taker should know allowing the client to take anything by mouth would be an inappropriate action, so options "1" and "2" could be eliminated. Deep breathing addresses the respiratory system, not the gastrointestinal system, so option "3" could also be eliminated.

115. 1. The JP bulb should be depressed, which indicates suction is being applied. A round bulb indicates the bulb is full and needs to be emptied, and suction reapplied.
2. The tube should be taped to the dressing to prevent accidentally pulling the drain out of the insertion site.
3. The insertion site should be pink and without any clinical manifestations of infection, which include drainage, warmth, and redness.
4. The JP bulb should be sunken in or depressed, indicating suction is being applied.

**TEST-TAKING HINT:** The stem is asking which data need intervention by the nurse. Option "2" can be ruled out because all tubes and drains should be secured. A pink insertion site with no drainage is expected, which would cause the test taker to eliminate option "3" as a possible correct answer.

116. 1. Medicating the client with an analgesic could increase the client's nausea unless the nausea is caused by pain. The nurse should assess the etiology to determine the interventions.
    2. The stem indicates the client has had abdominal surgery and gastric decompression is in place, which is a nasogastric (NG) tube. If the NG tube is not patent, this will cause nausea. Irrigating the NG tube may relieve nausea.
    3. Checking the temperature will not treat nausea.
    4. Hyperextending the neck will assist the client to breathe but will not treat nausea.

**TEST-TAKING HINT: Assessment is the first step in the nursing process. Checking the NG tube for patency and taking the temperature are the only assessment interventions. Temperature does not correlate with nausea. Medication may be administered, but it would be an antiemetic, not a narcotic analgesic.**

117. 1. The nurse cannot force the client to do anything; this would be considered assault.
    2. There are no data to support the need for a chest x-ray.
    3. Shallow respirations and refusal to deep breathe could be the result of abdominal pain. The nurse should assess the client for pain and determine the last time the PCA pump was used.
    4. Based on the information given, the client does not need oxygen.

**TEST-TAKING HINT: If the test taker is unsure of the answer, identifying keywords in the stem—"abdominal surgery" and "PCA"— should guide the test taker to select an option related to one of these keywords. "Determine" can be substituted for the word "assess," which is the first step of the nursing process.**

118. 170 mL/hr.
    The NG tube drainage of 45 mL must be added to the 125 mL/hr IV rate, which equals 170 (125 + 45 = 170). The nurse should infuse 170 mL in the next hour.

**TEST-TAKING HINT: The stem states the previous hour's NG tube output plus the baseline IV rate. The test taker must observe the keywords in the stem. Don't forget to use the drop-down calculator when taking the NCLEX-RN®.**

119. 1. A client not voiding within 4 hours after any surgery is not a priority. This is an acceptable occurrence, but if the client hasn't voided for 8 hours, then the nurse should assess further.
    2. A sudden cessation of pain may indicate a ruptured appendix, which could lead to peritonitis, a life-threatening complication; therefore, the nurse should assess this client first.
    3. Bowel sounds should return within 24 hours after abdominal surgery. Absent bowel sounds at 4 hours postoperative are not of great concern to the nurse.
    4. The client being discharged is stable and not a priority for the nurse.

**TEST-TAKING HINT: The stem is asking which client the nurse should see first. Therefore, the test taker should look for life-threatening or serious complications or abnormal assessment data for the disease process.**

120. 1. The last bowel movement does not help identify the cause of the client's right lower abdominal pain. This might be appropriate for a client with left lower abdominal pain.
    2. Information about a high-fat meal would be asked if the nurse suspected the client had a gallbladder problem.
    3. An older client may experience a ruptured appendix with minimal pain; therefore, the nurse should assess the characteristics of the pain.
    4. The passage of flatus (gas) does not help determine the cause of right lower abdominal pain.

**TEST-TAKING HINT: The test taker should go back to basics and assess the client.**

## Eating Disorders

121. 1. This client is 5'10" tall and weighs 99 pounds (45 kg × 2.2 = 99). Menses will cease if the client is severely emaciated. A 24-hour dietary recall is a step toward assessing the client's eating patterns.
    2. The type of birth control could be asked, but the client is asking about missing menstrual periods. Birth control does not interfere with having a period; if anything, some forms of birth control will make the cycles more regular.

3. The nurse can look at the client and see a very thin young woman, which should confirm more assessment is needed, not reweighing.
4. The pulse and BP will not provide the nurse any information as to why the client's menstrual cycles have ceased.

**TEST-TAKING HINT:** The stem of the question provides information about the client's height and weight, and the test taker must determine if this is important information. Information in the stem must be eliminated as not pertinent to the question or closely regarded to let the test taker know what the question is asking.

122. 1. Many clients jog 1 to 2 miles per day as part of their exercise program. This does not indicate bulimia.
2. Not gaining weight may be an end result of bulimia, but it does not identify bulimia.
3. Bulimia is characterized by bingeing and purging by inducing vomiting after a meal. Stomach contents are acidic, and the acid wears away the enamel on the teeth, leaving the teeth a green color.
4. The client has calluses on the knuckles from pushing them into the throat to induce vomiting.

**TEST-TAKING HINT:** The question requires the nurse to be knowledgeable regarding the clinical manifestations of bulimia. Vomiting should lead the test taker to green teeth secondary to hydrochloric acid.

123. 1. Clients diagnosed with bulimia will eat the entire meal and more food if available. This is not unusual behavior for a client diagnosed with bulimia.
2. By having someone stay with the client for 45 minutes to 1 hour after a meal, the client will be prevented from inducing vomiting and ridding the body of the meal before it can be metabolized.
3. Clients diagnosed with anorexia nervosa tend to overexercise to prevent weight gain and to lose imagined excess weight.
4. Bedrest is not needed for this client.

**TEST-TAKING HINT:** The test taker must be able to differentiate between bulimia and anorexia. It can be difficult to keep these processes separate, especially because some clients have both anorexia and bulimia.

124. 1. The goal is written in terms of client behavior; this option is a nursing intervention, not a client goal.
2. Eating 50% of meals provided does not address low self-esteem.
3. High-protein shakes are a dietary intervention.
4. The problem of "low self-esteem" requires the client to verbalize psychosocial feelings. Identifying one positive attribute is an appropriate goal.

**TEST-TAKING HINT:** The test taker could eliminate distracter "3" as a health-care discipline intervention. Psychosocial problems require goals addressing a nonphysiological need.

125. 1. The client is 67 inches tall (5′7″) and weighs 88 pounds (40 kg × 2.2 = 88). This client is severely underweight, and nutrition is the priority.
2. Clients diagnosed with anorexia have a chronic low self-esteem problem, but this is a psychosocial problem, and actual physical problems are the priority.
3. Disturbed body image is a psychosocial problem manifested in a physical one. The physical problem is the priority; this would be an appropriate long-term goal.
4. This client thinks her body is not appealing and this could be a problem, but it is a psychosocial issue and not the priority.

**TEST-TAKING HINT:** The test taker must decide which problem is the priority when all the problems could apply to the client. Unless the client is considering suicide and has a plan to carry it out, physical problems are the priority.

126. 1. The client diagnosed with anorexia will have muscle tissue wasting; liver function tests will not monitor for this.
2. Kidney function tests will not monitor nutrition or muscle wasting.
3. The heart is a muscle; in severe anorexia (more than 60% under ideal body weight), muscle tissue is catabolized to provide energy to the body. The client is at risk of death from cardiac complications.
4. The client's entire body will be involved in the process as a result of malnutrition, but bone density tests are not done.

**TEST-TAKING HINT:** The test taker needs to be aware of the complications associated with specific disease processes.

127. 1. The client does not owe the nurse an explanation.
2. If the HCP determines it is safe for the client to exercise, a gymnasium might be recommended, but walking is the best exercise, and this can be done in the neighborhood or at an enclosed shopping mall.
3. The client should set realistic weight loss goals. A realistic weight loss goal is 1 to 1½ pounds per week, but this should be done after assessing the client.
4. Determining the client's eating patterns and what triggers the client to eat—stress or boredom, for example—and where and when the client consumes most of the calories—snacking in front of the TV at night, for example—is needed to assist the client in changing eating behaviors.

**TEST-TAKING HINT: This question is an example of using the nursing process to arrive at the correct answer. Assessing the client has priority.**

128. 1. The morbidly obese client will have a large abdomen, preventing the lungs from expanding, which predisposes the client to respiratory complications.
2. The client may be weighed daily, but this is not the priority.
3. The client should be taught proper nutrition for weight loss, but this is not the priority in the immediate postoperative period.
4. This is very important for the long term, but respiratory status is the priority.

**TEST-TAKING HINT: Regardless of the procedure or the size of the client, respiratory status is the priority in the immediate postoperative period. The test taker should apply Maslow's hierarchy of needs.**

129. Correct answers are 2 and 5.
1. Exercise recommendations for weight loss are to exercise for 30 minutes at least three times per week, not three times a day.
2. The client should be aware of situations triggering the consumption of food when the client is not hungry, such as anger, boredom, and stress. Food-seeking behaviors are not associated only with hunger for obese clients.
3. The client should weigh about once a week. If weight loss is not observed, the

client becomes discouraged and feels powerless to control the weight. This can lead to diet failure.
4. Sodium is limited in clients diagnosed with hypertension, not obesity.
5. Weight loss support groups such as Weight Watchers or Take Off Pounds Sensibly (TOPS) are helpful in keeping the client participating in a weight loss program.

**TEST-TAKING HINT: This is an alternate-type question. The test taker must judge each answer option for itself; one option does not eliminate another. The NCLEX-RN® gives credit for the entire question. The test taker must identify all the right answers, or the answer will be counted as incorrect.**

130. Correct answers are 2 and 5.
1. Jogging is not an appropriate exercise for obese clients: there is too much stress on the heart and joints.
2. If lifestyle behaviors such as patterns of eating and daily exercise are not modified, the client losing weight will regain weight and usually more.
3. The client should eat frequent small meals during the day to keep from being hungry. Breakfast should not be skipped.
4. Diets containing fewer than 1,200 calories per day need to be supplemented with a multivitamin to provide the body with the nutrients needed to stay healthy.
5. Drinking water 30 minutes before each meal decreases calorie consumption and leads to greater weight loss (Dennis et al., 2010).

**TEST-TAKING HINT: The test taker could eliminate answer option "4" because health-care professionals should not discourage health promotion activities.**

131. 1. The client does not have to explain her actions to the nurse; the nurse should not ask "why."
2. Telling the client she is skinny is belittling the client.
3. The client is 36 years old and has the right to refuse to eat, even to the detriment of her body. Restraining the client could be considered assault unless the psychiatric team had a court order.
4. "Might cause physical problems" is a factual statement to the client about the possible results if the client refuses nourishment.

**TEST-TAKING HINT:** The test taker could eliminate answer option "1" based on "why." Option "2" is not therapeutic or factual information.

132. 1. Clients diagnosed with anorexia exercise excessively; clients diagnosed with bulimia do not.
   2. Clients diagnosed with bulimia frequently take cathartic laxatives to prevent the absorption of calories from the food consumed.
   3. Clients diagnosed with bulimia and anorexia have low self-esteem. The client feels ugly or unlovable if overweight (self-perception).
   4. High-fiber foods do help the body to produce larger stools, but this client would use a cathartic laxative.

**TEST-TAKING HINT:** The test taker must distinguish between bulimia and anorexia to answer this question. Clients diagnosed with anorexia are usually underweight, whereas clients diagnosed with bulimia may be of normal or slightly larger size.

## Constipation and Diarrhea Disorders

133. 1. An antidiarrheal medication would slow down the peristalsis in the colon, worsening the problem.
   2. The client has an immediate need to evacuate the bowel, not a need for bowel training.
   3. Oil retention enemas will help to soften the feces and evacuate the stool.
   4. A UGI series adds barium to the already hardened stool in the colon. Barium enemas x-ray the colon; a UGI series x-rays the stomach and jejunum.

**TEST-TAKING HINT:** If the test taker understands fecal impaction is the opposite of diarrhea, then answer option "1" can be eliminated. Knowledge of anatomy and physiology eliminates option "4" because stool is formed in the colon and transported to the anus, part of the lower gastrointestinal tract.

134. 1. Bananas are encouraged for clients diagnosed with potassium loss from diuretics; a banana is not needed for harsh laxative (cathartic) use. Harsh laxatives should be discouraged because they cause laxative dependence and a narrowing of the colon with long-term use.
   2. It is not necessary to have a bowel movement every day to have normal bowel functioning.

3. Limiting fluids will increase the problem; the client should be encouraged to increase the fluids in the diet.
   4. If the client is feeling "sluggish" from not being able to have a bowel movement, these foods increase constipation because they are low in residue (fiber).

**TEST-TAKING HINT:** The test taker must understand words such as "cathartic." Limiting fluids is used for clients diagnosed with renal disease or congestive heart failure, but increasing fluids is recommended for most other conditions.

135. 1. Blood may indicate a hemorrhoid, but it is not normal to expel blood when having a bowel movement.
   2. Nurses manually remove feces; it is not a self-care activity.
   3. Cathartic use on a daily basis creates dependence and a narrowing of the lumen of the colon, creating a much more serious problem.
   4. A high-fiber (residue) diet provides bulk for the colon to use in removing the waste products of metabolism. Bulk laxatives and fiber from vegetables and bran assist the colon to work more effectively.

**TEST-TAKING HINT:** Blood is not normal in any circumstance. It may be expected but is not "normal" unless inside a vessel.

136. 1. This is a symptom of diarrhea moving around an impaction higher up in the colon. The nurse should assess for an impaction when observing this finding.
   2. Encouraging the client to drink fluids should be done, but it is not the first intervention.
   3. The sodium level is usually not a problem for clients experiencing diarrhea, but the potassium level may be checked. However, again, this is not the first intervention.
   4. A protective cream can be applied to an excoriated perineum, but first, the nurse should assess the situation.

**TEST-TAKING HINT:** The first step of the nursing process is assessment, after which a nursing diagnosis and interventions follow. The nurse should assess first.

137. 1. This client is improving; semiformed stools are better than diarrhea.
   2. This client has just arrived, so the nurse does not know if the report is valid and needs intervention unless assessed. Older people have difficulty with constipation as a result of

decreased gastric motility, medications, poor diet, and immobility.
3. The client has diarrhea, but only 200 mL,
and has elastic tissue turgor, indicating
the client is not dehydrated.
4. This is not normal, but it is expected for a
client diagnosed with hemorrhoids.

**TEST-TAKING HINT: The test taker should notice
descriptive words such as "older," which should
alert the test taker to the age range having an
implication in answering the question. Answer
options "3" and "4" are expected for the disease processes.**

138. 1. Cheeseburgers and milkshakes are low-
residue foods and can make constipation
worse.
2. Canned peaches are soft and can be
chewed and swallowed easily while
providing some fiber; whole-wheat
bread is higher in fiber than white
bread. These foods will be helpful for
clients diagnosed with slowed gastric
motility as a result of a lack of exercise
or immobility.
3. Mashed potatoes and mechanically
ground meat do not provide high fiber.
4. Biscuits, gravy, and bacon are refined flour
foods or processed meat (fat). These will
not help clients to prevent constipation.

**TEST-TAKING HINT: The test taker must realize
the consequences of immobility include constipation.**

139. Correct answers are 1, 4, and 5.
1. It is important to keep track of the
amounts, color, and other characteristics of body fluids excreted.
2. Skin turgor should be assessed at least
every 6 to 8 hours, not daily.
3. Carbonated soft drinks increase flatus in
the GI tract, and the increased sugar will
act as an osmotic laxative and increase
diarrhea.
4. Daily weights are the best method of
determining fluid loss and gain.
5. Sitz baths will assist in keeping the
client's perianal area clean without
having to rub. The warm water is
soothing, providing comfort.

**TEST-TAKING HINT: The test taker should note
the time frame for any answer option. "Every
day" is not often enough to assess for dehydration in a client diagnosed with massive
("voluminous") fluid loss. If the test taker were
not aware of the definition, then an associated
word, "volume," would be a hint.**

140. 1. The RN will be responsible for signing
off on the UAP when competent to perform the blood glucose. The nurse should
do this to determine the competency of
the UAP.
2. The laboratory values may require the
nurse to interpret and act on the results.
The nurse cannot delegate tasks requiring
professional judgment.
3. The LPN can administer medications
such as a laxative.
4. The nurse cannot delegate assessment.

**TEST-TAKING HINT: Nurses cannot delegate
any activity requiring professional judgment,
assessment, teaching, or evaluation.**

141. 1. The client is tolerating the feeding
change, so there is no need for immediate
action.
2. The client has a PEG tube inserted into
the stomach through the abdominal wall.
The client does not have a nasogastric
feeding tube.
3. Reports of being thirsty should be
addressed; the client may require some
ice chips in the mouth or oral care, but
this is not a priority over assessing the client's ability to swallow.
4. This client needs to be cleaned immediately, the abdomen must be assessed,
and a determination must be made
regarding the type of feeding and
the additives and medications being
administered and skin damage occurring. This occurrence is the priority.

**TEST-TAKING HINT: The test taker must identify
assessment data indicating a complication secondary to the disease process when the stem
asks which occurrence warrants immediate
intervention.**

142. 1. This client may have developed an
infection from the undercooked meat.
The nurse should obtain a stool specimen for the laboratory to analyze.
2. Antibiotic therapy is initiated in only the
most serious cases of infectious diarrhea;
the diarrhea must be assessed first. A
specimen for culture should be obtained
before beginning medication.
3. A complete blood count will provide an
estimate of blood loss, but it is not the
first intervention.
4. The antidiarrheal medication diphe-
noxylate and atropine (Lomotil) would
be administered after the specimen
collection.

**TEST-TAKING HINT:** All options in a priority-setting question may be interventions the nurse could implement, but the right answer will be the one implemented first. Collecting a stool sample is assessment, which is the first step in the nursing process.

143. 1. The clinic nurse should not ask the client to measure stool at home; this is done in the acute care setting.
 2. Unless the client has had diarrhea for longer than 48 hours, the client does not need to be seen in the clinic.
 3. The BRAT (bananas, rice, applesauce, and toast) diet is recommended for a client diagnosed with diarrhea because it is low residue and produces nutrition while not irritating the GI system.
 4. Histamine-2 blockers decrease gastric acid production and would not be prescribed for a client diagnosed with diarrhea.

**TEST-TAKING HINT:** The test taker should realize diarrhea involves the gastrointestinal system, and selecting an intervention addressing the GI system would be an appropriate choice.

144. 1. Normal serum sodium levels are 135 to 145 mEq/L, so the client's 128 mEq/L value requires intervention.
 2. The client diagnosed with a fecal impaction is beginning to move the stool; this indicates an improvement.
 3. Normal potassium levels are 3.5 to 5.5 mEq/L. A level of 3.8 mEq/L is within normal limits and does not require intervention.
 4. This client has been having diarrhea and now is having semiliquid stools, so this client is getting better.

**TEST-TAKING HINT:** The test taker must determine if the client is experiencing a potentially life-threatening complication, such as the potential for seizures. Answer options "2," "3," and "4" are expected for the disease process and are normal or show improvement.

145. 1. This blood gas indicates metabolic alkalosis with partial compensation. The pH level is high, indicating alkalosis. The $HCO_3$ level is low, indicating an alkalosis problem. The $Paco_2$ is outside the normal range, indicating lungs are trying to retain acid to help correct the pH, but the pH is not in the normal range (partial compensation). The NG tube could be removing too much acid from the stomach. The nurse should assess the NGT output.
    2. This is a metabolic problem, not respiratory.
    3. This is a metabolic problem, not respiratory.
    4. The client has an NGT removing acidic contents from the stomach; stool specimen or observation is not indicated.

**TEST-TAKING HINT:** The nurse must be able to interpret common laboratory results. Part of the assessment of a symptom requires determining what therapies can impact the result.

146. Correct answers are 1, 2, 3, and 5.
    1. The client should remain NPO until the inflammation in the colon resolves.
    2. The client should have an IV to maintain hydration while being NPO.
    3. The nurse should assess the client for complications of a ruptured diverticulum.
    4. The client will be NPO to rest the bowel.
    5. The client is kept on bedrest with bathroom privileges to decrease colon activity. Ambulation increases peristalsis.

**TEST-TAKING HINT:** The test taker must make decisions based on basic principles. If the client has a diagnosis of gastrointestinal disease, the treatment will depend on allowing the bowel to rest. When choosing options for a "select all that apply" question, each option is treated as a true or false question.

147. Correct answers are 1, 2, 3, 4, and 5.
    1. The nurse should assess the client's intake; a 72-hour calorie count will allow the nurse to do this.
    2. Protein calorie malnutrition can result from several different diseases. Diarrhea can impact the ability to absorb calories and nutrition from food.
    3. Daily weights will monitor the client's weight loss or gain.

    4. The nurse should assess medications for drug and food interactions.
    5. The dietitian can be invaluable in assisting this client to gain or at least maintain weight.

**TEST-TAKING HINT:** To answer "select all that apply" questions, the test taker must read each option as a true or false question. One option does not rule out another one.

148. 12.06 BMI. This client is extremely underweight.
    To figure the BMI, the test taker must first multiply the height in inches times the height in inches. This client is 67 inches tall.

$$67 \times 67 = 4489$$

The next step is to divide the weight in pounds by the sum of the height times the height:

$$35 \times 2.2 = 77 \text{ pounds}$$
$$77 \div 4489 = 0.01715$$

Then multiply this number times the conversion of 703:

$$0.01715 \times 703 = 12.06$$

**TEST-TAKING HINT:** The nurse must be able to work common math problems to determine the client's needs.

149. 1. Sodium is retained by the body before potassium. The sodium level would be in the normal range after 2 days of diarrhea.
    2. Albumin is the protein level synthesized by the liver; the albumin level should not be affected.
    3. Potassium is excreted through diarrhea; the nurse should assess the client's potassium level.
    4. Glucose should not be affected.

**TEST-TAKING HINT:** The nurse must be able to interpret common laboratory results and how they affect the body. Part of the assessment of a symptom requires determining what therapies can impact the result.

150. 1. A 3 on the pain scale indicates mild pain. This would not be the first client for the nurse to return the call.
    2. A prescription refill would not be a reason for the nurse to make this client first.
    3. A client diagnosed with diabetes type 1 and vomiting is at risk for diabetes ketoacidosis. The nurse should have the client come in immediately.

4. This client needs a referral to a social worker. The client is not the first one to receive a return call.

**TEST-TAKING HINT:** The nurse must be able to interpret the implications of disease processes and comorbid conditions (vomiting). Part of the assessment of a symptom requires determining what other diseases can impact the result.

151. 1. This is a gastrointestinal issue, not a respiratory virus.
    2. Antibacterial soap will not affect a virus. A virus is not a bacterium.
    3. A hepatitis vaccine prevents hepatitis, but this is a gastrointestinal viral illness.
    4. Hand washing will prevent the spread of the virus and decrease the risk for the employees.

**TEST-TAKING HINT:** The test taker should remember basic infection control standards.

152. 1. This blood gas is metabolic acidosis, a potentially lethal situation. The nurse should notify the HCP immediately.
    2. These results for sodium and potassium are WNL. The glucose is at the edge of the normal.
    3. The results of the hemoglobin and hematocrit are not in the range to require more blood at this time. The nurse can give the results to the HCP on rounds.
    4. This pulse oximetry reading is WNL.

**TEST-TAKING HINT:** The nurse must be able to interpret common laboratory results. Part of the assessment of a symptom requires knowing the normal ranges.

153. 1. The usual diet is not a concern at this time. When the child goes home, the nurse will need to explain what the parents can offer the child to prevent dehydration.
    2. Assessing the skin turgor will give the nurse information about the hydration status of the toddler. The nurse should perform an assessment based on the presenting symptoms.
    3. Suckers are sugar-based and rarely given to children for "good behavior" anymore.
    4. The nurse should perform the assessment before notifying the HCP to see the child.

**TEST-TAKING HINT:** The nurse must assess the client. This is a professional responsibility regardless of other health-care professionals and their responsibilities.

154. Correct answers are 1, 2, 4, and 5.
    1. Knowledge of previous weight loss attempts will assist in planning a weight loss program.
    2. The dietitian will monitor the nutritional intake and help in planning a nutritionally balanced diet.
    3. The client should be encouraged to maintain an active lifestyle.
    4. The client's weight will be useful in determining the client's progress.
    5. Clients desiring weight loss frequently want a quick fix. The nurse should assist the client in determining a consistent weight loss goal in order to achieve behavior modification to maintain weight loss.

**TEST-TAKING HINT:** The test taker must read each option of a "select all that apply" question as a true or false question.

155. 1. The BMI is not low; these symptoms are associated with anorexia.
    2. The BMI is WNL but does not indicate the therapy is effective.
    3. The client diagnosed with bulimia binge eats and then induces vomiting or uses laxatives to prevent weight gain.
    4. The BMI is WNL.

**TEST-TAKING HINT:** The test taker will be required to interpret graphs on the NCLEX-RN® and associate the graph information with disease processes. (BMI graph from National Heart, Lung, and Blood Institute, 2020.)

156. 1. Weighing the food is no longer recommended, but if the client weighs the food, then it should be weighed after cooking because cooking changes the weight of the food.
    2. The client should eat some carbohydrates but also protein foods to maintain blood glucose levels.
    3. The client can be taught how to read food labels by looking at the serving size and total grams of carbohydrates (America Diabetes Association, 2019).
    4. Seventy-five percent of the diet being protein places a great burden on the kidneys and can result in acidosis. This is unhealthy.

**TEST-TAKING HINT:** The nurse must be able to provide basic teaching for diets.

# GASTROINTESTINAL DISORDERS COMPREHENSIVE EXAMINATION

1. The nurse is caring for the client diagnosed with *Clostridium difficile*. Which intervention should the nurse implement to **prevent** health-care-associated infection spread to other clients?
   1. Wash hands with Betadine for 2 minutes after giving care.
   2. Wear nonsterile gloves when handling GI excretions.
   3. Clean the perianal area with soap and water after each stool.
   4. Flush the commode twice when disposing of stool.

2. The client receiving antibiotic therapy reports white, cheesy plaques in the mouth. Which intervention should the nurse implement?
   1. Notify the HCP to obtain an antifungal medication.
   2. Explain the patches will go away naturally in about 2 weeks.
   3. Instruct to rinse the mouth with diluted hydrogen peroxide and water daily.
   4. Allow the client to verbalize feelings about having the plaques.

3. Which instructions should be discussed with the client diagnosed with GERD? **Select all that apply.**
   1. Eat a low-carbohydrate, low-sodium diet.
   2. Lie down for 30 minutes after eating.
   3. Do not eat spicy foods or acidic foods.
   4. Drink two glasses of water before bedtime.
   5. Do not wear tight-fitting clothes or belts.

4. Which data should the nurse report to the HCP when assessing the oral cavity of an older client?
   1. The client's tongue is rough and beefy red.
   2. The client's tonsils are +1 on a grading scale.
   3. The client's mucosa is pink and moist.
   4. The client's uvula rises with the mouth open.

5. Which report is significant for the nurse to assess in the adolescent male client using oral tobacco?
   1. The client reports clear to white sputum.
   2. The client has an episodic blister on the upper lip.
   3. The client reports a nonhealing sore in the mouth.
   4. The client has bilateral ducts at the second molars.

6. The client is diagnosed with ulcerative colitis. Which clinical manifestation **warrants immediate** intervention by the nurse?
   1. The client has 20 bloody stools a day.
   2. The client's oral temperature is 99.8°F.
   3. The client's abdomen is hard and rigid.
   4. The client reports urinating when coughing.

7. Which outcome should the nurse identify for the client diagnosed with aphthous stomatitis?
   1. The client will be able to cope with perceived stress.
   2. The client will consume a balanced diet.
   3. The client will deny any difficulty swallowing.
   4. The client will take antacids as prescribed.

8. The nurse is administering a proton pump inhibitor to a client diagnosed with peptic ulcer disease. Which statement supports the rationale for administering this medication?
   1. It prevents the final transport of hydrogen ions into the gastric lumen.
   2. It blocks receptors controlling hydrochloric acid secretion by the parietal cells.
   3. It protects the ulcer from the destructive action of the digestive enzyme pepsin.
   4. It neutralizes the hydrochloric acid secreted by the stomach.

9. Which task should the RN delegate to the UAP to improve the desire to eat in a 14-year-old client diagnosed with anorexia?
   1. Administer an antiemetic 30 minutes before the meal.
   2. Provide mouth care with lemon-glycerin swabs before the meal.
   3. Create a social atmosphere by interacting with the client.
   4. Encourage the client's parents to sit with the client during meals.

10. The client with a diagnosis of possible colon cancer is 2 hours post-sigmoidoscopy procedure. Which assessment data **warrant immediate** intervention by the nurse?
    1. The client has hyperactive bowel sounds.
    2. The client is eating a hamburger the family brought.
    3. The client is sleepy and wants to sleep.
    4. The client's BP is 96/60 and an apical pulse is 108.

11. The nurse identifies the client problem "alteration in gastrointestinal system" for the older client. Which statement reflects the **most appropriate** rationale for this problem?
    1. Older clients have the ability to chew food more thoroughly with dentures.
    2. Older clients have an increase in digestive enzymes, which helps with digestion.
    3. Older clients have an increased need for laxatives because of a decrease in bile.
    4. Older clients have an increase in bacteria in the GI system, resulting in diarrhea.

12. Which interventions should the nurse discuss regarding the prevention of an acute exacerbation of diverticulosis? **Select all that apply.**
    1. Eat a low-fiber diet.
    2. Drink 2,500 mL of water daily.
    3. Avoid eating foods with seeds.
    4. Walk 30 minutes a day.
    5. Take an antacid every 2 hours.

13. The clinic nurse is caring for a client 67 inches tall, weighing 100 kg. The client reports occasional pyrosis, which resolves with standing or taking antacids. Which treatment should the nurse expect the HCP to order?
    1. Place the client on a weight loss program.
    2. Instruct the client to eat three balanced meals.
    3. Tell the client to take an antiemetic before each meal.
    4. Discuss the importance of decreasing alcohol intake.

14. The client is being prepared for discharge after a laparoscopic cholecystectomy. Which intervention should the nurse implement?
    1. Discuss the need to change the abdominal dressing daily.
    2. Tell the client to check the T-tube output every 8 hours.
    3. Include the significant other in the discharge teaching.
    4. Instruct the client to stay off clear liquids for 2 days.

15. Which information should the nurse teach the client post-barium enema procedure?
    1. The client should not eat or drink anything for 4 hours.
    2. The client should remain on bedrest until the sedative wears off.
    3. The client should take a mild laxative to help expel the barium.
    4. The client will have a normal elimination color and pattern.

16. The client diagnosed with a hiatal hernia is scheduled for a laparoscopic Nissen fundoplication. Which statement indicates the nurse's teaching is **effective?**
    1. "I will have four to five small incisions."
    2. "I will be in the hospital for at least 1 week."
    3. "I will not have any pain because this is laparoscopic surgery."
    4. "I will be returning to work the day after my surgery."

17. The client is diagnosed with esophageal diverticula. Which lifestyle modification should be taught by the nurse?
    1. Raise the foot of the bed to 45 degrees to increase peristalsis.
    2. Eat the evening meal at least 2 hours before bed.
    3. Eat a low-fat, low-cholesterol, high-fiber diet.
    4. Wear an abdominal binder to strengthen the abdominal muscles.

18. The client weighs 160 pounds and is 5'1" tall. Calculate the BMI using the following formula and enter the results in the box.

$$BMI = \frac{703 \times weight\ in\ pounds}{(height\ in\ inches)^2}$$

19. Based on the client's BMI from the previous question, which category should the nurse document in the client's EHR?

**BMI**

| Category | BMI Lower Range | BMI Upper Range |
|---|---|---|
| Underweight | Less than 18.5 | — |
| Ideal weight | 18.5 | 24.9 |
| Overweight | 25 | 29.9 |
| Obese | 30 or greater | — |

    1. Underweight.
    2. Overweight.
    3. Ideal weight.
    4. Obese.

20. Which intervention should the nurse implement specifically for the client diagnosed with end-stage liver disease experiencing hepatic encephalopathy?
    1. Assess the client's neurological status.
    2. Prepare to administer a loop diuretic.
    3. Check the client's stool for blood.
    4. Assess for an abdominal fluid wave.

21. Which **priority** teaching information should the nurse discuss with the client to help **prevent** contracting hepatitis B?
    1. Explain the importance of good hand washing.
    2. Recommend the client take the hepatitis B vaccine.
    3. Tell the client not to ingest unsanitary food or water.
    4. Discuss how to implement standard precautions.

22. The emergency department nurse is working in a community hospital. During the past 2 hours, 15 clients have been admitted with *Salmonella* food poisoning. Which information should the nurse discuss with the clients?
    1. Explain the incubation period is 48 to 72 hours.
    2. Explain the source of this poisoning is contaminated water.
    3. Explain the sources of contamination are eggs and chicken.
    4. Explain the bacterial contaminant came from canned foods.

23. Which intervention should the nurse include when discussing ways to **prevent** food poisoning?
    1. Wash hands for 10 seconds after handling raw meat.
    2. Clean all cutting boards between meats and fruits.
    3. Maintain food temperatures at 140°F during extended servings.
    4. Explain that fruits do not require washing before eating or preparing.

24. Which problem is **most appropriate** for the nurse to identify for the client diagnosed with diarrhea?
    1. Alteration in skin integrity.
    2. Chronic pain perception.
    3. Fluid volume excess.
    4. Ineffective coping.

25. The nurse is assessing a client reporting abdominal pain. Which data support the diagnosis of a bowel obstruction?
    1. Steady, aching pain in one specific area.
    2. Sharp back pain radiating to the flank.
    3. Sharp pain increases with deep breaths.
    4. Intermittent colicky pain near the umbilicus.

26. The nurse is caring for the client scheduled for an abdominal perineal resection for Stage IV colon cancer. Which client problem should the nurse include in the intraoperative care plan?
    1. Fluid volume deficit.
    2. Impaired tissue perfusion.
    3. Infection of the surgical site.
    4. Risk for immunosuppression.

27. The nurse is assessing the client diagnosed with end-stage liver disease and portal hypertension. Which intervention should the nurse include in the plan of care?
    1. Assess the abdomen for a tympanic wave.
    2. Monitor the client's blood pressure.
    3. Percuss the liver for size and location.
    4. Weigh the client twice each week.

28. The nurse is caring for the client diagnosed with ascites secondary to hepatic cirrhosis. Which information should the nurse report to the HCP?
    1. A decrease in the client's daily weight of 1 pound.
    2. An increase in urine output after administration of a diuretic.
    3. An increase in abdominal girth of 2 inches.
    4. A decrease in the serum direct bilirubin to 0.6 mg/dL.

29. The nurse is caring for the client diagnosed with hepatic encephalopathy. Which clinical manifestation indicates the disease is progressing?
    1. The client has a decrease in serum ammonia level.
    2. The client is not able to circle choices on the menu.
    3. The client is able to take deep breaths as directed.
    4. The client is able to eat previously restricted food items.

30. The client is scheduled for a colostomy secondary to colon cancer, and the surgeon tells the client the stool will be a formed consistency. Where would the nurse teach the client the stoma will be located?

    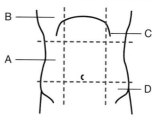

    1. A
    2. B
    3. C
    4. D

31. The nurse is facilitating a support group for clients diagnosed with Crohn's disease. Which information is **most important** for the nurse to discuss with the clients?
    1. Discuss coping skills to assist with the adaptation to lifestyle modifications.
    2. Teach about drug administration, dosages, and scheduled times.
    3. Teach dietary changes necessary to control symptoms.
    4. Explain the care of the ileostomy and necessary equipment.

32. The nurse is caring for a client diagnosed with ulcerative colitis. Which clinical manifestation(s) support this diagnosis?
    1. Increased appetite and thirst.
    2. Elevated hemoglobin.
    3. Multiple bloody, liquid stools.
    4. Exacerbations unrelated to stress.

33. The client is diagnosed with an acute exacerbation of IBD. Which food selection would be the **best choice** for a meal?
    1. Roast beef on wheat bread and a milkshake.
    2. Hamburger, french fries, and a cola.
    3. Pepper steak, brown rice, and iced tea.
    4. Roasted turkey, instant mashed potatoes, and water.

34. The nurse is caring for an older client diagnosed with acute gastritis. Which client problem is the **priority** for this client?
    1. Fluid volume deficit.
    2. Altered nutrition: less than body requirements.
    3. Impaired tissue perfusion.
    4. Alteration in comfort.

35. The nurse is assessing the client diagnosed with chronic gastritis. Which clinical manifestation(s) support this diagnosis?
    1. Rapid onset of midsternal discomfort.
    2. Epigastric pain relieved by eating food.
    3. Dyspepsia and hematemesis.
    4. Nausea and projectile vomiting.

36. The nurse identifies the problem of "fluid volume deficit" for a client diagnosed with gastritis. Which intervention should be included in the plan of care?
    1. Obtain permission for a blood transfusion.
    2. Prepare the client for TPN.
    3. Monitor the client's lung sounds every shift.
    4. Assess the client's intravenous site.

37. The nurse working in a skilled nursing facility is collaborating with the dietitian concerning the meals of an immobile client. Which foods are **most appropriate** for this client?
    1. Oatmeal and wheat toast.
    2. Cream of wheat and biscuits.
    3. Cottage cheese and canned peaches.
    4. Tuna on a croissant and applesauce.

38. Which intervention should the nurse implement when administering a potassium supplement?
    1. Determine the client's allergies.
    2. Ask the client about leg cramps.
    3. Monitor the client's blood pressure.
    4. Monitor the client's complete blood count.

39. The nurse is caring for the client 1 day post-upper gastrointestinal (UGI) series. Which assessment data **warrant intervention**?
    1. No bowel movement.
    2. Oxygen saturation 96%.
    3. Vital signs within normal baseline.
    4. Intact gag reflex.

40. The client is reporting painful swallowing secondary to mouth ulcers. Which statement indicates the nurse's teaching is **effective?**
    1. "I will brush my teeth with a soft-bristle toothbrush."
    2. "I will rinse my mouth with Listerine mouthwash."
    3. "I will swish with antifungal solution and then swallow."
    4. "I will avoid spicy foods, tobacco, and alcohol."

41. The nurse is assessing the integumentary system of the client diagnosed with anorexia nervosa. Which findings supports the diagnosis? **Select all that apply.**
    1. Preoccupation with calories.
    2. Thick body hair.
    3. Sore tongue.
    4. Dry, brittle hair.
    5. Acne.

42. The nurse is teaching the client scheduled for a colostomy and diagnosed with colon cancer. Which behavior indicates the nurse is utilizing adult learning principles?
    1. The nurse repeats the information as indicated by the client's questions.
    2. The nurse teaches in one session all the information the client needs.
    3. The nurse uses a video so the client can hear the medical terms.
    4. The nurse waits until the client asks questions about the surgery.

43. The nurse is caring for the client 1 day postoperative sigmoid colostomy. Which independent nursing intervention should the nurse implement?
    1. Change the infusion rate of the intravenous fluid.
    2. Encourage the client to verbalize feelings about body image.
    3. Administer opioid narcotic medications for pain management.
    4. Assist the client out of bed to sit in the chair twice daily.

44. The nurse is caring for the client recovering from intestinal surgery. Which assessment finding requires **immediate intervention**?
    1. Presence of thin, pink drainage in the Jackson Pratt.
    2. Guarding when the nurse touches the abdomen.
    3. Tenderness around the surgical site during palpation.
    4. Reports of chills and feeling feverish.

45. The nurse is caring for the client diagnosed with hemorrhoids. Which statement indicates **further teaching** is needed?
    1. "I should increase fruits, bran, and fluids in my diet."
    2. "I will use warm compresses and take sitz baths daily."
    3. "I must take a laxative every night and have a stool daily."
    4. "I can use an analgesic ointment or suppository for pain."

46. The nurse is preparing the postoperative nursing care plan for the client recovering from a hemorrhoidectomy. Which intervention should the nurse implement?
    1. Establish rapport with the client to decrease the embarrassment of assessing the site.
    2. Encourage the client to lie in the lithotomy position twice a day.
    3. Milk the tube inserted during surgery to allow the passage of flatus.
    4. Digitally dilate the rectal sphincter to express old blood.

47. The client is newly diagnosed with irritable bowel syndrome (IBS). Which interventions should the nurse teach the client to reduce symptoms? **Select all that apply.**
    1. Instruct the client to avoid drinking fluids with meals.
    2. Explain the need to decrease gluten and foods that contain FODMAPs.
    3. Teach the client how to perform gentle perianal care.
    4. Encourage the client to attend a support group meeting.
    5. Reinforce the need to take a probiotic tablet daily.

48. The nurse at the scene after a knife fight is caring for a young man with a knife protruding from an abdominal wound. Which action should the nurse implement?
    1. Stabilize the knife.
    2. Remove the knife gently.
    3. Turn the client on the side.
    4. Apply pressure to the insertion site.

49. The nurse writes the problem "risk for impaired skin integrity" for a client with a sigmoid colostomy. Which expected outcome would be **appropriate** for this client?
    1. The client will have intact skin around the stoma.
    2. The client will be able to change the ostomy bag.
    3. The client will express anxiety about body changes.
    4. The client will maintain fluid balance.

50. The client is admitted to the emergency department reporting acute epigastric pain and vomiting a large amount of bright red blood at home. Which interventions should the nurse implement? **Rank in order of priority.**
    1. Assess the client's vital signs.
    2. Insert a nasogastric tube.
    3. Begin iced saline lavage.
    4. Start an IV with an 18-gauge needle.
    5. Type and crossmatch for a blood transfusion.

**51.** The male client diagnosed with a peptic ulcer is being admitted to the surgical unit. The client admits to using multiple over-the-counter medications to control his symptoms, including omeprazole daily; ranitidine once or twice a day; and several different brands of antacids at least every 2 hours. Which ABG results should the nurse expect to find in the EHR?

1. Arterial Blood Gas Results

| Arterial Blood Gas | Client Results | Normal Values |
|---|---|---|
| pH | 7.34 | 7.35–7.45 |
| Pco$_2$ | 36 | 35–45 mmHg |
| Hco$_3$ | 21 | 22–26 mEq/L |
| O$_2$ saturation | 96 | 95%–99% |

2. Arterial Blood Gas Results

| Arterial Blood Gas | Client Results | Normal Values |
|---|---|---|
| pH | 7.4 | 7.35–7.45 |
| Pco$_2$ | 40 | 35–45 mmHg |
| Hco$_3$ | 24 | 22–26 mEq/L |
| O$_2$ saturation | 98 | 95%–99% |

3. Arterial Blood Gas Results

| Arterial Blood Gas | Client Results | Normal Values |
|---|---|---|
| pH | 7.49 | 7.35–7.45 |
| Pco$_2$ | 44 | 35–45 mmHg |
| Hco$_3$ | 28 | 22–26 mEq/L |
| O$_2$ saturation | 95 | 95%–99% |

4. Arterial Blood Gas Results

| Arterial Blood Gas | Client Results | Normal Values |
|---|---|---|
| pH | 7.25 | 7.35–7.45 |
| Pco$_2$ | 32 | 35–45 mmHg |
| Hco$_3$ | 23 | 22–26 mEq/L |
| O$_2$ saturation | 100 | 95%–99% |

# GASTROINTESTINAL DISORDERS COMPREHENSIVE EXAMINATION ANSWERS AND RATIONALES

1. 1. The nurse should use soap and water for 15 to 30 seconds before and after caring for the client. Betadine is a surgical scrub.
   2. Clean gloves should be worn when providing care to prevent the transfer of the bacteria found in the stool. This will prevent the spread of bacteria to other clients in the health-care facility (nosocomial). But this is not a substitute for good hand hygiene.
   3. The nurse should clean the perianal area or instruct the client to clean the area, but this will not prevent the spread of the bacteria to other clients.
   4. Flushing the commode twice is not necessary when disposing of stool and will not prevent a nosocomial infection.

2. 1. Candidiasis, or thrush, presents as white, cheesy plaques, which bleed when rubbed and is a side effect of antibiotic therapy. Candidiasis is treated with antifungal solution, swished around the mouth, held for at least 1 minute, and then swallowed. Candidiasis can be prevented if *Lactobacillus acidophilus* is administered concurrently with antibiotic therapy.
   2. White painless patches disappearing in approximately 2 weeks are leukoplakia, caused by tobacco use, which may be cancerous and should be evaluated by an HCP.
   3. A solution of hydrogen peroxide is not recommended to treat candidiasis.
   4. The nurse needs to treat the client's mouth, not use therapeutic communication.

3. Correct answers are 3 and 5.
   1. The client should eat a low-fat, high-fiber diet.
   2. The client should not lie down for at least 2 hours after each meal to prevent gastric reflux.
   3. The client should avoid irritants, such as spicy foods or acidic foods, as well as alcohol, caffeine, and tobacco, because they increase gastric secretions.
   4. The client should avoid food or drink 2 hours before bedtime or lying down after eating.

   5. The client should avoid wearing tight-fitting clothes or belts around the abdomen to prevent squeezing of the stomach and causing reflux.

4. 1. A rough, beefy-red tongue may indicate the client has pernicious anemia and should be evaluated by the HCP.
   2. A score of +1 on the tonsil grading scale shows the tonsils are extending to the haryngopalatine arch, which is normal.
   3. The mucosa should be pink and moist; therefore, the nurse would not need to notify the HCP.
   4. Symmetrical movement of the uvula is normal and should not be reported to the HCP.

5. 1. Clear to white sputum is not significant in the client using oral tobacco.
   2. Episodic blisters on the lips are herpes simplex 1 and are not specific to this client.
   3. The presence of any nonhealing sore on the lips or mouth may be oral cancer. Oral cancer risk increases by using oral tobacco.
   4. Bilateral Stensen's ducts visible at the site of the second molars are normal assessment data.

6. 1. The colon is ulcerated and unable to absorb water; 10 to 20 bloody diarrhea stools are the most common symptom of ulcerative colitis and do not warrant immediate intervention.
   2. This is not an elevated temperature and does not warrant immediate intervention by the nurse.
   3. A hard, rigid abdomen indicates peritonitis, a complication of ulcerative colitis, and warrants immediate intervention.
   4. Stress incontinence is not a symptom of colitis and does not warrant immediate intervention.

7. 1. The cause of canker sores (aphthous stomatitis) is unknown. The small ulcerations of soft oral tissue are linked to stress, trauma, allergies, viral infections, and metabolic disorders. Therefore, being able to cope with stress is the desired outcome.
   2. The client diagnosed with recurrent erythematous macule cankers will not have malnutrition; therefore, a balanced diet is not applicable to this client.
   3. The client diagnosed with cankers should not have difficulty swallowing.
   4. Antacids are not a treatment for canker sores.

8. 1. This statement is the rationale for proton pump inhibitors.
   2. This statement explains the rationale for histamine receptor antagonists.
   3. This statement describes how mucosal protective agents work in the body.
   4. This statement is the rationale for antacids.

9. 1. UAPs cannot administer medications, and this is not appropriate for a client diagnosed with anorexia.
   2. Mouth care should be provided before and after meals but not with alcohol-based mouth wash and lemon-glycerin swabs, which can decrease the appetite.
   3. The UAP assisting the client with meals should increase interaction to improve the client's appetite and make it an enjoyable occasion.
   4. Often the parents are the cause of the client's stress and anxiety, which may have led to the client's anorexia; therefore, the parents should not be asked to stay with the client.

10. 1. The client has been NPO and had laxatives; therefore, hyperactive bowel sounds do not warrant immediate intervention.
    2. The client is able to eat after the procedure, so this does not warrant immediate intervention.
    3. The client received sedation during the procedure and may have been up during the night having bowel movements, resulting in the client being exhausted and sleepy.
    4. These are clinical manifestations of hypovolemic shock requiring immediate intervention by the nurse.

11. 1. Dentures are not an improvement over the client's own teeth in mastication.
    2. The secretion of digestive enzymes and bile are decreased in older people, resulting in an alteration in nutrition and elimination.
    3. Bile does not affect the motility of the intestines. The older client's perception of the need for laxatives is caused by the client's misunderstanding about normal bowel function.
    4. When the motility of the gastrointestinal tract decreases, bacteria remain in the gut longer and multiply, which results in diarrhea.

12. Correct answers are 2, 3, and 4.
    1. A high-fiber diet will prevent constipation, the primary reason for diverticulosis and diverticulitis. A low-fiber (residue) diet is prescribed for acute diverticulitis.
    2. Increased fluids help to keep the stool soft and prevent constipation.
    3. It is controversial if seeds cause an exacerbation of diverticulosis, but this is an appropriate intervention to teach until proven otherwise.
    4. Exercise helps to prevent constipation, which can cause an exacerbation of diverticulitis.
    5. There are no medications used to help prevent an acute exacerbation of diverticulosis and diverticulitis. Antacids are used to neutralize hydrochloric acid in the stomach.

13. 1. Obesity increases the risk of pyrosis (heartburn); therefore, losing weight could help decrease the incidence.
    2. Eating small, frequent meals along with decreased intake of spicy foods have been linked to the prevention of heartburn (pyrosis).
    3. Antiemetics decrease nausea, which does not occur with heartburn. Antacids neutralize the acid of the stomach and are used to treat heartburn.
    4. Drinking alcoholic beverages increases heartburn and should be avoided, not decreased.

14. 1. The client has three to four incisions with adhesive bandages in the upper quadrant, not an abdominal dressing.
    2. The client will not have a T-tube with a laparoscopic cholecystectomy.
    3. A laparoscopic cholecystectomy is done in day surgery. The nurse must make sure the significant others taking care of the client are knowledgeable of postoperative care.

4. The client will be on a regular diet after being discharged from the day surgery clinic.

15. 1. The client may resume a regular diet.
    2. The client will not be sedated for this procedure; therefore, the client does not need to be on bedrest.
    3. **The nurse needs to teach the client to take a mild laxative to help evacuate the barium and return to the client's normal bowel routine. Failure to pass the barium could cause constipation when the barium hardens.**
    4. The client can expect to pass white- or light-colored stools until the barium has completely been evacuated.

16. 1. **In a laparoscopic Nissen fundoplication, there are four to five incisions approximately 1 inch apart, allowing for the passage of equipment to visualize the abdominal organs and perform the operation.**
    2. Many clients come through the day surgery department and go home the same day. Some clients may remain in the hospital for 1 or 2 days but not for a week.
    3. All surgeries will result in pain for the client.
    4. The client should not return to work the next day; the client should wait at least 1 week before returning to work.

17. 1. The client should elevate the head, not the foot, of the bed to prevent the reflux of stomach contents.
    2. **The evening meal should be eaten at least 2 hours before going to bed. Small, frequent meals and semisoft foods ease the passage of food, which decreases clinical manifestations of the disease process.**
    3. This diet is recommended for a client diagnosed with coronary artery disease, not for esophageal diverticula.
    4. Restrictive clothing should be avoided, and abdominal binders do not strengthen muscles and would not benefit this client.

18. **BMI of 30.2.**

    **Formula:** $BMI = \dfrac{703 \times \text{weight in pounds}}{(\text{height in inches})^2}$

    $BMI = \dfrac{703 \times 160}{3,721} = 30.2$

19. 1. A client with less than an 18.5 BMI is underweight.
    2. A BMI between 25 and 29.9 is considered overweight.
    3. The ideal weight for a client is a BMI between 18.5 and 24.9.
    4. **This client is obese, with a BMI greater than 30.**

20. 1. **The increased serum ammonia level associated with liver failure causes the hepatic encephalopathy, which, in turn, leads to neurological deficit.**
    2. Administering a loop diuretic is an appropriate intervention for ascites and portal hypertension.
    3. Checking the stool for bleeding is an appropriate intervention for esophageal varices and decreased vitamin K.
    4. Assessing the abdominal fluid wave is an appropriate intervention for ascites and portal hypertension.

21. 1. This intervention would be appropriate for the prevention of hepatitis A.
    2. **The hepatitis B vaccine will prevent the client from contracting this disease.**
    3. This intervention would be appropriate for the prevention of hepatitis A.
    4. The nurse uses standard precautions, not the client.

22. 1. The incubation period for *Salmonella* food poisoning is 8 to 48 hours.
    2. *Salmonellae* bacteria are not transmitted to humans via water.
    3. **Eggs, poultry, and some vegetables are sources of the *Salmonellae* bacteria, which cause food poisoning. Animals, particularly reptiles, amphibians, and birds, are also sources of *Salmonellae* (Foodsafety.gov, 2019).**
    4. *C. botulinum* is transmitted via improperly canned food.

23. 1. Hand washing for 10 seconds is not long enough to remove any bacteria. Hands should be washed for at least 30 seconds before handling food or eating.
    2. Cutting surfaces used for meats should be different from those used for fruits and vegetables to prevent contamination.
    3. **Foods being served for an extended time should be kept at 140°F because food sitting at less than this temperature allows for bacterial growth (Foodsafety.gov, 2019).**
    4. All fruits and vegetables should be washed before eating or preparing.

24. 1. When clients have multiple liquid stools, the rectal area can become irritated. The integrity of the skin can be impaired.
    2. Pain experienced by this client would be acute, rather than chronic.
    3. Fluid volume deficit is appropriate, rather than fluid volume excess.
    4. Ineffective coping is a psychosocial problem and is not appropriate for a client diagnosed with diarrhea.

25. 1. Steady, aching pain is associated with a peritoneal inflammation, which may be secondary to a ruptured spleen or perforated ulcer or other abdominal organs.
    2. Sharp pain in the back and flank indicate kidney involvement.
    3. Sharp pain increasing with deep breaths indicates muscular involvement.
    4. **Intermittent and colicky pain located near the umbilicus is indicative of a small bowel obstruction; lumbar pain is indicative of colon involvement.**

26. 1. Fluid deficit is a potential problem, not an actual problem. The client's fluid balance should be managed by intravenous fluids.
    2. **The perfusion of the surgical site is compromised as a result of the surgical incision, especially when a graft is used.**
    3. Infection is a potential problem, but not at the time of surgery.
    4. After surgery, not during surgery, the client may require chemotherapy, which can cause immunosuppression.

27. 1. **A client diagnosed with portal hypertension should be assessed for a tympanic (fluid) wave to check for ascites.**
    2. High BP is not the etiology of portal hypertension.
    3. In portal hypertension, percussion is difficult and will not provide pertinent information about the client's condition.
    4. Weighing the client should be done daily, not twice each week.

28. 1. A decrease in weight indicates a loss in fluid and is not data necessary to report to the HCP.
    2. An increase in urine output indicates the diuretic was effective.
    3. **An increase in abdominal girth indicates the ascites is increasing, meaning the client's condition is becoming more serious and should be reported to the HCP.**

    4. The normal serum direct bilirubin should be less than 1.2 mg/dL; therefore, a decrease in the value would not be reported.

29. 1. An increase in serum ammonia levels is seen in clients diagnosed with hepatic encephalopathy and coma.
    2. **The inability to circle food items on the menu may indicate deterioration in the client's cognitive status. The client's neurological status is impaired with hepatic encephalopathy; the nurse should investigate this behavior.**
    3. The client being able to follow commands indicates the client's neurological status is intact.
    4. Consuming foods providing adequate nutrition indicates the client is getting better and able to follow client teaching.

30. 1. Stools are liquid in the ascending colon.
    2. Stools are mushy in the right transverse colon.
    3. The left transverse colon has a semimushy stool.
    4. **The sigmoid colon is located in the left lower quadrant, and the client expels solid feces.**

31. 1. **The objectives for support groups are to help members cope with chronic diseases and help manage symptom control.**
    2. Drug administration, dosage, and scheduled times should be discussed in the hospital before discharge or in the HCP's office; therefore, this is not a priority at the support group meeting.
    3. Dietary changes should be taught at the time the disease is diagnosed, but this is not a priority at the support group meeting.
    4. An ileostomy may be the surgical option for clients unresponsive to medical treatment, but other nonsurgical treatments would be topics of discussions during support group meetings.

32. 1. Clients suffering from ulcerative colitis experience anorexia, not an increased appetite.
    2. The hemoglobin and hematocrit are decreased, not elevated, as a result of blood loss.
    3. Clients report as many as 10 to 20 liquid, bloody stools in a day.
    4. **Stressful events have been linked to an increase in symptoms. The nurse needs to assess for perceived stress in the client's life producing symptoms.**

33. 1. Wheat bread and whole grains should be avoided, and most clients cannot tolerate milk products.
2. Fried foods such as hamburgers and french fries should be avoided. Raw fruits and vegetables such as lettuce and tomatoes are usually not tolerated.
3. Whole grains such as brown rice should be avoided. White rice can be eaten. Spicy meats and foods should be avoided.
4. Meats can be eaten if prepared by roasting, baking, or broiling. Vegetables should be cooked, not raw, and skins should be removed. Instant mashed potatoes do not have the skin. A low-residue diet should be eaten.

34. 1. Pediatric and geriatric clients have an increased risk for fluid volume and electrolyte imbalances. The nurse should always be alert to this possible complication.
2. Altered nutrition may be appropriate, depending on how long the client has been unable to eat, but it is not a priority over fluid volume deficit.
3. Impaired tissue perfusion may be appropriate if the mucosal lining of the stomach is unable to heal, but it is not a priority over fluid volume deficit.
4. Alteration in comfort may be appropriate, but it is not a priority over fluid volume deficit.

35. 1. Acute gastritis is characterized by sudden epigastric pain or discomfort, not midsternal chest pain.
2. **Chronic pain in the epigastric area relieved by ingesting food is a clinical manifestation of chronic gastritis.**
3. Dyspepsia (heartburn) and hematemesis (vomiting blood) are frequent symptoms of acute gastritis.
4. Projectile vomiting is not a clinical manifestation of chronic gastritis.

** 36. 1. There are no data to suggest the client needs a blood transfusion.
2. TPN is not a treatment for a client diagnosed with a fluid volume deficit. TPN provides calories for nutritional deficits, not fluid deficits.
3. If the client's problem were fluid volume excess, assessing lung sounds would be appropriate.
4. **Fluid administration is the medical treatment for dehydration, so the nurse must monitor and ensure the IV site is patent.**

37. 1. Oatmeal and wheat toast are high-fiber foods and are recommended for immobile clients to help prevent constipation.
2. Cream of wheat and biscuits are low-fiber foods.
3. Cottage cheese and canned peaches are low-fiber foods.
4. Tuna is a good source of protein for the client, but croissants have a high fat content and are a factor in weight gain if consistently eaten. Applesauce is low in fiber.

38. 1. The nurse should inquire about drug allergies before administering all medications, not just potassium.
2. Leg cramps occur when serum potassium levels are too low or too high. If the client has leg cramps, this could indicate an imbalance, which could lead to cardiac dysrhythmias.
3. The BP does not evaluate for dysrhythmias, a possible result of abnormal potassium levels.
4. The complete blood count does not include the potassium level; a chemistry panel is needed.

39. 1. The nurse should monitor the client for the first bowel movement to document the elimination of barium, which should be eliminated within 2 days. If the client does not have a bowel movement, a laxative may be needed to help the client to eliminate the barium before it becomes too hard to pass.
2. An oxygen saturation of 96% is acceptable and does not require intervention.
3. Vital signs should be monitored to recognize and treat complications before the client is in danger. Baseline is a desired outcome.
4. The client's throat is not anesthetized for this procedure, so the gag reflex is not pertinent information in this procedure.

40. 1. A soft-bristle toothbrush will not affect painful swallowing.
2. An alcohol-based mouthwash (Listerine) is irritating to the oral cavity and can increase pain.
3. An antifungal medication should be used with candidiasis and is not an effective treatment for plain mouth ulcers.
4. **Irritating substances should be avoided during the outbreaks of ulcers in the mouth. Spicy foods, alcohol, and tobacco are common irritants the client should avoid.**

**41. Correct answers are 4 and 5.**
   1. The preoccupation with food, calories, and preparing meals are psychosocial behaviors suggesting the client has an eating disorder.
   2. Clients diagnosed with anorexia nervosa have thin, fine body hair.
   3. Iron-deficiency anemia causes clients to experience a sore tongue.
   4. **Thin, brittle hair occurs in clients diagnosed with anorexia.**
   5. **Acne is present in almost 50% of all diagnosed cases of anorexia nervosa.**

**42.** 1. **The nurse should realize the client is anxious about the diagnosis of cancer and the impending surgery. Therefore, the nurse should be prepared to repeat information as necessary. The learning principle the nurse needs to consider is "anxiety decreases learning."**
   2. Small manageable sessions increase learning, especially when the client is anxious.
   3. Videos are not the best teaching tool for adults. Short videos are useful for children.
   4. The nurse should assess the client's readiness and willingness to learn and not wait until the client asks questions about the surgery.

**43.** 1. The rate of the intravenous fluid is a collaborative nursing intervention because it requires an order from the HCP.
   2. **Encouraging the client to verbalize feelings about body changes assists the client to accept these changes. This is an independent intervention not requiring an HCP's order.**
   3. Medication administration is a collaborative intervention because it requires an order by the HCP.
   4. The activity level immediately postoperative requires an order by the HCP.

**44.** 1. Thin pink drainage is expected in the Jackson Pratt (JP) bulb.
   2. Guarding is a normal occurrence when touching a tender area on the abdomen and does not require immediate intervention.
   3. Tenderness around the surgical site is a normal finding and does not require intervention.
   4. **Reports of chills, sudden onset of fever, tachycardia, nausea, and hiccups are symptoms of peritonitis, which is a life-threatening complication.**

**45.** 1. Clients diagnosed with hemorrhoids need to eat high-fiber diets and increase fluid intake to keep the stools soft and prevent constipation; therefore, the teaching is effective.
   2. Warm compresses or sitz baths decrease pain; therefore, the teaching is effective.
   3. **Laxatives can be harsh to the bowel and are habit-forming; they should not be taken daily. Stool softeners soften stool and can be taken daily.**
   4. Analgesic ointments, suppositories, and astringents can be used to decrease pain and decrease edema; therefore, the teaching has been effective.

**46.** 1. **The site of the surgery can cause embarrassment when the nurse assesses the site; therefore, the nurse should establish a positive relationship.**
   2. The lithotomy position is with the client's legs in stirrups for procedures such as Pap smears and some surgeries such as transurethral resection of the prostate, not for the client postoperative hemorrhoidectomy.
   3. A tube is not placed in the client's rectum after this surgery.
   4. The rectal sphincter does not need to be digitally dilated.

**47. Correct answers are 1, 2, 4, and 5.**
   1. Avoidance of fluids during meals will help prevent abdominal distention, which causes symptoms of IBS. Do not confuse inflammatory bowel disease (IBD) and irritable bowel syndrome (IBS).
   2. Avoidance of gluten and foods that contain FODMAPs. Gluten, found in wheat, barley, and rye, can contribute to IBS symptoms. A low FODMAP diet is a special diet that reduces certain foods containing carbohydrates—apples, beans, dairy products, honey, and sweeteners ending in"-ol" that can improve symptoms (National Institute of Diabetes and Digestive and Kidney Diseases, 2017).
   3. Clients diagnosed with IBS do have altered bowel habits such as diarrhea and constipation, but perianal care will not prevent IBS.
   4. IBS does have a psychological component, a client newly diagnosed with IBS may find a support group meeting assists in coping with diet changes and IBS management to reduce symptoms.

5. Probiotics are encouraged by physicians and the efficacy is being researched (NIDDK, 2017).

48. 1. The nurse should not remove any penetrating object in the abdomen; removal could cause further internal damage.
   2. Removal of the knife could cause further internal damage.
   3. The client should be kept on the back, and the knife should be stabilized.
   4. The nurse should stabilize the knife and notify Emergency Medical Services as quickly as possible.

49. 1. Intact skin around the stoma is the most appropriate outcome for the problem of "impaired skin integrity."
   2. The client's ability to change the ostomy bag is a goal for a knowledge deficit problem or self-care.
   3. Expressing anxiety about body changes is a goal for an alteration in body image.
   4. Maintaining a balance in fluid is a goal for a nursing diagnosis of risk for a fluid deficit.

50. Correct order is 1, 4, 5, 2, 3.
   1. The nurse should assess the vital signs to determine if the client is in hypovolemic shock. The stem of the question does not provide information indicating the client is hypovolemic. The client's perception of a large amount of blood may differ from the nurse's assessment.
   4. The nurse should start the IV line to replace fluid volume.
   5. While the nurse is starting the IV, a blood sample for typing and cross-matching should be obtained and sent to the laboratory.
   2. An NG tube should be inserted so that direct iced saline can be instilled to cause constriction, which will decrease the bleeding.
   3. The iced saline lavage will help decrease bleeding.

51. 1. This is metabolic acidosis; the client taking many antacids would be in metabolic alkalosis.
   2. These are normal blood gas results.
   3. This is metabolic alkalosis, a result of taking multiple over-the-counter medications to control his symptoms, including omeprazole (Prilosec, a proton pump inhibitor) daily; ranitidine (Zantac, an $H_2$ receptor blocker) once or twice a day; and several different brands of antacids at least every 2 hours.
   4. This is respiratory alkalosis, a result of hyperventilation.

# Endocrine Disorders

8

*A little knowledge that acts is worth infinitely more than much knowledge that is idle.*

—Kahlil Gibran

The endocrine system, along with the nervous system, controls or influences the activities of other body systems. The major glands of the endocrine system—the pituitary, thyroid, parathyroid, adrenals, pancreas, and ovaries and testes—play a major role in regulating activities of the body, including metabolism, fluid balance, reaction to stress, and sexual function. As with organs in other systems, these glands are subject to many disorders, some relatively minor and easily treated and others life-threatening. This chapter focuses on diabetes mellitus, one of the most common and major endocrine system disorders; on other pancreatic disorders; and on adrenal, pituitary, and thyroid disorders. Disorders affecting the glands involved in reproduction and sexual functioning are discussed in Chapter 10.

## KEYWORDS

| | |
|---|---|
| Addisonian crisis | Hypoparathyroidism |
| Aldosteronism | Hypothyroidism |
| Androgen | Iatrogenic |
| Antidiuretic | Ketone |
| Endogenous | Kussmaul's respirations |
| Euthyroid | Mineralocorticoid |
| Exogenous | Pruritus |
| Fluid deprivation test | Tenesmus |
| Glucocorticoid | Turgor |
| Hyperparathyroidism | Vasopressin |
| Hyperthyroidism | Water challenge test |

## PRACTICE QUESTIONS

### Diabetes Mellitus

1. An 18-year-old female client, 5′4″ tall, weighing 113 kg, comes to the clinic for a nonhealing wound, which she has had for 2 weeks. Which disease process should the nurse suspect the client has developed?
    1. Type 1 diabetes.
    2. Type 2 diabetes.
    3. Gestational diabetes.
    4. Acanthosis nigricans.

2. The client diagnosed with type 1 diabetes has a glycosylated hemoglobin (A1c) of 8.1%. Which interpretation should the nurse make based on this result?
   1. This result is below normal levels.
   2. This result is within acceptable levels.
   3. This result is above the recommended levels.
   4. This result is dangerously high.

3. The nurse administered 28 units of insulin isophane to a client diagnosed with type 1 diabetes at 1600. Which intervention should the nurse implement?
   1. Ensure the client eats the bedtime snack.
   2. Determine how much food the client ate at lunch.
   3. Perform a glucometer reading at 0700.
   4. Offer the client protein after administering insulin.

4. The client diagnosed with type 1 diabetes is receiving insulin lispro by sliding scale. The unlicensed assistive personnel (UAP) reports to the nurse the client's glucometer reading is 189. How much insulin should the registered nurse (RN) administer to the client?

   [                    ]

| Client Name: Mr. A.G. | MR# 3456889 | Diagnosis: Diabetes Mellitus Type 1 |
|---|---|---|
| Age: 60 years | Allergies: NKDA | |
| Medication | 0701–1900 | 1901–0700 |
| Insulin lispro Subcutaneously a.c. and h.s.    0–150 = 0 units    151–200 = 3 units    201–250 = 6 units    Greater than 250 = Call HCP | 0730 1130 | 1630 2100 |

5. The nurse is discussing the importance of exercising with a client diagnosed with type 2 diabetes well controlled with diet and exercise. Which information should the nurse include in the teaching about diabetes?
   1. Eat a simple carbohydrate snack before exercising.
   2. Carry peanut butter crackers when exercising.
   3. Encourage the client to walk 20 minutes three times a week.
   4. Perform warm-up and cool-down exercises.

6. The nurse is assessing the feet of a client diagnosed with long-term type 2 diabetes. Which assessment data **warrant immediate** intervention by the nurse?
   1. The client has crumbling toenails.
   2. The client has athlete's foot.
   3. The client has a necrotic big toe.
   4. The client has thickened toenails.

7. The home health nurse is completing the admission assessment for a 76-year-old client diagnosed with type 2 diabetes controlled with 70/30 insulin.

Which intervention should be included in the plan of care?
   1. Assess the client's ability to read the small print.
   2. Monitor the client's serum prothrombin time (PT) level.
   3. Teach the client how to perform a hemoglobin $A_{1c}$ test daily.
   4. Instruct the client to check the feet weekly.

8. The client diagnosed with type 2 diabetes, controlled with biguanide medication, and a history of liver disease, is scheduled for a computed tomography (CT) scan with contrast of the abdomen to evaluate pancreatic function. Which intervention should the nurse implement?
   1. Provide a high-fat diet 24 hours before the test.
   2. Hold the biguanide medication for 48 hours before the test.
   3. Obtain an informed consent form for the test.
   4. Administer pancreatic enzymes before the test.

9. The diabetic educator is teaching a class on diabetes type 1 and is discussing sick-day rules. Which interventions should the diabetes educator include in the discussion? **Select all that apply.**
   1. Take diabetic medication even if unable to eat the client's normal diabetic diet.
   2. If unable to eat, drink liquids equal to the client's normal caloric intake.
   3. It is not necessary to notify the health-care provider (HCP) if ketones are in the urine.
   4. Test blood glucose levels and test urine ketones once a day and keep a record.
   5. Call the HCP if glucose levels are higher than 180 mg/dL.

10. The client received 10 units of regular insulin at 0700. At 1030 the UAP tells the nurse the client has a headache and is really acting "funny." Which intervention should the RN implement **first**?
    1. Instruct the UAP to obtain the blood glucose level.
    2. Have the client drink 8 ounces of orange juice.
    3. Go to the client's room and assess the client for hypoglycemia.
    4. Prepare to administer one ampule 50% dextrose intravenously.

11. The nurse at a freestanding health-care clinic is caring for a homeless 56-year-old male client diagnosed with type 2 diabetes controlled with insulin. Which action is an example of client advocacy?
    1. Ask the client if he has somewhere he can go and live.
    2. Arrange for someone to give him insulin at a local homeless shelter.
    3. Notify Adult Protective Services about the client's situation.
    4. Ask the HCP to take the client off insulin because he is homeless.

12. The nurse is developing a care plan for the client diagnosed with type 1 diabetes. The nurse identifies the problem "high risk for hyperglycemia related to noncompliance with the medication regimen." Which statement is an **appropriate** short-term goal for the client?
    1. The client will have a blood glucose level between 90 and 140 mg/dL.
    2. The client will demonstrate an appropriate insulin injection technique.
    3. The nurse will monitor the client's blood glucose levels four times a day.
    4. The client will maintain normal kidney function with 30 mL/hr urine output.

13. The client diagnosed with type 2 diabetes is admitted to the intensive care unit (ICU) with hyperosmolar hyperglycemic nonketotic syndrome (HHNS) coma. Which assessment data should the nurse expect the client to exhibit?
    1. Kussmaul's respirations.
    2. Diarrhea and epigastric pain.
    3. Dry mucous membranes.
    4. Ketone breath odor.

14. The older client is admitted to the intensive care unit diagnosed with severe HHNS. Which collaborative intervention should the nurse include in the plan of care?
    1. Infuse 0.9% normal saline intravenously.
    2. Administer intermediate-acting insulin.
    3. Perform blood glucometer checks daily.
    4. Monitor arterial blood gas (ABG) results.

15. Which electrolyte replacement should the nurse anticipate being ordered by the HCP for the client diagnosed with diabetic ketoacidosis (DKA) just admitted to the ICU?
    1. Glucose.
    2. Potassium.
    3. Calcium.
    4. Sodium.

16. The client diagnosed with HHNS was admitted yesterday with a blood glucose level of 780 mg/dL. The client's blood glucose level is now 300 mg/dL. Which intervention should the nurse implement?
    1. Increase the regular insulin IV drip.
    2. Check the client's urine for ketones.
    3. Provide the client with a therapeutic diabetic meal.
    4. Notify the HCP to obtain an order to decrease insulin.

17. The client diagnosed with type 1 diabetes is found lying unconscious on the floor of the bathroom. Which intervention should the nurse implement **first**?
    1. Administer 50% dextrose (IVP).
    2. Notify the health-care provider.
    3. Move the client to the ICU.
    4. Check the serum glucose level.

18. Which assessment data indicate the client diagnosed with diabetic ketoacidosis is **responding** to medical treatment?
    1. The client has tented skin turgor and dry mucous membranes.
    2. The client is alert and oriented to date, time, and place.
    3. The client's ABG results are pH 7.29, Pco$_2$ 44, HCO$_3$ 15.
    4. The client's serum potassium level is 3.3 mEq/L.

19. The UAP on the medical floor tells the nurse the client diagnosed with DKA wants something else to eat for lunch. Which intervention should the RN implement?
    1. Instruct the UAP to get the client some additional food.
    2. Notify the dietitian about the client's request.
    3. Request the HCP to increase the client's caloric intake.
    4. Tell the UAP the client cannot have anything else.

20. The emergency department nurse is caring for a client diagnosed with HHNS and a blood glucose of 680 mg/dL. Which question should the nurse ask the client to determine the cause of this acute complication?
    1. "When is the last time you took your insulin?"
    2. "When did you have your last meal?"
    3. "Have you had some type of infection lately?"
    4. "How long have you had diabetes?"

21. The nurse is discussing ways to prevent diabetic ketoacidosis with the client diagnosed with type 1 diabetes. Which instruction is **most important** to discuss with the client?
    1. Refer the client to the American Diabetes Association.
    2. Do not take any over-the-counter (OTC) medications.
    3. Take the prescribed insulin even when unable to eat because of illness.
    4. Explain the need to get the annual flu and pneumonia vaccines.

22. The charge nurse is making client assignments in the ICU. Which client should be assigned to the **most experienced** nurse?
    1. The client diagnosed with type 2 diabetes and a blood glucose level of 348 mg/dL.
    2. The client diagnosed with type 1 diabetes experiencing hypoglycemia.
    3. The client diagnosed with DKA having multifocal premature ventricular contractions.
    4. The client diagnosed with HHNS and a plasma osmolarity of 290 mOsm/L.

23. Which ABG results should the nurse expect in the client diagnosed with diabetic ketoacidosis?

    1.

    | Arterial Blood Gas | Client Results | Normal Values |
    | --- | --- | --- |
    | pH | 7.34 | 7.35–7.45 |
    | $Pco_2$ | 48 | 35–45 mm Hg |
    | $Hco_3$ | 24 | 22–26 mEq/L |
    | $Pao_2$ | 99 | 80–95 mm Hg |

    2.

    | Arterial Blood Gas | Client Results | Normal Values |
    | --- | --- | --- |
    | pH | 7.38 | 7.35–7.45 |
    | $Pco_2$ | 40 | 35–45 mm Hg |
    | $Hco_3$ | 22 | 22–26 mEq/L |
    | $Pao_2$ | 95 | 80–95 mm Hg |

    3.

    | Arterial Blood Gas | Client Results | Normal Values |
    | --- | --- | --- |
    | pH | 7.46 | 7.35–7.45 |
    | $Pco_2$ | 30 | 35–45 mm Hg |
    | $Hco_3$ | 26 | 22–26 mEq/L |
    | $Pao_2$ | 85 | 80–95 mm Hg |

    4.

    | Arterial Blood Gas | Client Results | Normal Values |
    | --- | --- | --- |
    | pH | 7.30 | 7.35–7.45 |
    | $Pco_2$ | 30 | 35–45 mm Hg |
    | $Hco_3$ | 18 | 22–26 mEq/L |
    | $Pao_2$ | 90 | 80–95 mm Hg |

24. The client is admitted to the ICU diagnosed with DKA. Which interventions should the nurse implement? **Select all that apply.**
    1. Maintain adequate ventilation.
    2. Assess fluid volume status.
    3. Administer intravenous potassium.
    4. Check for urinary ketones.
    5. Monitor intake and output.

## Pancreatitis

25. The client is admitted to the medical department with a diagnosis of possible acute pancreatitis. Which laboratory values should the nurse monitor to **confirm** this diagnosis?
    1. Creatinine and BUN.
    2. Troponin and CK-MB.
    3. Serum amylase and lipase.
    4. Serum bilirubin and calcium.

26. Which client problem has **priority** for the client diagnosed with acute pancreatitis?
    1. Risk for fluid volume deficit.
    2. Alteration in comfort.
    3. Imbalanced nutrition: less than body requirements.
    4. Knowledge deficit.

27. The nurse is preparing to administer morning medications to clients. Which medication should the nurse **question** before administering?
    1. Pancreatic enzymes to the client finished with breakfast.
    2. Morphine to the client with a respiratory rate of 20.
    3. A loop diuretic to the client with a serum potassium level of 3.9 mEq/L.
    4. A beta blocker to the client with an apical pulse of 68 bpm.

28. The client is diagnosed with acute pancreatitis. Which HCP's admitting order should the nurse **question**?
    1. Bedrest with bathroom privileges.
    2. Initiate IV therapy of LR at 200 mL/hr.
    3. Weigh the client daily.
    4. Low-fat, low-carbohydrate diet.

29. The nurse is completing discharge teaching to the client diagnosed with acute pancreatitis. Which instructions should the nurse discuss with the client? **Select all that apply.**
    1. Instruct the client to decrease alcohol intake.
    2. Explain the need to avoid all stress.
    3. Discuss the importance of stopping smoking.
    4. Teach the correct way to take pancreatic enzymes.
    5. Encourage the client to eat a low-fat diet.

30. The male client diagnosed with chronic pancreatitis calls and reports to the clinic nurse he has been having a lot of "gas," along with frothy and very foul-smelling stools. Which intervention should the nurse implement?
    1. Explain this is common for chronic pancreatitis.
    2. Ask the client to bring in a stool specimen to the clinic.
    3. Arrange an appointment with the HCP for today.
    4. Discuss the need to decrease fat in the diet, so this won't happen.

31. The nurse is discussing complications of chronic pancreatitis with a client diagnosed with the disease. Which complication should the nurse discuss with the client? **Select all that apply.**
    1. Diabetes insipidus (DI).
    2. Crohn's disease.
    3. Narcotic addiction.
    4. Peritonitis.
    5. Metabolic bone disease.

32. The client is **immediate** postprocedure endoscopic retrograde cholangiopancreatogram (ERCP). Which intervention should the nurse implement?
    1. Assess for rectal bleeding.
    2. Increase fluid intake.
    3. Assess gag reflex.
    4. Keep in the supine position.

33. The client diagnosed with acute pancreatitis is in pain. Which position should the nurse assist the client in assuming to help **decrease** the pain?
    1. Recommend lying in the prone position with legs extended.
    2. Maintain a tripod position over the bedside table.
    3. Place in a side-lying position with knees flexed.
    4. Encourage a supine position with a pillow under the knees.

34. The client diagnosed with an acute exacerbation of chronic pancreatitis has a nasogastric (NG) tube. Which interventions should the nurse implement? **Select all that apply.**
    1. Monitor the client's bowel sounds.
    2. Monitor the client's food intake.
    3. Assess the client's intravenous site.
    4. Provide oral and nasal care.
    5. Monitor the client's blood glucose.

35. The nurse is administering a pancreatic enzyme to the client diagnosed with chronic pancreatitis. Which statement **best explains** the rationale for administering this medication?
    1. It is an exogenous source of protease, amylase, and lipase.
    2. This enzyme increases the number of bowel movements.
    3. This medication breaks down in the stomach to help with digestion.
    4. Pancreatic enzymes help break down fat in the small intestine.

36. The client diagnosed with acute pancreatitis is being discharged home. Which statement by the client indicates the teaching has been **effective?**
    1. "I should decrease my intake of coffee, tea, and cola."
    2. "I will eat a low-fat diet and avoid spicy foods."
    3. "I will check my amylase and lipase levels daily."
    4. "I will return to work tomorrow, but take it easy."

## Cancer of the Pancreas

37. The nurse is assessing a client with reports of vague upper abdominal pain worse at night but relieved by sitting up and leaning forward. Which assessment question should the nurse ask **next**?
    1. "Have you noticed a yellow haze when you look at things?"
    2. "Does the pain get worse when you eat a meal or snack?"
    3. "Have you had your amylase and lipase checked recently?"
    4. "How much weight have you gained since you saw an HCP?"

38. The nurse caring for a client diagnosed with cancer of the pancreas writes the problem of "altered nutrition: less than body requirements." Which collaborative intervention should the nurse include in the plan of care?
    1. Continuous feedings via PEG tube.
    2. Have the family bring in food from home.
    3. Assess for food preferences.
    4. Refer to the dietitian.

39. The nurse is planning a program for clients at a health fair regarding the prevention and early detection of cancer of the pancreas. Which self-care activity should the nurse discuss as an example of a **primary** nursing intervention?
    1. Monitor for elevated blood glucose at random intervals.
    2. Inspect the skin and sclera of the eyes for a yellow tint.
    3. Limit meat in the diet and eat a diet low in fat.
    4. Instruct the client diagnosed with hyperglycemia about insulin injections.

40. The nurse and a UAP are caring for clients on an oncology floor. Which intervention should the RN delegate to the UAP?
    1. Assist the client with abdominal pain to turn to the side and flex the knees.
    2. Monitor the Jackson Pratt drainage tube to ensure it is draining properly.
    3. Check to see if the client is sleeping after pain medication is administered.
    4. Empty the bedside commode of the client having melena.

41. The client diagnosed with cancer of the pancreas is being discharged to start chemotherapy in the HCP's office. Which statement made by the client indicates the client **understands** the discharge instructions?
    1. "I will have to see the HCP every day for 6 weeks for my treatments."
    2. "I should write down all my questions so I can ask them when I see the HCP."
    3. "I am sure this is not going to be a serious problem for me to deal with."
    4. "The nurse will give me an injection in my leg and I will get to go home."

42. The client is being admitted to the outpatient department before an endoscopic retrograde cholangiopancreatogram (ERCP) to rule out cancer of the pancreas. Which instructions should the nurse teach? **Select all that apply.**
    1. Prepare to be admitted to the hospital after the procedure for observation.
    2. If something happens during the procedure, then emergency surgery will be done.
    3. Do not eat or drink anything after midnight the night before the test.
    4. If done correctly, this procedure will correct the blockage of the stomach.
    5. Expect a sore throat after the procedure that can last 1 to 2 days.

43. The client is diagnosed with cancer of the head of the pancreas. Which clinical manifestations should the nurse expect to assess?
    1. Clay-colored stools and dark urine.
    2. Night sweats and fever.
    3. Left lower abdominal cramps and tenesmus.
    4. Nausea and coffee-ground emesis.

44. The client diagnosed with cancer of the head of the pancreas is 2 days post-pancreatoduodenectomy (Whipple's procedure). Which nursing problem has the **highest priority**?
    1. Anticipatory grieving.
    2. Fluid volume imbalance.
    3. Alteration in comfort.
    4. Altered nutrition.

45. The client had a total pancreatectomy and splenectomy for cancer of the body of the pancreas. Which discharge instructions should the nurse teach? **Select all that apply.**
    1. Keep a careful record of intake and output.
    2. Use a stool softener or bulk laxative regularly.
    3. Use correct insulin injection technique.
    4. Take pain medication before the pain gets too bad.
    5. Sleep with the head of the bed on blocks.

46. The client admitted to rule out pancreatic islet tumors reports feeling weak, shaky, and sweaty. Which **priority** intervention should be implemented by the nurse?
    1. Start an IV with $D_5W$.
    2. Notify the health-care provider.
    3. Perform a bedside glucose check.
    4. Give the client some orange juice.

47. The home health nurse is admitting a client diagnosed with cancer of the pancreas. Which information is the **most important** for the nurse to discuss with the client?
    1. Determine the client's food preferences.
    2. Ask the client if there is an advance directive.
    3. Find out about insurance and Medicare reimbursement.
    4. Instruct the client to eat as much as possible.

48. The nurse caring for a client diagnosed with cancer of the pancreas writes the nursing diagnosis of "risk for altered skin integrity related to pruritus." Which intervention should the nurse implement?
    1. Assess tissue turgor.
    2. Apply antifungal creams.
    3. Monitor bony prominences for skin breakdown.
    4. Have the client keep the fingernails short.

## Adrenal Disorders

49. The nurse is admitting a client diagnosed with primary adrenal cortex insufficiency (Addison's disease). Which clinical manifestations should the nurse expect to assess?
    1. Moon face, buffalo hump, and hyperglycemia.
    2. Hirsutism, fever, and irritability.
    3. Bronze pigmentation, hypotension, and anorexia.
    4. Tachycardia, bulging eyes, and goiter.

50. The nurse is developing a plan of care for the client diagnosed with acquired immunodeficiency syndrome (AIDS) and an infection in the adrenal gland. Which client problem is the **highest priority?**
    1. Altered body image.
    2. Activity intolerance.
    3. Impaired coping.
    4. Fluid volume deficit.

51. The nurse is planning the care of a client diagnosed with Addison's disease. Which intervention should be included?
    1. Administer steroid medications.
    2. Place the client on fluid restriction.
    3. Provide frequent stimulation.
    4. Consult physical therapy for gait training.

52. The client is admitted to rule out Cushing's syndrome. Which laboratory tests should the nurse anticipate being ordered?
    1. Plasma drug levels of quinidine, digoxin, and hydralazine.
    2. Plasma levels of ACTH and cortisol.
    3. Twenty-four-hour urine for metanephrine and catecholamine.
    4. Spot urine for creatinine and white blood cells (WBCs).

53. The client has developed iatrogenic Cushing's disease. Which statement is the scientific rationale for the development of this diagnosis?
    1. The client has an autoimmune problem causing the destruction of the adrenal cortex.
    2. The client has been taking steroid medications for an extended period for another disease process.
    3. The client has a pituitary gland tumor causing the adrenal glands to produce too much cortisol.
    4. The client has developed an adrenal gland problem for which the HCP does not have an explanation.

54. The nurse is performing discharge teaching for a client diagnosed with Cushing's disease. Which statement by the client demonstrates an **understanding** of the instructions?
    1. "I will be sure to notify my health-care provider if I start to run a fever."
    2. "Before I stop taking the prednisone, I will be taught how to taper it off."
    3. "If I get weak and shaky, I need to eat some hard candy or drink some juice."
    4. "It is fine if I continue to participate in weekend games of tackle football."

55. The charge nurse of an ICU is making assignments for the night shift. Which client should be assigned to the **most experienced** intensive care nurse?
    1. The client diagnosed with respiratory failure is on a ventilator and requires frequent sedation.
    2. The client diagnosed with lung cancer and iatrogenic Cushing's disease with ABGs of pH 7.35, Pao$_2$ 88, Paco$_2$ 44, and HCO$_3$ 22.
    3. The client diagnosed with Addison's disease is lethargic and has a BP of 80/45, P 124, and R 28.
    4. The client diagnosed with hyperthyroidism has undergone a thyroidectomy 2 days ago and has a negative Trousseau's sign.

56. The nurse writes a problem of "altered body image" for a 34-year-old client diagnosed with Cushing's disease. Which intervention should be implemented?
    1. Monitor blood glucose levels before meals and at bedtime.
    2. Perform a head-to-toe assessment on the client every shift.
    3. Use therapeutic communication to allow the client to discuss feelings.
    4. Assess bowel sounds and temperature every 4 hours.

57. The client diagnosed with Addison's disease is admitted to the emergency department after a day at the lake. The client is lethargic, forgetful, and weak. Which intervention should the nurse implement?
    1. Start an IV with an 18-gauge needle and infuse NS rapidly.
    2. Have the client wait in the waiting room until a bed is available.
    3. Obtain a permit for the client to receive a blood transfusion.
    4. Collect urinalysis and blood samples for a CBC and calcium level.

58. The client diagnosed with Cushing's disease has developed 1+ peripheral edema. The client has received intravenous fluids at 100 mL/hr via IV pump for the past 79 hours. The client received intravenous piggyback (IVPB) medication in 50 mL of fluid every 6 hours for 15 doses. How many milliliters of fluid did the client receive?

    [                    ]

59. The nurse manager of a medical-surgical unit is asked to determine if the unit should adopt a new care delivery system. Which behavior is an example of an **autocratic** style of leadership?
    1. Call a meeting and educate the staff on the new delivery system being used.
    2. Organize a committee to investigate the various types of delivery systems.
    3. Wait until another unit has implemented the new system and see if it works out.
    4. Discuss with the nursing staff if a new delivery system should be adopted.

60. The client diagnosed with Cushing's disease has undergone a unilateral adrenalectomy. Which discharge instructions should the nurse discuss with the client?
    1. Instruct the client to take the glucocorticoid and mineralocorticoid medications as prescribed.
    2. Teach the client regarding sexual functioning and androgen replacement therapy.
    3. Explain the clinical manifestations of infection and when to call the HCP.
    4. Demonstrate turn, cough, and deep-breathing exercises the client should perform every 2 hours.

## Pituitary Disorders

61. The client diagnosed with a pituitary tumor developed syndrome of inappropriate antidiuretic hormone (SIADH). Which interventions should the nurse implement?
    1. Assess for dehydration and monitor blood glucose levels.
    2. Assess for nausea and vomiting and weigh daily.
    3. Monitor potassium levels and encourage fluid intake.
    4. Administer vasopressin IV and conduct a fluid deprivation test.

62. The nurse is admitting a client postoperative transsphenoidal hypophysectomy to the neurological ICU. Which data **warrant immediate** intervention?
    1. The client is alert to name but is unable to tell the nurse the location.
    2. The client has an output of 2,500 mL since surgery and an intake of 1,000 mL.
    3. The client's vital signs are T 97.6°F, P 88, R 20, and BP 130/80.
    4. The client has a 3-cm amount of dark-red drainage on the turban dressing.

63. Which laboratory value should be monitored by the nurse for the client diagnosed with diabetes insipidus?
    1. Serum sodium.
    2. Serum calcium.
    3. Urine glucose.
    4. Urine white blood cells.

64. The nurse is discharging a client diagnosed with diabetes insipidus. Which statement made by the client **warrants further** intervention?
    1. "I will keep a list of my medications in my wallet and wear a medical alert bracelet."
    2. "I should take my medication in the morning and leave it refrigerated at home."
    3. "I should weigh myself every morning and record any weight gain."
    4. "If I develop tightness in my chest, I will call my health-care provider."

65. The client is admitted to the medical unit with a diagnosis of possible diabetes insipidus (DI). Which instructions should the nurse teach regarding a fluid deprivation test?
    1. The client will be asked to drink 100 mL of fluid as rapidly as possible and then will not be allowed fluid for 24 hours.
    2. The client will be administered an injection of antidiuretic hormone (ADH), and urine output will be measured for 4 to 6 hours.
    3. The client will have nothing by mouth (NPO), and vital signs and weights will be done hourly until the end of the test.
    4. An IV will be started with normal saline, and the client will be asked to try to hold the urine in the bladder until a sonogram can be done.

66. The nurse is caring for clients on a medical floor. Which client should be assessed **first**?
    1. The client diagnosed with SIADH and weight gain of 1.5 pounds since yesterday.
    2. The client diagnosed with a pituitary tumor and diabetes insipidus with an intake of 1,500 mL and an output of 1,600 mL in the last 8 hours.
    3. The client diagnosed with SIADH having muscle twitches.
    4. The client diagnosed with DI, reporting feeling tired after having to get up at night.

67. The HCP has ordered 40 g/24 hr of intranasal vasopressin for a client diagnosed with diabetes insipidus. Each metered spray delivers 10 g. The client takes the medication every 12 hours. How many sprays are delivered at each dosing time?

    <br>

68. The nurse is planning the care of a client diagnosed with SIADH. Which interventions should be implemented? **Select all that apply.**
    1. Restrict fluids per HCP order.
    2. Assess level of consciousness every 2 hours.
    3. Provide an atmosphere of stimulation.
    4. Monitor urine and serum osmolality.
    5. Weigh the client every 3 days.

69. The nurse is caring for a client diagnosed with DI. Which intervention should be implemented?
    1. Administer sliding-scale insulin as ordered.
    2. Restrict caffeinated beverages.
    3. Check urine ketones if blood glucose is >250.
    4. Assess tissue turgor every 4 hours.

70. The UAP reports to the nurse she has filled the water pitcher four times during the shift for a client diagnosed with a closed head injury, and the client has asked for the pitcher to be filled again. Which intervention should the RN implement **first**?
    1. Tell the UAP to fill the pitcher with ice cold water.
    2. Instruct the UAP to start measuring the client's I&O.
    3. Assess the client for polyuria and polydipsia.
    4. Check the client's BUN and creatinine levels.

71. The nurse is admitting a client diagnosed with SIADH. Which clinical manifestations should be reported to the HCP?
    1. Serum sodium of 112 mEq/L and a headache.
    2. Serum potassium of 5.0 mEq/L and heightened awareness.
    3. Serum calcium of 10 mg/dL and tented tissue turgor.
    4. Serum magnesium of 1.6 mg/dL and large urinary output.

72. The male client diagnosed with SIADH secondary to cancer of the lung tells the nurse he wants to discontinue the fluid restriction and does not care if he dies. Which action by the nurse is an example of the ethical principle of **autonomy**?
    1. Discuss the information the client told the nurse with the HCP and significant other.
    2. Explain it is possible the client could have a seizure if he drank fluid beyond the restrictions.
    3. Notify the HCP of the client's wishes and give the client fluids as desired.
    4. Allow the client an extra drink of water and explain the nurse could get into trouble if the client tells the HCP.

## Thyroid Disorders

73. The client is diagnosed with hypothyroidism. Which clinical manifestations should the nurse expect the client to exhibit?
    1. Reports of extreme fatigue and hair loss.
    2. Exophthalmos and reports of nervousness.
    3. Reports of profuse sweating and flushed skin.
    4. Tetany and reports of stiffness of the hands.

74. The nurse identifies the client problem "risk for imbalanced body temperature" for the client diagnosed with hypothyroidism. Which intervention should be included in the plan of care?
    1. Discourage the use of an electric blanket.
    2. Assess the client's temperature every 2 hours.
    3. Keep the room temperature cool.
    4. Plan activity intervals to promote rest.

75. The client diagnosed with hypothyroidism is prescribed levothyroxine. Which assessment data indicate the medication has been **effective**?
    1. The client has a 3-pound weight gain.
    2. The client has a decreased pulse rate.
    3. The client's temperature is WNL.
    4. The client denies any diaphoresis.

76. Which nursing intervention should be included in the plan of care for the client diagnosed with hyperthyroidism?
    1. Increase the amount of fiber in the diet.
    2. Encourage a low-calorie, low-protein diet.
    3. Decrease the client's fluid intake to 1,000 mL/day.
    4. Provide six small, well-balanced meals a day.

77. The client is admitted to the ICU diagnosed with myxedema coma. Which assessment data **warrant immediate** intervention by the nurse?
    1. Serum blood glucose level of 74 mg/dL.
    2. Pulse oximeter reading of 90%.
    3. Telemetry reading showing sinus bradycardia.
    4. The client is lethargic and sleeps all the time.

78. Which medication order should the nurse **question** in the client diagnosed with untreated hypothyroidism?
    1. Thyroid hormones.
    2. Oxygen.
    3. Sedatives.
    4. Laxatives.

79. Which statement made by the client makes the nurse suspect the client is experiencing hyperthyroidism?
    1. "I just don't seem to have any appetite anymore."
    2. "I have a bowel movement about every 3 to 4 days."
    3. "My skin is really becoming dry and coarse."
    4. "I have noticed all my collars are getting tighter."

80. The 68-year-old client diagnosed with hyperthyroidism is being treated with radioactive iodine therapy. Which interventions should the nurse discuss with the client? **Select all that apply.**
    1. Explain that it will take up to a month for symptoms of hyperthyroidism to subside.
    2. Teach that the iodine therapy will have to be tapered slowly over 1 week.
    3. Discuss that the client will have to be hospitalized during the radioactive therapy.
    4. Inform the client after therapy the client will not have to take any medication.
    5. Tell the client they could experience a metallic taste in the mouth and nausea.

81. The nurse is teaching the client diagnosed with hyperthyroidism. Which information should be taught to the client? **Select all that apply.**
    1. Notify the HCP if a 3-pound weight loss occurs in 2 days.
    2. Discuss ways to cope with emotional lability.
    3. Notify the HCP if taking OTC medication.
    4. Carry a medical identification card or bracelet.
    5. Teach how to take thyroid medications correctly.

82. The nurse is providing an in-service on thyroid disorders. One of the attendees asks the nurse, "Why don't the people in the United States get goiters as often as those in other countries?" Which statement by the nurse is the **best response**?
    1. "It is because of the screening techniques used in the United States."
    2. "It is a genetic predisposition rare in North Americans."
    3. "The medications available in the United States decrease goiters."
    4. "Iodized salt helps prevent the development of goiters in the United States."

83. The nurse is preparing to administer the following medications. Which medication should the nurse **question** administering?
    1. The thyroid hormone to the client without a $T_3$, $T_4$ level.
    2. The regular insulin to the client with a blood glucose level of 210 mg/dL.
    3. The loop diuretic to the client with a potassium level of 3.3 mEq/L.
    4. The cardiac glycoside to the client with a digoxin level of 1.4 mg/dL.

84. Which clinical manifestations should make the nurse suspect the client is experiencing a thyroid storm?
    1. Obstipation and hypoactive bowel sounds.
    2. Hyperpyrexia and extreme tachycardia.
    3. Hypotension and bradycardia.
    4. Decreased respirations and hypoxia.

# CONCEPTS

The concepts covered in this chapter focus on metabolism and acid–base problems. Exemplars that are covered are diabetes mellitus types 1 and 2 and thyroid disorders. Interrelated concepts of the nursing process and clinical judgment are covered throughout the questions. The concept of clinical judgment is presented in prioritizing or "first" questions.

85. The nurse is administering morning medications. Which medications should the nurse **question** administering?
    1. The oral sucralfate to a client before the breakfast meal.
    2. The subcutaneous insulin to a client refusing blood glucose checks.
    3. The levothyroxine PO to a client diagnosed with hypothyroidism.
    4. The sliding scale insulin to a client with a 320 mg/dL blood glucose level.

86. The nurse is administering medications at the beginning of the day shift. Which should the nurse implement **first**?

| Client Name: Mr. C.A. | MR# 3456789 | Diagnosis: Diabetes Mellitus Type 2 |
|---|---|---|
| Age: 63 years | Allergies: NKDA | |
| | 0701–1900 | 1901–0700 |
| Regular insulin Subcutaneously a.c. and h.s. 0–60 = 1 amp D$_{50}$ 61–150 = 0 units 151–300 = 5 units 301–450 = 10 units Greater than 450 = Call HCP | 0730 1130 | 1630 2100 |
| Glargine 15 units SQ a.c. | 0730 | |
| Metformin 500 mg PO bid | 0800 | 1930 |
| Signature of Nurse: | Day Nurse RN/DN | Night Nurse RN/NN |

1. The nurse should determine the blood glucose level.
2. The nurse should combine the sliding scale insulin with the glargine.
3. The nurse should prepare to give both insulins and metformin.
4. The nurse should check the client's health record for new orders.

87. The nurse identified a concept of metabolism for a client diagnosed with diabetes mellitus type 1. Which interventions should the nurse include in the plan of care? **Select all that apply.**
    1. Teach the client to perform self-glucose monitoring.
    2. Instruct the client about complications of high glucose levels.
    3. Instruct the client to inspect the feet daily.
    4. Explain the need to carry a source of quick-acting proteins.
    5. Encourage the client to have regular eye examinations.

88. The client diagnosed with hyperthyroidism is reporting being hot and cannot sit still. Which should the RN do based on the assessment?
    1. Continue to monitor the client.
    2. Have the UAP take the client's vital signs.
    3. Request an order for a sedative.
    4. Insist the client lie down and rest.

89. The concepts of nutrition and metabolism have been identified for the client. Which referral should the nurse include in the plan of care?
    1. Physical therapy.
    2. Social work.
    3. Speech therapy.
    4. Dietary.

90. Which laboratory data would the nurse identify when discussing a client diagnosed with uncontrolled diabetes mellitus type 2?

1.

| Laboratory Test | Patient Results | Normal Values |
|---|---|---|
| Glucose | 89 | Fasting < 100 mg/dL Random < 200 mg/dL |
| Hemoglobin A1c | 5.5 | Non-diabetic 4%–5.5% Prediabetes 5.7%–6.4% Diabetes 6.5% or less |

2.

| Laboratory Test | Patient Results | Normal Values |
|---|---|---|
| Glucose | 134 | Fasting < 100 mg/dL Random < 200 mg/dL |
| Hemoglobin A1c | 5.8 | Non-diabetic 4%–5.5% Prediabetes 5.7%–6.4% Diabetes 6.5% or less |

3.

| Laboratory Test | Patient Results | Normal Values |
|---|---|---|
| Glucose | 112 | Fasting < 100 mg/dL<br>Random < 200 mg/dL |
| Hemoglobin A1c | 6.2 | Non-diabetic 4%–5.5%<br>Prediabetes 5.7%–6.4%<br>Diabetes 6.5% or less |

4.

| Laboratory Test | Patient Results | Normal Values |
|---|---|---|
| Glucose | 439 | Fasting < 100 mg/dL<br>Random < 200 mg/dL |
| Hemoglobin A1c | 9.3 | Non-diabetic 4%–5.5%<br>Prediabetes 5.7%–6.4%<br>Diabetes 6.5% or less |

91. The nurse identified a concept of metabolism for a client diagnosed with diabetes. Which antecedent would be identified as placing the client at **risk** for diabetes?
    1. Nutrition.
    2. Sensory perception.
    3. pH regulation.
    4. Medication.

92. The client is diagnosed with hypothyroidism. Which assessment data support this diagnosis?
    1. The client's vital signs are T 99.0, P 110, R 26, and BP 145/80.
    2. The client reports constipation and being constantly cold.
    3. The client has an intake of 780 mL and an output of 256 mL.
    4. The client reports a headache and has projectile vomiting.

93. The client diagnosed with diabetes reports a curtain being drawn across the eyes. Which should the nurse implement **first**?
    1. Assess the eyes using an ophthalmoscope.
    2. Tell the client to keep the eyes closed.
    3. Notify the health-care provider (HCP).
    4. Call the rapid response team (RRT).

94. The nurse is teaching the client diagnosed with diabetes. Which should the nurse teach to **limit** the complications of diabetes?
    1. Teach the client to keep the blood glucose under 140 mg/dL.
    2. Demonstrate how to test the urine for ketones.
    3. Instruct the client to apply petroleum jelly between the toes.
    4. Allow the client to eat meals as desired and then take insulin.

95. Which interrelated concepts could be identified as actual or potential for a 56-year-old male client diagnosed with diabetes mellitus type 2? **Select all that apply.**
    1. Nutrition.
    2. Metabolism.
    3. Infection.
    4. Male reproduction.
    5. Skin integrity.

96. Which client would the nurse identify as being **at risk** for developing diabetes?
    1. The client with a diet of mostly candy and potatoes.
    2. The 22-year-old client taking birth control pills.
    3. The client having a cousin diagnosed with diabetes 2 years ago.
    4. The 38-year-old female after delivering a 10-pound infant.

# PRACTICE QUESTIONS ANSWERS AND RATIONALES

## Diabetes Mellitus

1. 1. Type 1 diabetes usually occurs in young, underweight clients. In this disease, there is no production of insulin from the beta cells in the pancreas. People with type 1 diabetes are insulin-dependent with a rapid onset of symptoms, including polyuria, polydipsia, and polyphagia.
   2. **Type 2 diabetes is a disorder usually occurring around the age of 40, but it is now being detected in children and young adults as a result of obesity and sedentary lifestyles. Nonhealing wounds are a sign of type 2 diabetes (Salazar, Ennis, & Koh, 2016). This client weighs 248.6 pounds and is short.**
   3. Gestational diabetes occurs during pregnancy.
   4. Acanthosis nigricans (AN), dark pigmentation and skin creases in the neck, is a sign of hyperinsulinemia. The pancreas is secreting excess amounts of insulin as a result of excessive caloric intake. It is identified in young children and is a precursor to the development of type 2 diabetes.

   **TEST-TAKING HINT: The test taker must be aware of kilograms and pounds. The stem is asking about a disease process, and acanthosis nigricans is a clinical manifestation of a disease, not a disease itself. Therefore, the test taker should not select this as a correct answer.**

2. 1. The acceptable level for an A1c for a client diagnosed with diabetes is less than 7%, which corresponds to a 154 mg/dL average blood glucose level.
   2. This result is not within acceptable levels for the client diagnosed with diabetes, which is less than 7%.
   3. **This result parallels a serum blood glucose level of approximately 185 mg/dL. An A1c is a blood test reflecting average blood glucose levels over a period of 3 months; clients with elevated blood glucose levels are at risk for developing long-term complications (American Diabetes Association, 2020).**
   4. An A1c of 13% is dangerously high; it reflects a 326-mg/dL average blood glucose level over the past 3 months.

**TEST-TAKING HINT: The test taker must know normal and abnormal diagnostic laboratory values. Laboratory values may vary depending on which laboratory performs the test.**

3. 1. **Insulin isophane (Humulin N), intermediate-acting insulin, peaks in 4 to 6 hours (Vallerand & Sanoski, 2019). The client will be at risk for hypoglycemia before midnight, which is why the client should receive a bedtime snack. This snack will prevent nighttime hypoglycemia.**
   2. The food intake at lunch will not affect the client's blood glucose level at midnight.
   3. The client's glucometer reading should be done around 2100 to assess the effectiveness of insulin given at 1600.
   4. The onset of insulin isophane (Humulin N), intermediate-acting insulin, is 2 to 4 hours, but it does not peak until 4 to 6 hours.

**TEST-TAKING HINT: The test taker must be familiar with the five types of insulins (rapid-acting, short-acting, intermediate-acting, long-acting, and combinations); the peak, onset, and duration of the five types of insulins; and the generic names of the insulins in each category. In this case, memorization is required.**

4. **Three units.**
   The client's result is 189, which is between 151 and 200, so the nurse should administer 3 units of insulin lispro (Humalog), rapid-acting insulin, subcutaneously.

**TEST-TAKING HINT: The test taker must be aware of the way HCPs write medication orders. HCPs order insulin on a sliding scale according to a range of blood glucose levels.**

5. 1. The client diagnosed with type 2 diabetes, not taking insulin or oral agents, does not need extra food before exercise.
   2. The client diagnosed with diabetes at risk for hypoglycemia when exercising should carry a simple carbohydrate, but this client is not at risk for hypoglycemia.
   3. Clients with diabetes controlled by diet and exercise must exercise daily at the same time and in the same amount to control the glucose level.
   4. **All clients should perform warm-up and cool-down routines to help prevent muscle strain and injury while exercising.**

**TEST-TAKING HINT:** Options "1" and "2" apply directly to clients diagnosed with diabetes, and options "3" and "4" do not directly address clients diagnosed with diabetes. The reader could narrow the choices by either eliminating or including the two similar options.

6. 1. Crumbling toenails indicate tinea unguium, which is a fungus infection of the toenail.
   2. Athlete's foot is not a life-threatening fungal infection.
   3. A necrotic big toe indicates "dead" tissue. The client does not feel pain, does not realize the injury, and does not seek treatment. Increased blood glucose levels decrease the oxygen supply needed to heal the wound and increase the risk of developing an infection.
   4. Big, thick toenails are fungal infections and do not require immediate intervention by the nurse.

**TEST-TAKING HINT:** The test taker should select the option indicating this is possibly a life-threatening complication or some type of assessment data the health-care provider should be informed of immediately. Remember, "warrants immediate intervention."

7. 1. Age-related visual changes and diabetic retinopathy could cause the client to have difficulty in reading and drawing up insulin dosage accurately.
   2. The PT level is monitored for clients receiving warfarin (Coumadin), an anticoagulant, which is not ordered for clients diagnosed with diabetes, type 1 or 2.
   3. Glycosylated hemoglobin is a serum blood test usually performed in a laboratory, not in the client's home. The hemoglobin A1c is performed every 3 months. Self-monitoring blood glucose should be taught to the client.
   4. The client's feet should be checked daily, not weekly. In a week, the client could develop gangrene from an unnoticed injury.

**TEST-TAKING HINT:** Always notice the age of a client if it is provided because this is important when determining the correct answer for the question. Be sure to note the adverbs, such as "weekly" instead of "daily."

8. 1. High-fat diets are not recommended for clients diagnosed with diabetes, and food does not have an effect on a CT scan with contrast.

2. According to the Food and Drug Administration (FDA), biguanides, oral diabetic medications such as metformin, must be held for a test with contrast medium in clients with a glomerular filtration rate below 60 mL/min/1.73 m² or a history of liver disease, alcoholism, or heart failure. In these clients, biguanides combined with contrast mediums increase the risk of lactic acidosis, which leads to renal problems. Before 2016, the FDA required metformin to be discontinued for all clients, regardless of medical history (Lipska, Flory, Hennessy, & Inzucchi, 2016).
   3. Informed consent is not required for a CT scan. The admission consent covers routine diagnostic procedures.
   4. Pancreatic enzymes are administered when the pancreas cannot produce amylase and lipase, not when the beta cells cannot produce insulin.

**TEST-TAKING HINT:** The test taker could eliminate option "1" because high-fat diets are not recommended for any client. Because the stem specifically refers to the biguanide medication and CT contrast, a good choice addresses both of these. Option "2" discusses both the medication and the test.

9. Correct answers are 1, 2, and 5.
   1. The most important issue to teach clients is to take insulin, even if they are unable to eat. Glucose levels are increased with illness and stress.
   2. The client should drink liquids such as regular cola or orange juice or eat regular gelatin, which provides enough glucose to prevent hypoglycemia when receiving insulin.
   3. Ketones indicate a breakdown of fat and must be reported to the HCP because they can lead to metabolic acidosis.
   4. Blood glucose levels and ketones must be checked every 3 to 4 hours, not daily.
   5. The HCP should be notified if the blood glucose level is this high. Regular insulin may need to be prescribed to keep the blood glucose level within an acceptable range.

**TEST-TAKING HINT:** This is an alternate-type question having more than one correct answer. The test taker should read all options and determine if each is an appropriate intervention.

10. 1. The blood glucose level should be obtained, but it is not the first intervention.
    2. If it is determined the client is having a hypoglycemic reaction, orange juice is appropriate.
    3. **Regular insulin (Humulin R), fast-acting insulin, peaks in 2 to 4 hours. Therefore, the registered nurse (RN) should think about the possibility the client is having a hypoglycemic reaction and should assess the client. The nurse should not delegate nursing tasks to a UAP if the client is unstable.**
    4. Dextrose 50% is only administered if the client is unconscious, and the nurse suspects hypoglycemia.

**TEST-TAKING HINT: When answering a question requiring the nurse to decide which intervention to implement first, all four options are plausible for the situation, but only one answer should be implemented first. The test taker must apply the nursing process; assessment is the first step of the nursing process.**

11. 1. This is an example of interviewing the client; it is not an example of client advocacy.
    2. **Client advocacy focuses support on the client's autonomy. Even if the nurse disagrees with his living on the street, it is the client's right. Arranging for someone to give him his insulin provides for his needs and allows his choices.**
    3. Adult Protective Services is an organization investigating any actual or potential abuse in adults. This client is not being abused by anyone.
    4. The client needs the insulin to control diabetes, and talking to the HCP about taking him off a needed medication is not an example of advocacy.

**TEST-TAKING HINT: Remember, the test taker must understand what the question is asking and the definition of the terms.**

12. 1. The short-term goal must address the response part of the nursing diagnosis, which is "high risk for hyperglycemia," and this blood glucose level is within acceptable ranges for a noncompliant client.
    2. This is an appropriate goal for a knowledge-deficit nursing diagnosis. Noncompliance is not always the result of a knowledge deficit.

3. The nurse is implementing an intervention, and the question asks for a goal that addresses the problem of "high risk for hyperglycemia."
    4. The question asks for a short-term goal, and this is an example of a long-term goal.

**TEST-TAKING HINT: Remember, the nursing diagnosis consists of a problem related to an etiology. The goals must address the problem, and the interventions must address the etiology. The test taker should always remember a short-term goal is usually a goal met during the hospitalization, and the long-term goal may take weeks, months, or even years.**

13. 1. **Kussmaul's respirations occur with diabetic ketoacidosis (DKA) as a result of the breakdown of fat, resulting in ketones.**
    2. Diarrhea and epigastric pain are not associated with HHNS.
    3. **Dry mucous membranes are a result of the hyperglycemia and occur with both HHNS and DKA.**
    4. This occurs with DKA as a result of the breakdown of fat, resulting in ketones.

**TEST-TAKING HINT: The test taker must be able to differentiate between HHNS (type 2 diabetes) and DKA (type 1 diabetes), which primarily is the result of the breakdown of fat and results in an increase in ketones causing a decrease in pH, resulting in metabolic acidosis.**

14. 1. **The initial fluid replacement is 0.9% normal saline (an isotonic solution) intravenously, followed by 0.45% saline. The rate depends on the client's fluid volume status and physical health, especially of the heart.**
    2. Regular insulin, not intermediate, is the insulin of choice because of its quick onset and peak in 2 to 4 hours.
    3. Blood glucometer checks are done every 1 hour or more often for clients diagnosed with HHNS and receiving regular insulin drips.
    4. ABGs are not affected in HHNS because there is no breakdown of fat, resulting in ketones leading to metabolic acidosis.

**TEST-TAKING HINT: The test taker should eliminate option "3" based on the word "daily." In the ICU with a very ill client, most checks are more often than daily. Remember to look at adjectives; "intermediate" in option "2" is the word eliminating this as a possible correct answer.**

**15.** 1. Glucose is elevated in DKA; therefore, the HCP would not be replacing glucose.

2. **The client diagnosed with DKA loses potassium from increased urinary output, acidosis, catabolic state, and vomiting. Replacement is essential for preventing cardiac dysrhythmias secondary to hypokalemia.**

3. Calcium is not affected in the client diagnosed with DKA.

4. The prescribed IV for DKA—0.9% normal saline—has sodium, but it is not specifically ordered for sodium replacement. This is an isotonic solution.

**TEST-TAKING HINT: Option "1" should be eliminated because the problem with DKA is elevated glucose, so the HCP would not be replacing it. The test taker should use physiology knowledge and realize potassium is in the cell.**

**16.** 1. The regular intravenous insulin is continued because ketosis is not present, as with DKA.

2. The client diagnosed with type 2 diabetes does not excrete ketones in HHNS because there is enough insulin to prevent fat breakdown but not enough to lower blood glucose.

3. The client may or may not feel like eating, but it is not the appropriate intervention when the blood glucose level is reduced to 300 mg/dL.

4. **When the glucose level is decreased to around 300 mg/dL, the regular insulin infusion therapy is decreased. Subcutaneous insulin will be administered per sliding scale.**

**TEST-TAKING HINT: When two options are the opposite of each other, they can either be eliminated or can help eliminate the other two options as incorrect answers. Options "2" and "3" do not have insulin in the answer; therefore, they should be eliminated as possible answers.**

**17.** 1. **The nurse should assume the client is hypoglycemic and administer IVP dextrose, which will rouse the client immediately. If the collapse is the result of hyperglycemia, this additional dextrose will not further injure the client.**

2. The health-care provider may or may not need to be notified, but this is not the first intervention.

3. The client should be left in the client's room, and 50% dextrose should be administered first.

4. The serum glucose level requires a venipuncture, which will take too long. A blood glucometer reading may be obtained, but the nurse should first treat the client, not the machine. The glucometer only reads "low" after a certain point, and a serum level is needed to confirm the exact glucose level.

**TEST-TAKING HINT: The question is requesting the test taker to select which intervention should be implemented first. All four options could be possible interventions, but only one intervention should be implemented first. The test taker should select the intervention directly treating the client; do not select a diagnostic test.**

**18.** 1. This indicates the client is dehydrated, which does not indicate the client is getting better.

2. **The client's level of consciousness can be altered because of dehydration and acidosis. If the client's sensorium is intact, the client is getting better and responding to medical treatment.**

3. These ABGs indicate metabolic acidosis; therefore, the client is not responding to treatment.

4. This potassium level is low and indicates hypokalemia, which shows the client is not responding to medical treatment.

**TEST-TAKING HINT: The phrase "responding to medical treatment" is asking the test taker to determine which data indicate the client is getting better. The correct answer will be normal data, and the other three options will be clinical manifestations of the disease process or condition.**

**19.** 1. The client is on a special diet and should not have any additional food.

2. **The client will not be compliant with the diet if still hungry. Therefore, the nurse should request that the dietitian talk with the client and adjust the meals so the client will adhere to the diet.**

3. The nurse does not need to notify the HCP for an increase in caloric intake. The appropriate referral is to the dietitian.

4. The client is on a special diet. The nurse needs to help the client maintain compliance with the medical treatment and should refer the client to the dietitian.

**TEST-TAKING HINT: The test taker should select the option attempting to ensure the client maintains compliance. The test taker should remember to work with members of the multidisciplinary health-care team.**

20. 1. A client diagnosed with type 2 diabetes usually is prescribed oral hypoglycemic medications, not insulin.
    2. The client could not eat enough food to cause a 680 mg/dL blood glucose level; therefore, this question does not need to be asked.
    3. **The most common precipitating factor is infection. The manifestations may be slow to appear, with onset ranging from 24 hours to 2 weeks (Hoffman & Sullivan, 2020).**
    4. This does not help determine the cause of this client's HHNS.

**TEST-TAKING HINT: If the test taker does not know the answer to this question, the test taker could possibly relate to the phrase "acute complication," realizing a medical problem might cause this, and thus select infection, option "3."**

21. 1. The American Diabetes Association is an excellent referral, but the nurse should discuss specific ways to prevent DKA.
    2. The client should be careful with OTC medications, but this intervention does not help prevent the development of DKA.
    3. **Illness increases blood glucose levels; therefore, the client must take insulin and consume high-carbohydrate foods such as regular Jell-O, regular popsicles, and orange juice.**
    4. Vaccines are important to help prevent illness, but regardless of whether the client gets these vaccines, the client can still develop diabetic ketoacidosis.

**TEST-TAKING HINT: The words "most important" in the stem of the question indicate one or more options may be appropriate instructions, but only one is the priority intervention.**

22. 1. This blood glucose level is elevated, but not life-threatening, in the client diagnosed with type 2 diabetes. Therefore, a less experienced nurse could care for this client.
    2. Hypoglycemia is an acute complication of type 1 diabetes, but it can be managed by frequent monitoring, so a less experienced nurse could care for this client.
    3. **Multifocal PVCs, which are secondary to hypokalemia and can occur in clients diagnosed with DKA, are a potentially life-threatening emergency. This client needs an experienced nurse.**
    4. A plasma osmolarity of 275 to 295 mOsm/kg is within normal limits; therefore, a less experienced nurse could care for this client.

**TEST-TAKING HINT: The test taker must select the client with an abnormal, unexpected, or a life-threatening clinical manifestation for the disease process and assign this client to the most experienced nurse.**

23. 1. This ABG indicates respiratory acidosis, which is not expected.
    2. This ABG is normal, which is not expected.
    3. This ABG indicates respiratory alkalosis, which is not expected.
    4. **This ABG indicates metabolic acidosis, which is expected in a client diagnosed with diabetic ketoacidosis.**

**TEST-TAKING HINT: The test taker must know normal ABGs to be able to answer this question correctly. Normal ABGs are pH 7.35 to 7.45; $Pao_2$ 80 to 100; $Pco_2$ 35 to 45; $Hco_3$ 22 to 26.**

24. Correct answers are 1, 2, 3, 4, and 5.
    1. **The nurse should always address the airway when a client is seriously ill.**
    2. **The client must be assessed for fluid volume deficit, and then for fluid volume excess after the fluid replacement is started.**
    3. **The electrolyte imbalance of primary concern is the depletion of potassium.**
    4. **Ketones are excreted in the urine; levels are documented from negative to a large amount. Ketones should be monitored frequently.**
    5. **The nurse must ensure the client's fluid intake and output are equal.**

**TEST-TAKING HINT: The test taker must select all answer options that apply. Do not try to outguess the item writer. In some instances, all options are correct.**

## Pancreatitis

25. 1. These laboratory values are monitored for clients diagnosed with kidney failure.
    2. These laboratory values are elevated in clients diagnosed with myocardial infarction.
    3. **Serum amylase increases within 2 to 12 hours of the onset of acute pancreatitis to two to three times normal and returns to normal in 3 to 4 days; lipase elevates and remains elevated for 7 to 14 days.**
    4. Bilirubin may be elevated as a result of compression of the common duct, and hypocalcemia develops in up to 25% of clients diagnosed with acute pancreatitis, but these laboratory values do not confirm the diagnosis.

**TEST-TAKING HINT:** The test taker must be able to identify at least two laboratory values that reflect each organ function before taking the NCLEX-RN®. There is no test-taking hint to help select the correct answer; this is knowledge.

26. 1. The client will be NPO to help decrease pain, but it is not the priority problem because the client will have intravenous fluids.
    2. **Autodigestion of the pancreas results in severe epigastric pain, accompanied by nausea, vomiting, abdominal tenderness, and muscle guarding.**
    3. Nutritional imbalance is a possible client problem, but it is not a priority.
    4. Knowledge deficit is always a client problem, but it is not a priority over pain.

**TEST-TAKING HINT:** The test taker should apply Maslow's hierarchy of needs when selecting the priority problem for a client. After airway, pain is often a priority.

27. 1. Pancreatic enzymes must be administered with meals to enhance the digestion of starches and fats in the gastrointestinal tract.
    2. The client's respiratory rate is within normal limits; therefore, the pain medication, morphine, should be administered to the client having pain.
    3. This is a normal potassium level; therefore, the nurse does not need to question administering the loop diuretic medication.
    4. The apical pulse is within normal limits; therefore, the nurse should not question administering the beta blocker medication.

**TEST-TAKING HINT:** The test taker must determine if the assessment data provided in the option are abnormal, unexpected, or life-threatening to warrant questioning the administration of the medication.

28. 1. Bedrest will decrease metabolic rate, gastrointestinal secretion, pancreatic secretions, and pain; therefore, this HCP's order should not be questioned.
    2. The client will be NPO; therefore, initiating IV therapy is an appropriate order.
    3. Short-term weight gain changes reflect fluid balance because the client will be NPO and receiving IV fluids. Daily weight is an appropriate HCP's order.
    4. The client will be NPO, which will decrease the stimulation of the pancreatic enzymes, resulting in decreased autodigestion of the pancreas, therefore decreasing pain.

**TEST-TAKING HINT:** The test taker must determine which HCP's order is not expected for the diagnosis. Sometimes, if the test taker asks which order is expected, it is easier to identify the unexpected or abnormal HCP order.

29. Correct answers are 3 and 5.
    1. Alcohol must be avoided entirely because it can cause stones to form, blocking pancreatic ducts and the outflow of pancreatic juice, causing further inflammation and destruction of the pancreas.
    2. Stress stimulates the pancreas and should be dealt with, but it is unrealistic to think a client can avoid all stress. By definition, the absence of all stress is death.
    3. **Smoking stimulates the pancreas to release pancreatic enzymes and should be stopped.**
    4. The client has acute pancreatitis, and pancreatic enzymes are only needed for chronic pancreatitis.
    5. **The client should initially eat a high-carbohydrate, low-fat diet to decrease the stimulation of pancreatic enzyme production.**

**TEST-TAKING HINT:** The test taker should eliminate option "2" because of the word "all," which is an absolute, and there are few absolutes in health care. The test taker should note the adjective "acute" in the stem, which may help the test taker eliminate option "4" because enzymes are administered for a chronic condition.

30. 1. Any change in the client's stool should be a cause for concern to the clinic nurse.
    2. This is not necessary because the nurse knows changes in stool occur as a complication of pancreatitis, and the client needs to see the HCP.
    3. **Steatorrhea (fatty, frothy, foul-smelling stool) is caused by a decrease in pancreatic enzyme secretion and indicates impaired digestion and possibly an increase in the severity of the pancreatitis. The client should see the HCP.**
    4. Decreasing fat in the diet will not help stop this type of stool.

**TEST-TAKING HINT:** This question requires the test taker to have knowledge of the disease process, but if the test taker knows the exocrine function of the pancreas is part of the gastrointestinal system, the test taker might think altered stool is a cause for concern.

31. Correct answers are 3 and 5.
    1. The client is at risk for diabetes mellitus (destruction of beta cells), not diabetes insipidus, a disorder of the pituitary gland.
    2. Crohn's disease is an inflammatory disorder of the lining of the gastrointestinal system, especially of the terminal ileum.
    3. Narcotic addiction is related to frequent, severe pain episodes often occurring with chronic pancreatitis, which requires narcotics for relief.
    4. Peritonitis, an inflammation of the lining of the abdomen, is not a common complication of chronic pancreatitis.
    5. Metabolic bone disease, also known as chronic-pancreatitis-associated osteopathy, is a common complication of chronic pancreatitis and can increase the risk of low trauma fractures in clients (Ramsey, Conwell, & Hart, 2017).

**TEST-TAKING HINT:** The test taker may be able to delete options based on normal anatomical and physiological data. Diabetes insipidus is a complication of the pituitary gland; Crohn's disease is a disease of the gastrointestinal tract; and the peritoneum is the lining of the abdomen. Therefore, options "1," "2," and "4" can be eliminated.

32. 1. During this procedure, a scope is placed down the client's throat; therefore, assessing for rectal bleeding is not an intervention.
    2. The client's throat has been anesthetized to insert the scope; therefore, fluid and food are withheld until the gag reflex has returned.
    3. The gag reflex will be suppressed as a result of the local anesthesia applied to the throat to insert the endoscope into the esophagus; therefore, the gag reflex must be assessed before allowing the client to resume eating or drinking.
    4. The client should be in a semi-Fowler's or side-lying position to prevent aspiration.

**TEST-TAKING HINT:** The test taker should apply the nursing process and select an option that addresses assessment—either "1" or "3." The medical prefix *endo-* should help the test taker select option "3" as the correct answer.

33. 1. Lying on the stomach will not help to decrease the client's pain.
    2. This is a position used by clients diagnosed with chronic obstructive pulmonary disease to help lung expansion.
    3. This fetal position decreases pain caused by the stretching of the peritoneum as a result of edema.
    4. Laying supine causes the peritoneum to stretch, which increases the pain.

**TEST-TAKING HINT:** The test taker should think about where the pancreas is located in the abdomen to help identify the correct answer. The prone or supine position causes the abdomen to be stretched, which increases pain.

34. Correct answers are 1, 3, 4, and 5.
    1. The return of bowel sounds indicates the return of peristalsis, and the nasogastric suction is usually discontinued within 24 to 48 hours thereafter.
    2. The client will be NPO secondary to chronic pancreatitis, and the client cannot eat with a nasogastric tube.
    3. The nurse should assess for clinical manifestations of infection or infiltration.
    4. Fasting and the NG tube increase the client's risk for mucous membrane irritation and breakdown.
    5. Blood glucose levels are monitored because clients diagnosed with chronic pancreatitis can develop diabetes mellitus.

**TEST-TAKING HINT:** This alternative-type question requires the test taker to select all interventions appropriate for the client's diagnosis. The test taker should evaluate each answer independently as to whether it is appropriate or not.

35. 1. Pancreatic enzymes enhance the digestion of starches (carbohydrates) in the gastrointestinal tract by supplying an exogenous (outside) source of the pancreatic enzymes protease, amylase, and lipase.
    2. Pancreatic enzymes decrease the number of bowel movements.
    3. The enzymes are enteric-coated and should not be crushed because the hydrochloric acid in the stomach will destroy the enzymes; these enzymes work in the small intestine.
    4. Pancreatic enzymes help break down carbohydrates, and bile breaks down fat.

**TEST-TAKING HINT:** Remember: Enzymes break down other foods and the names end in *-ase*. The test taker must know the normal function of organs to identify correct answers.

36. 1. Coffee, tea, and cola stimulate gastric and pancreatic secretions and may precipitate pain, so these foods should be avoided, not decreased.
    2. **High-fat and spicy foods stimulate gastric and pancreatic secretions and may precipitate an acute pancreatic attack.**
    3. Amylase and lipase levels must be checked via venipuncture with laboratory tests, and there are no daily tests the client can monitor at home.
    4. The client will be fatigued as a result of decreased metabolic energy production and will need to rest and not return to work immediately.

**TEST-TAKING HINT: The test taker should be careful with words such as "decrease" because many times the client must avoid certain foods and situations completely, not decrease the intake of them. Only a few blood studies are monitored at home on a daily basis—mainly glucose levels—which should cause the test taker to eliminate option "3."**

## Cancer of the Pancreas

37. 1. A yellow haze is a sign of a toxic level of digoxin, with the client seeing through the yellow haze. Seeing a yellow haze is not the same as the client having jaundice. In jaundice, the skin and sclera are yellow, clinical manifestations of pancreatic cancer.
    2. **The abdominal pain is often made worse by eating and lying supine in clients diagnosed with cancer of the pancreas.**
    3. The client does not know these terms, and the HCP should check these laboratory values.
    4. Clients diagnosed with cancer of the pancreas lose weight; they do not gain weight.

**TEST-TAKING HINT: The test taker could arrive at the correct answer by correlating words in the stem of the question and words in the answer options—the abdomen with eating and pain with pain.**

38. 1. Tube feedings are collaborative interventions, but the stem did not say the client had a feeding tube.
    2. Having family members bring food from home is an independent intervention.
    3. Assessment is an independent intervention and the first step in the nursing process. No one should have to tell the nurse to assess the client.
    4. **A collaborative intervention is to refer to the nutrition expert, the dietitian.**

**TEST-TAKING HINT: The keyword in the stem is "collaborative," which means another health-care discipline must be involved. Only options "1" and "4" involve other members of the health-care team. The test taker could eliminate distracter "1" by rereading the stem and realizing the stem did not include the client having a feeding tube.**

39. 1. Monitoring the blood glucose at random intervals, as done at a health fair, could identify possible diabetes mellitus or the presence of a pancreatic tumor, but detecting disease at an early stage is secondary screening, not primary prevention.
    2. Inspecting the skin for jaundice is a secondary nursing intervention.
    3. **Limiting the intake of meat and fats in the diet is an example of primary interventions. Risk factors for the development of cancer of the pancreas are cigarette smoking and eating a high-fat diet. By changing these behaviors, the client could possibly prevent the development of cancer of the pancreas. Other risk factors include genetic predisposition and exposure to industrial chemicals.**
    4. Instructing a client diagnosed with hyperglycemia (diabetes mellitus) is an example of tertiary nursing care.

**TEST-TAKING HINT: Even if the test taker were not sure of the definition of primary, secondary, or tertiary nursing interventions, "primary" means first. Only one answer option is preventive, and preventing something comes before treating it.**

40. 1. **The UAP can help a client to turn to the side and assume the fetal position, which decreases some abdominal pain.**
    2. Monitoring a Jackson Pratt drain is a high-level nursing intervention, which the UAP is not qualified to implement.
    3. Evaluation of the effectiveness of a prn medication must be done by the RN.
    4. The nurse should empty the bedside commode to determine if the client is continuing to pass melena (blood in the stool).

**TEST-TAKING HINT: There are basic rules to delegation. The nurse cannot delegate assessment, teaching, evaluation, medications, unstable clients, or situations requiring nursing judgment.**

41. 1. This is routine for radiation therapy, but chemotherapy is given 1 to 3 or 4 days in a row, and then a period of 3 to 4 weeks will elapse before the next treatment. The schedule will vary based on the chemotherapy drug used. This is called intermittent pulse therapy.
    2. **The most important person in the treatment of cancer is the client. Research has proven the more involved a client becomes in the care, the better the prognosis. Clients should have a chance to ask questions.**
    3. Cancer of any kind is a serious problem.
    4. Most antineoplastic medications are administered intravenously. Many of the medications can cause severe complications if administered intramuscularly.

**TEST-TAKING HINT: The test taker can eliminate option "3" based on this statement being denial of the problem.**

42. Correct answers are 3 and 5.
    1. The client should stay in the outpatient department after the procedure for observation unless the HCP determines a more extensive work-up should be completed.
    2. This is not the type of procedure where the results warrant emergency surgery. Cardiac catheterization sometimes results in emergency surgery, and the client is prepared for this possibility, but this is not the case with an ERCP.
    3. **The client should be NPO after midnight to make sure the stomach is empty to reduce the risk of aspiration during the procedure.**
    4. The possible blockage is of the duodenum, common bile duct, or pancreatic outlet.
    5. **A sore throat is commonly reported by clients following an ERCP. It is treated with throat lozenges and resolves in 1 to 2 days (American College of Gastroenterology, n.d.).**

**TEST-TAKING HINT: The nurse should never preface any instruction with "if done correctly" because this sets the nurse, HCP, and facility up for a lawsuit. The client is NPO for any procedure or surgery where the client will receive general or twilight sleep anesthesia. An endoscope is inserted into the mouth and down the throat, so irritation of the throat would be a common occurrence.**

43. 1. **The client will have jaundice, claycolored stools, and tea-colored urine resulting from blockage of the bile drainage.**
    2. Night sweats and fevers are associated with lymphoma.
    3. Left lower abdominal cramps are associated with diverticulitis, and tenesmus is straining when defecating.
    4. Nausea and coffee-ground emesis are clinical manifestations of gastric ulcers.

**TEST-TAKING HINT: The test taker should remember anatomical placement of organs. This eliminates options "3" and "4." The pancreas empties pancreatic enzymes into the small bowel in close proximity to where the common bile duct enters the intestine to aid in the digestion of carbohydrates and fats.**

44. 1. Clients diagnosed with cancer of the pancreas have a poor prognosis, but this is not the priority problem at this time.
    2. **This is major abdominal surgery, and massive fluid volume shifts occur when this type of trauma is experienced by the body. Maintaining the circulatory system without overloading it requires extremely close monitoring.**
    3. Pain is a priority but not over fluid volume status.
    4. Altered nutrition is an appropriate problem but not a priority over fluid volume shift. The client will be NPO with a nasogastric tube to suction and will be receiving total parenteral nutrition.

**TEST-TAKING HINT: The nurse should identify all of the problems, but one—fluid volume imbalance—has the greatest priority because, if not addressed promptly and correctly, it could lead to severe complications.**

45. Correct answers are 2, 3, and 4.
    1. The client is being discharged. There is no need for the client to continue recording intake and output at home.
    2. **The client has undergone radical and extensive surgery and will need narcotic pain medication, and a bowel regimen should be in place to prevent constipation.**
    3. **Removal of the pancreas will create a diabetic state for the client. The client will need insulin and pancreatic enzyme replacement.**
    4. **The client should not allow pain to reach above a "5" before taking pain medication or it will be more difficult to get the pain under control.**
    5. There is no reason for the client to sleep with the head of the bed elevated.

**TEST-TAKING HINT:** The test taker might choose option "3" by remembering the pancreas secretes insulin. Option "4" is taught to all clients in pain.

46. 1. The client may need IV medication, but in this case, if it is needed, it is 50% dextrose.
    2. The HCP might be notified, but the nurse needs to assess the client first.
    3. These are clinical manifestations of an insulin reaction (hypoglycemia). A bedside glucose check should be done. Pancreatic islet tumors can produce hyperinsulinemia or hypoglycemia.
    4. Treating the client is done after the nurse knows the glucose reading.

**TEST-TAKING HINT:** The test taker should remember the function of the pancreas. This leads the test taker to look for interventions for hypoglycemia.

47. 1. Food preferences are important for the caregiver to know because this will be the person preparing meals for the client, but it is not the highest priority.
    2. Cancer of the pancreas has a poor prognosis; the nurse should determine if the client has executed an advance directive to outline a vision of care.
    3. This is important because of payment issues, but it is not the highest priority.
    4. Clients diagnosed with cancer frequently have anorexia, and explaining the client should eat does not mean the client will eat.

**TEST-TAKING HINT:** The test taker needs to know general information about the disease process to answer this question, but option "2" is a good choice for many terminal diseases. Remember to read the questions carefully. The home health nurse is not arranging meals for the client.

48. 1. The client is at risk for poor nutrition and malabsorption syndrome for which tissue turgor assessment is appropriate, but the client problem is pruritus or itching.
    2. The itching is associated with the cancer and not a fungus.
    3. The client should be monitored for skin breakdown, but pruritus is itching, and an intervention is needed to prevent skin problems as a result of scratching.
    4. Keeping the fingernails short will reduce the chance of breaks in the skin from scratching.

**TEST-TAKING HINT:** The problem is "risk for skin breakdown." The etiology is "pruritus." Interventions address the etiology. Goals address the problem.

## Adrenal Disorders

49. 1. A moon face, buffalo hump, and hyperglycemia result from Cushing's syndrome, hyperfunction of the adrenal gland.
    2. Hirsutism is hair growth where it normally does not occur, such as facial hair on women. Fever and irritability, along with hirsutism, are clinical manifestations of Cushing's syndrome.
    3. Bronze pigmentation of the skin, particularly of the knuckles and other areas of skin creases, occurs in Addison's disease. Hypotension and anorexia also occur with Addison's disease.
    4. Tachycardia, bulging eyes, and goiter are clinical manifestations occurring with thyroid disorders.

**TEST-TAKING HINT:** This question contains answer options referring to opposite diseases, Addison's disease and Cushing's syndrome. If two options—in this case, options "1" and "2"—are appropriate for one of the diseases, then these two can be ruled out as the correct answer.

50. 1. Altered body image is a psychosocial problem, which is not a priority over a potentially lethal physical complication, and physical changes occur over an extended period.
    2. Activity intolerance will occur with adrenal gland hypofunction, but this is not a priority over dehydration.
    3. Impaired coping can occur in clients diagnosed with adrenal gland disorders, but it is not a priority over dehydration.
    4. Fluid volume deficit (dehydration) can lead to circulatory impairment and hyperkalemia.

**TEST-TAKING HINT:** Assuming all of the problems listed apply to the client diagnosed with Addison's disease, two are psychosocial problems and two are physiological. Applying Maslow's hierarchy of needs, the two psychological problems can be ruled out as the highest priority. Of the two options remaining, activity intolerance is not life-altering or threatening.

51. 1. Clients diagnosed with Addison's disease have adrenal gland hypofunction. The hormones normally produced by the gland must be replaced. Steroids and androgens are produced by the adrenal gland.
    2. The client will have decreased fluid volume, and fluid restriction exacerbates a crisis.
    3. The client requires a quiet, calm, relaxed atmosphere.
    4. The client walks with a stooped posture from fatigue, but gait training is not needed.

**TEST-TAKING HINT: To answer this question, the test taker must have knowledge of adrenal gland function.**

52. 1. The drugs quinidine, digoxin, and hydralazine can interfere with adrenal gland secretions and cause hypofunction. Cushing's syndrome is adrenal gland hyperfunction.
    2. **The adrenal gland secretes cortisol and the pituitary gland secretes adrenocorticotropic hormone (ACTH), a hormone used by the body to stimulate the production of cortisol.**
    3. A 24-hour urine specimen for 17-hydroxycorticosterone and 17-ketosteroid may be collected. Metanephrines and catecholamines are urine collections for pheochromocytomas.
    4. Spot urinalysis and WBCs count will not provide information on adrenal gland functions.

**TEST-TAKING HINT: If the test taker is aware the adrenal gland produces cortisol, then there is only one answer option that refers to cortisol.**

53. 1. Cushing's disease is not an autoimmune problem.
    2. **"Iatrogenic" means a problem has been caused by a medical treatment or procedure—in this case, treatment with steroids for another problem. Clients taking steroids over a period of time develop the clinical manifestations of Cushing's disease. Disease processes for which long-term steroids are prescribed include chronic obstructive pulmonary disease, cancer, and arthritis.**
    3. This could be a cause for primary Cushing's syndrome.
    4. There is a known reason for the client to have iatrogenic Cushing's syndrome.

**TEST-TAKING HINT: This question requires the test taker to know basic medical terminology.**

54. 1. Cushing's syndrome and disease predispose the client to develop infections as a result of the immunosuppressive nature of the disease.
    2. The client has too much cortisol; this client should not be receiving prednisone, a steroid medication.
    3. These are clinical manifestations of hypoglycemia, which is not expected in this client because this client has high glucose levels.
    4. The client is predisposed to osteoporosis and fractures. Contact sports should be avoided.

**TEST-TAKING HINT: If the test taker is not aware of the disease problem, this question could be answered correctly because of common standard discharge instructions—namely, notify the HCP of a fever.**

55. 1. This client could be cared for by any nurse qualified to work in an ICU.
    2. These blood gases are within normal limits.
    3. **This client has low blood pressure and tachycardia. This client may be experiencing an Addisonian crisis, a potentially life-threatening condition. The most experienced nurse should care for this client.**
    4. A negative Trousseau's sign is normal for this client.

**TEST-TAKING HINT: The answer options "1," "2," and "4" have expected or normal data. Only one option has abnormal data. Even if the test taker is unaware of Addisonian crisis, these are vital signs indicating potential shock.**

56. 1. Blood glucose levels do not address the problem of altered body image.
    2. Head-to-toe assessments are performed to detect a physiological problem, not a psychosocial one.
    3. **Allowing the client to verbalize feelings about altered body image is the most appropriate intervention. The nurse cannot do anything to help the client's buffalo hump or moon face.**
    4. Bowel sounds and temperature are physical symptoms.

**TEST-TAKING HINT: The intervention must match the problem.**

57. 1. The client was exposed to wind and sun at the lake during the hours before being admitted to the emergency department. This predisposes the client to dehydration and an Addisonian crisis. Rapid IV fluid replacement is necessary.
    2. Sitting in the waiting area could cause the client to go into a coma and die.
    3. A blood transfusion is not an appropriate intervention for this client.
    4. Laboratory specimens are not priority and calcium is not a problem in clients diagnosed with Addison's disease.

**TEST-TAKING HINT:** This client is weak, lethargic, and forgetful, indicating a diminished level of consciousness. The nurse should choose an action addressing the problem.

58. The client has received 8,650 mL of intravenous fluid.

**TEST-TAKING HINT:** This is a basic addition problem. If the test taker has difficulty with this problem, then a math review course would be in order.

59. 1. An autocratic style is one in which the person in charge makes the decision without consulting anyone else.
    2. This behavior is an example of a democratic leadership style.
    3. This behavior is an example of a laissez-faire leadership style.
    4. This behavior is an example of a democratic leadership style.

**TEST-TAKING HINT:** The test taker could choose the correct answer if the test taker knew terms such as "autocratic" and "democratic."

60. 1. A unilateral adrenalectomy results in one adrenal gland still functioning. No hormone replacement will be required.
    2. The client can still have normal physiological functioning, including sexual functioning, with the remaining gland.
    3. Notifying the HCP if clinical manifestations of infection develop is an instruction given to all surgical clients on discharge.
    4. Turning and coughing are taught before surgery, not at discharge.

**TEST-TAKING HINT:** The test taker must notice the adjectives; "discharge" tells the reader a time frame for the instructions. This rules out option "4."

## Pituitary Disorders

61. 1. The client has excess fluid and is not dehydrated, and blood glucose levels are not affected.
    2. Early clinical manifestations are nausea and vomiting. The client has the syndrome of inappropriate secretion of antidiuretic (against allowing the body to urinate) hormone. In other words, the client is producing a hormone that will not allow the client to urinate.
    3. The client experiences dilutional hyponatremia, and the body has too much fluid already.
    4. Vasopressin is the name of the antidiuretic hormone. Giving more increases the client's problem. Also, a water challenge test is performed, not a fluid deprivation test.

**TEST-TAKING HINT:** The syndrome's name is confusing, with a double negative—"inappropriate" and "anti." It is helpful to put the situation in the test taker's own words to remember which way the fluids are being shifted in the body.

62. 1. Neurological status is monitored every 1 to 2 hours. This client's neurological status appears intact. Clients waking up in an intensive care area may not be aware of their surroundings.
    2. The output is more than double the intake in a short time. This client could be developing diabetes insipidus, a complication of trauma to the head.
    3. These vital signs are within normal limits.
    4. Transsphenoidal hypophysectomy is performed by surgical access above the gum line and through the nasal passage. There is no dressing. A drip pad is taped below the nares.

**TEST-TAKING HINT:** Two of the answer options contain normal data and would not warrant immediate intervention. Option "4" does not match the type of surgery.

63. 1. The client will have an elevated sodium level as a result of low circulating blood volume. The fluid is being lost through the urine. Diabetes means "to pass through" in Greek, indicating polyuria, a symptom shared with diabetes mellitus. Diabetes insipidus is a totally separate disease process.
    2. Serum calcium is not affected by diabetes insipidus.

3. Urine glucose is monitored for diabetes mellitus.
4. WBCs in the urine indicate the presence of a urinary tract infection.

**TEST-TAKING HINT:** The test taker should not confuse diabetes insipidus and diabetes mellitus.

64. 1. The client should keep a list of medications being taken and wear a Medic Alert bracelet.
2. **Medication for diabetes insipidus is usually taken twice a day (PO) or three times a day (intranasal), depending on the client (Vallerand & Sanoski, 2017). The client should keep the medication close at hand.**
3. The client is at risk for fluid shifts. Weighing every morning allows the client to follow the fluid shifts. Weight gain indicates too much medication.
4. Tightness in the chest could be an indicator the medication is not being tolerated; if this occurs, the client should notify the HCP.

**TEST-TAKING HINT:** This is an "except" question. This means all answers except one will be actions the client should do. If the test taker missed interpreting this from the stem, then the test taker could jump to the first action the client should do as the correct answer.

65. 1. The client is not allowed to drink during the test.
2. This test does not require any medications to be administered, and vasopressin will treat the DI, not help diagnose it.
3. **The client is deprived of all fluids, and if the client has DI, the urine production will not diminish. Vital signs and weights are taken every hour to determine circulatory status. If a marked decrease in weight or vital signs occurs, the test is immediately terminated.**
4. No fluid is allowed and a sonogram is not involved.

**TEST-TAKING HINT:** The name of the test is a fluid deprivation test. Two of the options require the administration of some type of fluid.

66. 1. Clients with SIADH have a problem with retaining fluid. This is expected.
2. This client's intake and output are relatively the same.
3. **Muscle twitching is a sign of early sodium imbalance. If an immediate**

intervention is not made, the client could begin to seize.
4. The client has to get up all night to urinate, so the client feeling tired is expected.

**TEST-TAKING HINT:** All of the answer options contain expected information except option "3."

67. **Two sprays per dose.**
Forty grams of medication every 24 hours is to be given in doses administered every 12 hours. First, determine the number of doses needed:

$$24 \div 12 = 2 \text{ doses}$$

Then, determine the amount of medication to be given in each of those two doses:

$$40 \div 2 = 20 \text{ g of medication per dose}$$

Finally, determine how many sprays are needed to deliver the 20 mg when each spray delivers 10 g:

$$20 \div 10 = 2 \text{ sprays}$$

**TEST-TAKING HINT:** The test taker should take each step of the problem one at a time and check the answer with the drop-down calculator if taking the examination on a computer.

68. **Correct answers are 1, 2, and 4.**
1. **Fluids are restricted to 500 to 600 mL per 24 hours.**
2. **Orientation to person, place, and time should be assessed every 2 hours or more often.**
3. A safe environment, not a stimulating one, is provided.
4. **Urine and serum osmolality are monitored to determine fluid volume status.**
5. The client should be weighed daily.

**TEST-TAKING HINT:** The test taker should notice numbers: Is assessing the client's level of consciousness every 2 hours enough, or is weighing the client every 3 days enough?

69. 1. Diabetes insipidus is not diabetes mellitus; sliding-scale insulin is not administered to the client.
2. There is no caffeine restriction for DI.
3. Checking urine ketones is not indicated.
4. **The client is excreting large amounts of dilute urine. If the client is unable to drink enough fluids, the client will quickly become dehydrated, so tissue turgor should be assessed frequently.**

**TEST-TAKING HINT:** Two of the answer options are appropriate for diabetes mellitus, not diabetes insipidus, and can be eliminated based on this alone.

70. 1. The client should have the water pitcher filled, but this is not the first action.
    2. This should be done but not before assessing the problem.
    3. **The first action should be to determine if the client is experiencing polyuria and polydipsia as a result of developing diabetes insipidus, a complication of the head trauma.**
    4. This could be done, but it will not give the nurse information about DI.

**TEST-TAKING HINT: The nurse must apply a systematic approach to answering priority questions. Maslow's hierarchy of needs should be applied if it is a physiological problem and the nursing process if it is a question of this nature. Assessment is the first step in the nursing process.**

71. 1. **A serum sodium level of 112 mEq/L is dangerously low, and the client is at risk for seizures. A headache is a symptom of a low-sodium level.**
    2. This is a normal potassium level, and a heightened level of awareness indicates drug usage.
    3. This is a normal calcium level, and the client is fluid overloaded, not dehydrated, so there would not be tented tissue turgor.
    4. This is a normal magnesium level, and a large urinary output is desired.

**TEST-TAKING HINT: The nurse must know common laboratory values.**

72. 1. Discussing the information with others is not allowing the client to decide what is best for himself.
    2. This could be an example of beneficence (to do good), so the client has information on which to base a decision on whether to continue the fluid restriction.
    3. **This is an example of autonomy (the client has the right to decide for himself).**
    4. This is an example of dishonesty and should never be tolerated in a health-care setting.

**TEST-TAKING HINT: The stem asks the test taker about autonomy. Even if the test taker did not know the ethical principle, autonomy means the right of self-governance. Only one of the answer options could fit the definition of autonomy.**

## Thyroid Disorders

73. 1. **A decrease in thyroid hormone causes decreased metabolism, which leads to fatigue and hair loss.**
    2. These are clinical manifestations of hyperthyroidism.
    3. These are clinical manifestations of hyperthyroidism.
    4. These are clinical manifestations of parathyroidism.

**TEST-TAKING HINT: Often, if the test taker does not know the specific clinical manifestations of the disease but knows the function of the system affected by the disease, some possible answers can be ruled out. Tetany and stiffness of the hands are related to calcium, the level of which is influenced by the parathyroid gland, not the thyroid gland; therefore, option "4" can be ruled out.**

74. 1. **External heat sources (heating pads, electric or warming blankets) should be discouraged because they increase the risk of peripheral vasodilation and vascular collapse.**
    2. Assessing the client's temperature every 2 hours is not needed because the temperature will not change quickly. The client needs thyroid hormones to help increase the client's temperature.
    3. The room temperature should be kept warm because the client will report of being cold.
    4. The client is fatigued, and this is an appropriate intervention but is not applicable to the client problem of "risk for imbalanced body temperature."

**TEST-TAKING HINT: The test taker must always know exactly what the question is asking. Option "4" can be ruled out because it does not address body temperature. If the test taker knows the normal function of the thyroid gland, this may help identify the answer; decreased metabolism will cause the client to be cold.**

75. 1. The thyroid hormone levothyroxine (Synthroid) will help increase the client's metabolic rate. A weight gain indicates not enough medication is being taken to put the client in a euthyroid (normal thyroid) state.
    2. A decreased pulse rate indicates there is not enough thyroid hormone level; therefore, the medication is not effective.
    3. **The client diagnosed with hypothyroidism frequently has a subnormal temperature, so a temperature WNL indicates the thyroid hormone levothyroxine (Synthroid) is effective.**
    4. Diaphoresis (sweating) occurs with hyperthyroidism, not hypothyroidism.

**TEST-TAKING HINT:** One way of determining the effectiveness of a medication is to determine if the clinical manifestations of the disease are no longer noticeable.

76. 1. Fiber should be increased in the client diagnosed with hypothyroidism because the client experiences constipation secondary to decreased metabolism.
    2. The client diagnosed with hyperthyroidism should have a high-calorie, high-protein diet.
    3. The client's fluid intake should be increased to replace fluids lost through diarrhea and excessive sweating.
    4. **The client diagnosed with hyperthyroidism has an increased appetite; therefore, well-balanced meals served several times throughout the day will help with the client's constant hunger.**

**TEST-TAKING HINT:** If the test taker knows the metabolism is increased with hyperthyroidism, then increasing the food intake is the most appropriate choice.

77. 1. Hypoglycemia is expected in a client diagnosed with myxedema; therefore, a 74 mg/dL blood glucose level is expected.
    2. **A pulse oximeter reading of less than 93% is significant. A 90% pulse oximeter reading indicates a Pao$_2$ of approximately 60 on an ABG gas test; this is severe hypoxemia and requires immediate intervention.**
    3. The client diagnosed with myxedema coma is in an exaggerated hypothyroid state; a low pulse is expected in a client diagnosed with hypothyroidism.
    4. Lethargy is an expected symptom in a client diagnosed with myxedema; therefore, this does not warrant immediate intervention.

**TEST-TAKING HINT:** The words "warrant immediate intervention" means the test taker should select an option that is abnormal for the disease process or a life-threatening clinical manifestation.

78. 1. Thyroid hormones are the treatment of choice for the client diagnosed with hypothyroidism; therefore, the nurse should not question this medication.
    2. In untreated hypothyroidism, medical management is aimed at supporting vital functions, so administering oxygen is an appropriate medication.
    3. Untreated hypothyroidism is characterized by an increased susceptibility to the effects of most hypnotic and sedative agents; therefore, the nurse should question this medication.
    4. Clients with hypothyroidism become constipated as a result of decreased metabolism, so laxatives should not be questioned by the nurse.

**TEST-TAKING HINT:** When a question asks which order the nurse should question, three of the options are medications the nurse expects to administer to the client. Sometimes saying, "The nurse administers this medication," may help the test taker select the correct answer.

79. 1. Decreased appetite is a symptom of hypothyroidism, not hyperthyroidism.
    2. Constipation is a symptom of hypothyroidism.
    3. Dry, coarse skin is a sign of hypothyroidism.
    4. **The thyroid gland (in the neck) enlarges as a result of the increased need for thyroid hormone production; an enlarged gland is called a goiter.**

**TEST-TAKING HINT:** If the test taker does not know the answer, sometimes thinking about the location of the gland or organ causing the problem may help the test taker select or rule out specific options.

80. Correct answers are 1 and 5.
    1. **Radioactive iodine therapy is used to destroy overactive thyroid cells. After treatment, the client is followed closely for 3 to 4 weeks until the euthyroid state is reached.**
    2. A single dose of radioactive iodine therapy is administered; the dosage is based on the client's weight.
    3. The colorless, tasteless radioiodine is administered by the radiologist, and the client may have to stay up to 2 hours after the treatment in the office.
    4. If too much of the thyroid gland is destroyed by the radioactive iodine therapy, the client may develop hypothyroidism and have to take thyroid hormone indefinitely.
    5. **The client may experience side effects from the radioactive iodine, including a metallic taste in the mouth, nausea, and swollen salivary glands. The side effects last from a few days to a few weeks following treatment (Milas, 2020).**

**TEST-TAKING HINT:** Some questions require the test taker to have knowledge of the information, especially medical treatments, and there are no specific hints to help the test taker answer the question.

81. Correct answers are 1, 2, 3, and 4.
    1. Weight loss indicates the medication may not be effective and will probably need to be increased.
    2. The client needs to know emotional highs and lows are secondary to hyperthyroidism. With treatment, this emotional lability will subside.
    3. Any OTC medications (for example, alcohol-based medications) may negatively affect the client's hyperthyroidism or medications being used for treatment.
    4. This will help any HCP immediately know of the client's condition, especially if the client is unable to tell the HCP.
    5. The client diagnosed with hyperthyroidism will be on antithyroid medications, not thyroid medications.

**TEST-TAKING HINT:** This alternate-type question instructs the test taker to select all the interventions that apply. The test taker must read and evaluate each option as to whether it applies or not.

82. 1. There is no screening for thyroid disorders, just serum thyroid levels.
    2. This is not a true statement.
    3. Medications do not decrease the development of goiters.
    4. Almost all of the iodine entering the body is retained in the thyroid gland. A deficiency in iodine will cause the thyroid gland to work hard and enlarge, which is called a goiter. Goiters are commonly seen in geographical regions having an iodine deficiency. Most table salt in the United States has iodine added.

**TEST-TAKING HINT:** The nurse must know about disease processes. There is no test-taking hint to help with knowledge.

83. 1. The thyroid hormone must be administered daily, and thyroid levels are drawn every 6 months or so.
    2. A blood glucose level of 210 mg/dL requires insulin administration; therefore, the nurse should not question administering this medication.
    3. This potassium level is below normal, which is 3.5 to 5.5 mEq/L. Therefore, the nurse should question administering this medication because loop diuretics cause potassium loss in the urine.
    4. The digoxin level is within therapeutic range—0.5 to 2 mg/dL; therefore, the nurse should administer this medication.

**TEST-TAKING HINT:** When administering medication, the nurse must know when to question the medication, how to know it is effective, and what must be taught to keep the client safe while taking the medication. The test taker may want to turn the question around and say, "I should give this medication."

84. 1. These are clinical manifestations of myxedema (hypothyroidism) coma. Obstipation is extreme constipation.
    2. Hyperpyrexia (high fever) and heart rate above 130 beats per minute are clinical manifestations of thyroid storm, a severely exaggerated hyperthyroidism.
    3. Decreased blood pressure and slow heart rate are clinical manifestations of myxedema coma.
    4. These are clinical manifestations of myxedema coma.

**TEST-TAKING HINT:** If the test taker does not have the knowledge to answer the question, the test taker should look at the options closely. Options "1," "3," and "4" all have clinical manifestations of "decrease"—hypoactive, hypotension, and hypoxia. The test taker should select the option that does not match.

85. 1. Sucralfate (Carafate) is a mucosal barrier agent and should be administered on an empty stomach so the medication can coat the mucosa. The nurse would not question administering this medication.
2. **The nurse cannot administer sliding-scale insulin without knowing the current blood glucose. The nurse should talk with the client to try and obtain the client's cooperation and, if not, then notify the HCP that the medication cannot be administered.**
3. Levothyroxine is an appropriate treatment for hypothyroidism.
4. The sliding scale usually begins at 150 mg/dL; the nurse would not question administering this medication.

**TEST-TAKING HINT: The test taker must know normal and abnormal diagnostic laboratory values. Medications are administered per sliding scale in response to blood glucose levels. The nurse must also recognize accepted treatments for diseases.**

86. 1. **The nurse should know the blood glucose level before making any decision about the administration of either insulin. Insulin is due at this time.**
2. Glargine (Lantus) insulin is not combined with any other insulin in the same syringe.
3. The nurse should prepare to give the insulins but not before knowing the current blood glucose.
4. This is not needed at this time.

**TEST-TAKING HINT: The nurse must know the rules of medication administration and must know the medications and when they are due.**

87. Correct answers are 1, 2, 3, and 5.
1. **The client diagnosed with diabetes should be taught to perform self-glucose monitoring.**
2. **In order to maintain a healthy lifestyle, the client should be aware of the consequences of not controlling blood glucose.**
3. **Diabetes affects all tissues in the body. The feet are particularly at risk for the development of foot sores.**
4. The client should carry sources of quick-acting carbohydrates, not protein.
5. **Diabetes can cause retinal changes and detachment.**

**TEST-TAKING HINT: The nurse should be able to teach common information to the client.**

88. 1. **The nurse should continue to monitor the client. The behavior is expected for a client diagnosed with hyperthyroidism.**
2. The client's vital signs are not indicated because of the symptoms.
3. This behavior is expected for a client diagnosed with hyperthyroidism. A sedative is not needed.
4. The nurse cannot insist the client do anything.

**TEST-TAKING HINT: The test taker must know expected clinical manifestations for disease processes.**

89. 1. Physical therapy is not indicated.
2. Social work is not indicated.
3. Speech therapy is not indicated.
4. **Metabolism involves the intake and utilization of nutrients; the dietitian should be consulted.**

**TEST-TAKING HINT: As a coordinator of care, the nurse must be aware of each discipline and how it affects the client's care.**

90. 1. These results are both WNL; they do not indicate type 2 diabetes.
2. These results are both slightly above normal, but they do not indicate type 2 diabetes.
3. These results are both slightly above normal, but they do not indicate type 2 diabetes.
4. **Both laboratory values are above the normal range. The A1c indicates a lengthy time (at least 2 to 3 months) that the blood glucose has been high. This would be supportive of uncontrolled type 2 diabetes.**

**TEST-TAKING HINT: The test taker must know normal and abnormal diagnostic laboratory values. Laboratory values vary depending on which laboratory performs the test.**

91. 1. **Nutrition encompasses obesity, and obesity is a risk factor for developing diabetes mellitus type 2.**
2. Sensory perception may be a problem for clients diagnosed with diabetes because ophthalmological issues occur as a result of high blood glucose levels for a prolonged period of time but are not antecedents.

3. The concept of pH is a situation that can occur as a result of DM1 but not DM2 because acidosis results from lactic acid buildup from no insulin production from the pancreas. Type 2 diabetes clients still produce some insulin. Insulin resistance is an issue in type 2 diabetes.

4. Medication is given to treat diabetes but not to cause it.

**TEST-TAKING HINT: The test taker must know risk factors for developing a disease process.**

92. 1. The client diagnosed with hypothyroidism has slowed body processes, so the temperature, pulse, and BP would be lower.
    2. All body processes slow as a result of decreased thyroid production. The client will be constipated, cold, have thicker skin, low temperature, and bradycardia.
    3. The intake and output would not be affected.
    4. Hypothyroidism does not cause headaches or projectile vomiting.

**TEST-TAKING HINT: The test taker must know basic clinical manifestations. The word "hypo" in the name of the disease would help the test taker eliminate option "1."**

93. 1. The HCP and not the nurse should perform this assessment. The nurse has an unusual and potentially life-changing issue identified.
    2. Keeping the eyes closed will not change the outcome of retinal detachment. This is an ophthalmological emergency.
    3. This is an emergency; this indicates retinal detachment. The nurse should notify the HCP.
    4. The RRT will help to prevent cardiac or respiratory arrest. The HCP should be notified to arrange for an ophthalmologist consult.

**TEST-TAKING HINT: The test taker should recognize life-changing or life-threatening complications of a disease process. Failure to intervene immediately can result in a "failure to rescue" situation.**

94. 1. To limit the complications of diabetes, the client should keep the blood glucose levels under 140 mg/dL. This can be done with medications, diet, and exercise. Self-monitoring of glucose allows the client to monitor glucose levels.
    2. Testing for urine ketones will not help to keep the blood glucose level controlled.
    3. Petroleum jelly is rubbed on the feet but not between the toes.
    4. The client should administer sliding-scale insulin when needed but not eat whatever the client wishes. The client should still attempt to control the number of carbohydrates.

**TEST-TAKING HINT: The nurse must recommend measures to control or treat disease processes.**

95. Correct answers are 1, 2, 3, 4, and 5.
    1. Obesity is included in the concept of nutrition. Obesity is an antecedent of diabetes mellitus type 2.
    2. Diabetes is a problem of glucose metabolism.
    3. The client is at greater risk for developing infections resulting from the high circulating glucose levels. Bacteria utilize glucose for energy, as do mammals.
    4. Diabetes affects the ability of the blood vessels to respond to the circulatory need. For a middle-aged male, this can result in erectile dysfunction.
    5. Skin integrity is an issue if a pressure sore or a blister occurs on the feet. If not noted and treated early, then an infection can result in amputation.

**TEST-TAKING HINT: The test taker must know the disease process and potential complications.**

96. 1. Eating sweets and high-carbohydrate foods can lead to obesity, but eating candy does not cause diabetes.
    2. Birth control pills do not increase the risk of developing diabetes.
    3. Type 2 diabetes can be more prevalent in families, but having one cousin with diabetes does not increase the risk of diabetes for the client.
    4. Research shows that women are at greater risk of developing diabetes after delivering a large infant.

**TEST-TAKING HINT: The test taker must know the antecedents of developing disease processes.**

# ENDOCRINE DISORDERS COMPREHENSIVE EXAMINATION

1. The nurse is teaching a community class to people with type 2 diabetes mellitus. Which **best** explains the development of type 2 diabetes?
   1. The islet cells in the pancreas stop producing insulin.
   2. The client eats too many foods high in sugar.
   3. The pituitary gland does not produce vasopressin.
   4. The cells become resistant to circulating insulin.

2. The nurse is teaching the client diagnosed with type 2 diabetes mellitus about diet. Which diet selection indicates the client **understands** the teaching?
   1. A submarine sandwich, potato chips, and diet cola.
   2. Four slices of a supreme thin-crust pizza and milk.
   3. Smoked turkey sandwich, celery sticks, and unsweetened tea.
   4. A roast beef sandwich, fried onion rings, and a cola.

4. Which clinical manifestations should the nurse expect to assess in the 31-year-old client diagnosed with a sustained release of growth hormone (GH)?
   1. An enlarged forehead, maxilla, and face.
   2. A 6-inch increase in the height of the client.
   3. The client reporting a severe headache.
   4. A systolic blood pressure of 200 to 300 mm Hg.

5. Which clinical manifestation indicates to the nurse the client is experiencing hypoparathyroidism?
   1. A negative Trousseau's sign.
   2. A positive Chvostek's sign.
   3. Nocturnal muscle cramps.
   4. Tented skin turgor.

6. Which laboratory data make the nurse suspect the client diagnosed with primary hyperparathyroidism is experiencing a complication?
   1. A serum creatinine level of 2.8 mg/dL.
   2. A calcium level of 9.2 mg/dL.
   3. A serum triglyceride level of 130 mg/dL.
   4. A sodium level of 135 mEq/L.

3. The nurse is preparing to administer sliding-scale insulin to a client diagnosed with type 2 diabetes. The MAR for this client is populated below. At 1130, the client has a blood glucometer level of 322. Which intervention should the nurse implement?
   1. Notify the health-care provider.
   2. Administer 10 units of regular insulin.
   3. Administer 5 units of insulin lispro.
   4. Administer 10 units of intermediate-acting insulin.

| Client Name: Ms. B.D. | MR# 2345678 | Diagnosis: Diabetes Mellitus Type 2 |
|---|---|---|
| **Age: 59 years** | **Allergies: NKDA** | |
| Medication | 0701–1900 | 1901–0700 |
| Regular insulin subcutaneously a.c. and h.s. 0–60 = 1 amp D$_{50}$ 61–150 = 0 units 151–300 = 5 units 301–450 = 10 units Greater than 450 = Call HCP | 0730 1130 | 1630 2100 |
| Metformin 500 mg PO bid | 0800 | 1930 |
| **Signature of Nurse:** | **Day Nurse RN/DN** | **Night Nurse RN/NN** |

7. The nurse is assessing a client in an outpatient clinic. Which assessment data are a risk factor for developing pheochromocytoma?
    1. A history of skin cancer.
    2. A history of high blood pressure.
    3. A family history of adrenal tumors.
    4. A family history of migraine headaches.

8. The client is 3 days postoperative unilateral adrenalectomy. Which discharge instructions should the nurse teach?
    1. Discuss the need for lifelong steroid replacement.
    2. Instruct the client on the administration of vasopressin.
    3. Teach the client to care for the suprapubic Foley catheter.
    4. Tell the client to notify the HCP if the incision is inflamed.

9. Which psychosocial problem should be included in the plan of care for a female client diagnosed with Cushing's syndrome?
    1. Altered glucose metabolism.
    2. Body image disturbance.
    3. Risk for suicide.
    4. Impaired wound healing.

10. The nurse is admitting a client with possible aldosteronism. Which assessment data support the client's diagnosis?
    1. Temperature.
    2. Pulse.
    3. Respirations.
    4. Blood pressure.

11. When diagnosed with iatrogenic Cushing's disease, which client history is **most significant** in the development of clinical manifestations?
    1. Long-term use of anabolic steroids.
    2. Extended use of inhaled steroids for asthma.
    3. History of long-term glucocorticoid use.
    4. Family history of increased cortisol production.

12. The client is 1 hour postoperative thyroidectomy. Which intervention should the nurse implement?
    1. Check the posterior neck for bleeding.
    2. Assess the client for Chvostek's sign.
    3. Monitor the client's serum calcium level.
    4. Change the client's surgical dressing.

13. Which clinical manifestations indicate the client diagnosed with hypothyroidism is not taking enough thyroid hormone?
    1. Reports of weight loss and fine tremors.
    2. Reports of excessive thirst and urination.
    3. Reports of constipation and being cold.
    4. Reports of delayed wound healing and belching.

14. Which client problem is the nurse's **priority concern** for the client diagnosed with acute pancreatitis?
    1. Impaired nutrition.
    2. Skin integrity.
    3. Anxiety.
    4. Pain relief.

15. Which laboratory data indicate to the nurse the client's pancreatitis is **improving**?
    1. The amylase and lipase serum levels are decreased.
    2. The white blood cell (WBC) count is decreased.
    3. The conjugated and unconjugated bilirubin levels are decreased.
    4. The blood urea nitrogen (BUN) serum level is decreased.

16. The client diagnosed with acute pancreatitis has a ruptured pseudocyst. Which procedure should the nurse anticipate the HCP prescribing?
    1. Paracentesis.
    2. Percutaneous drainage.
    3. Lumbar puncture.
    4. Biopsy of the pancreas.

17. Which clinical manifestations should the nurse expect to assess in the client diagnosed with an insulinoma?
    1. Nervousness, jitteriness, and diaphoresis.
    2. Flushed skin, dry mouth, and tented skin turgor.
    3. Polyuria, polydipsia, and polyphagia.
    4. Hypertension, tachycardia, and feeling hot.

18. Which risk factor should the nurse expect to find in the client diagnosed with pancreatic cancer?
    1. Chewing tobacco.
    2. Low-fat diet.
    3. Chronic alcoholism.
    4. Exposure to industrial chemicals.

19. The nurse is discussing the endocrine system with the client. Which endocrine gland secretes epinephrine and norepinephrine?
    1. The pancreas.
    2. The adrenal cortex.
    3. The adrenal medulla.
    4. The anterior pituitary gland.

20. Which question should the nurse ask when assessing the client for an endocrine dysfunction?
    1. "Have you noticed any pain in your legs when walking?"
    2. "Have you had any unexplained weight loss?"
    3. "Have you noticed any change in your bowel movements?"
    4. "Have you experienced any joint pain or discomfort?"

21. Which nursing instruction should the nurse discuss with the client receiving glucocorticoids for Addison's disease?
    1. Discuss the importance of tapering medications when discontinuing the medication.
    2. Explain the dose may need to be increased during times of stress or infection.
    3. Instruct the client to take medication on an empty stomach with a glass of water.
    4. Encourage the client to wear clean white socks when wearing tennis shoes.

22. The client diagnosed with chronic alcoholism has chronic pancreatitis and hypomagnesemia. Which data should the nurse assess when administering magnesium sulfate to the client?
    1. Deep tendon reflexes.
    2. Arterial blood gases.
    3. Skin turgor.
    4. Capillary refill time.

23. Which endocrine disorder should the nurse assess for the client diagnosed with a closed head injury and **increased** intracranial pressure?
    1. Pheochromocytoma.
    2. Diabetes insipidus.
    3. Hashimoto's thyroiditis.
    4. Gynecomastia.

24. Which clinical manifestation should the nurse expect in the client diagnosed with syndrome of inappropriate antidiuretic hormone (SIADH)?
    1. Excessive thirst.
    2. Orthopnea.
    3. Ascites.
    4. Concentrated urine output.

25. In which area should the nurse administer the regular insulin to ensure the **best absorption** of the medication?

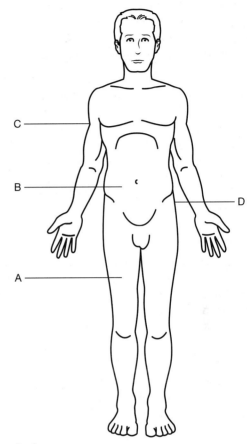

    1. A
    2. B
    3. C
    4. D

26. The client diagnosed with type 1 diabetes mellitus received regular insulin 2 hours ago. The client is reporting being jittery and nervous. Which interventions should the nurse implement? **Rank in order of priority.**
    1. Call the laboratory to confirm the blood glucose level.
    2. Administer a quick-acting carbohydrate.
    3. Have the client eat a bologna sandwich.
    4. Check the client's blood glucose level at the bedside.
    5. Determine if the client has had anything to eat.

27. The nurse in the ICU is caring for a client 20 hours postoperative Whipple's procedure for cancer of the pancreas. The client has two intravenous lines running via a central catheter and 1 unit of packed red blood cells in a peripheral line. The client's intake and output record from the previous day is as follows:

### Intake and Output Record

| Day 1 | Oral (in mL) | Intravenous (mL) | Urine (mL) | Nasogastric Tube (mL) | Other (Specify) (mL) |
|---|---|---|---|---|---|
| 0701–1900 | 1,450 | 1,800 | 2,800 | 950 | Emesis 400 |
| 1901–0700 | 765 | 1,325 | 1,700 | 1215 | |
| Total | 2,215 | 3,125 | 4,500 | 2,165 | 400 |

Based on these findings, which action should the nurse implement?
1. Slow down the intravenous rates and notify the HCP immediately.
2. Assess the client for change in sensorium daily and stay in the room.
3. Continue to assess intake and output every 1 hour.
4. Increase the blood rate to infuse rapidly and crossmatch for 2 more units.

1. 1. This is the cause of type 1 diabetes mellitus.
   2. This may be a reason for obesity, which may lead to type 2 diabetes, but eating too much sugar does not cause diabetes.
   3. This is the explanation for diabetes insipidus, which should not be confused with diabetes mellitus.
   4. Normally insulin binds to special receptors sites on the cell and initiates a series of reactions involved in metabolism. In type 2 diabetes, these reactions are diminished primarily as a result of obesity and aging.

2. 1. A submarine sandwich is on a bun-type bread and is usually 6 to 12 inches long, and potato chips add fat and more carbohydrates to the meal.
   2. Four slices of pizza contain excessive numbers of carbohydrates, plus cheese and meats, and whole milk is high in fat.
   3. Turkey is a low-fat meat. A sandwich usually means normal slices of bread, and the client needs at least 50% carbohydrates in each meal. Celery sticks are not counted as carbohydrates.
   4. The roast beef sandwich is high in carbohydrates, fried onion rings are high in fat, and a regular cola is high in carbohydrates.

3. 1. The client's blood glucose level does not warrant notifying the HCP.
   2. According to the sliding scale, any blood glucose reading between 301 and 450 requires 10 units of regular insulin, which is fast-acting insulin.
   3. Insulin lispro (Humalog) is rapid-acting insulin, but the order reads regular insulin.
   4. Intermediate-acting insulin, NPH or Humulin N, is not regular insulin.

4. 1. Acromegaly (enlarged extremities) occurs when sustained GH hypersecretion begins during adulthood, most commonly because of a pituitary tumor.
   2. Gigantism occurs when GH hypersecretion begins before puberty when the closure of the epiphyseal plates occurs. Note the age of the client.
   3. A severe headache is not a symptom of acromegaly.
   4. High blood pressure is a sign of pheochromocytoma.

5. 1. A carpopedal spasm occurs when the blood flow to the arm is decreased for 3 minutes with a blood pressure cuff; a positive Trousseau's sign indicates hypocalcemia, which is a sign of hypoparathyroid function. A normal Trousseau means the body is functioning as it should.
   2. When a sharp tapping over the facial nerve elicits a spasm or twitching of the mouth, nose, or eyes, the client is hypocalcemic, which occurs in clients diagnosed with hypoparathyroidism. This is known as a positive Chvostek's sign.
   3. Muscle cramps make the nurse suspect hypokalemia (low potassium).
   4. Tented skin turgor makes the nurse suspect dehydration, which occurs with hypernatremia.

6. 1. A serum creatinine level of 2.8 mg/dL indicates the client is in renal failure, which is a complication of hyperparathyroidism. The formation of stones in the kidneys related to the increased urinary excretion of calcium and phosphorus occurs in about 55% of clients diagnosed with primary hyperparathyroidism and can lead to renal failure.
   2. This calcium level is within the normal range of 8.2 to 10.2 mg/dL.
   3. This serum triglyceride level is within the normal range of less than 150 mg/dL.
   4. This sodium level is within the normal range of 135 to 145 mEq/L.

7. 1. A history of skin cancer is not a risk factor for pheochromocytoma.
   2. A history of high blood pressure is a sign of this disease, not a risk factor for developing it.
   3. There is a high incidence of pheochromocytomas in family members with adrenal tumors with the von Hippel-Lindau gene inherited in an autosomal dominant pattern (U.S. National Library of Medicine, 2019).
   4. Headaches are a symptom of this disease but not a risk factor for it.

8. 1. Because the client has one adrenal gland remaining, the client may not need lifelong supplemental steroids.
   2. Vasopressin is administered to clients diagnosed with diabetes insipidus.
   3. The client does not have a suprapubic catheter during this procedure.
   4. **Any inflammation of the incision indicates an infection, and the client will need to receive antibiotics, so the HCP must be notified.**

9. 1. This is not a psychosocial problem; it is a physiological problem in clients diagnosed with Cushing's syndrome.
   2. **The client diagnosed with Cushing's syndrome has body changes, including moon face, buffalo hump, truncal obesity, hirsutism, and striae and bruising, all of which affect the client's body image.**
   3. This is a psychosocial problem, but it is not one that commonly occurs in clients diagnosed with Cushing's syndrome.
   4. This is not a psychosocial problem; it is a physiological problem, which does occur in clients diagnosed with Cushing's syndrome.

10. 1. The temperature is not affected by aldosteronism.
    2. The pulse is not affected by this disorder.
    3. The respirations are not affected by this disorder.
    4. **Blood pressure is affected by aldosteronism, with hypertension being the most prominent and universal sign of aldosteronism.**

11. 1. Anabolic steroids are used by individuals to build muscle mass. Long-term use can lead to psychosis or heart attacks.
    2. Inhaled steroids do not have systemic effects, which is described by iatrogenic Cushing's disease.
    3. **Iatrogenic Cushing's disease is Cushing's disease caused by medical treatment—in this case, by taking excessive steroids resulting in the clinical manifestations of a moon face, buffalo hump, and other associated symptoms.**
    4. Family history does not cause iatrogenic problems.

12. 1. **The incision for a thyroidectomy allows the blood to drain dependently by gravity to the back of the client's neck. Therefore, the nurse should check this area for hemorrhaging, which is a possible complication of any surgery.**
    2. Chvostek's sign indicates hypocalcemia, which is too early to assess for in this client.
    3. Accidental removal of or damage to the parathyroid glands will not decrease the calcium level for at least 24 hours.
    4. Surgeons often prefer to remove the surgical dressing for the first time.

13. 1. Weight loss and fine tremors make the nurse suspect the client is taking too much thyroid hormone because these are clinical manifestations of hyperthyroidism.
    2. Excessive thirst and urination are symptoms of diabetes.
    3. **If the client were not taking enough thyroid hormone, the client would exhibit symptoms of hypothyroidism such as constipation and being cold.**
    4. This indicates Cushing's disease.

14. 1. The client is NPO and can live without food for a number of days if receiving fluids.
    2. The client is not on strict bedrest and can move about in the bed; therefore, skin integrity is not a priority problem. In pancreatitis, the tissue damage is internal.
    3. The client may be anxious, but psychosocial problems are not the priority.
    4. **The client diagnosed with pancreatitis is in excruciating pain because the enzymes are autodigesting the pancreas; severe abdominal pain is the hallmark clinical manifestation of pancreatitis.**

15. 1. **These laboratory data are used to diagnose and monitor pancreatitis because amylase and lipase are the enzymes produced by the pancreas.**
    2. Pancreatitis is not an infection of the pancreas resulting from bacteria; such an infection causes an elevation in the WBCs.
    3. Bilirubin is used to monitor liver problems.
    4. BUN monitors kidney function.

16. 1. A paracentesis is used to remove fluid from the abdominal cavity.
    2. **The pancreas lies immediately below the diaphragm. When the cyst ruptures, alkaline substances in the abdomen cause fluid leaks at the esophageal diaphragmatic opening into the thorax. The fluid must be removed to prevent lung collapse. CT or ultrasound-guided drainage is performed for draining pancreatic fluid (Matsusue et al., 2016).**
    3. Lumbar puncture is used to diagnose meningitis.
    4. Biopsies are performed to confirm a diagnosis; they are not used for treatment.

**17.** 1. Insulinoma is a tumor of the islet cells of the pancreas that produces insulin. The clinical manifestations of an insulinoma are signs of hypoglycemia.
   2. These are clinical manifestations of hyperglycemia.
   3. These are clinical manifestations of hyperglycemia.
   4. These are clinical manifestations of hyperthyroidism.

**18.** 1. A history of smoking cigarettes is pertinent, but a history of chewing tobacco is not.
   2. A diet high in fat, not low in fat, is a risk factor.
   3. Chronic alcoholism is not a risk factor, but chronic pancreatitis or cirrhosis is a risk factor.
   4. **Exposure to industrial chemicals or environmental toxins is a risk factor for pancreatic cancer.**

**19.** 1. The endocrine function of the pancreas is the secretion of insulin and amylin.
   2. The adrenal cortex secretes mineralocorticoids, glucocorticoids, and gonadotrophins.
   3. **The adrenal medulla secretes the catecholamines epinephrine and norepinephrine.**
   4. The anterior pituitary gland secretes the growth hormone.

**20.** 1. Leg pain when walking indicates intermittent claudication, which occurs with peripheral vascular disease.
   2. **Weight loss with normal appetite may indicate hyperthyroidism.**
   3. Changes in bowel movements may indicate colon cancer.
   4. Joint pain indicates a musculoskeletal or degenerative joint disease.

**21.** 1. The client will have to receive this medication indefinitely, so this should not be discussed with the client.
   2. **During times of stress, the medication may need to be increased to prevent adrenal insufficiency.**
   3. The medication should be taken with food to minimize its ulcerogenic effect.
   4. Wearing white socks with tennis shoes is not an intervention pertinent to a client diagnosed with Addison's disease.

**22.** 1. If deep tendon reflexes are hypoactive or absent, the nurse should hold the magnesium and notify the HCP.
   2. The ABGs are not affected by the serum magnesium level.
   3. The client's skin turgor will not be affected by the client's serum magnesium level.
   4. The client's capillary refill time is not affected by the client's serum magnesium level.

**23.** 1. This is a tumor of the adrenal medulla.
   2. **Diabetes insipidus can be caused by brain tumors or infections, pituitary surgery, cerebrovascular accidents, or renal and organ failure, or it may be a complication of a closed head injury with increased intracranial pressure. Diabetes insipidus is a result of antidiuretic hormone (ADH) insufficiency.**
   3. Hashimoto's thyroiditis causes hypothyroidism.
   4. Gynecomastia is the abnormal enlargement of breast tissue in men.

**24.** 1. Excessive thirst is a symptom of diabetes insipidus, which is a deficiency of antidiuretic (ADH) hormone.
   2. Orthopnea is difficulty breathing when in the supine position, which is not a clinical manifestation of SIADH.
   3. Ascites is excess fluid in the peritoneal cavity, which is not a clinical manifestation of SIADH.
   4. **Excess antidiuretic hormone (ADH) causes SIADH, which causes increased water reabsorption and leads to increased fluid volume and scant, concentrated urine.**

**25.** 1. The anterior thigh is an appropriate area, but it does not provide the best absorption.
   2. **The abdominal area allows for the most rapid absorption of insulin and is the recommended site.**
   3. The deltoid is an appropriate area, but it does not provide the most rapid absorption.
   4. The gluteal buttocks area is primarily the best area for intramuscular injections.

26. Correct order is 5, 2, 4, 1, 3.
    5. Regular insulin peaks in 2 to 4 hours; therefore, the nurse should suspect a hypoglycemic reaction if the client has not eaten anything.
    2. The antidote for insulin is glucose; therefore, the nurse should give the client some type of quick-acting food source.
    4. The nurse should obtain the client's blood glucose level as soon as possible; this can be done with a glucometer at the bedside.
    1. Most hospitals require a confirmatory serum blood glucose level. Do not wait for results to give food.
    3. A source of long-acting carbohydrate and protein should be given to prevent a reoccurrence of hypoglycemia.

27. 1. The IV rates are preventing the client from developing hypovolemic shock as a result of third spacing after major abdominal surgery. The ICU nurse must be vigilant for third spacing and fluid shifts following major trauma to the body.
    2. The sensorium must be assessed more frequently than daily, and the nurse does not have to remain with the client continuously.
    3. The intake and output should be assessed hourly to determine kidney perfusion and to determine when the fluids have stopped shifting to the surgical area.
    4. There is no evidence that the client has begun to bleed and requires faster infusion and another crossmatch.

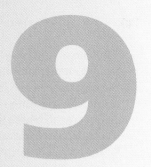

# Genitourinary Disorders

*The possession of knowledge does not kill the sense of wonder and mystery. There is always more mystery.*

—Anaïs Nin

The genitourinary system includes the kidneys; ureters; bladder; urethra; and the associated organ, the prostate gland. The urinary system organs are subject to acute or chronic infections, functioning disorders or diseases, and formation of calculi (stones). These disorders can lead to fluid and electrolyte disorders having wide-ranging effects throughout the body. The prostate is also subject to disorders, a very common one being benign prostatic hypertrophy. (Cancer of the prostate is discussed in Chapter 10.) The nurse must know the normal laboratory values of the many tests used to assess the function of these organs and recognize what independent and collaborative interventions are necessary.

## KEYWORDS

Anuria

Azotemia

Corrected output

Creatinine

Diffusion

Hyperkalemia

Intravesical

Oliguria

Osmolality

Osmosis

## PRACTICE QUESTIONS

### Acute Kidney Injury (AKI)

1. The nurse is admitting a client diagnosed with acute kidney injury (AKI). Which question is **most important** for the nurse to ask during the admission interview?
   1. "Have you recently traveled outside the United States?"
   2. "Did you recently begin a vigorous exercise program?"
   3. "Is there a chance you have been exposed to a virus?"
   4. "What over-the-counter medications do you take regularly?"

2. The nurse is caring for a client diagnosed with AKI. Which laboratory values are **most significant** for diagnosing AKI?
   1. BUN and creatinine.
   2. WBC and hemoglobin.
   3. Potassium and sodium.
   4. Bilirubin and ammonia level.

3. The nurse is caring for a client diagnosed with possible AKI. Which condition predisposes the client to develop prerenal AKI?
   1. Diabetes mellitus.
   2. Hypotension.
   3. Aminoglycosides.
   4. Benign prostatic hypertrophy.

4. The client is diagnosed with AKI. Which clinical manifestations indicate to the nurse the client is in the recovery period? **Select all that apply.**
   1. Increased alertness and no seizure activity.
   2. Increase in hemoglobin and hematocrit.
   3. Denial of nausea and vomiting.
   4. Decreased urine-specific gravity.
   5. Increased serum creatinine level.

5. The client diagnosed with AKI has a serum potassium level of 6.8 mEq/L. Which **collaborative** treatment should the nurse anticipate for the client?
   1. Administer a phosphate binder.
   2. Type and crossmatch for whole blood.
   3. Assess the client for leg cramps.
   4. Prepare the client for dialysis.

6. The nurse is developing a plan of care for a client diagnosed with AKI. Which statement is an **appropriate** outcome for the client?
   1. Monitor intake and output every shift.
   2. Decrease of pain by three levels on a 1-to-10 scale.
   3. Electrolytes are within normal limits.
   4. Administer enemas to decrease hyperkalemia.

7. The client diagnosed with AKI is admitted to the intensive care unit and placed on a therapeutic diet. Which diet is **most appropriate** for the client?
   1. A high-potassium and low-calcium diet.
   2. A low-fat and low-cholesterol diet.
   3. A high-carbohydrate and restricted-protein diet.
   4. A regular diet with six small feedings a day.

8. The client diagnosed with AKI is placed on bedrest. The client asks the nurse, "Why do I have to stay in bed? I don't feel bad." Which scientific rationale supports the nurse's response?
   1. Bedrest helps increase the blood return to the renal circulation.
   2. Bedrest reduces the metabolic rate during the acute stage.
   3. Bedrest decreases the workload of the left side of the heart.
   4. Bedrest aids in the reduction of peripheral and sacral edema.

9. The nurse and an unlicensed assistive personnel (UAP) are caring for clients on a medical floor. Which nursing task is **most appropriate** for the registered nurse (RN) to delegate?
   1. Collect a clean voided midstream urine specimen.
   2. Evaluate the client's 8-hour intake and output.
   3. Assist in checking a unit of blood before hanging.
   4. Administer a cation-exchange resin enema.

10. The client is admitted to the emergency department after a gunshot wound to the abdomen. Which nursing intervention should the nurse implement **first** to prevent AKI?
    1. Administer normal saline IV.
    2. Take vital signs.
    3. Place the client on telemetry.
    4. Assess abdominal dressing.

11. The client diagnosed with AKI is experiencing hyperkalemia. Which medication should the nurse prepare to administer to help **decrease** the potassium level?
    1. Erythropoietin.
    2. Calcium gluconate.
    3. Regular insulin.
    4. Osmotic diuretic.

## Chronic Kidney Disease (CKD)

12. The UAP tells the nurse the client diagnosed with CKD has a white crystal-like layer on top of the skin. Which intervention should the RN implement?
    1. Have the assistant apply a moisture barrier cream to the skin.
    2. Instruct the UAP to bathe the client in cool water.
    3. Tell the UAP not to turn the client in this condition.
    4. Explain this is normal and do not do anything for the client.

13. The nurse is caring for the client diagnosed with chronic kidney disease (CKD) experiencing metabolic acidosis. Which statement **best describes** the scientific rationale for metabolic acidosis in this client?
    1. There is an increased excretion of phosphates and organic acids, which leads to an increase in arterial blood pH.
    2. A shortened life span of red blood cells because of damage secondary to dialysis treatments in turn leads to metabolic acidosis.
    3. The kidney cannot excrete increased levels of acid because it cannot excrete ammonia or cannot reabsorb sodium bicarbonate.
    4. An increase in nausea and vomiting causes a loss of hydrochloric acid and the respiratory system cannot compensate adequately.

14. The nurse in the dialysis center is initiating the morning dialysis run. Which client should the nurse assess **first**?
    1. The client with hemoglobin of 9.8 g/dL and hematocrit of 30%.
    2. The client with no palpable thrill or auscultated bruit.
    3. The client reporting being exhausted and is sleeping.
    4. The client prescribed antihypertensive medication.

15. The male client diagnosed with CKD received the initial dose of erythropoietin 1 week ago. Which report by the client indicates the need to notify the health-care provider (HCP)?
    1. The client reports flu-like symptoms.
    2. The client reports being tired all the time.
    3. The client reports an elevation in his blood pressure.
    4. The client reports discomfort in his legs and back.

16. The nurse is developing a nursing care plan for the client diagnosed with CKD. Which nursing problem is a **priority** for the client?
    1. Low self-esteem.
    2. Knowledge deficit.
    3. Activity intolerance.
    4. Excess fluid volume.

17. The client diagnosed with CKD is placed on a fluid restriction of 1,500 mL/day. On the 7 a.m. to 7 p.m. shift, the client drank an 8-ounce cup of coffee, 4 ounces of juice, 12 ounces of tea, and 2 ounces of water with medications. What amount of fluid can the 7 p.m. to 7 a.m. nurse give to the client?

    _____

18. The client diagnosed with CKD has a new arteriovenous fistula in the left forearm. Which intervention should the nurse implement? **Select all that apply.**
    1. Teach the client to carry heavy objects with the right arm.
    2. Perform all laboratory blood tests on the left arm.
    3. Instruct the client to lie on the left arm during the night.
    4. Discuss the importance of not performing any hand exercises.
    5. Have the client wash the area with soap and warm water daily.

19. The male client diagnosed with CKD secondary to diabetes has been receiving dialysis for 12 years. The client is notified he will not be placed on the kidney transplant list. The client tells the nurse he will not be back for any more dialysis treatments. Which response by the nurse is **most therapeutic**?
    1. "You cannot just quit your dialysis. This is not an option."
    2. "You're angry at not being on the list, and you want to quit dialysis?"
    3. "I will call your nephrologist right now so you can talk to the HCP."
    4. "Make your funeral arrangements because you are going to die."

20. The nurse is discussing kidney transplants with clients at a dialysis center. Which type of donation is most common?
    1. Living, related donor.
    2. Nondirected, altruistic donor.
    3. Cadaver donor.
    4. Xenotransplantation donor.

21. The client receiving dialysis is reporting being dizzy and light-headed. Which action should the nurse implement **first**?
    1. Place the client in the Trendelenburg position.
    2. Turn off the dialysis machine immediately.
    3. Bolus the client with 500 mL of normal saline.
    4. Notify the health-care provider as soon as possible.

22. The nurse caring for a client diagnosed with CKD writes a client problem of "noncompliance with dietary restrictions." Which intervention should be included in the plan of care?
    1. Teach the client the proper diet to eat while undergoing dialysis.
    2. Refer the client and significant other to the dietitian.
    3. Explain the importance of eating the proper foods.
    4. Determine the reason for the client not adhering to the diet.

23. The client diagnosed with CKD is receiving peritoneal dialysis. Which assessment data **warrant immediate** intervention by the nurse?
    1. Inability to auscultate a bruit over the fistula.
    2. The client's abdomen is soft, is nontender, and has bowel sounds.
    3. The dialysate being removed from the client's abdomen is clear.
    4. The dialysate instilled was 1,500 mL and removed was 1,500 mL.

24. The client receiving hemodialysis is being discharged home from the dialysis center. Which instruction should the nurse teach the client?
    1. Notify the HCP if oral temperature is 102°F or greater.
    2. Apply ice to the access site if it starts bleeding at home.
    3. Maintain fluid and salt restrictions to decrease side effects.
    4. Encourage the significant other to make decisions for the client.

## Fluid and Electrolyte Disorders

25. The client is admitted to a nursing unit from a long-term care facility with the laboratory results populated in the chart below. Which condition is a cause for these findings?

| Client: Mr. L.T. | | |
|---|---|---|
| Laboratory Test | Client Results | Normal Values |
| Hematocrit (Hct) | 56 | Male: 42%–52% Female: 36%–48% |
| Sodium (Na⁺) | 152 | 135–145 mEq/L or mmol/L |
| Potassium (K) | 5.5 | 3.5–5.3 MEq/L or mmol/L |

1. Overhydration.
2. Anemia.
3. Dehydration.
4. Acute kidney injury.

26. The client, after undergoing an exploratory laparotomy with subsequent removal of a large intestinal tumor, has a nasogastric tube (NGT) in place and an IV running at 150 mL/hr via an IV pump. Which data should be reported to the HCP?
    1. The pump keeps sounding an alarm indicating the high pressure has been reached.
    2. Intake is 1,800 mL, NGT output is 550 mL, and Foley output is 950 mL.
    3. On auscultation, crackles and rhonchi in all lung fields are noted.
    4. The client has negative pedal edema and an increasing level of consciousness.

27. The client diagnosed with diabetes insipidus weighed 180 pounds when the daily weight was taken yesterday. This morning's weight is 175.6 pounds. One liter of fluid weighs approximately 2.2 pounds. How much fluid, in milliliters, has the client lost?

[                    ]

28. The nurse writes the client problem of "fluid volume excess" (FVE). Which intervention should be included in the plan of care? **Select all that apply.**
    1. Change the IV fluid from 0.9% NS to D₅W.
    2. Restrict the sodium in the client's diet.
    3. Monitor blood glucose levels.
    4. Prepare the client for hemodialysis.
    5. Weigh the client daily.

29. The client is admitted with a serum sodium level of 110 mEq/L. Which nursing intervention should be implemented?
    1. Encourage fluids orally.
    2. Administer 10% saline solution IVPB.
    3. Administer antidiuretic hormone intranasally.
    4. Place on seizure precautions.

30. The telemetry monitor technician notifies the nurse of the morning telemetry readings. Which client should the nurse assess **first**?
    1. The client in normal sinus rhythm with a peaked T wave.
    2. The client diagnosed with atrial fibrillation with a rate of 100.
    3. The client diagnosed with a myocardial infarction and occasional PVCs.
    4. The client diagnosed with a first-degree atrioventricular block and a rate of 92.

31. The client post-thyroidectomy reports numbness and tingling around the mouth and the tips of the fingers. Which intervention should the nurse implement **first**?
    1. Notify the health-care provider immediately.
    2. Tap the cheek about 2 cm anterior to the earlobe.
    3. Check the serum calcium and magnesium levels.
    4. Prepare to administer calcium gluconate IVP.

32. The nurse is caring for a client diagnosed with diabetic ketoacidosis (DKA). Which statement **best** explains the scientific rationale for the client's Kussmaul's respirations?
    1. The kidneys produce excess urine and the lungs try to compensate.
    2. The respirations increase the amount of carbon dioxide in the bloodstream.
    3. The lungs speed up to release carbon dioxide and increase the pH.
    4. The shallow and slow respirations will increase the HCO₃ in the serum.

33. The client is NPO and is receiving total parenteral nutrition (TPN) via a subclavian line. Which precautions should the nurse implement? **Select all that apply.**
    1. Place the solution on an IV pump at the prescribed rate.
    2. Monitor blood glucose every 6 hours.
    3. Weigh the client weekly, first thing in the morning.
    4. Change the IV tubing every 3 days.
    5. Monitor intake and output every shift.

34. The client has received IV solutions for 3 days through a 20-gauge IV catheter placed in the left cephalic vein. On morning rounds, the nurse notes the IV site is tender to palpation, and a red streak has formed. Which intervention should the nurse implement **first**?
    1. Start a new IV in the right hand.
    2. Discontinue the intravenous line.
    3. Complete an incident record.
    4. Place a warm washrag over the site.

35. The nurse and a UAP are caring for a group of clients. Which nursing intervention should the RN perform?
    1. Measure the client's output from the indwelling catheter.
    2. Record the client's intake and output on the I&O sheet.
    3. Instruct the client on appropriate fluid restrictions.
    4. Provide water for a client diagnosed with diabetes insipidus.

36. The client has been vomiting and has had numerous episodes of diarrhea. Which laboratory test should the nurse monitor?
    1. Serum calcium.
    2. Serum phosphorus.
    3. Serum potassium.
    4. Serum sodium.

## Urinary Tract Infection (UTI)

37. The client from a long-term care facility is admitted to the medical unit with a fever, hot flushed skin, and clumps of white sediment in the indwelling catheter. Which intervention should the nurse implement **first**?
    1. Start an IV with a 20-gauge catheter.
    2. Initiate antibiotic therapy IVPB.
    3. Collect a urine specimen for culture.
    4. Change the indwelling catheter.

38. The nurse is inserting an indwelling catheter into a female client. Which interventions should be implemented? **Rank in order of performance.**

1. Explain the procedure to the client.
2. Set up the sterile field.
3. Insert the catheter.
4. Place absorbent pads under the client.
5. Clean the perineum with povidone-iodine.

39. The nurse performs bladder irrigation through an indwelling catheter. The nurse instilled 90 mL of sterile normal saline. The catheter drained 710 mL. What is the client's output?

    [                    ]

40. The nurse is examining a 15-year-old female client reporting pain, frequency, and urgency when urinating. After asking the parent to leave the room, which question should the nurse ask the client?
    1. "When was your last menstrual cycle?"
    2. "Have you noticed any change in the color of the urine?"
    3. "Are you sexually active?"
    4. "What have you taken for the pain?"

41. The client is reporting chills, fever, and left costovertebral pain. Which diagnostic test should the nurse expect the HCP to prescribe **first**?
    1. A midstream urine for culture.
    2. A sonogram of the kidney.
    3. An intravenous pyelogram for renal calculi.
    4. A CT scan of the kidneys.

42. The nurse is caring for a 1-year-old client diagnosed with chronic pyelonephritis. Which assessment data support the diagnosis of chronic pyelonephritis? **Select all that apply.**
    1. Fever.
    2. Flank pain.
    3. Failure to thrive.
    4. Fifth disease.
    5. Hypertension.

43. The female client in an outpatient clinic is being sent home with a diagnosis of UTI. Which instruction should the nurse teach to **prevent** a recurrence of a UTI?
    1. Clean the perineum from back to front after a bowel movement.
    2. Take warm tub baths instead of hot showers daily.
    3. Void immediately preceding sexual intercourse.
    4. Avoid coffee, tea, colas, and alcoholic beverages.

44. The nurse is caring for a pregnant client diagnosed with acute pyelonephritis. Which scientific rationale supports the client being hospitalized for this condition?
    1. The client must be treated aggressively to prevent maternal and fetal complications.
    2. The nurse can force the client to drink fluids and avoid nausea and vomiting.

3. The client will be dehydrated, and there won't be sufficient blood flow to the baby.
4. Pregnant clients historically are afraid to take the antibiotics as ordered.

45. The nurse is discharging a client diagnosed with a catheter-associated urinary tract infection (CAUTI). Which information should the nurse include in the discharge teaching?
1. Limit fluid intake so the urinary tract can heal.
2. Collect a routine urine specimen for culture.
3. Take all the antibiotics as prescribed.
4. Tell the client to void every 5 to 6 hours.

46. The nurse is preparing a plan of care for the client diagnosed with acute glomerulonephritis. Which statement is an **appropriate** long-term goal?
1. The client will have a blood pressure within normal limits.
2. The client will show no protein in the urine.
3. The client will maintain normal renal function.
4. The client will have clear lung sounds.

47. The elderly client is diagnosed with chronic glomerulonephritis. Which laboratory value indicates to the nurse the condition has **become worse**?

| Client: E.C. | | Diagnosis: Glomerulonephritis |
|---|---|---|
| Laboratory Test | Client Results | Normal Values |
| BUN | 15 | 8–21 mg/dL Age ≥ 90 years: 10–31 mg/dL |
| Creatinine | 1.2 | Male: 0.61–1.21 mg/dL Female: 0.51–1.11 mg/dL |
| Glomerular filtration rate (GFR) | 40 | Over 60 mL/min/ 1.73 m² |
| Creatinine clearance (24 hr urine) | 100 | Male: 85–125 mL/ min/1.73 m² Female: 75–115 mL/ min/1.73 m² |

1. The blood urea nitrogen.
2. The creatinine level.
3. The glomerular filtration rate.
4. The 24-hour creatinine clearance.

48. The clinic nurse is caring for a client diagnosed with chronic pyelonephritis and prescribed trimethoprim-sulfamethoxazole twice a day for 90 days. Which statement is the scientific rationale for prescribing this medication?
1. The antibiotic will treat the bladder spasms that accompany a UTI.
2. If the urine cannot be made bacteria-free, the medication will suppress bacterial growth.
3. In 3 months, the client should be rid of all bacteria in the urinary tract.
4. The HCP is providing the client with enough medication to treat future infections.

## Benign Prostatic Hypertrophy (BPH)

49. The nurse emptied 2,000 mL from the drainage bag of a client's continuous irrigation after transurethral resection of the prostate (TURP). The amount of irrigation in the bag hanging was 3,000 mL at the beginning of the shift. There were 1,800 mL left in the bag 8 hours later. What is the correct urine output at the end of the 8 hours?

> [ ]

50. The nurse observes red urine and several large clots in the tubing of the normal saline continuous irrigation catheter for the client 1 day postoperative TURP. Which intervention should the nurse implement?
1. Remove the indwelling catheter.
2. Titrate the NS irrigation to run faster.
3. Administer protamine sulfate IVP.
4. Administer vitamin K slowly.

51. Which data support to the nurse the client's diagnosis of acute bacterial prostatitis? **Select all that apply.**
1. Terminal dribbling.
2. Urinary frequency.
3. Stress incontinence.
4. Sudden fever and chills.
5. Pelvic pain.

52. Which interventions should the nurse include when preparing a teaching plan for the client diagnosed with chronic prostatitis? **Select all that apply.**
1. Sit in a warm sitz bath for 10 to 20 minutes several times daily.
2. Sit in the chair with the feet elevated for 2 hours daily.

3. Drink at least 3,000 mL of oral fluids, especially tea and coffee, daily.
4. Stop broad-spectrum antibiotics as soon as the symptoms subside.
5. Take nonsteroidal anti-inflammatory medications for pain.

53. Which nursing diagnosis is a **priority** for the client after a TURP?
    1. Potential for sexual dysfunction.
    2. Potential for an altered body image.
    3. Potential for chronic infection.
    4. Potential for hemorrhage.

54. Which statement indicates discharge teaching has been **effective** for the postoperative TURP client?
    1. "I will call the surgeon if I experience any difficulty urinating."
    2. "I will take my finasteride daily, the same as before my surgery."
    3. "I will continue restricting my oral fluid intake."
    4. "I will take my pain medication routinely even if I do not hurt."

55. The client is 1 day postoperative TURP. Which task should the RN delegate to the UAP?
    1. Increase the irrigation fluid to clear clots from the tubing.
    2. Elevate the scrotum on a towel roll for support.
    3. Change the dressing on the first postoperative day.
    4. Teach the client how to care for the continuous irrigation catheter.

56. The client with a TURP and continuous irrigation catheter reports the need to urinate. Which intervention should the nurse implement **first**?
    1. Call the surgeon to inform the HCP of the client's report.
    2. Administer the client a narcotic medication for pain.
    3. Explain to the client this sensation happens frequently.
    4. Assess the continuous irrigation catheter for patency.

57. The client, postoperative TURP, asks the nurse, "When will I know if I will be able to have sex after my TURP?" Which response is **most appropriate** by the nurse?
    1. "You seem anxious about your surgery."
    2. "Tell me about your fears of impotency."

3. "Potency can return in 6 to 8 weeks."
4. "Did you ask your doctor about your concern?"

58. The client asks, "What does an elevated PSA test mean?" On which scientific rationale should the nurse base the response?
    1. An elevated PSA can result from several different causes.
    2. An elevated PSA can be only from prostate cancer.
    3. An elevated PSA can be diagnostic for testicular cancer.
    4. An elevated PSA is the only test used to diagnose BPH.

59. The client returned from surgery after having a TURP with cool and clammy skin, and the vitals populated in the flowsheet below. Which interventions should the nurse implement? **Select all that apply.**

| Vital Sign Flowsheet | Client Results | Normal Values |
|---|---|---|
| Blood Pressure | 90/40 | 100–119 mm Hg systolic 60–80 mm Hg diastolic |
| Temperature | 98°F | Oral: 98°F (36.7°F) |
| Pulse | 110 | 60–100 beats/min |
| Respirations | 24 | 12–20 breaths/min |

1. Assess the urine in the continuous irrigation drainage bag.
2. Decrease the irrigation fluid in the continuous irrigation catheter.
3. Lower the head of the bed while raising the foot of the bed.
4. Contact the surgeon to give an update on the client's condition.
5. Check the client's postoperative creatinine and BUN.

60. The nurse is caring for a client with a TURP. Which expected outcome indicates the client's condition is **improving**?
    1. The client is using the maximum amount allowed by the PCA pump.
    2. The client's bladder spasms are relieved by medication.
    3. The client's scrotum is swollen and tender with movement.
    4. The client has passed a large, hard, brown stool this morning.

# Renal Calculi

61. The laboratory data reveal a calcium phosphate renal stone for a client diagnosed with renal calculi. Which discharge teaching intervention should the nurse implement?
    1. Encourage the client to eat a low-purine diet and limit foods such as organ meats.
    2. Explain the importance of not drinking water 2 hours before bedtime.
    3. Discuss the importance of limiting vitamin D–enriched foods.
    4. Prepare the client for extracorporeal shock wave lithotripsy (ESWL).

62. The client diagnosed with renal calculi is admitted to the medical unit. Which intervention should the nurse implement first?
    1. Monitor the client's urinary output.
    2. Assess the client's pain and rule out complications.
    3. Increase the client's oral fluid intake.
    4. Use a safety gait belt when ambulating the client.

63. The client diagnosed with possible renal calculi is scheduled for a renal ultrasound. Which intervention should the nurse implement for this procedure?
    1. Ask if the client is allergic to shellfish or iodine.
    2. Keep the client NPO 8 hours before the ultrasound.
    3. Ensure the client has a signed informed consent form.
    4. Explain the test is noninvasive, and there is no discomfort.

64. Which clinical manifestations should the nurse expect to assess for the client diagnosed with a ureteral renal stone?
    1. Dull, aching flank pain, and microscopic hematuria.
    2. Nausea; vomiting; pallor; and cool, clammy skin.
    3. Gross hematuria and dull suprapubic pain with voiding.
    4. The client will be asymptomatic.

65. The client diagnosed with renal calculi is scheduled for a 24-hour urine specimen collection. Which interventions should the RN implement? **Select all that apply.**
    1. Check for the ordered diet and medication modifications.
    2. Instruct the client to urinate, and discard this urine when starting a collection.
    3. Collect all urine for 24 hours and place it in the appropriate specimen container.
    4. Insert an indwelling catheter in the client after having the client empty the bladder.
    5. Instruct the UAP to notify the nurse when the client urinates.

66. The client is diagnosed with an acute episode of ureteral calculi. Which client problem is the **priority** when caring for this client?
    1. Fluid volume loss.
    2. Knowledge deficit.
    3. Impaired urinary elimination.
    4. Alteration in comfort.

67. The client diagnosed with renal calculi is scheduled for lithotripsy. Which postprocedure nursing task is the **most appropriate** to delegate to the UAP?
    1. Monitor the amount, color, and consistency of urine output.
    2. Teach the client about the care of the indwelling Foley catheter.
    3. Assist the client to the car when being discharged home.
    4. Take the client's postprocedural vital signs.

68. Which statement indicates the client diagnosed with calcium phosphate renal calculi **understands** the discharge teaching for ways to **prevent** future calculi formation?
    1. "I should increase my fluid intake, especially in warm weather."
    2. "I should eat foods containing cocoa and chocolate."
    3. "I will walk about a mile every week and not exercise often."
    4. "I should take one vitamin a day with extra calcium."

69. Which intervention is **most important** for the nurse to implement for the client diagnosed with possible renal calculi?
    1. Assess the client's neurological status every 2 hours.
    2. Strain all urine and send any sediment to the laboratory.
    3. Monitor the client's creatinine and BUN levels.
    4. Take a 24-hour dietary recall during the client interview.

70. The client with a history of renal calculi calls the clinic and reports having burning on urination, chills, and an elevated temperature. Which instruction should the nurse discuss with the client?
    1. Increase water intake for the next 24 hours.
    2. Take two acetaminophen to help decrease the temperature.
    3. Come to the clinic and provide a urine specimen for urinalysis.
    4. Use a sterile 4 × 4 gauze to strain the client's urine.

71. The client had surgery to remove a kidney stone. Which laboratory assessment data **warrant immediate** intervention by the nurse?
    1. A serum potassium level of 3.8 mEq/L.
    2. A urinalysis shows microscopic hematuria.
    3. A creatinine level of 0.8 mg/dL.
    4. A white blood cell count of $14 \times 10^3$/microL.

72. The client is diagnosed with a uric acid stone. Which foods should the client eliminate from the diet to help **prevent** reoccurrence?
    1. Beer and colas.
    2. Asparagus and cabbage.
    3. Venison and sardines.
    4. Cheese and eggs.

## Cancer of the Bladder

73. The nurse is caring for clients in a renal surgery unit. After the afternoon report, which client should the nurse assess **first**?
    1. The male client just returned from a CT scan stating he left his glasses in the x-ray department.
    2. The client 1 day postoperative with a moderate amount of serous drainage on the dressing.
    3. The client scheduled for surgery in the morning and wants an explanation of the operative procedure before signing the permit.
    4. The client, after ileal conduit surgery this morning, has not had any drainage in the drainage bag.

74. Which modifiable **risk factor** should the nurse identify for the development of cancer of the bladder in a client?
    1. Previous exposure to chemicals.
    2. Pelvic radiation therapy.
    3. Cigarette smoking.
    4. Parasitic infections of the bladder.

75. The client diagnosed with cancer of the bladder is scheduled to have a cutaneous urinary diversion procedure. Which preoperative teaching intervention specific to the procedure should be included?
    1. Demonstrate turn, cough, and deep breathing.
    2. Explain a bag will drain the urine from now on.
    3. Instruct the client on the use of a PCA pump.
    4. Take the client to the ICU to become familiar with it.

76. The client diagnosed with cancer of the bladder is undergoing intravesical chemotherapy. Which instructions should the nurse provide the client about the procedure? **Select all that apply.**
    1. Instruct the client to restrict fluids 4 hours before the procedure.
    2. Teach not to empty the bladder for 1 to 2 hours after the procedure.
    3. Explain that the client will need to administer filgrastim at home.
    4. Have the client take acetaminophen before coming to the clinic.
    5. Tell the client to sit to avoid urine splashing after the procedure.

77. The nurse is planning the care of a postoperative client with an ileal conduit. Which intervention should be included in the plan of care?
    1. Provide meticulous skin care and pouching.
    2. Apply sterile drainage bags daily.
    3. Monitor the pH of the urine weekly.
    4. Assess the stoma site every day.

78. The RN and a licensed practical nurse (LPN) are caring for a group of clients. Which intervention should be assigned to the LPN?
    1. Assessment of the client after a Kock pouch procedure.
    2. Monitoring of the postoperative client with a WBC of $22 \times 10^3$/microL.
    3. Administration of the prescribed antineoplastic medications.
    4. Care for the client going for an MRI of the kidneys.

79. The male client diagnosed with metastatic cancer of the bladder is emaciated and refuses to eat. Which nursing action is an example of the ethical principle of paternalism?
    1. The nurse allows the client to talk about not wanting to eat.
    2. The nurse tells the client if he does not eat, a feeding tube will be placed.
    3. The nurse consults the dietitian about the client's nutritional needs.
    4. The nurse asks the family to bring favorite foods for the client to eat.

80. The client diagnosed with cancer of the bladder states, "I have young children. I am too young to die." Which statement is the nurse's **best** response?
    1. "This cancer is treatable, and you should not give up."
    2. "Cancer occurs at any age. It is just one of those things."
    3. "You are afraid of dying and what will happen to your children."
    4. "Have you talked to your children about your death?"

81. The client with a continent urinary diversion is being discharged. Which discharge instructions should the nurse include in the teaching?
    1. Have the client demonstrate catheterizing the stoma.
    2. Instruct the client on how to pouch the stoma.
    3. Explain the use of a bedside drainage bag at night.
    4. Tell the client to call the HCP if the temperature is 99°F or less.

82. Which information regarding the care of a cutaneous ileal conduit should the nurse discuss with the client?
    1. Teach the client to instill a few drops of vinegar into the pouch.
    2. Tell the client the stoma should be slightly dusky colored.
    3. Inform the client that large clumps of mucus are expected.
    4. Tell the client it is normal for the urine to be pink or red in color.

83. The client is 2 days post-ureterosigmoidostomy for cancer of the bladder. Which assessment data **warrants notification** of the HCP by the nurse?
    1. The client reports pain at a "3," 30 minutes after being medicated.
    2. The client reports it hurts to cough and deep breathe.
    3. The client ambulates to the end of the hall and back before lunch.
    4. The client is lying in a fetal position and has a rigid abdomen.

84. The female client diagnosed with bladder cancer has a cutaneous urinary diversion and states, "Will I be able to have children now?" Which statement is the nurse's **best response**?
    1. "Cancer does not make you sterile, but sometimes the therapy can."
    2. "Are you concerned you can't have children?"
    3. "You will be able to have as many children as you want."
    4. "Let me have the chaplain come to talk with you about this."

# CONCEPTS

The concepts covered in this chapter focus on urinary elimination and fluid and electrolyte balance. Exemplars that are covered are acute and chronic renal failure, UTI, and dehydration. Interrelated concepts of the nursing process and clinical judgment are covered throughout the questions. The concept of clinical judgment is presented in prioritizing or "first" questions.

85. The nurse is monitoring the client's laboratory values. Which laboratory report is **diagnostic** for a UTI?
    1. Complete Blood Count

**Date: Today**

| Laboratory Test | Client Value | Normal Values |
|---|---|---|
| Red Blood Cells (RBCs) | 3.8 | Male: 4.21–5.81 ($10^6$ cells/microL) Female: 3.61–5.11 ($10^6$ cells/microL) |
| Hemoglobin (Hgb) | 11 | Male: 14–17.3 g/dL Female: 11.7–15.5 g/dL |
| Hematocrit (Hct) | 33% | Male: 42%–52% Female: 36%–48% |
| Platelet | 250 | 140–400 × ($10^3$/microL) |
| White Blood Cells (WBCs) | 12.5 | 4.5–11.1 × ($10^3$/cells/microL) |

2. Urinalysis

|  | Client Values | Normal Values |
|---|---|---|
| pH | 5.5 | 4.5–8 |
| Color | Dark amber | Amber yellow |
| Clarity | Cloudy | Clear |
| Specific gravity | 1.029 | 1.005–1.03 |
| Osmolality | 450 | 50–1200 mOsm/kg (random) |
| Protein | 0 | Less than 20 mg/dL |
| Glucose | 0 | None |
| Ketones | 0 | None |
| RBC | 0 | Less than 5/hpf |
| WBC | 4 | Less than 5/hpf |

3. Urine Culture

| Urine Culture | Organism | Sensitivity |
|---|---|---|
| 48-hour result | Greater than $10^5$ *Escherichia coli* bacteria | Ceftriaxone Cefazolin Imipenem-Cilastatin |

4. Metanephrines

|  | Client Value | Normal Values |
|---|---|---|
| Metanephrines, total (24-hour urine) | 700 | 94–832 mcg/24 hr |

86. The nurse is caring for a client diagnosed with CKD. Which antecedents would the nurse assess? **Select all that apply.**
    1. Current diet.
    2. Diabetes.
    3. Hypertension.
    4. Fluid restriction.
    5. Race.

87. The client is in the intensive care unit (ICU) after a motor vehicle accident in which the client lost an estimated 3 units of blood. Which action by the nurse could **prevent** the client from developing AKI?
    1. Take and document the client's vital signs every hour.
    2. Assess the client's dressings every 2 hours.
    3. Check the client's urinary output every shift.
    4. Maintain the client's blood pressure greater than 100/60.

88. The nurse has identified the concept of urinary elimination for a client. Which information is **most important** for the nurse to provide to the HCP the next day?

**Intake and Output**

| Day 1 (Shift Time) | Oral (mL) | Intravenous (mL) | Urine (mL) | Nasogastric Tube (mL) | Other (Specify) (mL) |
|---|---|---|---|---|---|
| 0701–1900 | 2,200 | 1,600 | 735 |  | Emesis 40 |
| 1901–0700 | 1,600 | 1,400 | 575 |  |  |
| Total | 3,800 | 3,000 | 1,310 |  | 40 |

1. The client vomited 40 mL on the day shift.
2. The client has adequate oral intake, and IV fluids are not needed.
3. The client has had 6,800 mL intake and 1,350 mL output in the last 24 hours.
4. The client does not like to have to keep the urine for measurement.

89. The client diagnosed with CKD is prescribed hemodialysis on Monday, Wednesday, and Friday. Which interventions should the dialysis nurse implement? **Select all that apply.**
    1. Weigh the client before and after each treatment.
    2. Discuss the recommended fluid restriction.
    3. Provide potato chips or pretzels as a snack.
    4. Monitor the hemodialysis access site continuously.
    5. Keep up a lively conversation during the treatments.

90. The nurse is administering morning medications. Which medication should the nurse **question** administering?

| Client Name: ACC | MR# 678905 | Diagnosis: Acute Renal Failure |
|---|---|---|
| Age: 42 years | Allergies: Penicillin | |
| Medication | 0701–1900 | 1901–0700 |
| Furosemide 80 mg PO daily | 0900<br>K + 4.3 | |
| Erythropoietin Sub Q daily ×3 days | 0900 | |
| Multivitamin with iron PO daily | 0900 | |
| Levothyroxine 0.75 mcg PO daily | 0900 | |
| Signature of Nurse: | Day Nurse RN/DN | Night Nurse RN/NN |

1. Furosemide.
2. Erythropoietin.
3. Multivitamin with iron.
4. Levothyroxine.

91. The nurse identifies the concepts of elimination and immunity for a female client diagnosed with a UTI. Which discharge instructions should the nurse provide the client? **Select all that apply.**
    1. Teach the client to wipe from front to back after voiding.
    2. Encourage the client to drink cranberry juice each morning.
    3. Inform the client that frequent episodes of incontinence are expected.
    4. Discuss the clinical manifestations of a recurrent infection.
    5. Have the client fill a container of water to sip until at least 2,000 mL are consumed.
    6. Request that the client sit in a tub of warm water twice a day for 25 minutes.

92. The client diagnosed with CKD is prescribed a 60-gm protein, 2,000-mg sodium diet. Which food choices indicate the client **understands** the dietary restrictions?

1. A 4-ounce grilled chicken breast, broccoli, and small glass of unsweet tea.
2. Baked potato with chopped ham and sour cream, 12-ounce steak, and beer.
3. Double patty cheeseburger, french fries, and an artificially sweetened beverage.
4. Roast beef sandwich, potato chips, and soft drink.

93. The older client presents to the emergency department reporting burning on urination with an urgency to void, and a temperature of 99.8°F. Which intervention should the nurse implement **first**?
    1. Ask the client to provide a clean voided midstream urine for culture.
    2. Insert an 18-gauge peripheral IV catheter and start normal saline fluids.

3. Arrange for the client to be admitted to the medical unit.
4. Initiate the ordered intravenous antibiotic medication.

94. The client diagnosed with a UTI has a blood pressure of 83/56 mm Hg and a pulse of 122 bpm. Which should the nurse implement **first**?
    1. Notify the health-care provider (HCP).
    2. Hang the IVPB antibiotic at the prescribed rate.
    3. Check the laboratory work to determine if the urine culture has been completed.
    4. Increase the normal saline IV fluids from keep open to 150 mL/hour on the IV pump.

95. The nurse is developing a care map for a client diagnosed with chronic kidney disease (CKD) on hemodialysis. Which interrelated concepts should be included in the map? **Select all that apply.**
    1. Fluid and electrolytes.
    2. Hematologic regulation.
    3. Digestion.
    4. Metabolism.
    5. Mobility.
    6. Nutrition.

96. The telemetry nurse is reviewing the laboratory results for a client. Which **further assessment** data should the nurse determine **before** notifying the HCP?

| Laboratory Test | Client Values | Normal Values |
|---|---|---|
| Potassium | 2.3 | 3.5–5.3 mEq/L |
| Sodium | 139 | 135–145 mEq/L |
| Glucose | 143 | Fasting < 100 mg/dL Random < 200 mg/dL |
| Creatinine | 1.5 | M: 0.61–1.21 mg/dL F: 0.51–1.11 mg/dL |
| BUN | 20 | 8 to 21 mg/dL Age ≥ 90 years: 10 to 31 mg/dL |
| B-Type Natriuretic Peptide (BNP) | 80 | Less than 125 pg/mL |

1. Obtain the client's 24-hour urine output.
2. Ask the UAP to get a blood glucose reading.
3. Assess the client's telemetry reading.
4. Call the rapid response team (RRT).

### Acute Kidney Injury (AKI)

1. 1. Usually, there are no diseases or conditions warranting this question when discussing AKI.
   2. Vigorous exercise will not impede blood flow to the kidneys, leading to AKI.
   3. Usually, viruses do not cause AKI.
   4. Medications such as NSAIDs and some herbal remedies are nephrotoxic; therefore, asking about medications is appropriate (Thornburg & Gray-Vickrey, 2016).

   **TEST-TAKING HINT:** Asking about medications, especially over-the-counter and herbal remedies, during the admission interview is an important intervention because many medications are nephrotoxic and hepatotoxic.

2. 1. Blood urea nitrogen (BUN) levels reflect the balance between the production and excretion of urea from the kidneys. Creatinine is a by-product of the metabolism of the muscles and is excreted by the kidneys. Creatinine is the ideal substance for determining renal clearance because it is relatively constant in the body and is the laboratory value most significant in diagnosing kidney injury.
   2. WBCs (white blood cells) are monitored for infection, and hemoglobin is monitored for blood loss.
   3. Potassium (intracellular) and sodium (interstitial) are electrolytes and are monitored for a variety of diseases or conditions not specific to renal function. Potassium levels will increase with renal failure, but the level is not a diagnostic indicator for kidney injury.
   4. Bilirubin and ammonia levels are laboratory values determining the function of the liver, not the kidneys.

   **TEST-TAKING HINT:** The nurse must know specific laboratory tests for specific organ functioning or conditions. This is memorizing, but it must be done.

3. 1. Diabetes mellitus is a disease that may lead to CKD.
   2. Hypotension, which causes a decreased blood supply to the kidney, is one of the most common causes of prerenal AKI (before the kidney).
   3. Nephrotoxic medications are a cause of intrarenal (intrinsic) AKI (directly to the kidney).
   4. Benign prostatic hypertrophy (BPH) is a cause of postrenal (obstructive) AKI (after the kidney).

   **TEST-TAKING HINT:** The test taker must be cautious of adjectives (words describing something); "prerenal" is the key to selecting the correct answer. The prefix *pre-* means "before."

4. Correct answers are 1, 2, and 3.
   1. AKI affects almost every system in the body. Neurologically, the client may have drowsiness, headache, muscle twitching, and seizures. In the recovery period, the client is alert and has no seizure activity.
   2. In renal failure, levels of erythropoietin are decreased, leading to anemia. An increase in hemoglobin and hematocrit indicates the client is in the recovery period.
   3. Nausea, vomiting, and diarrhea are common in the client diagnosed with AKI; therefore, an absence of these indicates the client is in the recovery period.
   4. The client in the recovery period has an increased urine-specific gravity.
   5. The client in the recovery period has a decreased serum creatinine level.

   **TEST-TAKING HINT:** This is an alternate-type question in which the test taker may choose as many correct answers as warranted. The test taker should not immediately assume that the option mentioning urine is the correct answer. The nurse must realize kidney injury affects every body system.

5. 1. Phosphate binders are used to treat elevated phosphorus levels, not elevated potassium levels.
   2. Anemia is not the result of an elevated potassium level.
   3. Assessment is an independent nursing action, which is appropriate for the elevated potassium level, but the question asks for a collaborative treatment.
   4. Normal potassium level is 3.5 to 5.3 mEq/L. A level of 6.8 mEq/L is life-threatening and could lead to cardiac dysrhythmias. Therefore, the client may be dialyzed to decrease the potassium level quickly. This requires an HCP order, so it is a collaborative intervention.

**TEST-TAKING HINT:** Adjectives must be noted when reading the stem of the question and the answer options.

6. 1. This is a nursing intervention, not a client outcome.
   2. This is a measurable client outcome, but acute kidney injury does not cause pain.
   3. AKI causes an imbalance of electrolytes (potassium, sodium, calcium, phosphorus). Therefore, the desired client outcome is electrolytes within normal limits.
   4. A Kayexalate resin enema may be administered to help decrease the potassium level, but this is an intervention, not a client outcome.

**TEST-TAKING HINT:** The nurse must have knowledge of the nursing process. Client outcomes are used to evaluate the planning part of the nursing process. The outcomes must be measurable, client focused, and realistic.

7. 1. The diet is low potassium, and calcium is not restricted in AKI.
   2. This is a diet recommended for clients diagnosed with cardiac disease and atherosclerosis.
   3. Carbohydrates are increased to provide for the client's caloric intake, and protein is restricted to minimize protein breakdown and to prevent the accumulation of toxic waste products.
   4. The client must be on a therapeutic diet, and small feedings are not required.

**TEST-TAKING HINT:** The test taker must notice adjectives. A "therapeutic" diet should cause the test taker to eliminate option "4" because it is a regular diet.

8. 1. Kidney function is improved by about 40% when recumbent, but this is not the scientific rationale for bedrest in AKI.
   2. Bedrest reduces exertion and the metabolic rate, thereby reducing catabolism and subsequent release of potassium and accumulation of endogenous waste products (urea and creatinine).
   3. This is a scientific rationale for prescribing bedrest in clients diagnosed with heart failure.
   4. This is not the scientific rationale for prescribing bedrest. The foot of the bed may be elevated to help decrease peripheral edema, and bedrest causes an increase in sacral edema.

**TEST-TAKING HINT:** The test taker should not jump to conclusions and select the only option with "renal" in the sentence. The nurse must know the normal anatomy and physiology of the body and be aware that keeping someone in bed will not restore kidney function when the kidneys have failed.

9. 1. The UAP can collect specimens. Collecting a midstream urine specimen requires the client to clean the perineal area, to urinate a little, and then collect the rest of the urine output in a sterile container.
   2. The UAP can obtain the client's intake and output, but the nurse must evaluate the data to determine if interventions are needed or if interventions are effective.
   3. Two RNs must check the unit of blood at the bedside before administering it.
   4. This is a medication enema, and UAPs cannot administer medications. Also, for this to be ordered, the client must be unstable with an excessively high serum potassium level.

**TEST-TAKING HINT:** Nursing tasks not delegated to a UAP include any task requiring nursing judgment, medication administration, teaching, evaluating, or assessing.

10. 1. Preventing and treating shock with blood and fluid replacement will prevent AKI from hypoperfusion of the kidneys. Significant blood loss is expected in the client diagnosed with a gunshot wound.
   2. Taking and evaluating the client's vital signs is an appropriate action, but regardless of the results, this will not prevent AKI.
   3. Placing the client on telemetry is an appropriate action, but telemetry is an assessment tool for the nurse and will not prevent AKI.
   4. Assessment is often the first action, but assessing the abdominal dressing will not help prevent AKI.

**TEST-TAKING HINT:** The test taker must read the stem carefully and understand what the question is asking. Options "2," "3," and "4" are all forms of assessment and do not help prevent AKI because they are not treatments.

11. 1. Erythropoietin is a chemical catalyst produced by the kidneys to stimulate red blood cell production; it does not affect the potassium level.
   2. Calcium gluconate helps protect the heart from the effects of high potassium levels.

3. Regular insulin, along with glucose, will drive potassium into the cells, thereby lowering serum potassium levels temporarily.
4. A loop diuretic, not an osmotic diuretic, may be ordered to help decrease the potassium level.

**TEST-TAKING HINT:** The test taker must be familiar with medical terms such as "hyperkalemia" and know the rationale for administering medications.

## Chronic Kidney Disease (CKD)

12. 1. Moisture barrier cream will keep the crystals on the skin.
2. These crystals are uremic frost resulting from irritating toxins deposited in the client's tissues. Bathing in cool water will remove the crystals, promote client comfort, and decrease the itching resulting from uremic frost (Saardi & Schwartz, 2016).
3. The client should be turned every 2 hours or more frequently to prevent skin breakdown.
4. This may occur with CKD, and it does require a nursing intervention.

**TEST-TAKING HINT:** The nurse must know what is normal for specific disease processes, and something coming out of the skin requires some action even if the test taker is not familiar with the disease process. Option "4" could be eliminated based on this test-taking strategy. The test taker should eliminate option "3" because there are very few instances in which the client is not turned or moved; turning and movement are necessary to prevent the development of pressure ulcers.

13. 1. There is a decrease in the excretion of phosphates and organic acids, not an increase.
2. The red blood cell destruction does not affect the arterial blood pH.
3. This is the correct scientific rationale for metabolic acidosis occurring in the client diagnosed with CKD.
4. This compensatory mechanism occurs to maintain an arterial blood pH between 7.35 and 7.45, but it does not occur as a result of CKD.

**TEST-TAKING HINT:** In option "1," the test taker should note "increased excretion"; CKD does not have any type of increase in excretion,

so the test taker could eliminate option "1." Option "4" does not even mention the renal system, and a loss of hydrochloric acid results in metabolic alkalosis, not acidosis, so the test taker can eliminate this option.

14. 1. These laboratory findings are low but do not require a blood transfusion and often are expected for a client experiencing anemia secondary to ESRD.
2. The client's dialysis access is compromised, so this client should be assessed first.
3. It is not uncommon for a client undergoing dialysis to be exhausted and sleep through the treatment.
4. Clients are instructed not to take their antihypertensive medications before dialysis to help prevent episodes of hypotension.

**TEST-TAKING HINT:** The test taker must determine which client's situation is not normal or expected for the disease process, which in this question is CKD because all clients are in the dialysis unit.

15. 1. Flu-like symptoms are expected and tend to subside with repeated doses; the nurse should suggest acetaminophen (Tylenol) before the injections.
2. Erythropoietin, a biologic response modifier, takes 2 to 6 weeks to become effective in improving anemia and thereby reducing fatigue.
3. After the initial administration of erythropoietin, a client's antihypertensive medications may need to be adjusted. Therefore, this report requires notification of the HCP. Erythropoietin therapy is contraindicated in clients diagnosed with uncontrolled hypertension (Federal Drug Administration, 2012).
4. Long bone and vertebral pain is an expected occurrence because the bone marrow is being stimulated to increase the production of red blood cells.

**TEST-TAKING HINT:** The test taker should select the potentially life-threatening option or a report requiring the medication to be adjusted or discontinued. The nurse should notify the HCP if the medication is causing an adverse effect, not an expected side effect.

16. 1. Low self-esteem, related to dependency, role changes, and changes in body image, is a pertinent client problem, but psychosocial problems are not a priority over physiological problems.

2. Teaching is always an important part of the care plan, but it is not a priority over a physiological problem.
3. Activity intolerance related to fatigue, anemia, and retention of waste products is a physiological problem, but it is not a life-threatening problem.
4. **Excess fluid volume is the priority because of the stress placed on the heart and vessels, which could lead to heart failure, pulmonary edema, and death.**

**TEST-TAKING HINT:** The test taker must read the stem of the question and understand what the question is asking. This is a priority question. This means all the options are pertinent problems for CKD, but only one is the priority. Applying Maslow's hierarchy of needs is one way to determine priorities: physiological problems are priority over psychosocial problems, and life-threatening conditions take first priority.

17. **720 mL.**
    The nurse must add up how many milliliters of fluid the client drank during the 7 a.m. to 7 p.m. shift and then subtract that number from 1,500 mL to determine how much fluid the client can receive on the 7 p.m. to 7 a.m. shift. One ounce is equal to 30 mL. The client drank 26 ounces (8 + 4 + 12 + 2) of fluid, or 780 mL (26 × 30) of fluid. Therefore, the client can have 720 mL (1,500 − 780) of fluid during the 7 p.m. to 7 a.m. shift.

**TEST-TAKING HINT:** The test taker must have knowledge of basic conversion factors. Use the drop-down calculator on the computer examination to ensure accuracy in computations.

18. **Correct answers are 1 and 5.**
    1. **Carrying heavy objects in the left arm could cause the fistula to clot by putting undue stress on the site, so the client should carry objects with the right arm.**
    2. The fistula should only be used for dialysis access, not for routine blood draws.
    3. The client should not lie on the left arm because this may cause clotting by putting pressure on the site.
    4. Hand exercises are recommended for new fistulas to help mature the fistula.
    5. **The client should wash the area around the access daily with soap and warm water and observe for signs of infection (National Institute of Diabetes and Digestive and Kidney Diseases, n.d.).**

**TEST-TAKING HINT:** The test taker must notice the adjectives, such as "left" and "right." Options "2" and "3" have the nurse doing something to the arm with the fistula.

19. 1. The client does have the right to quit dialysis if desired.
    2. **Reflecting the client's feelings and restating them are therapeutic responses the nurse should use when addressing the client's issues.**
    3. This is passing the buck; the nurse should address the client's issues.
    4. This may be true, but it is not therapeutic in attempting to get the client to verbalize feelings.

**TEST-TAKING HINT:** When asked to select a therapeutic response, the test taker should select an option with some type of "feeling" in the response, such as "angry" in option "2."

20. 1. Living, related donors occur when a family member or someone close to the recipient donates their kidney to the client. This is not the most common form of kidney donation; however, the kidney is the most commonly given organ by a living donor.
    2. Nondirected, altruistic donors are living donors who are strangers to the transplant recipient. This is not the most common form of kidney donation.
    3. **The most common form of kidney donation is cadaveric or from a deceased donor.**
    4. Xenotransplantation is the use of healthy animal organs for transplantation into humans. Research is being conducted on transplanting genetically engineered pig kidneys into rhesus monkeys to prove the effectiveness of xenotransplantation for kidney transplants (Vagefi, 2018). Xenotransplants of the kidney are not performed in humans at this time.

**TEST-TAKING HINT:** The nurse must be aware of transplantation information and terminology in health care.

21. 1. **The nurse should place the client's chair with the head lower than the body, which will shunt blood to the brain; this is the Trendelenburg position.**
    2. The blood in the dialysis machine must be infused back into the client before the machine is turned off.

3. Normal saline infusion is the last resort because one of the purposes of dialysis is to remove excess fluid from the body.

4. Hypotension is an expected occurrence in clients receiving dialysis; therefore, the HCP does not need to be notified.

**TEST-TAKING HINT: The Trendelenburg position is often used as a distracter in questions, and the nurse needs to know it is only used in cases where blood needs to be shunted to the brain.**

22. 1. Teaching is an intervention for a knowledge deficit, not noncompliance.
    2. Referring the client does not address the issue of noncompliance.
    3. Noncompliance is a client's choice, and explaining interventions will not necessarily make the client choose differently.
    4. Noncompliance is a choice the client has a right to make, but the nurse should determine the reason for the noncompliance and then take appropriate actions based on the client's rationale. For example, if the client has financial difficulties, the nurse may suggest how the client can afford the proper foods along with medications, or the nurse may be able to refer the client to a social worker.

**TEST-TAKING HINT: The test taker must always clarify and understand exactly what the question is asking the nurse to do. Answer options "1," "2," and "3" have the nurse doing the talking; only option "4" is allowing the client to explain the lack of compliance.**

23. 1. Peritoneal dialysis is administered through a catheter inserted into the peritoneal cavity; a fistula is used for hemodialysis.
    2. Peritonitis, inflammation of the peritoneum, is a serious complication resulting in a hard, rigid abdomen. Therefore, a soft abdomen does not warrant immediate intervention.
    3. The dialysate return is normally colorless or straw-colored, but it should never be cloudy, which indicates an infection.
    4. Because the client is in ESRD, fluid must be removed from the body, so the output should be more than the amount instilled. These assessment data require intervention by the nurse.

**TEST-TAKING HINT: The words "warrant immediate intervention" should clue the test taker into selecting an option with abnormal or unexpected data for the client.**

24. 1. The client should not wait until the temperature is 102°F to call the HCP; the client should call when the temperature is 100°F or greater.
    2. The client should apply direct pressure and notify the HCP if the access site starts to bleed, not apply ice to the site.
    3. The client should maintain fluid and salt restrictions to avoid side effects related to excess salt and fluid accumulation between dialysis treatments (Berns, 2019).
    4. The nurse should encourage the client's independence, not foster dependence by encouraging the significant other to make the client's decision.

**TEST-TAKING HINT: The test taker must read the question carefully. A temperature of 102°F is usually not acceptable in any client. Fostering dependence in any chronic illness is not encouraged by the nurse, so the test taker could eliminate option "4."**

## Fluid and Electrolyte Disorders

25. 1. Clients with overhydration or who have FVE experience dilutional values of sodium (135 to 145 mEq/L) and red blood cells (44% to 52%). The levels are lower than normal, not higher.
    2. Anemia is a low red blood cell count for a variety of reasons.
    3. Dehydration results in concentrated serum, causing laboratory values to increase because the blood has normal constituents but not enough volume to dilute the values to within normal range or possibly lower.
    4. In AKI, the kidneys cannot excrete urine, and this results in too much fluid in the body.

**TEST-TAKING HINT: The test taker must decide first if the values are high or low and then determine what is happening with body fluids in each process. Overhydration and renal failure result in the same fluid shift, so these two options ("1" and "4") could be excluded.**

26. 1. The pump is alerting the nurse there is resistance distal to the pump; this does not require notifying the HCP.
    2. The client has a 1,800-mL intake and a total output of 1,500 mL. The body has an insensible loss of approximately 400 mL/day through the skin, respiration, and other body functions. This does not warrant notifying the HCP.

3. Crackles and rhonchi in all lung fields indicate the body is not able to process the amount of fluid being infused. This should be brought to the HCP's attention.

4. Negative pedal edema and an increasing level of consciousness indicate the client is not experiencing a problem.

**TEST-TAKING HINT: The question requires the test taker to distinguish nursing problems from client problems. Option "1" is a nursing problem, and options "2" and "4" are expected results, so the HCP does not need to be notified. Only one option, "3," contains abnormal or life-threatening information.**

27. **2,000 mL has been lost.**
   First, determine how many pounds the client has lost:

   $$180 - 175.6 = 4.4 \text{ pounds lost}$$

   Then, based on the fact that 1 liter of fluid weighs 2.2 pounds, determine how many liters of fluid have been lost:

   $$4.4 \div 2.2 = 2 \text{ liters lost}$$

   Then, because the question asks for the answer in milliliters, convert 2 liters into milliliters:

   $$2 \times 1,000 = 2,000 \text{ mL}$$

**TEST-TAKING HINT: The test taker must be able to work basic math problems. This problem has several steps. Sometimes it is helpful to write out what is occurring at each step, such as 4.4 divided by 2.2 kg per pound. This can help the test taker realize if a step has been overlooked. Remember, on the NCLEX-RN®, use the drop-down calculator on the computer.**

28. **Correct answers are 2 and 5.**
   1. The nursing plan of care does not include changing the HCP's orders.
   2. Fluid volume excess refers to an isotonic expansion of the extracellular fluid by an abnormal expansion of water and sodium. Therefore, sodium is restricted to allow the body to excrete the extra volume.
   3. High blood glucose levels result in viscous blood and cause the kidneys to try to fix the problem by excreting the glucose through increasing the urine output, which results in fluid volume deficits.
   4. If the FVE is the result of renal failure, then hemodialysis may be ordered, but this information was not provided in the stem of the question.

5. Obtaining a daily weight is essential to provide information about fluid loss or gain. Each kilogram of weight is equivalent to 1 L of fluid (Hoffman & Sullivan, 2020).

**TEST-TAKING HINT: Option "1" is not a nursing prerogative. The test taker should not read into the question.**

29. 1. The client probably will be placed on fluid restriction. Fluids should not be encouraged for a client with a low sodium level (normal: 135 to 145 mEq/L).
   2. Hypertonic solutions of saline are 3% to 5%, not 10%, because of the extreme nature of hypertonic solutions. Hypertonic solutions of saline may be used, but very cautiously; if the sodium levels are increased too rapidly, a massive fluid shift can occur in the body, resulting in neurological damage and heart failure.
   3. The antidiuretic hormone (vasopressin) causes water retention in the body and increases the problem.
   4. Clients with sodium levels less than 120 mEq/L are at risk for seizures as a complication. The lower the sodium level, the greater the risk of a seizure.

**TEST-TAKING HINT: The test taker must memorize certain common laboratory values and understand how deviations in the electrolytes affect the body.**

30. 1. A client diagnosed with a peaked T wave could be experiencing hyperkalemia. Changes in potassium levels can initiate cardiac dysrhythmias and instability.
   2. Fluctuations in rate are expected in clients diagnosed with atrial fibrillation, and a heart rate of 100 is at the edge of a normal rate.
   3. Most people experience an occasional premature ventricular contraction (PVC); this does not warrant the nurse assessing this client first.
   4. A first-degree block is not an immediate problem.

**TEST-TAKING HINT: The test taker must know the normal data so the abnormal will be apparent. The normal heart rate is 60 to 100 bpm. The nurse should assess the client with an abnormal or life-threatening condition first.**

**31.** 1. The HCP may need to be notified, but the nurse should perform an assessment first.
2. **These are clinical manifestations of hypocalcemia, and the nurse can confirm this by tapping the cheek to elicit the Chvostek's sign. If the muscles of the cheek begin to twitch, then the HCP should be immediately notified because hypocalcemia is a medical emergency.**
3. A positive Chvostek's sign can indicate a low calcium or magnesium level, but serum laboratory levels may have been drawn hours previously or may not be available.
4. If the client does have hypocalcemia, this may be ordered, but it is not implemented before assessment.

**TEST-TAKING HINT: Assessment is the first step in the nursing process and is an appropriate option to select if the test taker has difficulty when trying to decide between two options.**

**32.** 1. Kussmaul's respirations are the lung's attempt to maintain the narrow range of pH compatible with human life. The respiratory system reacts rapidly to changes in pH.
2. Respiration is the act of moving oxygen and carbon dioxide. Kussmaul's respirations are rapid and deep and allow the client to exhale carbon dioxide.
3. **The lungs attempt to increase the blood pH level by blowing off the carbon dioxide (carbonic acid).**
4. $HCO_3$ (sodium bicarbonate) is an alkaline (base) substance regulated by the kidneys and is part of the metabolic buffer system, not a respiratory system buffer. The excretion and retention of carbon dioxide ($CO_2$) are regulated by the lungs and therefore a part of the respiratory buffer system.

**TEST-TAKING HINT: Homeostasis is a delicate balance between acids and bases. The test taker can discard option "1" by realizing the production of urine does not affect the respirations.**

**33.** Correct answers are 1, 2, and 5.
1. **TPN is a hypertonic solution with enough calories, proteins, lipids, electrolytes, and trace elements to sustain life. It is administered via a pump to prevent too rapid infusion.**
2. **TPN contains a 50% dextrose solution; therefore, the client is monitored to ensure the pancreas is adapting to the high glucose levels.**
3. The client is weighed daily, not weekly, to monitor for fluid overload.
4. The IV tubing is changed with every bag because the high glucose level can cause bacterial growth.
5. **Intake and output are monitored to observe for fluid balance.**

**TEST-TAKING HINT: Options "3" and "5" refer to the same factor—namely, fluid level. The test taker should then determine if the time factors are appropriate. Weekly weighing is not appropriate, so option "3" can be eliminated.**

**34.** 1. A new IV will be started in the right hand after the IV is discontinued.
2. **The client has clinical manifestations of phlebitis, and the IV must be removed to prevent further complications.**
3. Depending on the health-care facility, this may or may not be done, but client care comes before documentation.
4. A warm washrag placed on an IV site sometimes provides comfort to the client. If this is done, it should be done for 20 minutes, four times a day.

**TEST-TAKING HINT: The question is asking for a first action, which means all of the options may be actions the nurse could implement, but only one is the priority. In general, priority actions are to stop the problem, continue treatment, treat the problem, and then document.**

**35.** 1. The UAP can empty the catheter and measure the amount.
2. The UAP can record intake and output on the I&O sheet.
3. **The RN cannot delegate teaching.**
4. The client has a disease, but all the UAP is being asked to do is take water to the client.

**TEST-TAKING HINT: This is an example of an "except" question. Frequently, questions ask which tasks can be assigned to the UAP, but this question asks which action the RN should implement. If the test taker does not read carefully, it is easy to jump to the first option for actions the UAP can perform.**

**36.** 1. Serum calcium is decreased in conditions such as osteoporosis or post–thyroid surgery but not in vomiting and diarrhea.
2. Serum phosphorus levels are altered in acute and chronic renal failure or diabetic ketoacidosis, among other conditions, but not with acute fluid losses from the gastrointestinal tract.

3. Clients lose potassium from the GI tract or through the use of diuretic medications. Potassium imbalances can lead to cardiac arrhythmias.
4. The body is not at risk of losing sodium from these sources as it is with potassium.

**TEST-TAKING HINT:** The nurse must recognize basic fluids and electrolytes in the body and the implications of excess or loss. The body holds on to sodium and releases potassium.

## Urinary Tract Infection (UTI)

37. 1. The first action is to get a viable urine culture, so the causative pathogen can be identified. An IV should be started, but this is not the first action.
2. Initiating an IV antibiotic is a priority, but obtaining a culture is done first to make sure the HCP can treat the causative organism.
3. This is not the first intervention because the culture will be obtained when the new catheter has been inserted.
4. Unless the nurse can determine the catheter has been inserted within a few days, the nurse should replace the catheter and then get a specimen. This will provide the most accurate specimen for analysis.

**TEST-TAKING HINT:** In a question requiring the test taker to choose a "first" action, the test taker usually can order the choices 1, 2, 3, 4. In this question, options "4," "3," "1," and "2" should be the order of interventions.

38. Correct order is 1, 4, 2, 5, 3.
1. The procedure should be explained to the client.
4. Incontinence pads should be placed under the client before beginning the sterile part of the procedure.
2. The sterile field must be set up before cleaning the client's perineum.
5. During the procedure, the perineum is swiped with povidone-iodine (Betadine) or antiseptic swabs from front to back and also down the middle, making only one stroke per swab and discarding after each area (Teas et al., 2018).
3. The catheter should be inserted and the balloon inflated.

**TEST-TAKING HINT:** This is an alternative-type question requiring the test taker to rank the options in the correct order. The test taker must have knowledge of the skills performed by the nurse.

39. 620 mL of urine.
The amount of sterile normal saline is subtracted from the total volume removed from the catheter. 710 − 90 = 620.

**TEST-TAKING HINT:** This is a simple subtraction problem, but the test taker must understand any fluid used to irrigate a body system must be subtracted from the total volume in the suction device or catheter bag to get accurate information of the client's fluid-balance status.

40. 1. This could be asked with a parent in the room, and the nurse should receive a truthful answer.
2. There is no reason the client should not answer this question in the presence of the parent.
3. These are clinical manifestations of cystitis, a bladder infection, which may be caused by sexual intercourse as a result of the introduction of bacteria into the urethra during the physical act. A teenager may not want to divulge this information in front of the parent.
4. This information could be obtained in front of the parent.

**TEST-TAKING HINT:** The test taker must analyze the client's age, 15, and determine which of the options might not be answered truthfully if the parents are present. In this question, "asking the parent to leave the room" is the key to choosing the correct option.

41. 1. Fever, chills, and costovertebral pain are clinical manifestations of a urinary tract infection (acute pyelonephritis), which requires a urine culture first to confirm the diagnosis.
2. A sonogram of the kidney might be ordered if the client has recurrent UTIs to determine if a physical obstruction is causing the recurrent infections but not as the first diagnostic procedure.
3. An intravenous pyelogram is rarely used to determine pyelonephritis because the results are negative 75% of the time in clients diagnosed with acute pyelonephritis.
4. A CT scan might be ordered if other tests have not been conclusive.

**TEST-TAKING HINT:** The question asks which test should be ordered first, and the test taker should determine what the clinical manifestations might be indicating. Fever and chills indicate an infection. The anatomical position of the costovertebral angle (the flank area between a rib and a vertebra) should alert the test taker to the kidney area of the body. A urine culture is most likely to determine if a kidney infection is present.

**42.** Correct answers are 1, 2, 3, and 5.
1. Fever can be noted in children diagnosed with chronic pyelonephritis.
2. Flank pain or dysuria are clinical manifestations of chronic pyelonephritis.
3. Failure to thrive may be noted in young children with a diagnosis of chronic pyelonephritis.
4. Fifths disease is not associated with chronic pyelonephritis.
5. Some children with chronic pyelonephritis can be hypertensive (Lohr, 2019).

**TEST-TAKING HINT:** The key to this question is the age of the client. The test taker must be aware of the clinical manifestations of disease processes in all ages of clients. Chronic pyelonephritis occurs more often in infants and children younger than 2 years old than in older children and adults.

**43.** 1. The perineum should be cleaned from front to back after a bowel movement to prevent fecal contamination of the urethral meatus.
2. The temperature of the water does not matter, but the client should take showers instead of baths to prevent bacteria in the bath water from entering the urethra.
3. Voiding immediately after, not before, sexual intercourse uses the action of the urine passing through the urethra to the outside of the body to flush bacteria from the urethra that might have been introduced during intercourse.
4. Coffee, tea, cola, and alcoholic beverages are urinary tract irritants.

**TEST-TAKING HINT:** The test taker might jump to option "3" as the correct answer if the test taker did not read the word "preceding."

**44.** 1. A pregnant client diagnosed with a UTI will be admitted for aggressive IV antibiotic therapy to decrease the risk of preterm labor and delivery, septic shock, and other complications. After symptoms subside, the client will be sent home to complete the course of treatment with oral medications.
2. The nurse cannot "force" a client to drink, and forcing fluids could result in nausea and vomiting, not prevent it.
3. The client may or may not be dehydrated.
4. Pregnant clients have a right to be concerned about taking medications, but most are comfortable taking medications prescribed by the obstetrician.

**TEST-TAKING HINT:** In option "2" the nurse is "forcing" a client to do something, which should be eliminated as a possible correct answer. Option "4" is a broad generalization about "all" pregnant clients and should be discarded as a possible correct answer.

**45.** 1. The function of the urinary tract is to process fluids and wastes from the body. Limiting its functioning will increase the problem, not help the problem.
2. A routine urine specimen is not a clean voided specimen and cannot be used for culture.
3. The client should be taught to take all the prescribed medication anytime a prescription is written for antibiotics.
4. The client should be taught to void every 2 to 3 hours and to empty the bladder completely. This prevents overdistension of the bladder wall and resulting compromised blood supply, either of which predisposes the client to develop a UTI.

**TEST-TAKING HINT:** Unless contraindicated by a disease process, it is recommended for all clients to drink six to eight glasses of water each day; therefore, option "1" should be eliminated as a possible correct answer. Option "2" has the adjective "routine," which could be eliminated because routine procedures are usually not implemented when the client is ill.

**46.** 1. Blood pressure within normal limits is a short-term goal.
2. Lack of protein in the urine is a short-term goal.
3. A long-term complication of glomerulonephritis is that it can become chronic if unresponsive to treatment, and this can lead to end-stage renal disease. Maintaining renal function is an appropriate long-term goal.
4. Clear lung sounds indicate the client has been able to process fluids and excrete them from the body. Preventing pulmonary edema is a short-term goal.

**TEST-TAKING HINT:** Answer options "1," "2," and "4" all refer to body processes controlled or treated immediately after assessment of the problem. The stem is requesting a long-term goal.

**47.** 1. Normal BUN levels are 8 to 21 mg/dL or 10 to 31 mg/dL for clients older than age 90 years (Van Leeuwen & Bladh, 2017).
2. Normal creatinine levels are male: 0.61 to 1.2 mg/dL, and Female: 0.51 to 1.11 mg/dL (Van Leeuwen & Bladh, 2017).

3. Glomerular filtration rate (GFR) in a normally functioning kidney is over 60 mL/min/1.73 m². If the GFR is decreased below 60 mL/min, it may indicate kidney disease. A GFR of 15 or lower may mean kidney failure (National Institute of Diabetes and Digestive and Kidney Diseases, n.d.).

4. Normal creatinine clearance is 85 to 125 mL/min/1.73 m² for males and 75 to 115 mL/min/1.73 m² for females (Van Leeuwen & Bladh, 2017).

**TEST-TAKING HINT: The nurse must memorize common laboratory values. BUN and creatinine levels are common laboratory values used to determine status in a number of diseases.**

48. 1. Antibiotics may indirectly treat bladder spasms if the spasms are caused by an infection, but this is not the reason for prescribing trimethoprim-sulfamethoxazole (Bactrim), a sulfa antibiotic, in this manner.

2. **Some clients develop a chronic infection and must receive antibiotic therapy as a routine daily medication to suppress bacterial growth. The prescription for trimethoprim-sulfamethoxazole (Bactrim), a sulfa antibiotic, will be refilled after the 90 days and continued.**

3. Clients with chronic infections may never be free of the bacteria.

4. HCPs do not usually prescribe prn prescriptions for antibiotics.

**TEST-TAKING HINT: The question is asking why an HCP prescribes long-term use of antibiotics for a client diagnosed with a chronic infection. Antibiotics treat bacterial infections. Based on this, option "1" can be eliminated. Option "3" promises "all," which is false reassurance and can be eliminated. Option "4" describes future infections, but the client currently has an infection, so this option can be eliminated.**

## Benign Prostatic Hypertrophy (BPH)

49. 800 mL.
First, determine the amount of irrigation fluid:

$$3,000 - 1,800 = 1,200 \text{ mL of irrigation fluid}$$

Then, subtract 1,200 mL of irrigation fluid from the drainage of 2,000 mL to determine the urine output:

$$2,000 - 1,200 = 800 \text{ mL of urine output}$$

**TEST-TAKING HINT: The test taker should use the drop-down calculator for the NCLEX-RN® examination.**

50. 1. **The indwelling catheter should not be removed because doing so may result in edema, which, in turn, may obstruct the urethra and not allow the client to urinate.**

2. Increasing the irrigation fluid will flush out the clots and blood.

3. Protamine is the reversal agent for heparin, an anticoagulant.

4. Vitamin K is the reversal agent for the anticoagulant warfarin (Coumadin).

**TEST-TAKING HINT: The test taker should eliminate options "3" and "4" because both are medications, and the problem is with continuous irrigation, which does not require medications.**

51. Correct answers are 2, 4, and 5.
1. Terminal dribbling is a symptom of BPH.

2. **Urinary frequency is a sign of an acute or a chronic bacterial prostatitis or a UTI.**

3. Stress incontinence occurs in women urinating when coughing, running, or jumping.

4. **Clients diagnosed with acute bacterial prostatitis will frequently experience a sudden onset of fever and chills. Clients diagnosed with chronic prostatitis have milder symptoms.**

5. **Pelvic pain is present in acute bacterial prostatitis. Pelvic pain may be present in chronic prostatitis, but the client will not appear acutely ill (Davis & Silberman, 2019).**

**TEST-TAKING HINT: The words "acute" and "bacterial" should cue the test taker into the specific clinical manifestations of infection. Symptoms for any infection are fever and chills. Urinary frequency and pelvic pain are signs of both acute and chronic prostatitis.**

52. Correct answers are 1 and 5.
1. **The client should sit in a warm sitz bath for 10 to 20 minutes several times each day to provide comfort and assist with healing.**

2. Clients should avoid sitting for extended periods because it increases the pressure.

3. Oral fluids should be consumed to satisfy thirst but not to push fluids to dilute the medication levels in the bladder.

4. Broad-spectrum antibiotics are administered for 10 to 14 days and should not be stopped until all medications are taken by the client.
5. Nonsteroidal anti-inflammatory medications such as ibuprofen or naproxen can relieve pain (Society of Urologic Nurses and Associates, 2013).

**TEST-TAKING HINT:** The test taker must know basic concepts when answering questions; this includes the need for the client to take all prescribed antibiotics. If the test taker is unsure of option "3," drinking plenty of tea and coffee should indicate this is an incorrect answer because these are high in caffeine.

53. 1. TURPs can cause sexual dysfunction, but if there were a sexual dysfunction, it is not a priority over a physiological problem such as hemorrhaging.
    2. This is not a life-threatening problem.
    3. This client has had this problem preoperatively.
    4. This is a potentially life-threatening problem.

**TEST-TAKING HINT:** A basic concept the test taker must know is, for most surgeries, the highest priority problem is hemorrhaging. Hemorrhaging is life-threatening.

54. 1. This indicates the teaching is effective.
    2. Clients do not need to take finasteride (Proscar) postoperatively.
    3. There is no reason to restrict the client's fluid intake.
    4. Pain medication should be taken as needed.

**TEST-TAKING HINT:** If the test taker is not sure of the correct answer, selecting an option addressing notifying an HCP is usually an appropriate choice.

55. 1. This intervention requires analysis and should not be delegated.
    2. Elevating the scrotum on a towel for support is a task that can be delegated to the UAP.
    3. The surgeon changes the first dressing; therefore, this cannot be delegated. A TURP does not have a dressing.
    4. The RN is responsible for teaching.

**TEST-TAKING HINT:** Teaching, assessing, evaluating, and intervening for unstable clients cannot be delegated to a UAP.

56. 1. The nurse should not call a surgeon until all assessment is completed.
    2. Pain medication should not be administered until the cause of the problem is determined and all complications are ruled out.

3. Telling a client that what he is experiencing is expected without assessing the situation is dangerous.
4. The nurse should always assess any report before dismissing it as a commonly occurring problem.

**TEST-TAKING HINT:** When the question requires the test taker to decide which intervention should be first, assessment is usually first. If the test taker has no idea which intervention is correct, the test taker should choose assessment.

57. 1. The client wants information, and the nurse should provide facts.
    2. The client wants information, and the nurse should provide facts.
    3. Usually, this is the length of time clients need to wait before having sexual intercourse; this is the information the client wants to know.
    4. The client may need to talk with his surgeon, but it should be after the nurse answers the client's question.

**TEST-TAKING HINT:** The client is asking for factual information, and the nurse should provide this information. Options "1" and "2" are therapeutic responses addressing feelings, and option "4" is passing the buck—the nurse can discuss this with the client.

58. 1. An elevated PSA can be from urinary retention, BPH, prostate cancer, or prostate infarct.
    2. An elevated PSA does not indicate only prostate cancer.
    3. PSA does not diagnose testicular cancer.
    4. An elevated PSA and digital examination are used in combination to diagnose BPH or prostate cancer.

**TEST-TAKING HINT:** Answer options "2" and "4" have the word "only"; an absolute word should cause the test taker to eliminate them as possible answers. Options with words such as "always," "never," and "only" are usually incorrect.

59. Correct answers are 1, 3, and 4.
    1. The nurse should assess the drain postoperatively.
    2. The client is hemorrhaging, so the nurse should increase the irrigation fluid to clear the red urine, not decrease the rate.
    3. The head of the bed should be lowered, and the foot should be elevated to shunt blood to the central circulating system.

4. The surgeon needs to be notified of the change in condition.
5. These laboratory values assess kidney function, not the circulatory system, so this is not an appropriate intervention.

**TEST-TAKING HINT:** When the test taker reads vital signs with the blood pressure decreased and the pulse and respiratory rate elevated, the test taker should recognize the clinical manifestations of shock. (Normal vital signs obtained from Teas et al., 2018.)

60. 1. Using the maximum amount of medication does not indicate the client is achieving pain management.
2. Bladder spasms are common, but since the spasms are relieved with medication, this indicates the condition is improving.
3. Scrotal edema and tenderness do not indicate improvement.
4. Clients are administered laxatives or stool softeners to prevent constipation, which could cause increased pressure.

**TEST-TAKING HINT:** The stem asks which option indicates the client is improving. Needing maximum medication (option "1") and scrotal edema (option "3") do not indicate the client is getting better. A bowel movement has nothing to do with the prostate.

## Renal Calculi

61. 1. This is appropriate for the client with uric acid stones.
2. The nurse should recommend drinking one to two glasses of water at night to prevent the concentration of urine during sleep.
3. Dietary changes for preventing renal stones include reducing the intake of the primary substance forming the calculi. In this case, limiting vitamin D will inhibit the absorption of calcium from the gastrointestinal tract.
4. This is a treatment for an existing renal stone, not a discharge teaching intervention after successfully passing a renal calculus.

**TEST-TAKING HINT:** The test taker should remember to read the question carefully. The question asks for a "discharge teaching" intervention. This rules out option "4," which is a treatment, as a potential answer.

62. 1. The client's urinary output should be monitored, but it is not the first nursing intervention.
2. Assessment is the first part of the nursing process and is a priority. The renal colic pain can be so intense it can cause a vasovagal response, with resulting hypotension and syncope.
3. Increased fluid increases urinary output, which will facilitate the movement of the renal stone through the ureter and help decrease pain, but it is not the first intervention.
4. Ambulation will help facilitate the movement of the renal stone through the ureter, and safety is important, but it is not the first intervention.

**TEST-TAKING HINT:** Remember, if the question asks which intervention is first, all four options may be appropriate for the client's diagnosis, but only one has priority. Assessment is the first part of the nursing process and it is the first intervention a nurse should implement if the client is not in distress.

63. 1. An ultrasound does not require the administration of contrast dye.
2. Food, fluids, and ordered medication are not restricted before this test.
3. This is not an invasive procedure, so a signed consent is not required.
4. No special preparation is needed for this noninvasive, nonpainful test. A conductive gel is applied to the back or flank and then a transducer is applied, which produces sound waves, resulting in a picture.

**TEST-TAKING HINT:** The nurse must be aware of preprocedure and postprocedure teaching and care. The test taker must know the invasive and noninvasive diagnostic tests in general. Ultrasound, computed tomography (CT), and magnetic resonance imaging (MRI) are a few of the noninvasive diagnostic tests.

64. 1. Dull flank pain and microscopic hematuria are manifestations of a renal stone in the kidney.
2. The severe flank pain associated with a stone in the ureter often causes a sympathetic response with associated nausea; vomiting; pallor; and cool, clammy skin.
3. Gross hematuria and suprapubic pain when voiding are manifestations of a stone in the bladder.

4. Kidney stones and bladder stones may produce no clinical manifestations, but a ureteral stone always causes pain on the affected side because a ureteral spasm occurs when the stone obstructs the ureter.

**TEST-TAKING HINT: Options "1" and "3" both have assessment data indicating bleeding. The test taker can usually eliminate these as possible answers or eliminate the other two options not addressing blood. Renal stones are painful; therefore, option "4" could be eliminated as a possible answer.**

65. Correct answers are 1, 2, and 3.
    1. The HCP may order certain foods and medications when obtaining a 24-hour urine collection to evaluate for calcium oxalate or uric acid.
    2. When the collection begins, the client should completely empty the bladder and discard this urine. The test is started after the bladder is empty.
    3. All urine for 24 hours should be saved and put in a container with preservative, refrigerated, or placed on ice as indicated. Not following specific instructions will result in an inaccurate test result.
    4. The urine is obtained in some type of urine collection device such as a bedpan, bedside commode, or commode hat. The client is not catheterized.
    5. The RN can delegate placing the urine output in the proper container to the UAP; therefore, the UAP does not need to notify the nurse when the client urinates.

**TEST-TAKING HINT: This is an alternate-type question that has more than one correct answer. The test taker must have knowledge of specific laboratory tests.**

66. 1. The client's fluid volume is increased, and there is usually not a fluid volume loss.
    2. Knowledge deficit is important to help prevent future renal calculi, but this is not a priority when the client is in pain, which will occur with an acute episode.
    3. Impaired urinary elimination may occur, but it is not a priority for the client diagnosed with an acute episode of calculi.
    4. Pain is the priority. The pain can be so severe a sympathetic response may occur, causing nausea; vomiting; pallor; and cool, clammy skin.

**TEST-TAKING HINT: Remember Maslow's hierarchy of needs: airway and pain are a priority. No option mentions possible airway problems, so pain is the priority.**

67. 1. The urine must be assessed for bleeding and cloudiness. Initially, the urine is bright red, but the color soon diminishes and cloudiness may indicate an infection. This assessment should not be delegated to a UAP.
    2. Teaching cannot be delegated to a UAP. The RN should teach and evaluate the effectiveness of the teaching.
    3. **The UAP could assist the client to the car once the discharge has been completed.**
    4. The kidney is highly vascular. Hemorrhaging and resulting shock are potential complications of lithotripsy, so the nurse should not delegate vital signs postprocedure.

**TEST-TAKING HINT: There are some basic rules about delegation: the nurse cannot delegate assessment, teaching, evaluation, or any task requiring judgment.**

68. 1. **An increased fluid intake ensuring 2 to 3 L of urine a day prevents the stone-forming salts from becoming concentrated enough to precipitate.**
    2. Cocoa and chocolate are high in calcium and should be avoided or the amount should be decreased to help prevent the formation of calcium phosphate renal stones.
    3. Physical activity prevents bone absorption and possible hypercalciuria; therefore, the nurse should instruct the client to walk daily to help retain calcium in bone.
    4. The renal calculi are caused by calcium; therefore, the client should not increase calcium intake.

**TEST-TAKING HINT: This is a urinary problem and fluid is a priority. Therefore, the test taker should select an option addressing fluid, and there is only one option addressing oral intake.**

69. 1. Assessment is important, but the neurological system is not the priority for a client diagnosed with a urinary problem.
    2. **Passing a renal stone may negate the need for the client to have lithotripsy or a surgical procedure. Therefore, all urine must be strained, and a stone, if found, should be sent to the laboratory to determine what caused the stone.**
    3. These are laboratory studies evaluating kidney function, but they are not pertinent when passing a renal stone. These values do not elevate until at least half the kidney function is lost.

4. A dietary recall can be done to determine what types of foods the client is eating that may contribute to the stone formation, but it is not the most important intervention.

**TEST-TAKING HINT: Remember, if the question asks for "most important," more than one of the options could be appropriate, but only one is most important. Assessment is a priority if the client is not in distress, but the test taker should make sure it is appropriate for the situation.**

70. 1. The client needs to be evaluated for a possible UTI, which may accompany renal calculi. Therefore, the clinic nurse should not give advice without knowing what is wrong with the client.
    2. The nurse should not recommend any medication, even acetaminophen (Tylenol), unless the nurse is absolutely sure what is wrong with the client.
    3. A urinalysis can assess for hematuria, the presence of WBCs, crystal fragments, or all three, which can determine if the client has a urinary tract infection or possibly a renal stone, with accompanying clinical manifestations of UTI.
    4. The client needs to strain the urine if there is a possibility of renal calculi, which these clinical manifestations do not support. Further diagnostic testing is needed to determine the presence of renal calculi.

**TEST-TAKING HINT: Fever, chills, and burning on urination require some type of assessment. Therefore, the test taker should select an option that helps determine what is wrong with the client and "3" is the only such option.**

71. 1. This potassium level is within normal limits, 3.5 to 5.3 mEq/L.
    2. Hematuria is not uncommon after the removal of a kidney stone.
    3. A normal creatinine level is a male: 0.61 to 1.21 mg/dL, female: 0.51 to 1.11 mg/dL.
    4. The white blood cell count is elevated; normal is 4.5 to $11.1 \times 10^3$/microL.

**TEST-TAKING HINT: The nurse must know normal laboratory data and be able to apply the normal and abnormal results to specific diseases and disorders.**

72. 1. Beer and colas are foods high in oxalate, which can cause calcium oxalate stones.
    2. Asparagus and cabbage are foods high in oxalate, which can cause calcium oxalate stones.

3. Venison, sardines, goose, organ meats, and herring are high-purine foods, which should be eliminated from the diet to help prevent uric acid stones.
4. Cheese and eggs are foods that help acidify the urine and do not cause the development of uric acid stones.

**TEST-TAKING HINT: The nurse has to have knowledge of foods included in specific diets. This is memorizing, but the test taker must have this knowledge to answer questions evaluating types of diets for specific diseases and disorders.**

## Cancer of the Bladder

73. 1. This client does not need to be assessed first. A unit secretary can call the department and check on the glasses.
    2. A moderate amount of serous drainage is expected after surgery. *Serous* drainage is a pale yellow body fluid. *Sanguineous* is the term used to describe bloody drainage.
    3. The nurse is not responsible for informing the client about operative procedures. The surgeon should be notified to see this client and provide the explanation.
    4. An ileal conduit is a procedure diverting urine from the bladder and provides an alternate cutaneous pathway for urine to exit the body. Urinary output should always be at least 30 mL/hr. This client should be assessed to make sure the stents placed in the ureters have not become dislodged or blocked.

**TEST-TAKING HINT: Basic care of any postoperative client is to ensure urinary output. Two of the options involve tasks that can be delegated or are not in the realm of the nurse.**

74. 1. The client has already been exposed; this cannot be undone.
    2. Pelvic radiation is prescribed for cancer in the abdomen. It is a life-saving procedure, but one of the risks of radiation therapy is the development of a secondary cancer.
    3. Cigarette smoke contains more than 400 chemicals, 17 of which are known to cause cancer. The risk is directly proportional to the amount of smoking.
    4. Clients may be unaware of a parasitic infection of the bladder for some time before diagnosis, but it is not a risk factor for cancer of the bladder.

**TEST-TAKING HINT: The question asks for a modifiable risk factor. Modifiable factors involve lifestyle changes, weight loss, tobacco use, and eating habits.**

75. 1. Any client undergoing general anesthesia should be taught to turn, cough, and deep breathe to prevent pulmonary complications. This is not specific to a urinary diversion procedure.
    2. A urinary diversion procedure involves the removal of the bladder. In a cutaneous procedure, the ureters are implanted in some way to allow for stoma formation on the abdominal wall, and the urine drains into a pouch. There are numerous methods used for creating the stoma.
    3. Many clients with multiple types of procedures use PCA pumps to control pain after surgery.
    4. This should be done for any client expected to need intensive care postoperatively.

**TEST-TAKING HINT:** The test taker must notice the phrase "specific to the procedure" to be able to answer this question correctly. All of the options are standard interventions for major surgeries, but only one is specific to the procedure.

76. Correct answers are 1, 2, and 5.
    1. The client should restrict fluid intake, caffeinated beverages, and the use of diuretics 4 hours prior to the procedure.
    2. The client will need to avoid emptying the bladder for 1 to 2 hours after the procedure.
    3. The advantage of administering chemotherapy intravesically is that the systemic side effects of bone marrow suppression are avoided. Filgrastim (Neupogen), a biologic response modifier, is used to stimulate the production of WBCs, so a client is not at risk for developing an infection and is not necessary.
    4. The procedure is not painful, so acetaminophen (Tylenol), an analgesic, is not needed. The client may use acetaminophen or ibuprofen for postprocedure body aches or fever.
    5. After the procedure, for the first void and the next 6 hours, the client should sit to avoid urine splashing, avoid public toilets or urinating outside, and should be taught the use of bleach to clean the toilet after voiding at home (American Urological Association, 2019).

**TEST-TAKING HINT:** If the test taker is not aware of the term "intravesical," then dividing the word into its components may be useful. *Intra-* means "into" and *vesical* means "bladder." The test taker should choose options that have a direct effect on urine production and elimination.

77. 1. Urine is acidic, and the abdominal wall tissue is not designed to tolerate acidic environments. The stoma is pouched so the urine will not touch the skin.
    2. Urinary diversion drainage bags are changed every 4 to 5 days so the skin can remain intact; the bags should be clean but not sterile.
    3. The urine will have a normal pH of all urine; it is not necessary to monitor the pH.
    4. The stoma should be assessed a minimum of every 2 hours initially, then every 4 hours.

**TEST-TAKING HINT:** The test taker should look at time frames—daily and weekly. If the time frame is not sufficient, then the option can be eliminated as a possible correct answer.

78. 1. Assessment cannot be assigned to an LPN, no matter how knowledgeable the LPN.
    2. This client has the laboratory clinical manifestations of infection; therefore, the nurse should assess and care for this client.
    3. Antineoplastic medication is administered only by a qualified RN.
    4. It is in the scope of practice for the LPN to care for this client.

**TEST-TAKING HINT:** The client least ill or having the least invasive procedure should be the client assigned to the LPN.

79. 1. This is therapeutic communication and is allowing the client autonomy, but it is not an example of paternalism.
    2. Paternalism is deciding for the client what is best, similar to a parent making decisions for a child. Feeding a client, as with a feeding tube, without the client wishing to eat is paternalism.
    3. Consulting with a dietitian about the nutritional needs of a client is an appropriate nursing intervention, but it does not represent any ethical principle.
    4. This is an excellent intervention, but it does not represent any ethical principle.

**TEST-TAKING HINT:** The question asks for an ethical principle, and only two of the options could be considered to represent ethical principles. Option "1" is allowing the client a voice in the situation; the term "paternalism" eliminates this option.

80. 1. This is advising the client, a nontherapeutic technique.
    2. This statement does not address the client's feelings.
    3. **This is an example of restating, a therapeutic technique used to clarify the client's feelings and encourage a discussion of those feelings.**
    4. The stem did not say the client was dying. The stem said the client feels too young to die. A conversation to discuss the client's death with the children may be premature.

**TEST-TAKING HINT: When the question requires a therapeutic response, the test taker should select an option addressing the client's feelings.**

81. 1. A continent urinary diversion is a surgical procedure in which a reservoir is created to hold urine until the client can self-catheterize the stoma. The nurse should observe the client's technique before discharge.
    2. The purpose of creating a continent diversion is so the client will not need a pouch.
    3. Clients with cutaneous diversions that drain constantly use a bedside drainage bag at night, not those with continent diversions.
    4. The client should be taught to notify the HCP if the temperature is 100°F or greater.

**TEST-TAKING HINT: Options "2" and "3" are related to continuous drainage and could be eliminated on this basis. The word "continent" in the stem should key the test taker to the fact this diversion is a procedure in which there is no continuous drainage of urine.**

82. 1. Vinegar will act as a deodorizing agent in the pouch and help prevent a strong urine smell.
    2. **The stoma should be pink and moist at all times. A dusky color indicates a compromised blood supply to the stoma, and the HCP should be notified immediately.**

3. There will be mucus in the urine because of the tissue used to create the diversion, but large clumps of mucus could occlude the stoma or ureters.
    4. Urinary drainage should be a pale yellow to amber color. The procedure does not change the color of the urine.

**TEST-TAKING HINT: A dusky color is never normal when discussing body functioning. There are very few procedures for which bloody urine is a normal expectation.**

83. 1. A report of a "3" on a 1-to-10 pain scale is expected after medication and does not warrant notifying the HCP.
    2. Pain on coughing and deep breathing after surgery is expected.
    3. This indicates the client is able to ambulate and is doing activities needed to recover.
    4. **The client is drawn up in a position that relieves pressure off the abdomen; a rigid abdomen is an indicator of peritonitis, a medical emergency.**

**TEST-TAKING HINT: When the test taker is deciding on a priority question, the test taker should decide if the situation is expected or if it is life-threatening.**

84. 1. **This client is asking for information and should be provided with factual information. The surgery will not make the client sterile, but chemotherapy can induce menopause and radiation therapy to the pelvis can render a client sterile.**
    2. This is a therapeutic response, but the client asked for information.
    3. This is a false statement and lying to the client.
    4. This is outside the realm of a chaplain.

**TEST-TAKING HINT: When the stem has the client asking for specific information, then the nurse should provide the correct information. It is easy to confuse these questions with ones requiring therapeutic responses.**

85. 1. This client has an elevated WBC, but it only informs the nurse that an infection may be present in the body. It is not diagnostic for a UTI.
    2. Cloudy urine may indicate a UTI, but the culture is definitive. Cloudy urine may contain protein, WBCs, RBCs, bacteria, or noncellular casts.
    3. **The urine culture has identified an infectious organism. This is the diagnostic test for a UTI.**
    4. Twenty-four-hour urine specimens for metanephrines indicate the presence of other diseases but not a UTI. Mild increases in catecholamines in urine can be caused by stress, such as operations, burns, or childbirth. A marked increase in metanephrines indicates a pheochromocytoma (a hereditary tumor on the adrenal medulla or from certain neuroblastomas).

**TEST-TAKING HINT: The test taker must pay attention to specific words. "Diagnostic" means a test that specifically indicates, without a doubt, the cause of the disease process.**

86. Correct answers are 2, 3, and 5.
    1. The current diet should be one that limits the complications of CKD; it is current, not an antecedent.
    2. Diabetes is a leading cause of CKD caused by the microvascular changes that occur when the blood glucose levels are high.
    3. Hypertension is also a leading cause of CKD because hypertension narrows the renal artery and decreases the blood flow to the kidney.
    4. Fluid restriction is a recommended treatment for CKD, not an antecedent.
    5. Race is an antecedent because genetics are a risk factor for CKD. Non-whites are more at risk for developing CKD, especially when the client has a comorbid condition such as diabetes or hypertension.

**TEST-TAKING HINT: When answering a "Select all that apply" question, the test taker must look at each option independently of the other options. Each option becomes a true or false question. The NCLEX-RN® can test several diseases or concepts in any multiple-choice question, but this is especially true of "Select all that apply" questions.**

87. 1. The nurse taking vital signs and documenting them will not prevent AKI because an action is not initiated that will directly affect the client's health status because of the results of the data. The nurse must always initiate an intervention based on abnormal data assessed.
    2. Assessing the client's dressing will allow the nurse to be aware of bleeding but does not prevent AKI.
    3. The urinary output is checked to ensure the kidneys are being perfused, but there is no action that will maintain the perfusion in this option.
    4. **Maintaining the client's blood pressure to greater than 100/60 ensures perfusion of the kidneys. AKI occurs when the kidneys have not been adequately perfused. Vasopressor drips are used to maintain BP.**

**TEST-TAKING HINT: The test taker must be aware of the purpose behind medications and the results of inadequate administration of certain critical medications.**

88. 1. The client had a small emesis 24 hours ago, which has not been repeated; this is not pertinent information at this time.
    2. Whether or not IV fluids are indicated depends on more than the oral intake. The recommendation to discontinue the IV fluids might be indicated because the client is not able to process all the fluid.
    3. **The client has a deficit output of almost 5,500 mL. This should be brought to the HCP's attention to determine if renal insufficiency is present.**
    4. Clients are frequently requested to do things that give the health-care personnel information to assess what is occurring with the client. It is not necessary for the client to "like" saving the urine.

**TEST-TAKING HINT: The test taker must be able to read and interpret information from graphs to determine important information to report.**

89. Correct answers are 1, 2, and 4.
    1. These are called the pre- and post-weights. The pre-weight is used to determine the amount of fluid to be removed during the treatment, and the post-weight is used to determine if the goal was met.

2. Clients experiencing renal failure are not processing the fluids in their bodies. Fluid restrictions are prescribed to allow for some fluid so the client does not become dehydrated but limited so the heart is not overtaxed, causing the client to go into heart failure.

3. Potato chips and pretzels are high in sodium content and could increase a problem with fluid retention.

4. The client's entire blood supply is being removed from the body and then returned after being filtered. The client could bleed to death in a matter of minutes if the access becomes dislodged.

5. Most clients develop a routine of resting during the treatments. The nurse should not keep the client from being able to rest, read, or watch television.

**TEST-TAKING HINT:** This is an alternative format question requiring the test taker to identify each intervention performed by the nurse during hemodialysis. The test taker should be familiar with the basic steps of the dialysis process.

90. 1. Clients diagnosed with renal failure are frequently placed on a diuretic such as furosemide (Lasix). The potassium level is WNL. The nurse would not question administering this medication.

2. Erythropoietin (Epogen) is frequently prescribed for the anemia associated with renal failure; however, this is an incomplete order because no dosage is prescribed. The nurse should contact the HCP to determine the dose to be administered. The dose is determined by units/kilogram/dose.

3. The nurse would not question administering this medication. The client should receive the multivitamin, and iron will assist in the production of red blood cells.

4. The nurse would not question administering levothyroxine (Synthroid). Nothing in the question would lead the nurse to think that the order was incorrect.

**TEST-TAKING HINT:** The test taker and nurse should always remember the five rights of medication administration. An incomplete medication order cannot be implemented until all the requirements of the order are present.

91. Correct answers are 1, 2, 4, and 5.
1. A female client should be taught to wipe the meatus and vaginal area from front to back to avoid contaminating the urethra (urinary orifice) with fecal matter.

2. Cranberry juice is acidic and changes the pH of the urine, making the environment less conducive to bacterial growth.

3. Incontinence is not expected for a client diagnosed with a UTI.

4. The client should be taught about the clinical manifestations of a UTI so she can know when to notify the HCP.

5. The client should increase the intake of water to at least 2000 mL/24 hours in order to flush the bacteria from the urinary system.

6. Sitting in a tub of water increases the risk of bacteria entering the urethra.

**TEST-TAKING HINT:** The test taker must remember basic nursing care. Several options are basic nursing interventions.

92. 1. This meal has a small portion of protein and does not contain sodium if the client does not add salt.

2. Ham and sour cream are high in sodium content, and 12 ounces of protein is too much for the client.

3. Double burger patties are too much protein, and cheese is high in sodium.

4. Potato chips are high in sodium, and the roast beef could be too much protein.

**TEST-TAKING HINT:** Dietary menus and questions are some of the least favorites of many test takers. Basic rules include, if a choice exists between grilled or fried foods, choose grilled, between chicken or beef, choose chicken. Fresh vegetables are usually better than canned or frozen.

93. 1. Before the other options are performed, the nurse should have a urine culture specimen sent to the laboratory for culture. A culture is indicated from the symptoms.

2. The IV catheter will be required before being able to initiate the antibiotic, but getting the urine culture is first.

3. The urine culture is first.

4. The urine culture is first so that treatment can be initiated.

**TEST-TAKING HINT:** Basic nursing principles are applied in test questions, such as the results of cultures will be skewed if the sample is collected after antibiotics have been initiated.

**94.** 1. The HCP should be notified, but this delay could cost the client's life; this client is in septic shock.
2. The IVPB will not treat the client as quickly as increasing the IV fluids. This would be the second action to be performed by the nurse.
3. This is not the time to check the EHR for information; it is the time for action.
4. This is septic shock and not fluid volume shock, but the circulatory system is still compromised. Increasing the fluid volume will support the client's BP until the IVPB is infused.

**TEST-TAKING HINT:** The test taker must remember: "If in stress, do not assess; do something that will treat the client."

**95.** Correct answers are 1, 2, and 6.
1. The balance of fluids and electrolytes is regulated by the kidneys.
2. Hematologic regulation is an interrelated concept because the client on dialysis does not have a functioning kidney to produce erythropoietin to stimulate the bone marrow to produce red blood cells. In addition, removal of the entire circulating blood three times a week through the dialysis machine places stress on the red blood cells, and they do not last as long as in a nondialyzed body.
3. The CKD client does not have an issue with digestion unless there is a comorbid condition that involves a lack of mobility.
4. The CKD client does not have an issue with metabolism unless there is a comorbid condition that involves a lack of mobility.
5. The CKD client does not have an issue with mobility unless there is a comorbid condition that involves a lack of mobility.
6. Nutrition is an issue because the client must adhere to a restricted diet to decrease the number of toxic metabolites not being eliminated through the kidneys.

**TEST-TAKING HINT:** The test taker must remember the entire client when determining the client's needs and problems, including knowing the pathology of the disease process and how it affects other systems in the body.

**96.** 1. The urine output would not be affected by laboratory results.
2. The blood glucose is higher than normal but would not require the RN to notify the HCP. The HCP can note the level during rounds. The UAP does not need to collect a blood glucose reading.
3. The potassium level is at a critical level. Low potassium levels impact the cardiac rhythm by causing a dysrhythmia. The nurse should assess the telemetry reading to determine if this is occurring.
4. At this time, the RRT is not needed.

**TEST-TAKING HINT:** The test taker must be able to read and interpret laboratory results.

# GENITOURINARY DISORDERS COMPREHENSIVE EXAMINATION

1. The older client being seen in the clinic reports urinary frequency, urgency, and "leaking." Which **priority intervention** should the nurse implement when interviewing the client?
   1. Ensure communication is nonjudgmental and respectful.
   2. Set the temperature for comfort in the examination room.
   3. Speak loudly to ensure the client understands the nurse.
   4. Ensure the examining room has adequate lighting.

2. The client is experiencing urinary incontinence. Which intervention should the nurse implement?
   1. Teach the client to drink prune juice weekly.
   2. Encourage the client to eat a high-fiber diet.
   3. Discuss the need to urinate every 6 hours.
   4. Explain the importance of wearing cotton underwear.

3. Which information indicates to the nurse the client teaching about the treatment of urinary incontinence has been **effective**?
   1. The client prepares a scheduled voiding plan.
   2. The client verbalizes the need to increase fluid intake.
   3. The client explains how to perform pelvic floor exercises.
   4. The client attempts to retain the vaginal cone in place the entire day.

4. Which intervention should the RN implement **first** for the client having incontinence?
   1. Palpate the client's bladder to assess for urinary retention.
   2. Obtain a bedside commode for the client.
   3. Assist the client with changing the wet clothes.
   4. Request the UAP to change the client's linens.

5. The older client recovering from a prostatectomy has been experiencing stress incontinence. Which independent nursing intervention should the nurse discuss with the client?
   1. Establish a set voiding frequency of every 2 hours while awake.
   2. Encourage a family member to assist the client to the bathroom to void.
   3. Apply a transurethral electrical stimulator to relieve symptoms of urinary urgency.
   4. Discuss the use of a "bladder drill," including a timed voiding schedule.

6. The nurse is preparing the plan of care for the client diagnosed with a neurogenic flaccid bladder. Which expected outcome is **appropriate** for this client?
   1. The client has conscious control over bladder activity.
   2. The client's bladder does not become overdistended.
   3. The client has bladder sensation and no discomfort.
   4. The client demonstrates how to check for bladder distention.

7. Which nursing intervention is **most important** before attempting to catheterize a client?
   1. Determine the client's history of catheter use.
   2. Evaluate the level of anxiety of the client.
   3. Verify the client is not allergic to latex.
   4. Assess the client's sensation level and ability to void.

8. Which clients should the RN assign to a UAP working on a surgical floor? **Select all that apply.**
   1. The client with a suprapubic catheter inserted yesterday.
   2. The client with an indwelling catheter for the past week.
   3. The client on a bladder-training regimen.
   4. The client being discharged after catheter removal this morning.
   5. The client with frequent urinary incontinence.

9. The nurse is caring for an older client with an indwelling catheter. Which data **warrant further** investigation?
   1. The client's temperature is 98°F.
   2. The client has become confused and irritable.
   3. The client's urine is clear and light yellow.
   4. The client feels the need to urinate.

10. The RN is observing the UAP providing direct care to a client with an indwelling catheter. Which data **warrant immediate** intervention by the nurse?
    1. The UAP secures the tubing to the client's leg with tape.
    2. The UAP provides catheter care with the client's bath.
    3. The UAP puts the collection bag on the client's bed.
    4. The UAP cares for the catheter after thorough hand washing.

11. Which intervention should the nurse implement when caring for the client with a nephrostomy tube?
    1. Change the dressing only if soiled by urine.
    2. Clean the end of the connecting tubing with povidone-iodine.
    3. Clean the drainage system every day with bleach and water.
    4. Assess the tube for kinks to prevent obstruction.

12. The client is 12 hours postoperative renal surgery. Which data **warrant immediate** intervention by the nurse?
    1. The abdomen is soft, nontender, and rounded.
    2. Pain is not felt with dorsal flexion of the foot.
    3. The urine output is 60 mL for the past 2 hours.
    4. The client's trough vancomycin level is 24 mcg/mL.

13. The nurse is teaching the female client diagnosed with urinary tract tuberculosis (UTTB) before discharge. Which information should the nurse include specific to this diagnosis?
    1. Instruct the client to take the medication with food.
    2. Explain condoms should be used for intercourse during treatment.
    3. Discuss the need for follow-up chest x-rays.
    4. Encourage a well-balanced diet and fluid intake.

14. The nurse is assessing a client diagnosed with urethral strictures. Which data support the diagnosis?
    1. Reports of frequency and urgency.
    2. Clear yellow drainage from the urethra.
    3. Reports of burning during urination.
    4. A diminished force and stream during voiding.

15. The nurse is providing discharge teaching to the client diagnosed with polycystic kidney disease. Which statement made by the client indicates the teaching has been **effective**?
    1. "I need to monitor my diet carefully to prevent complications."
    2. "I should avoid taking medications for high blood pressure."
    3. "When I urinate, there may be blood streaks in my urine."
    4. "I may have occasional burning when I urinate with this disease."

16. Which intervention should the nurse include when assessing the client for urinary retention? **Select all that apply.**
    1. Inquire if the client has the sensation of fullness.
    2. Percuss the suprapubic region for a dull sound.
    3. Scan the bladder with the ultrasound scanner.
    4. Palpate from the umbilicus to the suprapubic area.
    5. Auscultate the two lower abdominal quadrants.

17. The RN is discussing how to prioritize care with the UAP. Which client should the RN instruct the UAP to see **first**?
    1. The immobile client needing sequential compression devices removed.
    2. The older woman requiring assistance ambulating to the bathroom.
    3. The surgical client needing help changing the gown after bathing.
    4. The male client requiring the intravenous catheter be discontinued.

18. The nurse is caring for the client recovering from a percutaneous renal biopsy. Which data indicate the client **is complying** with client teaching?
    1. The client is lying flat in the supine position.
    2. The client continues oral fluids restriction while on bedrest.
    3. The client uses the bedside commode to urinate.
    4. The client refuses to ask for any pain medication.

19. Which intervention should the nurse implement for the client after an ileal conduit?
    1. Pouch the stoma with a 1-inch margin around the stoma.
    2. Refer the client to the United Ostomy Association for discharge teaching.
    3. Report to the HCP any decrease in urinary output.
    4. Monitor the stoma for clinical manifestations of infection every shift.

20. The nurse is preparing the plan of care for a client diagnosed with fluid volume deficit. Which interventions should the nurse include in the plan of care? **Select all that apply.**
    1. Monitor vital signs every 2 hours until stable.
    2. Measure the client's oral intake and urinary output daily.
    3. Administer mouth care when bathing the client.
    4. Weigh the client weekly in the same clothing at the same time.
    5. Assess skin turgor and mucous membranes every shift.

21. Which outcome should the nurse identify for the client diagnosed with fluid volume excess?
    1. The client will void a minimum of 30 mL per hour.
    2. The client will have elastic skin turgor.
    3. The client will have no adventitious breath sounds.
    4. The client will have a serum creatinine of 1.4 mg/dL.

22. The nurse is caring for a client diagnosed with possible nephrotic syndrome. Which intervention should be included in the plan of care?
    1. Monitor the urine for bright-red bleeding.
    2. Evaluate the calorie count of the 500-mg protein diet.
    3. Assess the client's sacrum for dependent edema.
    4. Monitor for a high serum albumin level.

23. The nurse is preparing a teaching care plan for the client diagnosed with nephrotic syndrome. Which intervention should the nurse include?
    1. Stop steroids if a moon face develops.
    2. Provide teaching for taking diuretics.
    3. Increase the intake of dietary sodium.
    4. Report a decrease in daily weight.

24. Which intervention is **most important** for the nurse to implement for the client with a left nephrectomy?
    1. Assess the intravenous fluids for rate and volume.
    2. Change the surgical dressing every day at the same time.
    3. Monitor the client's PT/PTT/INR level daily.
    4. Monitor the percentage of each meal eaten.

25. The nurse is preparing the discharge teaching plan for the male client with a left-sided nephrectomy. Which statement indicates the teaching is **effective**?
    1. "I can't wait to start back to work next week; I really need the money."
    2. "I will take my temperature, and if it is above 100.5°F, I will call my doctor."
    3. "I am glad I won't have to keep track of how much I urinate in the day."
    4. "I am happy I will be able eat what I usually eat; I don't like this food."

26. The client diagnosed with a fluid and electrolyte disturbance in the emergency department is exhibiting peaked T waves on the STAT electrocardiogram (EKG). Which interventions should the nurse implement? **Rank in order of priority.**
    1. Assess the client for leg and muscle cramps.
    2. Check the serum potassium level.
    3. Notify the health-care provider.
    4. Arrange for a transfer to the telemetry floor.
    5. Administer polystyrene sulfonate.

1. 1. Clients with urinary incontinence are often embarrassed, so it is the responsibility of the nurse to approach this subject with respect and consideration.
   2. The temperature of the room is not pertinent to the nurse interviewing the client.
   3. The nurse should not assume elderly clients have hearing difficulties. If the client is "hard of hearing," the nurse should speak clearly and concisely but should not shout.
   4. The lighting of the room is not pertinent to interviewing the client about incontinence.

2. 1. Prune juice is given to prevent constipation but should be taken daily, not weekly.
   2. Clients experiencing incontinence should eat a high-fiber diet to avoid constipation, which increases pressure on the bladder, which may increase incontinence.
   3. Bladder training is used to assist with urinary incontinence by voiding every 2 to 3 hours, not every 6 hours.
   4. Cotton underwear may help decrease UTIs but does not affect urinary incontinence.

3. 1. Scheduled voiding allows the client to void every 2 to 3 hours, and when the client has remained consistently dry, the interval is increased by about 15 minutes.
   2. The fluid intake should not be increased but should be adequate to prevent dehydration. The majority of the fluid should be drunk early in the day to prevent nocturia.
   3. Pelvic floor (Kegel) exercises should be performed two to three times daily, with repetitions of 10 to 30 each session, but this is recommended for stress incontinence, not urinary incontinence.
   4. A series of vaginal weights can be used to increase muscle tone. The time is usually only 15 minutes, not all day.

4. 1. The nurse may assess the bladder to determine if urine is being retained but not before changing the client's wet clothes.
   2. Having a bedside commode may or may not be helpful for the client with incontinence.
   3. The nurse should first assist the client in getting out of the wet clothes before any other action. Wet clothes are embarrassing to the client and can lead to skin breakdown.
   4. The client's linens need to be changed, but not before changing the client's wet clothes.

5. 1. Timed voiding is more helpful with neurogenic disorders, such as those related to diabetes.
   2. A prompted voiding is useful for a client without the cognitive ability to recognize the need.
   3. The use of transvaginal or transurethral electrical stimulation to stimulate the pelvic floor muscles to contract is a collaborative intervention.
   4. The use of the bladder-training drill is helpful in stress incontinence. The client is instructed to void at scheduled intervals. After consistently being dry, the interval is increased by 15 minutes until the client reaches an acceptable interval.

6. 1. In the neurogenic flaccid bladder, the client has lost the ability to recognize the need to void; therefore, this is not a realistic expected outcome.
   2. The treatment goal of the flaccid bladder is to prevent overdistention.
   3. The sensation has been lost as a result of a lower motor neuron problem; therefore, there is no sensation to maintain and no discomfort, so this is not a realistic goal.
   4. The client does not have to assess the bladder; this is a nursing intervention.

7. 1. To determine if the client has had a catheter in place previously assists with teaching and alleviating anxiety, but it is not the most important intervention.
   2. Assessing the level of anxiety is helpful in assisting the client but does not endanger the client; therefore, it is not the most important intervention.
   3. The nurse should always assess for allergies to latex before inserting a latex catheter or using a drainage system because, if the client is allergic to latex, use of it could cause a life-threatening reaction.
   4. There are many reasons the client is catheterized regardless of the sensation and ability to void. The nurse should not assess this until the catheter is removed.

8. **Correct answers are 2, 3, 4, and 5.**
   1. This client requires the most skill and knowledge because this client has the greatest potential for infection; therefore, the client should not be assigned to a UAP.
   2. **The UAP can care for a client with an indwelling catheter because adherence to standard precautions is the only requirement for safe client care.**
   3. **The UAP cannot teach bladder training but can implement the strategies for the client on a bladder-training program, such as taking the client to the bathroom at scheduled times.**
   4. **The UAP can care for this client because noting if the client voided after removal of the catheter is within the realm of the UAP's ability.**
   5. **The UAP can care for a client with urinary incontinence.**

9. 1. This temperature, 98°F, is within normal limits and does not require further investigation.
   2. **When an older client's mental status changes to confused and irritable, the nurse should seek the etiology, which may be a UTI secondary to an indwelling catheter. Older clients often do not present with classic clinical manifestations of infection.**
   3. The client's urine should be clear and light yellow; therefore, this does not warrant further investigation.
   4. The client often has a feeling of the need to void when having an indwelling catheter, but this comment does not warrant further intervention.

10. 1. The client's catheter should be secured on the leg to prevent manipulation, which increases the risk of a UTI. This action does not require intervention.
   2. The client with an indwelling catheter should receive catheter care with the bath and as needed.
   3. **The drainage bag should be kept below the level of the bladder to prevent the reflux of urine into the renal system; it should not be placed on the bed.**
   4. Hand hygiene is important before and after handling any portion of the drainage system.

11. 1. The dressing should be routinely changed as often as daily or weekly.
   2. When connecting the tubing to the drainage bag, both ends should be cleaned with alcohol, not povidone-iodine (Betadine).
   3. The drainage system can be cleaned daily with soap and water.
   4. **The nephrostomy tube should never be clamped or have kinks because an obstruction can cause pyelonephritis.**

12. 1. The client, after renal surgery, is at risk for paralytic ileus from the manipulation of the colon. A soft, rounded, and nontender abdomen does not require intervention.
   2. Pain felt with dorsal flexion of the foot indicates a deep vein thrombosis; therefore, an asymptomatic client does not require intervention.
   3. A minimum of 30 mL/hr does not require intervention by the nurse.
   4. **The client with restricted kidney function after surgery should be monitored for damage as a result of the use of aminoglycoside antibiotics, such as vancomycin, which are nephrotoxic. This level is high and warrants notifying the HCP.**

13. 1. Antitubercular medications (rifampin and INH) should be taken 1 hour before or 2 hours after a meal.
   2. **Clients diagnosed with tuberculosis of the renal tract should use condoms to prevent transmission of the mycobacterium. If the infection is located in the penis or urethra, abstaining from sexual activity is recommended.**
   3. Follow-up chest x-rays are important for the client diagnosed with tuberculosis of the lung.
   4. Maintaining a well-balanced diet and fluid intake is important for recovery from any illness and for a healthy lifestyle, but it is not specifically for this diagnosis.

14. 1. Frequency and urgency are clinical manifestations of a UTI.
   2. Clear yellow urethral drainage is urine.
   3. A report of burning during voiding is a clinical manifestation of UTI.
   4. **The client diagnosed with urethral strictures will report a decrease in force and stream during voiding. The stricture is treated by dilation using small filiform bougies.**

15. 1. Diet modification in clients diagnosed with polycystic kidney disease is important to prevent complications from eating foods high in protein, potassium, and phosphorus that are difficult for the kidney to excrete (Hoffman & Sullivan, 2020).
    2. Antihypertensive medications should be taken to protect the kidneys from further damage.
    3. Blood should always be reported to the HCP, and hematuria is a sign of polycystic kidney disease. Further evaluation is needed.
    4. Burning during urination should be treated to prevent further damage to the kidneys and renal system.

16. Correct answers are 1, 2, 3, and 4.
    1. **The nurse needs to assess the client's sensation of needing to void or feeling of fullness.**
    2. **A dull sound heard when percussing the bladder indicates it is filled with urine.**
    3. **A portable bladder scan is used to assess for the presence of urine rather than using a straight catheter.**
    4. **A distended bladder can be palpated.**
    5. Auscultation cannot assess the client's bladder.

17. 1. The client needing a sequential compression device removed is not urgent.
    2. **The older woman may have age-related changes (decreased bladder capacity, weakened urinary sphincter, shortened urethra) causing urinary urgency or incontinence. The older client is at risk for falling while attempting to get to the bathroom, so this client should be seen first.**
    3. Changing a gown does not affect the client's safety.
    4. In many facilities, this task cannot be delegated, but the client's safety is not affected if the IV catheter is not immediately discontinued.

18. 1. The client needs to lie flat on the back to apply pressure to prevent bleeding.
    2. The client has oral intake withheld before the biopsy, not after the client is awake.
    3. The client must lie flat on the back, so using a bedside commode is not maintaining bedrest.
    4. The client should request pain medication if the client is in pain. This indicates the client is not compliant with the client's teaching.

19. 1. The nurse should maintain the drainage bag with a 1/8-inch border around the stoma.
    2. The United Ostomy Association is an excellent referral for information but not for discharge teaching. The nurse retains the responsibility to teach information the client needs to know before discharge.
    3. **The output should be monitored to detect a decreased amount, indicating an obstruction from edema or ureteral stenosis. Any decrease should be reported to the HCP.**
    4. The stoma should be monitored much more frequently than once a shift.

20. Correct answers are 1 and 5.
    1. **Vital signs should be monitored every 2 hours until stable and more frequently if the client is unstable.**
    2. Intake and output should be monitored more frequently than every 24 hours. Depending on the client's condition, the frequency may vary from every hour to every 4 hours.
    3. Mouth care should be given as often as needed. A minimum of care should be every 8 hours, not once a day when bathing the client.
    4. The client should be weighed daily, not weekly, at the same time, wearing the same clothing to ensure the reliability of this indicator.
    5. **Skin turgor and mucous membranes should be assessed every shift or more often depending on the client's condition.**

21. 1. Voiding a minimum of 30 mL of urine each hour is appropriate for a client diagnosed with fluid volume deficit.
    2. Elastic skin turgor indicates the client has adequate fluid volume status. This is an expected outcome for the client diagnosed with fluid volume deficit.
    3. **The client diagnosed with FVE has too much fluid. Excess fluid is reflected by adventitious breath sounds. Therefore, an expected outcome is to have no excess fluid, as evidenced by normal, clear breath sounds.**
    4. The creatinine is elevated in a client diagnosed with dehydration. The normal male should have a creatinine of 0.6 to 1.2 mg/dL, and a female client's normal creatinine is between 0.5 and 1.1 mg/dL.

22. 1. Hematuria is not a symptom of nephrotic syndrome.
2. A calorie count may be helpful in the treatment of this client, but a calorie count monitors what the name implies—calories. The dietitian can calculate the amount of protein the client consumes, but this is a protein count.
3. **The classic clinical manifestation of nephrotic syndrome is dependent edema located on the client's sacrum and ankles.**
4. A low serum albumin level is expected for a client diagnosed with nephrotic syndrome.

23. 1. Steroid therapy should not be stopped abruptly if clinical manifestations of toxicity occur, such as moon face, because it may result in adrenal insufficiency.
2. **Treatment includes diuretics to eliminate dependent edema, usually in the ankles and sacrum. Medication teaching is an appropriate intervention.**
3. Sodium is restricted to prevent fluid retention.
4. A decrease in weight is expected if a diuretic is administered; this indicates the medication is effective.

24. 1. **Assessing the rate and volume of intravenous fluid is the most important intervention for the client with one kidney because an overload of fluids can result in pulmonary edema.**
2. A daily dressing change can be performed at any time and is not the priority intervention.
3. A client after surgery should not be receiving any type of anticoagulant therapy, so the nurse should not have to monitor this laboratory data.
4. The nurse assesses the amount of food eaten, but it is not the most important intervention.

25. 1. The client recovering from a nephrectomy needs to refrain from strenuous or heavy activities, and normal activities should not be resumed until the client is given permission by the surgeon.
2. **The client or family needs to contact the surgeon if the client develops chills, flank pain, decreased urinary output, or fever (U.S. National Library of Medicine, 2019).**
3. The client needs to be informed of how to monitor the urinary output and which parameters should be reported to the surgeon.
4. The client needs to follow any dietary or fluid restriction the surgeon prescribes.

26. **Correct order is 1, 2, 3, 5, 4.**
1. The nurse should assess to determine if the client is symptomatic of hyperkalemia.
2. A peaked T wave is indicative of hyperkalemia; therefore, the nurse should obtain a potassium level.
3. Hyperkalemia is a life-threatening situation because of the risk of cardiac dysrhythmias; therefore, the nurse should notify the HCP.
5. Polystyrene sulfonate (Kayexalate), a cation resin, will help remove potassium through the gastrointestinal system and should be administered to decrease the potassium level.
4. The client should be monitored continuously for cardiac dysrhythmias, so a transfer to the telemetry unit is warranted.

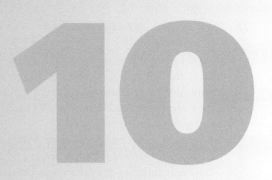

# Reproductive Disorders

*The aim of education is the knowledge not of fact, but of values.*

—Dean William R. Inge

The organs of the male and female reproductive systems are subject to many disorders and diseases. Some are hereditary, some are related to the endocrine system and may involve an underproduction or overproduction of hormones, and others may be the result of infections or neoplastic growths. Whatever the etiology, the nurse must be well informed about all the possible disorders and diseases and how to monitor and treat them.

## KEYWORDS

Aneuploid
Brachytherapy
Chancre
Colporrhaphy
DNA ploidy

Dysmenorrhea
Dyspareunia
Nulliparity
Pessary
Phimosis

## PRACTICE QUESTIONS

### Breast Disorders

1. The client frequently finds lumps in her breasts, especially around her menstrual period. Which information should the nurse teach the client regarding breast self-care?
   1. This is a benign process, which does not require follow-up.
   2. The client should eliminate chocolate and caffeine from the diet.
   3. The client should practice breast self-examination monthly.
   4. This is the way breast cancer begins, and the client needs surgery.

2. The client is diagnosed with breast cancer and is considering whether to have a lumpectomy or a more invasive procedure, a modified radical mastectomy. Which information should the nurse discuss with the client? **Select all that apply.**
   1. Ask if the client is afraid of having general anesthesia.
   2. Determine how the client feels about radiation and chemotherapy.
   3. Tell the client she will need reconstruction with either procedure.
   4. Find out if the client has any history of breast cancer in her family.
   5. Inform the client of no difference in overall survival rate between procedures.

3. The client has undergone a partial mastectomy for cancer of the left breast. Which discharge instruction should the nurse teach?
   1. Don't lift more than 5 pounds with the left hand until released by the HCP.
   2. The cancer has been totally removed and no follow-up therapy will be required.
   3. The client should empty the closed wound suction evacuator drain about every 12 hours.
   4. The client should arrange an appointment with a plastic surgeon for reconstruction.

4. Which recommendation is the American Cancer Society's (ACS) 2015 guideline for the early detection of breast cancer?
   1. Beginning at age 18, have a biannual clinical breast examination by an HCP.
   2. Beginning at age 30, perform monthly breast self-examinations.
   3. At age 45 through 54, receive a yearly mammogram.
   4. Beginning at age 50, have a breast sonogram every 5 years.

5. The client had a mastectomy for cancer of the breast and asked the nurse about a TRAM flap procedure. Which information should the nurse explain to the client?
   1. The surgeon will insert a saline-filled sac under the skin to simulate a breast.
   2. The surgeon will pull the client's own tissue under the skin to create a breast.
   3. The surgeon will use tissue from inside the mouth to make a nipple.
   4. The surgeon can make the breast any size the client wants the breast to be.

6. The nurse is teaching a class on breast health to a group of women at a senior citizen's center. Which risk factor is the **most important** to emphasize to this group?
   1. The clients should find out about their family history of breast cancer.
   2. Men at this age can get breast cancer also and should be screened.
   3. Monthly breast self-examination is the key to early detection.
   4. The older a woman gets, the greater the chance of developing breast cancer.

7. The client scheduled to have a breast biopsy with sentinel node dissection states, "I don't understand. What does a sentinel node biopsy do?" Which scientific rationale should the nurse use to base the response?
   1. A dye is injected into the tumor and traced to determine the spread of cells.
   2. The surgeon removes the nodes that drain the diseased portion of the breast.

   3. The nodes felt manually will be removed and sent to pathology.
   4. A visual inspection of the lymph nodes will be made while the client is sleeping.

8. The client is 4 months pregnant and finds a lump in her breast. The biopsy is positive for stage II cancer of the breast. Which treatment should the nurse anticipate the HCP recommending to the client?
   1. A lumpectomy to be performed after the baby is born.
   2. A modified radical mastectomy.
   3. Radiation therapy to the chest wall only.
   4. Chemotherapy only until the baby is born.

9. The client had a right modified radical mastectomy 4 years before and is now being admitted for a cardiac work-up for chest pain. Which intervention is **most important** for the nurse to implement?
   1. Determine when the client had chemotherapy last.
   2. Ask the client if she received doxorubicin.
   3. Post a sign at the head of bed for staff not to use the right arm for venipunctures or BPs.
   4. Examine the chest wall for cancer sites.

10. The client is being discharged after a left partial mastectomy. Which discharge instructions should the nurse include? **Select all that apply.**
    1. Notify the HCP of a temperature of 100°F.
    2. Carry large purses and bundles with the right hand.
    3. Do not go to church or anywhere with crowds.
    4. Try to keep the arm as still as possible until seen by the HCP.
    5. Have a mammogram of the right and left breasts yearly.

11. The client, who has had a mastectomy, tells the nurse, "My spouse will leave me now because I am not a whole woman anymore." Which response by the nurse is **most therapeutic**?
    1. "You're afraid your spouse will not find you sexually appealing?"
    2. "Your spouse should be grateful you will be able to live and be with him."
    3. "Maybe your spouse would like to attend a support group for spouses."
    4. "You don't know that is true. You need to give your spouse a chance."

12. The client has been diagnosed with cancer of the breast. Which referral is **most important** for the nurse to make?
    1. The hospital social worker.
    2. CanSurmount.
    3. Reach to Recovery.
    4. I Can Cope.

## Pelvic Floor Relaxation Disorders

13. Which question is **most important** for the nurse to ask the client diagnosed with a cystocele and scheduled to have a pessary inserted?
    1. "Do you know if you are allergic to latex?"
    2. "When did you start having incontinence?"
    3. "When was your last bowel movement?"
    4. "Are you experiencing any pelvic pressure?"

14. Which intervention should the nurse include when teaching the client having an anterior colporrhaphy to repair a cystocele?
    1. Discuss the need to perform perineal care every 4 hours.
    2. Discuss the care of an indwelling catheter for at least 1 month.
    3. Instruct the client how to care for the pessary inserted in surgery.
    4. Teach the client how to perform Kegel exercises.

15. The nurse is assessing the client diagnosed with a rectocele. Which clinical manifestations should the nurse expect? **Select all that apply.**
    1. Rectal pressure.
    2. Flatus.
    3. Fecal incontinence.
    4. Constipation.
    5. Urinary frequency.

16. What intervention should the nurse implement for a client diagnosed with a rectocele? **Select all that apply.**
    1. Limit oral intake to decrease voiding.
    2. Encourage a low-residue diet.
    3. Administer a stool softener daily.
    4. Arrange for the client to take sitz baths.
    5. Recommend pelvic floor exercises.

17. Which statement indicates **further instruction** is needed for the client diagnosed with a cystocele?
    1. "I need to have a sonogram to diagnose this problem."
    2. "I need to practice Kegel exercises to help strengthen my muscles."
    3. "I lose my urine when I sneeze because of my cystocele."
    4. "I can never have sexual intercourse again."

18. Which specific complication should the nurse assess for in the client diagnosed with a uterine prolapse recovering from an anterior and posterior repair?
    1. Orthostatic hypotension.
    2. Atelectasis.
    3. Allen sign.
    4. Deep vein thrombosis.

19. Which information should the nurse include in the discharge teaching for the client recovering from a laparoscopic hysterectomy? **Select all that apply.**
    1. The client should report any bright red vaginal bleeding to the surgeon.
    2. The client should start a vigorous exercise routine to restore her muscle tone.
    3. The client should continue sitting in the bedside chair at least 6 hours daily.
    4. The client should soak in a warm tub bath each night for 1 hour.
    5. The client should drink six to eight glasses of water a day.

20. Which nursing task could be delegated to the unlicensed assistive personnel (UAP) for the client after a total vaginal hysterectomy?
    1. Observe the color and amount of drainage on the client's perineal pad.
    2. Maintain a current intake and output for the client each shift.
    3. Provide the client with a plan of pharmacological pain management.
    4. Prepare the client for her discharge scheduled for the next day.

21. The nurse is formulating a care plan for a client who had an abdominal hysterectomy. Which nursing diagnosis is **appropriate** for the client developing a complication?
    1. Potential for urinary retention.
    2. Potential for nerve damage.
    3. Potential for intestinal obstruction.
    4. Potential for fluid imbalance.

22. The nurse is teaching the client diagnosed with uterine prolapse. Which information should the nurse include in the discussion?
    1. Increase fluids and daily exercise to prevent constipation.
    2. Explain there is only one acceptable treatment for uterine prolapse.
    3. Instruct the client to check the uterine prolapse visually every day.
    4. Discuss limiting coughing and lifting heavy objects.

23. The nurse is preparing the client for the insertion of a pessary. Which information should the nurse teach the client? **Select all that apply.**
    1. The pessary does not need to be changed.
    2. The client should clean the pessary routinely.
    3. The pessary must be inserted in surgery.
    4. Estrogen cream is necessary for effective use of a pessary.
    5. Routine follow-up visits are recommended every 3 months.

24. An older woman is diagnosed with pelvic relaxation disorder secondary to age-related changes. Which medication should the nurse expect to administer?
    1. Estrogen.
    2. Dinoprostone.
    3. Progesterone.
    4. Oxytocin.

## Uterine Disorders

25. The nurse is caring for a 30-year-old nulliparous client reporting severe dysmenorrhea. Which diagnostic test should the nurse prepare the client to undergo to determine the diagnosis?
    1. A bimanual vaginal exam.
    2. A pregnancy test.
    3. An exploratory laparoscopy.
    4. An ovarian biopsy.

26. The client in the gynecology clinic asks the nurse, "What are the risk factors for developing cancer of the cervix?" Which statement is the nurse's **best response**?
    1. "The earlier the age of sexual activity and the more partners, the greater the risk."
    2. "Eating fast foods high in fat and taking birth control pills are risk factors."
    3. "A *Chlamydia trachomatis* infection can cause cancer of the cervix."
    4. "Having yearly Pap smears will protect you from developing cancer."

27. The nurse is admitting a client diagnosed with stage Ia cancer of the cervix to an outpatient surgery center for a conization. Which data would the client **most likely** report?
    1. Diffuse watery discharge.
    2. No symptoms.
    3. Dyspareunia.
    4. Intense itching.

28. The client diagnosed with cancer of the uterus is scheduled to have radiation brachytherapy. Which precautions should the nurse implement? **Select all that apply.**
    1. Place the client in a private room.
    2. Wear a dosimeter when entering the room.
    3. Encourage visitors to come and stay with the client.
    4. Plan to spend extended time with the client.
    5. Notify the nuclear medicine technician.

29. The postmenopausal client reveals it has been several years since her last gynecological examination and states, "Oh, I don't need examinations anymore. I am beyond having children." Which statement should be the nurse's response?

1. "As long as you are not sexually active, you don't have to worry."
2. "You should be taking hormone replacement therapy now."
3. "You are beyond bearing children. How does that make you feel?"
4. "There are situations other than pregnancy that should be checked."

30. The client had a total abdominal hysterectomy and tumor debulking for endometrial cancer. Which discharge instruction should the nurse teach? **Select all that apply.**
    1. The client should take hormone replacement therapy every day to prevent bone loss.
    2. The client should practice pelvic rest until seen by the HCP.
    3. The client can drive a car as soon as she is discharged from the hospital.
    4. The client should expect some bleeding after this procedure.
    5. The client should notify the HCP of fever or severe pain.

31. The client diagnosed with uterine cancer is reporting lower back pain and unilateral leg edema. Which statement **best explains** the scientific rationale for these clinical manifestations?
    1. This is the expected pain for this type of cancer.
    2. This means the cancer has spread to other areas of the pelvis.
    3. The pain is a result of the treatment of uterine cancer.
    4. Radiation treatment always causes some type of pain in the region.

32. The client diagnosed with endometriosis experiences pain rated a "5" on a 1-to-10 pain scale during her menses. Which intervention should the nurse teach the client?
    1. Teach the client to take a stool softener when taking morphine.
    2. Instruct the client to soak in a tepid bath for 30 to 45 minutes when the pain occurs.
    3. Explain the need to take NSAIDs with food.
    4. Discuss the possibility of a hysterectomy to help relieve the pain.

33. The client is diagnosed with benign uterine fibroid tumors. Which question should the nurse ask to determine if the client is experiencing a complication?
    1. "How many periods have you missed?"
    2. "Do you get short of breath easily?"
    3. "How many times have you been pregnant?"
    4. "Where is the location of the pain you are having?"

34. The HCP has prescribed two IV antibiotics for the female client diagnosed with diabetes and pneumonia. Which order should the nurse request from the HCP?
    1. Request written information on antibiotic-caused vaginal infections.
    2. Request yogurt to be served on the client's meal trays.
    3. Request a change of one of the antibiotics to an oral route.
    4. Request *Lactobacillus acidophilus* three times a day.

35. The registered nurse (RN) and a UAP are caring for clients on a gynecology surgery floor. Which intervention can be delegated to the UAP? **Select all that apply.**
    1. Empty the indwelling catheter on the 3-hour postoperative client.
    2. Assist the client 2 days post-hysterectomy to the bathroom.
    3. Monitor the peri-pad count on a client diagnosed with fibroid tumors.
    4. Encourage the client refusing to get out of bed to walk in the hall.
    5. Record the breakfast intake of the client preparing for discharge.

36. The nurse is caring for a client diagnosed with uterine cancer receiving systemic therapy for 6 months. Which intervention should the nurse implement **first**?
    1. Determine which antineoplastic medication the client has received.
    2. Ask the client if she has had any problems with mouth ulcers at home.
    3. Administer filgrastim to the client diagnosed with uterine cancer.
    4. Encourage the client to discuss feelings about having cancer.

## Ovarian Disorders

37. The 24-year-old female client presents to the clinic with lower abdominal pain on the left side rated as a "9" on a 1-to-10 scale. Which diagnostic procedure should the nurse prepare the client for?
    1. A computed tomography scan.
    2. A lumbar puncture.
    3. An appendectomy.
    4. A pelvic sonogram.

38. The nurse is caring for a client newly diagnosed with stage IV ovarian cancer. What is the scientific rationale for detecting the tumors at this stage?
    1. The client's ovaries lie deep within the pelvis and early symptoms are vague.
    2. The client has regular gynecological examinations and this helps with detection.
    3. The client had a history of dysmenorrhea and benign ovarian cysts.
    4. The client had a family history of breast cancer and was being checked regularly.

39. The female client presents to the gynecologist's office for the fifth time with an ovarian cyst and is scheduled for an exploratory laparoscopy. The client asks the nurse, "Why do I need to have another surgery? The other cysts have all been benign." Which statement is the nurse's **best response**?
    1. "Because eventually, the cysts will become cancerous."
    2. "All abnormal findings in the ovary should be checked out."
    3. "The surgery will not be painful and you will have peace of mind."
    4. "Are you afraid of having surgery? Would you like to talk about it?"

40. The client has had an exploratory laparotomy to remove an ovarian tumor. The pathology report classifies the tumor as a "low malignancy potential" tumor. Which statement explains the scientific rationale for this pathology report?
    1. The client does not have cancer but will need adjuvant therapy.
    2. The client would have developed cancer if the tumor had not been removed.
    3. These borderline tumors resemble ovarian cancer but have better outcomes.
    4. The client has a very poor prognosis and has less than 6 months to live.

41. The 50-year-old female client reports bloating and indigestion and tells the nurse she has gained 2 inches in her waist recently. Which question should the nurse ask the client?
    1. "What do you eat before you feel bloated?"
    2. "Have you had your ovaries removed?"
    3. "Are your stools darker in color lately?"
    4. "Is the indigestion worse when you lie down?"

42. The nurse writes a problem of "anticipatory grieving" for a client diagnosed with ovarian cancer. Which nursing intervention is a **priority** for this client?
    1. Request the HCP to order an antidepressant medication.
    2. Refer the client to a CanSurmount volunteer for counseling.
    3. Encourage the client to verbalize feelings about having cancer.
    4. Give the client an advance directive form to fill out.

43. The client diagnosed with ovarian cancer has had eight courses of chemotherapy. Which laboratory data **warrant immediate** intervention by the nurse?

| Laboratory Test | Client Value | Normal Values |
|---|---|---|
| Red blood cell count (RBC) | 5 | Male: 4.21–5.81 (10⁶ cells/microL) Female: 3.61–5.11 (10⁶ cells/microL) |
| Absolute neutrophil count (ANC) | 3,500 | 1,500–8,000/mm³ |
| Platelets | 150 | 140–400 × (10³/microL) |
| White blood cells (urinalysis) | 100 | Less than 5/hpf |

1. Absolute neutrophil count.
2. Platelet count.
3. Red blood cell count.
4. Urinalysis report white blood cells.

44. The client diagnosed with ovarian cancer is prescribed radiation therapy for regional control of the disease. Which statement indicates the client **requires further** teaching?
1. "I will not wash the marks off my abdomen."
2. "I will have a treatment every day for 6 weeks."
3. "Nausea caused by radiation therapy cannot be controlled."
4. "I need to drink a nutritional shake if I don't feel like eating."

45. The female client's mother died from ovarian cancer, and her sister is now diagnosed with ovarian cancer. Which recommendations should the nurse make regarding early detection of ovarian cancer?
1. The client should consider having a prophylactic bilateral oophorectomy.
2. The client should have a transvaginal ultrasound and a CA-125 laboratory test every 6 months.
3. The client should have yearly magnetic resonance imaging (MRI) scans.
4. The client should have a biannual gynecological examination with flexible sigmoidoscopy.

46. The client has had a total abdominal hysterectomy for cancer of the ovary. Which diet should the nurse discuss when providing discharge instructions?
1. A low-residue diet without seeds.
2. A low-sodium, low-fat diet with skim milk.
3. A regular diet with fruits and vegetables.
4. A full liquid-only diet with milkshake supplements.

47. The nurse is preparing an educational presentation for women in the community. Which primary nursing intervention should the nurse discuss regarding the development of ovarian cancer?
1. Instruct the clients not to use talcum powder on the perineum.
2. Encourage clients to consume diets with high-fat content.
3. Teach the women to have a lower pelvic sonogram yearly.
4. Discuss the need to be aware of the family history of cancer.

48. The nurse is caring for a client 1 day postoperative hysterectomy for cancer of the ovary. Which nursing interventions should the nurse implement? **Select all that apply.**
1. Assess for calf enlargement and tenderness.
2. Turn, cough, and deep breathe every 6 hours.
3. Assess pain on a 1-to-10 pain scale.
4. Apply sequential compression devices to legs.
5. Assess bowel sounds every 4 hours.

## Prostate Disorders

49. Which is the American Cancer Society's recommendation for the early detection of cancer of the prostate?
1. A yearly PSA level and digital rectal exam (DRE) beginning at age 50.
2. A biannual rectal examination beginning at age 40.
3. A semiannual alkaline phosphatase level beginning at age 45.
4. A yearly urinalysis to determine the presence of prostatic fluid.

50. The client is diagnosed with early cancer of the prostate. Which assessment data would the client report?
1. Urinary urgency and frequency.
2. Retrograde ejaculation during intercourse.
3. Low back and hip pain.
4. No problems have been noticed.

51. The 80-year-old male client has been diagnosed with cancer of the prostate. Which treatment should the nurse discuss with the client?
1. Radiation therapy every day for 4 weeks.
2. Radical prostatectomy with lymph node dissection.
3. Gonadotropin-releasing hormone agonists (GnRH).
4. Penile implants to maintain sexual functioning.

52. The nurse writes a client problem of urinary retention for a client diagnosed with stage IV cancer of the prostate. Which intervention should the nurse implement **first**?
    1. Catheterize the client to determine the amount of residual.
    2. Encourage the client to assume a normal position for urinating.
    3. Teach the client to use the Valsalva maneuver to empty the bladder.
    4. Determine the client's normal voiding pattern.

53. The client has undergone a bilateral orchiectomy for cancer of the prostate. Which intervention should the nurse implement?
    1. Support the scrotal sac with a towel and apply ice.
    2. Administer testosterone replacement hormone orally.
    3. Encourage the client to place sperm in a sperm bank.
    4. Have the client talk to another man with ejaculation dysfunction.

54. The client diagnosed with cancer of the prostate has been placed on luteinizing hormone-releasing hormone (LHRH) agonist therapy. Which statement indicates the client **understands** the treatment?
    1. "I will be able to function sexually as always."
    2. "I may have hot flashes while taking this drug."
    3. "This medication will cure prostate cancer."
    4. "There are no side effects with this medication."

55. The client is diagnosed with metastatic prostate cancer to the bones. Which nursing intervention should the nurse implement?
    1. Prepare for a transurethral resection of the prostate.
    2. Keep the foot of the bed elevated at all times.
    3. Place the client on a scheduled bowel regimen.
    4. Discuss the client's altered sexual functioning.

56. Which could be a complication of cryotherapy surgery for cancer of the prostate?
    1. The urethra could become scarred and cause retention.
    2. The client could have ejaculation difficulties and be impotent.
    3. Bone marrow suppression could occur from the chemotherapy.
    4. Chronic vomiting and diarrhea causing electrolyte imbalance.

57. The client is 8 hours post-transurethral prostatectomy for cancer of the prostate. Which nursing intervention is **a priority** at this time?
    1. Control postoperative pain.
    2. Assess abdominal dressing.
    3. Encourage early ambulation to prevent DVT.
    4. Monitor fluid and electrolyte balance.

58. The client scheduled for a radical prostatectomy surgical procedure has an intravenous antibiotic medication ordered on call to surgery. The antibiotic is prepared in 100 mL of sterile normal saline. At what rate should the nurse infuse, via the IV pump, the medication in 30 minutes?

    ┌─────────────┐
    │             │
    └─────────────┘

59. The client diagnosed with cancer of the prostate tells the nurse, "I caused this by being promiscuous when I was young and now I have to pay for my sins." Which statement is the nurse's **most therapeutic** response?
    1. "Why would you think prostate cancer is caused by sex?"
    2. "You feel guilty about some of your actions when you were young?"
    3. "Well, there is nothing you can do about that behavior now."
    4. "Have you told the HCP and been checked for an HIV infection?"

60. The nurse is preparing the care plan for a 45-year-old client after a radical prostatectomy. Which **psychosocial and physiological** problem should be included in the plan?
    1. Altered coping.
    2. High risk for hemorrhage.
    3. Sexual impotence.
    4. Risk for electrolyte imbalance.

## Testicular Disorders

61. The school nurse is preparing a class on testicular cancer for male high school seniors. Which information regarding testicular self-examination should the nurse include?
    1. Perform the examination in a cool room under a fan.
    2. Any lump should be examined by an HCP as soon as possible.
    3. Discuss having a second person confirm a negative result.
    4. The procedure will cause mild discomfort if done correctly.

62. The nurse enters the room of a 24-year-old client diagnosed with testicular cancer. The fiancée of the client asks the nurse, "Will we be able to have children?" Which is the nurse's **best response**?
    1. "Your fiancée will be able to father children like always."
    2. "You will have to adopt children because he will be sterile."
    3. "You and he should consider sperm banking before treatment."
    4. "Have you discussed this with your fiancée? I can't discuss this with you."

63. The client diagnosed with testicular cancer is scheduled for a unilateral orchiectomy. Which information is **important** to teach regarding sexual functioning?
    1. The client will have ejaculation difficulties after the surgery.
    2. The client will be prescribed male hormones following the surgery.
    3. The client may need to have a penile implant to be able to have intercourse.
    4. Libido and orgasm usually are unimpaired after this surgery.

64. Which client has the **highest risk** for developing cancer of the testicles?
    1. The client diagnosed with epididymitis.
    2. The client born with cryptorchidism.
    3. The client diagnosed with an enlarged prostate.
    4. The client diagnosed with hypospadias.

65. The nurse is caring for a client 8 hours postoperative unilateral orchiectomy for cancer of the testes. Which interventions should the nurse implement? **Select all that apply.**
    1. Provide an athletic supporter before ambulating.
    2. Encourage the client to delay the use of pain medications.
    3. Place the client on a clear liquid diet for the first 48 hours.
    4. Monitor the PT/INR levels and have vitamin K ready.
    5. Use ice packs to the scrotum and around the incision.

66. The RN and an UAP are caring for clients on a genitourinary floor. Which nursing task can be delegated to the UAP?
    1. Increase the drip rate on a continuous bladder irrigation set.
    2. Check the suprapubic catheter insertion site for infection.
    3. Encourage the 2-hour postoperative client to turn and cough.
    4. Document the amount of red drainage in the catheter.

67. The nurse is caring for a client diagnosed with epididymitis secondary to a chlamydia infection. Which discharge instruction should the nurse discuss?
    1. The sexual partner must be prescribed antibiotics.
    2. Delay sexual intercourse for a minimum of 3 months.
    3. Expect the urine to have white clumps for 1 to 2 months.
    4. Drainage from the scrotum is fine as long as there is no fever.

68. The nurse is assessing a client admitted for possible testicular cancer. Which assessment data support the client having testicular cancer?
    1. The client reports pain when urinating.
    2. There is a chancre sore on the shaft of the penis.
    3. The client reports heaviness in the scrotum.
    4. There is a red, raised rash on the testes.

69. The 30-year-old male client diagnosed with germinal cell carcinoma of the testes asks the nurse, "What chance do I have? Should I end it all now?" Which response by the nurse indicates an **understanding** of the disease process?
    1. "God does not want you to give up hope and end it all now."
    2. "There is a good chance for survival with standard treatment options."
    3. "There may be little hope, but ending it all is not the answer."
    4. "You have a 50/50 chance of living for at least 5 years."

70. Which tumor marker information is used to follow the progress of a client diagnosed with testicular cancer?
    1. CA-125.
    2. Carcinogenic embryonic antigen (CEA).
    3. DNA ploidy test.
    4. Human chorionic gonadotropin (hCG).

71. The client diagnosed with cancer of the testes calls and tells the nurse he is having low back pain that does not go away with acetaminophen. Which action should the nurse implement?
    1. Ask the client to come in to see the HCP for an examination.
    2. Tell the client to use an NSAID instead.
    3. Inform the client this means the cancer has metastasized.
    4. Encourage the client to perform lower back strengthening exercises.

72. The RN charge nurse is making rounds on the genitourinary surgery floor. Which action by the primary nurse **warrants immediate** intervention?
    1. The nurse elevates the scrotum of a client after an orchiectomy.
    2. The nurse encourages the client to cough, although he reports pain.
    3. The nurse empties the client's JP drain and leaves it rounded.
    4. The nurse asks the UAP to empty a catheter drainage bag.

## Sexually Transmitted Infections

73. The occupational health nurse is preparing a class regarding sexually transmitted infections (STIs) for employees at a manufacturing plant. Which **high-risk** behavior information should be included in the class information?
    1. Engaging in oral or anal sex decreases the risk of getting an STI.
    2. Using a sterile needle guarantees the client will not get an STI.
    3. The more sexual partners, the greater the chance of developing an STI.
    4. If a condom is used, the client will not get a sexually transmitted infection.

74. The female client diagnosed with human papillomavirus (HPV) asks the nurse, "What other problems can HPV lead to?" Which statement is the **most appropriate** response by the nurse?
    1. "HPV is transmitted during sexual intercourse."
    2. "HPV infection can cause cancer of the cervix."
    3. "It has been known to lead to ovarian problems."
    4. "Regular Pap smears can help prevent problems."

75. The male client presents to the public health clinic reporting joint pain and malaise. On assessment, the nurse notes a rash on the trunk, palms of the hands, and soles of the feet. Which action should the nurse implement **next**?
    1. Determine if the client has had a chancre sore within the last 2 months.
    2. Ask the client how many sexual partners he has had in the past year.
    3. Refer the client to a dermatologist for a diagnostic work-up.
    4. Have the client provide a clean, voided midstream urine specimen.

76. The nurse is caring for a young adult client diagnosed with gonorrhea. Which statement reflects an **understanding** of the transmission of STIs?
    1. Only lower socioeconomic income people are at risk for gonorrhea and syphilis.
    2. The longer a client waits to become sexually active, the greater the risk for an STI.
    3. Females can transmit infectious diseases more rapidly than males.
    4. If a client is diagnosed with an STI, the client should be evaluated for other STIs.

77. The young female client is admitted with pelvic inflammatory disease secondary to a chlamydia infection. Which discharge instruction should be taught to the client?
    1. The client will develop antibodies to protect against future infection.
    2. This infection will not have any long-term effects for the client.
    3. Both the client and the sexual partner must be treated simultaneously.
    4. Once the infection subsides, the pain will go away and not be a problem.

78. The nurse is assessing a male client for clinical manifestations of gonorrhea. Which data support the diagnosis?
    1. Presence of a chancre sore on the penis.
    2. No symptoms.
    3. A CD4 count of less than 200.
    4. Pain in the testes and scrotal edema.

79. The nurse is working in a health clinic. Which condition is **required** to be reported to the public health department?
    1. Pelvic inflammatory disease.
    2. Epididymitis.
    3. Syphilis.
    4. Ectopic pregnancy.

80. The nurse is planning the care of a client diagnosed with pelvic inflammatory disease secondary to an STI. Which **collaborative** diagnosis is appropriate for this client?
    1. Risk for infertility.
    2. Knowledge deficit.
    3. Fluid volume deficit.
    4. Noncompliance.

81. Which laboratory test should the nurse expect for the client to **rule out** the diagnosis of syphilis?
    1. Vaginal cultures.
    2. Rapid plasma reagin card test (RPR-CT).
    3. Gram-stained specimen of the urethral meatus.
    4. Immunological assay.

82. The client is diagnosed with tertiary syphilis. Which clinical manifestations should the nurse expect the client to exhibit?
    1. Lymphadenopathy and hair loss.
    2. Warts in the genital area.
    3. Dementia and psychosis.
    4. Raised rash covering the body.

83. Which statement **best describes** the responsibility of the public health nurse regarding STIs?
    1. Notify the sexual partners of clients diagnosed with an STI.
    2. Determine the course of treatment for clients diagnosed with an STI.
    3. Explain the legal aspects of STI reporting to a client diagnosed with an STI.
    4. Analyze the statistics regarding STI transmission and reporting the findings.

84. The nurse is admitting a client diagnosed with trichomoniasis. Which assessment data support this diagnosis?
    1. Odorless, white, curdlike vaginal discharge.
    2. Strawberry spots on the vaginal surface and itching.
    3. Scant white vaginal discharge and dyspareunia.
    4. Purulent discharge from the endocervix and pelvic pain.

# CONCEPTS

The concepts covered in this chapter focus on reproduction and sexuality. Exemplars that are covered are pregnancy and newborns, breast and prostate disorders, and sexually transmitted illnesses. Interrelated concepts of the nursing process and clinical judgment are covered throughout the questions. The concept of clinical judgment is presented in prioritizing or "first" questions.

85. The outpatient clinic nurse is working with clients diagnosed with STIs. Which long-term complication should the nurse discuss with the clients about STIs?
    1. Stress the need for clients to finish all antibiotic prescriptions completely.
    2. Inform the clients that, legally, many STIs must be reported to the health department.
    3. Sexually transmitted infections can result in reproductive problems.
    4. Discuss the myth that acquired immunodeficiency syndrome is an STI.

86. The gravida 7 para 6 client delivered a 9-pound 4-ounce infant 2 hours ago. Which intervention is a **priority** for the nurse to implement?
    1. Assess the client's fundus every hour.
    2. Assess the client's voiding pattern every shift.
    3. Discuss birth control options with the client.
    4. Discuss breastfeeding methods with the client.

87. The nurse in the gynecology clinic is assessing a 14-year-old client reporting being sexually active. Which information should the nurse teach the client? **Select all that apply.**
    1. Inform the client that the nurse must tell the parents of her being sexually active.
    2. Teach the client about possible birth control options.
    3. Instruct the client regarding sexually transmitted infections.
    4. Demonstrate how a condom is applied correctly.
    5. Tell the client about the importance of finishing all antibiotics.
    6. Discuss the importance of attending parenting classes.

88. The 67-year-old male client reports difficulty initiating a urinary stream, urinary frequency, and inability to completely empty the bladder. Which procedure would the nurse anticipate the HCP performing **first**?
    1. Digital rectal examination (DRE).
    2. Prostate-specific surface antigen (PSA).
    3. Prostate ultrasound.
    4. Biopsy of the prostate.

89. The nurse is instructing a 2-week postpartum client with red, tender breasts after trying to breastfeed the infant. Which should the nurse teach the client?
    1. Be sure the baby empties each breast when feeding.
    2. Apply a warm, moist pack to the breasts for comfort.
    3. Apply rubbing alcohol to the breast to treat the infection.
    4. The baby must be given formula because the mother cannot breastfeed.

**90.** The nurse is assessing a 34-year-old female client diagnosed with fibrocystic breasts. Which question should the nurse ask the client during the assessment?
1. "Are your breasts more tender during your period?"
2. "Have you ever developed an allergy to chocolate?"
3. "Can you tell me more about your feelings of having fibrocystic breast changes?"
4. "Have you considered having a prophylactic mastectomy?"

**91.** The day nurse is administering the initial dose of medications to a newly admitted client at 0900. Which medication should the nurse administer **first**?

| Client Name: Mr. D.S. | MR# 654231 | Diagnosis: Prostatitis |
|---|---|---|
| DOB: 7/10/1953 | Allergies: NKDA | |
| Medication | 0701–1900 | 1901–0700 |
| Digoxin 0.125 mg PO every day | 0900 | |
| Furosemide 40 mg every 12 hours | 0900 | |
| Gentamycin 80 mg IVPB every 6 hours | 1000<br>1600 | 2200<br>0400 |
| Acetaminophen 650 mg every 4 hours prn | | |
| Signature of Nurse: | Day Nurse RN/DN | Night Nurse RN/NN |

1. Digoxin.
2. Furosemide.
3. Gentamycin.
4. Acetaminophen.

**92.** The client scheduled for chemotherapy is diagnosed with inflammatory breast cancer. Which intervention should the nurse implement based on the complete blood count (CBC) report?

| Complete Blood Count | Client Values | Normal Values |
|---|---|---|
| Red blood cell count (RBC) | 4.8 | Male: 4.21–5.81 $\times$ 10$^6$ cells/microL<br>Female: 3.61–5.11 $\times$ 10$^6$ cells/microL |
| Hemoglobin (Hgb) | 12.4 | Male: 14–17.3 g/dL<br>Female: 11.7–15.5 g/dL |
| Hematocrit (Hct) | 40 | Male: 42%–52%<br>Female: 36%–48% |
| White blood cell count (WBC) | 7.8 | 4.5–11.1 $\times$ 10$^3$ cells/microL |
| Platelets | 192 | 140–400 $\times$ 10$^3$/microL |
| Absolute neutrophil count (ANC) | 1500 | 1,500–8,000/mm$^3$ |

1. Administer the chemotherapy as prescribed.
2. Notify the oncologist immediately.
3. Request urine and blood cultures.
4. Prepare to administer 1 unit of packed red blood cells.

**93.** The nurse is teaching men about early detection of prostate cancer according to the American Cancer Society (ACS) guidelines. Which should the nurse teach the clients?
1. Beginning at age 39, men should have a digital rectal examination (DRE) followed by a prostate-specific antigen (PSA).
2. Beginning at age 45, men should have a rectal sonogram, and if positive, a DRE.
3. Beginning at age 50, men should have a prostate-specific antigen (PSA) followed by a DRE.
4. Beginning at age 60, men should have a PSA followed, if positive, by a prostate biopsy.

94. The client diagnosed with gestational diabetes delivered a 10-pound 5-ounce infant. Which is a **priority** for the nursery nurse to monitor?
    1. Failure to latch on to the breast during feeding.
    2. Jaundice and clay-colored stools.
    3. Parchment-like skin and lack of lanugo.
    4. Low blood glucose readings.

95. Which steps should the nurse provide clients choosing to perform breast self-examination (BSE) according to the American Cancer Society (ACS) guidelines? **Rank in order of performance.**
    1. Lie flat on the bed with a rolled towel placed under the scapula; perform palpation of each breast.
    2. Pinch each nipple to see if fluid can be expressed.
    3. With the breasts exposed, stand in front of a mirror and examine the breasts from the front and each side.
    4. In the shower, soap the breasts, and perform palpation in a systematic manner on each breast.
    5. Find a private place where the self-examination can be performed.

96. Which should the nurse teach the client regarding Breast Health Awareness (BHA) according to the American Cancer Society (ACS). **Select all that apply.**
    1. Women at high risk should talk to the HCP about when to have a mammogram.
    2. Beginning at age 45, the client should have a yearly mammogram.
    3. The client should perform a breast self-examination (BSE) bimonthly.
    4. The client should get a sonogram of the breasts semiannually.
    5. The client should have an MRI of the breasts every 5 years.

## Breast Disorders

1. 1. This is symptomatic of benign fibrocystic disease, but follow-up is always needed if the lumps do not go away when the hormone levels change.
   2. Some practitioners suggest eliminating caffeine and chocolate from the diet if the breasts become tender from the changes, but there is no research supporting this to be effective in controlling the discomfort associated with fibrocystic breasts.
   3. The American Cancer Society (2015) no longer recommends breast self-examination (BSE) for all women, but it is advisable for women with known breast conditions to perform BSE monthly to detect potential cancer.
   4. The client may need a breast biopsy for potential breast cancer at some point, but breast cancer develops when there is an alteration in the DNA of a cell.

   **TEST-TAKING HINT:** The test taker could eliminate option "1" because of the clause "does not require follow-up." The question is asking about self-care, and only two options—"2" and "3"—involve the client doing something. The test taker should choose between these.

2. Correct answers are 2 and 5.
   1. General anesthesia is used for either procedure.
   2. The client should understand the treatment regimen for follow-up care. A lumpectomy requires follow-up with radiation therapy to the breast and then systemic chemotherapy. In a modified radical mastectomy, radiation therapy is not always required, but systemic chemotherapy is the usual treatment (Komen. org, 2011).
   3. A lumpectomy removes only the tumor and a small amount of tissue surrounding the tumor; reconstruction is not needed.
   4. A history of breast cancer in the family is immaterial because this client *has* breast cancer.
   5. If the cancer is in its early stages, this regimen has results equal to those with a modified radical mastectomy (Komen. org, 2011).

**TEST-TAKING HINT:** The test taker should use the nursing process to answer this question and select an assessment intervention, which eliminates option "3" as a correct answer. Option "1" uses the word "afraid," which is an assumption; therefore, this option could be eliminated.

3. 1. A partial mastectomy or excisional biopsy is a type of surgery on this side of the body. Pressure on the incision should be limited until the client is released by the HCP to perform normal daily activities.
   2. This is providing the client with false hope. Cancer cells characteristically move easily in the lymph or bloodstream to other parts of the body. Microscopic disease cannot be determined by the naked eye.
   3. A client after a mastectomy might be discharged with a closed wound suction evacuator (Hemovac) drain, but a partial mastectomy should not require one.
   4. The breast has not been removed; reconstruction is not needed.

**TEST-TAKING HINT:** If the test taker did not know this answer, option "1" is information provided to any client after surgery on the upper chest or arm.

4. 1. Unless there is a personal history of breast cancer or strong family history, clinical breast examinations are not recommended for average risk women at any age (American Cancer Society, 2015).
   2. If the client is going to perform breast self-examination (BSE), it should begin at age 18. The ACS no longer includes monthly BSE as part of its guidelines.
   3. The ACS recommends a yearly mammogram for the early detection of breast cancer beginning at age 45 to age 54 and approximately every 2 years at the age of 55 and older. Before age 45 and after age 54 it should be a discussion between the woman and her HCP to determine if more frequent mammograms are warranted. A mammogram can detect disease that will not be large enough to feel.
   4. Breast sonograms are performed to diagnose specific breast disease when a screening mammogram has shown a suspicious area.

**TEST-TAKING HINT:** This is a knowledge-based question. The test taker might be swayed by the option about BSE, but the age must be considered.

5. 1. This is done for reconstruction of a breast or augmentation of breast size, but it is not a TRAM flap procedure, which uses the client's own tissue.
   2. The TRAM flap procedure is one in which the client's own tissue is used to form the new breast. Abdominal tissue, fat, skin, and blood vessels are moved under the skin to rebuild the breast.
   3. The plastic surgeon can rebuild a nipple from pigmented skin donor sites or can tattoo the nipple in place.
   4. This is true of saline implants but not of TRAM flaps.

**TEST-TAKING HINT:** If the test taker is taking a standard pencil-and-paper test and is not familiar with this procedure, then skipping the question and returning to it at a later time is advisable. Another question might give a clue about the procedure. This is not possible on the NCLEX-RN® computerized examination.

6. 1. Most women diagnosed with breast cancer have no family history of the disease. Specific genes—*BRCA-1* and *BRCA-2*—implicated in the development of breast cancer have been identified, but most women with breast cancer do not have these genes.
   2. Approximately 1,000 men are diagnosed every year with breast cancer, but as with women, it can occur at any age. Breast cancer in men frequently goes undetected because men consider this a woman's disease.
   3. Mammograms can detect breast cancer earlier than BSE and are the current recommendation by the American Cancer Society.
   4. The greatest risk factor for developing breast cancer is being female. The second greatest risk factor is being older. By age 80, one in every eight women develops breast cancer.

**TEST-TAKING HINT:** The test taker cannot overlook the age when it is given in a question. "Senior citizen's center" should alert the test taker to the older age group. The test taker should decide what age has to do with the answer.

7. 1. A sentinel node biopsy is a procedure in which a radioactive dye is injected into the tumor and then traced by instrumentation and color to try to identify the exact lymph nodes the tumor could have shed into. The sentinel node is removed and tested for cancer cells (National Cancer Institute, 2019).
   2. This is the older procedure in which the surgeon removed the nodes thought to drain the tumor. There was no way of knowing if the surgeon was actually removing the affected nodes.
   3. The purpose of the procedure is not to rely on guesswork in determining the extent of tumor involvement.
   4. Microscopic disease cannot be seen by the naked eye.

**TEST-TAKING HINT:** The test taker could eliminate options "3" and "4" if aware of the *sentinel* definition, which means "to watch over as a sentry." This might lead the test taker to determine what specific areas would have to be identified.

8. 1. Waiting until the baby is born allows the cancer to continue to develop and spread. This might be an option if the client were in the third trimester, but not at this early stage.
   2. A modified radical mastectomy is recommended for this client because the client is not able to begin radiation or chemotherapy, which are part of the regimen for a lumpectomy or wedge resection. Many breast cancers developed during pregnancy are hormone sensitive and have the ideal grounds for growth. The tumor should be removed as soon as possible.
   3. Radiation therapy cannot be delivered to a pregnant client because of possible harm to the fetus.
   4. Chemotherapy is not given to the client while she is pregnant because of potential harm to the fetus.

**TEST-TAKING HINT:** The test taker should eliminate options "3" and "4" because of potential harm to the fetus but also because each option has the word "only." There are very few "onlys" in health care.

9. 1. A client 4 years post-mastectomy should be finished with adjuvant therapy, which lasts from 6 months to 1 year.
   2. The client may have received doxorubicin (Adriamycin), an antineoplastic agent that is a cardiotoxic medication, but knowing this will not change the tests performed or preparation for the tests.

3. The nurse should post a message at the head of the client's bed to not use the right arm for blood pressures or laboratory draws. This client is at risk for lymphedema, and this is a lymphedema precaution.
4. The chest wall is sometimes involved in breast cancer, but the most important intervention is to prevent harm to the client.

**TEST-TAKING HINT: The question is asking for an intervention common in the health-care industry. There are many breast cancer survivors with unrelated problems and comorbidities, but the nurse must still be aware of the lingering needs of the client.**

10. Correct answers are 1, 2, and 5.
    1. It is a common instruction for any client after surgery to notify the HCP if a fever develops. This could indicate a postoperative infection.
    2. The client after a mastectomy is at risk for lymphedema in the affected arm because the lymph nodes are removed during the surgery. The client should protect the arm from injury and carry heavy objects with the opposite arm.
    3. The client can attend church services and large gatherings. This client had surgery, not chemotherapy, which would make the client immunosuppressed.
    4. The client should be taught arm-climbing exercises before leaving the hospital to facilitate maintaining range of motion.
    5. The client has developed a malignancy in one breast and is at a higher risk for developing another tumor in the remaining breast area.

**TEST-TAKING HINT: The test taker must determine if the option of keeping the arm still is recommended. Most postoperative recommendations require the client to move as much as possible.**

11. 1. This is restating the client's feelings and is a therapeutic response.
    2. This is not recognizing the client's concerns and putting the nurse's expectations on the spouse.
    3. This is problem-solving and could be offered, but the therapeutic response is to restate the client's feelings and encourage a conversation.
    4. The client may know this is true. The nurse is telling the client she has no reason for her feelings. Feelings are what they are and should be accepted as such.

**TEST-TAKING HINT: When the question asks for a therapeutic response, the test taker should choose an option encouraging the client to verbalize her feelings.**

12. 1. The social worker assists clients in finding a nursing home placement and financial arrangements and does some work with clients to discuss feelings, but this is not the best referral.
    2. CanSurmount volunteers work with all types of clients diagnosed with cancer, not just clients diagnosed with breast cancer.
    3. Reach to Recovery is a specific referral program for clients diagnosed with breast cancer.
    4. I Can Cope is a cancer education program for all clients diagnosed with cancer and their significant others.

**TEST-TAKING HINT: The question asks for the most appropriate referral, and the test taker should choose the one specific to breast cancer.**

## Pelvic Floor Relaxation Disorders

13. 1. The client should be assessed for allergies to latex as a result of the composition of the pessary.
    2. These clients frequently have incontinence, which is assessed before recommending a pessary.
    3. A pessary is manually inserted to keep a prolapsed uterus in place. Asking about a bowel movement is not an appropriate question.
    4. This is a symptom experienced by a client diagnosed with a cystocele.

**TEST-TAKING HINT: If the test taker has no idea what the answer is, then the test taker should apply Maslow's hierarchy of needs, which in this question is safety. Only option "1" addresses a safety issue. Allergies are a safety issue.**

14. 1. Perineal care is given every shift or as needed.
    2. The client may have an indwelling catheter for 2 to 4 days postoperative but not for a month.
    3. A pessary is used in place of surgery.
    4. The client should be taught how to perform Kegel exercises to strengthen the muscles.

**TEST-TAKING HINT: When selecting a correct answer, the test taker should always look at the adjectives, especially numbers such as four in option "1" or one in option "2."**

15. Correct answers are 1, 2, 3, and 4.
    1. A rectocele causes the rectum to be pouched upward, causing rectal pressure.
    2. When the rectum pushes against the posterior wall of the vagina, the result is flatus.
    3. Clients diagnosed with a rectocele experience fecal incontinence.
    4. Clients diagnosed with a rectocele frequently are constipated.
    5. A client diagnosed with a rectocele does not experience urinary frequency.

**TEST-TAKING HINT:** The test taker should learn the terms. If the test taker does not know the answer, the test taker can eliminate urinary frequency because it is different from the other options. It refers to the urinary tract, whereas the others refer to bowel elimination.

16. Correct answers are 3 and 5.
    1. There is no reason to limit oral intake or to decrease voiding.
    2. The client should be eating a high-fiber diet to prevent constipation.
    3. Stool softeners and laxatives are used to prevent and treat constipation, which is common with a rectocele. Because of the positioning of the rectum, the stool can stay in the rectal pouch, causing constipation (American Society of Colon and Rectal Surgeons, n.d.).
    4. Sitz baths are not used to treat a rectocele.
    5. Pelvic floor exercises, also known as Kegel exercises, can strengthen the pelvic floor muscles to decrease symptoms.

**TEST-TAKING HINT:** The test taker knowledgeable of medical terminology could eliminate option "1," which has the word "voiding" because "rectocele" refers to the rectum.

17. 1. Sonograms and pelvic examinations are used to diagnose cystoceles.
    2. Kegel exercises strengthen the pelvic floor muscles.
    3. Clients diagnosed with cystoceles frequently have urinary incontinence when they cough, sneeze, laugh, lift heavy items, or make sudden jarring motions.
    4. Clients diagnosed with cystoceles may have sexual intercourse unless contraindicated by another medical reason.

**TEST-TAKING HINT:** This type of question is confusing to test takers because the correct option provides incorrect information. Most of the time absolutes such as "never," "only," and "always" make the option incorrect. Option "4"

has an absolute—"never"—but it is the correct answer because all of the other options contain correct information the client has learned.

18. 1. Orthostatic hypotension is not a surgery-specific complication.
    2. Atelectasis is a complication of general anesthesia, not an A & P repair.
    3. An Allen test is a physical examination evaluating the arterial blood supply to the radial and ulnar arteries.
    4. Assessing for deep vein thrombosis (DVT) is performed on all clients having a vaginal hysterectomy. After any surgery requiring the client to be placed in the lithotomy position, the client should be assessed for DVT. These clients are at a higher risk for this complication.

**TEST-TAKING HINT:** The test taker must have knowledge of this surgical procedure to be able to answer this question. A good choice is to choose an option assessed for most immobile clients.

19. Correct answers are 1 and 5.
    1. The client should report any bright red vaginal bleeding or bleeding that soaks more than one sanitary pad an hour.
    2. Clients should rest and not start a vigorous exercise program until the surgeon gives permission.
    3. Clients should avoid prolonged sitting to prevent blood clots.
    4. Clients should avoid taking baths to help prevent infection of the incision site.
    5. The client should drink 6 to 8 glasses of water a day to avoid constipation.

**TEST-TAKING HINT:** When the test taker is selecting possible correct answers, the test taker should carefully consider the descriptive words. In option "2," the adjective "vigorous" should cause the test taker to eliminate it, and in option "3" the words "6 hours" should help eliminate it.

20. 1. Observation is assessment, which cannot be delegated.
    2. This nursing task can be delegated, but evaluation is the responsibility of the nurse.
    3. Teaching cannot be delegated.
    4. Teaching cannot be delegated.

**TEST-TAKING HINT:** The RN cannot delegate assessment, teaching, evaluation, or an unstable client to a UAP.

21. 1. Urinary retention is a complication of a vaginal hysterectomy.
2. Nerve damage is a possible complication of improper positioning during surgery, but the client is "post" surgery.
3. Clients after a total abdominal hysterectomy are at risk for intestinal obstruction.
4. An imbalance of fluid is a complication of several surgeries, not specifically a total abdominal hysterectomy.

TEST-TAKING HINT: When the test taker does not know the answer, the test taker should consider the similarities and the differences in surgeries. A total abdominal hysterectomy has complications similar to all types of abdominal surgeries.

22. 1. Uterine prolapse is not caused by constipation; it is caused by a weakening of the pelvic muscles. It is a protrusion of the uterus through the vagina. It can pull on the vaginal wall, bladder, and rectum.
2. There are multiple treatment modalities for uterine prolapse. The selection of treatment is determined by the degree of the prolapse and the medical history of the client.
3. The protrusion from the vagina can be seen in some cases, but this is not so with all clients.
4. Symptoms can be aggravated by coughing, sneezing, lifting heavy objects, standing for prolonged periods, and climbing stairs.

TEST-TAKING HINT: The test taker should eliminate options containing words such as "only," "never," "always," "all," or "most of the time." If the test taker does not have a clue, "uterine" is not in the same body system as constipation, so option "1" can be eliminated.

23. Correct answers are 2 and 5.
1. Pessaries need to be changed to prevent complications.
2. Clients do need to clean the pessary routinely.
3. Pessaries are not only inserted in surgery, but also in such places as an HCP's office.
4. Hormone cream may be used and prescribed by the HCP.
5. Routine follow-up visits are required to evaluate the health of the vaginal tissue.

TEST-TAKING HINT: The test taker should realize any removable device inserted into the body requires routine changing at some time; therefore, option "1" can be eliminated. Option "4" is a medication and a pessary is a device, so option "4" can be eliminated.

24. 1. Estrogen, a hormone, changes the pelvic floor muscles and lining of the uterus and may help improve a pelvic relaxation disorder.
2. Dinoprostone (Cervidil), a cervical ripening agent, is used to prepare the cervix for the delivery of a baby. It causes the cervix to shorten, soften, and dilate.
3. Progesterone, a hormone, is given for implantation of a fertilized ovum.
4. Oxytocin (Pitocin), an oxytocic agent, causes the uterus to contract. It is used during the labor and delivery process.

TEST-TAKING HINT: Options "2," "3," and "4" are similar because they are all used during pregnancy or delivery. If the test taker doesn't have a clue as to the correct answer, the test taker should attempt to determine what answer is different from all the others.

## Uterine Disorders

25. 1. A vaginal examination does not provide a definitive diagnosis to determine the cause of the pain.
2. A pregnancy test is not usually ordered unless the client has a reason to think she may be pregnant. Pregnancy temporarily alleviates the symptoms of endometriosis because neither ovulation nor menses occur during pregnancy.
3. There is a high incidence of endometriosis among women with no biological children (nulliparity) and those having children later in life. The most common way to diagnose this condition is through an exploratory laparoscopy.
4. The ovaries lie deep within the pelvic cavity. Some form of abdominal procedure must be performed, such as laparoscopy, to reach the ovaries. However, the symptoms are not those of an ovarian cyst.

TEST-TAKING HINT: The test taker could eliminate answer option "1" because "diagnosis" is in the stem. The stem is asking for a procedure providing a definitive diagnosis. Option "2" could be eliminated because, if the client is menstruating (*dysmenorrhea* means "painful menstruation"), then the client is usually not pregnant.

26. 1. Risk factors for cancer of the cervix include sexual activity before the age of 20 years; multiple sexual partners; early childbearing; exposure to the human papillomavirus; HIV infection; smoking; and nutritional deficits of folates, beta carotene, and vitamin C.
2. High-fat diets place clients at risk for some cancers but not for cervical cancer. The use of birth control pills may allow increased sexual freedom because of the protection from pregnancy, but it does not increase the risk for cancer of the cervix.
3. Infections with the human papillomavirus are a risk factor for cancer of the cervix.
4. Having a yearly Pap smear increases the chance of detecting cellular changes early, but it does not decrease the risk of developing cancer.

**TEST-TAKING HINT:** The test taker could discard option "4" as a possible answer because it is a yearly test for the early detection of cervical cancer, not a risk factor.

27. 1. Diffuse, watery, foul-smelling discharge occurs at a much later stage.
2. At this stage the client is asymptomatic and cancer has been determined by a Pap smear.
3. Dyspareunia is painful sexual intercourse; the client is asymptomatic.
4. Intense itching occurs with vaginal yeast infections.

**TEST-TAKING HINT:** The test taker could either choose option "2" because it is the least presenting symptom or discard it. Staging for all cancers starts with "0" or "1," indicating the least detectable cancer.

28. Correct answers are 1, 2, and 5.
1. Brachytherapy is the direct implantation of radioactive seeds through the vagina into the uterus. The client should be in a private room at the end of the hall to prevent radiation exposure to the rest of the unit.
2. Nurses wear a dosimeter registering the amount of radiation they have been exposed to. When a certain level is reached, the nurse is no longer allowed to care for clients undergoing internal radiation therapy.
3. Visitors are limited while the radiation is in place.
4. In this case, spending extra time with a client is not done. The nurse only does what must be done and leaves the room.

5. The nuclear medicine technician will assist with the placement of the implants and will deliver the implants in a lead-lined container. The technician will also scan any items (linens and wastes) leaving the room for radiation contamination.

**TEST-TAKING HINT:** This is an alternate-type question, which requires the test taker to select more than one correct answer. The test taker must select all the correct answers to receive credit for the question.

29. 1. This client is at risk for cancer of the ovary and uterus because of advancing age, regardless of sexual activity, and should see an HCP yearly.
2. Hormone replacement therapy (HRT) is not recommended for most postmenopausal clients because research has shown HRT increases the risk of myocardial infarctions and cerebrovascular accidents (strokes).
3. This is a therapeutic response, and the client did not state a feeling.
4. The client should have a yearly clinical examination of the breasts and pelvic area for the detection of cancer.

**TEST-TAKING HINT:** If the stem is not asking for a therapeutic response, then factual information should be provided to the client. This eliminates option "3" as a possible answer.

30. Correct answers are 2 and 5.
1. Clients diagnosed with cancer of the uterus have the ovaries removed to reduce hormone production. The client will not be taking HRT.
2. Pelvic rest means nothing is placed in the vagina. The client does not need a tampon at this time, but sexual intercourse should be avoided until the vaginal area has healed.
3. The sitting position a client assumes when driving a vehicle places stress on the lower abdomen. The client should wait until the HCP releases her to drive.
4. The client should not have any vaginal bleeding.
5. Clients should be instructed about signs of complications that should be reported including fever, severe pain, and urinary burning or frequency.

**TEST-TAKING HINT:** The test taker should apply basic postoperative concepts when answering questions and realize bleeding is not expected postoperatively and safety should always be addressed.

31. 1. This pain indicates metastasis in the retroperitoneal region. If caught early, a complete hysterectomy is usually the only therapy recommended. This type of pain indicates the cancer is advanced and the prognosis is poor.
 2. This pain indicates the cancer is in the retroperitoneal region and the prognosis is poor.
 3. Pain is not part of the treatment of cancer. Surgery may cause pain, but most treatments do not.
 4. Radiation therapy does not always result in pain; it depends on the area irradiated.

**TEST-TAKING HINT:** Option "4" has the absolute word "always" and should be eliminated as a correct answer. The stem is describing symptoms in regions other than the lower pelvis, so an educated choice is option "2."

32. 1. The client taking a narcotic medication should be placed on a bowel regimen, but this client would not be prescribed morphine, a narcotic medication.
 2. A tepid bath for 30 to 45 minutes is not appropriate because the lukewarm water gets cold. A heating pad to the abdomen sometimes helps with the pain.
 3. The medication of choice for mild to moderate dysmenorrhea is an NSAID. NSAIDs cause gastrointestinal upset and should be taken with food.
 4. This may be an option eventually, but the stem did not give an age nor state the client has decided she does not want to get pregnant.

**TEST-TAKING HINT:** The test taker should not read into the question. Option "4" is only correct when more information is provided. The test taker must know about the scales used to rate pain, nausea, or depression. The client's report of midrange symptoms does not indicate the need for routine narcotic administration.

33. 1. Benign fibroid tumors in the uterus cause the client to bleed longer with a heavier flow, not miss periods.
 2. Many women delay surgery until anemia has occurred from the heavy menstrual flow. A symptom of anemia is shortness of breath.
 3. The number of pregnancies does not matter at this time; the client has a different problem.
 4. The pain is in the pelvic region to the low back, where the uterus lies.

**TEST-TAKING HINT:** This is a high-level question requiring the test taker to make several judgments before arriving at the answer. First, the test taker must decide what happens when a client has fibroid tumors and then which symptoms the client will exhibit.

34. 1. The nurse does not require an order to teach. Teaching is an independent nursing function.
 2. The nurse can request the dietitian to include yogurt in the client's calorie restrictions without an order.
 3. If the HCP has ordered an IV antibiotic, then there is no reason to request a change to an oral route.
 4. Female clients on antibiotics are at risk for killing the good bacteria, which keep yeast infections in check. This is especially true in clients diagnosed with diabetes. *L. acidophilus,* a probiotic, is a yeast replacement medication.

**TEST-TAKING HINT:** The test taker must be aware of independent nursing functions. This eliminates options "1" and "2."

35. Correct answers are 1, 2, 4, and 5.
 1. The UAP can empty the indwelling catheter and record the output.
 2. This is an appropriate assignment.
 3. Monitoring a peri-pad count is done to determine if the client is bleeding excessively; the nurse should do this as part of the assessment.
 4. All personnel should encourage the client to ambulate.
 5. This is an appropriate assignment.

**TEST-TAKING HINT:** The RN cannot delegate assessment. The nurse must be aware of the tasks a UAP can perform.

36. 1. This can be done to determine specific problems resulting from the specific side effects of the medication, but it is not the first action. The nurse can ask general assessment questions to determine how the client is tolerating the treatments.
 2. The systemic side effects of chemotherapy are not always apparent, and the development of stomatitis can be extremely distressing for the client. The nurse should assess the client's tolerance to treatments.
 3. The biologic response modifier filgrastim (Neupogen) is administered if the white blood cell count is low. The nurse assesses the WBC count and then obtains an order from the HCP.
 4. This is an appropriate action, but not before assessing physical problems.

**TEST-TAKING HINT:** When prioritizing nursing interventions, the test taker should apply the nursing process, and assessment is the first step.

## Ovarian Disorders

37. 1. The client has symptoms of an ovarian cyst, usually diagnosed by a pelvic sonogram.
    2. The client has abdominal pain, not back or neurological pain, which is when a lumbar puncture is performed.
    3. The appendix is in the right lower abdomen, not the left.
    4. Ovarian cysts are fluid-filled sacs located on the surface of the ovary. A lower pelvic sonogram is the preferred diagnostic tool. It is not invasive and usually not painful.

**TEST-TAKING HINT:** The test taker could eliminate options "2" and "3" by using knowledge of basic anatomy and physiology. The age of the client places this client in the typical age range for a benign ovarian cyst; before age 29 years, 98% of ovarian cysts are benign.

38. 1. The ovaries are anatomically positioned deep within the pelvis, and because of this, clinical manifestations of cancer are vague and nonspecific. Clinical manifestations include increased abdominal girth, pelvic pressure, indigestion, bloating, flatulence, and pelvic and leg pain. Increasing abdomen size as a result of the accumulation of fluid is the most common clinical manifestation. Many women ignore the clinical manifestations because they are so nonspecific.
    2. Regular gynecological examinations are recommended, but this is an advanced disease.
    3. Dysmenorrhea is not a risk factor for developing ovarian cancer. Any enlarged ovary should be evaluated, especially if the client is postmenopausal, when the ovaries shrink in size.
    4. A family history of breast cancer is a cause for the client to be assessed regularly for breast and ovarian cancer, but this is a late disease.

**TEST-TAKING HINT:** "Stage IV" should help the test taker to eliminate options "2" and "4" because this client has advanced disease and it is hoped regular checkups find problems early.

39. 1. All cysts do not become cancerous; 98% of ovarian cysts in clients younger than age 29 are benign, whereas in women older than age 50, about half are benign.
    2. Any abnormal ovary that cannot be diagnosed with a transvaginal ultrasound should be examined laparoscopically.
    3. Any time the client has surgery, she should be prepared to experience some pain. This is a false statement and could cause a breach in the nurse-client relationship.
    4. This is a therapeutic statement and the client is asking for information.

**TEST-TAKING HINT:** The test taker should read the stem of the question carefully. Option "1" has a form of absolute, "eventually will become," so it can be eliminated. Option "3" is a false statement. Option "4" is a therapeutic response and the stem asks the nurse to provide information.

40. 1. The client has low-grade cancer occurring in a small percentage of ovarian tumors. The affected ovary usually is removed, and the client may or may not require additional treatment. Women with this type of tumor are usually younger than age 40 years.
    2. The tumor is classified as cancer. The follow-up care is not as extensive because of the characteristics the tumor displays.
    3. Ovarian low malignant potential tumors have abnormal cells in the tissues covering the ovary. These tumors are low-grade cancers with fewer propensities for metastasis than most ovarian cancers (National Cancer Institute, 2018).
    4. This client has a better prognosis than 85% of clients diagnosed with ovarian cancer.

**TEST-TAKING HINT:** The test taker could eliminate option "4" because "low malignancy potential" and "poor prognosis" do not match. The statement in option "1" says the client does not have cancer but will need therapy for cancer, so the test taker could eliminate this option.

41. 1. This statement would be appropriate if not for the abdominal girth change. This should alert the nurse to some internal reason for the change in girth. Ascites causes a change in abdominal girth.

2. Ovarian cancer has vague clinical manifestations of abdominal discomfort, but increasing abdominal girth is the most common symptom. If the client has had the ovaries removed, then the nurse could assess for another cause.

3. This could be an assessment for a peptic ulcer, but ulcers do not cause increasing abdominal girth.

4. This is a question to determine if the client has gastroesophageal reflux, but this does not cause an increased waist size.

**TEST-TAKING HINT:** The test taker must notice all the symptoms the client is reporting. Flatulence and bloating could be associated with a number of problems, but these clinical manifestations, along with increased waist size, narrow the possibilities.

42. 1. An antidepressant may be needed at some time, but at this point the nurse should offer time, interest, and encouragement for the client to discuss the feeling of having cancer.

2. CanSurmount volunteers are extremely helpful in talking about having cancer with the client, but they do not provide counseling. The programs work based on the fact a cancer survivor after going through treatment can relate to the client beginning treatment.

3. **The nurse should plan to spend time with the client and allow the client to discuss the feelings of having cancer, dying, fear of the treatments, and any other concerns.**

4. The client will need to complete an advance directive, but this action does not address the client's grieving process.

**TEST-TAKING HINT:** The test taker could eliminate option "2" because a client is not referred to a volunteer for counseling. Only one option directly addresses the problem and requires the nurse to interact with the client.

43. 1. An absolute neutrophil count of 3,500 indicates the client has sufficient mature white blood cells, or granulocytes, to act as a defense against infections.

2. A platelet count of 150,000 is within normal range $(150 \times 10^3 [1,000] = 150,000)$. Thrombocytopenia is less than 100,000.

3. A red blood cell count of 5,000,000 is within normal limits $(5 \times 10^6 [1,000,000] = 5,000,000)$.

4. A normal urinalysis contains one to two WBCs. A report of 100 WBCs indicates the presence of an infection. A clean voided specimen should be obtained, and a urine culture should be done. This client should be prescribed antibiotics immediately.

**TEST-TAKING HINT:** The test taker should memorize normal values for common laboratory tests. Urine will not have a large number of white blood cells unless there is a pathological process occurring. The kidneys filter the blood but do not process the destruction of blood cells.

44. 1. The radiation markings on a client are there to guide the technician to irradiate only the area within the marks. The marks must remain until the client has completed the treatments.

2. Radiation therapy is administered in fractionated (divided) doses to allow for the regeneration of normal cells. Cancer cells do not regenerate as rapidly as normal cells.

3. There are many medications prescribed for cancer or treatment-induced nausea. The client should notify the HCP if adequate relief is not obtained.

4. Cancer treatments frequently interfere with the client's appetite, but supporting the nutritional status of the client is important.

**TEST-TAKING HINT:** The question is an "except" question. All options except one will be statements indicating the client does understand the teaching. If the test taker missed the information making this an "except" question, finding two options with correct answers might clue the test taker to reread the stem.

45. 1. This is appropriate information if the client is in her mid- to late-30s and has completed her family, but this is not discussing early detection of ovarian cancer.

2. A transvaginal ultrasound is a sonogram in which the sonogram probe is inserted into the vagina and sound waves are directed toward the ovaries. The CA-125 tumor marker is elevated in several cancers. It is nonspecific, but coupled with the sonogram, can provide information about ovarian cancer for early diagnosis.

3. Yearly MRI scans will not provide the information the two tests will, and every 12 months is too long an interval.
4. A flexible sigmoidoscopy provides the HCP with a visual examination of the sigmoid colon, not the ovaries.

**TEST-TAKING HINT:** The test taker could eliminate option "4" because of the anatomical site and option "3" because of the time factor. The test taker should ask, "If looking for early detection, at what interval should the client see the HCP?"

46. 1. This diet is appropriate for a client diagnosed with diverticulitis.
2. This diet applies to a client diagnosed with coronary artery disease and hypertension.
3. The client is not placed on a specific diet, but it is always a good recommendation to include fruits and vegetables in the diet.
4. There is no reason to limit the consistency of the foods consumed to full liquids.

**TEST-TAKING HINT:** The test taker should recognize option "3" as a recommended diet for all clients without a specific disease process limiting the types of foods consumed.

47. 1. Research has shown the use of talcum powder perineally increases the risk for developing ovarian cancer, although there is no explanation known for this occurrence (Zuckerman & Shapiro, 2019). Other risk factors include a high-fat diet, nulliparity, infertility, older age (70 to 80 years), mumps before menarche, and family history of ovarian cancer.
2. Nurses should never encourage a high-fat diet.
3. Only clients in a high-risk category should have routine sonograms. The time frame for the high-risk group of clients is 6 months. This is not a primary intervention; early detection is secondary intervention.
4. This alerts the client to participate in activities detecting cancer early, a secondary intervention.

**TEST-TAKING HINT:** The test taker could eliminate options "3" and "4" because of the word "primary" in the stem. Option "2" could be eliminated because of the recommendation of a high-fat diet.

48. Correct answers are 1, 3, 4, and 5.
1. All clients after surgery are at risk for developing DVT, and an enlarged, tender calf is a clinical manifestation of DVT.

2. The client should be turned and encouraged to cough and deep breathe at least every 2 hours.
3. Clients after surgery should be assessed for pain on a pain scale and by observing for physiological markers indicating pain.
4. Sequential compression hose are used prophylactically to prevent DVT.
5. The client should be assessed for the return of bowel sounds.

**TEST-TAKING HINT:** Option "2" has a time frame in it, and the test taker should ask if the time frame is correct for the intervention.

## Prostate Disorders

49. 1. The American Cancer Society recommends all men have a yearly PSA blood level test, followed by a DRE beginning at age 50. Men in the high-risk group, including all African American men, should begin at age 45.
2. A biannual (every 6 months) examination is not recommended.
3. Alkaline phosphatase levels are performed on men with known prostate cancer to determine bone involvement. This is not a screening test.
4. This test is done if the client has clinical manifestations of prostatitis.

**TEST-TAKING HINT:** The nurse must be aware of recommended screening guidelines for a number of diseases. The test taker should carefully look at the time frame for the tests and the age of the client.

50. 1. Urgency and frequency are obstructive symptoms and are late clinical manifestations.
2. Retrograde ejaculation occurs when sperm are ejaculated into the urine; it occurs in some cases of male infertility.
3. Low back pain and hip pain are clinical manifestations of metastasis to the bone and are late symptoms.
4. In early-stage prostate cancer, the man will not be aware of the disease. Early detection is achieved by screening for cancer.

**TEST-TAKING HINT:** The test taker should notice the word "early" in the stem of the question and choose the option with the least amount of symptoms.

51. 1. Radiation therapy is considered aggressive therapy and is not recommended for the older client unless needed to alleviate pain from bony metastasis.
    2. A radical prostatectomy with lymph node dissection is extensive surgery and only recommended for clients with a life expectancy of greater than 10 years.
    3. Gonadotropin-releasing hormone agonists (GnRH) such as leuprolide (Lupron) lower the amount of testosterone made by the testicles and slows the growth of the tumor. Some men with a life expectancy of fewer than 10 years choose not to treat cancer at all and will usually die from causes other than prostate cancer.
    4. Penile implants do not treat prostate cancer. Sexual functioning may or may not be impaired, depending on whether the client is treated surgically by radical prostatectomy. If so, then the client may be prescribed Viagra or Cialis. Eighty-year-old men are not candidates for a radical prostatectomy.

**TEST-TAKING HINT: The test taker should notice the age of the client. When an age is provided in the question, it is significant. Older clients do not tolerate many treatments well, so the test taker should choose the least invasive treatment.**

52. 1. The nurse should assess the client's normal voiding pattern before taking any action.
    2. This is a good intervention, but it comes after assessment.
    3. The Valsalva maneuver will help the client to empty the bladder, but assessment comes before teaching.
    4. Determining the client's normal voiding patterns provides a baseline for the nurse and client to use when setting goals.

**TEST-TAKING HINT: Assessment is the first step of the nursing process. In any question requiring the test taker to choose the first action, an answer option with the words "check," "assess," or "determine" should be considered as a possible answer.**

53. 1. Elevating a surgical site and applying ice will reduce edema to the area.
    2. The testes have been excised to remove the majority of male hormones. Replacing the hormones negates the purpose of the surgery.

3. Sperm banking is encouraged for younger men wanting children in the future. Prostate cancer is a cancer diagnosed in older men, and sperm banking is not normally recommended.
4. Bilateral orchiectomy will render the client impotent but not with ejaculation dysfunction.

**TEST-TAKING HINT: The test taker should try to match the procedure to the answer option. The procedure removes hormone-producing ability, so option "2" could be eliminated because it reverses the effects of the procedure.**

54. 1. This hormone will suppress the production of male hormones, and the client will not function sexually as usual.
    2. The client may have hot flashes because these drugs increase hypothalamic activity, which stimulates the thermoregulatory centers of the body.
    3. The medication decreases the growth rate of the cancer, but it does not cure the cancer.
    4. There are side effects with all medications. These medications can cause gynecomastia, hot flashes, cardiovascular effects, and decreased sexual functioning. The LHRH agonists have fewer side effects than the estrogens.

**TEST-TAKING HINT: The test taker could eliminate options "3" and "4" because of the promise of no side effects or a cure.**

55. 1. This intervention addresses the prostate cancer but not the metastatic process of bone involvement.
    2. There is no reason to keep the foot of the bed elevated.
    3. Bone metastasis is very painful, and the client should be placed on a scheduled regimen of pain medication. Pain medication slows peristalsis and causes constipation. The client should be placed on a routine bowel management program to prevent impactions.
    4. This does not address the metastasis to the bone.

**TEST-TAKING HINT: The test taker must decide which intervention addresses both the cancer and the metastasis to the bone. Only one option does this.**

56. 1. Cryotherapy involves placing freezing probes into the prostate to freeze the cancer cells. An indwelling catheter is placed into the urethra, and warm water is circulated through the catheter to try to prevent the urethra from freezing. If the urethra scars, then the lumen will constrict, causing retention of urine.
2. Ejaculation difficulties are caused by obstruction from tumor growth.
3. Bone marrow suppression is caused by radiation or chemotherapy.
4. Cryotherapy does not cause chronic vomiting or diarrhea.

**TEST-TAKING HINT:** The test taker should dissect the word "cryotherapy." *Cryo-* means "to freeze," so cryotherapy indicates some form of cold therapy. Then the test taker should decide what cold therapy could cause to happen in the area being treated.

57. 1. Pain does not have priority over a fluid and electrolyte imbalance.
2. There is no dressing for a transurethral resection. The body cavity is entered through the penis.
3. Early ambulation prevents several complications, but the immediate complication is electrolyte imbalance and fluid overload.
4. With irrigation of the surgical site through the indwelling three-way catheter to prevent blood clots, fluids may be absorbed through the open surgical site and retained. This can lead to fluid volume overload and electrolyte imbalance (hyponatremia).

**TEST-TAKING HINT:** This client is 8 hours postoperative, so the test taker could eliminate preventing DVT (option "3"). Option "2" could be eliminated if the test taker looks at the surgical approach described in the procedure. Pain is a priority, but the test taker should read to see if another option has a higher priority.

58. 200 mL/hr.
IV pumps work on the principle of the number of milliliters per hour to infuse, and unless otherwise specified, IVPB medications are infused over a 30-minute time frame. Sixty minutes in 1 hour divided by 30 = 2. Two times the volume of 100 mL = 200 mL, the rate at which the nurse should set the pump.

**TEST-TAKING HINT:** The test taker must know basic rules for medication administration and be able to compute simple math equations.

59. 1. The nurse should never ask "why." The client does not owe the nurse an explanation.
2. The question asks for a therapeutic response from the nurse. This response is restating and clarifying.
3. This is dismissive of the client's feelings and appears to agree with the client. There is no evidence cancer of the prostate is caused by promiscuous behavior.
4. This is a problem-solving statement and does not address the client's feelings.

**TEST-TAKING HINT:** Because the question is asking for a therapeutic response, the test taker should address the client's feelings. However, the test taker should not use this test-taking hint as an absolute because each question should be answered on its own merit.

60. 1. This is a psychosocial problem.
2. This is a physiological problem.
3. This problem has both physiological and psychosocial implications.
4. This is a physiological problem.

**TEST-TAKING HINT:** The test taker should read the stem carefully. The stem asks for a physiological *and* psychosocial problem. Options "1," "2," and "4" can be sorted into only one of the categories.

## Testicular Disorders

61. 1. The body temperature should be warm for the scrotum to relax. The best place to perform testicular self-examination is in a warm or hot shower.
2. The client may note a cordlike structure; this is the spermatic cord and is normal. Any lump or mass felt is abnormal and should be checked by an HCP as soon as possible.
3. The client can confirm his own negative result; a negative result is no masses felt.
4. The procedure is painless. If pain is elicited, then an HCP should examine the client. Cancer is usually painless; the presence of pain may indicate an infection.

**TEST-TAKING HINT:** The test taker might choose option "2" as an answer because any abnormality should be examined by an HCP.

62. 1. The usual treatment for testicular cancer is the removal of the involved testicle followed by radiation to the area and chemotherapy. Every attempt is made to shield the remaining testicle from the radiation, but sterility sometimes occurs.

2. With artificial insemination, the client may be able to father children, if the client has banked his sperm.

3. Sperm banking will allow the client to father children through artificial insemination with the client's sperm.

4. The nurse is in the client's room. The client's presence implies consent for the nurse to discuss his case with the fiancée.

**TEST-TAKING HINT: The nurse must abide by HIPAA rules. It is important for the nurse to know and understand the confidentiality laws. Options "1" and "2" are opposites, so only one could be correct or neither may be correct. Option "3" actually gives an option that lies between the extremes.**

63. 1. The client usually will be able to maintain normal sexual functioning with the remaining testicle. If not, testosterone may be prescribed to improve functioning. Ejaculation is not the problem; it is impotence (erectile dysfunction).

2. This will not be done until the HCP determines the remaining testicle is not able to maintain adequate hormone production.

3. The client will be able to function sexually with the remaining testicle alone or with prescribed male hormones.

4. Sex drive (libido) and orgasms usually are unimpaired because the client still has one testicle.

**TEST-TAKING HINT: The key to this question is "unilateral." The client will still have one functioning testicle.**

64. 1. Epididymitis is inflammation of the epididymis, usually caused by bacteria descending from the prostate or bladder. This does not increase the risk of developing cancer of the testes.

2. *Cryptorchidism* is the medical term for an undescended testicle. The testicles may be in the abdomen or inguinal canal at birth. This condition places the client at higher risk for testicular cancer.

3. Prostate enlargement occurs as men age, whereas the most common age range for testicular cancer is age 15 to 35.

4. Hypospadias is a congenital abnormality in which the urethral meatus is on the underside of the penis. This does not increase the risk of cancer.

**TEST-TAKING HINT: This is a knowledge-based question, but answer options "3" and "4" could be eliminated based on anatomical position.**

65. Correct answers are 1 and 5.

1. The scrotum will require support during ambulation. An athletic supporter is designed to provide support in this area.

2. The client should be encouraged to take pain medications before the pain is at a high level to help the pain medication be more effective.

3. The client can be on a regular diet as soon as the client is not nauseated from the anesthesia.

4. This surgery does not increase bleeding times.

5. Ice packs will help to reduce swelling in the scrotum and alleviate pain.

**TEST-TAKING HINT: Option "2" can be eliminated because it states the opposite of the instructions given to clients about pain medication.**

66. 1. Increasing the drip rate on a continuous bladder (Murphy) irrigation requires nursing judgment and cannot be delegated.

2. In this situation, checking for infection is an assessment situation. The nurse cannot delegate assessment.

3. **The UAP can be asked to help a client turn, cough, and deep breathe. This requires the UAP to perform an action only, not to use judgment or to assess.**

4. Red drainage in the catheter implies bleeding. The nurse should assess the amount of bleeding occurring.

**TEST-TAKING HINT: The test taker should choose the lowest level activity when choosing an action to have UAP perform. Blood should always be assessed.**

67. 1. Chlamydia is a sexually transmitted infection usually silent in the male partner, but it can cause epididymitis. If both sexual partners are not treated, then the partner can reinfect the client.

2. Sexual intercourse can be resumed within a couple of weeks as long as both partners have been treated for the infection.

3. This indicates a urinary tract infection. A UTI is another cause of epididymitis.

4. The scrotum is a closed cavity. There should not be any drainage from the scrotum. If there is drainage, this could indicate a fistula and requires immediate notification of the HCP.

**TEST-TAKING HINT: The test taker should always look at the time frame provided in either the stem or the answer options as a clue to**

answering the question correctly. The test taker should look closely at any option that has a "month" time frame.

68. 1. Pain when urinating indicates a urinary tract infection.
    2. A chancre sore on the shaft of the penis indicates syphilis, a sexually transmitted infection.
    3. Classic clinical manifestations of cancer of the testes are a mass on the testicle, painless enlargement of the testes, and heaviness of the scrotum or lower abdomen.
    4. There is no rash associated with cancer of the testes.

**TEST-TAKING HINT:** The test taker could eliminate option "2" because the penis and testes are separate body parts. The testicles lie within the scrotum. Only one option concerns that part of the body.

69. 1. The nurse should not impose any personal religious beliefs on the client.
    2. Testicular cancers have very good prognoses, and even if the tumor returns, there is a good prognosis for extended survival.
    3. There is a great deal of hope to offer these clients.
    4. This is giving the client incorrect information.

**TEST-TAKING HINT:** This is a question in which the test taker must know the information. Rarely can a nurse provide a specific percentage of survival.

70. 1. CA-125 is a tumor marker used for a number of cancers but not for testicular cancer.
    2. CEA is a nonspecific tumor marker used for a number of cancers, but it does not apply to testicular cancer.
    3. The DNA ploidy test is used to determine the number of chromosomes and the arrangement of chromosomes in a tumor cell. It is used for prognosis in some cancers, such as breast cancer, but not as a tumor marker to determine response to treatment.
    4. Tumor markers are substances synthesized by the tumor and released into the bloodstream. They can be used to follow the progress of the disease. Testicular cancers secrete hCG and alpha-fetoprotein.

**TEST-TAKING HINT:** This is a knowledge-based question. If the test taker were aware of what the test tells the HCP, then the DNA ploidy test could be eliminated. The other options are all tumor markers.

71. 1. This information could signal the onset of clinical manifestations of metastasis to the retroperitoneum. The HCP should see the client and discuss follow-up diagnostic tests.
    2. This information should be investigated and not put off.
    3. This may or may not have occurred. Only diagnostic tests can confirm metastasis.
    4. Low back exercises will not help the client if this is metastatic cancer, and they could increase the pain.

**TEST-TAKING HINT:** The nurse cannot diagnose the client as having metastasis, so option "3" can be eliminated. As a rule, any pain unrelieved with pain medication requires the client to see the HCP.

72. 1. This should be done for clients after scrotal surgery.
    2. Postoperative clients do not want to perform deep-breathing and coughing exercises because it hurts, but they should be encouraged to do so to prevent complications.
    3. The Jackson Pratt (JP) drain is a drain attached to a bulb, and the bulb should remain compressed to apply gentle suction to the surgical site.
    4. This is an appropriate delegation.

**TEST-TAKING HINT:** The test taker could eliminate option "4" by knowing the rules of delegation. The RN did not ask the UAP to perform anything requiring nursing judgment or assessment. Option "2" is just good nursing practice and could be eliminated. The charge nurse does not need to stop this action.

## Sexually Transmitted Infections

73. 1. Engaging in oral and anal sex increases the risk of contracting an STI.
    2. Using a sterile needle for drug abuse ensures the client will not get an STI from needle sharing, but the client can still contract an STI from other risky behaviors.
    3. The more sexual partners, the greater the risk of contracting an STI.
    4. Condom use provides a barrier to contracting an STI, but it is not a guarantee. The condom can break or come off during intercourse.

**TEST-TAKING HINT:** In option "2" the word "guarantees" appears, and the nurse cannot guarantee anything in dealing with health-care issues. Option "4" is an absolute statement—"will not get"—and can be eliminated on this basis.

**74.** 1. This is a true statement, but it does not answer the client's question.
2. **An untreated HPV infection is a cause for developing cancer of the cervix.**
3. HPV infection does not invade the abdominal cavity and therefore does not cause ovarian cancer.
4. The Pap test was developed to note early cell changes in the cervix. It indirectly monitors the effects of HPV, but it does not help prevent problems.

**TEST-TAKING HINT: The test taker should choose the answer for the question the client is asking. Option "1" discusses transmission and option "4" discusses prevention; therefore, these two options could be eliminated based on the stem of the question.**

**75.** 1. **These are clinical manifestations of second-stage syphilis. The nurse should ask about the development of a chancre sore, one of the first signs of a syphilis infection.**
2. This may be required of the public health nurse for notification of the partners, but it is not required to assess this problem.
3. This client does not need a dermatologist to determine an STI infection. The HCP can treat this infection.
4. A urine culture will not diagnose this disease.

**TEST-TAKING HINT: If the test taker is aware the clinical manifestations are those of an STI, options "3" and "4" can be eliminated.**

**76.** 1. All socioeconomic levels of clients contract STIs.
2. The longer the client abstains from sexual activity and the fewer partners the client has, the less the risk of an STI.
3. **Females and males can spread STIs equally. Specific diseases may be asymptomatic in the sexes (in females, gonorrhea; in males, chlamydia) and they can transmit them unknowingly.**
4. If the client has one STI, there is a great likelihood the client has another disease also. If one STI is found, the client should be monitored for others.

**TEST-TAKING HINT: Option "2" does not make sense: If sexual activity is put off, there cannot be an increased risk. Socioeconomic reasons may be a reason for delaying the treatment of a disease, but diseases are not financially based and occur in all socioeconomic levels.**

**77.** 1. Chlamydia does not cause an antigen–antibody reaction.
2. **There are long-term problems associated with any STI. Chlamydia may have the long-term effects of chronic pain and increased risk for ectopic pregnancy, postpartum endometritis, and infertility.**
3. **If both the client and the sexual partner are not treated simultaneously, the sexual partner can reinfect the client.**
4. The client may develop chronic pelvic pain as a result of the infection.

**TEST-TAKING HINT: Options "2" and "4" have a form of absolute. The words "any," "will," or "will not" are absolutes, and in health care, there are very few absolutes.**

**78.** 1. A chancre sore is a symptom of syphilis, not gonorrhea.
2. Gonorrhea is more likely to be asymptomatic in females.
3. A CD4 count of less than 200 is a diagnostic indicator for AIDS.
4. **Pain in the testes and scrotal edema can indicate epididymitis, an inflammatory process of the epididymis. This and urethritis are the most common presenting symptoms in a male with gonorrhea.**

**TEST-TAKING HINT: Two answer options mention male anatomy. If the test taker did not know the information, then choosing between these two options might be the appropriate method of elimination.**

**79.** 1. Pelvic inflammatory disease (PID) does not have to be reported, but the cause of the PID may need to be reported.
2. There are causes for epididymitis other than an STI.
3. **Syphilis is an STI and therefore must be reported to the appropriate health department.**
4. An ectopic pregnancy may have numerous causes.

**TEST-TAKING HINT: Only one answer option is an STI. The other diseases and conditions may be caused by STIs, but they all have other causes as well.**

**80.** 1. **Determining and diagnosing the risk for infertility problems requires collaboration between the nurse and the HCP.**
2. The nurse is required to teach a client. This is an independent action.
3. Fluid volume deficit is not an appropriate nursing diagnosis for this client.
4. Noncompliance is an independent nursing problem.

**TEST-TAKING HINT:** The question requires the test taker to determine which are autonomous functions of the nurse. The nurse does not have the capability to prescribe fertility medications or treatments.

81. 1. Vaginal cultures are obtained to assess for gonorrhea and chlamydia.
    2. **The RPR-CT test and the Venereal Disease Research Laboratory (VDRL) test are diagnostic tests for syphilis.**
    3. Gram stains of the vagina or urethral meatus of a male may be done for gonorrhea but not for syphilis.
    4. An immunological assay may be done for chlamydia but not for syphilis.

**TEST-TAKING HINT:** The test taker must memorize the tests used to diagnose specific STIs and the clinical manifestations differentiating one STI from another.

82. 1. Lymphadenopathy and hair loss are clinical manifestations of secondary syphilis, not tertiary syphilis.
    2. Genital warts are not signs of tertiary syphilis.
    3. **Aortitis and neurosyphilis (dementia, psychosis, stroke, paresis, and meningitis) are the most common manifestations of tertiary syphilis.**
    4. A rash covering the body is a symptom of gonorrhea.

**TEST-TAKING HINT:** The keyword in this question is "tertiary." The test taker must decide which disease has three distinct phases and then which clinical manifestations accompany each phase.

83. 1. **The public health nurse is responsible for attempting to notify the sexual partners of a client diagnosed with an STI of potential infection and urging the partner to be tested for the disease and to receive treatment. Health departments offer confidential testing and treatment.**

2. An HCP will determine the course of treatment for a client diagnosed with an STI.
3. The nurse can teach some information about reporting, but the nurse is not qualified to discuss all the legal aspects of reporting an STI.
4. The nurse is not responsible for analyzing statistics.

**TEST-TAKING HINT:** Answer options "2," "3," and "4" ask the nurse to take on roles not within the nurse's expertise. The nurse must know the Nurse Practice Act of the state where the nurse practices. No state allows the nurse to give legal or medical advice.

84. 1. An odorless, white, curdlike vaginal discharge is a symptom of *Candida albicans*, a vaginal yeast infection.
    2. **A strawberry spot on the vaginal wall or cervix, a fishy smelling vaginal discharge, and itching are clinical manifestations of trichomonas.**
    3. Scant white vaginal discharge and dyspareunia are clinical manifestations of atrophic vaginitis.
    4. Purulent discharge from the endocervix and pelvic pain are clinical manifestations of cervicitis.

**TEST-TAKING HINT:** When studying for a test covering similar diseases, the test taker should concentrate on the information that makes one different from another. Only one STI has a characteristic strawberry spot.

85. 1. A general rule when discussing antibiotics is to teach clients to finish all of the prescription, but this is not specific information related to STIs.
    2. Most STIs must be reported to comply with public health laws, but this is not a long-term complication of having an STI.
    3. Because of the scarring of reproductive tissue, infertility may be an issue resulting from STI infection.
    4. AIDS is a sexually transmitted infection and can also be transmitted by non-sexual blood and body fluid exposure.

**TEST-TAKING HINT:** The test taker can rule out option "1" because of the generalized nature of the option; it is not specific to STIs. Option "2" does not address a long-term complication for the client. And option "4" requires the test taker to know the transmission of the disease.

86. 1. A gravida 7 para 6 client has had seven pregnancies and carried six of those pregnancies to 20 weeks or longer. This woman is at risk of having the fundus remain boggy and not diminishing in size, resulting in excessive bleeding. The nurse should assess the fundus hourly.
    2. Voiding should be assessed related to the delivery time and position of the fundus, not just every 12 hours (a normal shift).
    3. It is not a priority immediately postdelivery to discuss birth control options.
    4. If the client wishes to breastfeed her infant at this time, with her history she can perform this without teaching.

**TEST-TAKING HINT:** The test taker could eliminate option "2" because of the words "every shift." Timing words such as "hourly," "every day," "every 2 hours" can make an option correct or incorrect. The stem of the question said the delivery was 2 hours ago; this requires the nurse to determine which intervention should be performed immediately postdelivery.

87. Correct answers are 2, 3, and 4.
    1. The nurse does not have to inform the parents of the teenager's disclosure of information.
    2. The nurse should discuss birth control and STIs with the client. She is at risk for pregnancy and STIs.
    3. The nurse should discuss birth control and STIs with the client. She is at risk for pregnancy and STIs.
    4. The male wears the most commonly used condoms, but both partners are responsible for contraception and prevention of STIs. This information will assist the client in knowing if the device is correctly applied and will have the best chance of preventing both pregnancy and STIs.
    5. This would be information to provide if the client had an STI but is not needed at this time.
    6. The client is not pregnant at this time.

**TEST-TAKING HINT:** The test taker could eliminate options "5" and "6" because the client is not currently pregnant.

88. 1. The DRE is performed after the PSA to avoid false elevation of the PSA from the manipulation of the prostate during DRE.
    2. The PSA is drawn before the DRE to prevent a false elevation due to the prostate being massaged during the DRE.
    3. Prostate ultrasound is performed if a nodule is found or suspected and cannot be localized on DRE. It would not be anticipated as the first action by the HCP.
    4. A biopsy would be done if all the other data are positive, but not first.

**TEST-TAKING HINT:** The test taker could eliminate options "3" and "4" because they are more invasive than a laboratory test or a digital examination.

89. 1. Failure to have the baby to express all of the milk produced will result in less milk produced at future feedings and for the breasts to become sore and inflamed.
    2. Ice packs are usually applied to decrease the discomfort.
    3. Rubbing alcohol will dry out the breast tissues and the infant should not feed after alcohol has been applied to the breast because of absorption into the infant's system.
    4. The mother should be taught correct breastfeeding techniques, not to avoid breastfeeding.

**TEST-TAKING HINT:** The test taker could eliminate option "3" because the infant could ingest the alcohol during feeding.

90. 1. Mastalgia (breast pain and tenderness) is common during the menstrual cycle. This question assists the nurse in determining if the mastalgia is from the fibrocystic disease.
    2. Some women find that avoiding chocolate and stimulants (caffeine) reduces the discomfort of fibrocystic breasts, but it is not considered an allergy.
    3. This is a therapeutic response, not an interviewing question to be asked during the assessment of the disease.
    4. This is not precancerous; there is no reason for a mastectomy.

**TEST-TAKING HINT:** The test taker could eliminate option "3" because a therapeutic response was not needed; the nurse needs to ask a question that assists in gaining information about the disease being assessed.

91. 1. Digoxin is a routine maintenance medication, and the nurse can begin the medication from 0800 to 1000, an hour before or after the 0900 time scheduled.
    2. Furosemide is a routine maintenance medication, and the nurse can begin the medication from 0800 to 1000, an hour before or after the 0900 time scheduled.
    3. An initial dose of IV antibiotics should be considered a STAT or Now medication. The nurse should make sure that any ordered cultures are obtained and the medication initiated within 1 hour of the prescription being written.
    4. Acetaminophen is a mild analgesic or antipyretic medication; this could be administered if needed after the antibiotic.

**TEST-TAKING HINT:** The test taker could eliminate options "1" and "2" because the guidelines allow up to 1 hour after the scheduled time to administer these medications.

92. 1. The nurse should administer the chemotherapy as ordered because all listed laboratory values are within normal limits (WNL).
    2. The laboratory data are WNL; the oncologist can see the laboratory report on rounds.
    3. The laboratory data are WNL; there is no need for cultures because infection is not indicated.
    4. The laboratory data are WNL; no blood is needed.

**TEST-TAKING HINT:** The test taker should be able to read and interpret reports so appropriate nursing decisions can be made.

93. 1. According to the ACS, beginning at age 50, a PSA level followed by a DRE should be done yearly.
    2. According to the ACS, beginning at age 50, a PSA level followed by a DRE should be done yearly.
    3. According to the ACS, beginning at age 50, a PSA level followed by a DRE should be done yearly.
    4. According to the ACS, beginning at age 50, a PSA level followed by a DRE should be done yearly.

**TEST-TAKING HINT:** The test taker must have a level of knowledge concerning basic nursing activities and information to teach a client.

94. 1. Failure of the baby to latch onto the breasts is not the priority for the nurse to assess.
    2. There is nothing that indicates this baby will have jaundice and clay-colored stools.
    3. The baby would have parchment-like skin and lack lanugo if the baby were over 40 weeks gestation. This is not stated in the stem.
    4. The neonate is a high birth weight, and the mother had gestational diabetes. This infant had a high glucose content passing through the placenta in utero, and the infant's pancreas has been producing insulin to take care of the glucose content of the blood. The infant's pancreas must adjust to lower levels of glucose in the system.

**TEST-TAKING HINT:** The test taker could eliminate option "2" because this is associated with liver or gallbladder issues, and basic knowledge of the pathophysiology of post-maturity gestation could eliminate option "3."

95. Correct order is 5, 3, 4, 1, 2.
    5. BSE should be performed in a private area with good lighting and a comfortable temperature so the woman is warm and can be consistent in the steps.
    3. The first part of BSE is performed in front of a mirror. The breasts are examined from the front and each side, then with arms down by the side, then raised, next with the arms on the hips and bending over. The woman is looking for dimpling and irregularity in size or shape.
    4. The woman then gets into a warm shower and palpates each breast when the breasts are soapy and slippery.

1. The last position the woman assumes is lying flat on the bed with a towel behind each scapula and palpation is performed.
2. After each breast is palpated, the last thing done is to pinch the nipples to see if there is a discharge.

**TEST-TAKING HINT:** The test taker must remember basic guidelines for procedures and which steps are involved.

96. Correct answers are 1 and 2.
    1. Women at high risk for breast cancer should have the opportunity to have mammograms beginning earlier than recommended for routine screening.
    2. According to 2015 guidelines, routine screening mammograms should begin at age 45 and be performed yearly until age 55. At age 55, mammograms should be performed biennially.
    3. Beginning in their 20s, women should be told about the benefits and limitations of breast self-examination (BSE). Even those choosing not to do BSE should be aware of how their breasts normally look and feel and report any new breast changes to a health professional as soon as they are found. Finding a breast change does not necessarily mean there is cancer. BSE is performed monthly, not bimonthly.
    4. Ultrasound or sonogram of the breast may be used to evaluate a breast change seen on a mammogram but are not performed semiannually on a routine basis.
    5. MRIs are performed on women with special needs (breast implants, etc.) but are not performed on a routine basis.

**TEST-TAKING HINT:** The test taker could eliminate option "3" based on the timing "bimonthly."

# REPRODUCTIVE DISORDERS COMPREHENSIVE EXAMINATION

1. The nurse is reviewing the laboratory data on a male client. Which interpretation should the nurse make regarding the prostate-specific antigen (PSA)?

| Laboratory Test | Client Value | Normal Value |
|---|---|---|
| Prostate-specific antigen (PSA) | 6 mcg/L | Male: less than 4 mcg/L |
| | | Female: less than 0.5 mcg/L |

   1. The client has early-stage prostate cancer.
   2. The client should have more tests.
   3. The client does not have prostate cancer.
   4. The client has benign prostatic hypertrophy.

2. The nurse is performing the admission assessment on a 78-year-old female client and observes bilateral pendulous breasts with a stringy appearance. Which intervention should the nurse implement?
   1. Request a mammogram.
   2. Notify the HCP of the finding.
   3. Continue with the examination.
   4. Assess for *peau d'orange* skin.

3. The client is scheduled for a right breast biopsy for a mass found in the tail of Spence. While the client is waiting in the holding area, the client asks the nurse, "Which lymph nodes will my surgeon take from my body?" Which area should the nurse identify?

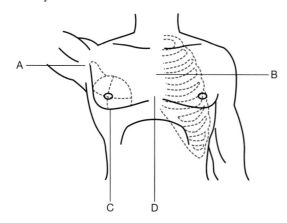

   1. A
   2. B
   3. C
   4. D

4. The client is diagnosed with left mastitis. Which assessment findings should the nurse observe?
   1. Dimpling of the left breast when the client raises the arm.
   2. A round lump in the left breast that is tender during menses.
   3. Dull pain in the left breast and tough, doughy feeling skin.
   4. Bloody discharge from the nipple and a hard, palpable mass.

5. The client has a diagnosis of rule out Paget's disease. Which test provides a **definitive diagnosis** of the disease?
   1. A breast biopsy.
   2. A diagnostic mammogram.
   3. Ultrasound of the breast.
   4. Magnetic resonance imaging.

6. The nurse in the gynecology clinic is assessing the 50-year-old biological mother of four children reporting lower abdominal pressure and fatigue along with some urinary incontinence. Which instruction should the nurse teach the client?
   1. Wear a peri-pad to keep from having an accident.
   2. Try not to laugh or sneeze unless at home.
   3. Discuss the pros and cons of a vaginal hysterectomy.
   4. Instruct to perform Kegel exercises.

7. The client is diagnosed with a rectovaginal fistula to be managed medically. Which information should the nurse teach the client before discharge?
   1. Douche with normal saline.
   2. Eat a low-residue diet.
   3. Keep ice packs on the area.
   4. Use an abdominal binder.

8. The client was diagnosed with an infected Bartholin's cyst, and the HCP performed an incision and drainage (I&D) of the area. Which discharge instructions should the nurse teach the client?
   1. Complete all antibiotics as ordered.
   2. Report any drainage immediately.
   3. Keep all water away from the area.
   4. Lie prone as much as possible.

9. The client is diagnosed with vulvar cancer. Which are the **most common** symptoms of cancer of the vulva?
   1. Red, painful lesions.
   2. Vulvar itching.
   3. Thin, white vulvar skin.
   4. Vaginal dryness.

10. The nurse is teaching a class to older women concerning cancer of the uterus. Which is a **risk factor** for developing endometrial cancer?
    1. Age 40 years or younger.
    2. Perimenopausal bleeding.
    3. Progesterone given with estrogen.
    4. Truncal obesity.

11. The nurse is caring for a client diagnosed with uterine cancer. The client has received afterload intracavitary radiation. Which precaution should the nurse implement?
    1. Wear rubber gloves to protect the nurse from all exposure.
    2. Allow any visitor the client wishes to see.
    3. Minimize the amount of time spent with the client.
    4. Encourage the client to ambulate in the hallway.

12. The nurse is caring for client A after a breast biopsy. The pathology report is posted in the EHR. Which statement is the interpretation of the DNA ploidy pathology report?

    | Client A | Client Number: 001234567 |
    | --- | --- |

    A 0.5 × 1.2-cm specimen of tissue from the right breast was evaluated with a microscope examination. Margins were not clear. Tissue sample indicates high-grade invasive ductal cell carcinoma. DNA ploidy by flow cytometry reveals aneuploid characteristics.
    Findings: Invasive ductal cell carcinoma of the right breast with aneuploid findings.

    1. This is stage IV breast cancer with a poor prognosis.
    2. The cancer will respond to hormonal therapy.
    3. The chromosomes do not resemble normal human DNA.
    4. The client should have a mastectomy as soon as possible.

13. The nurse is discharging a client diagnosed with PID. Which statement by the client indicates an **understanding** of the discharge instructions?
    1. "I should expect pelvic pain after intercourse."
    2. "I need to douche every day to prevent PID."
    3. "I will have a vaginal examination every 2 years."
    4. "My partner should use a condom if he is infectious."

14. The client has failed to conceive after many attempts over a 3-year time period and says to the nurse, "I have tried everything. What should I do now?" Which statement is the nurse's **best response**?

    1. "By 'everything' do you mean you have consulted an infertility specialist?"
    2. "You have tried everything. This must be hard for you. Would you like to talk?"
    3. "You should get on an adoption list because it can take a long time."
    4. "You need to relax and not try so hard. It is your nerves preventing conception."

15. The nurse writes a problem of "potential for complications related to ovarian hyperstimulation" for a client taking clomiphene. Which intervention should be included in the plan of care?
    1. Instruct the client to delay intercourse until menses.
    2. Schedule the client for frequent pelvic sonograms.
    3. Explain the infusion therapy will take 21 days.
    4. Discuss that this may cause an ectopic pregnancy.

16. The HCP orders cultures of the urethral urine, bladder urine, and prostatic fluid. Which instructions should the nurse teach to achieve the **first** two specimens?
    1. Collect the first 15 mL in one jar and then the next 50 mL in another.
    2. Collect three early-morning, clean voided urine specimens.
    3. Collect the specimens after the HCP massages the prostate.
    4. Collect a routine urine specimen for analysis.

17. The nurse writes a client problem of "anxiety related to potential sexual dysfunction" for a client diagnosed with cancer of the prostate. Which intervention should the nurse implement?
    1. Tell the client to discuss his fears with the HCP.
    2. Talk to the spouse about the client's concerns.
    3. Inform the client that sexual functioning will not be altered.
    4. Provide a private area for the client to discuss his concerns.

18. The male client is considering a vasectomy for birth control. Which information should the nurse teach the client?
    1. Instruct the client to use hot packs to relieve scrotal edema after the surgery.
    2. Tell the client to wear loose-fitting boxer underwear after the surgery.
    3. Explain that an alternate form of birth control will be required initially.
    4. Discuss that potency will be diminished by about 20% after a vasectomy.

19. The 45-year-old male client has had a circumcision secondary to phimosis. Which intervention should the nurse include in the plan of care?
    1. Teach how to care for the glans to prevent the recurrence of the phimosis.
    2. Assess for pain on a scale of 1 to 10.
    3. Perform wet-to-dry dressing changes daily.
    4. Instruct the client to perform a monthly penis check for cancer.

20. Which vaccination should the nurse recommend to the post-pubertal male to **prevent** orchitis?
    1. Yearly flu vaccinations.
    2. Herpes varicella inoculations.
    3. Mumps vaccination.
    4. Rubella inoculation.

21. The nurse is instructing a group of workers at an industrial plant regarding the transmission of STIs. Which information should be included in the presentation? **Select all that apply.**
    1. The same behaviors causing one STI could lead to another.
    2. Once clients have had an STI, they develop immunity to it.
    3. Infection with syphilis protects the client from being infected with HIV.
    4. Herpes simplex 1 is a totally different disease from herpes simplex 2.
    5. Condoms do not provide protection against all STIs.

22. The male client reports mucus-like drainage from the rectum accompanied by rectal pain and diarrhea. Which interview question should the nurse ask the client?
    1. "Do you have difficulty trying to urinate?"
    2. "Have you had rectal sexual intercourse?"
    3. "Do you eat a high-fiber diet and drink lots of fluids?"
    4. "Does the diarrhea alternate with constipation?"

23. The client is diagnosed with primary syphilis. Which clinical manifestations should the nurse observe?
    1. A chancre sore in the perineal area.
    2. A rash on the trunk and extremities.
    3. Blistering of the palms of the hands.
    4. Confusion and disorientation.

24. The nurse is discussing pelvic floor exercises with a client. Which information should the nurse teach?
    1. Perform exercises four times per day.
    2. The exercises will prevent stress incontinence.
    3. Contract the perineal muscles and hold for 10 seconds.
    4. Contract the abdominal and buttock muscles to increase strength.

25. The county health department nurse is reviewing a client record and notes the RPR-CT laboratory results. Which question should the nurse ask the client?

| Laboratory Test | Client Result | Normal Finding |
|---|---|---|
| Rapid plasma reagin card test (RPR-CT) | Reactive for *T. pallidum* | Nonreactive |

    1. "When was your last tetanus shot?"
    2. "Have you had a cold recently?"
    3. "Do you have diabetes mellitus?"
    4. "Are you allergic to penicillin?"

26. The nurse is teaching a class on Breast Health Awareness. Which are the American Cancer Society's recommended guidelines for the performance of breast self-examination (BSE)? **Rank in order of performance.**
    1. Visualize the breast from the front while standing before a mirror.
    2. Gently squeeze the nipple to express any fluid.
    3. Turn to each side and view each breast in the mirror.
    4. Palpate each breast in a circular motion while lying on the back.
    5. Palpate each breast in a circular motion while in the shower.

27.  The 32-year-old client diagnosed with an ovarian cyst is reporting acute pain. Which picture depicts the area where the client would be experiencing pain?

1.

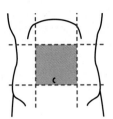

3.

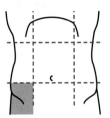

2.

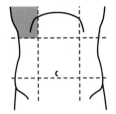

4.

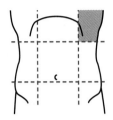

1. 1. The client may have cancer of the prostate, but this test does not provide conclusive results. There are several reasons for the PSA to be elevated, not just cancer.
   2. **The PSA is elevated, and more tests should be completed to determine the cause. PSA levels are increased in benign prostatic hypertrophy, urinary retention, prostatic infarct, and prostate cancer.**
   3. Cancer cannot be eliminated as a diagnosis until other tests have been completed.
   4. This may be the actual diagnosis, but the client should undergo more tests to confirm a diagnosis.

2. 1. These are normal findings in a postmenopausal breast and do not require a mammogram. The client should have a mammogram yearly.
   2. These are normal findings in the postmenopausal breast so there is no need to notify the HCP.
   3. **These are normal findings in the postmenopausal breast. Glandular tissue is replaced with fibrous tissue, the breasts become pendulous, and the Cooper's ligaments become prominent.**
   4. *Peau d'orange* skin occurs in advanced breast cancer.

3. 1. **The tail of Spence is the upper outermost part of the breast, which extends toward the arm. The most likely lymph nodes to biopsy are the axillary nodes.**
   2. This is the mediastinal node area, which is on the opposite side of the breast.
   3. The internal mammary nodes are under the breast, and the tail of Spence is at the top of the breast.
   4. The parasternal nodes are on the opposite side of the breast from the tail of Spence.

4. 1. The dimpling of the breast indicates a tumor has attached itself to the chest wall.
   2. This indicates fibrocystic changes in the left breast.
   3. **Mastitis is an infection of the breast occurring most often in lactating women. The breast becomes red and warm to the touch. The skin becomes doughy and tough in consistency, and the client develops a dull pain in the affected breast.**
   4. Bloody discharge indicates a tumor, benign or malignant.

5. 1. **Biopsy of the lesion is the only definitive test for Paget's disease, a form of breast cancer accounting for about 1% of all breast cancers.**
   2. Mammography is the only test that routinely screens for breast cancer, but a definitive diagnosis is made by tissue identification.
   3. Ultrasound of the breasts can diagnose fluid-filled cysts.
   4. MRI can be done to determine the extent of tumor involvement, but tissue identification is the definitive test for tumor diagnosis.

6. 1. The client would have determined the need for protection without the nurse having to tell her to do so.
   2. It is unrealistic to tell a client not to laugh or sneeze.
   3. The client probably has a cystocele resulting from childbirth. The corrective surgical repair is a bladder suspension.
   4. **Kegel exercises help to strengthen the pelvic muscles. They are recommended for all women and should be performed 30 to 80 times per day.**

7. 1. Cleansing douches are prescribed with tepid water, not normal saline.
   2. **Measures to assist the client in healing without surgical interventions include proper nutrition with a low-residue diet to minimize contamination of the tissues with feces, cleansing douches, enemas, and rest.**
   3. Warm perineal irrigations and controlled heat-lamp applications promote healing; ice vasoconstricts the area and delays wound healing.
   4. The client should wear perineal pads but not an abdominal binder.

8. 1. **The client has an infection and should complete the ordered antibiotics.**
   2. The client should be taught to expect some drainage from the area because the area has been opened to allow for exudate to escape the body.
   3. Routine hygiene is encouraged.
   4. The client can assume any position of comfort.

9. 1. Red, painful lesions are symptoms of lichen planus, which is benign, although uncomfortable.
   2. **Cancer of the vulva may be asymptomatic, but the client usually presents with persistent long-term itching.**
   3. Thin, white vulvar skin indicates lichen sclerosis.
   4. Vaginal dryness is not associated with cancer of the vulva.

10. 1. Clients at risk for uterine cancer are usually 55 years old or older.
    2. Postmenopausal bleeding places the client at risk, but perimenopausal bleeding is expected as the ovaries begin to slow the production of eggs.
    3. Unopposed estrogen replacement therapy predisposes women to develop uterine cancer, but progesterone offsets the risk.
    4. **Truncal obesity is one of the risk factors for developing endometrial cancer, although it has not been determined how this occurs.**

11. 1. Rubber gloves should be worn to dispose of any soiled material, but they will not protect the nurse from sealed radiation sources.
    2. Pregnant visitors and visitors younger than 18 years old should not be allowed in the client's room.
    3. **Afterload intracavitary radiation therapy treatments are completed in the client's room after prepared applicators are placed in surgery. This minimizes the exposure of the health-care workers to radiation. The nurse should plan care to minimize exposure to the client and the radiation.**
    4. The client is placed in a room at the far end of the hallway, and in some facilities, clients on either side of the client's room may have to be moved to limit exposure to radiation. The client is not allowed to leave the room until the radiation safety department clears the client for discharge.

12. 1. Staging for breast cancer is completed using a variety of measurements, including the size of the tumor and metastasis sites, but staging does not involve the DNA characteristics.
    2. The DNA ploidy tests are performed to determine the response to all types of treatments. The more the cell represents normal human DNA pairings (euploid), the better the prognosis for the client.

    3. Aneuploid means the cells do not have human pairing characteristics. This finding indicates the cells cannot be expected to respond as normal human cells respond and the prognosis is not good for the client.
    4. The choice of surgical approach is determined between the client and HCP. The tumor should be removed with enough tissue to have clear margins. Whether the client chooses a modified radical mastectomy, lumpectomy, or wedge resection depends on the choice of follow-up treatment.

13. 1. **Any pelvic pain after sexual exposure, childbirth, or pelvic surgery should be evaluated as soon as possible.**
    2. Douching reduces the natural flora, which combats infecting organisms and may help infecting bacteria move upward into the uterus, but douching will not prevent PID.
    3. The client should have a vaginal examination at least once a year.
    4. **The client and partner should consistently use a condom if there is any chance of transmission of any organism.**

14. 1. **The nurse should investigate which fertility measures have been attempted. There are many reasons for infertility, and only a specialist in the area can identify the cause.**
    2. This is a therapeutic response, but the client is asking for information.
    3. This is advising and not answering the client's question.
    4. The nurse cannot know this to be true, and this does not address the client's concern.

15. 1. Clomiphene (Clomid), an ovarian stimulant, is begun on the fifth day of the menstrual cycle and is taken for 5 days; ovulation should occur 4 to 8 days after—approximately from day 9 to day 13 of the cycle. Intercourse should be planned for the optimum chance of conception.
    2. **Frequent sonograms are needed to monitor follicular stimulation. The ovaries are monitored to prevent overstimulation, which can cause ascites, pleural effusions, and acute respiratory distress syndrome (ARDS).**
    3. Clomiphene (Clomid), an ovarian stimulant, is not given by infusion. GnRH is given by infusion.
    4. Ovarian stimulation does not cause ectopic pregnancy.

16. 1. After cleansing the penis and retracting the foreskin (if present), the client voids the first 15 mL in a sterile specimen cup; this is the urethral urine specimen. Then, the client voids the next 50 to 75 mL into another sterile specimen cup; this is the bladder urine. If the client does not have acute prostatitis, the HCP can massage the prostate and collect prostate fluid for culture, but if the fluid is not expressed with massage, the next urine is sent for analysis.
2. Early morning has no bearing on collecting prostatitis specimens.
3. This is the third specimen and is obtained by the HCP.
4. A routine specimen will not provide the information needed.

17. 1. This is not an appropriate referral. The nurse should discuss the client's fears.
2. The spouse may need to be encouraged to talk about the concerns, but this does not address the client's concerns.
3. The client's sexual functioning may be impaired depending on the treatment options chosen.
4. **Because the client may be sensitive and embarrassed about discussing problems related to genitalia and sexual functioning, the nurse should provide a private area in which to discuss these concerns.**

18. 1. Ice packs, not hot packs, should be applied after surgery to reduce edema.
2. The client should wear cotton, jockey-type underwear to provide support and added comfort.
3. **The client will not be sterile until the sperm stored distal to the surgery site in the tubules have been ejaculated or reabsorbed by the body. Therefore, an alternate form of birth control is needed for a certain period of time following the vasectomy.**
4. There is no effect on the client's potency after a bilateral vasectomy.

19. 1. Phimosis is a tightness of the prepuce of the penis preventing retraction of the foreskin over the glans. Once the foreskin has been surgically removed, this is not a problem.
2. **There is considerable pain after an adult circumcision, and the nurse should assess for the pain.**
3. A petroleum-saturated gauze is wrapped around the penis, not a wet-to-dry dressing.

4. Circumcision in infancy may prevent cancer of the penis. The older client after a circumcision should be aware of the potential for cellular changes, but the risk is greatly reduced after the surgery.

20. 1. The flu vaccine will not prevent orchitis.
2. This is the chickenpox vaccine and will not prevent orchitis.
3. **When post-puberty males contract mumps, one in five develops some form of orchitis (infection of the testes) within 4 to 7 days after the neck and jaw swell. The testes may show atrophy after the infection, and the client may become sterile.**
4. Rubella (measles) does not cause orchitis.

21. Correct answers are 1 and 5.
1. **The behaviors leading to the development of one STI could also lead to the development of another.**
2. There is no antigen–antibody reaction development with STIs. A client can be reinfected multiple times.
3. There is no protection provided by one STI from developing another, and, frequently, clients will have more than one STI simultaneously.
4. Herpes simplex 1 and 2 are caused by the same virus. Herpes simplex 1 refers to orolabial lesions and herpes simplex 2 refers to genital lesions, which can be transferred from one area to the other.
5. **Condoms are effective against most STIs if used correctly; however, some STIs can be spread from skin to skin contact (Centers for Disease Control and Prevention, 2013)**

22. 1. The client has rectal symptoms, not urinary tract symptoms.
2. **The client has described the clinical manifestations of proctitis (inflammation of the rectum). Proctitis is commonly associated with anal-receptive intercourse with an infected partner. The pathogens most frequently associated with proctitis are gonorrhea, chlamydia, herpes simplex, and *Treponema pallidum*.**
3. A high-fiber diet does not cause these symptoms.
4. Diarrhea alternating with constipation indicates a possible rectal tumor and does not cause these symptoms.

23. 1. A chancre sore on the perineal area is a symptom of primary syphilis.
    2. A rash on the trunk and extremities occurs in secondary syphilis.
    3. Blistering of the palms of the hand occurs in secondary syphilis.
    4. Tertiary syphilis occurs over a prolonged period and includes clinical manifestations of dementia, psychosis, paresis, stroke, and meningitis.

24. 1. Pelvic floor (Kegel) exercises should be performed 30 to 80 times per day.
    2. The exercises will help reduce stress incontinence, but they may not relieve all stress incontinence.
    3. **Perineal muscles should be contracted and held for 10 seconds followed by 10 seconds of rest.**
    4. The pelvic floor muscles are contracted without contracting the abdominal, buttock, or inner-thigh muscles.

25. 1. This is a test for syphilis and does not require a tetanus injection.
    2. Having a cold does not affect the diagnosis of syphilis.
    3. Diabetes places a client at risk for many illnesses, but sexual behavior places the client at risk for a sexually transmitted infection.
    4. **The test is positive for syphilis, and the nurse anticipates the HCP ordering an antibiotic; penicillin is the antibiotic of choice for syphilis. Syphilis is caused by the *T. pallidum* bacteria.**

26. Correct order is 1, 3, 5, 4, 2.
    1. The first step in BSE is to visualize the breasts for symmetry while looking at a frontal view before the mirror.
    3. The next step is to turn from side to side, looking for any dimpling, puckering, or asymmetry, in front of a mirror.
    5. The client should palpate the breasts in a warm shower with the breasts soaped to allow for the fingers to glide over the breast tissue.
    4. After the shower, the client should lie on the bed with a towel rolled up and placed under the shoulder to flatten the breast tissue and palpate the breast.
    2. The last step in BSE is to gently squeeze the nipple to determine if there is expressed fluid.

27. 1. The midabdominal area is where clients diagnosed with peptic ulcers report pain.
    2. The right upper quadrant is where clients diagnosed with gallbladder problems report pain.
    3. The lower abdominal quadrants are where a client diagnosed with an ovarian cyst will report pain. The appendix is also located in the right lower quadrant.
    4. The left upper abdominal quadrant is where clients diagnosed with spleen infarcts or rupture, stomach problems, or pancreas problems report pain.

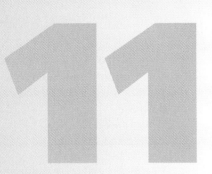

# Musculoskeletal Disorders

*Education is not the filling of a pail but the lighting of a fire.*

—William Butler Yeats

Musculoskeletal injuries and disorders are common. Many, such as fractures, result from accidents; others, such as osteoarthritis, osteoporosis, and joint replacement, are often associated with the aging process; and still others, such as amputation, may result as a complication of a specific disease process such as diabetes. Nurses must know how to assess these clients, when to notify the health-care providers, and how to carry out the proper procedures and administer the medications ordered.

## KEYWORDS

| | |
|---|---|
| Abduction | Laminectomy |
| Avulsion | Oblique |
| Collaborative | Paresthesia |
| Comminuted | Pathological |
| Compound | Primary care |
| Degenerative | Prostheses |
| Epiphyseal | Rhinitis |
| Greenstick | Secondary care |
| Herniated nucleus pulposus | Tertiary care |
| Impacted | |

## PRACTICE QUESTIONS

### Degenerative and Herniated Disk Disease

1. The nurse is caring for an older client diagnosed with a herniated nucleus pulposus of L4-5. Which scientific rationale explains the incidence of a ruptured disk in the older clients?
   1. The client did not use good body mechanics when lifting an object.
   2. There is an increased blood supply to the back as the body ages.
   3. Older clients develop atherosclerotic joint disease as a result of fat deposits.
   4. Clients develop intervertebral disk degeneration as they age.

2. The 34-year-old male client presents to the outpatient clinic reporting numbness and pain radiating down the left leg. Which **further** data should the nurse assess?
   1. Posture and gait.
   2. Bending and stooping.
   3. Leg lifts and arm swing.
   4. Waist twists and neck mobility.

3. The occupational health nurse is preparing an in-service for a group of workers in a warehouse. Which information should be included to help **prevent** on-the-job injuries?
   1. Increase sodium and potassium in the diet during the winter months.
   2. Use the large thigh muscles when lifting and hold the weight near the body.
   3. Use soft-cushioned chairs when performing desk duties.
   4. Have the employee arrange for assistance with household chores.

4. The occupational health nurse is planning health promotion activities for a group of factory workers. Which activity is an example of primary **prevention** for clients at risk for low back pain?
   1. Teach back exercises to workers after returning from an injury.
   2. Place signs in the work area about how to perform first aid.
   3. Start a weight-reduction group to meet at lunchtime.
   4. Administer a nonnarcotic analgesic to a client reporting back pain.

5. The client diagnosed with a cervical neck injury as a result of a motor-vehicle accident (MVA) is reporting unrelieved pain after the administration of a narcotic analgesic. Which alternative method of pain control is an **independent** nursing action?
   1. Medicate the client with a muscle relaxant.
   2. Heat alternating with ice applied by a physical therapist.
   3. Watch television or listen to music.
   4. Discuss surgical options with the health-care provider.

6. The client diagnosed with cervical disk degeneration has undergone a laminectomy. Which interventions should the nurse implement?
   1. Position the client prone with the knees slightly elevated.
   2. Assess the client for difficulty speaking or breathing.
   3. Measure the drainage in the Jackson Pratt bulb every day.
   4. Encourage the client to postpone the use of narcotic medications.

7. The client is 12-hours post–lumbar laminectomy. Which nursing interventions should be implemented?
   1. Assess the ability to void and log roll the client every 2 hours.
   2. Medicate with IV steroids and keep the bed in a Trendelenburg position.
   3. Place sandbags on each side of the head and give cathartic medications.
   4. Administer IV anticoagulants and place on $O_2$ at 8 L/min.

8. The registered nurse (RN) is working with an unlicensed assistive personnel (UAP). Which action by the UAP **warrants immediate** intervention?
   1. The UAP feeds a client a regular diet 2 days postoperative cervical laminectomy.
   2. The UAP calls for help when turning to the side a client postoperative lumbar laminectomy.
   3. The UAP is helping the client weighing 300 pounds, diagnosed with back pain, return to the chair.
   4. The UAP places the call light within reach of the client postoperative disk fusion.

9. The nurse is caring for clients on an orthopedic floor. Which client should be assessed **first**?
   1. The client diagnosed with back pain reporting a "4" on a 1-to-10 scale.
   2. The client after a myelogram reporting a slight headache.
   3. The client 2 days postoperative disk fusion with T 100.4, P 96, R 24, and BP 138/78.
   4. The client diagnosed with back pain being discharged and the ride home is here.

10. The nurse is administering 0730 medications to clients on a medical orthopedic unit. Which medication should be administered **first**?
    1. The daily cardiac glycoside to a client diagnosed with back pain and heart failure.
    2. The routine insulin to a client diagnosed with neck strain and type 1 diabetes.
    3. The oral proton pump inhibitor to a client scheduled for a laminectomy this morning.
    4. The fourth dose of IV antibiotic for a client diagnosed with a surgical infection.

11. The nurse writes the problem of "pain" for a client diagnosed with lumbar strain. Which nursing interventions should be included in the plan of care? **Select all that apply**.
    1. Assess pain on a 1-to-10 scale.
    2. Administer pain medication prn.
    3. Provide a regular bedpan for elimination.
    4. Assess surgical dressing every 4 hours.
    5. Perform a position change by the log roll method every 2 hours.

12. The nurse working on a medical-surgical floor feels a pulling in the back when lifting a client up in the bed. Which should be the **first** action taken by the nurse?
    1. Continue working until the shift is over and then try to sleep on a heating pad.
    2. Go immediately to the emergency department for treatment and muscle relaxants.
    3. Inform the charge nurse and nurse manager on duty and document the occurrence.
    4. See a private health-care provider on the nurse's off time but charge the hospital.

## Osteoarthritis (OA)

13. The occupational health nurse is teaching a class on the risk factors for developing osteoarthritis (OA). Which is a **modifiable** risk factor for developing OA?
    1. Being overweight.
    2. Increasing age.
    3. Previous joint damage.
    4. Genetic susceptibility.

14. The client is diagnosed with OA. Which clinical manifestations should the nurse expect the client to exhibit? **Select all that apply**.
    1. Severe bone deformity.
    2. Joint stiffness.
    3. Waddling gait.
    4. Swan-neck fingers.
    5. Crepitus.

15. The client diagnosed with OA is a resident in a long-term care facility. The resident is refusing to bathe because she is hurting. Which instruction should the RN give the UAP?
    1. Allow the client to stay in bed until the pain becomes bearable.
    2. Tell the UAP to give the client a bed bath this morning.
    3. Try to encourage the client to get up and go to the shower.
    4. Notify the family the client is refusing to be bathed.

16. The client has been diagnosed with OA for the last 7 years and has tried multiple medical treatments and alternative treatments but still has significant joint pain. Which **psychosocial** client problem should the nurse identify?
    1. Severe pain.
    2. Body image disturbance.
    3. Knowledge deficit.
    4. Depression.

17. The client diagnosed with OA is prescribed an NSAID. Which instructions should the nurse teach the client? **Select all that apply**.
    1. Take the medication on an empty stomach.
    2. Make sure to taper the medication when discontinuing.
    3. Apply the medication topically over the affected joints.
    4. Notify the health-care provider if vomiting blood.
    5. Avoid taking acetylsalicylic acid with this medication.

18. Which client goal is **most appropriate** for a client diagnosed with OA?
    1. Perform passive range-of-motion exercises.
    2. Maintain optimal functional ability.
    3. Client will walk 3 miles every day.
    4. Client will join a health club.

19. To which member of the health-care team should the nurse refer the client diagnosed with OA who reports not being able to get in and out of the bathtub?
    1. Physiatrist.
    2. Social worker.
    3. Physical therapist.
    4. Counselor.

20. The nurse is discussing the importance of an exercise program for pain control to a client diagnosed with OA. Which intervention should the nurse include in the teaching?
    1. Wear supportive tennis shoes with white socks when walking.
    2. Carry a complex carbohydrate while exercising.
    3. Alternate walking briskly and jogging when exercising.
    4. Walk at least 30 minutes three times a week.

21. The client diagnosed with OA is taking glucosamine and chondroitin supplements. What is the scientific rationale for taking this medication?
    1. It will help decrease the inflammation in the joints.
    2. It improves tissue function and retards the breakdown of cartilage.
    3. It is a potent medication that decreases the client's joint pain.
    4. It increases the production of synovial fluid in the joint.

22. The nurse is admitting the client diagnosed with OA to the medical floor. Which statement by the client indicates an **alternative** form of treatment for OA?
    1. "I take medication every 2 hours for my pain."
    2. "I use a heating pad when I go to bed at night."
    3. "I wear a copper bracelet to help with my OA."
    4. "I always wear my ankle splints when I sleep."

23. The client is reporting joint stiffness, especially in the morning. Which diagnostic tests should the nurse expect the health-care provider to order to rule out OA?
    1. Full-body magnetic resonance imaging scan.
    2. Serum studies for synovial fluid amount.
    3. X-ray of the affected joints.
    4. Serum erythrocyte sedimentation rate (ESR).

24. The nurse is caring for the following clients. After receiving the shift report, which client should the nurse assess **first**?
    1. The client with a total knee replacement reporting a cold foot.
    2. The client diagnosed with osteoarthritis reporting stiff joints.
    3. The client needing to receive a scheduled intravenous antibiotic.
    4. The client diagnosed with back pain scheduled for a lumbar myelogram.

## Osteoporosis

25. The nurse is discussing osteoporosis with a group of women. Which factors will the nurse identify as nonmodifiable risk factors? **Select all that apply**.
    1. Calcium deficiency.
    2. Tobacco use.
    3. Female sex.
    4. High alcohol intake.
    5. European ancestry.

26. The client diagnosed with osteoporosis asks the nurse, "Why does smoking cigarettes cause my bones to be brittle?" Which response by the nurse is **most appropriate**?
    1. "Smoking causes nutritional deficiencies, which contribute to osteoporosis."
    2. "Tobacco causes an increase in blood supply to the bones, causing osteoporosis."
    3. "Smoking low-tar cigarettes will not cause your bones to become brittle."
    4. "Nicotine impairs the absorption of calcium, causing decreased bone strength."

27. Which clinical manifestations indicate to the nurse the client has developed osteoporosis?
    1. The client has lost 1 inch in height.
    2. The client has lost 12 pounds in the last year.
    3. The client's hands are painful to the touch.
    4. The client's serum uric acid level is elevated.

28. The client is being evaluated for osteoporosis. Which diagnostic test is the **most accurate** when diagnosing osteoporosis?
    1. X-ray of the femur.
    2. Serum alkaline phosphatase.
    3. Dual-energy x-ray absorptiometry (DEXA).
    4. Serum bone Gla-protein test.

29. Which foods should the nurse recommend to a client when discussing sources of dietary calcium?
    1. Yogurt and dark-green, leafy vegetables.
    2. Oranges and citrus fruits.
    3. Bananas and dried apricots.
    4. Wheat bread and bran.

30. Which intervention is an example of a **secondary** nursing intervention when discussing osteoporosis?
    1. Obtain a bone density evaluation test.
    2. Perform non–weight-bearing exercises regularly.
    3. Increase the intake of dietary calcium.
    4. Refer clients to a smoking cessation program.

31. The female client diagnosed with osteoporosis tells the nurse she is going to perform swim aerobics for 30 minutes every day. Which response is **most appropriate** by the nurse?
    1. Praise the client for committing to do this activity.
    2. Explain to the client walking 30 minutes a day is a better activity.
    3. Encourage the client to swim every other day instead of daily.
    4. Discuss with the client how sedentary activities help prevent osteoporosis.

32. The client diagnosed with osteoporosis is prescribed alendronate. Which information should the nurse teach the client about this medication? **Select all that apply**.
    1. Take this medication at the same time every night.
    2. Drink 6 to 8 ounces of water with each dose.
    3. Wait 30 minutes before taking other medications, fluids, or food.
    4. Notify the HCP if experiencing pain or difficulty swallowing.
    5. Lie down for 30 minutes after taking medication.

33. The nurse is teaching a class to pregnant teenagers. Which information is most important when discussing ways to **prevent** osteoporosis?
    1. Take at least 1,300 mg of calcium a day.
    2. Eat foods low in calcium and high in phosphorus.
    3. Osteoporosis does not occur until around age 50 years.
    4. Remain as active as possible until the baby is born.

34. The 84-year-old client is a resident in a long-term care facility. Which intervention should be implemented to help **prevent** complications secondary to osteoporosis?
    1. Keep the bed in the high position.
    2. Perform passive range-of-motion exercises.
    3. Turn the client every 2 hours.
    4. Provide nighttime lights in the room.

35. The client is taking calcium carbonate to help **prevent** further development of osteoporosis. Which teaching should the nurse implement?
    1. Encourage the client to take calcium carbonate with at least 8 ounces of water.
    2. Teach the client to take calcium carbonate with the breakfast meal only.
    3. Instruct the client to take calcium carbonate 30 to 60 minutes before a meal.
    4. Discuss the need to get a monthly serum calcium level.

36. The client must take 3 grams of calcium supplement a day. The medication comes in 500-mg tablets. How many tablets will the client need to take daily?

    [                    ]

## Amputation

37. The nurse instructs the client with a right below-the-knee amputation (BKA) to lie on the stomach for at least 30 minutes twice a day. The client asks the nurse, "Why do I need to lie on my stomach?" Which statement is the **most appropriate** statement by the nurse?
    1. "This position will help your lungs expand better."
    2. "Lying on your stomach will help prevent contractures."
    3. "Many times this will help decrease pain in the limb."
    4. "The position will take the pressure off your backside."

38. The recovery room nurse is caring for a client after a left BKA. Which interventions should the nurse implement? **Select all that apply**.
    1. Assess the client's surgical dressing every 2 hours.
    2. Allow the client to see the residual limb.
    3. Keep a large tourniquet at the client's bedside.
    4. Perform passive range-of-motion exercises to the right leg.
    5. Wrap the limb with a compression dressing.

39. The 62-year-old client diagnosed with type 2 diabetes and a gangrenous right toe is being admitted for a BKA. Which nursing intervention should the nurse implement?
    1. Assess the client's nutritional status.
    2. Refer the client to an occupational therapist.
    3. Determine if the client is allergic to IVP dye.
    4. Start a 22-gauge angiocatheter in the right arm.

40. The male nurse is helping his friend cut wood with an electric saw. His friend cuts two fingers off his left hand with the saw. Which action should the nurse implement **first**?
    1. Wrap the left hand with towels and apply pressure.
    2. Instruct the friend to hold his hand above his head.
    3. Apply pressure to the radial artery of the left hand.
    4. Go into the friend's house and call 911.

41. A person's right thumb was accidentally severed with an ax. The amputated right thumb was recovered. Which action by the nurse preserves the thumb so it could possibly be reattached in surgery?
    1. Place the right thumb directly on some ice.
    2. Put the right thumb in a glass of warm water.
    3. Wrap the thumb in a clean piece of material.
    4. Secure the thumb in a plastic bag and place it on ice.

42. The Jewish client diagnosed with peripheral vascular disease is scheduled for a left above-the-knee amputation (AKA). Which question is **most important** for the operating room nurse to ask the client?
    1. "Have you made any special arrangements for your amputated limb?"
    2. "What types of food would you like to eat while you're in the hospital?"
    3. "Would you like a rabbi to visit you while you are in the recovery room?"
    4. "Will you start checking your other foot at least once a day for cuts?"

43. The client is 3 hours postoperative left AKA. The client tells the nurse, "My left foot is killing me. Please do something." Which intervention should the nurse implement?
    1. Explain to the client his left leg has been amputated.
    2. Medicate the client with a narcotic analgesic immediately.
    3. Instruct the client on how to perform bio-feedback exercises.
    4. Place the client's residual limb in the dependent position.

44. The nurse is caring for a client with a right BKA. There is a large amount of bright red blood on the client's residual limb dressing. Which intervention should the nurse implement **first**?
    1. Notify the client's surgeon immediately.
    2. Assess the client's blood pressure and pulse.
    3. Reinforce the dressing with additional dressing.
    4. Check the client's last hemoglobin and hematocrit levels.

45. The nurse is caring for clients on a surgical unit. Which nursing task is **most appropriate** for the RN to delegate to an UAP?
    1. Help the client with the 2-day postoperative amputation put on a prosthesis.
    2. Request the UAP double-check a unit of blood to be hung.
    3. Change the surgical dressing on the client with a Syme's amputation.
    4. Ask the UAP to take the client to the physical therapy department.

46. The client with a right AKA is being taught how to toughen the residual limb. Which intervention should the nurse implement?
    1. Instruct the client to push the residual limb against a pillow.
    2. Demonstrate how to apply an elastic bandage around the residual limb.
    3. Encourage the client to apply vitamin B12 to the surgical incision.
    4. Teach the client to elevate the residual limb at least three times a day.

47. The 27-year-old client has a right above-the-elbow amputation secondary to a boating accident. Which statement to the rehabilitation nurse indicates the client has accepted the amputation?
    1. "I am going to sue the guy for hitting my boat."
    2. "The therapist is going to help me get retrained for another job."
    3. "I decided not to get a prosthesis. I don't think I need it."
    4. "My spouse is so worried about me, and I wish my spouse wasn't."

48. The 32-year-old male client with a traumatic left AKA is being discharged from the rehabilitation department. Which discharge instructions should be included in the teaching? **Select all that apply**.
    1. Report any pain not relieved with analgesics.
    2. Eat a well-balanced diet and increase protein intake.
    3. Be sure to attend all outpatient rehabilitation appointments.
    4. Encourage the client to attend a support group for amputees.
    5. Stay at home as much as possible for the first couple of months.

## Fractures

49. The client is taken to the emergency department with an injury to the left arm. Which intervention should the nurse implement **first**?
    1. Assess the nailbeds for capillary refill time.
    2. Remove the client's clothing from the arm.
    3. Call radiology for a STAT x-ray of the extremity.
    4. Prepare the client for the application of a cast.

50. The nurse is preparing the plan of care for the client diagnosed with a closed fracture of the right arm. Which problem is **most appropriate** for the nurse to identify?
    1. Risk for ineffective coping related to the inability to perform ADL.
    2. Risk for compartment syndrome–related injured muscle tissue.
    3. Risk for infection related to exposed bone and tissue.
    4. Risk for complications related to compromised neurovascular status.

51. Which interventions should the nurse implement for the client diagnosed with an open fracture of the left ankle? **Select all that apply**.
    1. Apply an immobilizer snugly to prevent edema.
    2. Apply an ice pack for 10 minutes and remove for 20 minutes.
    3. Place the extremity in the dependent position to allow drainage.
    4. Obtain an x-ray of the ankle after applying the immobilizer.
    5. Administer tetanus toxoid, 0.5 mL intramuscularly, in the deltoid.

52. The nurse is caring for a client diagnosed with a fractured left tibia and fibula. Which data should the nurse report to the health-care provider **immediately**?
    1. Localized edema and discoloration occurring hours after the injury.
    2. Generalized weakness and increasing sensitivity to touch.
    3. Dorsalis pedal pulse cannot be located with a Doppler and increasing pain.
    4. Pain relieved after taking 4 mg hydromorphone.

53. The UAP reports a client diagnosed with a fractured femur has "fatty globules" floating in the urinal. Which intervention should the RN implement **first**?
    1. Assess the client for dyspnea and altered mental status.
    2. Obtain an arterial blood gas and order a portable chest x-ray.
    3. Call the HCP for a ventilation and perfusion scan.
    4. Instruct the UAP to keep the client on strict bedrest.

54. The nurse is caring for an 80-year-old client admitted with a fractured right femoral neck and oriented × 1. Which intervention should the nurse implement **first**?
    1. Check for a positive Homans' sign.
    2. Encourage the client to take deep breaths and cough.
    3. Determine the client's normal orientation status.
    4. Monitor the client's skin traction.

55. The client admitted with a diagnosis of a fractured hip is in skin traction and reporting severe pain. Which intervention should the nurse implement?
    1. Adjust the patient-controlled analgesia (PCA) machine for a lower dose.
    2. Ensure the weights of the skin traction are off the floor and hanging freely.
    3. Raise the head of the bed to 45 degrees and the foot to 15 degrees.
    4. Turn the client on the affected leg using pillows to support the other leg.

56. The nurse is providing discharge teaching to the parents and 12-year-old with a fractured humerus. Which information should the nurse include regarding cast care? **Select all that apply**.
    1. Keep the fractured arm at heart level.
    2. Use a wire hanger to scratch inside the cast.
    3. Apply an ice pack to any itching area.
    4. Explain foul smells are expected occurrences.
    5. Prevent the cast from getting wet.

57. Which statement by the client diagnosed with a fractured ulna indicates to the nurse the client **needs further** teaching?
    1. "I need to eat a high-protein diet to ensure healing."
    2. "I need to wiggle my fingers every hour to increase circulation."
    3. "I need to take my pain medication before my pain is too bad."
    4. "I need to keep this immobilizer on when lying down only."

58. The nurse is preparing the care plan for a client newly diagnosed with a fractured lower extremity. Which outcome is **most appropriate** for the client?
    1. The client will maintain the function of the leg.
    2. The client will ambulate with assistance.
    3. The client will be turned every 2 hours.
    4. The client will have no infection.

59. The nurse is caring for a client diagnosed with a fracture of the right distal humerus. Which data indicate a complication? **Select all that apply**.
    1. Numbness and mottled cyanosis.
    2. Paresthesia and paralysis.
    3. Proximal pulses and point tenderness.
    4. Coldness of the extremity and crepitus.
    5. Palpable radial pulse and functional movement.

60. An 88-year-old client is admitted to the orthopedic floor with the diagnosis of a fractured pelvis. Which intervention should the nurse implement **first**?
    1. Insert an indwelling catheter.
    2. Administer a sodium phosphate enema.
    3. Assess the abdomen for bowel sounds.
    4. Apply skin traction.

## Joint Replacements

61. The nurse is caring for the client after a total hip replacement (THR). Which interventions should the nurse implement postoperatively? **Select all that apply**.
    1. Keep an abduction pillow in place between the legs at all times.
    2. Cough and deep breathe at least every 4 to 5 hours.
    3. Turn to both sides every 2 hours to prevent pressure ulcers.
    4. Sit in a high-seated chair for a flexion of less than 90 degrees.
    5. Apply the sequential compression device to prevent blood clots.

62. The client, 1 day postoperative THR, reports hearing a "popping sound" when turning. Which assessment data should the nurse report **immediately** to the surgeon?
    1. Dark red-purple discoloration.
    2. Equal length of lower extremities.
    3. Groin pain in the affected leg.
    4. Edema at the incision site.

63. The nurse is discharging a client after a THR. Which statement indicates **further** teaching is needed?
    1. "I should not cross my legs because my hip may come out of the socket."
    2. "I will call my HCP if I have a sudden increase in pain."
    3. "I will sit on a chair with arms and a firm seat."
    4. "After 3 weeks, I don't have to worry about infection."

64. The nurse finds small, fluid-filled lesions on the margins of the client's surgical dressing. Which statement is the **most appropriate** scientific rationale for this occurrence?
    1. These were caused by the cautery unit in the operating room.
    2. These are papular wheals from herpes zoster.
    3. These are blisters from the tape used to anchor the dressing.
    4. These macular lesions are from a latex allergy.

65. Which interventions should be included in the discharge teaching for a client after THR? **Select all that apply**.
    1. Discuss the client's weight-bearing limits.
    2. Request the client demonstrate the use of assistive devices.
    3. Explain the importance of increasing activity gradually.
    4. Instruct the client not to take medication before ambulating.
    5. Tell the client to ambulate with open-toed house shoes.

66. The nurse is caring for the client after THR. Which data indicate the surgical treatment is **effective**?
    1. The client states the pain is at a "3" on a 1-to-10 scale.
    2. The client has a limited ability to ambulate.
    3. The client's left leg is shorter than the right leg.
    4. The client ambulates to the bathroom.

67. The nurse is caring for a client 6 hours postoperative right total knee replacement. Which data should the nurse report to the surgeon?
    1. A total of 100 mL of red drainage in the autotransfusion drainage system.
    2. Pain relief after using the patient-controlled analgesia (PCA) pump.
    3. Cool toes, distal pulses palpable, and pale nailbeds bilaterally.
    4. Urinary output of 60 mL of clear yellow urine in 3 hours.

68. The client is being discharged home after total knee replacement. The nurse should refer the client to which multidisciplinary team member?
    1. The occupational therapist.
    2. The physiatrist.
    3. The recreational therapist.
    4. The home health nurse.

69. The nurse is caring for a client with a right total knee replacement. Which intervention should the nurse implement? **Select all that apply**.
    1. Monitor the continuous passive motion machine.
    2. Apply thigh-high TED hose bilaterally.
    3. Place the abductor pillow between the legs.
    4. Encourage the family to perform ADLs for the client.
    5. Assist the client to the chair 6 hours after surgery.

70. The nurse is caring for the client after right shoulder replacement. Which data **warrant immediate** intervention?

| Laboratory Test | Client Value | Normal Values |
|---|---|---|
| Potassium (K⁺) | 4.2 | 3.5–5.3 mEq/L or mmol/L |
| Hemoglobin (Hgb) | 7.8 | M: 14–17.3 g/dL<br>F: 11.7–15.5 g/dL |
| Creatinine | 0.8 | M: 0.61–1.21 mg/dL<br>F: 0.51–1.11 mg/dL |
| White Blood Cells (WBCs) | 9.0 | 4.5–11.1 × (10³/cells/microL) |

1. The client's hemoglobin.
2. The client's white blood cell count.
3. The client's creatinine level.
4. The client's potassium level.

71. The nurse is assessing the client postoperative total knee replacement. Which assessment data **warrant immediate** intervention?
    1. T 99°F, HR 80, RR 20, and BP 128/76.
    2. Pain in the unaffected leg during dorsiflexion of the ankle.
    3. Bowel sounds heard intermittently in four quadrants.
    4. Diffuse, crampy abdominal pain.

72. The nurse is working on an orthopedic floor. Which client should the nurse assess **first** after the change-of-shift report?
    1. The 84-year-old female with a fractured right femoral neck in skin traction.
    2. The 64-year-old female with confusion after left total knee replacement.
    3. The 88-year-old male post–right total hip replacement with an abduction pillow.
    4. The 50-year-old postoperative client with a continuous passive motion (CPM) device.

## CONCEPTS

The concepts covered in this chapter focus on mobility and functional ability. Exemplars that are covered are arthritis, fractures, amputation, joint replacement, and degenerative disk disease. Interrelated concepts of the nursing process and clinical judgment are covered throughout the questions. The concept of clinical judgment is presented in the prioritizing or "first" questions.

73. The nurse identifies the concept of impaired functional ability for a client diagnosed with rheumatoid arthritis. Which intervention should the nurse implement?
    1. Teach the client to apply antiembolism (TED) hose.
    2. Administer the nonsteroidal medication before the morning meal.
    3. Encourage the client to perform low-impact exercises daily.
    4. Refer the client to occupational therapy for gait training.

74. The client diagnosed with osteomyelitis of the left foot and ankle is being prepared for a BKA. Which intervention to improve the client's functional ability is a **priority** after rehabilitation?
    1. Keep a large tourniquet at the bedside to stop potential bleeding from the amputation site.
    2. Place a pillow in the bed for the client to push the stump against many times per day.
    3. Take and document the client's vital signs every 4 hours.
    4. Have the dietary department send high-protein, high-carbohydrate meals six times a day.

75. The client in the rehabilitation hospital refuses to participate in physical therapy following surgery for repair of a fractured right femur sustained in an MVA. The client also fractured the left forearm. Which should the nurse implement **first** when encouraging the client to participate in therapy?

    1. Medicate the client for pain 30 minutes before the therapy.
    2. Have the health-care provider make the client go to therapy.
    3. Explain that insurance will not pay if the client does not participate in therapy daily.
    4. Determine why the client refuses to participate in therapy sessions.

76. The nurse is admitting a client diagnosed with rheumatoid arthritis (RA) and the hands have the appearance shown. Which concept would the nurse identify as a **priority**?

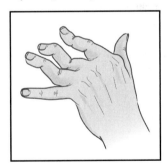

    1. Mobility.
    2. Functional ability.
    3. Coping.
    4. Rehabilitation.

77. Which medication should the nurse **question** administering to a client diagnosed with RA with a comorbid condition of non-Hodgkin's lymphoma?

| Client Name: Ms. J.S. | MR#: 654321 | Diagnosis: RA and Non-Hodgkin's Lymphoma |
|---|---|---|
| Age: 73 years | Allergies: NKDA | |
| Medication | 0701–1900 | 1901–0700 |
| Celecoxib 200 mg orally daily | 0900 | |
| Filgrastim 300 mg subcutaneous daily times 7 days | 0900 | |
| Adalimumab 40 mg subcutaneous every other week | 0900 | |
| Acetaminophen 650 mg orally every 4 hours prn | | |
| Signature of Nurse: | Day Nurse RN/DN | Night Nurse RN/NN |

1. Celecoxib.
2. Filgrastim.
3. Adalimumab.
4. Acetaminophen.

78. The nurse identifies the concept of impaired mobility for a male client diagnosed with degenerative disk disease. Which assessment data **best** support this concept?
    1. The client reports a history of chronic back pain and multiple back surgeries.
    2. The client reports that taking NSAIDs caused the development of peptic ulcers.
    3. The client reports a 3-year history of difficulty initiating a urinary stream.
    4. The client states he fell a year ago and had to have a cast on the right arm for a month.

79. The nurse is caring for a client diagnosed with a fracture of the right hip. Which data should be reported to the orthopedic surgeon **before** surgery?

| Complete Blood Count | Client Value | Normal Values |
|---|---|---|
| Red Blood Cells (RBCs) | 4.78 | M: 4.21–5.81 ($10^6$ cells/microL)<br>F: 3.61–5.11 ($10^6$ cells/microL) |
| Hemoglobin (Hgb) | 14 | M: 14–17.3 g/dL<br>F: 11.7–15.5 g/dL |
| Hematocrit (Hct) | 42 | M: 42%–52%<br>F: 36%–48% |
| Platelet | 98 | 140–400 × ($10^3$/microL) |
| White Blood Cells (WBCs) | 7.8 | 4.5–11.1 × ($10^3$/cells/microL) |
| Erythrocyte Sedimentation Rate (ESR) | 17 | Adult < 50 yr: M: 0–15 mm/hr<br>F: 0–25 mm/hr<br>Adult ≥ 50 yr: M: 0–20 mm/hr<br>F: 0–30 mm/hr |

1. The red blood cell count of 4.78.
2. The hemoglobin of 14 g/dL.
3. The platelet count of 98.
4. The sedimentation rate of 17 mm/hr.

80. The client after a left AKA as a result of uncontrolled diabetes asks the nurse, "Why did this happen to me? I have always been a good person." Which is the nurse's **most therapeutic** response?
    1. "How does it feel knowing you could have prevented this?"
    2. "I know how you feel; having your leg cut off is sad."

3. "Why do you think that you had to have your leg amputated?"

4. "I can see you are hurting. Would you like to talk?"

81. The nurse writes a concept of "impaired mobility" for a client diagnosed with a fractured right hip. Which would the nurse include in the plan of care? **Select all that apply**.
    1. Request a physical therapy referral.
    2. Administer enoxaparin subcutaneously.
    3. Utilize a gait belt when ambulating the client.
    4. Assess the client's pain levels on a 1-to-10 scale.
    5. Provide a high-carbohydrate, high-fat, high-sodium diet.

82. The nurse is admitting a female client reporting severe back pain radiating down the left leg whenever she tries to ambulate. The concepts of impaired mobility and comfort are implemented on the care map. Which nursing interventions should the nurse implement?
    1. Assist the client when ambulating to the bathroom and administer medications based on the pain scale.
    2. Place the client on strict bedrest and have the client use a regular bedpan for the elimination of urine and feces.
    3. Ambulate the client in the hallway at least 4 times per day and discourage the use of pharmacological pain relief.
    4. Request the HCP to assist the client in ambulating in the hallway so the HCP can observe the client's pain.

83. The client diagnosed with a left-sided cerebrovascular accident (stroke) has residual right-sided paralysis. The nurse identifies a concept of impaired functional ability. Which should be included in the care map? **Select all that apply**.
    1. Refer to the occupational therapist.
    2. Assess the client for neglect of the right side.
    3. Place the client in a room where the door is on the left side.
    4. Teach the client to call for assistance before getting out of bed.
    5. Encourage the client to participate in physical therapy daily.

84. The 35-year-old client diagnosed with a crushing injury to the left hand and forearm is being discharged. Which referral should the nurse implement?
    1. Physical therapy at home.
    2. An assistive living facility.
    3. A workforce commission for job training.
    4. A dietitian.

## Degenerative and Herniated Disk Disease

1. 1. Back pain occurs in 80% to 90% of the population at different times in their lives. Although not using good body mechanics when lifting an object may be a reason for younger clients to develop a herniated disk, it is not the reason most older people develop back pain.
   2. There is a decreased blood supply as the body ages.
   3. Older clients develop degenerative joint disease. Fat does not deposit itself in the nucleus pulposus.
   4. Less blood supply, degeneration of the disk, and arthritis are reasons older people develop back problems.

**TEST-TAKING HINT:** The clue in this question is "older." The answer must address a problem occurring as a result of aging.

2. 1. Posture and gait will be affected if the client is experiencing sciatica (pain radiating down a leg resulting from pressure on the sciatic nerve).
   2. The client with pain and numbness is not able to bend or stoop and should not be asked to do so.
   3. Leg lifts will not give the nurse the needed information and could cause this client pain; also, the lower extremity, not the upper extremity, is being assessed.
   4. Waist twists will not assess the mobility of the lower extremity, and neck mobility is assessed if a cervical neck problem is suspected.

**TEST-TAKING HINT:** Anatomical positioning and the function of spinal nerves rule out options "3" and "4."

3. 1. Increased calcium, not potassium or sodium, is helpful in preventing orthopedic injuries. Increasing sodium intake could prevent water loss in a non–air-conditioned warehouse in the summer months, not the winter months.
   2. These are instructions to prevent back injuries as a result of poor body mechanics.
   3. Soft-cushioned chairs are not ergonomically designed. Soft-cushioned chairs promote poor body posture.
   4. This might help the client prevent back injuries at home, but it does not prevent job-related injuries.

**TEST-TAKING HINT:** The question is asking for information that will prevent on-the-job back injuries. Option "4" can be ruled out because of this. The two electrolytes in option "1" are not associated with orthopedic injuries or bones, thus ruling out this option.

4. 1. Teaching back exercises to a client already experiencing a problem is tertiary care.
   2. Placing signs with instructions about how to render first aid is a secondary intervention, not primary prevention.
   3. Excess weight increases the workload on the vertebrae. Weight-loss activities help to prevent back injury.
   4. Administering a nonnarcotic analgesic to a client with back pain is an example of secondary or tertiary care, depending on whether the client has a one-time problem or a chronic problem with back pain.

**TEST-TAKING HINT:** Primary care is any activity that will prevent an illness or injury.

5. 1. This is an example of collaborative care.
   2. This is an example of collaborative care.
   3. This is a distraction and is an alternative method often recommended for the promotion of client comfort.
   4. Surgery is collaborative care.

**TEST-TAKING HINT:** The question asks for an alternative, independent type of care. Options "1," "2," and "4" are all collaborative care. If the test taker can find a common thread among three of the options, then the correct answer will be the other option.

6. 1. "Prone" means on the abdomen. On the abdomen with the knees flexed is an uncomfortable position, placing the spine in an unnatural position.
   2. The surgical position of the wound places the client at risk for edema of tissues in the neck. Difficulty speaking or breathing should alert the nurse to a potentially life-threatening problem.
   3. The drainage from a JP drain should be emptied and monitored every shift.
   4. The client should be kept as comfortable as possible.

**TEST-TAKING HINT:** The nurse must know the meaning of the common medical term prone and realize this would be uncomfortable for the client, thus eliminating option "1." The time frame of "every day" makes option "3" wrong.

7. 1. The lumbar nerves innervate the lower abdomen. The bladder is in the lower abdomen. The client will be required to lie flat, and this is a difficult position for many clients, especially males, in which to void. Clients are log rolled every 2 hours.
   2. The client should be receiving IV pain medication, not steroids. A Trendelenburg position is head down.
   3. Sandbags keep the neck still, but the surgical area is in the lumbar region, so there is no reason the client cannot turn the head; also, cathartic medications are harsh laxatives.
   4. The client will be receiving subcutaneous anticoagulant medications to prevent deep vein thrombosis, but IV anticoagulant therapy is not warranted. Eight liters per minute of oxygen is high-flow oxygen and is used for a client diagnosed with respiratory distress but without carbon dioxide narcosis.

**TEST-TAKING HINT:** The test taker must note the adjective "lumbar"; this can rule out option "3." Knowledge of medication classifications would rule out options "2" and "4."

8. 1. A client 2 days postoperative laminectomy should be eating a regular diet.
   2. The client, after undergoing a lumbar laminectomy, is log rolled. It requires four people or more to log roll a client.
   3. The legs of any client diagnosed with back pain can give out and collapse at any time, but a large client diagnosed with back pain is at increased risk of injuring the UAP as well as the client. The RN should intervene before the client or UAP becomes injured.
   4. This action helps ensure safety for the client.

**TEST-TAKING HINT:** This question is an "except" question. All the options but one contain interventions that should be implemented.

9. 1. Mild back pain is expected with this client.
   2. Lumbar myelograms require access to the spinal column. A small amount of cerebrospinal fluid may be lost, causing a mild headache. The client should stay flat in bed to prevent this from occurring.

3. This client is postoperative and now has a fever. This client should be assessed, and the health-care provider should be notified.
4. A discharged client does not have priority over a surgical infection.

**TEST-TAKING HINT:** Options "1" and "2" contain assessment data expected for the procedure.

10. 1. This could be administered after breakfast, if necessary. There is nothing in the action of the medication requiring before breakfast medication administration.
    2. Clients diagnosed with type 1 diabetes are insulin dependent. This medication should be administered before the client eats.
    3. This medication should be held until after surgery.
    4. The client has already received three doses of the IV antibiotic. This medication could be given after insulin.

**TEST-TAKING HINT:** The nurse must decide which medication has priority by determining the action of the medication, the route of administration, and the diagnosis of the client.

11. Correct answers are 1 and 2.
    1. An objective method of quantifying the client's pain should be used.
    2. Once the nurse has determined the client is stable and not experiencing complications, the nurse can medicate the client.
    3. A regular bedpan is high and could cause pain for a client diagnosed with back pain. The client should be given a fracture pan.
    4. There is no surgical dressing.
    5. The client has not been to surgery, so log rolling is not necessary.

**TEST-TAKING HINT:** Two of the options, "4" and "5," apply to postsurgical cases and could be eliminated.

12. 1. The nurse should not continue working, and this is self-diagnosing and treating.
    2. The nurse may go to the emergency department, but this is not the first action.
    3. The first action is to notify the charge nurse so a replacement can be arranged to take over the care of the clients. The nurse should notify the nurse manager or house supervisor. An occurrence report should be completed, documenting the situation. This provides the nurse with the required documentation to begin a worker's compensation case for payment of medical bills.

4. The nurse has the right to see a private health-care provider in most states, but this is not the first action.

**TEST-TAKING HINT:** When the test taker is determining a priority, then all of the answers may be appropriate interventions, but only one is implemented first. The test taker should read the full stem, identify the important words, and be certain what the question is asking.

## Osteoarthritis (OA)

13. 1. Obesity is a well-recognized risk factor for the development of OA, and it is modifiable because the client can lose weight.
    2. Increasing age is a risk factor, but there is nothing the client can do about getting older.
    3. Previous joint damage is a risk factor, but it is not modifiable, which means the client cannot do anything to change it.
    4. Genetic susceptibility is a result of family genes, which the client cannot change; it is a nonmodifiable risk factor.

**TEST-TAKING HINT:** The adjective "modifiable" is the key to selecting the correct answer. Only option "1" contains anything the client has control over changing or modifying.

14. Correct answers are 2 and 5.
    1. Severe bone deformity is seen in clients diagnosed with rheumatoid arthritis.
    2. Pain, stiffness, and functional impairment are the primary clinical manifestations of OA. Stiffness of the joints is commonly experienced after resting but usually lasts less than 30 minutes and decreases with movement.
    3. A waddling gait is usually seen in women in their third trimester of pregnancy or in older children with congenital hip dysplasia.
    4. Swan-neck fingers are seen in clients diagnosed with rheumatoid arthritis.
    5. Crepitus, a crackling or grating sensation, is common in clients with OA (Hoffman & Sullivan, 2020).

**TEST-TAKING HINT:** The test taker can have difficulty distinguishing clinical manifestations of two similar sounding diseases, osteoarthritis and RA. Both diseases involve the joints and cause pain and stiffness. Remember, RA can permanently disfigure the client, leading to "bone deformity" and "swan-neck fingers."

15. 1. Clients diagnosed with OA should be encouraged to move, which will decrease the pain.
    2. A bed bath does not require as much movement from the client as getting up and walking to the shower.
    3. The pain will decrease with movement, and warm or hot water will help decrease the pain. The worst thing the client can do is not move.
    4. Notifying the family will not address the client's pain, and the client has a right to refuse a bath, but the nursing staff must explain why moving and bathing will help decrease the pain.

**TEST-TAKING HINT:** Allowing clients to stay in bed only increases complications of immobility and will increase the client's pain secondary to OA. Clients diagnosed with chronic illnesses should be encouraged to be as independent as possible. The family should only be notified if a significant situation has occurred.

16. 1. Pain is a physiological problem, not a psychosocial problem.
    2. A client diagnosed with OA does not have bone deformities; therefore, body image disturbance is not appropriate.
    3. After 7 years of OA and multiple treatment modalities, knowledge deficit is not appropriate for this client.
    4. The client experiencing chronic pain often experiences depression and hopelessness.

**TEST-TAKING HINT:** The adjective "psychosocial" should help the test taker rule out option "1." The test taker needs to read the stem carefully. This client has had a problem for years, and, therefore, option "3" could be ruled out as a correct answer.

17. Correct answers are 4 and 5.
    1. This medication should be taken with food to prevent gastrointestinal distress.
    2. Glucocorticoids, not NSAIDs, must be tapered when discontinuing.
    3. Topical analgesics are applied to the skin; NSAIDs are oral or intravenous medications.
    4. NSAIDs are well known for causing gastric upset and increasing the risk for peptic ulcer disease, which could cause the client to vomit blood.
    5. Acetylsalicylic acid (aspirin) should not be taken with other NSAIDs to avoid increased side effects such as bleeding (Hoffman & Sullivan, 2020).

**TEST-TAKING HINT:** The worst-scenario option is "4," which has blood in the answer. If the test taker did not know the answer, then selecting an option with blood in it is most appropriate. Acetylsalicylic acid is an NSAID and should not be taken with another NSAID.

18. 1. This is an intervention, not a goal, and "passive" means the nurse performs the range of motion, which should not be encouraged.
    2. **The two main goals of treatment for OA are pain management and optimizing the functional ability of the joints to ensure movement of the joints.**
    3. Most clients diagnosed with OA are older, are overweight, and have a sedentary lifestyle, so walking 3 miles every day is not a realistic or safe goal.
    4. Joining a health club is an intervention, and the fact the client joins the health club doesn't mean the client will exercise.

**TEST-TAKING HINT:** The test taker must remember a goal is the measurable outcome of nursing interventions based on the client's problem and diagnosis. Interventions are not goals; therefore, the test taker could eliminate options "1" and "4" as possible answers.

19. 1. A physiatrist is a physician specializing in physical medicine and rehabilitation, but the nurse should not refer the client to this person just because the client is having difficulty with transfers.
    2. The social worker does not address this type of physical problem. Social workers address issues concerning finances, placement, and acquiring assistive devices.
    3. **The physical therapist is able to help the client with transferring, ambulation, and other lower extremity difficulties.**
    4. A counselor is not able to help the client learn how to get in and out of the bathtub.

**TEST-TAKING HINT:** The nurse must know the roles of all the health-care team members.

20. 1. **Safety should always be discussed when teaching about exercises. Supportive shoes will prevent shin splints. Colored socks have dye and may cause athlete's foot, which is why white socks are recommended.**
    2. Clients diagnosed with diabetes mellitus should carry complex carbohydrates with them.
    3. Osteoarthritis occurs most often in weight-bearing joints. Exercise is encouraged, but jogging increases stress on these joints.

4. For exercising to help pain control, the client must walk daily, not three times a week. Walking at least 30 minutes 3 times a week is appropriate for weight loss.

**TEST-TAKING HINT:** The test taker can rule out option "3" as an answer because the stem says "pain control"; option "1" is correct for any exercise program.

21. 1. NSAIDs or glucocorticoids help decrease inflammation of the joints.
    2. **This is the rationale for administering these medications, although experts disagree on the efficacy of these medications in the treatment of pain from osteoarthritis (National Center for Complementary and Integrative Health, 2017).**
    3. Narcotic and nonnarcotic analgesics help decrease the client's pain.
    4. There is no medication at this time to help increase synovial fluid production, but surgery can increase the viscosupplementation in the joint.

**TEST-TAKING HINT:** There are some questions that require the test taker to have the knowledge, and there are no test-taking hints to help with selecting the right answer.

22. 1. Medication is standard therapy and is not considered an alternative therapy.
    2. A heating pad is an accepted medical recommendation for the treatment of pain for clients diagnosed with OA.
    3. **Alternative forms of treatment have not been proved efficacious in the treatment of a disease. The nurse should be nonjudgmental and open to discussions about alternative treatment unless it interferes with the medical regimen.**
    4. Conservative treatment measures for OA include splints and braces to support inflamed joints.

**TEST-TAKING HINT:** The test taker needs to read the stem carefully to be able to determine what the question is asking. There is only one option with alternative-type treatment, which is option "3"; options "1," "2," and "4" are accepted treatment options listed in a textbook.

23. 1. MRIs are not routinely ordered for diagnosing OA.
    2. There is no serum laboratory test to measure synovial fluid in the joints.
    3. **X-rays reveal loss of joint cartilage, which appears as a narrowing of the joint space in clients diagnosed with OA.**
    4. An ESR is a diagnostic laboratory test for rheumatoid arthritis, not osteoarthritis.

**TEST-TAKING HINT:** If the test taker is guessing which answer is correct and knows osteo- means "bone," the only option with any specific connection to bones is an x-ray. This selection is an educated guess.

24. 1. A cold foot in a client after surgery may indicate a neurovascular compromise and must be assessed first.
 2. A client diagnosed with osteoarthritis is expected to have stiff joints.
 3. A routine medication is not a priority over a potential complication of surgery.
 4. A routine diagnostic procedure does not have priority over a potential complication of surgery.

**TEST-TAKING HINT:** The test taker must take a systematic approach when answering prioritizing questions. First, the test taker must determine if any client is experiencing a life-threatening or life-altering complication such as loss of a limb. The test taker must determine if the clinical manifestation is expected for the disease or condition.

## Osteoporosis

25. Correct answers are 3 and 5.
 1. Calcium deficiency is a modifiable risk factor, which means the client can do something about this factor—namely, increase the intake of calcium—to help prevent the development of osteoporosis.
 2. Smoking is a modifiable risk factor because the client can quit smoking.
 3. A nonmodifiable risk factor is a factor the client cannot do anything to alter or change. Approximately 50% of all women will experience an osteoporosis-related fracture in their lifetime.
 4. The client can quit drinking alcohol; therefore, this is a modifiable risk factor.
 5. Another nonmodifiable risk factor is ancestry. All individuals can be affected by osteoporosis but individuals of non-Hispanic, European, and Asian ancestry are at higher risk.

**TEST-TAKING HINT:** The keyword to answering this question is "nonmodifiable," which means the client cannot do anything to modify or change behavior to help prevent developing osteoporosis.

26. 1. This is the rationale for heavy alcohol use leading to the development of osteoporosis.
 2. Smoking decreases, not increases, the blood supply to the bone.
 3. Cigarette smoking has long been identified as a risk factor for osteoporosis, and it doesn't matter if the cigarettes are low tar.
 4. Nicotine slows the production of osteoblasts and impairs the absorption of calcium, contributing to decreased bone density.

**TEST-TAKING HINT:** The test taker must always be aware of the words "increase" and "decrease" when selecting a correct answer.

27. 1. The loss of height occurs as vertebral bodies collapse.
 2. Weight loss is not a sign of osteoporosis.
 3. This may indicate rheumatoid arthritis but not osteoporosis.
 4. This is a sign of gout.

**TEST-TAKING HINT:** If the test taker is not sure of the answer and knows osteo- means "bone," the only answer related to bones is the height of the client related to the spine.

28. 1. Osteoporotic changes do not occur in the bone until more than 30% of the bone mass has been lost.
 2. This serum blood study may be elevated after a fracture, but it does not help diagnose osteoporosis.
 3. This test measures bone mineral density in the lumbar spine or hip and is considered to be highly accurate (National Institute of Arthritis and Musculoskeletal and Skin Diseases, n.d).
 4. This test is most useful to evaluate the effects of treatment, rather than as an indicator of the severity of the bone disease.

**TEST-TAKING HINT:** Option "2" does not have bone or x-ray in it; therefore, if the test taker did not know the correct answer, eliminating this option is appropriate. If the test taker knew osteoporosis is secondary to poor absorption of calcium, option "3" is an appropriate selection for the correct answer.

29. 1. The best dietary sources of calcium are milk and other dairy products. Other sources include oysters; canned sardines or salmon; beans; cauliflower; and dark-green, leafy vegetables.
 2. These foods are high in vitamin C.
 3. These foods are high in potassium.
 4. These foods are recommended for a high-fiber diet.

**TEST-TAKING HINT: A question about special diets is a knowledge-based question, and the test taker must know which foods are in which type of diets. Foods high in calcium should be associated with milk products such as yogurt.**

30. 1. This is an example of a secondary nursing intervention, which includes screening for early detection.
    2. The client should perform weight-bearing exercises, which promote osteoblast activity, helping to maintain bone strength and integrity. This is a primary nursing intervention.
    3. Increasing dietary calcium may be a primary intervention to help prevent osteoporosis or a tertiary intervention, which helps treat osteoporosis.
    4. Smoking cessation is a primary intervention, which will help prevent the development of osteoporosis.

**TEST-TAKING HINT: The nurse must be knowledgeable of primary, secondary, and tertiary nursing interventions. Primary interventions are those that prevent the disease; secondary interventions are interventions such as screening the client for the disease with the goal of detecting it early, and tertiary interventions are interventions implemented when the client has the disease.**

31. 1. Swimming is not as beneficial as walking in maintaining bone density because of the lack of weight-bearing activity.
    2. Weight-bearing activity, such as walking, is beneficial in preventing or slowing bone loss. The mechanical force of weight-bearing exercises promotes bone growth.
    3. Swimming is not as beneficial in maintaining bone density because of the lack of weight-bearing activity.
    4. A sedentary lifestyle is a risk factor for the development of osteoporosis.

**TEST-TAKING HINT: Sedentary activities include sitting and very low-activity exercises, which are risk factors in developing many diseases and disorders; therefore, option "4" can be eliminated.**

32. Correct answers are 2, 3, and 4.
    1. Alendronate (Fosamax) should be taken first thing in the morning, not at night.
    2. The client should be sure to drink 6 to 8 ounces of water (not coffee, juice, or other beverages) to increase the absorption of alendronate (Fosamax).
    3. Waiting 30 minutes before taking other medications, fluids, or food will increase the absorption of alendronate (Fosamax).
    4. The client should be instructed to notify the HCP if experiencing pain, difficulty swallowing, or new or worsening heartburn. The medication may need to be discontinued.
    5. The client should not lay down but remain upright after taking alendronate (Fosamax) to decrease the risk of irritation to the esophagus.

**TEST-TAKING HINT: The test taker should be familiar with medications such as alendronate (Fosamax), a bone reabsorption inhibitor, used to treat osteoporosis. This is a knowledge-based question.**

33. 1. The National Institutes of Health (NIH) recommends a daily calcium intake of 1,300 mg/day for adolescents, young adults, and pregnant and lactating women (National Institutes of Health, 2019).
    2. The pregnant teenager should eat foods high in calcium.
    3. Osteoporosis may not occur before age 50 years, but taking calcium throughout the life span will help prevent it. Remember, teenagers tend to focus on the present, not the future, so the most important intervention to teach them is to take calcium supplements.
    4. Activity will not help prevent osteoporosis in the teenager; the teenager must take calcium supplements.

**TEST-TAKING HINT: The age of the client is important when answering questions; developmental stages will help rule out or help select the correct answer.**

34. 1. The bed should be kept in the low position. Preventing falls is a priority for a client diagnosed with osteoporosis.
    2. Range-of-motion (ROM) exercises will help prevent deep vein thrombosis or contractures, but they do not help prevent osteoporosis.
    3. Turning the client will help prevent pressure ulcers but does not help prevent osteoporosis.
    4. Nighttime lights will help prevent the client from falling; fractures are the number one complication of osteoporosis.

**TEST-TAKING HINT:** The test taker should realize the bed should be kept in a low position at all times and should eliminate option "1" as a possible answer; ROM exercises and turning will help prevent complications of immobility, not osteoporosis.

35. 1. There is no reason to take calcium carbonate (Tums) with 8 ounces of water. Tums are usually chewed.
    2. Tums should not be taken with meals.
    3. Free hydrochloric acid is needed for calcium absorption; therefore, calcium carbonate (Tums) should be taken on an empty stomach.
    4. To determine the effectiveness of calcium supplements, the client must have a bone density test, not a serum calcium level measurement.

**TEST-TAKING HINT:** If unsure of the answer, the test taker should not select an option with an absolute-type word such as "only," "always," or "never." There are very few absolutes in health care.

36. **Six tablets.**
    One thousand milligrams is equal to 1 gram. Therefore, 3 grams is equal to 3,000 mg. If one tablet is 500 mg, the client will need six tablets to get the total amount of calcium needed daily:

    $$3,000 \div 500 = 6$$

**TEST-TAKING HINT:** The test taker must know how to perform math calculations and must be knowledgeable regarding conversions. Remember to use the drop-down calculator on the NCLEX-RN® examination.

## Amputation

37. 1. This position will decrease lung expansion.
    2. The prone position will help stretch the hamstring muscles, which will help prevent flexion contractures leading to problems when fitting the client for a prosthesis.
    3. Lying on the back will not help decrease actual or phantom pain.
    4. This will help take the pressure off the client's buttocks area, but it is not why it is recommended for a client with a lower extremity amputation.

**TEST-TAKING HINT:** The test taker can eliminate option "1" if visualizing the client in a prone position. This position will limit the expansion

of the lung more than increase it. When trying to allow for expansion of the lungs, clients are placed with the head elevated, a position the client in a prone position cannot achieve.

38. **Correct answers are 2 and 3.**
    1. The client is in the recovery room, and the dressing must be assessed more frequently than every 2 hours.
    2. The client must come to terms with the amputation; therefore, the nurse should encourage the client to look at the residual limb.
    3. The large tourniquet can be used if the residual limb begins to hemorrhage either internally or externally.
    4. The nurse should encourage active, not passive, range-of-motion exercises.
    5. The limb is wrapped with a compression dressing to decrease edema, but this is not performed until 1 to 3 days after the surgery.

**TEST-TAKING HINT:** Remember to look at the phrases describing the intervention, such as "every 2 hours" and "passive."

39. 1. For wound healing, a balanced diet with adequate protein and vitamins is essential, along with meals appropriate for type 2 diabetes.
    2. An occupational therapist addresses activities of daily living and usually addresses upper extremity amputations. A referral to a physical therapist is most appropriate to address ambulating and transfer concerns.
    3. There is no type of intravenous dye used in this surgical procedure, so this answer is not appropriate.
    4. An 18-gauge catheter should be started because the client is going to surgery; the client may need a blood transfusion, which should be administered through an 18-gauge catheter.

**TEST-TAKING HINT:** The nurse must take into account all the client's comorbid conditions (diabetes type 2) when selecting the correct answer.

40. 1. Wrapping the hand with towels is appropriate, but it is not the first intervention.
    2. Holding the arm above the head will help decrease the bleeding, but it is not the first intervention.
    3. Applying direct pressure to the artery above the amputated parts will help decrease the bleeding immediately and is the first intervention the nurse

should implement. Then the nurse should instruct the client to hold the hand above the head, apply towels, and call 911.

4. Calling 911 should be done, but it is not the first intervention.

**TEST-TAKING HINT: Remember, when the stem asks the test taker to identify the first intervention, all four options will be probable interventions, but only one is the first intervention.**

41. 1. Placing the amputated part directly on ice will cause vasoconstriction and necrosis of viable tissue.
2. Warm water will cause the amputated part to disintegrate and lose viable tissue.
3. Wrapping the amputated part in a piece of material will not help preserve the thumb so it can be reconnected.
4. Placing the thumb in a plastic bag will protect it, and then placing the plastic bag on ice will help preserve the thumb so it may be reconnected in surgery. Do not place the amputated part directly on ice because this will cause necrosis of viable tissue.

**TEST-TAKING HINT: The test taker should make sure to know what the question is asking before selecting the option. The question is asking "what will help preserve the thumb?"—which is the key to answering this question.**

42. 1. Some members of the Jewish faith believe all body parts must be buried together. Therefore, many synagogues will keep amputated limbs until death occurs. Or, a burial plot may be purchased and the severed limb buried (Shiva.com, 2019).
2. Specific foods are important, but not while the client is in the operating room.
3. Spiritual issues are important for the nurse to discuss with the client, but the operating room should be concerned with the disposition of the amputated limb.
4. Addressing teaching issues is important, but the most important concern is the disposition of the amputated limb.

**TEST-TAKING HINT: The nurse must always address the cultural needs of the client, and when the test taker sees a specific culture in the stem of a question, it is a prompt indicating this will be important when selecting the answer.**

43. 1. The client is 3 hours postoperative and needs medical intervention.
2. Phantom pain is caused by severing the peripheral nerves. The pain is real to the client, and the nurse needs to medicate the client immediately.
3. Biofeedback exercises will not help address the client's postoperative surgical pain.
4. Placing the residual limb below the heart (dependent) will not help address the client's pain and could actually increase the pain.

**TEST-TAKING HINT: The test taker needs to be aware of adjectives such as "dependent." The nurse must know medical terms for positioning a client.**

44. 1. If the client is hemorrhaging, the surgeon needs to be notified, but hemorrhaging has not been determined.
2. Determining if the client is hemorrhaging is the first intervention. The nurse should check for clinical manifestations of hypovolemic shock: decreased BP and increased pulse.
3. Reinforcing the dressing helps decrease bleeding, but the nurse must assess first.
4. Checking the client's laboratory results is an appropriate intervention, but it is not the first intervention.

**TEST-TAKING HINT: Remember, when the stem asks the test taker to identify the first intervention, all four options will be probable interventions, but only one is the first intervention. Also, the nurse should always assess first. Remember the nursing process.**

45. 1. A client just 2 days postoperative amputation is not putting on a prosthesis.
2. Two RNs must double-check a unit of blood before infusing the blood.
3. The surgical dressing is changed by the surgeon or the RN; Syme's amputation is above the ankle, just removing the foot.
4. The UAP could take a client to another department in the hospital.

**TEST-TAKING HINT: Remember, teaching, assessing, and evaluating cannot be delegated.**

46. 1. Applying pressure to the end of the residual limb will help toughen the limb. Gradually pushing the residual limb against harder and harder surfaces is done in preparation for prosthesis training.
2. An Ace bandage applied distal to proximal will help decrease edema and help shape the residual limb into a conical shape.

3. Vitamin E oil will help decrease the angriness of the scar, but it will not help with residual limb toughening.
4. Elevating the residual limb will help decrease edema, but it will also cause a contracture if the residual limb is elevated after the first 24 hours.

**TEST-TAKING HINT:** The stem of the question asks the test taker to choose a method of toughening the residual limb. Demonstrating how to apply an elastic bandage or elevating the limb would not accomplish this, so options "2" and "4" could be eliminated from consideration.

47. 1. This statement does not indicate acceptance; the client is still in the anger stage of grieving.
   2. **Looking toward the future and problem-solving indicates the client is accepting the loss.**
   3. At this young age, a client with an upper extremity prosthesis needs to be thinking about obtaining employment and living a full life. Getting a prosthesis is important to pursue this goal.
   4. This statement does not indicate acceptance; his spouse will worry about the client's life, which has been changed dramatically.

**TEST-TAKING HINT:** Always notice when the age is given for the client. This will help guide the test taker to the correct answer.

48. **Correct answers are 1, 2, 3, and 4.**
   1. **Pain not relieved with analgesics could indicate complications or could be phantom pain.**
   2. **A well-balanced diet promotes wound healing, especially a diet high in protein.**
   3. **The client must keep appointments in outpatient rehabilitation to continue to improve physically and emotionally.**
   4. **A support group may help the client adjust to life with an amputation.**
   5. The client should be encouraged to get out as much as possible and live as normal a life as possible.

**TEST-TAKING HINT:** The test taker needs to select all appropriate options.

## Fractures

49. 1. The nurse should assess the nailbeds for the capillary refill time. A prolonged time (greater than 3 seconds) indicates impaired circulation to the extremity.

2. Clothing may need to be removed but not before assessment.
3. An x-ray will be done but is not the highest priority action.
4. A cast may or may not be applied, depending on the type and location of the fracture.

**TEST-TAKING HINT:** When the question asks to prioritize nursing care, usually, assessment is first. Assessment is an independent nursing intervention.

50. 1. The client may experience difficulty coping depending on how much mobility the client has after medical treatment, but it is not the most appropriate nursing diagnosis at this time.
   2. Compartment syndrome (edema within a muscle compartment) may occur, but there are multiple complications the nurse should be assessing for, so this is not the most appropriate nursing intervention.
   3. The client has a closed fracture, so there is no exposed bone or tissue.
   4. **Assessing and preventing complications related to the neurovascular compromise is the most appropriate intervention because, if there are no complications, a closed fracture should heal without problems.**

**TEST-TAKING HINT:** Physiological problems are a priority over psychosocial problems, so the test taker could rule out option "1."

51. **Correct answers are 2 and 5.**
   1. An immobilizer should not be applied snugly. There should be enough room to allow for edema and adequate perfusion of the tissues.
   2. **Ice packs should be applied 10 minutes on and 20 minutes off. This allows for vasoconstriction and decreases edema. Ice is a nonpharmacological pain management technique.**
   3. An injured extremity should be elevated above the level of the heart to decrease edema and pain.
   4. An x-ray should be done before the immobilizer is in place, not after.
   5. **Anytime trauma occurs, tetanus should be considered. In an open fracture, this is an appropriate treatment.**

**TEST-TAKING HINT:** This is an alternative-type question. When selecting all that apply, it is important to consider the descriptive words which make the options incorrect. Read adjectives and adverbs carefully. The terms "snugly," "dependent," and "after" make options "1," "3," and "4" incorrect.

52. 1. Localized edema and discoloration hours after the injury are normal occurrences after a fracture.
    2. Generalized weakness and increasing tenderness are common and not life-threatening.
    3. If the nurse cannot hear the pedal pulse with a Doppler and the client's pain is increasing, the nurse should notify the HCP. These are clinical manifestations of neurovascular compromise.
    4. Pain management is a desired outcome demonstrated by pain relieved after hydromorphone, a narcotic analgesic, administration.

**TEST-TAKING HINT: The nurse should notify the HCP of abnormal or unexpected assessment data; no pulse indicates a neurovascular complication. All the other options contain normal or expected data.**

53. 1. The nurse should assess the client for clinical manifestations of hypoxia from a fat embolism, which is what the nurse should anticipate from "fatty globules" in the urine.
    2. Arterial blood gases and portable chest x-ray will be done, but they will not be done first.
    3. A ventilation and perfusion scan is not the highest priority for the client. Assessment for complications is a priority.
    4. The UAP should keep the client on strict bedrest, but the RN's first intervention is to assess the client. The client is unstable and the nurse should assess the client first, then maintain strict bedrest.

**TEST-TAKING HINT: If the test taker is unsure of the correct answer, always apply the nursing process. Assessment is the first part of the nursing process.**

54. 1. There is controversy over assessing for a positive Homans' sign, but it is not the first intervention for a client oriented to person only.
    2. Encouraging the client to take deep breaths and cough aids in the exchange of gases. Mental changes are early signs of hypoxia in the elderly client, but the nurse must first determine if mental changes have occurred.
    3. The nurse is not aware of the client's usual mental status, so before taking any further action the nurse should determine what is normal or usual for this client.

4. Checking the client's skin (Buck's) traction will not address the problem of confusion. This will not address taking care of the orientation of the client.

**TEST-TAKING HINT: The test taker needs to understand what the question is asking. Although the client has a fractured hip, the orientation status is the unexpected symptom that requires assessment.**

55. 1. The HCP orders the dosage on a PCA. Unless a range of dosages or a new order is obtained, a lower dose will not help the pain.
    2. **Weights from traction should be off the floor and hanging freely. Skin (Buck's) traction is used to reduce muscle spasms preoperatively in clients diagnosed with fractured hips.**
    3. Raising the head of the bed or the foot will alter the traction.
    4. Turning the client to the affected side could increase pain rather than relieve it.

**TEST-TAKING HINT: This intervention is a form of assessment, assessing the equipment being used for the client's condition. Remember to apply the nursing process.**

56. Correct answers are 3 and 5.
    1. The arm should be elevated above the heart, not at heart level.
    2. The nurse should instruct the child not to insert anything under the cast because it could cause a break in the skin, leading to an infection.
    3. **Applying ice packs to the cast will relieve itching, and nothing should be placed down a cast to scratch. Skin becomes fragile inside the cast and is torn easily. Alteration in the skin's integrity can become infected.**
    4. Smells indicate infection and should be reported to the HCP.
    5. **Keep the cast clean and dry at all times. The cast can be covered with a plastic bag or cast cover for bathing and showering.**

**TEST-TAKING HINT: A concept for any injury is elevating it above the heart to decrease edema. Many times the test taker must apply basic concepts to a variety of client conditions. Any foul smell is not expected in any disease or condition.**

57. 1. Protein is necessary for healing.
    2. By wiggling the fingers of the affected arm, the client can improve the circulation.
    3. Pain medication should be taken before the perception of severe pain. Pain relief will require more medication if allowed to become severe.
    4. The immobilizer should be kept on at all times. This indicates the client does not understand the teaching and needs the nurse to provide more instruction.

**TEST-TAKING HINT: When selecting an answer for questions such as this, the test taker should remember to look for an untrue statement. This indicates teaching is needed.**

58. 1. The expected outcome for a client diagnosed with a fracture is maintaining the function of the extremity.
    2. Ambulation with assistance is not the best goal.
    3. This is a nursing intervention, not a client goal.
    4. Infection is not the highest priority problem for a client diagnosed with a fracture.

**TEST-TAKING HINT: The test taker must note the words "most appropriate" and look at the client as a whole entity. With musculoskeletal problems, maintaining normal function or anatomical function is the desired outcome. Remember, independence is a priority for the client.**

59. Correct answers are 1, 2, and 4.
    1. The nurse should assess for numbness and mottled cyanosis, which might indicate nerve damage.
    2. The presence of paresthesia and paralysis indicates impaired circulation.
    3. Pulses should be assessed but not proximal to the fracture. Pulses distal to the fracture should be assessed. Point tenderness should be expected.
    4. Coldness indicates decreased blood supply. Crepitus indicates air in the subcutaneous tissue and is not expected.
    5. Palpable radial pulses and functional movement do not indicate a complication has occurred.

**TEST-TAKING HINT: This is an alternate-type question in which the test taker must select all options that apply. The test taker should remember the neuromuscular assessment, which includes the 6 Ps—pulse, pain, paresthesia, paralysis, pallor, polar (cold).**

60. 1. Inserting an indwelling catheter is a good intervention, but it is not the first intervention. A tear or injury to the bladder should be suspected.
    2. Administering a sodium phosphate (Fleet's) enema should not be implemented until internal bleeding has been ruled out.
    3. Assessing the bowel sounds should be the first intervention to determine if an ileus has occurred. This is a common complication of a fractured pelvis.
    4. Skin (Buck's) traction is not used to treat a fractured pelvis. It is used to treat a fractured hip.

**TEST-TAKING HINT: When prioritizing two equal options, usually, assessing is the answer.**

## Joint Replacements

61. Correct answers are 4 and 5.
    1. The abduction pillow should be kept between the legs while in bed to maintain a neutral position and prevent internal rotation.
    2. The client should deep breathe and cough at least every 2 hours to prevent atelectasis and pneumonia.
    3. The client will need to turn every 2 hours but should not turn to the affected side.
    4. Using a high-seated toilet and chair will help prevent dislocation by limiting the flexion to less than 90 degrees.
    5. Compression devices such as antiembolism stockings or mechanical sequential compression devices are used to improve blood circulation and prevent blood clots (Topfer, 2016).

**TEST-TAKING HINT: Option "1" has the word "all"; an absolute word such as this usually eliminates the option as a possible correct answer. Nursing usually does not have situations involving absolutes.**

62. 1. Bruising is common after a total hip replacement.
    2. When a dislocation occurs, the affected extremity will be shorter.
    3. Groin pain or increasing discomfort in the affected leg and the "popping sound" indicate the leg was dislocated, which should be reported immediately to the HCP for a possible closed reduction.
    4. Edema at the incision site is common, but an increase in edema or redness should be reported.

**TEST-TAKING HINT:** The nurse should notify the surgeon of abnormal, unexpected, or life-threatening assessment data; if the test taker did not have an idea of the answer, pain is always a good choice because pain means something is wrong—it may be expected pain, but it may mean a complication.

63. 1. Clients should not cross their legs because the position increases the risk of dislocation.
    2. If the client experiences a sudden increase in pain, redness, edema, or stiffness in the joint or surrounding area, the client should notify the HCP.
    3. Clients should sleep on firm mattresses and sit on chairs with firm seats and high arms. These will decrease the risk of dislocating the hip joint.
    4. Infections are possible months after surgery. Clients should monitor temperatures and report any clinical manifestations of infection.

**TEST-TAKING HINT:** Note the stem is asking about the need for "further teaching." This means the test taker is looking for an unexpected option. This is an "except" question. Sometimes, if the test taker will change the question and say, "the client understands the teaching," then the option with an incorrect statement is the answer.

64. 1. These are not burns from the cautery unit. Such burns are located in or near the incision site and are usually black.
    2. Herpes simplex lesions occur in a linear pattern along a dermatome.
    3. Fluid-filled blisters are from a reaction to the tape and usually occur along the margins of the dressing where the tape was applied.
    4. Skin reactions to latex are local irritations or generalized dermatitis, not blisters.

**TEST-TAKING HINT:** If the test taker does not know the answer, the test taker might think about the dressing because the lesions are on the side of the dressing. How is a dressing anchored to the skin? Answer: with tape. The test taker should choose the option having the word "tape."

65. Correct answers are 1, 2, and 3.
    1. Clients need to understand the amount of weight-bearing to prevent injury.
    2. Teaching the safe use of assistive devices is necessary before discharge.
    3. Increases in activity should occur slowly to prevent complications.
    4. Using medication therapy, including analgesics, anti-inflammatory agents, or muscle relaxants, should be taught, so the client is comfortable while ambulating.
    5. The client should ambulate with well-fitted, supported, closed-toed shoes such as tennis shoes or walking shoes.

**TEST-TAKING HINT:** The test taker should apply basic concepts to all surgeries. Many times the test taker may not be familiar with the specific surgery, but by using discharge teaching applicable to all clients, a choice can be made.

66. 1. Minimal pain is expected in a postoperative client, but it does indicate surgical treatment is effective.
    2. The client should be able to ambulate with almost full mobility.
    3. A shorter leg indicates a dislocation of the hip.
    4. The hip should have functional motion, and the client should be able to ambulate to the bathroom. This indicates surgical treatment has been effective.

**TEST-TAKING HINT:** With musculoskeletal problems, functional movement is a priority. Also note option "2" has the word "limited" and "3" has "one leg shorter than the other," both of which are negative outcomes, so the test taker could eliminate these options.

67. 1. Drainage in the first 24 hours can be expected to be 200 to 400 mL. When using an autotransfusion drainage system, the client's blood will be filtered and returned to the client.
    2. Pain relief with the PCA does not require notifying the surgeon.
    3. Bilateral coolness of the toes is not a concern because both feet are cool. Circulation is not restricted if pulses are present. Seeing pale pink nailbeds indicates blood loss during surgery.
    4. The urinary output is not adequate; therefore, the surgeon needs to be notified. This is only 20 mL/hr. The minimum should be 30 mL/hr.

**TEST-TAKING HINT:** A concept the test taker will see throughout testing and throughout the nurse's practice is 30 mL of urine output per hour is necessary to maintain kidney function.

68. 1. The occupational therapist addresses upper extremity activities of daily living, swallowing issues, and cognition. This is not an appropriate referral.
    2. The physiatrist is a physician specializing in rehabilitation medicine practicing in a rehabilitation setting.

3. The recreational therapist is used in psychiatric settings, rehabilitation hospitals, and long-term care facilities. The discipline is not seen in the home.

4. The home health-care nurse will be able to assess the client in the home and make further referrals if necessary.

**TEST-TAKING HINT:** The nurse should always think about safety; therefore, the test taker should select options addressing safety issues.

69. Correct answers are 1 and 5.

1. The CPM machine is used to ensure the client has an adequate range of motion in the knee postoperatively.

2. The TED hose are only applied to the unaffected leg, not the leg with the incision.

3. Adductor pillows are used in clients with total hip replacements to maintain function hip alignment.

4. The client should perform as many ADLs as possible. The client should maintain independence as much as possible.

5. The client should begin moving from bed to chair within 6 to 8 hours after the procedure to strengthen muscles and facilitate recovery (Hoffman & Sullivan, 2020).

**TEST-TAKING HINT:** The test taker should remember to think about basic concepts of surgical care: Would an elastic hose be placed over a new incision? Sometimes trying to imagine what is actually occurring at the bedside helps to eliminate some options.

70. 1. The client's hemoglobin is 7.8 g/dL, which indicates the client requires a blood transfusion (Franchini et al., 2017). This information warrants intervention by the nurse.

2. This white blood cell count is within normal limits, so it does not warrant immediate intervention.

3. The creatinine level is within normal limits and does not warrant intervention.

4. The potassium level is within normal limits and does not require intervention by the nurse.

**TEST-TAKING HINT:** The test taker must be knowledgeable of laboratory values. There is no test-taking hint except memorizing the values.

71. 1. These vital signs are within normal limits.

2. Pain with dorsiflexion of the ankle indicates deep vein thrombosis. This can be from immobility or surgery; therefore, pain should be assessed in both legs.

3. Bowel sounds are normally intermittent.

4. This type of pain should make the nurse suspect the client has flatus, which is not a life-threatening complication and does not warrant immediate intervention.

**TEST-TAKING HINT:** "Warrant immediate intervention" means life-threatening, abnormal, or unexpected for the client's condition. Pain with dorsiflexion of the ankle, the Homans' sign, may be life-threatening if not treated immediately.

72. 1. This is a normal treatment of a fractured femoral neck.

2. This is an abnormal occurrence from this information. This client should be seen first because confusion is a symptom of hypoxia.

3. This is a common treatment of a total hip replacement.

4. This is a treatment used for total knee replacement.

**TEST-TAKING HINT:** When deciding the answer for this type of question, the test taker not knowing the answer should realize three choices have normal treatments for the disease process and one option contains different information, such as a symptom, and choose the option that is different.

**73.** 1. Antiembolism hose are to prevent venous stasis, a circulatory issue, not for functional ability.
2. NSAIDs are given with meals or food to prevent gastric distress and risk of bleeding ulcers. They are not administered on empty stomachs.
3. Low-impact exercises improve the client's range of motion in the joints and help to maintain functional ability. They should be performed on a daily basis.
4. Occupational therapists work on upper body activities and activities of daily living. Physical therapists work on the lower body and gait training as well as large muscle functioning.

**TEST-TAKING HINT:** The test taker could eliminate option "4" by knowing the function of the different therapies, "1" can be eliminated by knowing the purpose of antiembolism hose, and "2" can be eliminated by knowing basic nursing interventions for classifications of medications.

**74.** 1. The tourniquet is used to prevent hemorrhage from the residual limb. It does not improve functional ability.
2. The client should push against a pillow to toughen the stump and prepare it for a prosthesis. This will assist the client in regaining functional ability and mobility.
3. Taking and documenting vital signs provides the nurse with data to determine the stability of the client but does not improve functional ability.
4. A diet high in protein improves wound healing. The client's diet should have sufficient calories for wound healing but not particularly high carbohydrates. These interventions help with tissue integrity and wound healing, not functional ability.

**TEST-TAKING HINT:** The test taker should read the question carefully; the question is asking about what helps with functional ability. In this question, the test taker can eliminate the other three options based on the fact that they do not address functional ability. Even if the test taker does not "like" option "2," it is the odd man out, so it should be the one chosen.

**75.** 1. The nurse should medicate the client for pain before therapy if that is determined to be the cause for the client refusing to participate in therapy.
2. The client can make decisions. The HCP cannot make the client do anything.
3. The nurse should explain the rules of rehabilitation coverage, but this is not first.
4. The nurse should first assess the situation to determine the reason the client does not wish to participate in therapy.

**TEST-TAKING HINT:** The test taker should remember the first step of the nursing process is assessment. There are many words that can be used to indicate an assessment step.

**76.** 1. This picture does not indicate any deformity except the hands.
2. This is a picture of swan-neck fingers associated with RA. The function of the client's hands is a priority.
3. The client may have an issue with coping with the RA, but a psychosocial need is not a priority over an actual physiological need.
4. Rehabilitation would be an interrelated concept needed for this client, but determining the extent of functional impairment is a priority.

**TEST-TAKING HINT:** The test taker should not read into the question; in option "1" mobility refers to the ability of the client to move the body, not just the hands. The hands are the only body parts pictured. If an option exists that is more specific to the picture (functional ability), then the test taker should choose the one that is most closely related to the issue.

**77.** 1. Celecoxib (Celebrex) is approved for the routine treatment of arthritis and bone and joint diseases. The nurse would not question this medication.
2. Clients undergoing treatment for cancer frequently require filgrastim (Neupogen) to promote the production of WBCs due to the suppression of the bone marrow. The nurse would not question this medication.
3. An adverse effect of adalimumab (Humira) is the development of lymphoma. Because this client has a lymphoma, suppressing the immune system even further could have disastrous results for the client. The nurse would question administering this medication.

**435**

4. Acetaminophen (Tylenol) would not be questioned; the client has pain, and the dose is a recommended dose.

**TEST-TAKING HINT: The test taker must know basic medication guidelines.**

78. 1. A history of low back pain and multiple back surgeries indicates a history of disk and back issues.
    2. The use of NSAIDS could have happened for reasons other than degenerative disk disease.
    3. Difficulty initiating a urinary stream usually indicates a male client has benign prostatic hypertrophy. The prostate is blocking the urethra.
    4. A fall and wearing a cast on the arm do not indicate degenerative disk (vertebra of the back) disease.

**TEST-TAKING HINT: The test taker could eliminate option "4" if familiar with medical terminology; disks refer to the back, not the arm. Option "2" is nonspecific as to the reason for taking the NSAIDs and could be eliminated.**

79. 1. The RBC is within normal limits (WNL); there is no reason for the nurse to notify the surgeon.
    2. The hemoglobin is WNL; there is no reason for the nurse to notify the surgeon.
    3. The client is going to surgery, and bone surgeries result in blood loss. This client's platelet count is below 100,000, impairing the client's ability to clot. The nurse should immediately notify the surgeon.
    4. The sedimentation rate is WNL; there is no reason for the nurse to notify the surgeon.

**TEST-TAKING HINT: When reading a graph or a laboratory report, the test taker should read the normal ranges carefully in order to identify what is abnormal.**

80. 1. Placing blame is not therapeutic.
    2. If the nurse has not experienced the exact same situation, then the nurse cannot make this statement. It is not therapeutic.
    3. Asking why is not therapeutic; the nurse is requesting the client to defend personal feelings.
    4. This is a broad opening statement and offering self. Both are therapeutic techniques. The client needs an opportunity to verbalize the feeling associated with loss.

**TEST-TAKING HINT: When a question asks for a therapeutic response by the nurse, the nurse must give a response that does NOT lay blame or advise in any way and MUST encourage the client to discuss feelings.**

81. Correct answers are 1, 2, 3, and 4.
    1. A physical therapist will assist the client in ambulating safely while protecting the hip from being displaced.
    2. The client's mobility is compromised, placing the client at risk for developing a deep vein thrombosis (DVT). Enoxaparin (Lovenox) will assist in preventing a DVT.
    3. Health-care workers should use gait belts to provide support and stability when ambulating clients.
    4. Fractures of any bone are painful; pain scales are useful in qualifying the amount and type of pain being experienced by the client.
    5. The client's diet should be a well-balanced diet with an emphasis on protein for wound healing.

**TEST-TAKING HINT: Knowledge of basic nursing care is required when answering this question. The use of a gait belt for ambulating and assessing pain are basic nursing skills.**

82. 1. The nurse or nursing staff should assist the client in ambulating to the bathroom, and pain medication should be administered using the pain scale to quantify and qualify the pain level.
    2. The client should have bathroom privileges; strict bedrest will place the client at risk for pneumonia and DVT development. Movement should be encouraged within safe guidelines. A regular bedpan would place the client's back in an awkward position and increase the pain.
    3. Pain is whatever the client says it is and occurs whenever the client says it does. The nurse should not discourage the use of pain medications in the light of "severe" pain.
    4. The HCP does not need to assist the client in ambulating in the hallway to observe the effect of ambulation on the client's pain. The HCP can ask the client to ambulate in the room with the assistance of the UAP, RN, or PT.

**TEST-TAKING HINT:** The test taker should read words in the stem of a question and in the options—words matter. In option "2" "strict" and "regular" make this an incorrect option; in option "3" "discourage" makes it incorrect. In option "4," HCPs do not do the nurse's job of ambulating.

83. Correct answers are 1, 2, 3, 4, and 5.
    1. Occupational therapists work on upper body ability and activities of daily living as well as increasing cognitive ability. This is an excellent referral.
    2. Clients no longer having use of a side of the body will not realize when the arm or leg moves, and this can be a safety issue.
    3. The client may not realize that one-half of the visual field has been impaired as a result of the stroke. If this has happened, the client will not see things in the left visual fields. Remember that the nerve pathways cross over at the base of the skull, so a left-sided stroke produces issues for the body below the neck on the opposite side of the stroke, but in the brain (visual fields), it would be on the side of the stroke.
    4. For safety, this should be done for all clients.

5. The nurse should encourage the client to participate in an activity that increases the client's functional ability.

**TEST-TAKING HINT:** When answering "Select all that apply" questions, each option is read independently of the others. Each option becomes a true or false question.

84. 1. The client should be able, at age 35, to perform exercises independently.
    2. The client is 35 and should prepare to live life with the new limitations, not go into an assistive living facility.
    3. The client needs to gain new skills to become a productive member of society with the new limitations. All states have opportunities for clients with issues to be able to access training and assistance.
    4. The client has a functional disability, not a dietary need.

**TEST-TAKING HINT:** The test taker must read the words in the question and options. The ages matter. This 35-year-old client should be in Erikson's stage of generativity versus stagnation.

# MUSCULOSKELETAL DISORDERS COMPREHENSIVE EXAMINATION

1. The 50-year-old female client is being evaluated for osteoporosis. Which data should the nurse assess? Select all that apply.
   1. Family history of osteoporosis.
   2. Estrogen or androgen deficit.
   3. Exposure to secondhand smoke.
   4. Level and amount of exercise.
   5. Alcohol intake.

2. Which intervention should the nurse include for a client diagnosed with carpal tunnel syndrome?
   1. Teach hyperextension exercises to increase flexibility.
   2. Monitor safety during occupational hazards.
   3. Prepare for the insertions of pins or screws.
   4. Monitor dressing and drain after the fasciotomy.

3. Which staff nurse should the charge nurse assign to the client recovering from a repair of the hallux valgus?
   1. A new graduate nurse.
   2. An experienced nurse.
   3. A nurse practitioner.
   4. An unlicensed assistive personnel.

4. The client is scheduled for a computed tomography (CT) scan. Which question is most important for the nurse to ask before the procedure?
   1. "On a scale of 1 to 10, how do you rate your pain?"
   2. "Do you feel uncomfortable in enclosed spaces?"
   3. "Are you allergic to seafood or iodine?"
   4. "Have you signed a permit for this procedure?"

5. Two UAPs are using the transfer board to move the client from the bed to the wheelchair. Which action should the RN take?
   1. Take no action because this is the correct procedure for transferring a client.
   2. Instruct the UAPs not to use a transfer board when moving the client.
   3. Tell the UAPs to use the bed scale sling to move the client to the chair.
   4. Request the UAPs to stop and come to the nurse's station immediately.

6. Which priority intervention should the day surgery nurse implement for a client after right knee arthroscopy?
   1. Encourage the client to perform ROM exercises.
   2. Monitor the amount and color of the urine.

3. Check the client's pulses distally and assess the toes.
4. Monitor the client's vital signs.

7. The client is prescribed alendronate. Which information should the nurse teach?
   1. Take this medication with a full glass of water.
   2. Take with breakfast to prevent gastrointestinal upset.
   3. Use sunscreen to prevent sensitivity to sunlight.
   4. This medication increases calcium reabsorption.

8. The school nurse is completing spinal screenings. Which data require a referral to an HCP?
   1. Bilateral arm lengthening while bending over at the waist.
   2. A deformity that resolves when the head is raised.
   3. Equal spacing of the arms and body at the waist.
   4. A right arm lower than the left while bending over at the waist.

9. The clinic nurse assesses a client with reports of pain and numbness in the left hand and fingers. Which question should the nurse ask the client?
   1. "Do you smoke or use any type of tobacco products?"
   2. "Do you have to wear gloves when you are out in the cold?"
   3. "Do you do repetitive movements with your left fingers?"
   4. "Do you have tremors or involuntary movements of your hand?"

10. Which statement by the client prescribed calcitonin indicates to the nurse the teaching has been effective?
    1. "I should administer the mediation in a different nostril each day."
    2. "I need to drink a lot of water when I take my medicine."
    3. "I have to dilute the medication with vitamin D before I take it."
    4. "This medication will help the calcium leave my bones."

11. The client diagnosed with rule out osteosarcoma asks the nurse, "Why am I having a bone scan?" Which statement is the nurse's best response?
    1. "You seem anxious. Tell me about your anxieties."
    2. "Why are you concerned? Your HCP ordered it."
    3. "I'll have the radiologist come back to explain it again."
    4. "A bone scan looks for cancer, infection, or injury inside the bones."

12. The client is scheduled for a magnetic resonance imaging (MRI) scan. Which intervention should the RN delegate to the UAP?
    1. Prepare the client by removing all metal objects.
    2. Inject the contrast into the intravenous site.
    3. Administer a sedative to the client to decrease anxiety.
    4. Explain why the client cannot have any breakfast.

13. A client sustained a fractured femur in an MVA. Which data require immediate intervention by the nurse? Select all that apply.
    1. The client requests pain medication to sleep.
    2. The client has eupnea and normal sinus rhythm.
    3. The client has petechiae over the neck and chest.
    4. The client has a high arterial oxygen level.
    5. The client has yellow globules floating in the urine.

14. The nurse is caring for the client diagnosed with fat embolism syndrome. Which HCP order should the nurse question?
    1. Maintain heparin to achieve a therapeutic level.
    2. Initiate and monitor intravenous fluids.
    3. Keep the $O_2$ saturation higher than 93%.
    4. Administer an intravenous loop diuretic.

15. The client is postoperative open reduction and internal fixation (ORIF) of a fractured femoral neck. Which long-term goal should the nurse identify for the client?
    1. The client will maintain vital signs within normal limits.
    2. The client will have a decrease in muscle spasms in the affected leg.
    3. The client will have no clinical manifestations of infection.
    4. The client will be able to ambulate down to the nurse's station.

16. The nurse is preparing to administer subcutaneous enoxaparin. Which intervention should the nurse implement?
    1. Monitor the client's serum aPTT.
    2. Encourage oral and intravenous fluids.
    3. Do not eat foods high in vitamin K.
    4. Administer in the anterolateral upper abdomen.

17. Which intervention should the nurse implement for a client diagnosed with a fractured hip in skin traction?
    1. Assess the insertion sites for clinical manifestations of infection.
    2. Monitor for drainage or odor from under the plaster covering the pins.
    3. Check the condition of the skin beneath the Velcro boot frequently.
    4. Take weights off for 1 hour every 8 hours and as needed.

18. The nurse is caring for a client in a hip spica cast. Which intervention should the nurse include in the plan of care?
    1. Assess the client's popliteal pulses every shift.
    2. Elevate the leg on pillows and apply ice packs.
    3. Teach the client how to ambulate with a tripod walker.
    4. Assess the client for distention and vomiting.

19. The nurse is providing discharge teaching for a client with a short leg cast. Which statement indicates the client understands the discharge teaching?
    1. "I need to keep my leg elevated on two pillows for the first 24 hours."
    2. "I must wear my sequential compression device all the time."
    3. "I can remove the cast for 1 hour so I can take a shower."
    4. "I will be able to walk on my cast and not have to use crutches."

20. Which psychosocial problem should the nurse identify for a client with an external fixator device?
    1. Ineffective coping.
    2. Alteration in body image.
    3. Grieving.
    4. Impaired communication.

21. A client recovering from a THR has developed a DVT. The HCP has ordered a continuous infusion of heparin to infuse at 1,200 units per hour. The bag comes with 20,000 units of heparin in 500 mL of 0.9% normal saline. At what rate should the nurse set the pump?

22. The nurse is caring for a client diagnosed with a left fractured humerus. Which data warrant intervention by the nurse?
    1. Capillary refill time is less than 3 seconds.
    2. Pain is not relieved by the patient-controlled analgesia.
    3. Left fingers are edematous and the left hand is purple.
    4. Warm and dry skin on left fingers distal to the elastic bandage.

23. The client with a long arm cast is reporting unrelenting severe pain and feeling as if the fingers are asleep. Which complication should the nurse suspect the client is experiencing?
    1. Fat embolism.
    2. Compartment syndrome.
    3. Pressure ulcer under the cast.
    4. Surgical incision infection.

24. The older client is admitted to the hospital for severe back pain. Which data should the nurse assess first during the admission assessment?
    1. The client's use of herbs.
    2. The client's current pain level.
    3. The client's sexual orientation.
    4. The client's ability to care for self.

25. Which information should the nurse teach the client regarding sports injuries? Select all that apply.
    1. Apply heat intermittently for the first 48 hours.
    2. An injury is not serious if the extremity can be moved.
    3. Only return to the HCP if the foot becomes cold.
    4. Keep the injury immobilized and elevated for 24 to 48 hours.
    5. Avoid exercise and reduce activity until healed.

26. The emergency department nurse is caring for a client diagnosed with a compound fracture of the right ulna. Which interventions should the nurse implement? Rank in order of priority.
    1. Apply sterile, normal saline-soaked gauze to the arm.
    2. Send the client to radiology for an x-ray of the arm.
    3. Assess the fingers of the client's right hand.
    4. Stabilize the arm at the wrist and the elbow.
    5. Administer a tetanus toxoid injection.

27. The emergency department nurse is caring for a 6-year-old child diagnosed with a fractured forearm and suspects the injury is the result of abuse. Which x-ray would confirm the suspicions for the nurse?

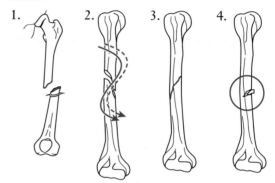

1. Correct answers are 1, 2, 4, and 5.
   1. Clients are more prone to have osteoporosis if there is a genetic predisposition.
   2. Clients deficient in either estrogen or androgen are at risk for osteoporosis.
   3. Smokers are more at risk for osteoporosis. Research does not show a correlation between osteoporosis and secondhand smoke.
   4. Regular, weight-bearing exercise promotes healthy bones.
   5. Alcohol consumption and diets low in calcium put clients at higher risk for osteoporosis.

2. 1. Treatment for carpal tunnel syndrome does not include hyperextension of the wrist.
   2. The nurse should monitor for potential injuries resulting from the alterations in motor, sensory, and autonomic function of the first three digits of the hand and palmar surface of the fourth.
   3. Surgery may be needed to release the compression of the medial nerve, but pins and screws are used to hold the position.
   4. Fasciotomy refers to the surgical excision of strips of connective tissue. This is not applicable to clients diagnosed with carpal tunnel syndrome.

3. 1. A new graduate (GN) is the best choice for this client. The client's surgery (correction of a hammer toe) is not a high-risk procedure but requires assessment and pain management.
   2. This client does not need a more experienced nurse.
   3. A nurse practitioner does not need to be assigned to this client.
   4. The UAP is not assigned the responsibility of managing the care of a client; the UAP works under the guidance of the RN.

4. 1. The assessment of the pain is important in order that the client will be able to tolerate the procedure. Pain is not a life-threatening problem but is a quality-of-care issue.
   2. This is an appropriate question for a client having a closed MRI, not a CT scan.
   3. This is the most important information the nurse should obtain. Any client allergic to seafood cannot be injected with the iodine-based contrast. This contrast could cause an allergic response, endangering the client's life.
   4. The general consent for admission to the hospital covers this procedure. A separate informed consent is not required.

5. 1. The UAPs are transferring the client correctly and safely, so no action should be taken. The UAPs are adhering to the Patient Care Safety Standards by using approved equipment.
   2. The RN should encourage the use of appropriate equipment designed to protect the client and the staff from injury.
   3. The bed scale sling is inappropriate to use when moving the client from the bed to a wheelchair.
   4. There is no reason for the RN to stop the UAPs because the task is being performed correctly.

6. 1. The nurse should not encourage range of motion until the surgeon gives permission for flexion of the knee.
   2. Urinary output is important postoperatively, but monitoring is not a priority over a neurovascular assessment.
   3. The neurovascular assessment is a priority because this surgery has two to three small incisions in the knee area. The nurse needs to make sure circulation is getting past the surgical site.
   4. Vital signs should be assessed, but the priority is to maintain the neurovascular status of the limb.

7. 1. The client needs to take alendronate (Fosamax), a bisphosphonate, with a full glass of water and remain upright for at least 30 minutes to reduce the risk of esophagitis.
   2. This medication should be taken before breakfast on an empty stomach.
   3. This medication does not cause photosensitivity.
   4. Alendronate (Fosamax), a bisphosphonate, decreases calcium reabsorption by decreasing the activity of osteoclasts.

8. 1. These are normal data and do not require intervention.
   2. If the screener suspects the client has scoliosis while the client is bending over, the screener asks the client to raise the head. An abnormality caused by scoliosis will not resolve.
   3. This indicates a normal occurrence and does not need to be referred.
   4. Unequal arm length may indicate scoliosis, and further assessment is needed by an HCP.

9. 1. Assessing for smoking is an evaluation for Raynaud's disease.
   2. Exposure to cold is appropriate to assess for Raynaud's disease.
   3. Repetitive movements are appropriate to assess for carpal tunnel syndrome. Clients diagnosed with this disorder experience pain and numbness.
   4. Tremors or involuntary movements could indicate Parkinson's disease.

10. 1. Calcitonin, a thyroid hormone, is administered intranasally. Alternating nostrils will decrease the risk of nasal irritation.
    2. This intervention should be implemented for alendronate (Fosamax), a bisphosphonate, not calcitonin, a thyroid hormone.
    3. Clients do not dilute their medication. Vitamin D is not used as a diluent for medication.
    4. Calcium should be retained in the bone to maintain bone strength; medications are not administered to encourage loss from the bone.

11. 1. This is a therapeutic technique, but the client is asking for information. When a client seeks information, the nurse should give information first. A discussion of feelings should follow.
    2. This nontherapeutic technique blocks communication between the client and the nurse. The nurse should avoid a response with the word "why," which asks the client to explain or justify feelings to the nurse.
    3. When the client requests information, the nurse needs to provide accurate information, not pass the buck.
    4. This statement answers the client's question.

12. 1. Metal objects such as jewelry and zippers can interfere with the magnetic imaging and pose a danger to the client as a result of the magnetic properties of the equipment. This intervention can be delegated to the UAP.
    2. Injection of contrast is given in the radiology department.
    3. UAPs are unable to administer medications in hospitals.
    4. The RN cannot delegate teaching to a UAP.

13. Correct answers are 3 and 5.
    1. The client requesting something for sleep is expected and does not require notifying the HCP.
    2. Normal respiration and heart rate do not require notifying the HCP.
    3. Petechiae are macular, red-purple pinpoint bleeding under the skin. The appearance of petechiae is a classic sign of fat embolism syndrome.
    4. The arterial oxygen level would be low, not elevated. This sign does not warrant immediate intervention.
    5. Yellow globules in the urine are fat globules released from the bone as it breaks. This should be reported immediately.

14. 1. The HCP should prescribe heparin to treat a fat embolism.
    2. The client should be hydrated to prevent platelet aggregation.
    3. The nurse should monitor oxygen levels and administer oxygen as needed to prevent further complications.
    4. The nurse should question this order. This will decrease the client's hydration and may result in further embolism.

15. 1. Vital signs remaining stable is a short-term goal, not a long-term goal.
    2. This is an expected short-term outcome for a preoperative client diagnosed with a fractured femoral neck.
    3. No clinical manifestations of infection is a short-term goal for the nurse to identify in the hospital.
    4. The discharge goal or long-term goal for this client is to return the client to ambulatory status.

16. 1. An aPTT is used to determine therapeutic levels of unfractionated heparin. Laboratory studies such as aPTT are not monitored when administering subcutaneous enoxaparin (Lovenox), a low molecular weight heparin. A therapeutic level will not be achieved as a result of a short half-life.
    2. Oral fluids do not need to be increased because of this medication.
    3. Vitamin K is the antidote for warfarin (Coumadin), an oral anticoagulant. It does not affect enoxaparin (Lovenox).
    4. **Administering the medication in the prescribed areas, the "love handles," ensures safety and decreases the risk of abdominal trauma.**

17. 1. Skeletal traction has a pin, screws, tongs, or wires inserted into the bone. There is no insertion site in skin (Buck's) traction.
    2. Plaster traction is a combination of skeletal traction using pins and a plaster brace to maintain alignment of any deformities.
    3. **In skin (Buck's) traction, a Velcro boot is used to attach the ropes to weights to maintain alignment. Skin covered by the boot can become irritated and break down.**
    4. Buck's traction is applied preoperatively to prevent muscle spasms and maintain alignment, and the weights should not be removed unless assessing for skin breakdown.

18. 1. The client's popliteal pulse will be under the cast and cannot be assessed by the nurse; circulation is assessed by the 6 Ps of the neurovascular assessment.
    2. Elevation should be used with an arm cast or a leg cast, but this is not possible with a spica cast.
    3. Clients with spica casts will not be able to ambulate because the cast covers the entire lower half of the body.
    4. **The nurse should assess the client for clinical manifestations of cast syndrome—vomiting after meals, epigastric pain, and abdominal distention. This is caused by a partial bowel obstruction from compression and can lead to complete obstruction. The client may still have bowel sounds present with this syndrome.**

19. 1. **This is a correct intervention. The leg should be elevated for at least the first 24 hours. If edema is present, the client needs to keep it elevated longer.**

2. Sequential compression devices work to prevent DVT, and the client does not wear one of these at home.
3. The client will not be able to remove the cast for any reason. The cast must be cut off.
4. Clients with casts can only ambulate if they have a walking cast or boot. This information is not in the stem of the question.

20. 1. The client problem of ineffective coping is usually not indicated for a client with an external fixator device, unless the stem provides more information about the client.
    2. **Many clients with an external fixator have alterations in body image because the large, bulky frame makes dressing difficult and because of scarring, which occurs from the trauma and treatment. The length of healing is prolonged, so returning to the client's normal routine is delayed.**
    3. The client problem of grieving is usually not indicated for a client with an external fixator device, unless the stem of the question provides more information about the client.
    4. The client problem of impaired communication is usually not indicated for a client with an external fixator device, unless the stem provides more information about the client.

21. 30 mL/hr.
    Divide the amount of heparin, an anticoagulant, by the volume of fluid to get the concentration:

    20,000 units ÷ 500 mL = 40 units of heparin per 1 mL

    Divide the dose ordered by the concentration for the amount of milliliters per hour to set the pump:

    1,200 units/hr ÷ 40 units/mL = 30 mL/hr

22. 1. This is a normal assessment finding and does not require immediate action.
    2. **Unrelieved pain should warrant intervention by the nurse. Pain may indicate a complication or the need for pain medication, but either way, it warrants intervention.**
    3. Edema and a hematoma as a result of the injury are expected and do not warrant intervention by the nurse.
    4. The fingers distal to the Ace bandage indicate adequate circulation and require no intervention.

23. 1. These are not clinical manifestations of a fat embolism.
    2. These are the classic clinical manifestations of compartment syndrome.
    3. Clients in casts rarely develop pressure ulcers, and usually, they are not painful.
    4. Hot spots on the cast usually indicate an infection of the surgical incision under the cast.

24. 1. This is a question the admitting nurse asks all clients, but it is not the most important.
    2. Pain assessment and management are the most important issues if the client is breathing and has circulation. Lack of pain management decreases the attention of the client during the admission process. Pain is called the fifth vital sign.
    3. Sexual practices are included in the admission forms, but they are not as important as pain management.
    4. Assessing the client's ability to perform activities of daily living and self-care is important to prepare this client for discharge, which begins on admission, but this is not the most important at this time.

25. Correct answers are 4 and 5.
    1. Ice should be applied intermittently for the first 48 hours. Heat can be used later in the recovery process.
    2. Severe injury can be present even with some range of motion.
    3. The client needs to return if the injury does not improve, and if the foot gets cold.
    4. The leg should be iced, elevated, and immobilized for 48 hours.
    5. The client should avoid exercise and reduce daily physical activity until the injury is healed.

26. Correct order is 4, 1, 3, 2, 5.
    4. The nurse first should stabilize the arm to prevent further injury.
    1. A compound fracture is one in which the bone protrudes through the skin. The nurse should apply sterile, saline-soaked gauze to protect the area from the intrusion of bacteria.
    3. The nurse should assess the client's circulation to the part distal to the injury. This is done after the first two interventions because life-threatening complications could occur if stabilization and protection from infection are not addressed first.
    2. An x-ray will be needed to determine the extent of the injury.
    5. A tetanus toxoid injection should be administered, but this can be done last.

27. 1. A compound fracture is a fracture in which the bone protrudes through the skin; it is also called an open fracture, and the nurse would not suspect child abuse based on only the type of fracture.
    2. A spiral fracture is a fracture that involves twisting around the shaft of the bone, such as when an adult twists the arm of a child. The nurse should suspect child abuse.
    3. An oblique fracture is a fracture that remains contained and does not break the skin. There are many reasons the child could have this type of fracture other than child abuse.
    4. A greenstick fracture is a fracture in which one side of the bone is broken and the other side is bent. There are many reasons other than child abuse that could account for this type of fracture.

# Integumentary Disorders

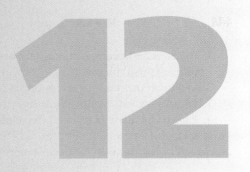

*Success is the sum of small effort, repeated day-in and day-out.*

—Robert Collier

The integument, or skin—the largest organ in the body—is subject to many disorders. Some, like the diseases and disorders that affect other body systems, are infectious; included are bacterial, viral, and fungal infections of the skin. Burns and pressure injury also affect the skin. This chapter discusses these disorders and other problems, including psoriasis, seborrheic dermatosis, and contact dermatitis.

## KEYWORDS

Escharotomy
Keloid

Paraplegia
Quadriplegia

## PRACTICE QUESTIONS

### Burns

1. The client comes into the emergency department in severe pain and reports that a pot of boiling hot water accidentally spilled on his lower legs. The assessment reveals blistered, mottled red skin, and both feet are edematous. Which depth of burn should the nurse document?
   1. Superficial partial thickness.
   2. Deep partial-thickness.
   3. Full-thickness.
   4. First degree.

2. The client diagnosed with full-thickness burns to 40% of the body, including both legs, is being transferred from a community hospital to a burn center. Which measure should be instituted **before** the transfer?

**Rule of Nines for Establishing Extent of Body Surface Burned**

| Anatomic Surface | Total Body Surface |
|---|---|
| Head and neck | 9% |
| Anterior trunk | 18% |
| Posterior trunk | 18% |
| Arms, including hands | 9% each |
| Legs, including feet | 18% each |
| Genitalia | 1% |

U.S. Department of Health & Human Services, Chemical Hazards Emergency Medical Management (CHEMM), 2019.

1. A 22-gauge intravenous line with normal saline infusing.
2. Wounds covered with moist sterile dressings.
3. No intravenous pain medication.
4. Ensure adequate peripheral circulation to both feet.

3. The client has full-thickness burns to 65% of the body, including the chest area. After establishing a patent airway, which collaborative intervention is a **priority** for the client?
    1. Replace fluids and electrolytes.
    2. Prevent contractures of extremities.
    3. Monitor urine output hourly.
    4. Prepare to assist with an escharotomy.

4. The nurse is applying mafenide acetate 10% cream to a client's lower extremity burn. Which assessment data would **require immediate** attention from the nurse?
    1. The client reports pain when the medication is administered.
    2. The client's potassium level is 3.9 mEq/L and the sodium level is 137 mEq/L.
    3. The client's ABGs are pH 7.34, $PO_2$ 98, $PCO_2$ 38, and $HCO_3$ 20.
    4. The client is able to perform active range-of-motion exercises.

5. The client is scheduled to have a xenograft to a left lower-leg burn. The client asks the nurse, "What is a xenograft?" Which statement by the nurse would be the **best** response?
    1. "The doctor will graft skin from your back to your leg."
    2. "The skin from a donor will be used to cover your burn."
    3. "The graft will come from an animal, probably a pig."
    4. "I think you should ask your doctor about the graft."

6. The intensive care unit (ICU) burn nurse is developing a nursing care plan for a client diagnosed with severe full-thickness and deep partial-thickness burns over half the body. Which client problem has **priority**?
    1. High risk for infection.
    2. Ineffective coping.
    3. Impaired physical mobility.
    4. Knowledge deficit.

7. The nurse writes the nursing diagnosis "impaired skin integrity related to open burn wounds." Which intervention would be **appropriate** for this nursing diagnosis?
    1. Provide analgesia before the pain becomes severe.
    2. Clean the client's wounds, body, and hair daily.

3. Screen visitors for respiratory infections.
4. Encourage visitors to bring plants and flowers.

8. Which nursing interventions should be included for the client diagnosed with full-thickness and deep partial-thickness burns to 50% of the body? **Select all that apply.**
    1. Perform meticulous hand hygiene.
    2. Use sterile gloves for wound care.
    3. Wear gown and mask during procedures.
    4. Change the central lines once a week.
    5. Administer antibiotics as prescribed.

9. The nurse is caring for a client diagnosed with deep partial-thickness and full-thickness burns to the chest area. Which assessment data would **warrant** notifying the health-care provider (HCP)?
    1. The client is reporting severe pain.
    2. The client's pulse oximeter reading is 95%.
    3. The client has T 100.4°F, P 100, R 24, and BP 102/60.
    4. The client's urinary output is 50 mL in 2 hours.

10. The client is admitted with full-thickness and partial-thickness burns to more than 30% of the body. The nurse is concerned with the client's nutritional status. Which intervention should the nurse implement?
    1. Encourage the client's family to bring favorite foods.
    2. Provide a low-fat, low-cholesterol diet for the client.
    3. Monitor the client's weight weekly in the same clothes.
    4. Make a referral to the hospital social worker.

11. The client sustained a hot grease burn to the right hand and calls the emergency department for advice. Which information should the nurse provide to the client?
    1. Apply an ice pack to the right hand.
    2. Place the hand in cool water.
    3. Be sure to rupture any blister formation.
    4. Go immediately to the doctor's office.

12. The client is being discharged after being in the burn unit for 6 weeks. Which strategies should the nurse identify to promote the client's mental health?
    1. Encourage the client to stay at home as much as possible.
    2. Discuss the importance of not relying on the family for needs.
    3. Tell the client to remember that changes in lifestyle take time.
    4. Instruct the client to discuss feelings only with the therapist.

## Pressure Injuries

13. The registered nurse (RN) in a long-term care facility is teaching a group of new unlicensed assistive personnel (UAP). Which information regarding skincare should the nurse include in the teaching? **Select all that apply.**
    1. Keep the skin moist by leaving the skin damp after the bath.
    2. Do not rub any lotion into the skin.
    3. Turn immobile clients at least every 2 hours.
    4. Only the licensed nursing staff may care for the client's skin.
    5. Avoid using talc powder or strong soaps.

14. The nurse is caring for a client diagnosed with stage IV pressure injury on the left trochanter and coccyx. Which collaborative problem has the **highest priority**?
    1. Impaired cognition.
    2. Altered nutrition.
    3. Self-care deficit.
    4. Altered coping.

15. The nurse is caring for clients in a long-term care facility. Which is a **modifiable** risk factor for the development of pressure injuries?
    1. Constant perineal moisture.
    2. Ability of the clients to reposition themselves.
    3. Decreased elasticity of the skin.
    4. Impaired cardiovascular perfusion of the periphery.

16. What is the scientific rationale for placing lift pads under an immobile client?
    1. The pads will absorb any urinary incontinence and contain stool.
    2. The pads will prevent the client from being diaphoretic.
    3. The pads will keep the staff from workplace injuries such as a pulled muscle.
    4. The pads will help prevent friction shearing when repositioning the client.

17. The client diagnosed with paraplegia is being admitted to a medical unit from home with a stage IV pressure injury over the right ischium. Which assessment tool should be completed on admission to the hospital?
    1. Complete the Braden Scale.
    2. Monitor the Glasgow Coma Scale.
    3. Assess for Babinski's sign.
    4. Initiate a Brudzinski flow sheet.

18. The wound care nurse documented a client's pressure injury on admission as 3.3 cm × 4 cm stage II on the coccyx. Which information would alert the nurse that the client's pressure injury is getting worse?

1. The skin is not broken and is 2.5 × 3.5 cm with erythema that does not blanch.
2. There is a 3.2 × 4.1 cm blister that is red and drains occasionally.
3. The skin covering the coccyx is intact, but the client reports pain in the area.
4. The coccyx wound extends to the subcutaneous layer and there is drainage.

19. The RN and a UAP on a medical floor are caring for older and immobile clients. Which action by the UAP **warrants immediate** intervention by the RN?
    1. The UAP elevates the head of the bed for a client able to self-feed with minimal assistance.
    2. The UAP asks to take a meal break before turning the clients at the 2-hour time limit.
    3. The UAP restocks the rooms that need unsterile gloves before clocking out for the shift.
    4. The UAP mixes a beverage thickener into a glass of water for the client diagnosed with difficulty swallowing.

20. The nurse is caring for clients on a medical unit. After the shift report, which client should the nurse assess **first**?
    1. The 34-year-old client diagnosed with quadriplegia, unable to move his arms.
    2. The older client diagnosed with a CVA and weakness on the right side.
    3. The 78-year-old client diagnosed with pressure injuries and a temperature of 102.3°F.
    4. The young adult who is unhappy with the care that was provided last shift.

21. The nurse is developing a plan of care for a client diagnosed with left-sided paralysis secondary to a right-sided cerebrovascular accident (stroke). Which should be included in the interventions?
    1. Use a pillow to keep the heels off the bed when supine.
    2. Order a low air-loss therapy bed immediately.
    3. Prepare to insert a nasogastric feeding tube.
    4. Order an occupational therapy consult for strength training.

22. The client diagnosed with a debilitating illness has developed multiple pressure injuries and reports to the nurse during a dressing change that he is "tired of it all." Which is the nurse's **best** therapeutic response?
    1. "These wounds can heal if we get enough protein into you."
    2. "Are you tired of the treatments and needing to be cared for?"

3. "Why would you say that? We are doing our best."

4. "Have you made out an advance directive to let the HCP know your wishes?"

23. The nurse writes the problem "impaired skin integrity" for a client diagnosed with stage IV pressure injuries. Which interventions should be included in the plan of care? **Select all that apply.**
    1. Turn the client every 3 to 4 hours.
    2. Ask the dietitian to consult.
    3. Have the client sign a consent for pictures of the wounds.
    4. Obtain an order for a low air-loss bed.
    5. Elevate the head of the bed at all times.

24. The client diagnosed with stage IV infected pressure injuries on the coccyx is scheduled for a fecal diversion operation. The nurse knows that client teaching has been **effective** when the client makes which statement?
    1. "This surgery will create a skin flap to cover my wounds."
    2. "This surgery will get all the old black tissue out of the wound so it can heal."
    3. "The surgery is important to allow oxygen to get to the tissue for healing to occur."
    4. "Stool will come out of an opening in my abdomen so it won't get in the sore."

## Skin Cancer

25. The school nurse is preparing to teach a health promotion class for high school seniors. Which information regarding self-care should be included in the teaching? **Select all that apply.**
    1. Apply a sunscreen with a protection factor of 10 or less when in the sun.
    2. Try to stay out of the sun between 0300 and 0500 daily.
    3. Perform a thorough skin check monthly.
    4. Remember, caps and long sleeves do not help prevent skin cancer.
    5. Wear sunglasses that block 99% to 100% of UVA and UVB rays.

26. The female client admitted for an unrelated diagnosis asks the nurse to check her back because "it itches all the time in that one spot." When the nurse assesses the client's back, the nurse notes an irregular-shaped lesion with some scabbed-over areas surrounding the lesion. Which action should the nurse implement **first**?
    1. Notify the HCP to check the lesion on rounds.
    2. Measure the lesion and note the color.

3. Apply lotion to the lesion.
4. Instruct the client to have the HCP check the lesion.

27. The nurse is caring for clients in an outpatient surgery clinic. Which client should be assessed **first**?
    1. The crying client scheduled for a skin biopsy.
    2. The client 3 hours postoperation now sleeping.
    3. The client needing to void before discharge.
    4. The client receiving discharge instructions and ready to go home.

28. Which client is at the greatest risk for the development of skin cancer?
    1. The African American male living in the northeast.
    2. The older Hispanic female who immigrated from Mexico as a child.
    3. The client with a family history of basal cell carcinoma.
    4. The client with fair complexion and unable to tan.

29. The middle-aged client has had two lesions diagnosed as basal cell carcinoma removed. Which discharge instruction should the nurse include?
    1. Teach the client that there is no more risk for cancer.
    2. Refer the client to a prosthesis specialist for a prosthesis.
    3. Instruct the client on how to apply sunscreen to the area.
    4. Demonstrate care of the surgical site.

30. The nurse is caring for a client diagnosed with squamous cell skin cancer and writes a psychosocial problem of "fear." Which nursing interventions should be included in the plan of care?
    1. Explain to the client that the fears are unfounded.
    2. Encourage the client to verbalize the feeling of being afraid.
    3. Have the HCP discuss the client's fear with the client.
    4. Inform the client regarding all planned procedures.

31. The RN and a UAP are caring for clients in a dermatology clinic. Which task should be delegated to the UAP? **Select all that apply.**
    1. Stock the rooms with the equipment needed.
    2. Weigh the clients and position the clients for the examination.
    3. Discuss the problems the client has experienced since the previous visit.
    4. Identify any teaching needs the clients may have at this visit.
    5. Take the biopsy specimens to the laboratory.

32. The client is admitted to the outpatient surgery center for the removal of a malignant melanoma. Which assessment data indicate the lesion is malignant melanoma?
    1. The lesion is asymmetrical and has irregular borders.
    2. The lesion has a waxy appearance with pearl-like borders.
    3. The lesion has a thickened and scaly appearance.
    4. The lesion appeared as a thickened area after an injury.

33. The client has had a squamous cell carcinoma removed from the lip. Which discharge instructions should the nurse provide?
    1. Notify the HCP if a nonhealing lesion develops around the mouth.
    2. Squamous cell carcinoma tumors do not metastasize.
    3. Limit foods to liquid or soft consistency for 1 month.
    4. Apply heat to the area for 20 minutes every 4 hours.

34. Which client physiological outcome (goal) is appropriate for a client diagnosed with skin cancer after surgery to remove the lesion?
    1. The client will express feelings of fear.
    2. The client will ask questions about the diagnosis.
    3. The client will state a diminished level of pain.
    4. The client will demonstrate care of the operative site.

35. The male client diagnosed with acquired immunodeficiency syndrome (AIDS) states that he has developed a purple-brown spot on his calf. Which action should the nurse do **first**?
    1. Refer the client to an HCP for a biopsy of the area.
    2. Assess the lesion for size, color, and symmetry.
    3. Discuss end-of-life decisions with the client.
    4. Report the sexually transmitted illness to the health department.

36. The nurse participating in a health fair is discussing malignant melanoma with a group of clients. Which information regarding the use of sunscreen should the nurse include? **Select all that apply.**
    1. Sunscreen is needed only during the hottest hours of the day.
    2. Check the expiration date to make sure the sunscreen is still effective.
    3. Sunscreen does not help prevent skin cancer.
    4. The higher the SPF number of sunscreen, the more UV rays it blocks.
    5. Reapply sunscreen every 6 to 8 hours.

## Bacterial Skin Infection

37. The client comes to the emergency department reporting pain in the left lower leg following a puncture wound from a nail in a plywood board. The left lower leg is reddened with streaks, edematous, and hot to the touch, and the client has a temperature of 100.8°F. Which condition would the nurse suspect the client is experiencing?
    1. Cellulitis.
    2. Lyme disease.
    3. Impetigo.
    4. Deep vein thrombosis.

38. The client comes to the clinic reporting the sudden onset of high fever, chills, and a headache. The nurse assesses a patchy macular rash on the trunk and a circular type of rash that looks like an insect bite. Which question would be **most appropriate** for the nurse to ask during the interview?
    1. "Do you live in an area where animals roam the street?"
    2. "Have you been working in your garden lately?"
    3. "Have you been deer hunting in the last week?"
    4. "Do you use sunscreen when you are outside?"

39. The school nurse is discussing impetigo with the teachers in an elementary school. One of the teachers asks the nurse, "How can I prevent getting impetigo?" Which statement would be the **most appropriate** response?
    1. "Wash your hands after using the bathroom."
    2. "Do not touch any affected areas without gloves."
    3. "Apply a topical antibiotic to your hands."
    4. "Keep the child with impetigo isolated in the room."

40. The client is admitted to the medical floor diagnosed with cellulitis of the left arm. Which assessment data would **warrant immediate** intervention by the nurse?
    1. The client has bilaterally weak radial pulses.
    2. The client is able to move the left fingers.
    3. The client has a CRT less than 3 seconds.
    4. The client is unable to remove the wedding ring.

41. The nurse writes the client problem of "acute pain and itching secondary to bacterial skin lesions." Which interventions should be included in the care plan? **Select all that apply.**
    1. Keep humidity at less than 20%.
    2. Maintain a cool environment.
    3. Use a mild soap for sensitive skin.
    4. Keep lesions covered at all times.
    5. Apply skin lotion after bathing.

42. The nurse observes the UAP squeezing the "blackheads" on an elderly client. Which action should the RN implement **first**?
    1. Notify the unit manager of witnessing this activity.
    2. Instruct the assistant to stop this behavior.
    3. Demonstrate the correct way to care for the skin.
    4. Complete an incident report regarding the action.

43. The client is diagnosed with acne vulgaris. Which psychosocial problem is a **priority**?
    1. Impaired skin integrity.
    2. Ineffective grieving.
    3. Body image disturbance.
    4. Knowledge deficit.

44. Which individual would **most** likely experience the skin disorder pseudofolliculitis barbae (shaving bumps)?
    1. A male African American soldier.
    2. A female white hairdresser.
    3. A male Asian food server.
    4. A female Hispanic schoolteacher.

45. The female client calls the clinic and tells the nurse that she has a really big "boil" in the perineal area that is causing a lot of pain. Which intervention should the nurse implement?
    1. Schedule an emergency appointment for the client.
    2. Instruct the client to apply warm, moist compresses to the area.
    3. Determine if someone can squeeze the boil.
    4. Explain that this will resolve on its own.

46. Which client would **most** likely be at risk for the development of a carbuncle?
    1. The young male just beginning to shave.
    2. The female with a fair complexion.
    3. The male with a daily gym workout routine.
    4. The female diagnosed with diabetes mellitus.

47. The female teacher comes to the school nurse's office and shows the nurse a rash on her hands. The nurse tells the teacher she has probably contracted impetigo from one of the students. Which intervention should the nurse implement?
    1. Instruct the teacher to go to her HCP today.
    2. Tell the teacher to wash her hands with soap and water.
    3. Encourage the teacher to rub vitamin E oil on the lesions.
    4. Explain that the rash will go away in a few days.

48. The nurse is teaching a class on how to prevent Lyme disease. Which interventions should be included in the discussion? **Select all that apply.**
    1. Instruct the clients to wear dark clothes when hunting.
    2. Use a sunscreen of at least SPF 30 when outside.
    3. Avoid dense undergrowth when in a wooded area.
    4. Do not use any type of insect repellant when deer hunting.
    5. Treat clothing and gear before going outdoors.

## Viral Skin Infection

49. The nurse is discussing the prevention of herpes simplex 2. Which intervention should the nurse discuss with the client?
    1. Encourage the client to get the chickenpox immunization.
    2. Do not engage in oral sex if you have a cold sore on the mouth.
    3. Wear nonsterile gloves when cleaning the genital area.
    4. Do not share any type of towel or washcloth with another person.

50. The client is reporting a burning, stabbing pain that radiates around the left rib cage area. The nurse cannot find any type of skin abnormality. Which action should the nurse implement?
    1. Transfer the client to the ED for a cardiac work-up.
    2. Inform the client that the nurse can't see anything.
    3. Administer a nonnarcotic analgesic to the client.
    4. Ask if the client ever had chickenpox.

51. The client is diagnosed with herpes simplex 2 and prescribed valacyclovir. Which instructions should the nurse teach?
    1. This medication will prevent pregnancy and treat the virus.
    2. This medication must be tapered when discontinuing the medication.
    3. This medication will suppress symptoms but does not cure the disease.
    4. This medication may cause the client's urine to turn orange.

52. The nurse administered morphine sulfate IVP 45 minutes ago to a client diagnosed with herpes zoster. On reassessment, the client reports the pain **decreased** to a "5" on a 1-to-10 scale. Which intervention should the nurse implement?

1. Turn on soft music and shut the blinds.
2. Apply warm, moist heat to the lesions.
3. Notify the HCP for more pain medication.
4. Encourage the client to ambulate with assistance.

53. The client is diagnosed with disseminated herpes zoster secondary to AIDS. Which interventions should the nurse implement? **Select all that apply.**
    1. Place the client in contact isolation.
    2. Administer a corticosteroid IVP.
    3. Assess the client's pain on a 1-to-10 scale.
    4. Request that the client not have any visitors.
    5. Ensure nurses with prior chickenpox infection care for this client.

54. Which statement by the client diagnosed with chickenpox indicates that the client **understands** the teaching?
    1. "I should put rubbing alcohol on the lesions twice a day."
    2. "I should not scratch myself if at all possible. It might lead to scarring."
    3. "I can go to work when my lesions have all disappeared."
    4. "I need to take all my antibiotics no matter how I feel."

55. The client diagnosed with viral skin lesions is experiencing pruritus. Which statement would be an appropriate **long-term** goal?
    1. The client will refrain from scratching the skin.
    2. The client will maintain intact skin integrity.
    3. The client will have relief from itching.
    4. The client will not develop a secondary bacterial infection.

56. The RN is admitting an 88-year-old client diagnosed with a viral skin infection. Which nursing task could the nurse delegate to the UAP?
    1. Measure and document the client's skin lesions.
    2. Apply the antihistamine cream to the lesions.
    3. Set up the isolation equipment for the client.
    4. Determine if the client has prepared an advance directive.

57. The client is diagnosed with a viral infection and the HCP has prescribed an antiviral medication to be administered by weight. The client weighs 220 pounds and the order reads 10 mg per kilogram per day to be administered in equally divided doses every 6 hours. How many milligrams will be administered in one dose?

[_____]

58. The 55-year-old client contracted chickenpox from his grandchild. The client had to be hospitalized because of the seriousness of the condition. Which complication is the client **at risk** for developing secondary to chickenpox?
    1. Deep vein thrombosis.
    2. Varicella pneumonia.
    3. Pericarditis.
    4. Scarring of the skin.

59. The nurse is assessing a young mother in the clinic reporting sores on her skin. Which assessment data would support that the client has chickenpox?
    1. Crops of lesions that have pus and reddened base.
    2. Oval scaling lesions that occur on the legs and arms.
    3. Severe itching of the scalp with tiny eggs visible.
    4. Ringed red lesions on the face, neck, trunk, and extremities.

60. The long-term care nurse has received the morning shift report. Which client should the nurse assess **first**?
    1. The client with no bowel movement today.
    2. The client needing an indwelling catheter changed.
    3. The client diagnosed with periorbital skin lesions.
    4. The client diagnosed with a stage I pressure injury.

## Fungal and Parasitic Skin Infection

61. The school nurse is assessing a teacher with pediculosis. Which statement by the teacher makes the nurse suspect that the teacher complied with the instructions discussed in the classroom? **Select all that apply.**
    1. "I used the comb to remove all the nits."
    2. "I washed my hair with pyrethrin shampoo."
    3. "I removed all the sheets from my bed."
    4. "I had to fix my daughter's hair with my brush."
    5. "I sealed my favorite fur-lined hat in a plastic bag."

62. The RN clinic nurse is reviewing information submitted by the UAP that states the presence of pediculosis pubis. Which area of the client's body should the nurse assess?

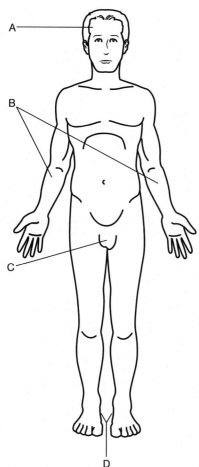

1. A
2. B
3. C
4. D

63. The school nurse is discussing how to prevent tinea cruris with the football players. Which intervention should the nurse implement?
    1. Instruct the football players to wear tight, snug-fitting jockstraps.
    2. Explain the importance of wearing white socks.
    3. Teach the football players not to share brushes or combs.
    4. Discuss the need to dry the groin area thoroughly after bathing.

64. The older client is admitted from the long-term care facility diagnosed with congestive heart failure. The client reports severe itching on both hands and the nurse notes wavy, brown, thread-like lesions between the client's fingers. Which comorbid condition would the nurse suspect the client of having based on these assessment data?
    1. Tinea capitis.
    2. Herpes simplex 2.
    3. Scabies.
    4. Psoriasis.

65. The HCP prescribed malathion lotion to be applied to the head. Which instructions should the nurse teach the client concerning this medication? **Select all that apply.**
    1. Leave the lotion on for 8 hours after applying it to the hair.
    2. Make sure that the hair is dry before applying the lotion.
    3. Repeat the hair lotion application daily for at least 1 week.
    4. Put the lotion in the bathwater and soak for at least 20 minutes.
    5. Avoid hair dryers, cigarettes, or open flames during treatment.

66. The RN in the long-term care facility must delegate a nursing task to a UAP. Which nursing task would be **most appropriate** to delegate?
    1. Comb the nits out of the client's hair.
    2. Massage the reddened area on the hip.
    3. Scrape the burrows to remove the scabies mite.
    4. Apply antifungal lotion to the groin area.

67. The client has tinea pedis. Which intervention should the nurse teach to the client?
    1. Soak feet in a vinegar-and-water solution.
    2. Wear shoes without any type of socks.
    3. Alternate shoes on a monthly basis.
    4. Cut toenails straight across.

68. The client with thick, crusty, yellow toenails is diagnosed with tinea unguium (onychomycosis) and asks the clinic nurse what happens if he can't afford to take the medication the physician prescribed. The nurse's response will be based on which scientific rationale?
    1. The toes will become gangrenous and may have to be amputated.
    2. Over-the-counter antifungal creams can be substituted for oral medication.
    3. The toenail plate will separate and the entire toenail may be destroyed.
    4. Take all the prescribed antibiotics or the infection may return.

69. There is an outbreak of scabies in a long-term care facility. Which instruction should the infection control nurse provide to all client care staff concerning the transmission of this parasitic infection?
    1. Use only hand-washing foam when caring for clients diagnosed with scabies.
    2. Wear gloves when providing hands-on care for a client diagnosed with scabies.
    3. Wash all linen and clothes in cold water and dry them outside in the sun.
    4. Instruct clients to use plastic eating utensils for meals.

70. The nurse in a dermatology clinic is taking the history of a client. Which questions should the dermatology nurse ask the client? **Select all that apply.**
    1. When did you first notice the skin problem?
    2. What cosmetics or skin products do you use?
    3. Have you experienced any loss of sensation?
    4. What is your current and previous occupation?
    5. Do you experience any itching, burning, or tingling?

71. The nurse is assessing the client diagnosed with scabies. Which assessment technique would be **most appropriate**?
    1. Gently palpate the affected area using sterile gloves.
    2. Apply vinegar to the affected area to identify scabies.
    3. Use a magnifying glass and a penlight to visualize the skin.
    4. Obtain a Doppler to assess the movement of the mites.

72. The public health nurse is providing a class on skin disorders in the African American community. Which information should the nurse include in the presentation?
    1. People with dark skin suffer the same skin conditions as people with light skin.
    2. African American men are more likely to have skin cancer than women.

    3. Dark-skinned individuals are less likely to form keloids after any type of surgery.
    4. Buccal mucosa of dark-skinned individuals is usually a bluish-tinged color.

73. Which skin condition would **most** likely occur in the highlighted areas?

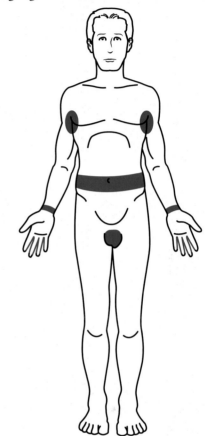

    1. Contact dermatitis.
    2. Herpes zoster.
    3. Seborrheic dermatitis.
    4. Scabies.

# CONCEPTS

The concepts covered in this chapter focus on tissue integrity. Exemplars that are covered are pressure injuries, skin cancers, and skin infections. Interrelated concepts of the nursing process and clinical judgment are covered throughout the questions. The concept of clinical judgment is presented in prioritizing or "first" questions.

74. The nurse is staging a pressure injury on a newly admitted client. Which would the nurse document for this client?

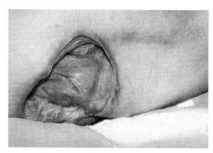

1. Stage I.
2. Stage II.
3. Stage III.
4. Stage IV.

75. The nurse has written the concept of impaired skin integrity for a client diagnosed with diabetes mellitus type 2 and an acute, infected wound on the left heel. Which interventions should the nurse implement? **Select all that apply.**
1. Administer antibiotics via IVPB method.
2. Perform wound dressing changes using unsterile gloves.
3. Monitor blood glucose levels.
4. Assess the client's culture daily.
5. Encourage the client to comply with the recommended diet.

76. The nurse is assessing a client's skin for melanoma. The example below illustrates which of the A, B, C, D, E's of skin cancer detection? **Select all that apply.**

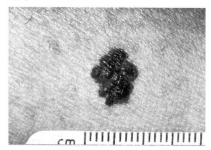

1. Asymmetry.
2. Borders.
3. Color.
4. Diameter.
5. Evolving.

77. The nurse is admitting the male client stating that he is having a lot of pain in his right chest and side. The nurse observes the client's side and chest area and notes the vesicles seen below. Which should the nurse implement?

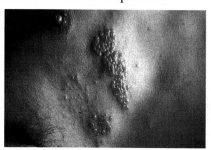

1. Allow the client's preschool-aged grandchildren to visit if they have not had the varicella vaccine.
2. Do not assign a nurse to care for the client if the nurse has never had chickenpox or the varicella vaccine.
3. Place the client in airborne precautions and have nuclear medicine decontaminate the trays before sending them to be washed.
4. Request a prescription for vancomycin so the client's infection will heal faster.

78. The nurse is presenting an in-service to participants in a local health fair. Which information regarding the development of skin cancers should the nurse teach?
1. The fairer the skin, the less the risk of developing skin cancer.
2. Eating a diet high in fiber helps to minimize the risk of skin cancer development.
3. Sun exposure at a beach is less dangerous than at a stadium.
4. The participants should avoid sun exposure in the middle of the day.

79. The nurse identifies the concept of impaired skin integrity for a pediatric client diagnosed with impetigo on the arms. Which interventions should the nurse implement?
1. Teach the parents to ensure the child takes all the prescribed antibiotics.
2. Give the parents a written excuse so the child can go back to school.
3. Encourage the parents to bathe the child in an oatmeal bath for the itching.
4. Apply topical lidocaine before debriding the crusts from the lesions.

80. The nurse admitting a client to a medical-surgical unit notes the lesion shown on the right. Which intervention should the nurse implement **first**?
    1. Measure the lesion with a ruler.
    2. Document the finding in the client's EHR.
    3. Determine if the client has noticed the lesion before.
    4. Notify the health-care provider (HCP) of the lesion.

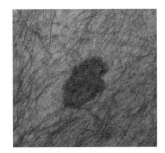

81. The clinic nurse is preparing to administer medications. Which safety precautions should the nurse employ when administering the client's medications?

| Client Name: Ms. I. L. Sun | MR#: 111 152 | Diagnosis: Basal Cell Carcinoma of the Lip |
|---|---|---|
| Age: 47 years | Allergies: Caine Drugs | |
| Medication | 0701–1900 | 1901–0700 |
| 5-fluorouracil cream apply topically to lip | 1000 | |
| Signature of Nurse: | Day Nurse RN/DN | Night Nurse RN/NN |

    1. Keep the head of the bed or chair elevated for 30 minutes after the application.
    2. Teach the client not to eat solid foods for 24 hours after the medication is applied.
    3. Have the client expose the area to sunlight for 30 minutes after the application.
    4. Wear unsterile gloves when applying the 5-fluorouracil cream to the client's lip.

## Burns

1. 1. Sunburn is an example of this depth of burn; a superficial partial-thickness burn affects the epidermis and the skin is reddened and blanches with pressure.
   2. Deep partial-thickness burns are scalds and flash burns that injure the epidermis, upper dermis, and portions of the deeper dermis. This causes pain, blistered and mottled red skin, and edema (Hoffman & Sullivan, 2020).
   3. Full-thickness burns are caused by flame, electric current, or chemical burns and include the epidermis, entire dermis, and sometimes subcutaneous tissue and may also involve connective tissue, muscle, and bone.
   4. A first-degree burn is another name for a superficial partial-thickness burn.

   **TEST-TAKING HINT: The adjectives in the stem are the most important words that assist the test taker when selecting a correct answer.**

2. 1. An 18-gauge catheter with lactated Ringer's infusion should be initiated to maintain a urine output of at least 30 mL/hr.
   2. Wounds should be covered with a clean, dry sheet.
   3. The client should be transferred with adequate pain relief, which requires intravenous morphine.
   4. The client's legs should have pedal pulses and be warm to the touch, and the client must be able to move the toes.

   **TEST-TAKING HINT: Note the adjectives "22-gauge" and "moist." If the test taker is unsure of the correct answer, then the test taker should determine which system is affected and see if that will help determine the right answer. A client's extremities and a neurovascular assessment are similar; therefore, the test taker should select option "4."**

3. 1. After the airway, the most urgent need is preventing irreversible shock by replacing fluids and electrolytes.
   2. This is important, but it is not a priority over fluid volume balance, and this is not a collaborative intervention because the nurse can do this independently.
   3. Output must be monitored, but this is an independent intervention.

4. An escharotomy, an incision that releases scar tissue that prevents the body from being able to expand, enables chest excursion in circumferential chest burns. The client has not had time to develop eschar.

**TEST-TAKING HINT: A collaborative intervention is an intervention that requires an HCP's order or working with another discipline. Therefore, options "2" and "3" should be eliminated immediately.**

4. 1. The client should be premedicated with an analgesic because mafenide acetate (Sulfamylon), a sulfa antibiotic cream, causes severe burning pain for up to 20 minutes after application.
   2. Silver nitrate solution is hypotonic and acts as a wick for sodium and potassium. Also, these electrolytes are WNL and would not require immediate intervention.
   3. Mafenide acetate (Sulfamylon), a sulfa antibiotic cream, is a strong carbonic anhydrase inhibitor that may reduce renal buffering and can cause metabolic acidosis. These arterial blood gases (ABGs) indicate metabolic acidosis and therefore require immediate intervention.
   4. The client being able to perform range-of-motion exercises does not warrant immediate intervention; this is a very good result.

**TEST-TAKING HINT: "Require immediate attention" means that the nurse must intervene independently or notify another HCP. The test taker must know how to interpret ABGs, and even if the test taker is not familiar with the medication, metabolic acidosis requires intervention.**

5. 1. This is the explanation for an autograft.
   2. This is the description of a homograft.
   3. A xenograft or heterograft consists of skin taken from animals, usually porcine (Vig et al., 2017).
   4. This is "passing the buck"; the nurse can and should answer this question with factual information.

**TEST-TAKING HINT: The test taker should eliminate options to help determine the correct answers. Option "1" can be eliminated because skin from self would be *auto-*, not *xeno-*. Option "4" should be eliminated because the nurse should answer the question and not pass the buck.**

6. 1. Although this is a potential problem, it is a priority because the body's protective barrier, the skin, has been compromised and there is an impaired immune response.
   2. This psychosocial client problem is important, but in the ICU, the first priority is preventing infection so wound healing can occur.
   3. Burn wound edema, pain, and potential joint contractures can cause mobility deficits, but the first priority is preventing infection so wound healing can occur.
   4. Teaching is always important, but in the ICU, the priority is the physiological integrity of the client.

**TEST-TAKING HINT: The adjectives "intensive care" mean the client is critically ill; therefore, a physiological problem is a priority and options "2" and "4" can be eliminated. Although actual problems are usually higher priority than potential problems, in the case of a burn, the risk for infection has to be the priority.**

7. 1. Addressing pain will not address impaired skin integrity.
   2. Daily cleaning reduces bacterial colonization.
   3. This intervention would be appropriate for a "risk for infection" nursing diagnosis.
   4. Plants and flowers in water should be avoided because stagnant water is a source of bacterial growth.

**TEST-TAKING HINT: The intervention addresses the etiology of the nursing diagnosis "open burn wounds," and the goal addresses the response "impaired skin integrity."**

8. Correct answers are 1, 2, 3, and 5.
   1. Hand washing is the number-one intervention used to prevent infection, which is a priority for the client diagnosed with a burn.
   2. Aseptic techniques minimize the risk of cross-contamination and the spread of bacteria.
   3. Aseptic techniques minimize the risk of cross-contamination and the spread of bacteria.
   4. Central lines are not changed unless they are no longer needed or the client has developed an infection related to the line. The central line catheter hubs, connectors, injection ports, and dressings are changed every 2 days for gauze dressings or every 7 days for semipermeable dressings. Dressings are changed if wet or visibly soiled (The Joint Commission, 2019).
   5. Antibiotics reduce bacteria.

**TEST-TAKING HINT: Alternative-type questions require the test taker to choose all options that apply. Infection is a priority for clients diagnosed with burns.**

9. 1. Severe pain would be expected in a client diagnosed with these types of burns; therefore, it would not warrant notifying the HCP.
   2. A pulse oximeter reading greater than 93% is WNL. Therefore, a 95% reading would not warrant notifying the HCP.
   3. The client's vital signs show an elevated temperature, pulse, and respiration, along with low blood pressure, but these vital signs would not be unusual for a client diagnosed with severe burns.
   4. Fluid and electrolyte balance is the priority for a client diagnosed with a severe burn. Fluid resuscitation must be maintained to keep a urine output of 30 mL/hr. Therefore, a 25 mL/hr output would warrant immediate intervention.

**TEST-TAKING HINT: The test taker must select an answer that is not expected for the client's disease or condition when being asked which data warrant immediate nursing intervention.**

10. 1. The client needs sufficient nutrients for wound healing and increased metabolic requirements, and homemade nutritious foods are usually better than hospital food. This also allows the family to feel part of the client's recovery (Clark, Imran, Madni, & Wolf, 2017).
    2. The client should be provided a high-calorie, high-protein diet along with vitamins.
    3. The client should be weighed daily, and the goal is that the client loses no more than 5% of the preburn weight.
    4. The nurse would make a referral to a dietitian, not a social worker.

**TEST-TAKING HINT: The nurse needs to be knowledgeable regarding different types of diets; this requires memorization.**

11. 1. Ice should never be applied to a burn because this will worsen the tissue damage by causing vasoconstriction.
    2. Cool water gives immediate and striking relief from pain and limits local tissue edema and damage.
    3. Blisters should be maintained intact to prevent infection.
    4. The client should be told to go to the ED, not the doctor's office, for burn care.

**TEST-TAKING HINT:** The test taker should select an answer that directly cares for the client's body. This eliminates options "3" (blisters have not formed yet) and "4." Therefore, the test taker has to decide between cool water and ice.

12. 1. The client should resume previous activities gradually and should not stay home; the client should go out and begin to live again.
    2. The client should be honest with self, family, and friends about needs, hopes, and fears.
    3. The client needs to know that it will take time to adjust to life after burns and that returning to work, family role, sexual intimacy, and body image will take time.
    4. The client should feel free to discuss feelings with family, friends, and the therapist.

**TEST-TAKING HINT:** Even if the test taker is not familiar with the disease process, there are certain interventions that go with any chronic problem, such as getting back to normal life as soon as possible and being independent, but also getting help when needed and not expecting too much too soon.

## Pressure Injuries

13. Correct answers are 3 and 5.
    1. The skin should be kept dry. The skin should be patted completely dry after each bath.
    2. Older people have decreased moisture in the skin. Applying lotion restores moisture.
    3. Clients should be turned at least every 1 to 2 hours to prevent pressure areas on the skin.
    4. All employees in any health-care facility are responsible for providing care within their scope of services.
    5. Talc powder and strong soaps dry the skin's natural oils and should not be used.

**TEST-TAKING HINT:** Option "2" has an absolute "any" in it. The test taker can eliminate this as an answer on this basis. Option "4" has the absolute "only," so this option can be eliminated. Of the remaining options, option "3" can apply to all immobile clients.

14. 1. This can be an independent nursing problem or a collaborative one, but it does not relate to pressure injuries.
    2. Altered nutrition is a collaborative problem involving the nurse, dietitian,

and HCP. The client will need a diet high in protein and vitamins if there is a chance for the client to heal.
    3. Self-care deficit is an independent nursing problem.
    4. Altered coping is an independent nursing problem and does not relate to skin integrity.

**TEST-TAKING HINT:** The stem gives two clues to the answer—"collaborative" and "pressure injuries." Collaborative means that some other members of the health-care team must be involved and pressure injuries are the client's problem. The correct answer must consider both of these variables.

15. 1. All the skin should be kept free of moisture. It is within the realm of nursing to provide this service. Clients with constant moisture on the skin are at high risk for impaired skin integrity.
    2. The clients able to reposition themselves would have decreased chances of developing pressure injuries. This would not be a risk factor.
    3. Decreased elasticity occurs with aging, and it is not modifiable.
    4. Impaired cardiovascular perfusion of the skin in the periphery is not modifiable.

**TEST-TAKING HINT:** The test taker must read the stem carefully. Which situation can the nurse modify with nursing care? The nurse cannot modify the changes that occur with aging or the sequelae that occur with disease processes.

16. 1. The pads will absorb moisture and will protect the bed, but they also will keep the moisture next to the client's skin, which increases the risk of skin breakdown.
    2. The pads are made with plastic liners, which tend to contain heat next to the client's body, thereby increasing diaphoresis.
    3. The pads are a help to lift the client but are not used to prevent workplace injuries. To prevent workplace injuries, the staff must practice good body mechanics.
    4. Lifting the client with a "lift" pad rather than pulling the client against the sheets helps to prevent skin damage from friction shearing.

**TEST-TAKING HINT:** The stem asks for the rationale for using "lift" pads. Lifting a client involves repositioning the client (option "4"). None of the other options mentions any kind of repositioning.

17. 1. The Braden and Norton scales are tools that identify clients at risk for skin problems. This client should be ranked on this scale, and appropriate measures should be initiated for controlling further damage to the skin.
2. The Glasgow Coma Scale is a neurological coma scale used to determine the depth of neurological damage.
3. Assessment for Babinski's sign would not be attempted with a client paralyzed from the waist down. The nerve pathways are not working.
4. Brudzinski's sign is used to assess for meningitis.

**TEST-TAKING HINT: The test taker must memorize the specific diagnostic tools used to assess clients.**

18. 1. This describes a stage I pressure injury, which would be an improvement of the client's wound.
2. This is a stage II pressure injury and is not a significant change in the wound.
3. This implies that the skin has healed and is not at stage I.
4. This is a stage III pressure injury and is a worsening of the client's condition.

**TEST-TAKING HINT: The test taker could look at the description in the stem and then at the descriptions in the options. Only one option appears to have a more involved skin condition.**

19. 1. The head of a client eating in bed should be elevated. This is a correct action on the part of the UAP.
2. It is important to turn bedfast clients every 1 to 2 hours and to encourage them, if they are able, to make minor readjustments to their position at least every 15 minutes. Allowing the client to lie in the same position for at least another 30 minutes before being turned should not be allowed.
3. It is a courtesy to the oncoming staff to leave the rooms equipped to care for the clients.
4. Beverage thickener (Thick-It) frequently is added to the liquids of a client diagnosed with difficulty swallowing.

**TEST-TAKING HINT: This is an "except" question. All but one option will be actions that are encouraged on the part of UAP. The test taker could jump to the conclusion that option "1" is correct if the test taker did not pay attention to the phrase "warrants immediate intervention."**

20. 1. The client diagnosed with quadriplegia cannot move arms or legs. "Quad" means four, and none of the four extremities moves. This is expected for the client's problem.
2. Weakness on one side of the body is expected in clients diagnosed with a CVA (stroke).
3. The client has a fever indicating an infection. Clients diagnosed with pressure injuries frequently develop infections in the wounds, which can lead to further complications.
4. This is a psychological problem and should be addressed, but not before assessing the infection.

**TEST-TAKING HINT: The test taker must decide if the situation is expected for the disease process or if it is life-threatening. Physiological problems come before psychological problems, according to Maslow.**

21. 1. Using a pillow to suspend the heels off the bed when a client is supine prevents the development of pressure injuries on the heels.
2. Low air-loss therapy beds are expensive and normally are provided only for clients diagnosed with stage III or stage IV impaired skin integrity. An egg-crate mattress may be applied to the bed for pressure relief, but many hospitals now have changed all of their regular mattresses for ones that provide the same pressure reduction surface as an egg-crate mattress.
3. There is no indication that the client requires tube feeding.
4. Physical therapists, not occupational therapists, work with clients on strength training. Occupational therapists address activities of daily living deficits.

**TEST-TAKING HINT: The test taker should not read into the question. The stem did not mention any swallowing problem, only a mobility problem. The correct answer must relate to the information provided in the stem.**

22. 1. The question asks for a therapeutic response. This response addresses a physiological problem and does not address the client's concerns.
2. This is restating and clarifying; both are therapeutic responses.
3. The client does not owe the nurse an explanation for the client's feelings. "Why" is not therapeutic.
4. This does not address the client's feelings.

**TEST-TAKING HINT:** When the stem asks the test taker for a therapeutic response, the correct answer must address the client's feelings.

23. Correct answers are 2 and 4.
    1. The client must be turned every 1 to 2 hours.
    2. Clients diagnosed with pressure injuries usually are debilitated and have a poor nutritional base for healing. An increase in protein and vitamins is needed in the diet to promote healing.
    3. Clients must sign consent if they are recognizable in the pictures. It is standard practice to document wounds by taking digital pictures and uploading the pictures into the EHR for reference by all concerned staff. In this instance, consent is not needed.
    4. A client diagnosed with a stage IV pressure injury needs a higher level of pressure reduction than a normal hospital mattress can provide.
    5. The head of the bed can be in any position of comfort for the client, but the head should not be elevated at "all" times because of the pressure applied to the lower body region.

**TEST-TAKING HINT:** The test taker must notice time frames. Is 3 to 4 hours the correct time frame for turning a client diagnosed with impaired skin integrity? Option "5" can be eliminated because of the word "all."

24. 1. A skin flap to graft an open wound is not a fecal diversion.
    2. This statement describes a débridement, not a fecal diversion.
    3. Hyperbaric chambers are used to increase oxygenation to nonhealing wounds, but surgery does not increase oxygenation.
    4. A fecal diversion is changing the normal exit of the stool from the body. A colostomy is created to keep stool from contaminating the wounds and causing infection.

**TEST-TAKING HINT:** The word *fecal* means "stool." Only one option mentions anything to do with the stool.

## Skin Cancer

25. Correct answers are 3 and 5.
    1. The lower the SPF number of sunscreen, the less protection. A sunscreen of SPF 15 is a minimum.
    2. Clients should avoid sunlight in the middle of the day, between 10 a.m. and 4 p.m, when the UV light is the strongest. "Between 0300 and 0500" refers to morning, the middle of the night.
    3. The American Cancer Society (2019) recommends a monthly skin check using mirrors to identify any suspicious skin lesion for early detection.
    4. Anything that prevents UV rays from reaching the skin helps to prevent skin cancer. Hats with a full brim are preferred to baseball caps, which leave the ears and back of the neck exposed.
    5. Sunglasses should be worn to protect the skin around the eyes, and the eyes from UV exposure. Labels that say "UV absorption up to 400 nm" or "Meets ANSI UV Requirements" means the glasses block at least 99% of UV rays. Those labeled "cosmetic" block about 70% of UV rays (American Cancer Society, 2019).

**TEST-TAKING HINT:** The test taker must notice time frames. In option "2," the use of "between 0300 and 0500" instead of "between 1500 and 1700" makes this option incorrect. In option "1" the number of the sunscreen makes this option wrong, and in option "4," the word "not" is an absolute word that could eliminate this option.

26. 1. The nurse should complete an assessment of the lesion before notifying the HCP to check it.
    2. This is part of assessing the lesion and should be completed. The ABCDEs of skin cancer detection include the following: (1) Asymmetry—Is the lesion balanced on both sides with an even surface? (2) Borders—Are the borders rounded and smooth or notched and indistinct? (3) Color—Is the color a uniform light brown or is it variegated and darker or reddish-purple? (4) Diameter—A diameter exceeding 4 to 6 mm is considered suspicious. (5) Evolving—Has the lesion changed during the past few weeks or months? (CDC, 2019c).
    3. This may help as a comfort measure, but it is not the first and most important action.
    4. Instructing the client to notify the HCP to assess the lesion also, should be done but does not have priority.

**TEST-TAKING HINT:** Assessment is the first step in the nursing process. The test taker should have a systematic decision-making model when determining a priority action.

27. 1. This client has an unexpected situation occurring and should be assessed before any stable client.
    2. This client's surgery was 3 hours ago, and the client should be stable and allowed to rest.
    3. This client can be seen after assessing the client in option "1."
    4. This client could be escorted to the door by a UAP; another nurse has already prepared the client for discharge.

**TEST-TAKING HINT: Physiological problems usually have priority over psychological ones, but none of the other clients has a life-threatening or life-altering situation. The only unexpected situation is the crying client.**

28. 1. Darker-skinned individuals have a lower risk of developing skin cancer. It is living in the southwestern regions of the United States, where sun exposure is the greatest, that increases skin cancer risk.
    2. Hispanic clients have more melanin in the skin than white clients, and moving from Mexico would have decreased the UV exposure.
    3. A family history of malignant melanoma increases the risk of developing malignant melanoma. Basal cell carcinoma is directly related to sun exposure and does not have an increased familial risk.
    4. Clients with very little melanin in the skin (fair-skinned) have an increased risk as a result of the UV damage to the underlying membranes. Damage to the underlying membranes never completely reverses itself; a lifetime of damage causes changes at the cellular level that can result in the development of cancer.

**TEST-TAKING HINT: If the test taker noticed the similarities in the clients in options "1" and "2"—darker skin and living in an area with less sun exposure or moving from an area with greater sun exposure to an area with less—the test taker could eliminate these two options. Based on skin color, the fair-skinned client would be most at risk.**

29. 1. The client should be taught to complete monthly skin checks to detect any future lesions.
    2. Basal cell lesions grow slowly and do not metastasize until the lesion has become very large. Prostheses are usually not needed.

    3. The area may need to have an antibiotic ointment, but sunscreen should not be applied until after the operative area has healed and then only when the client is going to be in the sun.
    4. On discharge, all clients should receive instructions in the care of surgical incisions.

**TEST-TAKING HINT: If the test taker did not know the specific information regarding this type of cancer surgery, then choosing an answer that is appropriate for all surgeries is a good option.**

30. 1. The diagnosis of cancer is concerning for clients; this is belittling the client's concerns and gives false reassurance.
    2. This is the most commonly written therapeutic communication goal. This addresses the client's concerns.
    3. The nurse is capable of discussing the client's concerns. Many clients feel more comfortable discussing fears with the nurse than with the HCP.
    4. This should be done but does not directly address the client's problem.

**TEST-TAKING HINT: The test taker must read the question carefully to decide what the question is asking. The answer must address the problem of fear.**

31. Correct answers are 1, 2, and 5.
    1. The UAP can restock rooms.
    2. These activities can be performed by a trained UAP.
    3. This is part of assessing the client and cannot be delegated.
    4. This is part of assessing the client and cannot be delegated.
    4. This is an appropriate delegation.

**TEST-TAKING HINT: This is an alternative format question. The test taker must be careful to read the question and determine which activities the UAP can perform.**

32. 1. Malignant melanomas are the most deadly of skin cancers. Asymmetry, irregular borders, variegated color, and rapid growth are characteristics of them.
    2. A waxy appearance and pearl-like borders are characteristic of basal cell carcinoma.
    3. A thickened and scaly appearance describes squamous cell carcinoma.
    4. A thickened area after an injury describes a benign condition called a keloid.

**TEST-TAKING HINT:** This is a knowledge-based question, but it does indicate the differences in the types of skin lesions. The test taker should concentrate on the differences when studying for an examination.

33. 1. The client should be aware of clinical manifestations that indicate the development of another skin cancer. Squamous cell carcinoma can develop in areas of the skin and mucous membranes.
    2. Of deaths from squamous cell carcinomas, 75% occur because of metastasis. Even basal cell carcinoma can metastasize but is usually so slow-growing that surgical excision removes cancer if the client does not delay treatment.
    3. The surgery was on the lip, not in the mouth. Food can be of a regular consistency.
    4. Applying heat to the area would increase circulation and edema, increasing the client's discomfort.

**TEST-TAKING HINT:** Anatomical positioning ("lip") could eliminate option "3." An HCP should be notified of any nonhealing wound.

34. 1. This is a psychological goal, not a physiological goal.
    2. This is a knowledge-deficit goal, not a physiological goal.
    3. Pain is a physiological problem; this is an appropriate physiological goal.
    4. This is a teaching goal, not a physiological goal.

**TEST-TAKING HINT:** The test taker must read the question carefully to determine what the stem is asking. All of the goals are appropriate for the client diagnosed with skin cancer, but only one is a physiological goal.

35. 1. The client may need a biopsy, but the nurse should assess the area before deciding to refer the client.
    2. This is the first step in deciding how to help the client. The nurse should assess the lesion to determine if it could be a Kaposi's sarcoma tumor or a healing contusion.
    3. This is important for all clients, even those without a chronic illness, but the question asks what should be done first. This is not the priority at this time.
    4. AIDS is a reportable disease, but reporting is not the priority intervention.

**TEST-TAKING HINT:** Assessment is the first step in the nursing process.

36. Correct answers are 2 and 4.
    1. Sunscreen should be used whenever the client is going to be exposed to UV rays.
    2. Most sunscreen is good for 2 to 3 years, but if it has been exposed to heat for long periods, it may be less effective (American Cancer Society, 2019).
    3. Sunscreen blocks the absorption of UV rays, which, when allowed to penetrate the skin, cause damage to the layers of the skin. This, in turn, causes cellular changes, which, over time, can develop into skin cancer.
    4. Sunscreen products range in numerical value from 4 to 100+; the higher the number of the sunscreen, the greater the UV protection (American Cancer Society, 2019).
    5. Sunscreen should be reapplied at least every 2 hours to maintain protection, more often if swimming or sweating.

**TEST-TAKING HINT:** Option "1" has the absolute word "only" and could be eliminated.

## Bacterial Skin Infection

37. 1. Cellulitis is a bacterial infection of the subcutaneous tissue usually associated with a break in the skin, and the nurse would suspect this with these clinical manifestations.
    2. Lyme disease is caused by the bite of a tick, resulting in a bull's-eye–appearing lesion.
    3. Impetigo is characterized by large, fluid-filled blisters and is very contagious.
    4. Deep vein thrombosis clinical manifestations are a reddened, warm calf, and pain on ambulation, but this condition is not caused by a nail puncture; it is caused by immobility.

**TEST-TAKING HINT:** If the test taker does not know the answer, the test taker should look at the stem and identify that redness and fever are clinical manifestations of inflammation; *-itis* means "inflammation" and option "1" would be an appropriate selection.

38. 1. Animals roaming the streets is not as important to ask as if the client has been to an area where there is a likelihood of being exposed.
    2. The client would most likely not be exposed to deer ticks while working in the garden.

3. Deer ticks (*Ixodes scapularis*) are responsible for the spread of Lyme disease, which is what this client is experiencing based on the clinical manifestations (CDC, 2019a).
4. Sunscreen is important, but it will not protect the client from any type of insect bites.

**TEST-TAKING HINT:** Option "4" could be eliminated as a possible answer if the test taker realized that the other three options all deal with some type of insect bite, which is stated in the stem of the question.

39. 1. Cleanliness and good hygiene prevent the spread of impetigo, but washing hands after going to the bathroom will not prevent the spread.
2. Lesions are extremely contagious and should not be touched, except when wearing gloves.
3. The topical antibiotic ointment is applied after impetigo has developed. It will not help prevent impetigo. Usually, the client diagnosed with impetigo is given systemic antibiotics.
4. The child is kept at home until after taking antibiotics for at least 48 hours; the child is not isolated in the room.

**TEST-TAKING HINT:** The test taker needs to think about what the options are saying. Option "4" can be eliminated because a child cannot be isolated in a room with many other children in the room. Washing hands after using the bathroom (option "1") is a general hygiene tip encouraged for all individuals and is not specific to impetigo. The test taker should look at the word "prevent" in the stem; antibiotic ointment is only prescribed for bacterial infections, so option "3" should be ruled out as an answer.

40. 1. As long as the client has bilateral pulses, there is no need for the nurse to intervene.
2. As long as the client is able to move the fingers, there is no need for the nurse to intervene.
3. A capillary refill time (CRT) less than 3 seconds is normal and would not require immediate intervention.
4. The client being unable to remove the wedding ring indicates that the arm is edematous, and the ring must be removed immediately or it may cause impaired circulation to the left ring finger. This is a dangerous situation.

**TEST-TAKING HINT:** When the stem asks the test taker to identify data that warrant immediate intervention, the test taker must select the option that is abnormal for the disease process.

All the options except "4" are normal neurovascular assessment data.

41. Correct answers are 2, 3, and 5.
1. Humidity should be kept high, around 60%, to prevent the skin from drying.
2. Coolness deters itching.
3. Mild soaps contain no detergents, dyes, or fragrances to cause an increase in itching.
4. Lesions should be left open to air as much as possible; cloth rubbing the lesions is irritating.
5. Effective hydration of the stratum corneum prevents compromise of the barrier layer of the skin.

**TEST-TAKING HINT:** "Select all that apply" questions require the test taker to make a determination for each option individually. Choosing one answer will not exclude another.

42. 1. The RN is responsible for providing correct information to the UAPs. This intervention would be appropriate if confronting the person has not altered the behavior.
2. This action could result in the client developing a skin infection and should be stopped immediately; therefore, stopping the behavior is the first intervention.
3. The RN must be a role model for the UAP and demonstrate the correct way to care for the client's skin, but it is not the first intervention.
4. An incident report may need to be completed to document the situation, but it is not the first intervention.

**TEST-TAKING HINT:** When the question asks the test taker to select the first intervention, all four options may be possible actions, but only one should be done first. In this situation, the behavior must be stopped before performing any other interventions.

43. 1. Impaired skin integrity is a physiological problem, not a psychosocial problem.
2. The nurse does not know if the client is grieving over the acne. Do not read more into the question than is available.
3. Acne occurs on the face and neck. This is the first impression that people get when looking at the client; therefore, body image disturbance is the priority.
4. Knowledge deficit is appropriate for this client, but it does not have priority over body image. Acne can be devastating to a client's self-image.

**TEST-TAKING HINT:** The test taker must remember to observe adjectives. "Psychosocial" is the keyword for answering this question.

44. 1. This disease is a bacterial inflammatory reaction that occurs predominantly on the faces and necks of curly-haired men as a result of shaving. The sharp in-growing hairs have a curved root that grows at a more acute angle and pierces the skin. The treatments are to apply creams and not to shave.
    2. This person will not get this disease.
    3. This person will not get this disease.
    4. This person will not get this disease.

**TEST-TAKING HINT:** If the answer to this question is not known, the test taker could examine the root words and endings: Follicle refers to "hair" and -*itis* is an inflammation. The test taker should think about what type of hair each individual has and realize that African Americans typically have curly hair.

45. 1. A furuncle (boil) is not a life-threatening emergency, and an appointment is not needed for this client.
    2. Warm, moist compresses increase vascularization and hasten the resolution of the furuncle.
    3. With staphylococcal infections, such as a boil, it is important not to rupture the protective wall of induration that localizes the infection.
    4. The client called the clinic to get help, and this response does not help the client. A nurse can recommend heat, ice, elevation, or some type of independent treatment.

**TEST-TAKING HINT:** The test taker can always rule out options that don't address the client's needs, such as option "4." Option "3" can also be ruled out: There are very few "never," answers, but one is never squeezing or popping a boil or pimple.

46. 1. This client is not at increased risk for developing a carbuncle.
    2. This client is not at increased risk for developing a carbuncle.
    3. This client is not at increased risk for developing a carbuncle.
    4. A carbuncle is an abscess of the skin and subcutaneous tissue and is an extension of a furuncle. These are more likely to occur in clients diagnosed with underlying systemic diseases such as diabetes, hematologic malignances, and immunosuppression.

**TEST-TAKING HINT:** If the definition of a carbuncle was not known, the test taker could look at the options and note that only one has a disease process, which might be the best choice for the correct answer.

47. 1. Systemic antibiotics are the treatment of choice for impetigo. Therefore, the teacher must go to the HCP to get the prescription today because impetigo is highly contagious.
    2. Washing hands is always a good practice, but the teacher needs medication for this bacterial infection.
    3. Vitamin E oil does help prevent scarring, but it will not treat this bacterial infection.
    4. Impetigo is not a rash; it is raised, crusty lesions.

**TEST-TAKING HINT:** The test taker must know that impetigo is a bacterial infection requiring medical treatment. Vitamins do not treat skin infections. Washing with an antiseptic solution may help, but antibiotics are the treatment of choice.

48. Correct answers are 3 and 5.
    1. To help prevent deer tick bites, which spread Lyme disease, the individual should wear light-colored, tightly woven clothing with long pants and long-sleeved shirts. These allow the person to see the tick better.
    2. Sunscreen will not help prevent the spread of Lyme disease.
    3. Staying on paths and avoiding dense undergrowth will help the person keep away from tick-infested areas where the person is more likely to be bitten by a tick and perhaps subsequently develop Lyme disease.
    4. Insect repellant should be used; there are special repellants, Environmental Protection Agency (EPA)–registered insect repellents, such as diethyltoluamide (DEET), that are used to help prevent Lyme disease.
    5. Clothing and outdoor gear can be treated with 0.5% permethrin or bought already treated with 0.5% permethrin to protect from tick bites (CDC, 2019a).

**TEST-TAKING HINT:** The test taker should be able to rule out sunscreen as an answer because the stem says "disease" and sunscreen cannot prevent infectious disease. Not wearing insect repellant (option "4") would not be appropriate for any teaching except teaching about infants.

## Viral Skin Infection

49. 1. The virus that causes chickenpox is the varicella-zoster virus (human herpesvirus 3), not the herpes simplex virus.
2. Herpes simplex 1 and 2 are caused by the same virus. Herpes simplex 1 refers to orolabial lesions and herpes simplex 2 refers to genital lesions, which can be transferred from one area to the other.
3. The question is asking which intervention the nurse should teach the client, and there is no reason for the client to have to wear nonsterile gloves for self-care. That is appropriate for the nursing personnel.
4. Herpes simplex is not transmitted via towels or washcloths.

**TEST-TAKING HINT: In some instances, the test taker simply must know about the disease process. Sexually transmitted diseases are common, and the nurse should know about how to prevent, discuss, and treat them.**

50. 1. The left rib cage area is not considered an area for revealing cardiac problems. The client diagnosed with a cardiac problem would have chest pain radiating to the left arm, sweating, and nausea.
2. This negates the client's reports and does not address the client's concerns. The nurse should always further assess when the client is in pain.
3. The nurse should not administer pain medication unless the cause of the pain is known. The client is reporting severe pain, and Tylenol (a nonnarcotic) will not be effective.
4. The client's description of the pain suggests shingles. Shingles is caused by herpes zoster, which is the same virus as varicella-zoster, which causes chickenpox. This virus is a retrovirus that never dies; it becomes dormant and lives in the body along nerve pathways. During times of stress, it can erupt as herpes zoster or shingles. The pain usually occurs before the eruption of the vesicles.

**TEST-TAKING HINT: If the test taker does not know the answer, then the test taker should apply the nursing process. Option "4" is the only option involving assessment, which is the first part of the nursing process.**

51. 1. The antiviral medication valacyclovir (Valtrex) is not a birth control medication.
2. (Valtrex) is usually prescribed for a set amount of time and does not need to be tapered.

3. Valacyclovir (Valtrex) is an antiviral medication that suppresses the virus replication, but herpes is a retrovirus, which means it never dies as long as the host body is alive.
4. This medication does not cause the urine to turn orange.

**TEST-TAKING HINT: Medications are frequently advertised to the public; therefore, the nurse must know about medications that laypeople may be asking about.**

52. 1. Diversionary techniques, including music and television, are often used in conjunction with medication to manage pain. Shutting the blinds will help provide a calm, quiet atmosphere.
2. Warm, moist heat will exacerbate the pain from the lesions; cool compresses would help.
3. The client was medicated 45 minutes ago and would not be able to have more morphine sulfate, a narcotic analgesic; therefore, there is no reason to notify the HCP.
4. Ambulating will not help decrease the client's pain and could aggravate it. In addition, the client has been given morphine, which causes drowsiness and could lead to a safety issue.

**TEST-TAKING HINT: The test taker could rule out option "4" with no knowledge of the disease process because the nurse does not ambulate clients on morphine. The nurse often uses diversionary interventions when addressing pain issues.**

53. Correct answers are 1, 2, 3, and 5.
1. The zoster lesions are contagious, so the client should be in contact isolation.
2. Corticosteroids decrease the inflammation, which helps with the healing process.
3. Assessment is always an appropriate intervention.
4. The client can have visitors as long as they do not have an infection that the client could get and the visitors comply with isolation protocol. Only visitors with prior chickenpox infection should be allowed to visit.
5. Herpes zoster is the same virus that causes chickenpox. It was thought for years that there were two separate viruses. Research has proven that the varicella virus and zoster are the same; therefore, only nurses with prior chickenpox infection should care for this client.

**TEST-TAKING HINT:** This is an alternate-type question where the test taker must select all the interventions that are pertinent. If the test taker is aware that corticosteroid medications decrease inflammation, then option "2" should be selected as a correct answer. Assessment (option "3") is always an appropriate selection if the assessment data apply to the situation.

54. 1. Rubbing alcohol will cause tremendous pain and will not help the lesions disappear.
    2. The lesions are very irritating, and the client will want to scratch them. Clients diagnosed with chickenpox should use calamine lotion, soak in oatmeal baths, and apply Benadryl topical cream or take oral Benadryl.
    3. The lesions are considered contagious until they are dry and crusted over, usually in 5 to 7 days. The client does not have to wait until they have disappeared; this may take up to 2 or 3 weeks.
    4. Chickenpox is a virus, and antibiotics are effective only with bacterial infections; antibiotics are not prescribed.

**TEST-TAKING HINT:** The test taker may realize that options with absolutes such as "all" should not be selected as the right answer, but the test taker should notice that the "all" in option "2" is not used in the same manner as to mean "always."

55. 1. This would be a short-term goal, but it is unrealistic to expect a client not to scratch when experiencing severe itching.
    2. The client currently has lesions; therefore, skin integrity is already compromised. The keyword is "maintain."
    3. Relief of itching is a short-term goal for this client. For a long-term goal, the nurse needs to recognize potential complications.
    4. A major complication of pruritus (itching) is the development of a bacterial skin infection, which is secondary to the client scratching and allowing bacteria from the dirty hands or nails to enter compromised tissue.

**TEST-TAKING HINT:** The test taker must recognize what clinical manifestations the client is experiencing. Lesions are open wounds; therefore, option "2" could be eliminated even if the test taker did not know what the word "pruritus" means. Furthermore, the test taker must look at adjectives; the question asks for long-term goals, and the test taker should realize immediate behavior change (refrain from scratching) and pain relief are short-term goals.

56. 1. The nurse cannot delegate assessment, which is what measuring the lesions is doing, and the nurse must document the assessment.
    2. This is a medication, and the nurse cannot delegate medication administration.
    3. The nurse can delegate the setup of equipment to the assistant.
    4. Determining if a client has an advance directive should not be delegated to the assistant because, if the client has questions, the nurse must provide factual information.

**TEST-TAKING HINT:** The nurse must know which nursing tasks can be delegated; assessment, teaching, evaluating, and medication administration cannot be delegated to UAP.

57. 250 mg per dose.
    First, determine the client's weight in kilograms; there are 2.2 pounds per kilogram, so:

    $$220 \text{ pounds} \div 2.2 = 100 \text{ kilograms}$$

    Then, determine the total dosage to be given per day based on the HCP order of 10 mg per kilogram per day:

    $$100 \times 10 = 1{,}000 \text{ milligrams per day}$$

    Then, determine how many doses are given in a day if a dose is to be given every 6 hours:

    $$24 \div 6 = 4 \text{ doses}$$

    Finally, determine how many milligrams per each dose to administer 1,000 mg in 24 hours:

    $$1{,}000 \div 4 = 250 \text{ mg per dose}$$

**TEST-TAKING HINT:** Math problems frequently require multiple steps. The test taker should replace each number as the conversion is made. The test taker must know conversion factors and how to use the drop-down calculator on the computer.

58. 1. This is a complication of immobility, not specifically chickenpox.
    2. Varicella-zoster (human herpesvirus 3) is the causative agent for chickenpox, and pneumonia is a potential complication in adults.
    3. Pericarditis (inflammation of the sac surrounding the heart) is not a complication of chickenpox.
    4. Scarring of the skin is an expected sequela of chickenpox, but it is not a complication.

**TEST-TAKING HINT:** The question asks for a complication; therefore, option "4" could be ruled out because it is expected; if the test taker knows that chickenpox is caused by varicella-zoster, then the most obvious answer is option "2."

59. 1. Chickenpox starts out with a macular rash. The lesions appear in crops first on the trunk and scalp, and then lesions move to the extremities. Then, they change to teardrop vesicles with an erythematous base and become pustular. Finally, they dry.
    2. Oval scaling indicates fungal infections.
    3. Severe itching of the scalp with tiny eggs visible supports the diagnosis of lice.
    4. Ringed red lesions support the diagnosis of ringworm.

**TEST-TAKING HINT:** This is primarily a knowledge-based question. The test taker either knows the clinical manifestations of different skin disorders or does not. One way to help identify the answer is to try to determine what condition each option describes. For example, "tiny eggs" should make the test taker think of a parasite (lice).

60. 1. This client would not be a priority; elderly clients frequently think they need a daily bowel movement.
    2. A catheter change would not be a priority.
    3. Periorbital lesions may extend into the client's eyes, which is an ophthalmic emergency, especially if it is herpes zoster.
    4. A stage I pressure injury requires changing the client's position, which can be delegated.

**TEST-TAKING HINT:** If the test taker knows medical terminology, then "periorbital" (around the eye) would be a priority.

## Fungal and Parasitic Skin Infection

61. Correct answers are 1, 2, 3, and 5.
    1. This statement indicates the teacher understands the teaching about the spread of lice (pediculosis).
    2. Pyrethrin (Rid) is a recommended over-the-counter medication to use when lice are found in the hair. Lindane (Kwell) shampoo is no longer recommend by the American Academy of Pediatrics as a pediculicide (CDC, 2019b).
    3. All linens and pertinent clothing should be washed in hot water to help destroy the eggs.

    4. Sharing brushes is one of the main ways that lice are spread. Therefore, this statement indicates the teacher did not comply with the instructions.
    5. Any items that cannot be laundered may be dry-cleaned or sealed in a plastic bag for 2 weeks to destroy the lice (CDC, 2019b).

**TEST-TAKING HINT:** This is an alternative format question. Therefore, more than one of the options will be correct actions for the problem. The test taker should always read all the options thoroughly.

62. 1. Pediculosis capitus is found on the head. Head lice are found commonly in children in elementary schools.
    2. Scabies are found on the forearms, and around the waist and elastic lines of underwear.
    3. The pubic lice are found in the pubic area and are commonly transmitted during sexual intercourse.
    4. The feet are not an area normally associated with body lice.

**TEST-TAKING HINT:** The nurse should be familiar with medical terminology, which can often help rule out incorrect options. Pubis, for example, pertains to the groin; therefore, option "3" near the groin should be chosen as the answer.

63. 1. To prevent tinea cruris (jock itch), the football players should avoid wearing nylon underwear, tight-fitting clothing, and wet bathing suits.
    2. This would be appropriate advice for tinea pedis (athlete's foot).
    3. This would be appropriate advice to help prevent lice.
    4. Tinea cruris (jock itch) results from a fungal infection in warm, moist areas of the body. When such an infection occurs in the groin area, it is called tinea cruris.

**TEST-TAKING HINT:** All the options discuss prevention of something; therefore, the test taker must know about disease processes. Test-taking hints do not substitute for studying and understanding the material. Remember that perfect test scores are few and far between.

64. 1. Tinea capitis is ringworm of the scalp, which does not support this client's clinical manifestations.
    2. A herpes simplex 2 lesion is in the genital area.
    3. Scabies is an infestation of the skin by the itch mite (*Sarcoptes scabiei*). The female burrows into the superficial layer of skin and burrows are found between the fingers and on the wrist.
    4. Psoriasis is a chronic, noninfectious inflammatory disorder of the skin, which results in scales.

**TEST-TAKING HINT:** The nurse should be familiar with medical terminology, which can often help rule out incorrect options. Capitus, for example, pertains to the head or scalp; therefore, option "1" could be eliminated as a possible answer.

65. Correct answers are 1, 2, and 5.
    1. The malathion (Ovide) lotion should be left on for at least 8 to 12 hours to be effective.
    2. The manufacturer recommends that malathion (Ovide) lotion be applied to dry hair until the scalp and hair are wet and thoroughly coated.
    3. One application may cure the infestation of lice or scabies, but another application may be needed in 1 week; daily administration is contraindicated.
    4. This medication must be applied to dry hair, not introduced into bathwater.
    5. Malathion (Ovide) lotion is flammable. The lotion and wet hair should not be exposed to heat sources or open flames (CDC, 2019b).

**TEST-TAKING HINT:** The test taker should always be aware of time frames, notice "8 hours," "20 minutes," and "daily." These are all terms that may help the test taker to choose the correct answer.

66. 1. The assistant could use a fine-toothed comb dipped in vinegar to remove any nits in the hair of the client with lice.
    2. Reddened areas should not be massaged; that will lead to further damage.
    3. Scraping the burrows is a diagnostic test and cannot be delegated to an assistant.
    4. Assistants cannot administer medication.

**TEST-TAKING HINT:** The test taker must apply universal delegation rules. Nurses cannot delegate medication administration or diagnostic tests. Some states allow medication aides to administer routine medications to clients in long-term care facilities, but the stem does not identify this employee as a medication aide. Do not read into the question.

67. 1. Soaking the feet will help remove the crust, scales, and debris to reduce the inflammation in a client diagnosed with athlete's foot. Vinegar is mildly acidic, which helps remove crusts, although the efficacy of home remedies has not been completely evaluated (National Center for Biotechnology Information, 2018).
    2. White cotton socks should be recommended to help prevent athlete's foot. Colored socks have dyes that irritate the skin, and cotton socks absorb moisture.
    3. Several pairs of shoes should be alternated so that shoes can be completely dry before wearing them again.
    4. Cutting toenails straight across is correct, but it will not prevent or treat athlete's foot.

**TEST-TAKING HINT:** There are basic interventions that are taught about foot care in general, and trimming toenails is one of them. This could apply to many foot conditions. Wearing socks is always advisable because feet perspire. Not very many interventions are done on a monthly basis—usually daily or weekly—so option "3" can be eliminated.

68. 1. This sequela may occur for a client diagnosed with diabetes and a foot ulcer.
    2. Oral antifungal agents must be taken for 12 weeks because the fungal infection is underneath the nail; topical medications would not reach the infection.
    3. This is a condition of ringworm of the toenail. The nurse must tell the client that the toenail will fall off if the client does not take the medication, and it might fall off anyway.
    4. This is not a bacterial infection; therefore, oral antibiotics will not be administered. It is a fungal infection and antifungal medication will be administered.

**TEST-TAKING HINT:** Gangrene is usually a circulation problem, not a toenail problem; therefore, option "1" could be eliminated as a possible answer. Option "2" should be eliminated because nurses cannot prescribe or change physicians' orders. Of the two remaining options, only "3" has the word toenail in it; therefore, the test taker should select option "3" as the correct answer.

69. 1. Foam or soap and water can be used to clean the hands.
    2. Because of the close living quarters, clients in long-term care facilities are at

high risk of developing scabies. Clients may have poor hygiene as a result of limited physical ability, and the nursing staff may transmit the parasite. Therefore, the nursing staff should wear gloves to provide a barrier to the mites.

3. Linens and clothing should be washed in hot water and dried in a hot dryer cycle because the mites can survive up to 36 hours in linens.
4. Plastic eating utensils will not help prevent the spread of scabies.

**TEST-TAKING HINT:** If the test taker has no idea what the correct answer is, then the test taker should eliminate options "1" and "3" because of the words "only" and "all." There are very few absolutes in the health-care profession.

70. Correct answers are 1, 2, 3, 4, and 5.
    1. Dermatology is the study of the skin. Therefore, asking about skin problems is appropriate.
    2. The nurse must differentiate between dermatitis, which could result from a cosmetic or other skin product, and skin infection.
    3. The skin is responsible for sensation, so any loss would be significant.
    4. Many occupations, including those involved in working with chemicals, predispose a client to abnormal skin conditions.
    5. These are hallmark clinical manifestations of skin abnormality.

**TEST-TAKING HINT:** In "Select all that apply" questions, each option stands or falls on its own. The test taker should not try to second-guess the item writer by thinking that there is no way that all five options will be correct.

71. 1. This technique will not help diagnose scabies.
    2. Vinegar will not help visualize and identify scabies.

3. A magnifying glass and a penlight are held at an oblique angle to the skin while a search is done for small raised burrows, which indicate scabies.
4. A Doppler is used to obtain faint pulses, but it will not help find a mite, which causes scabies.

**TEST-TAKING HINT:** The nurse must know about diagnostic equipment, and a Doppler is commonly used in clients diagnosed with a non-palpable pulse. Therefore, option "4" could be eliminated.

72. 1. This is the correct information.
    2. Dark-skinned people are less likely to have skin cancer.
    3. Dark-skinned people are more likely to have keloids (hypertrophied scar tissue) after surgery.
    4. Bluish-tinged buccal mucosa in anyone indicates decreased oxygenation.

**TEST-TAKING HINT:** The nurse should know that any blue color on the body is abnormal, thus ruling out option "4." The test taker should notice that options "2" and "3" have "more likely" and "less likely," which may encourage the test taker to rule out both answers and select option "1."

73. 1. Contact dermatitis usually occurs where cosmetics or perfume are applied or specific clothing items touch the skin.
    2. Herpes zoster in clients not immunocompromised occurs along the nerve roots around the rib cage and back.
    3. Seborrheic dermatitis occurs in the midline front and back of the body.
    4. Scabies occurs around the waist, around the wrist, between the fingers, and in the axilla area.

**TEST-TAKING HINT:** There may be questions that require the test taker to identify body parts when selecting the correct answer. The test taker must know about skin conditions to be able to answer the question.

74. 1. Stage I pressures are characterized by intact skin with unblanchable redness.
    2. Stage II pressure injuries are characterized by partial-thickness loss of the dermis as a shallow open ulcer with a red-pink wound bed without slough or as an intact unruptured serum-filled blister.
    3. Stage III pressure injuries are characterized by full-thickness tissue loss, subcutaneous fat may be visible, but bone, tendon, and muscle are not exposed. Slough may be present but does not obscure the depth of tissue loss.
    4. Stage IV pressure injuries are characterized by full-thickness tissue loss with exposed bone, tendon, or muscle. Slough or eschar may be present on some parts of the wound bed, often includes undermining and tunneling.

**TEST-TAKING HINT:** The test taker should concentrate on the stages I through IV. Usually, in health care, stage I will be minimal disease and stage IV will show an increase in the disease clinical manifestations. This wound has depth and exposed muscle tissue.

75. Correct answers are 1, 3, and 5.
    1. The wound is infected so antibiotics should be administered. In the hospital, most antibiotics are administered via IVPB.
    2. Dressing changes should be performed with sterile, not unsterile gloves due to the "acute" nature of the injury. Dressing changes for some chronic wounds may be done with unsterile gloves, but even a chronic wound in an immunosuppressed client should be performed as a sterile procedure (Treas, Wilkinson, Barnett, & Smith, 2018).
    3. High blood glucose levels impair wound healing and encourage bacterial growth.
    4. The client will not have daily cultures, and after an antibiotic is initiated, the culture will be skewed.
    5. Controlling the glucose levels will assist the client in promoting wound healing and disease stabilization.

**TEST-TAKING HINT:** When answering a "Select all that apply" question, the test taker must look at each option independently of the other options. Each option becomes a true or false question.

76. Correct answers are 1, 2, 3, and 4.
    1. Asymmetry means one-half of the area is not identical to the other half.
    2. Borders describe irregular edges to the lesion.
    3. Color means that various shades or colors are in the same lesion, including tan, brown, black, or purple.
    4. Diameter refers to a lesion that is greater than 6 mm (the diameter of a pencil eraser). This lesion from top to bottom would be more than 6 mm and from side to side would be at least 6 mm.
    5. Evolving is not correct because there is no way to see an evolving lesion from one static picture.

**TEST-TAKING HINT:** When looking at a picture or diagram, the test taker must carefully observe exactly what is being pictured. "Evolving" cannot be shown with one picture.

77. 1. Shingles, herpes zoster, is the same virus as herpes varicella, the chickenpox virus. Unvaccinated children are at risk of contracting chickenpox from the client.
    2. Only nurses with immunity from varicella (zoster) virus should care for the client.
    3. The virus can be spread by droplets but does not require a negative airflow room (airborne precautions), and no nuclear wastes are involved so decontamination is not needed.
    4. Acyclovir or another antiviral medication may hasten recovery, but vancomycin, an aminoglycoside antibiotic, is not needed.

**TEST-TAKING HINT:** The test taker should be able to recognize common skin ailments and make appropriate interventions based on the assessment of the problem.

**78.** 1. The fairer the skin, the greater the risk of developing skin cancer.
2. Dietary fiber does not impact the development of skin cancer.
3. Sun exposure is not less dangerous at a beach—the exposure is basically the same. It depends on the length of time and amount of exposure to the UV rays.
4. **The middle of the day, between 10 a.m. and 4 p.m., is when the UV rays are the strongest. UV rays are also stronger in the spring and summer, at higher elevations, and locations closest to the equator (American Cancer Society, 2019).**

**TEST-TAKING HINT:** The test taker must be aware of basic principles such as when the sun is hottest, resulting in greatest skin exposure, and that people at a beach usually are exposing more skin to the damaging rays of the sun.

**79.** 1. **Impetigo is a group A beta-hemolytic streptococci or staphylococci infection treated with antibiotics; the parents should make sure that all medication is taken as directed.**
2. The child has a contagious infection and is not allowed to return to school until the infection has resolved itself.
3. Oatmeal baths are useful to treat the pruritus of poison ivy or oak but are not used for bacterial infections.
4. The nurse would not débride the lesions. Sometimes soap and water are used to soften the crusts from the lesions.

**TEST-TAKING HINT:** Standard instructions to all clients regarding antibiotics are to finish them all to treat the infection and prevent regrowth of resistant bacteria from partially treated infection.

**80.** 1. **The nurse should completely assess the lesion before proceeding to document the finding or notify the HCP.**
2. Documenting the lesion would follow a full assessment of the lesion.
3. The lesion is present at this time, assessing it is first.
4. The nurse should completely assess the lesion before notifying the HCP.

**TEST-TAKING HINT:** When answering a "first" question, the test taker should put the options in the order of how a nurse would perform the tasks. First, the nurse would assess the lesion. Second (possible), determine the length of time the client has been aware of its presence. Third or fourth is documentation and notifying the HCP.

**81.** 1. The cream should not be affected by the position of the head.
2. Once the 5-fluorouracil cream has absorbed into the skin, the client can eat solid or liquid foods.
3. Exposure to sunlight is the most common reason for developing skin cancer; sun exposure is not recommended. Clients receiving 5-fluorouracil orally or intravenously can become photosensitive.
4. **The nurse should protect against coming into contact with the 5-fluorouracil cream.**

**TEST-TAKING HINT:** The test taker should remember basic medication administration guidelines. Unsterile gloves are required whenever a nurse is applying topical medications to prevent personal exposure to the medication.

# INTEGUMENTARY DISORDERS COMPREHENSIVE EXAMINATION

1. The nurse is caring for a client with reports of a rash and itching on the face for 1 week. Which intervention should the nurse implement **first?**
   1. Check for the presence of hirsutism on the face.
   2. Use the ultraviolet examination light to visualize the rash under the black light.
   3. Determine what OTC medications the client has used on the rash.
   4. Ask the client to describe when the rash first appeared.

2. The nurse is assessing the client diagnosed with psoriasis. Which data would support that diagnosis?
   1. Appearance of red, elevated plaques with silvery-white scales.
   2. A burning, prickling row of vesicles located along the torso.
   3. Raised, flesh-colored papules with a rough surface area.
   4. An overgrowth of tissue with an excessive amount of collagen.

3. The nurse is preparing the plan of care for a client diagnosed with psoriasis. Which intervention should the nurse include in the plan of care?
   1. Apply a thin dusting with nystatin powder over the area.
   2. Cover the area with an occlusive dressing after applying a steroid cream.
   3. Administer acyclovir to the affected areas six times a day.
   4. Teach the client the risks and hazards of implanted radiation therapy.

4. The nurse has completed the teaching plan for the client diagnosed with psoriasis. Which statement indicates the need for **further teaching?**
   1. "I will check my skin every day for redness with tenderness."
   2. "I must take my psoralen medication 2 hours before my treatment."
   3. "I will wear dark glasses during my treatment and the rest of the day."
   4. "The coal tar ointments and lotions will not stain my clothes."

5. The nurse is planning the care of a client diagnosed with psoriasis. Which psychosocial problem should be included in the plan?
   1. Alteration in comfort.
   2. Altered body image.
   3. Anxiety.
   4. Altered family processes.

6. The older client diagnosed with poison ivy is prescribed a methylprednisolone dose pack. Which intervention should the nurse teach the client?
   1. Tell the client to return to the office in 1 week for blood levels.
   2. Instruct the client to take the medication exactly as prescribed.
   3. Explain the medication should be taken on an empty stomach.
   4. Teach to stop the medication immediately if side effects occur.

7. The nurse is teaching clients at a community center about skin diseases. Which information about pruritus should the nurse include? **Select all that apply.**
   1. Cool environments increase itching.
   2. Using soap increases itching.
   3. Use hot water to rinse off the soap.
   4. Apply mild skin lotion for hydration.
   5. Blot gently, but completely dry the skin.

8. Which laboratory test should the nurse monitor to identify an allergic reaction for the client diagnosed with contact dermatitis?

| Laboratory Test | Normal Values (Adult) |
|---|---|
| Immunoglobulin A (IgA) | 40–350 mg/dL |
| Immunoglobulin D (IgD) | Less than 15 mg/dL |
| Immunoglobulin E (IgE) | Less than 100 units/L |
| Immunoglobulin G (IgG) | 650–1,600 mg/dL |

   1. IgA.
   2. IgD.
   3. IgE.
   4. IgG.

9. Which client's clinical manifestations indicate contact dermatitis to the nurse?
   1. Erythema and oozing vesicles.
   2. Pustules and nodule formation.
   3. Varicosities and edema.
   4. Telangiectasia and flushing.

10. The nurse is caring for the client diagnosed with contact dermatitis. Which **collaborative** intervention should the nurse implement?
    1. Encourage the use of support stockings.
    2. Administer a topical anti-inflammatory cream.
    3. Remove scales frequently by shampooing.
    4. Shampoo with pyrethrin weekly.

11. The client had an allergic reaction to poison oak 2 weeks ago. He has returned to the clinic with severe itching and weeping vesicles on the arms and legs. Which intervention should the nurse implement?
    1. Obtain a sample of the drainage for culture and sensitivities.
    2. Determine any allergic reactions to any medications taken recently.
    3. Inquire how the poison ivy or oak plants were destroyed.
    4. Assess for any temperature elevation since the last visit to the clinic.

12. The client is reporting severe itching following a course of antibiotics. Which independent nursing action should the nurse implement?
    1. Refer to an allergy specialist to begin desensitization.
    2. Use a tar-preparation gel after each shower or bath.
    3. Keep the covers tightly around the client at night.
    4. Take baths with an OTC colloidal oatmeal preparation.

13. The home health nurse is visiting an older client with concern for an area of rough skin having a greasy feel and multiple papules. Which information should the nurse provide the client?
    1. Contact the HCP immediately for an appointment.
    2. Tell the client this is a normal aging change and no action should be taken.
    3. Tell the client to discuss this with the HCP at the next appointment.
    4. Have the client buy a wart remover kit at the store.

14. The nurse is preparing the plan of care for a client diagnosed with Stevens-Johnson syndrome. Which interventions should the nurse include? **Select all that apply.**
    1. Monitor intake and output every 8 hours.
    2. Assess breath sounds and rate every 4 hours.
    3. Assess vesicles, erosions, and crusts frequently.
    4. Perform the whisper test for auditory changes daily.
    5. Assess orientation to person, place, and time every shift.

15. Which expected outcome should the nurse include in the plan of care for the client diagnosed with seborrheic dermatitis?
    1. The client will have no further outbreaks.
    2. The client will follow medical protocol.
    3. The client will shampoo three times a week.
    4. The client will apply bacitracin twice daily.

16. The public health nurse is caring for a client diagnosed with leprosy (Hansen's disease). Which intervention should the nurse implement?
    1. Explain the need for admission to the hospital.
    2. Administer dapsone for 1 month only.
    3. Instruct to use skin moisturizing lotion to control the symptoms.
    4. Discuss the ways leprosy is transmitted to other individuals.

17. The health department nurse is caring for the client diagnosed with leprosy (Hansen's disease). Which assessment data indicate the client is experiencing a complication of the disease?
    1. Elevated temperature at night.
    2. Brownish-black discoloration to the skin.
    3. Reduced skin sensation in the lesions.
    4. A high count of mycobacteria in the culture.

18. Which problem should the nurse identify for the client recently diagnosed with leprosy (Hansen's disease)?
    1. Social isolation.
    2. Altered body image.
    3. Potential for infection.
    4. Alteration in comfort.

19. The nurse is teaching the client diagnosed with atopic dermatitis. Which information should the nurse include in the teaching?
    1. Discuss skincare using hydrating lotions and minimal soap.
    2. Tell the client the methods of treating secondary infection.
    3. Explain there are no adverse effects to using topical corticosteroids daily.
    4. Instruct the client that inhaled allergens have never been linked to exacerbations.

20. The nurse is working with clients in an aesthetic surgery center. Which intervention should the nurse implement for a client undergoing a chemical peel?
    1. Teach the client to expect extreme swelling after the procedure.
    2. Apply the chemical mixture directly to the skin after the face is cleansed.
    3. Administer general anesthesia to the client before the procedure.
    4. Explain that there will be no pain or discomfort during the procedure.

21. The nurse is preparing the client scheduled for a dermabrasion. Which information should the nurse include while teaching the client?
    1. Erythema will go away within 24 hours.
    2. Do not change the dressing until seen by the HCP.
    3. Stay out of extreme cold or heat situations.
    4. Avoid direct sunlight for 3 days.

22. The nurse is caring for a client preoperative for facial reconstruction. Which client problem should the nurse include in the preoperative plan of care?
    1. Loss of self-esteem.
    2. Alteration in comfort.
    3. Ineffective airway clearance.
    4. Impaired communication.

23. The nurse is caring for a client 1 day postoperative for facial reconstruction. Which intervention should the nurse implement?
    1. Provide all activities of daily living.
    2. Allow the client to voice fears and concerns.
    3. Monitor nutritional food and fluid intake.
    4. Assess clinical manifestations of infection.

24. The RN and a UAP are caring for a client diagnosed with a stage IV pressure injury. Which action by the UAP **warrants intervention** by the RN?
    1. The UAP turns the client every 2 hours.
    2. The UAP keeps the sheets wrinkle-free.
    3. The UAP encourages the client to drink high-protein drinks.
    4. The UAP places multiple diapers on the client.

25. The nurse is caring for a male client diagnosed with folliculitis barbae. Which information should the nurse teach to **prevent** a reoccurrence?
    1. Tell the client to not shave the face.
    2. Instruct the client to rub on astringent after-shave lotion.
    3. Recommend the client apply hot packs for 20 minutes before shaving.
    4. Teach the client to use an antibacterial soap on the face.

26. The ED nurse is caring for a client admitted with extensive, deep partial-thickness and full-thickness burns. Which interventions should the nurse implement? **Rank in order of priority.**
    1. Estimate the amount of burned area using the rule of nines.
    2. Insert two 18-gauge catheters and begin fluid replacement.
    3. Apply sterile saline dressings to the burned areas.
    4. Determine the client's airway status.
    5. Administer morphine sulfate, IV.

1. 1. Hirsutism is an excessive amount of hair growth in unexpected areas. This is not associated with itching or a rash.
   2. An ultraviolet examination light (Wood's light) or black light is used to examine certain infections. This would be used during the physical examination portion of the assessment.
   3. The nurse should determine the previous treatment the client used, but it is not the first intervention.
   4. **It is important to assess the rash as it appeared. If the client treated the rash with an ointment or cream, its appearance might have changed. Many times the appearance has changed from the first onset and from the treatment. Assessment is the first part of the nursing process.**

2. 1. **Most clients diagnosed with psoriasis have red, raised plaques with silvery-white scales.**
   2. A burning, prickling row of vesicles located along the torso is the description of herpes zoster.
   3. Raised, flesh-colored papules with a rough surface area is a description of warts.
   4. An overgrowth of tissue with an excessive amount of collagen is the definition of a keloid.

3. 1. Nystatin (Mycostatin), an antifungal powder, would not be useful to treat psoriasis.
   2. **Covering the affected area with an occlusive dressing enhances the steroid's effectiveness. This intervention should be limited to 12 hours to reduce systemic and local side effects.**
   3. Acyclovir is an antiviral medication and is used for viral diseases. It would not be used for psoriasis.
   4. Implanted radiation is a treatment for some forms of cancer but not for psoriasis. Radiation in the form of UV light therapy is sometimes used to treat psoriasis.

4. 1. The client needs to perform a complete inspection of the skin to identify clinical manifestations of generalized redness and tenderness. Treatments will be discontinued if they occur. The client understands the teaching.
   2. Psoralen, a photosensitizing agent, is administered 2 hours before the ultraviolet light therapy to enhance the effects. The client understands the teaching.
   3. The client will wear dark glasses to protect the eyes during the treatments and for the remainder of the day. Before the treatment, dark glasses are not needed. The client understands the teaching.
   4. **Coal tar comes in lotions, ointments, shampoos, and gels. They are used more in the hospital setting than in home settings because of the staining and mess associated with their use. The client needs more teaching.**

5. 1. Psoriasis can cause discomfort, itching, and pain, but it is not a psychosocial issue.
   2. **Altered body image is a problem the nurse should assess in clients diagnosed with psoriasis. Any chronic skin disease affecting appearance can cause psychosocial problems.**
   3. Anxiety is not usually a problem in a client diagnosed with psoriasis. The main concern is body image and discomfort.
   4. The condition of psoriasis does not affect family processes.

6. 1. Clients taking a steroid dose pack do not require laboratory testing for a therapeutic level.
   2. **The client should take the methylprednisolone (Solu-Medrol), a steroid, exactly as instructed. The number of pills should be taken in a descending (tapering) manner.**
   3. Steroids by mouth can cause gastrointestinal bleeding. They should be taken with food or after eating.
   4. Steroids should not be stopped suddenly; they need to be tapered off.

7. Correct answers are 2, 4, and 5.
   1. A cool environment makes itching decrease, not increase.
   2. **Soaps cause itching to increase. The client should avoid soap when experiencing pruritus.**
   3. Tepid, cool water is better for the client with itching.

4. Mild lotion can help the skin stay hydrated.
5. The client should dry off completely after bathing and blot gently rather than rub vigorously.

8. 1. Immunoglobulin A (IgA) protects against respiratory, gastrointestinal, and genitourinary infections.
2. IgD is a protein that is activated in collagen disease.
3. **IgE is a protein responsible for allergic reactions.**
4. IgG is the major antibody for viruses, bacteria, and toxins.

9. 1. **Contact dermatitis presents with erythema and small oozing vesicles.**
2. Pustules and nodule formation indicate acne.
3. Stasis dermatitis presents with varicosities and edema.
4. Clients diagnosed with rosacea present with telangiectasia and periodic flushing.

10. 1. Support stockings are used for stasis dermatitis, which is caused by impaired circulation.
2. **Topical corticosteroids are administered to treat contact dermatitis, which comes from an allergic response to irritants. The irritant should be eliminated and topical anti-inflammatory creams should be administered.**
3. Seborrheic dermatitis is treated by frequent cleaning with medicated shampoos and soaps to remove the yellow scales.
4. Pyrethrin (Rid) shampoo is used to treat lice. The client shampoos the hair and rinses after 10 minutes.

11. 1. Collecting a sample for culture does not diagnose poison oak or ivy. This is a reoccurrence of the allergic reaction to the poison oak.
2. These are the clinical manifestations of exposure to poison oak, not to medication.
3. **Many people dispose of the poison oak plant in ways that spread the sap. Burning or pulling the plant without gloves can cause another allergic reaction. Pets can spread the allergen on fur. Tools should be cleaned before touching the skin.**
4. Clients do not have temperature elevation unless there is a secondary infection present.

12. 1. There is no indication of the need for the client to be desensitized to the medication. The client should inform HCPs of any previous reactions to medications before taking any medication.
2. Tar solutions are used for psoriasis, not pruritus. The use of tar solutions would be a collaborative intervention rather than an independent intervention.
3. Cool sleeping environments decrease itching. Warmth increases itching and should be avoided.
4. **Soothing baths, such as colloidal baths or emollient baths, are helpful in treating pruritus. *Balneotherapy* is a term used to refer to therapeutic baths.**

13. 1. An area that has a greasy, rough feel and multiple papules does not require an immediate appointment with the HCP.
2. Seborrheic keratosis is a common occurrence in the elderly, but the skin lesion should be assessed by an HCP.
3. **The client should discuss any suspicious area with the HCP. This is not an emergency, but it should be assessed.**
4. An area wartlike in appearance, varying in color from flesh tones to black, and having a greasy, rough feel is probably a seborrheic keratosis. The home health nurse does not have the authority to diagnose as an HCP, and, therefore, the nurse should not encourage the client to self-treat.

14. Correct answers are 1, 2, and 3.
1. **The client diagnosed with Stevens-Johnson syndrome must be assessed for fluid volume deficit, the need for fluid replacement, and renal failure. Intake and output monitor both.**
2. **Breath sounds and respiratory status should be assessed because many clients develop respiratory failure and require mechanical ventilation.**
3. **The client diagnosed with Stevens-Johnson syndrome has a combination of vesicles, erosions, and crusts at the same time. The skin should be assessed every 8 hours.**
4. Hearing is not affected by Stevens-Johnson syndrome, but blindness can be a complication; vision should be assessed for any changes.
5. Neurological status is not compromised.

15. 1. Seborrheic dermatitis is a chronic skin disorder with remissions and exacerbations. To have an expected outcome of no further outbreaks would not be realistic.
  2. **To control the disorder by following the medical protocols would be realistic and appropriate.**
  3. The client needs to shampoo daily or a minimum of three times each week for treatment. This is an intervention, not an outcome.
  4. To apply bacitracin would treat a bacterial infection. This is an intervention, not a goal or expected outcome.

16. 1. Clients are treated on an outpatient basis by specialized clinics. In the United States, it is the health department's responsibility to care for these clients and ensure that the clients are taking their medications.
  2. Dapsone, a sulfone, will be used to treat leprosy for several years up to the remainder of the client's life.
  3. Moisturizing lotions will not treat the infectious process and therefore cannot control the symptoms.
  4. **Contrary to popular thought, leprosy, although contagious, usually requires prolonged exposure for the infection to spread to another person. Directly touching the lesions will increase the potential for infection.**

17. 1. The client does not usually have an elevated temperature.
  2. A side effect of the medication dapsone is a discoloration of the skin from pink to brownish-black.
  3. **The decrease in sensation of the lesions is the result of peripheral nerve damage. Leprosy is a peripheral nervous system disease.**
  4. A high mycobacterium count would be expected from the disease but would not be a complication.

18. 1. **The client diagnosed with leprosy (Hansen's disease) may feel ostracized because of the stigma of the disease. Historically, people have been isolated from society when diagnosed. Leprosy colonies were sites of treatment for those diagnosed. Today much of the public is unaware of the presence of the disease. Clients are treated on an outpatient basis by health departments.**
  2. Altered body image would occur in the late stages of leprosy and may not occur at all if treated in the early stages.

3. The client diagnosed with leprosy already has an infection, so it is not potential.
  4. Clients diagnosed with leprosy have a decreased sensation from peripheral nerve damage and have no discomfort.

19. 1. **Skincare must be meticulous. Minimal soap and tepid water should be used when showering or bathing. Lotions that do not irritate should be used to keep the skin hydrated.**
  2. The client needs to know the clinical manifestations indicating the need to notify the HCP, not the methods of treatment.
  3. There are adverse effects of the topical use of corticosteroids.
  4. Research supports a link between inhaled allergens and atopic dermatitis exacerbations (Celakovska and Bukac, 2017).

20. 1. **After the first 6 to 8 hours, the client will have extreme edema, causing the eyes to swell. This is expected.**
  2. The dermatologist will apply the chemical to begin the peeling procedure.
  3. The client will be awake during the procedure, but an analgesic and a tranquilizer can be administered for sedation. Only certified registered nurse anesthetists (CRNAs) administer general anesthesia.
  4. There is a sensation of burning during the application of the chemical and for several days after the procedure.

21. 1. Erythema can last from 1 week to a month.
  2. After 24 hours, the serum oozes from the dressing, and the client needs to apply a prescribed ointment to keep the area soft and flexible.
  3. **Extreme cold and heat and straining and lifting heavy objects should be avoided.**
  4. Direct sunlight should be avoided for 3 to 6 months. Clients should be taught to wear sunscreen.

22. 1. **A loss of self-esteem can occur after a change in facial appearance through injury, disease, or age-related changes.**
  2. Edema and pain would be appropriate postoperatively.
  3. The airway has not been compromised preoperatively.
  4. Communication may be a problem postoperatively but not before surgery.

**23.** 1. The client should be able to perform most activities of daily living. The nurse must encourage independence in the client.
2. On the first day postoperative, the nurse's priority would be physiological needs.
3. **Monitoring the client's nutritional intake and fluid balance is important for healing.**
4. Assessing for infection is the responsibility of the nurse but would occur later than 1 day postoperative. This is an elective procedure, which means the client would not have had an infection before surgery.

**24.** 1. The client should be turned every 2 hours, so this would not warrant intervention by the nurse.
2. Keeping the sheets wrinkle-free helps with preventing skin breakdown. This would not warrant intervention by the nurse.
3. Protein is needed for wound healing, so this intervention is appropriate for the UAP.
4. **Placing extra diapers saves the UAP from changing the linens, but it keeps wet plastic against the skin, leading to further skin breakdown. This action would warrant intervention by the RN.**

**25.** 1. **Shaving is the cause of this condition, and refraining from shaving and lotions is the only cure. Special brushes are used. If the client must shave, he should use a depilatory cream or electric razor.**
2. Aftershave will not prevent folliculitis.
3. Hot packs will not prevent folliculitis.
4. Antibacterial soap is too strong for use on the face. Shaving is the cause of folliculitis.

**26.** Correct order is 4, 2, 3, 1, 5.
4. **The airway is always the first priority for any process in which the airway might be compromised.**
2. **The nurse should start fluid resuscitation as soon as possible before the client's blood pressure makes it more difficult to establish an IV route.**
3. **Covering the open burns will prevent further intrusion of bacteria.**
1. **Estimating the extent of the burned area should be done but does not have priority over the airway, fluid replacement, and the prevention of infection.**
5. **Pain is a priority but not over determining the airway and fluid status and prevention of infection.**

# Immune System Disorders

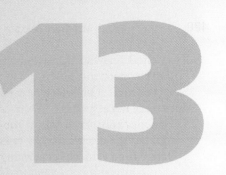

*The secret of joy in work is contained in one word—*
*excellence. To know how to do something well is to enjoy it.*

—Pearl S. Buck

The immune system, which involves many tissues throughout the body, is subject to several inflammatory disorders. Some involve genetic predisposition, some result from infectious processes, and many are of uncertain etiology. This chapter includes questions on the most common immune disorders—multiple sclerosis, Guillain-Barré syndrome, rheumatoid arthritis, AIDS, systemic lupus erythematosus, and allergies—and on other disorders affecting the body's immune system.

## KEYWORDS

| | |
|---|---|
| Alopecia | Hirsutism |
| Arthralgia | Ocular |
| Astringent | Plasmapheresis |
| Cogwheel rigidity | Polymyositis |
| Cutaneous | Pruritus |
| Demyelination | Raynaud's phenomenon |
| Diplopia | Rhinitis |
| Dysarthria | Scleroderma |
| Dysmetria | Scotomas |
| Eradicated | Spasticity |
| Erythema | Wheal |
| Exacerbation | |

## PRACTICE QUESTIONS

### Multiple Sclerosis (MS)

1. The nurse is assessing a 48-year-old client diagnosed with multiple sclerosis (MS). Which clinical manifestation **warrants immediate** intervention?
   1. The client has scanning speech and diplopia.
   2. The client has dysarthria and scotomas.
   3. The client has muscle weakness and spasticity.
   4. The client has a congested cough and dysphagia.

2. The client newly diagnosed with MS states, "I don't understand how I got multiple sclerosis. Is it genetic?" On which statement should the nurse base the response?
   1. Genetics may play a role in susceptibility to MS, but the disease may be caused by a virus.
   2. There is no evidence suggesting there is any chromosomal involvement in developing MS.
   3. MS is caused by a recessive gene, so both parents had to have the gene for the client to get MS.
   4. MS is caused by an autosomal dominant gene on the Y chromosome, so only fathers can pass it on.

3. The 30-year-old female client is admitted with reports of numbness, tingling, a crawling sensation affecting the extremities, and double vision, which has occurred two times in the month. Which question is **most important** for the nurse to ask the client?
   1. "Have you experienced any difficulty with your menstrual cycle?"
   2. "Have you noticed a rash across the bridge of your nose?"
   3. "Do you get tired easily and sometimes have problems swallowing?"
   4. "Are you taking birth control pills to prevent conception?"

4. The nurse enters the room of a client diagnosed with acute exacerbation of MS and finds the client crying. Which statement is the **most therapeutic** response for the nurse to make?
   1. "Why are you crying? The medication will help the disease."
   2. "You seem upset. I will sit down, and we can talk for a while."
   3. "Multiple sclerosis is a disease that has good times and bad times."
   4. "I will have the chaplain come and stay with you for a while."

5. The client diagnosed with MS is scheduled for a magnetic resonance imaging (MRI) scan of the head. Which information should the nurse teach the client about the test?
   1. The client will have wires attached to the scalp, and lights will flash off and on.
   2. The machine will be loud, and the client must not move the head during the test.
   3. The client will drink a contrast medium 30 minutes to 1 hour before the test.
   4. The test will be repeated at intervals during a 5- to 6-hour period.

6. The 45-year-old client is diagnosed with primary progressive MS, and the nurse writes the nursing diagnosis "anticipatory grieving related to progressive loss." Which intervention should be implemented **first**?
   1. Consult the physical therapist for assistive devices for mobility.
   2. Determine if the client has a legal power of attorney.
   3. Ask if the client would like to talk to the hospital chaplain.
   4. Discuss the client's wishes regarding end-of-life care.

7. The home health nurse is caring for the client newly diagnosed with MS. Which client issue is of **most importance**?
   1. The client refuses to have a gastrostomy feeding.
   2. The client wants to discuss if she should tell her fiancé.
   3. The client tells the nurse life is not worth living anymore.
   4. The client needs the flu and pneumonia vaccines.

8. The registered nurse (RN) and a licensed practical nurse (LPN) are caring for a group of clients. Which nursing tasks should be assigned to the LPN? **Select all that apply.**
   1. Administer a skeletal muscle relaxant to a client diagnosed with low back pain.
   2. Discuss bowel regimen medications with the HCP for the client on strict bedrest.
   3. Draw morning blood work on the client diagnosed with bacterial meningitis.
   4. Teach self-catheterization to the client diagnosed with multiple sclerosis.
   5. Collect a sputum sample from the client diagnosed with tuberculosis.

9. The male client diagnosed with MS states he has been investigating alternative therapies to treat his disease. Which intervention is **most appropriate** by the nurse?
   1. Encourage the therapy if it is not contraindicated by the medical regimen.
   2. Tell the client that only the health-care provider should discuss this with him.
   3. Ask how his significant other feels about this deviation from the medical regimen.
   4. Suggest the client research an investigational therapy instead.

10. The client diagnosed with an acute exacerbation of MS is placed on high-dose intravenous injections of corticosteroid medication. Which nursing intervention should be implemented?
    1. Discuss discontinuing the proton pump inhibitor with the HCP.
    2. Hold the medication until after all cultures have been obtained.
    3. Monitor the client's serum blood glucose levels frequently.
    4. Provide supplemental dietary sodium with the client's meals.

11. The nurse writes the client problem of "altered sexual functioning" for a male client diagnosed with MS. Which intervention should be implemented?
    1. Encourage the couple to explore alternative ways of maintaining intimacy.
    2. Make an appointment with a psychotherapist to counsel the couple.
    3. Explain daily exercise will help increase libido and sexual arousal.
    4. Discuss the importance of keeping physically calm during sexual intercourse.

12. The nurse is admitting a client diagnosed with MS. Which clinical manifestation should the nurse assess? **Select all that apply.**
    1. Muscle flaccidity.
    2. Epistaxis.
    3. Dysmetria.
    4. Fatigue.
    5. Dysphagia.

## Guillain-Barré Syndrome

13. Which clinical manifestations should the nurse assess in the client diagnosed with Guillain-Barré syndrome?
    1. An exaggerated startle reflex and memory changes.
    2. Cogwheel rigidity and inability to initiate voluntary movement.
    3. Sudden severe unilateral facial pain and inability to chew.
    4. Progressive ascending paralysis of the lower extremities and numbness.

14. Which statement by the client supports the diagnosis of Guillain-Barré syndrome?
    1. "I just returned from a short trip to Japan."
    2. "I had a really bad cold just a few weeks ago."
    3. "I think one of the people I work with had this."
    4. "I have been taking some herbs for more than a year."

15. Which assessment intervention should the nurse implement specifically for the diagnosis of Guillain-Barré syndrome?
    1. Assess deep tendon reflexes.
    2. Complete a Glasgow Coma Scale.
    3. Check for Babinski's reflex.
    4. Take the client's vital signs.

16. The health-care provider (HCP) scheduled a lumbar puncture for a client admitted with rule-out Guillain-Barré syndrome. Which preprocedure intervention has **priority**?
    1. Keep the client NPO.
    2. Instruct the client to void.
    3. Place in the lithotomy position.
    4. Assess the client's pedal pulse.

17. Which **priority** client problem should be included in the care plan for the client diagnosed with Guillain-Barré syndrome?
    1. High risk for injury.
    2. Fear and anxiety.
    3. Altered nutrition.
    4. Ineffective breathing pattern.

18. The nurse caring for the client diagnosed with Guillain-Barré syndrome writes the client problem "impaired physical mobility." Which long-term goal should be written for this problem?
    1. The client will have no skin irritation.
    2. The client will have no muscle atrophy.
    3. The client will perform range-of-motion exercises.
    4. The client will turn every 2 hours while awake.

19. The client diagnosed with Guillain-Barré syndrome is on a ventilator. Which intervention will assist the client in communicating with the nursing staff?
    1. Provide an erase slate board for the client to write on.
    2. Instruct the client to blink once for "no" and twice for "yes."
    3. Refer to a speech therapist to help with communication.
    4. Leave the call light within easy reach of the client.

20. The client diagnosed with Guillain-Barré syndrome asks the nurse, "Will I ever get back to normal? I am so tired of being sick." Which statement is the **best response** by the nurse?
    1. "You should make a full recovery within a few months to a year."
    2. "Most clients diagnosed with this syndrome have some type of residual disability."
    3. "This is something you should discuss with the health-care team."
    4. "The rehabilitation is short, and you should be fully recovered within a month."

21. The client admitted with rule-out Guillain-Barré syndrome has just had a lumbar puncture. Which intervention should the nurse implement postprocedure?
    1. Monitor the client for hypotension.
    2. Apply pressure to the puncture site.
    3. Test the client's cerebrospinal fluid.
    4. Increase the client's fluid intake.

22. The client diagnosed with Guillain-Barré syndrome is having difficulty breathing and is placed on a ventilator. Which situation **warrants immediate** intervention by the nurse?
    1. The ventilator rate is set at 14 breaths per minute.
    2. A manual resuscitation bag is at the client's bedside.
    3. The client's pulse oximeter reading is 85%.
    4. The ABG results are pH 7.4, $Po_2$ 88, $Pco_2$ 35, and $Hco_3$ 24.

23. The client diagnosed with Guillain-Barré syndrome is on a ventilator. When the wife comes to visit, she starts crying uncontrollably, and the client starts fighting the ventilator because his wife is upset. Which action should the nurse implement?
    1. Tell the wife she must stop crying.
    2. Escort the wife out of the room.
    3. Medicate the client immediately.
    4. Acknowledge the wife's fears.

24. The client diagnosed with Guillain-Barré syndrome is admitted to the rehabilitation unit after 23 days in the acute care hospital. Which interventions should the nurse implement? **Select all that apply.**
    1. Refer the client to the physical therapist.
    2. Include the speech therapist in the team.
    3. Request a social worker consult.
    4. Implement a regimen to address pain control.
    5. Refer the client to the Guillain-Barré Syndrome Foundation.

## Myasthenia Gravis

25. Which ocular or facial clinical manifestations should the nurse expect to assess for the client diagnosed with myasthenia gravis?
    1. Weakness and fatigue.
    2. Ptosis and diplopia.
    3. Breathlessness and dyspnea.
    4. Weight loss and dehydration.

26. The client is being evaluated to rule out myasthenia gravis and being administered the edrophonium chloride test. Which response to the test indicates the client has myasthenia gravis?
    1. The client has no apparent change in the assessment data.
    2. There is increased amplitude of electrical stimulation in the muscle.
    3. The circulating acetylcholine receptor antibodies are decreased.
    4. The client shows a marked improvement of muscle strength.

27. Which surgical procedure should the nurse anticipate the client diagnosed with myasthenia gravis undergoing to help prevent the clinical manifestations of the disease process?
    1. There is no surgical option.
    2. Transsphenoidal hypophysectomy.
    3. Thymectomy.
    4. Adrenalectomy.

28. The client diagnosed with myasthenia gravis is being discharged home. Which intervention has **priority** when teaching the client's significant others?
    1. Discuss ways to help prevent choking episodes.
    2. Explain how to care for a client on a ventilator.
    3. Teach how to perform passive range-of-motion exercises.
    4. Demonstrate how to care for the client's feeding tube.

29. Which collaborative health-care team member should the nurse refer the client to in the late stages of myasthenia gravis?
    1. Occupational therapist.
    2. Recreational therapist.
    3. Vocational therapist.
    4. Speech therapist.

30. The client diagnosed with myasthenia gravis is undergoing plasmapheresis at the bedside. Which assessment data **warrant immediate** intervention?
    1. The client's BP is 94/60 and AP is 112.
    2. Negative Chvostek's and Trousseau's signs.
    3. The serum potassium level is 3.5 mEq/L.
    4. Ecchymosis at the vascular site access.

31. Which statement by the female client diagnosed with myasthenia gravis indicates the client **needs more** discharge teaching?
    1. "I will not have any menstrual cycles because of this disease."
    2. "I should avoid people with respiratory infections."
    3. "I should not take a hot bath or swim in cold water."
    4. "I will drink at least 2,500 mL of water a day."

32. The client diagnosed with myasthenia gravis is admitted to the emergency department with a sudden exacerbation of motor weakness. Which assessment data indicate the client is experiencing a cholinergic crisis?
    1. The serum assay of circulating acetylcholine receptor antibodies is increased.
    2. The client's clinical manifestations improve when administering a cholinesterase inhibitor.
    3. The client's blood pressure, pulse, and respirations improve after IV fluid.
    4. The edrophonium chloride test does not show improvement in the client's muscle strength.

33. The client diagnosed with myasthenia gravis is admitted with an acute exacerbation. Which interventions should the nurse implement? **Select all that apply.**
    1. Assist the client to turn and cough every 2 hours.
    2. Place the client in a high or semi-Fowler's position.
    3. Assess the client's pulse oximeter reading every shift.
    4. Plan meals to promote medication effectiveness.
    5. Monitor the client's serum anticholinesterase levels.

34. The wife of a client diagnosed with myasthenia gravis is crying and shares with the nurse she just doesn't know what to do. Which response is the **best action** by the nurse?
    1. Discuss the Myasthenia Foundation with the client's wife.
    2. Refer the client to a local myasthenia gravis support group.
    3. Ask the client's wife if she would like to talk to a counselor.
    4. Sit down and allow the wife to verbalize her feelings to the nurse.

35. The client diagnosed with myasthenia gravis is prescribed neostigmine. Which data indicate the medication is **effective**?
    1. The client is able to feed self independently.
    2. The client is able to blink the eyes without tearing.
    3. The client denies any nausea or vomiting when eating.
    4. The client denies any pain when performing ROM exercises.

36. The client is diagnosed with myasthenia gravis. Which intervention should the nurse implement when administering pyridostigmine?
    1. Administer the medication 30 minutes before meals.
    2. Instruct the client to take with 8 ounces of water.
    3. Explain the importance of sitting up for 1 hour after taking medication.
    4. Assess the client's blood pressure before administering medication.

## Systemic Lupus Erythematosus (SLE)

37. The 26-year-old female client is reporting a low-grade fever, arthralgias, fatigue, and a facial rash. Which laboratory tests should the nurse expect the HCP to order if SLE is suspected?
    1. Comprehensive metabolic panel and liver function tests.
    2. Complete blood count and antinuclear antibody tests.
    3. Cholesterol and lipid profile tests.
    4. Blood urea nitrogen and glomerular filtration tests.

38. The client diagnosed with SLE is being discharged from the medical unit. Which discharge instructions are **most important** for the nurse to include? **Select all that apply.**
    1. Use a sunscreen of SPF 30 or greater when in the sunlight.
    2. Notify the HCP immediately when developing a low-grade fever.
    3. Some dyspnea is expected and does not need immediate attention.
    4. The hands and feet may change color if exposed to cold or heat.
    5. Explain that the client can be cured with continued therapy.

39. The nurse is developing a care plan for a client diagnosed with SLE. Which goal is a **priority** for this client?
    1. The client will maintain reproductive ability.
    2. The client will verbalize feelings of body-image changes.
    3. The client will have no deterioration of organ function.
    4. The client's skin will remain intact and have no irritation.

40. The nurse is admitting a client diagnosed with possible SLE. Which assessment data observed by the nurse support the diagnosis of SLE?
    1. Pericardial friction rub and crackles in the lungs.
    2. Muscle spasticity and bradykinesia.
    3. Hirsutism and clubbing of the fingers.
    4. Somnolence and weight gain.

41. The client diagnosed with an acute exacerbation of SLE is prescribed high-dose steroids. Which statement **best** explains the scientific rationale for using high-dose steroids in treating SLE?
    1. The steroids will increase the body's ability to fight the infection.
    2. The steroids will decrease the chance of the SLE spreading to other organs.
    3. The steroids will suppress tissue inflammation, which reduces damage to organs.
    4. The steroids will prevent scarring of skin tissues associated with SLE.

42. The nurse enters the room of a female client diagnosed with SLE and finds the client crying. Which statement is the **most** therapeutic response?
    1. "I know you are upset, but stress makes the SLE worse."
    2. "Please explain to me why you are crying."
    3. "I recommend going to an SLE support group."
    4. "I see you are crying. We can talk if you would like."

43. The nurse is assessing a client diagnosed with cutaneous lupus erythematosus. Which intervention should be implemented?
    1. Use astringent lotion on the face and skin.
    2. Inspect the skin weekly for open areas or rashes.
    3. Dry the skin thoroughly by patting.
    4. Apply anti-itch medication between the toes.

44. The nurse is caring for clients on a medical floor. Which client should be assessed **first**?
    1. The client diagnosed with SLE reporting chest pain.
    2. The client diagnosed with MS reporting pain at a "10."
    3. The client diagnosed with myasthenia gravis having dysphagia.
    4. The client diagnosed with GB syndrome barely able to move his toes.

45. The nurse and a female unlicensed assistive personnel (UAP) are caring for a group of clients on a medical floor. Which action by the UAP **warrants immediate** intervention by the RN?
    1. The UAP washes her hands before and after performing vital signs on a client.
    2. The UAP dons sterile gloves before removing an indwelling catheter from a client.
    3. The UAP raises the head of the bed to a high Fowler's position for a client about to eat.
    4. The UAP uses a fresh plastic bag to get ice for a client's water pitcher.

46. The client recently diagnosed with SLE asks the nurse, "What is SLE and how did I get it?" Which statement **best** explains the scientific rationale for the nurse's response?
    1. SLE occurs because the kidneys do not filter antibodies from the blood.
    2. SLE occurs after a viral illness as a result of damage to the endocrine system.
    3. There is no known identifiable reason for a client to develop SLE.
    4. This is an autoimmune disease that may have a genetic or hormonal component.

47. The client diagnosed with an acute exacerbation of SLE is being discharged with a prescription for an oral steroid, which will be discontinued gradually. Which statement is the scientific rationale for this type of medication dosing?
    1. Tapering the medication prevents the client from having withdrawal symptoms.
    2. The thyroid gland starts working again, because this medication stops it from working.
    3. Tapering the dose allows the adrenal glands to begin to produce cortisol again.
    4. This is the health-care provider's personal choice in prescribing the medication.

48. The nurse is discussing autoimmune diseases with a class of nursing students. Which clinical manifestations are shared by rheumatoid arthritis (RA) and SLE?
    1. Nodules in the subcutaneous layer and bone deformity.
    2. Renal involvement and pleural effusions.
    3. Joint stiffness and pain.
    4. Raynaud's phenomenon and skin rash.

## Acquired Immunodeficiency Syndrome (AIDS)

49. The school nurse is preparing to teach a health class to ninth graders regarding sexually transmitted infections. Which information regarding AIDS should be included?
    1. Females taking birth control pills are protected from becoming infected with HIV.
    2. Protected sex is no longer an issue because there is an approved vaccine for the HIV virus.
    3. Adolescents with a normal immune system are not at risk for developing AIDS.
    4. Abstinence is the only guarantee of not becoming infected with sexually transmitted HIV.

50. The nurse is admitting a client diagnosed with protein-calorie malnutrition secondary to AIDS. Which intervention(s) should the nurse implement **first**?
    1. Assess the client's body weight and ask what the client has been able to eat.

2. Place in contact isolation and don a mask and gown before entering the room.
3. Check the HCP's orders and determine what laboratory tests will be done.
4. Teach the client about total parenteral nutrition and monitor the subclavian IV site.

51. The client diagnosed with AIDS is reporting a sore mouth and tongue. When the nurse assesses the buccal mucosa, the nurse notes white, patchy lesions covering the hard and soft palates and the right inner cheek. Which interventions should the nurse implement?
    1. Teach the client to brush the teeth and patchy area with a soft-bristle toothbrush.
    2. Notify the HCP for an order of antifungal swish-and-swallow medication.
    3. Have the client gargle with an antiseptic-based mouthwash several times a day.
    4. Determine what types of food the client has been eating for the last 24 hours.

52. Which type of isolation technique is designed to decrease the risk of transmission of recognized and unrecognized sources of infections?
    1. Contact precautions.
    2. Airborne precautions.
    3. Droplet precautions.
    4. Standard precautions.

53. The nurse is describing HIV infection to a client diagnosed with HIV. Which information regarding the virus is important to teach?
    1. HIV is a retrovirus, which means it never dies as long as it has a host to live in.
    2. HIV can be eradicated from the host body with the correct medical regimen.
    3. It is difficult for HIV to replicate in humans because it is a monkey virus.
    4. HIV uses the client's own red blood cells to reproduce the virus in the body.

54. The client engaging in needle-sharing activities has developed a flu-like infection. An HIV antibody test is negative. Which statement **best** describes the scientific rationale for this finding?
    1. The client is fortunate not to have contracted HIV from an infected needle.
    2. The client must be repeatedly exposed to HIV before becoming infected.
    3. The client may be in the primary infection phase of an HIV infection.
    4. The antibody test is negative because the client has a different flu virus.

55. The nurse caring for a client diagnosed with HIV is stuck with the stylet used to start an IV. Which intervention should the nurse implement **first**?
    1. Flush the skin with water and try to get the area to bleed.

2. Notify the charge nurse and complete an incident report.
3. Report to the employee health nurse for prophylactic medication.
4. Follow up with the infection control nurse to have laboratory work done.

56. The client on a medical floor is diagnosed with HIV encephalopathy. Which client problem is the **priority**?
    1. Altered nutrition, less than body requirements.
    2. Anticipatory grieving.
    3. Knowledge deficit, procedures, and prognosis.
    4. Risk for injury.

57. The client diagnosed with *Pneumocystis* jiroveci (carinii) pneumonia (PJP) is being admitted to the intensive care unit. Which HCP's order should the nurse implement **first**?
    1. Draw a serum for CD4+ and complete blood count STAT.
    2. Administer oxygen to the client via nasal cannula.
    3. Administer trimethoprim-sulfamethoxazole IVPB.
    4. Obtain a sputum specimen for culture and sensitivity.

58. Which intervention is an important psychosocial consideration for the client diagnosed with AIDS?
    1. Perform a thorough head-to-toe assessment.
    2. Maintain the client's ideal body weight.
    3. Complete an advance directive.
    4. Increase the client's activity tolerance.

59. The nurse on a medical floor is caring for clients diagnosed with AIDS. Which client should be seen **first**?
    1. The client with flushed, warm skin with tented turgor.
    2. The client reporting the staff ignores the call light.
    3. The client with vital signs of T 99.9°F, P 101, R 26, and BP 110/68.
    4. The client unable to provide a sputum specimen.

60. The client diagnosed with AIDS is angry and yells at everyone entering the room, and none of the staff members want to care for the client. Which intervention is **most appropriate** for the nurse manager to use in resolving this situation?
    1. Assign a different nurse every shift to the client.
    2. Ask the HCP to tell the client not to yell at the staff.
    3. Call a team meeting and discuss options with the staff.

4. Tell one staff member to care for the client a week at a time.

## Allergies and Allergic Reactions

61. The charge nurse observes the primary nurse interacting with a client. Which action by the primary nurse **warrants immediate** intervention by the RN charge nurse?
    1. The nurse explains the IVP diuretic will make the client urinate.
    2. The nurse dons nonsterile gloves to remove the client's dressing.
    3. The nurse administers a medication without checking for allergies.
    4. The nurse asks the UAP for help moving a client up in bed.

62. The nurse in the emergency department is allergic to latex. Which intervention should the nurse implement regarding the use of nonsterile gloves?
    1. Use only sterile, nonlatex gloves for any procedure requiring gloves.
    2. Do not use gloves when starting an IV or performing a procedure.
    3. Keep a pair of nonsterile, nonlatex gloves in the pocket of the uniform.
    4. Wear white cotton gloves at all times to protect the hands.

63. The client diagnosed with a bee sting allergy is being discharged from the emergency department. Which **priority** discharge instruction should be taught to the client?
    1. Demonstrate how to use an epinephrine auto injector.
    2. Teach the client to never go outdoors in the spring and summer.
    3. Have the client buy diphenhydramine over the counter to use when stung.
    4. Discuss wearing a medical alert bracelet when going outside.

64. The client comes to the emergency department reporting dyspnea and wheezing after eating at a seafood restaurant. The client cannot speak and has a bluish color around the mouth. Which intervention should the nurse implement **first**?
    1. Initiate an IV with normal saline.
    2. Prepare to intubate the client.
    3. Administer oxygen at 100%.
    4. Ask the client about an iodine allergy.

65. The client in the HCP's office is reporting allergic rhinitis. Which assessment question is important for the nurse to ask the client?
    1. "What time of year do the symptoms occur?"

2. "Which over-the-counter medications have you tried?"
3. "Do other members of your family have allergies to animals?"
4. "Why do you think you have allergies?"

66. The client asks the nurse, "Which time of the year is allergic rhinitis least likely to occur?" Which statement is the nurse's **best response**?
    1. "It is least likely to occur during the springtime."
    2. "Allergic rhinitis is not likely to occur during the summer."
    3. "It is least likely to occur in the early fall."
    4. "Allergic rhinitis is least likely to occur in early winter."

67. The client is highly allergic to insect venom and is prescribed venom immunotherapy. Which statement is the scientific rationale for this treatment?
    1. Immunotherapy is effective in preventing anaphylaxis following a future sting.
    2. Immunotherapy will prevent all future insect stings from harming the client.
    3. This therapy will cure the client from having any allergic reactions in the future.
    4. This therapy is experimental and should not be undertaken by the client.

68. The client in the HCP's office has a red, raised rash covering the forearms, neck, and face and is experiencing extreme itching, which is diagnosed as an allergic reaction to poison ivy. Which discharge instructions should the nurse teach? **Select all that apply.**
    1. Tell the client never to scratch the rash.
    2. Instruct the client in administering IM diphenhydramine.
    3. Explain how to take a steroid dose pack.
    4. Have the client soak in an oatmeal bath.
    5. Apply cool compresses to itchy skin.

69. The nurse is developing a care plan for a client diagnosed with allergic rhinitis. Which independent problem has **priority**?
    1. Ineffective breathing pattern.
    2. Knowledge deficit.
    3. Anaphylaxis.
    4. Ineffective coping.

70. The nurse on a medical unit has received the morning shift report. Which client should the nurse assess **first**?
    1. The client with a 0730 sliding-scale insulin order.
    2. The client having received an initial dose of IV antibiotic at 0645.
    3. The client having back pain at a "4" on a 1-to-10 scale.

4. The client with dysphagia and needing to be fed.

71. The nurse in the holding area of the operating room is assessing the client before surgery. Which information **warrants immediate** intervention by the nurse?
    1. The client is able to mark the correct site for the surgery.
    2. The client can only tell the nurse about the surgery in lay terms.
    3. The client is allergic to iodine and does not have an allergy bracelet.
    4. The client has signed a consent form for surgery and anesthesia.

72. The client in the emergency department begins to experience a severe anaphylactic reaction after an initial dose of IV penicillin. Which interventions should the nurse implement? **Select all that apply.**
    1. Prepare to administer methylprednisolone IV.
    2. Request and obtain a STAT chest x-ray.
    3. Initiate the rapid response team.
    4. Administer epinephrine IM STAT.
    5. Assess for the client's pulse and respirations.

## Rheumatoid Arthritis (RA)

73. The client diagnosed with RA is being seen in the outpatient clinic. Which **preventive** care should the nurse include in the regularly scheduled clinic visits?
    1. Perform joint x-rays to determine the progression of the disease.
    2. Send blood to the laboratory for an erythrocyte sedimentation rate.
    3. Recommend the flu and pneumonia vaccines.
    4. Assess the client for increasing joint involvement.

74. The client diagnosed with RA has nontender, movable nodules in the subcutaneous tissue over the elbows and shoulders. Which statement is the scientific rationale for the nodules?
    1. The nodules indicate a rapidly progressive destruction of the affected tissue.
    2. The nodules are small amounts of synovial fluid that have become crystallized.
    3. The nodules are lymph nodes that have proliferated to try to fight the disease.
    4. The nodules present a favorable prognosis and mean the client is better.

75. The nurse is assessing a client diagnosed with RA. Which assessment findings **warrant immediate** intervention?
    1. The client reports joint stiffness and the knees feel warm to the touch.
    2. The client has experienced 1-kg weight loss and is very tired.
    3. The client requires a heating pad applied to the hips and back to sleep.
    4. The client is crying, has a flat facial affect, and refuses to speak to the nurse.

76. The client diagnosed with RA then prescribed etanercept shows marked improvement. Which instructions regarding the use of this medication should the nurse teach? **Select all that apply.**
    1. Explain the medication loses its efficacy after a few months.
    2. Continue to have checkups and laboratory work while taking the medication.
    3. Have yearly magnetic resonance imaging to follow the progress.
    4. Discuss the drug is taken for 3 weeks and then stopped for a week.
    5. May take analgesics, NSAIDs, and corticosteroids during medication therapy.

77. The client diagnosed with RA has developed swan-neck fingers. Which referral is **most appropriate** for the client?
    1. Physical therapy.
    2. Occupational therapy.
    3. Psychiatric counselor.
    4. Home health nurse.

78. The nurse is planning the care for a client diagnosed with RA. Which interventions should be implemented? **Select all that apply.**
    1. Plan a strenuous exercise program.
    2. Order a mechanical soft diet.
    3. Maintain a keep-open IV.
    4. Obtain an order for a sedative.
    5. Keep current with immunizations.

79. The 20-year-old female client diagnosed with advanced unremitting RA is being admitted to receive a regimen of immunosuppressive medications. Which question should the nurse ask during the admission process regarding the medications?
    1. "Are you sexually active, and, if so, are you using birth control?"
    2. "Have you discussed taking these drugs with your parents?"
    3. "Which arm do you prefer to have an IV in for 4 days?"
    4. "Have you signed an informed consent for investigational drugs?"

80. Which client problem is a **priority** for a client diagnosed with RA?
    1. Activity intolerance.
    2. Fluid and electrolyte imbalance.
    3. Alteration in comfort.
    4. Excessive nutritional intake.

81. The nurse is caring for clients on the medical floor. Which client should the nurse assess **first**?
    1. The client diagnosed with RA reporting pain at a "3" on a 1-to-10 scale.
    2. The client diagnosed with SLE and has a rash across the bridge of the nose.
    3. The client diagnosed with advanced RA receiving antineoplastic drugs IV.
    4. The client diagnosed with scleroderma and has hard, waxlike skin near the eyes.

82. The RN and an LPN are caring for clients in a rheumatologist's office. Which task can the nurse assign to the LPN?
    1. Administer methotrexate IV.
    2. Assess the lung sounds of a client diagnosed with RA now coughing.
    3. Demonstrate how to use clothing equipped with hook and loop fasteners.
    4. Discuss methods of birth control compatible with treatment medications.

83. The client diagnosed with early-stage RA is being discharged from the outpatient clinic. Which discharge instruction should the nurse teach regarding the use of NSAIDs?
    1. Take with an over-the-counter medication for the stomach.
    2. Drink a full glass of water with each pill.
    3. If a dose is missed, double the medication at the next dosing time.
    4. Avoid taking the NSAID on an empty stomach.

84. The nurse is preparing to administer morning medications. Which medication should the nurse administer **first**?
    1. The pain medication to a client diagnosed with RA.
    2. The diuretic medication to a client diagnosed with SLE.
    3. The steroid to a client diagnosed with polymyositis.
    4. The appetite stimulant to a client diagnosed with OA.

# CONCEPTS

The concepts covered in this chapter focus on immunity. Exemplars that are covered are systemic inflammatory response syndrome (SIRS), multiple organ dysfunction syndrome (MODS), and AIDS. Interrelated concepts of the nursing process and clinical judgment are covered throughout the questions. The concept of clinical judgment is presented in prioritizing or "first" questions.

85. The nurse is caring for a client diagnosed with systemic inflammatory response syndrome (SIRS) following major abdominal surgery. Which clinical manifestations would the nurse observe that indicate SIRS? **Select all that apply.**
    1. Bleeding times increased and platelet counts decreased.
    2. Increased urine osmolality and decreased urine output.
    3. Four-plus pitting edema of the lower extremities.
    4. Confusion, disorientation, delirium.
    5. Heart rate 78, blood pressure 124/84, and RR of 20.

86. The client diagnosed with multi-organ dysfunction syndrome is admitted to the intensive care department. Which assessment data are **most important** for the nurse to collect and monitor?

    1. Lung sounds, heart sounds, and blood pressure.
    2. The client's psychological response to the illness.
    3. The client's family's expectations of the hospitalization.
    4. Amount of emesis, bile secretions, and mouth ulcers.

87. The nurse is caring for a client diagnosed with systemic inflammatory response syndrome after extensive abdominal surgery. Which nursing interventions could prevent the development of multi-organ dysfunction syndrome?
    1. Place the client on strict intake and output.
    2. Administer pain medication via patient-controlled analgesia.
    3. Keep the head of the bed elevated at all times.
    4. Practice therapeutic communication.

88. The nurse is explaining systemic inflammatory response syndrome (SIRS) to the client's significant other. Which statement **best** describes SIRS?
    1. SIRS is a response of the body when it has sustained a major burn or crushing injury in a motor-vehicle accident.
    2. SIRS is a response by the body to some type of injury or insult; the insult can be infectious or noninfectious in nature.
    3. SIRS only occurs when the body is overwhelmed with an infectious organism such as streptococcus bacteria.
    4. SIRS occurs when the body is allergic to the prescribed antibiotic and the body tries to recover from the allergic response.

89. The client is known to be HIV positive. Which data indicate to the nurse that the client has now progressed to the diagnosis of AIDS?
    1. The client's CD4+ count is 189.
    2. The client has an Hgb of 9.4 and Hct of 29.1.
    3. The client's chest x-ray shows infiltrate.
    4. The client reports a headache unrelieved by acetaminophen.

90. The concept of impaired immunity has been identified by the nurse as it applies to the client diagnosed with AIDS. Which interventions should the RN implement?
    1. Keep fresh flowers and raw vegetables out of the client's room.
    2. Have the UAP assist with ADLs.
    3. Encourage the client to perform active range of motion.
    4. Teach the client about cardiovascular medications.

91. The female client is homeless and pregnant. The client supports an IV drug habit by prostitution. Which data would be considered antecedents (risk factors) for becoming HIV positive? **Select all that apply.**
    1. The client is pregnant.
    2. The client is an intravenous drug abuser.
    3. The client has multiple sexual partners.
    4. The client does not have available health care.
    5. The client does not have adequate bathroom facilities.
    6. The client spends her money on nonessential items.

92. The client is diagnosed with multi-organ dysfunction syndrome. Which is the **most appropriate** goal for the nurse to write when planning the client's care?
    1. The client will maintain vital signs within normal limits during the next 24 hours.
    2. The client's urine output will be maintained to achieve an output of 600 mL in the next 24 hours.
    3. The client will have elevated ALT, AST, and GGT liver enzymes within the next 24 hours.
    4. The client's blood glucose reading will be 200 to 240 mg/dL for the next 24 hours.

93. The client diagnosed with multi-organ dysfunction syndrome (MODS) has renal, cardiovascular, and pulmonary dysfunction issues. Which statement by the nurse indicates an understanding of the client's prognosis?
    1. "As long as the client is maintained on a ventilator, then the prognosis can be up to 60% recovery."
    2. "The client will have less than a 2% potential for recovery from the MODS."
    3. "When three or more body systems fail, the mortality rate can be 80% to 90%."
    4. "More than one body system in failure reduces the recovery rate to 70% to 80%."

94. The client diagnosed with systemic inflammatory response syndrome (SIRS) asks the nurse what the diagnosis means. Which is the nurse's **best** response?
    1. SIRS is a localized response to major trauma that has occurred within the last 3 months.
    2. SIRS is a syndrome of potential responses to illness that has an optimum prognosis.
    3. SIRS is a respiratory response to the client having had a myocardial infarction or pneumonia.
    4. SIRS is a systemic response to a variety of insults, including infection, ischemia, and injury.

95. The nurse caring for a client diagnosed with multi-organ dysfunction syndrome is preparing to administer morning medications. Which medication would the nurse **question**?

| Client Name: Mr. W.M. | MR#: 1257739 | Diagnosis: MODS |
|---|---|---|
| Age: 56 years | Allergies: NKDA | |
| Medication | 0701–1900 | 1901–0700 |
| Cefazolin sodium 2 g IVPB q 6 hours | 0900 1500 | 2100 0300 |
| Furosemide 40 mg PO twice daily | 0900 | 2100 |
| Metoprolol 5 mg IVP q 8 hours and PRN | 0900 1700 | 0100 |
| Acetaminophen 650 mg PO every 4 hours PRN | | |
| Signature of Nurse: | Day Nurse RN/DN | Night Nurse RN/NN |

1. Cefazolin sodium.
2. Furosemide.
3. Metoprolol.
4. Acetaminophen.

96. The nurse is preparing to administer medications to a client at 1600. Which medication would the nurse administer **first**?

| Client Name: Mr. James J. | MR#: 1258639 | Diagnosis: AIDS |
|---|---|---|
| Age: 36 years | Allergies: Penicillin | |
| Medication | 0701–1900 | 1901–0700 |
| Vancomycin 1,000 mg IVPB daily | 1800 | |
| Furosemide 40 mg IVP twice daily | 0900, 1600 | |
| Pantoprazole 40 mg oral daily | 0900 | |
| Acetaminophen 650 mg PO every 4 hours PRN | | |
| Signature of Nurse: | Day Nurse RN/DN | Night Nurse RN/NN |

1. Vancomycin.
2. Furosemide.
3. Pantoprazole.
4. Acetaminophen.

## Multiple Sclerosis (MS)

1. 1. These are clinical manifestations of multiple sclerosis and are expected.
   2. These are expected clinical manifestations of MS.
   3. These are expected clinical manifestations of MS.
   4. Dysphagia is a common problem of clients diagnosed with MS, and this places the client at risk for aspiration pneumonia. Some clients diagnosed with MS eventually become immobile and are at risk for pneumonia.

   **TEST-TAKING HINT:** This question is asking the test taker to identify the assessment data unexpected for the disease process. Respiratory problems are a high priority, according to Maslow, and often warrant immediate intervention.

2. 1. The exact cause of MS is not known, but research indicates it is an issue with the regulation of the immune system. Causes may include autoimmune response, an immune response to an infectious agent (such as a virus), and genetic predispositions (National Institute of Neurological Disorders and Stroke, 2019).
   2. There is some evidence supporting a genetic component involved in developing MS.
   3. A specific gene has not been identified to know if the gene is recessive or dominant.
   4. The X chromosome, not the Y chromosome, may be involved.

   **TEST-TAKING HINT:** Option "2" has the word "no" in it. Unless the test taker has absolute knowledge this is true, then an absolute word such as "no," "never," "all," or "always" should rule out the option.

3. 1. MS does not affect the menstrual cycle.
   2. A rash across the bridge of the nose suggests systemic lupus erythematosus.
   3. These are clinical manifestations of MS and can go undiagnosed for years because of the remitting-relapsing nature of the disease. Fatigue and difficulty swallowing are other clinical manifestations of MS.
   4. Taking birth control medications should not produce these clinical manifestations or the pattern of occurrence.

   **TEST-TAKING HINT:** This stem is somewhat involved. The test taker must be sure to understand the important parts, which are the client's age, reports, and occurrence of reports. This should cause the test taker to think about what these have in common.

4. 1. "Why" is requesting an explanation, and the client does not owe the nurse an explanation.
   2. This is stating a fact and offering self. Both are therapeutic techniques for conversations.
   3. The client did not ask about the nature of MS. The client needs to be able to verbalize feelings.
   4. This is "passing the buck." Therapeutic communication is an integral part of nursing.

   **TEST-TAKING HINT:** The question is asking for a therapeutic response. Therapeutic responses address feelings.

5. 1. This describes an evoked potential electroencephalogram (EEG).
   2. MRI scans require the client to lie still and not move the body; the client should be warned about the loud clicking or beeping noise (National Institute of Biomedical Imaging and Bioengineering, n.d.).
   3. The client does not drink any contrast medium. If contrast is used, it will be given IVP for a CT scan.
   4. The test is performed at one time.

   **TEST-TAKING HINT:** The test taker must be knowledgeable about different tests and procedures and be able to teach about them to the client. There are no test-taking hints to help remember protocols for procedures and tests.

6. 1. The problem is grieving related to loss of functioning. Assistive devices will not prevent the loss of functioning and do not address grieving.
   2. A legal power of attorney is for personal property and control of financial issues, which is not the focus of the nurse's care. A legal power of attorney for health care may be appropriate.
   3. The nurse should and must discuss end-of-life issues with the client and does not need to contact the hospital chaplain. If or when the client reveals spiritual needs, then the nurse could contact the chaplain.

4. The client should make personal choices about end-of-life issues while it is possible to do so. This client is progressing toward immobility and all the complications related to it.

**TEST-TAKING HINT:** This is a psychological problem requiring a psychological answer. Option "1" is a physical intervention and therefore should be eliminated as a correct answer. The test taker should remember adjectives ("legal") are important when answering questions. Option "3" is "passing the buck"; the test taker should be careful if thinking of selecting this type of option.

7. 1. This issue is not a priority concern of a newly diagnosed client with MS.
   2. This is not a priority over a potential suicide statement.
   3. A potential suicide statement is a priority for the nurse when caring for the client diagnosed with MS.
   4. Flu and pneumonia vaccines are not a priority.

**TEST-TAKING HINT:** When the test taker is prioritizing, a systematic approach must be used. Safety is a priority, and a threat to a client's life is a priority.

8. Correct answers are 1, 2, 3, and 5.
   1. The licensed practical nurse can administer a muscle relaxant.
   2. The licensed practical nurse can talk with a health-care provider about medication the LPN can give.
   3. The licensed practical nurse can draw blood.
   4. The RN should not assign assessing, teaching, or evaluation to the LPN. Evaluating the client's ability to perform self-catheterization should not be assigned to the LPN.
   5. The LPN can collect a sputum sample.

**TEST-TAKING HINT:** When deciding on assigning tasks, the test taker must be aware of the capabilities of each classification of staff by licensure.

9. 1. The nurse should listen without being judgmental about any alternative therapy the client is considering. Alternative therapies, such as massage and relaxation, are frequently beneficial and enhance the medical regimen.
   2. The nurse can discuss alternative therapy with the client.

3. This is not addressing the client's concern about using an alternative treatment.
4. Investigational therapies are treatments that may have efficacy if proved by scientific methods. It is the health-care provider's responsibility to discuss these therapies with the client.

**TEST-TAKING HINT:** Two options—"3" and "4"—don't address the issue. The answer must address the client's concern.

10. 1. Steroid medications increase gastric acid; therefore, a proton pump inhibitor is an appropriate medication for the client.
    2. Cultures are ordered before administering antibiotics, not steroids.
    3. Steroids interfere with glucose metabolism by blocking the action of insulin; therefore, blood glucose levels should be monitored.
    4. Steroid medications cause the client to retain sodium; therefore, a low-sodium diet should be encouraged.

**TEST-TAKING HINT:** Steroid medications are some of the most common medications administered by nurses. They are also among the most dangerous; therefore, the test taker must know about steroids, their actions, side effects, and adverse effects.

11. 1. This will assist the client and significant other to maintain a close relationship without putting undue pressure on the client.
    2. This is a real physical problem, not a psychological one.
    3. The problem is impotence, not libido.
    4. The problem is not psychosocial. It is a physical problem, and staying calm will not help.

**TEST-TAKING HINT:** The test taker must differentiate physical and psychological problems.

12. Correct answers are 1, 3, 4, and 5.
    1. Muscle flaccidity is a hallmark clinical manifestation of MS.
    2. Epistaxis, nosebleed, is not associated with MS.
    3. Dysmetria is the inability to control muscular action characterized by overestimating or underestimating range of movement.
    4. Fatigue is a clinical manifestation of MS.
    5. Dysphagia, or difficulty swallowing, is associated with MS.

**TEST-TAKING HINT:** These alternative-type questions are difficult because there are several correct answers. The test taker gets credit only if the entire question is answered correctly. The test taker should read each answer option carefully and rule it out as a potentially correct answer before moving on to the next option.

## Guillain-Barré Syndrome

13. 1. These clinical manifestations, along with sleep disturbances and nervousness, support the diagnosis of Creutzfeldt-Jakob disease.
    2. These clinical manifestations support the diagnosis of Parkinson's disease.
    3. These are clinical manifestations of trigeminal neuralgia.
    4. Ascending paralysis is the classic clinical manifestation of Guillain-Barré syndrome.

**TEST-TAKING HINT:** The test taker should try to remember at least one or two clinical manifestations of disease processes, and ascending paralysis is an unusual symptom specific to this syndrome.

14. 1. Visiting a foreign country is not a risk factor for contracting this syndrome.
    2. This syndrome is usually preceded by a respiratory or gastrointestinal infection 1 to 4 weeks before the onset of neurological deficits (National Institute of Neurological Disorders and Stroke, 2019).
    3. This syndrome is not a contagious or communicable disease.
    4. Taking herbs is not a risk factor for developing Guillain-Barré syndrome.

**TEST-TAKING HINT:** There are some questions requiring the test taker to be knowledgeable of the disease process. Herbs may aggravate a disease process, but as a rule, they do not cause disease processes, so option "4" can be eliminated.

15. 1. Hyporeflexia of the lower extremities is the classic clinical manifestation of this syndrome. Therefore, assessing deep tendon reflexes is appropriate.
    2. A Glasgow Coma Scale is used for clients diagnosed with potential neurologic deficits and used to monitor for increased intracranial pressure.
    3. Babinski's reflex evaluates the central nervous system neurologic status, which is not affected by this syndrome.

4. Vital signs are a part of any admission assessment but are not a specific assessment intervention for this syndrome.

**TEST-TAKING HINT:** Vital signs are general assessment skills and really do not help specifically diagnose a disease, except for blood pressure, which helps diagnose hypertension. The test taker should know the Glasgow Coma Scale is for head or brain injuries.

16. 1. The client does not need to be NPO before this procedure.
    2. The client should void before this procedure to avoid the discomfort of a full bladder during the procedure.
    3. The lithotomy position has the client lying flat with the legs in stirrups, such as when Pap smears are obtained.
    4. The pedal pulses should be assessed post-procedure, not before the procedure.

**TEST-TAKING HINT:** The adjective "pre-procedure" helps rule out option "4" as a possible correct answer; assessing pedal pulse is priority postprocedure. The test taker must know the terminology which describes positioning, such as lithotomy, side-lying, supine, Trendelenburg, or prone.

17. 1. Safety is an important issue for the client, but this is not the priority client problem.
    2. The client's psychological needs are important, but psychosocial problems are not a priority over physiological problems.
    3. Clients diagnosed with this syndrome may have choking episodes and are at risk for the inability to swallow as a result of the disease process, but this is not the priority nursing problem because weight loss is not an expected complication of this syndrome.
    4. Guillain-Barré syndrome has ascending paralysis causing respiratory failure. Therefore, the breathing pattern is a priority.

**TEST-TAKING HINT:** Knowledge of the disease process causes the test taker to select option "4," but applying Maslow's hierarchy of needs and choosing a client problem addressing the airway is always a good option if the test taker is not sure of the correct answer.

18. 1. This is an appropriate long-term goal for the client problem "impaired skin integrity."
    2. The client diagnosed with Guillain-Barré syndrome will not be able to move the extremities; therefore, preventing muscle atrophy is an appropriate long-term goal.

3. The client will not be able to move the extremities. Therefore, the nurse will have to do passive range-of-motion exercises; this is an intervention, not a goal.

4. This is a nursing intervention, not a goal, and the client should be turned while sleeping unless the client is on a special immobility bed.

**TEST-TAKING HINT: The adjective "long-term" should make the test taker eliminate option "4" because the words "2 hours" are in the goal. The word "perform" is an intervention, which is not a goal; therefore, option "3" could be eliminated as the correct answer.**

19. 1. The ascending paralysis has reached the client's respiratory muscles; therefore, the client will not be able to use the hands to write.

2. **The client will not be able to use the arms as a result of the paralysis but can blink the eyes as long as the nurse asks simple "yes-or-no" questions.**

3. A speech therapist will not be able to help the client communicate while the client is on the ventilator.

4. The ascending paralysis has reached the respiratory muscles; therefore, the client will not be able to use the hands to push the call light.

**TEST-TAKING HINT: The test taker must realize all the options except option "3" are ways to communicate with a client on the ventilator. Options "1" and "4" both involve the use of the hands, which might lead the test taker to eliminate these two options.**

20. 1. **Clients diagnosed with this syndrome usually have a full recovery, but it may take up to 1 year.**

2. Only about 10% of clients are left with permanent residual disability.

3. This is "passing the buck." The nurse should answer the client's question honestly, which helps establish a trusting nurse-client relationship.

4. This indicates the nurse does not understand the typical course for a client diagnosed with Guillain-Barré syndrome.

**TEST-TAKING HINT: The test taker could eliminate option "3" because this is "passing the buck" and is usually not the best action of a nurse. The test taker needs to be knowledgeable of the typical course of this syndrome to be able to answer this question.**

21. 1. Very little cerebrospinal fluid is removed from the client. Therefore, hypotension is not a potential complication of this procedure.

2. A bandage is placed over the puncture site, and pressure does not need to be applied to the site.

3. The laboratory staff, not the nurse, complete tests on the cerebrospinal fluid; the nurse could label the specimens and take them to the laboratory.

4. **Increased fluid intake will help prevent a postprocedure headache, which may occur after a lumbar puncture.**

**TEST-TAKING HINT: The test taker could eliminate option "3" because nurses usually do not perform tests on bodily fluids at the bedside. A basic concept in many procedures is, if a fluid is removed, it usually must be replaced, which might cause the test taker to select option "4."**

22. 1. The rate of ventilation is usually 12 to 15 breaths per minute in adults on ventilators, so this rate does not require immediate intervention.

2. **A manual resuscitation (Ambu) bag must be at the client's bedside in case the ventilator malfunctions; the nurse must bag the client.**

3. A pulse oximeter reading of less than 93% warrants immediate intervention; a 90% peripheral oxygen saturation indicates a $Pao_2$ of about 60 (normal, 80 to 100). When the client is placed on the ventilator, this should cause the client's oxygen level to improve.

4. These ABGs are within normal limits and do not warrant immediate intervention.

**TEST-TAKING HINT: The test taker must know specific norms for frequently performed tests for the client. Even if the test taker were not knowledgeable of the ventilator-based decisions based on norms, the test taker could ask, "Is a client with a respiratory rate of 14 in respiratory failure or compromise?" Equipment at the bedside probably does not warrant immediate intervention.**

23. 1. This action does not address the wife's fears, and telling her to stop crying will not help the situation.

2. Making the wife leave the room will further upset the client and the client's wife.

3. Medicating the client will not help the wife, but if the nurse can calm the wife, then it is hoped the client will calm down.

4. It is scary for a wife to see her loved one with a tube down his mouth and all the machines around him. The nurse should help the wife by acknowledging her fears.

**TEST-TAKING HINT:** The test taker should select the option addressing the wife's needs first. By addressing the wife's needs, the client will calm down. The test taker should not automatically select the option which medicates the client.

24. Correct answers are 1, 3, 4, and 5.
    1. The physical therapist is an important part of the rehabilitation team, addressing the client's muscle deterioration resulting from the disease process and immobility.
    2. There is no residual speech deficit from Guillain-Barré syndrome; therefore, this referral is not appropriate.
    3. The social worker could help with financial concerns, job issues, and issues concerning the long rehabilitation time for this syndrome.
    4. Pain may or may not be an issue with this syndrome. Each client is different, but a plan needs to be established to address pain if it occurs.
    5. This is an excellent resource for the client and the family.

**TEST-TAKING HINT:** The physical therapist and social worker are two members of the rehabilitation team, always appropriate in long-term rehabilitation. Physical therapy addresses complications of immobility; social workers help the client get back home. Any resource referral is an appropriate intervention.

## Myasthenia Gravis

25. 1. These are musculoskeletal manifestations of myasthenia gravis.
    2. These are ocular clinical manifestations of MG. Ptosis is drooping of the eyelid, and diplopia is unilateral or bilateral blurred vision.
    3. These are respiratory manifestations of myasthenia gravis.
    4. These are nutritional manifestations of myasthenia gravis.

**TEST-TAKING HINT:** The keys to answering this question are the adjectives "ocular" and "facial." This information should make the test taker rule out options "1," "3," and "4," even if the test taker doesn't know what "ptosis" or "diplopia" means.

26. 1. No change in the client's muscle strength indicates it is not MG.
    2. There is a reduced amplitude in an electromyogram (EMG) in a client diagnosed with MG.
    3. The serum assay of circulating acetylcholine receptor antibodies is increased, not decreased, in MG, and this test is only 80% to 90% accurate in diagnosing MG.
    4. Clients diagnosed with MG show a significant improvement of muscle strength lasting approximately 5 minutes when edrophonium chloride (Tensilon) is injected (American Academy of Ophthalmology, 2019).

**TEST-TAKING HINT:** There are some knowledge-based questions, such as diagnostic tests.

27. 1. There is a surgical option available.
    2. This surgery is performed in clients diagnosed with pituitary tumors and is accomplished by going through the client's upper lip through the nasal passage.
    3. In about 75% of clients diagnosed with MG, the thymus gland (which is usually inactive after puberty) continues to produce antibodies, triggering an autoimmune response in MG. After a thymectomy, the production of autoantibodies is reduced or eliminated, and this may resolve the clinical manifestations of MG.
    4. Adrenalectomy is a surgery for a client diagnosed with Cushing's disease, a disease in which there is an increased secretion of glucocorticoids and mineralocorticoids.

**TEST-TAKING HINT:** This is a knowledge-based question, but the test taker may be able to eliminate options "2" and "4" if the test taker has a basic understanding of anatomy and physiology and knows surgery involving the pituitary or adrenal glands does not help prevent clinical manifestations of a muscular disorder.

28. 1. The client is at risk for choking; knowing specific measures to help the client helps decrease the client's, as well as the significant other's, anxiety and promotes confidence in managing potential complications.
    2. Clients diagnosed with MG may end up on a ventilator at the end stage of the disease, but these clients would not be cared for at home; this would be a very unusual situation.

3. The client should be encouraged to perform active range-of-motion exercises, but the most important intervention is treating choking episodes.
4. The client diagnosed with MG doesn't necessarily have a feeding tube, and this information is not in the stem.

**TEST-TAKING HINT:** The test taker should only consider the information in the stem of the question, which causes the test taker to eliminate option "4." If the test taker could not decide between options "1" and "3," the test taker should apply Maslow's hierarchy of needs; the airway is a priority.

29. 1. The occupational therapist assists the client with ADLs, but with MG the client has no problems with performing them if the client takes the medication correctly (30 minutes before performing ADLs).
2. A recreational therapist is usually in a psychiatric unit or rehabilitation unit.
3. A vocational therapist or counselor helps the client with finding a job that accommodates the disease process; clients diagnosed with MG are usually not able to work in the late stages.
4. **Speech therapists address swallowing problems, and clients diagnosed with MG are dysphagic and at risk for aspiration. The speech therapist can help match food consistency to the client's ability to swallow, which enhances client safety.**

**TEST-TAKING HINT:** The test taker must be aware of the responsibilities of the other health-care team members. "Collaborative" means working with another health-care team discipline.

30. 1. **Hypovolemia is a complication of plasmapheresis, especially during the procedure when up to 15% of the blood volume is in the cell separator.**
2. Positive Chvostek's and Trousseau's signs (not negative signs) warrant intervention and indicate hypocalcemia, which is a complication of plasmapheresis.
3. This is a normal serum potassium level (3.5 to 5.5 mEq/L), which does not warrant intervention, but the level should be monitored because plasmapheresis could cause hypokalemia.
4. Ecchymosis (bruising) does not warrant immediate intervention. Clinical manifestations of infiltration or infection warrant immediate intervention.

**TEST-TAKING HINT:** If the test taker has no idea of the answer, then selecting clinical manifestations of hypovolemia—hypotension and tachycardia—is an appropriate selection if the question asks which data warrant immediate intervention.

31. 1. MG has no effect on the ovarian function; and the uterus is an involuntary muscle, not a skeletal muscle, so the menstrual cycle is not affected.
2. Infections can result in an exacerbation and extreme weakness.
3. An extremely hot or cold environment may cause an exacerbation of MG.
4. This will help the client mobilize and expectorate sputum.

**TEST-TAKING HINT:** This question is an "except" question and is asking the test taker to select the option that is not appropriate for the client's disease process. Three answers will be appropriate; sometimes, if the test taker rethinks the question and asks, "Which statements indicate the client understands the teaching?," this will help identify the correct answer.

32. 1. This is a diagnostic test done to diagnose MG.
2. These assessment data indicate the client is experiencing a myasthenic crisis, which is the result of undermedication, missed doses of medication, or the development of an infection.
3. The vital signs do not indicate if the client is experiencing a cholinergic crisis.
4. **The injection of edrophonium chloride (Tensilon test) not only diagnoses MG but helps to determine which type of crisis the client is experiencing. In a myasthenic crisis, the test is positive (the client's muscle strength improves), but in a cholinergic crisis, the test is negative (there is no improvement in muscle strength) or the client will actually get worse and emergency equipment must be available.**

**TEST-TAKING HINT:** This question requires the test taker to be knowledgeable of the disease process, but this is an important concept the test taker must understand about myasthenia gravis.

33. Correct answers are 1, 2, and 4.
1. Position changes promote lung expansion, and coughing helps clear secretions from the tracheobronchial tree.
2. This position expands the lungs and alleviates pressure from the diaphragm.

3. The respiratory system and pulse oximeter reading should be assessed more frequently than every shift; it should be done every 4 hours or more often.

4. **The medications should be administered 30 minutes before the meal to provide optimal muscle strength for swallowing and chewing.**

5. There is no serum level available for medications used to treat MG; the client's clinical manifestations are used to determine the effectiveness of this medication.

**TEST-TAKING HINT: An alternative-type question requests the test taker to select more than one option as the correct answer. The test taker must evaluate each option individually to determine if it is correct. The priority concerns for a client diagnosed with MG are respiration and eating.**

34. 1. This is an appropriate action by the nurse, but it is not the best action.
    2. Support groups are helpful to the client's significant others, but in this situation, it is not the best action for the nurse.
    3. A counselor is an appropriate intervention, but it is not the best action.
    4. **Directly addressing the wife's feelings is the best action for the nurse in this situation. All the other options can be done, but the best action is to address the wife's feelings.**

**TEST-TAKING HINT: The test taker should select the option directly addressing and helping the client or significant other. Remember, if the word "best," "most important," or "first" is in the stem, then all four options could be possible interventions, but only one is the highest priority.**

35. 1. **The cholinesterase inhibitor neostigmine (Prostigmin) promotes muscle contraction, which improves muscle strength, which in turn allows the client to perform ADLs without assistance.**
    2. This medication does not affect the secretions of the eye.
    3. This medication does not help with the digestion of food.
    4. This medication does not help with pain; clients diagnosed with MG do not have muscle pain.

**TEST-TAKING HINT: The test taker must know about the disease process to be able to answer this question. Remember, when answering pharmacology questions, the effectiveness of**

the medication is based on what clinical manifestation the client is experiencing.

36. 1. **The anticholinesterase pyridostigmine (Mestinon) will increase muscle strength to help enhance swallowing and chewing during meals (Vallerand & Sanoski, 2019).**
    2. There is no need for the client to take this medication with 8 ounces of water.
    3. The client does not have to sit up after taking the anticholinesterase pyridostigmine (Mestinon).
    4. These assessment data would not cause the nurse to question administering this medication.

**TEST-TAKING HINT: There are very few medications given specifically on time, but this medication is one of them. The blood pressure is checked before administering antihypertensive medications.**

## Systemic Lupus Erythematosus (SLE)

37. 1. SLE can affect any organ system, and these tests are used to determine the possibility of the liver being involved, but they are not used to diagnose SLE.
    2. **No single laboratory test diagnoses SLE, but the client usually presents with moderate to severe anemia, thrombocytopenia, leukopenia, and a positive antinuclear antibody.**
    3. Female clients diagnosed with SLE develop atherosclerosis at an earlier age, but cholesterol and lipid profile tests are not used to diagnose the disease.
    4. These tests may be done to determine SLE infiltration in the kidneys but not to diagnose the disease itself.

**TEST-TAKING HINT: A comprehensive metabolic panel is ordered for many different diseases; cholesterol and lipid panels are usually ordered for atherosclerosis, and BUN and glomerular filtration tests are specific to the kidneys. Options "1," "3," and "4" could be ruled out because they are specific to other diseases or not specific enough.**

38. Correct answers are 1, 2, and 4.
    1. Sunlight or UV light exposure has been shown to initiate an exacerbation of SLE, so the client should be taught to protect the skin when in the sun.
    2. A fever may be the first indication of an exacerbation of SLE.

3. Dyspnea is not expected and could signal respiratory involvement.
4. Raynaud's phenomenon is a condition in which the digits of the hands and feet turn red, blue, or white in response to heat or cold and stress. It occurs with some immune inflammatory processes.
5. SLE is a chronic disease, and there is no known cure.

**TEST-TAKING HINT: Dyspnea is an uncomfortable sensation of not being able to breathe. Usually, clients are not told this is normal regardless of the disease process.**

39. 1. SLE is frequently diagnosed in young women and reproduction is a concern for these clients, but it is not the most important goal.
2. The client's body image is important, but this is not the most important.
3. SLE can invade and destroy any body system or organ. Maintaining organ function is the primary goal of SLE treatment.
4. Measures are taken to prevent breakdown, but skin breakdown is not life-threatening.

**TEST-TAKING HINT: When the question asks for "priority," the test taker should determine if one of the options has life-threatening information or could result in a serious complication for the client.**

40. 1. SLE can affect any organ. It can cause pericarditis and myocardial ischemia as well as pneumonia or pleural effusions.
2. Muscle spasticity occurs in MS, and bradykinesia occurs in Parkinson's disease.
3. Hirsutism is an overgrowth of hair. Spotty areas of alopecia occur in SLE, and clubbing of the fingers occurs in chronic pulmonary or cardiac diseases.
4. Weight loss and fatigue are experienced by clients diagnosed with SLE.

**TEST-TAKING HINT: The test taker must know the clinical manifestations of disease processes.**

41. 1. Steroid medications mask the development of infections because steroids suppress the immune system's response.
2. SLE does not metastasize, or "spread"; it does invade other organ systems, but steroids do not prevent this from happening.
3. The main function of steroid medications is to suppress the inflammatory response of the body.
4. Steroid medications can delay the healing process, theoretically making scarring worse.

**TEST-TAKING HINT: Steroids are a frequently administered medication class. The test taker must know the common actions, side effects, adverse effects, and how to administer the medications safely.**

42. 1. Unless the nurse has SLE and has been through the exact same type of tissue involvement, then the nurse should not tell a client, "I know." This does not address the client's feelings.
2. The nurse should never ask the client "why?" The client does not owe the nurse an explanation of personal feelings.
3. Support groups should be recommended, but this is not the best response when the client is crying.
4. The nurse stated a fact, "You are crying," and then offered self by saying, "Would you like to talk?" This addresses the nonverbal cue, crying, and is a therapeutic response.

**TEST-TAKING HINT: The question asks for a therapeutic response, which means a feeling must be addressed. Therapeutic responses do not ask "why," so the test taker could rule out option "2."**

43. 1. Moisturizing lotions, not astringents, are applied. Astringent lotions have an alcohol base, which is drying to the client's skin.
2. The skin should be inspected daily for any breakdown or rashes.
3. The skin should be washed with mild soap, rinsed, and patted dry. Rubbing can cause abrasions and skin breakdown.
4. The stem does not tell the test taker the client is itching, and SLE does not have itching as a clinical manifestation. Lotions are not usually applied between the toes because this fosters the development of fungal infections between the toes.

**TEST-TAKING HINT: If the test taker did not know what "astringent" meant, then the test taker should skip this option and continue looking for a correct answer. In option "2," the time frame of weekly makes this option wrong.**

44. 1. Chest pain should be considered a priority regardless of the admitting diagnosis. Clients diagnosed with SLE can develop cardiac complications.
2. Pain at a "10" is a priority but not above chest pain.
3. Dysphagia is expected in clients diagnosed with MG.

4. Clients diagnosed with GB syndrome have ascending muscle weakness or paralysis, which could eventually result in the client being placed on a ventilator, but the problem currently is in the distal extremities (the feet) and is not a priority over chest pain.

**TEST-TAKING HINT: When the test taker is deciding on which client has priority, a potentially life-threatening condition is always the top priority.**

45. 1. The UAP should wash the hands before and after client care.
    2. **The UAP can remove an indwelling catheter with nonsterile gloves. This is a waste of expensive equipment. The RN is responsible for teaching UAPs appropriate use of equipment and supplies and cost containment.**
    3. Raising the head of the bed to a 90-degree angle (high Fowler's position) during meals helps to prevent aspiration.
    4. Using a clean plastic bag to access the ice machine indicates the assistant is aware of infection control procedures.

**TEST-TAKING HINT: This is really an "except" question—there will be three options with desired actions, and only one needs to change.**

46. 1. The kidneys filter wastes, not antibodies, from the blood.
    2. The problem is an overactive immune system, not damage to the endocrine system. There is no research supporting a virus as an initiating factor.
    3. SLE is an autoimmune disease characterized by exacerbations and remission. There is empirical evidence indicating hormones may cause the development of the disease, and some drugs can initiate the process.
    4. **There is evidence for familial and hormonal components to the development of SLE. SLE is an autoimmune disease process in which there is an exaggerated production of autoantibodies.**

**TEST-TAKING HINT: The test taker could eliminate options "1" and "2" by referring to basic anatomy and physiology and the function of the kidneys and endocrine system.**

47. 1. Steroids are not addicting.
    2. The adrenal gland, not the thyroid gland, produces the glucocorticoid cortisol.
    3. **Tapering steroids is important because the adrenal gland stops producing cortisol, a glucocorticosteroid, when the exogenous administration of steroids exceeds what normally is produced. The**

functions of cortisol in the body are to regulate glucose metabolism and maintain blood pressure.
    4. Tapering the dose is standard medical practice, not a whim of the HCP.

**TEST-TAKING HINT: Basic knowledge of anatomy and physiology eliminates option "2." Tapering steroid medication is basic knowledge for the nurse administering a steroid.**

48. 1. Nodules and bony deformity are clinical manifestations of RA but not of SLE.
    2. Organ involvement occurs in SLE but not RA.
    3. **Joint stiffness and pain are clinical manifestations occurring in both diseases.**
    4. Raynaud's phenomenon and skin rashes are associated with SLE.

**TEST-TAKING HINT: There are a number of illnesses sharing the same clinical manifestations. The test taker must be aware of the symptoms that distinguish one illness from another.**

## Acquired Immunodeficiency Syndrome (AIDS)

49. 1. Birth control pills provide protection against unwanted pregnancy, but they do not protect females from getting sexually transmitted infections. In fact, because of the reduced chance of becoming pregnant, some women may find it easier to become involved with multiple partners, increasing the chance of contracting a sexually transmitted infection.
    2. There is a preventive HIV vaccine being researched by the Food and Drug Administration (FDA), but it is not approved. Only participants in a clinical trial have access to the preventive HIV vaccine. There is no cure for AIDS (U.S. Department of Health and Human Services, 2019).
    3. **Adolescents are among the fastest-growing population to be newly diagnosed with HIV and AIDS.**
    4. Abstinence is the only guarantee the client will not contract a sexually transmitted infection, including AIDS. An HIV-negative individual in a monogamous relationship with another HIV-negative individual, committed to a monogamous relationship, is the safest sexual relationship.

**TEST-TAKING HINT: Answer option "1" is a form of an absolute, which could cause the test taker to eliminate this option. Option "4" is also an**

absolute—"only"—but it is a true statement. There are some absolutes in the health-care profession.

50. 1. The client has malnutrition syndrome. The nurse assesses the body and what the client has been able to eat.
   2. Standard precautions are used for clients diagnosed with AIDS, the same as for every other client.
   3. The nurse should check the orders but not before assessing the client.
   4. The client will probably be placed on total parenteral nutrition and will need to be taught these things, but this is not the first action.

**TEST-TAKING HINT:** Assessment is the first step in the nursing process. The nursing process is a good place to start when setting priorities for the nurse's actions.

51. 1. This client probably has oral candidiasis, a fungal infection of the mouth and esophagus. Brushing the teeth and patchy areas will not remove the lesions and will cause considerable pain.
   2. **This most likely is a fungal infection known as oral candidiasis, commonly called thrush. An antifungal medication is needed to treat this condition.**
   3. Antiseptic-based mouthwashes usually contain alcohol, which is painful for the client.
   4. The foods the client has eaten did not cause this condition.

**TEST-TAKING HINT:** The client is reporting a "sore mouth." The test taker must notice all the important information in the stem before attempting to choose an answer. How are brushing the area, an antiseptic mouthwash, or the foods eaten going to alleviate the pain?

52. 1. Contact precautions are a form of transmission-based precautions used when the infectious organism is known to be spread by contact with a substance.
   2. Airborne precautions are used for bacteria, which are very small organisms carried at some distance from the client on air currents. The bacterium that causes tuberculosis is an example of such bacteria. A special isolation mask is required to enter the client's negative air pressure room.
   3. Droplet precautions are used for organisms causing flu or some cases of pneumonia. The organisms have a larger molecule and "drop" within 3 to 4 feet. A normal isolation mask is used with this client.
   4. **Standard precautions are used for all contact with blood and body secretions.**

**TEST-TAKING HINT:** Isolation procedures are basic nursing knowledge, and the test taker must know, understand, and be able to comply with all of the procedures.

53. 1. Retroviruses never die; the virus may become dormant, only to be reactivated at a later time.
   2. "Eradicated" means to be completely cured or done away with. HIV cannot be eradicated.
   3. HIV originated in the green monkey, in which it is not deadly. HIV in humans replicates readily using the CD4+ cells as reservoirs.
   4. HIV uses the CD4+ cells of the immune system as reservoirs to replicate itself.

**TEST-TAKING HINT:** If the test taker is not aware of the definition of a word, the individual monitoring the test may be able to define the word, but this is not possible on the NCLEX-RN® examination. Of the answer options, option "1" has the most important information regarding prognosis and potential spread to noninfected individuals.

54. 1. The client may be in the primary infection stage when the body has not had time to develop antibodies to the HIV virus.
   2. Repeated exposure to HIV increases the risk of infection, but it only takes one exposure to develop an infection.
   3. **The primary phase of infection ranges from being asymptomatic to severe flu-like symptoms, but during this time, the test may be negative although the individual is infected with HIV.**
   4. The client may or may not have a different virus, but this is not the reason the test is negative.

**TEST-TAKING HINT:** Answer options "1" and "4" assume the client is negative for the HIV virus. Therefore, these options should be eliminated as correct answers unless the test taker is completely sure the statement is correct.

55. 1. The nurse should attempt to flush the skin and get the area to bleed. It is hoped this will remove contaminated blood from the body before infecting the nurse.
   2. The nurse should notify the charge nurse after flushing the area and trying to get it to bleed.
   3. This should be done within 4 hours of the exposure, not before trying to rid the body of the potential infection.
   4. This is done at 3 months and 6 months after initial exposure.

**TEST-TAKING HINT:** In questions asking the test taker to select the first action, all the options could be appropriate interventions, but the test taker must decide which has the most immediate need and the most benefit. Directly caring for the wound is of the most benefit.

56. 1. Altered nutrition may be a priority for a client diagnosed with malnutrition, but HIV encephalopathy is a cognitive deficit.
   2. The client might grieve if the client still has enough cognitive ability to understand the loss is occurring, but this is not the most important consideration.
   3. A client diagnosed with encephalopathy may not have the ability to understand instructions. The nurse should teach the significant others.
   4. **Safety is always an issue with a client diagnosed with diminished mental capacity.**

**TEST-TAKING HINT:** The test taker must have a basis for deciding priority. Maslow's hierarchy of needs lists safety as a high priority.

57. 1. Serum blood work, although ordered STAT, does not have priority over oxygenation of the client.
   2. **Oxygen is a priority, especially with a client diagnosed with a respiratory illness.**
   3. It is extremely important to initiate IV antibiotic therapy to a client diagnosed with an infection as quickly as possible, but this does not have priority over oxygen.
   4. Culture specimens should be obtained before initiating antibiotic therapy, but oxygen administration is still the first action.

**TEST-TAKING HINT:** Airway, breathing, and providing oxygen to the tissues is the top priority in any nursing situation. If the cells are not oxygenated, they die.

58. 1. Performing the head-to-toe assessment is a nursing consideration, not a client consideration. This is a physiological intervention, not a psychosocial one.
   2. Maintaining body weight is physical.
   3. **Clients diagnosed with AIDS should be encouraged to discuss their end-of-life issues with the significant others and to put those wishes in writing. This is important for all clients, not just those diagnosed with AIDS.**
   4. Activity tolerance is a physical problem.

**TEST-TAKING HINT:** All of the options except one focus on the physical care of the client. The stem asked the test taker to consider a psychosocial need.

59. 1. Flushed warm skin with tented turgor indicates dehydration. The HCP should be notified immediately for fluid orders or other orders to correct the reason for the dehydration.
   2. This is a concern, but it can be taken care of after the client with the physical problem.
   3. The temperature is slightly elevated and the pulse is one beat higher than normal. This client could wait to be seen.
   4. Many clients with sputum specimens orders are unable to produce sputum, but it does not warrant immediate intervention.

**TEST-TAKING HINT:** This is an "except" question asking the test taker to identify abnormal data indicating a life-threatening situation or a complication.

60. 1. This does not provide continuity of care for the client. It does recognize the nurse's position, but it is not the best care for the client.
   2. The HCP should be asked to attend the care plan meeting to assist in deciding how to work with the client, but asking the HCP to "tell" the client to behave is not the best way to handle the situation. The client can always refuse to behave as requested.
   3. **The health-care team should meet to discuss ways to best help the client deal with the anger being expressed, and the staff should be consistent in working with the client.**
   4. Telling a staff member to care for the client for a week could result in a buildup of animosity and make the situation worse.

**TEST-TAKING HINT:** The test taker is being asked for the most appropriate method. Option "4" can be discarded because of the word "tell." Option "3" gives the option for multiple individuals to work together toward an outcome.

## Allergies and Allergic Reactions

61. 1. This is appropriate anytime the nurse is administering a diuretic medication.
   2. A nurse uses nonsterile gloves to remove old dressings, then washes the hands and sets up the sterile field before donning sterile gloves to reapply the dressing.

3. Checking for allergies is one of the five rights of medication. Is it the right drug? Even if the drug is the one the HCP ordered, it is not the right drug if the client is allergic to it. The nurse should always assess a client's allergies before administering any medication.

4. The nurse should ask for assistance in moving a client in bed to prevent on-the-job injuries.

**TEST-TAKING HINT:** The stem asks the test taker to determine which is an incorrect action. This is an "except" question. Three answers are actions the nurse should take.

62. 1. The nurse should use nonlatex gloves because of the latex allergy, but the gloves do not have to be sterile.

2. The nurse must use gloves during procedures and starting an IV. Not using gloves is a violation of Occupational Safety and Health Administration standards and places the nurse at risk for developing illnesses.

3. The nurse should be prepared to care for a client at all times and should not be placed at risk because the facility does not keep nonlatex gloves available in the rooms. The nurse should carry the needed equipment (nonlatex gloves) in a pocket.

4. White cotton gloves are made of cloth and do not provide the barrier against wet substances.

**TEST-TAKING HINT:** The test taker must be aware of adjectives such as "sterile" in option "1." Basic concepts such as standard precautions should cause the test taker to eliminate option "2." Option "4" has the word "all" in it and could be eliminated as an answer because this is an absolute.

63. 1. Clients allergic to bee sting venom should be taught to keep an epinephrine auto injector (EpiPen), an adrenergic agonist, with them at all times and how to use the device. This could save their lives.

2. It is unrealistic to think the client will never go outdoors, but the client should be taught to avoid exposure to bees whenever possible.

3. Over-the-counter diphenhydramine (Benadryl) is a histamine-1 blocker, but it is oral and not useful in this situation.

4. The client should wear a medical alert bracelet (Medic Alert), but it is not a priority over ensuring the client knows how to treat a bee sting. Wearing the bracelet does not ensure the correct treatment of the bee sting.

**TEST-TAKING HINT:** Answer option "2" is an absolute and should be eliminated as a possible correct answer.

64. 1. This intervention should be implemented, but it is not the first action.

2. This does address oxygenation but will take time to accomplish, so this intervention is not the first action.

3. The client is cyanotic with dyspnea and wheezing. The nurse should administer oxygen first.

4. The client may be allergic to iodine, a component of many shellfish, but the first need of the client is oxygenation.

**TEST-TAKING HINT:** The test taker must apply some decision-making standard to determine what to do first. Maslow's hierarchy of needs ranks oxygen as first. Of the two options addressing oxygen, option "3" immediately attempts to provide oxygen to the client.

65. 1. The clinical manifestations are occurring at this time, so asking what time of the year the symptoms occur is not an appropriate question.

2. There are many over-the-counter remedies available. Therefore, the nurse should assess which medications the client has tried and what medications the client is currently taking.

3. The client being allergic to animals was not in the stem. Many clients diagnosed with allergic rhinitis are allergic to seasonal environmental allergens such as pollen and mold.

4. The client probably does not have any explanation for developing allergies.

**TEST-TAKING HINT:** The test taker should not read into a question. Because animals were not mentioned in the stem, option "3" can be eliminated. Many over-the-counter medications and herbal remedies are available to clients, and it is important for the nurse to determine what the client has been taking.

66. 1. Tree pollen is abundant in early spring.

2. Rose and grass pollen are prevalent in early summer.

3. Ragweed and other pollens are prevalent in early fall.

4. Early winter is the beginning of deciduous plants becoming dormant. Therefore, allergic rhinitis is least prevalent during this time of year.

**TEST-TAKING HINT:** The test taker could eliminate the three options based on the plant growing season if the test taker realized allergic rhinitis could be caused by environmental plant pollens and molds.

67. 1. Immunotherapy does not cure the problem. However, if immunotherapy is done following a reaction, it is effective in preventing the potentially life-threatening systemic reaction in subsequent insect stings (Kolaczek et al., 2017).
    2. This is an untrue statement.
    3. There is no cure for allergies to insect venom.
    4. This therapy is a standard procedure for clients with severe allergies to insect venom.

**TEST-TAKING HINT:** Answer options "2" and "3" contain forms of absolutes such as "all" and "cure." Rarely is anything absolute in health care. The test taker should be absolutely sure of the correct answer before choosing any answer containing an absolute descriptive word or passage. The stem asks for the rationale, and option "4" is giving advice, so it can be eliminated.

68. Correct answers are 3, 4, and 5.
    1. This is an unrealistic expectation for a client diagnosed with poison ivy. The pruritus is intense. However, the client should be instructed that scratching can cause an infection.
    2. The client would not be discharged with the expectation to administer IM diphenhydramine (Benadryl), a histamine-1 blocker, at home.
    3. Clients diagnosed with poison ivy are frequently prescribed a steroid dose pack. The dose pack has the steroid provided in descending doses to help prevent adrenal insufficiency.
    4. Clients can get relief from the itching by soaking in a lukewarm oatmeal bath.
    5. Cool compresses applied to itchy skin can reduce the itch (American Academy of Dermatology, 2019).

**TEST-TAKING HINT:** Option "1" has the word "never," which is an absolute word and can be eliminated on this basis. Very few conditions require the nurse to teach the client to take intramuscular (IM) injections; therefore, option "2" could be eliminated as a possible answer.

69. 1. This can be an independent or collaborative nursing problem. It is an airway problem and has priority.
    2. Knowledge deficit is not a priority over the client diagnosed with breathing problems.
    3. Anaphylaxis is a collaborative problem. The nurse will need to start IVs, administer medications, and possibly place the client on a ventilator if the client is to survive.
    4. Ineffective coping is a psychosocial problem; it does not have priority over breathing.

**TEST-TAKING HINT:** The test taker must apply some problem-solving and decision-making standards. In this case, Maslow's hierarchy of needs is a good option. Airway has priority.

70. 1. This client should be seen but not before assessing for a possible anaphylactic reaction.
    2. This client has received an initial dose of antibiotic IV and should be assessed for tolerance to the medication within 30 minutes.
    3. Pain is a priority but not over a potentially life-threatening emergency.
    4. This client can be seen last. A delayed meal is not life-threatening.

**TEST-TAKING HINT:** The test taker should determine which client has the most pressing need and rank the options in order. Life-threatening situations have priority.

71. 1. By the Joint Commission standards, clients must mark any surgical site to make sure the operation is not done on the incorrect site, such as the right arm instead of the left arm.
    2. The client should understand the surgery in basic terms.
    3. Iodine is the basic ingredient in Betadine (povidone-iodine), which is a common skin prep used for surgeries. Therefore, the nurse should notify the surgeon if the client has an allergy to iodine.
    4. The client should have signed consent for the surgery and the anesthesia before surgery.

**TEST-TAKING HINT:** The options involve basic concepts for surgical preparation, and allergies must be identified on the client as well as in the client's EHR.

72. Correct answers are 1, 3, 4, and 5.
    1. Steroid medications decrease inflammation, and therefore methylprednisolone (Solu-Medrol), a glucocorticoid, is one of the treatments for anaphylaxis.
    2. A STAT chest x-ray is not indicated at this time.
    3. The Rapid Response Team should be called because this client will be in respiratory and cardiac arrest very shortly.
    4. Because of its ability to cause blood vessel constriction and act as a beta-2 agonist for bronchial smooth muscle relaxation, epinephrine, an adrenergic blocker, is the treatment of choice for anaphylactic shock (Hoffman & Sullivan, 2020).
    5. The first step in initiating cardiopulmonary resuscitation is to assess for a pulse and respiration.

**TEST-TAKING HINT:** This is an alternative-type question. If the test taker did not read the sentence "Select all that apply," the fact there are five, not four, options should alert the test taker to go back and read the stem more closely. Each option must be decided on for itself. The test taker cannot eliminate one option based on the fact another option is correct.

## Rheumatoid Arthritis (RA)

73. 1. This is done, but it will not prevent any disease from occurring.
    2. This will follow the progression of the disease of RA, but it is not preventive.
    3. RA is a disease with many immunological abnormalities. The clients have increased susceptibility to infectious diseases, such as the flu or pneumonia, and therefore, vaccines, which are preventive, should be recommended.
    4. Assessing the client does not address preventive care.

**TEST-TAKING HINT:** The stem requires the test taker to determine what action is preventive care for the client diagnosed with RA. Only option "3" addresses preventive care.

74. 1. The nodules may appear over bony prominences and resolve spontaneously. They appear in clients diagnosed with the rheumatoid factor and are associated with the rapidly progressive and destructive disease.
    2. There is a proliferation of the synovial membrane in RA, which leads to the formation of pannus and the destruction of cartilage and bone, but synovial fluid does not crystallize to form the nodules.
    3. The nodules are not lymph nodes. Lymph nodes may enlarge in the presence of disease, but they do not proliferate (multiply).
    4. The nodes indicate a progression of the disease, not an improving prognosis.

**TEST-TAKING HINT:** The test taker can rule out option "3" with knowledge of anatomy or physiology. Lymph nodes do not multiply; they do form chains throughout the body.

75. 1. Joint stiffness and joints warm to the touch are expected in clients diagnosed with RA.
    2. Clients diagnosed with RA have bilateral and symmetrical stiffness, edema, tenderness, and temperature changes in the joints. Other clinical manifestations include sensory changes, lymph node enlargement, weight loss, fatigue, and pain. A 1-kg weight loss and fatigue are expected.
    3. The use of heat is encouraged to provide comfort for a client diagnosed with RA.
    4. The client has the clinical manifestations of depression. The nurse should attempt to intervene with therapeutic conversation and discuss these findings with the HCP.

**TEST-TAKING HINT:** The test taker should not automatically assume only physiological data require immediate intervention. There will be times when a psychological need will have priority. Because options "1," "2," and "3" are all expected in a client diagnosed with RA, the psychological need warrants intervention by the nurse.

76. Correct answers are 2 and 5.
    1. The drug does not lose efficacy, and clients are removed from the drug when the body cannot tolerate the side effects.
    2. Etanercept, a tumor necrosis factor alpha inhibitor, requires close monitoring to prevent organ damage.
    3. MRI scans are not used to determine the progress of RA.
    4. There is no "off" period for etanercept, a tumor necrosis factor alpha inhibitor.
    5. Analgesics, NSAIDs, corticosteroids, methotrexate, and salicylates may be continued during etanercept therapy (Vallerand & Sanoski, 2019).

**TEST-TAKING HINT:** If the test taker is not aware of the medication being discussed, option "2" is information that could be said of most medications.

77. 1. Physical therapists work with gait training and muscle strengthening. Generally, the physical therapist works on the lower half of the body.
2. **The occupational therapist assists the client in the use of the upper half of the body, fine motor skills, and activities of daily living. This is needed for the client diagnosed with abnormal fingers.**
3. A counselor can help the client discuss feelings about body image, loss of function, and role changes, but the best referral is to the occupational therapist.
4. The client may need a home health nurse eventually, but first, the client should be assisted to remain as functional as possible.

**TEST-TAKING HINT:** The test taker must be aware of the roles of all the health-care team members. The counselor (option "3") can be ruled out as a possible correct answer because swan-neck fingers are a physical problem.

78. Correct answers are 4 and 5.
1. The client diagnosed with RA is generally fatigued, and strenuous exercise increases the fatigue, places increased pressure on the joints, and increases pain.
2. The client should be on a balanced diet high in protein, vitamins, and iron for tissue building and repair and should not require a mechanically altered diet.
3. There is no specific reason for the client to be ordered a keep-open IV; the client can swallow needed medications.
4. **Sleep deprivation resulting from pain is common in clients diagnosed with RA. A mild sedative can increase the client's ability to sleep, promote rest, and increase the client's tolerance of pain.**
5. **The client diagnosed with RA is at risk for infections due to treatment but should not receive live vaccines if on immunosuppressive therapy.**

**TEST-TAKING HINT:** The test taker should be aware of adjectives leading to an option being eliminated—for example, the word "strenuous" in option "1."

79. 1. **Immunosuppressive medications are considered class C drugs and should not be taken while pregnant. These drugs are teratogenic and carcinogenic, and the client is only 20 years old.**
2. Any individual older than age 18 years is considered an adult and does not need to discuss treatment with her parents unless she chooses to do so.
3. The medications can be administered on an outpatient basis, but if an inpatient has intravenous therapy, then IV sites are changed every 72 hours, and there is no guarantee an IV will last for 4 days.
4. These are not investigational drugs and are standard therapy approved by the American College of Rheumatology and the Food and Drug Administration.

**TEST-TAKING HINT:** The age of the client and the fact the client is female could give the test taker an idea of the correct answer. This is a client in the childbearing years.

80. 1. Activity intolerance is an appropriate client problem, but it is not a priority over pain.
2. The client diagnosed with RA does not experience fluid and electrolyte disturbance.
3. **The client diagnosed with RA has chronic pain; therefore, alteration in comfort is a priority problem.**
4. Clients diagnosed with RA usually experience anorexia and weight loss unless they are taking long-term steroids.

**TEST-TAKING HINT:** The question is asking for the priority problem, and pain is a priority according to Maslow's hierarchy of needs.

81. 1. The client in pain should receive medication as soon as possible to keep the pain from becoming worse, but the client is not at risk for a serious complication.
2. A butterfly rash across the bridge of the nose occurs in approximately 50% of the clients diagnosed with SLE.
3. **Antineoplastic drugs can be caustic to tissues; therefore, the client's IV site should be assessed. The client should be assessed for any untoward reactions to the medications first.**
4. Scleroderma is a disease characterized by waxlike skin covering the entire body. This is expected for this client.

**TEST-TAKING HINT:** Pain is a priority, but the test taker must determine that another client may experience complications if not seen immediately.

82. 1. Methotrexate, an antineoplastic medication, can be administered only by an RN trained in the administration and disposal of these medications.

2. Assessment cannot be assigned to a licensed practical nurse.
3. The LPN can demonstrate how to use adaptive clothing such as hook and loop fasteners (Velcro).
4. This is teaching requiring knowledge of medications and interactions and should not be assigned to an LPN.

**TEST-TAKING HINT:** The nurse cannot assign assessment, evaluation, or teaching or any medication requiring specialized knowledge or skills to administer safely.

83. 1. This is prescribing, and the nurse is not licensed to do this unless the nurse has become a nurse practitioner.
   2. NSAIDs do not require a specific amount of water to be effective, unlike bulk laxatives.
   3. The medication should be taken in the usual dose when the client realizes a dose has been missed.
   4. NSAID medications decrease prostaglandin production in the stomach, resulting in less mucus production, which creates a risk for the development of ulcers. The client should take the NSAID with food.

**TEST-TAKING HINT:** Knowledge of medication administration is a priority for every nurse. It is especially important for the nurse to be familiar with commonly used medications such as NSAIDs, which can be purchased over the counter and may be taken by the client in addition to prescription medications.

84. 1. Pain medication is important and should be given before the client's pain becomes worse.
   2. Unless the client is in a crisis, such as pulmonary edema, this medication can wait.
   3. Steroids do not have precedence over pain medication and should be administered with food.
   4. Clients diagnosed with OA are usually overweight and do not require appetite stimulants. The nurse should question this medication before administering the medication.

**TEST-TAKING HINT:** When determining priorities, the test taker must employ some criteria to use as a guideline. According to Maslow, pain is a priority.

85. Correct answers are 1, 2, 3, and 4.
    1. SIRS involvement in the hematopoietic system includes prolonged bleeding times and thrombocytopenia.
    2. In the prerenal phase and intrarenal phase of SIRS affecting the renal system, urine osmolality increases, but urine production decreases because of decreased glomerular filtration.
    3. The capillary membranes have a systemic response to the insult, resulting in increased permeability and leaking of fluid into the interstitial spaces (pitting edema).
    4. The brain responds poorly to the increased interstitial fluid and can result in confusion, disorientation, and delirium.
    5. These vital signs are within normal limits. This indicates a stable client, not one diagnosed with SIRS.

**TEST-TAKING HINT:** This question is asking the test taker to identify the assessment data unexpected for the disease process. In "Select all that apply" questions, each option should be answered as a true or false question.

86. 1. Lung sounds assess the respiratory system; heart sounds and blood pressure assess the circulatory and cardiovascular system.
    2. Psychological responses do not assess for MODS.
    3. The family's expectations do not assess for MODS.
    4. Emesis is not particularly associated with MODS, and bile secretions and mouth ulcers have no correlation with MODS.

**TEST-TAKING HINT:** This question is asking the test taker to identify the assessment data expected for the disease process. Physiological problems are a high priority according to Maslow and often warrant immediate intervention.

87. 1. The intake and output will alert the nurse to potential renal and cardiovascular involvement in the inflammatory response system.
    2. Pain control would be under a pain or comfort concept, not immunity.
    3. Keeping the head of the bed elevated is to allow for lung expansion, not to decrease an immune system response, and at "all times" is not realistic.

4. Therapeutic communication addresses a psychosocial problem, not a physiological one.

**TEST-TAKING HINT:** This question is asking the test taker to identify the assessment data unexpected for the disease process. The test taker should be very careful about choosing an option with an absolute in the wording. "Every" means there is no exception to the situation that might apply.

88. 1. SIRS can occur from a burn, but it can also occur as a result of any insult that has a great impact on the body systems.
    2. This is the definition of SIRS.
    3. SIRS can occur from an infection, but it can also occur as a result of any insult that has a great impact on the body systems.
    4. SIRS can occur from an allergic response, but it can also occur as a result of any insult that has a great impact on the body systems.

**TEST-TAKING HINT:** This question is a basic knowledge level definition. The test taker should not refuse to choose an option because it seems too easy.

89. 1. The diagnosis of AIDS is determined by predefined criteria: Positive HIV, a CD4+ count less than 200, and one or more AIDS-defining illnesses, such as a fungal infection candidiasis of the bronchi, lungs, esophagus or *Pneumocystis jiroveci* (carinii) pneumonia (PJP), disseminated extrapulmonary coccidioidomycosis, disseminated extrapulmonary histoplasmosis, cytomegalovirus (CMV) disease other than liver, spleen, or nodes, toxoplasmosis, bacterial *Mycobacterium avium* complex (MAC) or *Mycobacterium kansasii*, or one of the following opportunistic cancers: invasive cervical cancer, Kaposi sarcoma, Burkitt's lymphoma, immunoblastic lymphoma, and primary lymphoma of the brain.
    2. See answer A.
    3. See answer A.
    4. See answer A.

**TEST-TAKING HINT:** This question is asking the test taker to identify the criteria for diagnosing AIDS, which is long and complicated. The test taker should remember any issue that occurs as a result of a failing immune system, opportunistic infections, and cancers.

90. 1. Raw fruits and vegetables and fresh flowers can harbor parasites and bacteria and should be kept out of the client's room.
    2. This addresses the concept of functional ability, not immunity.
    3. This addresses the concept of functional ability, not immunity.
    4. This addresses the concept of perfusion, not immunity.

**TEST-TAKING HINT:** This question is asking the test taker to identify the assessment data unexpected for the disease process. Respiratory problems are a high priority according to Maslow and often warrant immediate intervention.

91. Correct answers are 2 and 3.
    1. Pregnancy is a co-related condition, but being pregnant is not an antecedent for having an HIV infection.
    2. Intravenous drug use does create a risk of becoming HIV positive. When the drug user shares the needle used to inject the drugs, then body fluids are directly injected into the next person using the syringe and needle.
    3. Unprotected sex involves the sharing of body fluids. If using a condom, there is no guarantee the condom will not break, resulting in shared fluids. The more partners, the greater the risk.
    4. Lack of available health care may delay treatment but is not a risk factor for developing an HIV infection.
    5. Adequate bathroom facilities is not an antecedent for HIV infections. HIV dies 6 minutes outside of a host body or growth environment (petri dish).
    6. Many people spend their money on non-essential items; it is not an antecedent for HIV infection.

**TEST-TAKING HINT:** The test taker should answer each option as a true or false question. One option does not eliminate another.

92. 1. Vital signs within normal limits indicate the client is stable and is a realistic and measurable goal.
    2. Six hundred mL of urine in 24 hours average 25 mL per hour, an inadequate amount of urine to indicate renal perfusion (30 mL per hour).
    3. Liver enzymes indicating proper liver function would be to maintain enzymes within normal limits, not elevated.
    4. These blood glucose readings are not within normal limits, indicating the need for intervention to bring the glucose down to a normal range with a sliding scale.

**TEST-TAKING HINT:** This question is asking the test taker to identify the assessment data expected for the stabilization or improvement of the client. The test taker should work out the math to determine if the client's renal output falls within expected guidelines for adequate renal perfusion.

93. 1. This client is at high risk for a negative outcome, including death.
    2. This client has a 20% to 30% chance for survival.
    3. The prognosis for clients diagnosed with MODS is poor, with mortality rates between 80% and 90% if three or more systems fail (Hoffman & Sullivan, 2020).
    4. The rate of recovery is reduced to 20% to 30%.

**TEST-TAKING HINT:** This question is asking the test taker to identify data describing the potential outcomes for a client. In order to answer this question, the test taker must have a working knowledge of the disease process; however, if the test taker is not aware of the information, reading "Multiorgan" could help to eliminate option "1" because ventilators do maintain life; but the longer a client remains on a ventilator, the worse the prognosis. Hospital-acquired infections frequently occur with ventilator clients.

94. 1. This is a systemic problem, not a localized response.
    2. SIRS untreated or unresponsive to treatment progresses to MODS.
    3. SIRS is not limited to myocardial or pulmonary issues.
    4. This is the definition of SIRS.

**TEST-TAKING HINT:** This question is asking the test taker to know the definition of a disease process. The test taker may be able to answer the question by identifying words in the name that describe what is occurring in the body; localized versus the name "systemic" could eliminate option "1."

**95.** 1. MODS is frequently a result of sepsis; the nurse would not question cefazolin, an antibiotic.

2. MODS can involve the development of capillary permeability that allows fluids to "leak" from the capillaries into the interstitial space; the nurse would not question a medication such as furosemide that encourages the fluid to return to the circulatory system for excretion by the kidneys.

3. MODS' effect on the circulatory system includes a decreased blood pressure. The nurse would question administering a medication that decreases blood pressure, such as metoprolol.

4. This is not a high dose of acetaminophen and could be administered for mild pain. The nurse would not question this medication.

**TEST-TAKING HINT:** This question is asking the test taker to identify actions and side effects of medications. It is important for the nurse to recognize when medication would have untoward effects on the client.

**96.** 1. It is 1600, and the vancomycin is not due for 2 hours. Vancomycin is nephrotoxic and ototoxic; the nurse has a 1-hour window before and after the time due, but 1600 is too close to the previous dose.

2. **Furosemide is due now; it should be the medication given first. A diuretic is administered to help the client excrete urine; it is scheduled for this time so that the effects have subsided before bedtime.**

3. Pantoprazole should have been administered in the morning. Because it has not been acknowledged as given, the nurse must research the reason for the client not receiving the medication before administering a potential second dose.

4. Acetaminophen is for mild pain; it could be administered second.

**TEST-TAKING HINT:** This question is asking the test taker to identify actions and side effects of medications. It is important for the nurse to recognize when medication would have untoward effects on the client.

# IMMUNE SYSTEM DISORDERS COMPREHENSIVE EXAMINATION

1. The client is prescribed a prick epicutaneous test to determine the cause of hypersensitivity reactions. Which result indicates the client is hypersensitive to the allergen?
   1. The client reports shortness of breath.
   2. The skin is dry, intact, and without redness.
   3. The pricked blood tests positive for allergens.
   4. A pruritic wheal and erythema occur.

2. Which area of the body should the nurse assess to identify clinical manifestations to support the early diagnosis of Guillain-Barré syndrome?

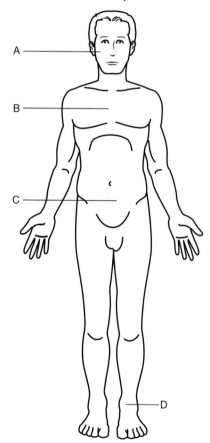

   1. A
   2. B
   3. C
   4. D

3. Which referral should the nurse implement for a client diagnosed with multiple severe allergies?
   1. Registered dietitian.
   2. Occupational therapist.
   3. Recreational therapist.
   4. Social worker.

4. The client diagnosed with an anaphylactic reaction is admitted to the emergency department. Which assessment data indicate the client is not responding to the treatment?
   1. The client has a urinary output of 120 mL in 2 hours.
   2. The client has an AP of 110 and a BP of 90/60.
   3. The client has clear breath sounds and an RR of 26.
   4. The client has hyperactive bowel sounds.

5. Which clinical manifestations should the nurse expect to assess in the client diagnosed with Sjögren's syndrome?
   1. Reports of dry mouth and eyes.
   2. Reports of peripheral joint pain.
   3. Reports of muscle weakness.
   4. Reports of severe itching.

6. Which intervention should the nurse implement for the client diagnosed with systemic sclerosis (scleroderma)?
   1. Instill artificial tears four times a day.
   2. Apply moisturizers to the skin frequently.
   3. Instruct the client on how to apply braces.
   4. Encourage the client to decrease smoking.

7. The nurse is caring for a client with suspected fibromyalgia. Which diagnostic test **confirms** the diagnosis of fibromyalgia?
   1. There is no diagnostic test to confirm fibromyalgia.
   2. A positive antinuclear antibody test.
   3. Magnetic resonance imaging (MRI) shows fibrosis.
   4. A negative erythrocyte sedimentation rate (ESR).

8. The primary nurse is administering medications to the assigned clients. Which client situation **requires immediate** intervention by the charge nurse?
   1. The client diagnosed with congestive heart failure, an apical pulse of 64, and received 0.125 mg digoxin.
   2. The client diagnosed with essential hypertension received a beta blocker, now has a blood pressure of 114/80.
   3. The client diagnosed with myasthenia gravis, 30 minutes late receiving anticholinesterase medication.
   4. The client diagnosed with AIDS having a CD4+ cell count of less than 200 after trimethoprim-sulfamethoxazole administration.

9. Which interventions should the nurse discuss with the female client diagnosed with HIV? **Select all that apply.**
   1. Recommend the client not engage in unprotected sexual activity.
   2. Instruct the client not to inform past sexual partners of HIV status.
   3. Tell the client not to donate blood.
   4. Suggest the client not get pregnant.
   5. Explain the client does not have to tell healthcare personnel of HIV status.

10. Which clinical manifestation should the nurse expect to assess for a client in the recovery stage of Guillain-Barré syndrome?
    1. Decreasing deep tendon reflexes.
    2. Drooping of the eyelids has resolved.
    3. A positive Babinski's reflex.
    4. Descending increase in muscle strength.

11. The client is diagnosed with SLE. Which area of the body in the figure below should the nurse assess for a butterfly rash?

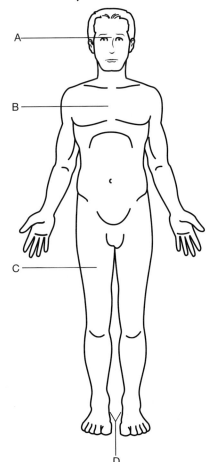

    1. A
    2. B
    3. C
    4. D

12. Which nursing intervention should the nurse include when teaching the client diagnosed with polymyositis? **Select all that apply.**
    1. Explain the care of a percutaneous endoscopic gastrostomy tube.
    2. Discuss the need to take corticosteroids every day.
    3. Instruct to wear long-sleeved shirts when exposed to sunlight.
    4. Teach the importance of strict hand washing.
    5. Encourage daily range-of-motion exercises.

13. The client recently diagnosed with rheumatoid arthritis is prescribed acetylsalicylic acid (ASA). Which comment by the client **warrants immediate** intervention by the nurse?
    1. "I always take the ASA with food."
    2. "If I have dark stools, I will call my HCP."
    3. "Acetylsalicylic acid will not cure my arthritis."
    4. "I have some ringing in my ears."

14. Which clinical manifestation makes the nurse suspect the client has ankylosing spondylitis?
    1. Low back pain at night relieved by activity in the morning.
    2. Ascending paralysis of the lower extremities up to the spinal cord.
    3. A deep ache and stiffness in the hip joints radiating down the legs.
    4. Difficulty changing from lying to sitting position, especially at night.

15. The client diagnosed with multiple sclerosis is having trouble maintaining balance. Which intervention should the nurse discuss with the client?
    1. Discuss obtaining a motorized wheelchair for the client.
    2. Teach the client to stand with the feet slightly apart.
    3. Encourage the client to narrow the base area of support.
    4. Explain the need to balance activity with rest.

16. The nurse is caring for the client diagnosed with AIDS dementia. Which action by the UAP **requires** intervention by the RN?
    1. The UAP is helping the client to sit on the bedside chair.
    2. The UAP is wearing sterile gloves when bathing the client.
    3. The UAP is helping the client shave and brush the teeth.
    4. The UAP is providing a back massage to the client.

17. Which assessment data should make the nurse suspect the client has chronic allergies?
    1. Jaundiced sclera and jaundiced palms of hands.
    2. Pale, boggy, edematous nasal mucosa.
    3. Lacy white plaques on the oral mucosa.
    4. Purple or blue patches on the face.

18. The client has had an anaphylactic reaction to insect venom, a bee sting. Which discharge instruction should the nurse discuss with the client?
    1. Take a corticosteroid dose pack when stung by a bee.
    2. Take antihistamines prior to outdoor activities.
    3. Use a cromolyn sodium inhaler prophylactically.
    4. Carry a bee sting kit, especially when going outside.

19. The client diagnosed with AIDS dementia is referred to hospice. Which intervention has the **highest priority** when caring for the client in the home?
    1. Assess the client's social support network.
    2. Identify the client's usual coping methods.
    3. Have consistent uninterrupted time with the client.
    4. Discuss and complete an advance directive.

20. The client diagnosed with multiple sclerosis is prescribed baclofen. Which statement by the client indicates the client **needs more** teaching?
    1. "This medication may cause drowsiness, so I need to be careful."
    2. "I should not drink any type of alcohol or take any antihistamines."
    3. "I will increase the fiber in my diet and increase fluid intake."
    4. "I stopped taking the medication because I can't afford it."

21. Which intervention has the **highest priority** when caring for a client diagnosed with rheumatoid arthritis?
    1. Encourage the client to verbalize feelings about the disease process.
    2. Discuss the effects this disease has on the client's career and life roles.
    3. Instruct the client to perform the most important activities in the morning.
    4. Teach the client proper use of hot and cold therapy to provide pain relief.

22. Which statement indicates the female client diagnosed with SLE **understands** the discharge instructions?
    1. "I should wear sunscreen with at least a 5 SPF."
    2. "I am not going to any activities with large crowds."
    3. "I should not get pregnant because I have SLE."
    4. "I must avoid using hypoallergenic products."

23. Which is the **highest priority** nursing intervention for the client having an anaphylactic reaction?
    1. Administer parenteral epinephrine.
    2. Prepare for immediate endotracheal intubation.
    3. Provide a calm assurance when caring for the client.
    4. Establish and maintain a patent airway.

24. Which discharge instruction should the nurse implement for the client newly diagnosed with myasthenia gravis (MG)? **Select all that apply.**
    1. Identify specific measures to help avoid fatigue and undue stress.
    2. Instruct the client to pad bony prominences, especially the sacral area.
    3. Discuss complementary therapies to help manage pain.
    4. Explain that having a splenectomy may help control the clinical manifestations.
    5. Refer the client to the Myasthenia Gravis Foundation of America.

25. Which clinical manifestations make the nurse suspect the **most common** opportunistic infection in the female client diagnosed with AIDS?
    1. Fever, cough, and shortness of breath.
    2. Oral thrush, esophagitis, and vaginal candidiasis.
    3. Abdominal pain, diarrhea, and weight loss.
    4. Painless violet lesions on the face and tip of the nose.

26. The client is experiencing an anaphylactic reaction to bee venom. Which interventions should the nurse implement? **Rank in order of priority.**
    1. Establish a patent airway.
    2. Administer epinephrine IVP.
    3. Start an IV with 0.9% saline.
    4. Teach the client to carry an epinephrine auto-injector when outside.
    5. Administer diphenhydramine IVP.

1. 1. This is a sign of an anaphylactic reaction to an allergen and will not happen during this test because of the small amount of allergen used.
   2. This indicates a negative test, and the client is not sensitive to the allergen.
   3. The skin reaction, not the blood pricked, indicates a positive or negative test.
   4. **During this test, a drop of a diluted allergenic extract is placed on the skin and then the skin is punctured through the drop. A positive test causes a localized pruritic wheal and erythema, which occurs in 5 to 20 minutes.**

2. 1. Head clinical manifestations are not found early in the diagnosis.
   2. Chest clinical manifestations are not found early in the diagnosis.
   3. Abdominal clinical manifestations are not found early in the diagnosis.
   4. **The presenting clinical manifestation of a client diagnosed with Guillain-Barré syndrome is ascending paralysis starting in the lower extremities.**

3. 1. **A dietitian could help the client with any necessary dietary changes for food allergies and with ways to continue to meet nutritional needs.**
   2. An occupational therapist addresses the client's ability to perform activities of daily living.
   3. A recreational therapist works in a psychiatric setting or rehabilitation setting and assists with the client's therapeutic recreational activities.
   4. A social worker addresses the client's financial needs.

4. 1. Urinary output of greater than 30 mL/hr is within normal limits and indicates the client is responding to treatment.
   2. **These vital signs indicate shock, which is a medical emergency and requires immediate intervention.**
   3. Clear breath sounds indicate response to treatment, and although the RR is increased, this could be the result of anxiety or fear.
   4. The client's bowel sounds are not significant data to determine the client's response to treatment.

5. 1. **Sjögren's syndrome is an autoimmune disorder causing inflammation and dysfunction of exocrine glands throughout the body. Dry mouth and eyes are some of the clinical manifestations.**
   2. Peripheral joint pain may be a clinical manifestation of rheumatoid arthritis.
   3. Muscle weakness is a clinical manifestation of a variety of disease processes and syndromes but not of Sjögren's syndrome.
   4. Severe itching is not a clinical manifestation of this syndrome.

6. 1. Artificial tears are appropriate for a client diagnosed with Sjögren's syndrome.
   2. **Nursing care addresses measures to maintain skin integrity and moisturizers help prevent dryness and cracking; once skin elasticity is lost, it cannot be regained.**
   3. Braces are not prescribed for the client diagnosed with scleroderma.
   4. The client should stop smoking, not just decrease smoking, because of the vasoconstrictive effect of nicotine and the respiratory effects of the disease.

7. 1. **The diagnosis of fibromyalgia is based on history and physical assessment. There is no laboratory or diagnostic test for fibromyalgia. However, tests may be performed to rule out other diagnoses.**
   2. This test is not used to diagnose fibromyalgia.
   3. An MRI is not used to diagnose fibromyalgia.
   4. An ESR does not support the diagnosis of fibromyalgia.

8. 1. An apical heart rate of fewer than 60 bpm warrants intervention if the primary nurse gave the digoxin, a cardiac glycoside.
   2. A blood pressure of less than 90/60 warrants intervention if the primary nurse gave the beta blocker medication.
   3. **The anticholinesterase medication must be administered exactly on time, so increased strength can occur during an activity such as eating or grooming. There are very few medications administered exactly on time, but this is one of them.**

4. The client diagnosed with AIDS receives prophylactic antibiotic treatment, trimethoprim-sulfamethoxazole, for *Pneumocystis* pneumonia (PCP) when the CD4+ count is less than 200 to 300.

9. **Correct answers are 1, 3, 4, and 5.**
   1. HIV is transmitted via sexual activity.
   2. HIV is transmitted via sexual activity, and the client may have been HIV positive for up to a year and not aware of it, so all past sexual partners should be informed of the HIV status.
   3. Blood donations are screened and excluded for this virus from a client diagnosed with HIV. This is because the virus can be transmitted to clients receiving the blood.
   4. HIV can be transmitted to the fetus from the pregnant woman with HIV.
   5. The client *should* tell the HCP, especially dentists, about the HIV status, but the client does not have to tell health-care personnel about the HIV status. Health-care personnel should always follow standard precautions.

10. 1. This occurs in the acute stage of Guillain-Barré syndrome.
    2. This indicates the client diagnosed with myasthenia gravis is getting better.
    3. A positive Babinski's reflex in an adult client is abnormal and indicates neurological deficits.
    4. The recovery stage may take from several months to 2 years, and muscle strength and function return in descending order.

11. 1. The client diagnosed with SLE often has a reddened area over both cheeks known as a butterfly rash; it is diagnostic of a client with SLE.
    2. The client does not have a butterfly rash on the chest area.
    3. The client does not have a butterfly rash on the upper thigh area.
    4. The client diagnosed with SLE does not have a butterfly rash on the feet.

12. **Correct answers are 2 and 5.**
    1. The client is at risk for aspiration as a result of muscle weakness, but modifications of dietary needs address this concern. The client does not require a PEG tube.
    2. Polymyositis is a systemic connective tissue disorder characterized by inflammation of connective tissues and muscle

fibers and is treated with long-term corticosteroid therapy. Adrenal insufficiency may occur if the client quits taking the corticosteroid.
    3. Sunlight does not cause an exacerbation or irritation of polymyositis.
    4. The client is not at risk for developing an infection, and an infection will not exacerbate the client's medical condition.
    5. Daily range-of-motion exercises, particularly of the shoulders and gentle exercises in a swimming pool, are helpful in keeping the joints supple (Muscular Dystrophy Association, 2019).

13. 1. Acetylsalicylic acid, or ASA (aspirin), a nonsteroidal anti-inflammatory medication, should be taken with food to prevent gastrointestinal upset.
    2. Daily aspirin is used as an anticoagulant; therefore, abnormal bleeding should be reported to the HCP.
    3. ASA, a nonsteroidal anti-inflammatory medication, is used to reduce the inflammatory process and manage the clinical manifestations, but it does not stop the disease process.
    4. Tinnitus (ringing in the ears) is a sign of aspirin toxicity, and the client should be instructed to decrease the aspirin dosage or stop taking ASA, a nonsteroidal anti-inflammatory medication, altogether. The client should be instructed to contact the HCP.

14. 1. Ankylosing spondylitis is a chronic inflammatory arthritis that primarily affects the spinal cord. The client reports intermittent bouts of low back pain with the pain worse at night, followed by morning stiffness relieved by activity.
    2. Ascending paralysis makes the nurse suspect Guillain-Barré syndrome.
    3. A deep ache and stiffness may indicate osteoarthritis, which occurs in weight-bearing joints.
    4. This is not a clinical manifestation of ankylosing spondylitis.

15. 1. Walkers or canes may be weighted to provide support and balance for the client; a wheelchair should be used as a last resort.
    2. Standing with the feet slightly apart widens the client's base of support and helps decrease balance problems.

3. The client should widen the base area of support by standing with the feet slightly apart. Narrowing the base of support does not help.

4. This intervention addresses fatigue, which does not cause balance problems.

16. 1. This action is appropriate and does not require any intervention by the RN.
   2. **The UAP should wear nonsterile gloves, not sterile gloves. Wearing sterile gloves is not cost-effective.**
   3. The client has dementia, so helping the client with activities of daily living is appropriate to enable the client to maintain as much independence as possible.
   4. This is an excellent intervention to help prevent skin breakdown; it is relaxing for the client and does not require intervention from the RN.

17. 1. This may indicate a hemolytic reaction.
   2. **Pale, boggy, edematous nasal mucosa indicates chronic allergies.**
   3. This may indicate hemolysis or immune deficiency.
   4. This may indicate Kaposi's sarcoma.

18. 1. Corticosteroids may be used in both systemic and topical forms for many types of hypersensitivity responses but must be ordered by an HCP and are not automatically taken after a bee sting.
   2. Antihistamines are the major class of drugs used to treat hypersensitivity responses, but they are not taken prophylactically. They are used when a reaction occurs.
   3. Cromolyn sodium (Intal) inhaler treats allergic rhinitis and asthma prophylactically. It does not help bee stings or insect bites.
   4. **The kit usually includes an auto-injectable epinephrine (EpiPen) and an epinephrine nebulizer, which allows prompt self-treatment for any future exposures to insect venom or other potential allergen exposure.**

19. 1. This will identify some people able to help support the client, but it is not the highest priority.
   2. This will help the nurse identify methods that worked previously in stressful situations and may help the client deal with this disease.
   3. **Developing a therapeutic relationship with the client is a priority because the client probably has less than 6 months**

to live. All the other interventions can be implemented, but establishing a therapeutic relationship will allow the nurse to discuss and implement additional interventions.
   4. An advance directive is important, and unless the client is declared legally incompetent in a court of law, the client can complete an advance directive, but establishing a therapeutic relationship with the client is the priority.

20. 1. Muscle relaxants have sedative effects, so appropriate safety measures should be taken.
   2. The client should avoid central nervous system depressants because they can increase the sedative effects of the muscle relaxant baclofen (Lioresal).
   3. This will help prevent constipation, which is a side effect of this medication.
   4. **The muscle relaxant baclofen (Lioresal) must be tapered over 1 to 2 weeks when discontinuing because sudden withdrawal may cause seizures and paranoid ideation.**

21. 1. Rheumatoid arthritis is a chronic illness, and verbalization of feelings is helpful in dealing with disease processes, but it is not the highest priority intervention.
   2. This helps the client accept the disease process and body changes and helps the client to begin to identify strategies for coping with them, but it is not the highest priority intervention.
   3. Helping the client prioritize activities helps the client maintain independence as long as possible.
   4. **Pain is a priority over psychological problems and activity; remember Maslow's hierarchy of needs.**

22. 1. A sunscreen with an SPF of at least 30 should be used by the client diagnosed with SLE.
   2. **The client diagnosed with SLE is at risk for infections and should avoid large crowds.**
   3. Pregnancy is not contraindicated in most women diagnosed with SLE.
   4. The client diagnosed with SLE *should* use hypoallergenic products and should not use irritating soaps, shampoos, or chemicals.

23. 1. Epinephrine, an adrenergic agonist, is the drug of choice for an anaphylactic reaction. It is a potent vasoconstrictor and bronchodilator, counteracting the effects of histamine, but this is not the priority intervention.
2. This is an important intervention, but it is not the priority intervention.
3. Decreasing the client's anxiety is important, but it is not the priority intervention.
4. Establishing a patent airway is a priority because facial angioedema, bronchospasm, and laryngeal edema occur with an anaphylactic reaction. Inserting a nasopharyngeal or oropharyngeal airway is the priority intervention to save the client's life.

24. Correct answers are 1 and 5.
1. The client must use measures to help prevent fatigue, which increases the depletion of acetylcholine and causes muscle weakness.
2. The client diagnosed with MG is not on strict bedrest, and impaired skin integrity is not an expected complication of this disease process, especially in the early stages.
3. Pain is not an expected report of clients diagnosed with MG.
4. A thymectomy, not a splenectomy, may be recommended. Approximately 75% of clients diagnosed with MG have dysplasia of the thymus gland.
5. The Myasthenia Gravis Foundation of America (MYGFA) provides education and resources for clients and their families (Myasthenia Gravis Foundation of America, 2019).

25. 1. *Pneumocystis* pneumonia occurs in approximately 75% to 80% of clients diagnosed with AIDS. Clinical manifestations include fever, cough, and shortness of breath.
2. This is an opportunistic infection, but it is not the most common infection.
3. These are clinical manifestations of *Mycobacterium avium* complex, which affects up to 25% of clients with AIDS, but it is not the most common opportunistic infection.
4. These are clinical manifestations of Kaposi's sarcoma, which is the most common cancer associated with AIDS; it is not an infectious disease.

26. Correct order is 1, 3, 2, 5, 4.
1. The airway is always the first priority for any process in which the airway might be compromised.
3. The nurse should start an IV so medications can be administered to treat the anaphylactic reaction.
2. Epinephrine, an adrenergic agonist, is the drug of choice for the treatment of anaphylaxis. The medication is administered every 10 to 15 minutes until the reaction has subsided. Epinephrine is given for its vasoconstrictive action.
5. Diphenhydramine (Benadryl), an antihistamine, is given to block histamine release, reducing capillary permeability.
4. Teaching about epinephrine autoinjector (EpiPen) use is important to prevent or treat further reactions, but this will be done after the crisis is over.

# Sensory Deficits

**14**

*The eye sees what the mind is prepared to comprehend.*

—Henri Bergson

Some sensory deficits occur with normal aging, whereas others are the result of specific disease processes. Problems involving the senses—sight, hearing, smell, taste, touch—arise from many sources. Some are inflammatory or infectious, or both (otitis); some are the result of a specific disease process (cataract, glaucoma); and still others are the result of the normal aging process (decreased peripheral vision, decreased sense of smell). Many of these diseases and disorders can be treated with appropriate medical-surgical interventions. Still others can be addressed through safety precautions (smoke alarms) and assistive devices (hearing aids). The nurse must be familiar with how to assess the sensory system, identify specific problems, and help in the care of clients diagnosed with these problems.

## KEYWORDS

| | |
|---|---|
| Amsler grid | Otoscope |
| Cataract | Ototoxic |
| Enucleation | Perforation |
| Glaucoma | Presbycusis |
| Intraocular | Ptosis |
| Macular degeneration | Retrobulbar |
| Ménière's disease | Snellen chart |
| Myopia | Stapedectomy |
| Nystagmus | Tinnitus |
| Otitis | Tympanic membrane |
| Otorrhea | Vertigo |

## PRACTICE QUESTIONS

### Eye Disorders

1. The client is diagnosed with glaucoma. Which symptom should the nurse expect the client to report?
   1. Loss of peripheral vision.
   2. Floating spots in the vision.
   3. A yellow haze around everything.
   4. A curtain coming across the vision.

2. The client is scheduled for a right-eye cataract removal surgery in 5 days. Which **preoperative** instruction should be discussed with the client?
   1. Administer dilating drops to both eyes for 72 hours before surgery.
   2. Before surgery do not lift or push any objects heavier than 15 pounds.
   3. Make arrangements for being in the hospital for at least 3 days.
   4. Avoid taking any type of medication which may cause bleeding, such as aspirin.

3. The client is postoperative retinal detachment surgery with pneumatic retinopexy. Which intervention should the nurse implement **first**?
   1. Teach the signs of increased intraocular pressure.
   2. Position the client as prescribed by the surgeon.
   3. Assess the eye for findings of complications.
   4. Explain the importance of follow-up visits.

4. The 65-year-old client is diagnosed with macular degeneration. Which statements by the client indicate the client **understands** the discharge teaching? **Select all that apply.**
   1. "I should use magnification devices as much as possible."
   2. "I will look at my Amsler grid at least twice a week."
   3. "I need to use low-watt light bulbs in my house."
   4. "I am going to contact a low-vision center to evaluate my home."
   5. "I will take my ordered nutritional supplements daily."

5. The nurse is at a local park and sees a young man on the ground after falling with a stick lodged in his eye. Which intervention should the nurse implement at the scene?
   1. Carefully remove the stick from the eye.
   2. Stabilize the stick as best as possible.
   3. Flush the eye with water if available.
   4. Place the young man in a high-Fowler's position.

6. The employee health nurse is teaching a class titled "Preventing Eye Injury." Which information should be discussed in the class?
   1. Read instructions thoroughly before using tools and working with chemicals.
   2. Wear some type of glasses when working around flying fragments.
   3. Always wear a protective helmet with eye shield around dust particles.
   4. Pay close attention to the surroundings so eye injuries will be prevented.

7. The 65-year-old male client is describing blurred vision and reports his glasses need to be cleaned all the time. The client denies any eye pain. Which eye disorder should the nurse suspect the client has?
   1. Corneal dystrophy.
   2. Conjunctivitis.
   3. Diabetic retinopathy.
   4. Cataracts.

8. The nurse is administering eyedrops to the client. Which guidelines should the nurse adhere to when instilling the drops into the eye? **Select all that apply.**
   1. Do not touch the tip of the medication container to the eye.
   2. Apply gentle pressure on the outer canthus of the eye.
   3. Apply sterile gloves before instilling eyedrops.
   4. Hold the lower lid down and instill drops into the conjunctiva.
   5. Gently pat the skin to absorb excess eyedrops on the cheek.

9. The client has had an enucleation of the left eye. Which intervention should the nurse implement?
   1. Discuss the need for special eyeglasses.
   2. Refer the client for an ocular prosthesis.
   3. Help the client obtain a guide dog.
   4. Teach the client how to instill eyedrops.

10. The client diagnosed with glaucoma is prescribed a miotic cholinergic medication. Which data indicate the medication has been **effective**?
    1. No redness or irritation of the eyes.
    2. A decrease in intraocular pressure.
    3. The pupil reacts briskly to light.
    4. The client denies any type of floaters.

11. The client is scheduled for laser-assisted in situ keratomileusis (LASIK) surgery for severe myopia. Which instructions should the nurse discuss before the client's discharge from the clinic? **Select all that apply.**
    1. Wear bilateral eye patches for 3 days.
    2. Wear sunglasses if outside in the daytime.
    3. Do not read any material for at least 1 week.
    4. Instill ophthalmic drops as demonstrated.
    5. Avoid swimming in pools or lakes for 1 week.

12. The client comes to the emergency department after splashing chemicals into the eyes. Which intervention should the nurse implement **first**?
    1. Have the client move the eyes in all directions.
    2. Administer a broad-spectrum antibiotic.
    3. Irrigate the eyes with normal saline solution.
    4. Determine when the client had a tetanus shot.

## Ear Disorders

13. Which statement indicates to the nurse the client is experiencing some hearing loss?
    1. "I clean my ears every day after I take a shower."
    2. "I keep turning up the sound on my television."
    3. "My ears hurt, especially when I yawn."
    4. "I get dizzy when I get up from the chair."

14. Which risk factors should the nurse discuss with the client concerning reasons for hearing loss? **Select all that apply.**
    1. Perforation of the tympanic membrane.
    2. Chronic exposure to loud noises.
    3. Recurrent ear infections.
    4. Use of nephrotoxic medications.
    5. Multiple piercings in the auricle.

15. The nurse is caring for a client diagnosed with acute otitis media. Which findings support this medical diagnosis?
    1. Unilateral pain in the ear.
    2. Green, foul-smelling drainage.
    3. Sensation of congestion in the ear.
    4. Reports of hearing loss.

16. The client diagnosed with chronic otitis media is scheduled for a mastoidectomy. Which discharge teaching should the nurse discuss with the client?
    1. Instruct the client to blow the nose with the mouth closed.
    2. Explain the client will never be able to hear from the ear.
    3. Instill ophthalmic drops in both ears and then insert a cotton ball.
    4. Do not allow water to enter the ear for 6 weeks.

17. The client is diagnosed with Ménière's disease. Which statement indicates the client **understands** the medical management for this disease?
    1. "After intravenous antibiotic therapy, I will be cured."
    2. "I will have to use a hearing aid for the rest of my life."
    3. "I must adhere to a low-sodium diet, 2,000 mg/day."
    4. "I should sleep with the head of my bed elevated."

18. The client is reporting ringing in the ears. Which data are **most appropriate** for the nurse to document in the client's EHR?
    1. Reports of vertigo.
    2. Reports of otorrhea.
    3. Reports of tinnitus.
    4. Reports of presbycusis.

19. Which statement **best** describes the scientific rationale for the nurse holding the otoscope with the hand in a pencil-hold position when examining the client's ear?

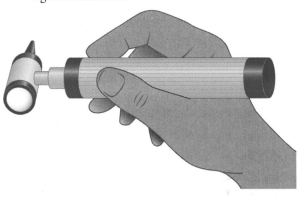

    1. It is usually the most comfortable position to hold the otoscope.
    2. This allows the best visualization of the tympanic membrane.
    3. This prevents inserting the otoscope too far into the external ear.
    4. It ensures the nurse will not cause pain when examining the ear.

20. The nurse is preparing to administer otic drops into an adult client's right ear. Which intervention should the nurse implement?
    1. Grasp the earlobe and pull back and out when putting drops in the ear.
    2. Insert the eardrops without touching the outside of the ear.
    3. Instruct the client to close the mouth and blow before instilling drops.
    4. Pull the auricle down and back before instilling drops.

21. Which medication should the nurse recognize as potentially ototoxic for the client?

| Client: Mr. A.C. | MR#: 1234567 | Date: Today |
|---|---|---|
| Medication | 0701–1900 | 1901–0700 |
| Amlodipine 5 mg po | 0900 | |
| Gentamicin 80 mg IVPB q 8 hours | 0900 1700 | 0100 |
| Methylprednisolone 40 mg IV push q 6 hours | 0900 1500 | 2100 0300 |
| Furosemide 40 mg po daily | 0900 | |

1. Amlodipine.
2. Gentamicin.
3. Methylprednisolone.
4. Furosemide.

22. Which teaching instruction should the nurse discuss with students on the high school swim team when discussing how to prevent external otitis?
1. Do not wear tight-fitting swim caps.
2. Avoid using silicone earplugs while swimming.
3. Use a drying agent in the ear after swimming.
4. Insert a bulb syringe into each ear to remove excess water.

23. The client comes to the clinic and is diagnosed with otitis media. Which intervention should the clinic nurse include in the discharge teaching?
1. Instruct the client not to take any over-the-counter pain medication.
2. Encourage the client to apply cold packs to the affected ear.
3. Tell the client to call the HCP if an abrupt relief of ear pain occurs.
4. Wear a protective earplug in the affected ear.

24. The client is scheduled for ear surgery. Which statement indicates the client **needs more** preoperative teaching concerning the surgery?
1. "If I have to sneeze or blow my nose, I will do it with my mouth open."
2. "I may get dizzy after the surgery, so I must be careful when walking."
3. "I will probably have some hearing loss after surgery, but my hearing will return."
4. "I can shampoo my hair the day after surgery as long as I am careful."

# CONCEPTS

The concepts covered in this chapter focus on sensory perception. Exemplars that are covered are eye and ear disorders. Interrelated concepts of the nursing process, assessment, and critical thinking are covered throughout the questions.

25. The nurse is observing the client administer the prescribed eye drops. Which intervention should the nurse implement?
1. Praise the client for instilling the eyedrops as recommended.
2. Remind the client to instill the eyedrops from 0.5 to 0.8 inches above the eye.
3. Ask the client if the eye drops have been warmed to room temperature.
4. Teach the client to instill the eyedrops in the upper conjunctival sac.

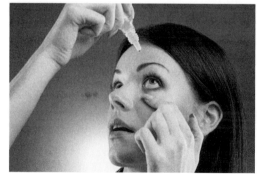

26. The nurse is administering eardrops to a 6-year-old client. Which indicates the nurse is aware of the correct method for instilling eardrops to a child?
    1. Pull the pinna upward only to instill the eardrops.
    2. Pull the pinna to a neutral position to instill the eardrops.
    3. Pull the pinna upward and backward before instilling the drops.
    4. Pull the pinna downward and forward to instill the drops.

27. The nurse is instilling eye ointment. Which should the nurse perform before instilling the medication depicted in the image?

    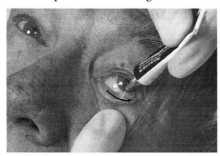

    1. Have the client close the eye tightly to rid the eye of tears.
    2. Place the nurse's nondominant hand on the client's eyebrow.
    3. Discard the first bead of ointment, then instill the ointment.
    4. Ask the client to look down toward the floor.

28. The nurse is assessing a client and performs a whisper test. Which should the nurse implement? **Rank in order of performance.**
    1. Have the client cover the ear not being tested.
    2. Stand 12 to 24 inches to the side of the client.
    3. Explain to the client to repeat what the nurse says.
    4. Repeat the test for the opposite ear.
    5. Determine the client's willingness to participate in the test.

29. The nurse is caring for a client diagnosed with a cerebrovascular accident (CVA). Which assessment information should the nurse determine **first** when placing the client in the assigned room?

1. Determine if the client has a loss of vision in the same half of each visual field.
2. Find out if the client prefers the bed by the window or by the bathroom.
3. Request dietary to place the meat at 1200 on each plate and vegetables at 0900 and 1500.
4. Request a physical therapy consult to assess the client's mobility issues.

30. The elderly client has undergone a right-eye cataract removal with an intraocular implant. Which discharge instructions should the nurse teach the client?
    1. Have the client demonstrate placing the otic drops in the ear.
    2. Teach the client to instill the eyedrops as prescribed.
    3. Remind the client to keep the lights in the home low at all times.
    4. Encourage the client to sleep on two pillows at night.

31. The nurse is assessing a client with a "pinpoint" pupil reaction bilaterally and no constriction of the pupils when a light is shined on the eye. Which should the nurse document in the client's EHR?

    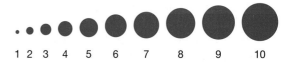

    1. The pupillary response is poor.
    2. Pupils 1 mm, equal and nonreactive to light.
    3. Pupils 2 to 3 mm and nonconstrictive to light.
    4. Pupils are barely open and don't constrict to light.

32. The emergency department nurse is assessing a client with a needle in the sclera of the right eyeball just below the iris. Which should the nurse implement **first**?
    1. Remove the needle with tweezers.
    2. Notify an ophthalmologist to care for the client.
    3. Stabilize the right eye and place a patch over the left eye.
    4. Irrigate the right eye to wash the needle out of the eye.

## Eye Disorders

1. 1. In glaucoma, the client is often unaware of the disease until the client experiences blurred vision, halos around lights, difficulty focusing, or loss of peripheral vision. Glaucoma is often called the "silent thief."
   2. Floating spots in the vision is a symptom of retinal detachment.
   3. A yellow haze around everything is a report of clients diagnosed with digoxin toxicity.
   4. The report of a curtain coming across vision is a symptom of retinal detachment.

**TEST-TAKING HINT:** The findings of eye disorders are confusing. The test taker must know which reports will be made by the client diagnosed with a specific eye disorder.

2. 1. Dilating drops are administered every 10 minutes for four doses 1 hour before surgery, not for 3 days before surgery.
   2. Lifting and pushing objects should be avoided after surgery, not before surgery.
   3. All types of cataract removal surgery are usually done in day surgery.
   4. Anticoagulation therapy is withheld, including aspirin, NSAIDs, and warfarin (Coumadin) to reduce retrobulbar hemorrhage.

**TEST-TAKING HINT:** The test taker must notice the adjectives; these descriptors are important when selecting a correct answer. The test taker should notice "preoperative" and "before surgery."

3. 1. This should be done, but it is not the first intervention the nurse should implement.
   2. The client will have to be specifically positioned to make the gas bubble float into the best position; some clients must lie face down or on their side for days, but it is not the first intervention.
   3. The nurse's priority must be the assessment of complications, which include increased intraocular pressure, endophthalmitis, development of another retinal detachment, or loss of turgor in the eye (Stewart & Chan, 2018).
   4. Follow-up visits are important, but this is not the first intervention the nurse should implement.

**TEST-TAKING HINT:** When the question asks which intervention should be implemented first, all four answer options are possible interventions, but only one should be implemented first. Remember to apply the nursing process to help select the correct answer. Assessment is the first part of the nursing process.

4. Correct answers are 1, 2, 4, and 5.
   1. Magnifying devices used with activities such as threading a needle will help the client's vision; therefore, this statement indicates the client understands the teaching.
   2. An Amsler grid is a tool to assess macular degeneration, often providing the earliest sign of a worsening condition. If the lines of the grid become distorted or faded, the client should call the ophthalmologist.
   3. Macular degeneration is the most common cause of visual loss in people older than age 60 years. Any intervention that helps increase vision should be included in the teaching, such as bright lighting, not decreased lighting.
   4. Low-vision centers will send representatives to the client's home or work to make recommendations about improving lighting, thereby improving the client's vision and safety.
   5. Taking nutritional supplements such as a combination of certain high-dose vitamins and minerals (vitamin C and E, beta-carotene, zinc, and copper) can protect against age-related macular degeneration or slow the progression (National Eye Institute, 2018).

**TEST-TAKING HINT:** This question is asking which statements indicate the client understands the teaching. It is an alternative format question. The test taker should select more than one option as correct and must select all appropriate options to receive credit for a correct answer. There are no partially correct answers.

5. 1. A foreign object should never be removed at the scene of the accident because this may cause more damage.
   2. The foreign object should be stabilized to prevent further movement, which could cause more damage to the eye.

3. Flushing with water may cause further movement of the foreign object and should be avoided.
4. The person should be kept flat and not in a sitting position because it may dislodge or cause movement of the foreign object.

**TEST-TAKING HINT:** In an emergency situation, the first responder should first "do no harm." The test taker should examine each option and decide what will happen if this option is performed—will it help, harm, or stabilize the client? If the test taker determines one action may not help, then stabilization becomes the priority.

6. 1. Instructions provide precautions and steps to take if eye injuries occur secondary to the use of tools or chemicals.
2. The employee must wear safety glasses, not just any type of glasses, and especially not regular prescription glasses.
3. A protective helmet is used to help prevent sports eye injuries, not work-related injuries.
4. Eye injuries will not be prevented by paying close attention to their surroundings. They are prevented by wearing protective glasses or eye shields.

**TEST-TAKING HINT:** The test taker must make sure what the question is asking and must pay close attention to adjectives. An "employee health nurse" is in the workplace. If the test taker is going to select an option with a word such as "always," "never," or "only," be absolutely sure it is an intervention never questioned. In health care, there are very few absolutes.

7. 1. Corneal dystrophy is an inherited eye disorder occurring at about age 20 and results in decreased vision and the development of blisters; it is usually associated with primary open-angle glaucoma.
2. Conjunctivitis is an inflammation of the conjunctiva, which results in a scratching or burning sensation, itching, and photophobia.
3. Diabetic retinopathy results from deterioration of the small blood vessels nourished by the retina; it leads to blindness.
4. A cataract is a lens opacity or cloudiness, resulting in the findings discussed in the stem of the question.

**TEST-TAKING HINT:** The test taker must know the findings of eye disorders, especially those commonly occurring in the elderly. Option "2" could be ruled out because -*itis* means inflammation, and none of the findings are inflammatory.

8. Correct answers are 1, 4, and 5.
1. Touching the tip of the container to the eye may cause eye injury or an eye infection.
2. Gentle pressure should be applied on the inner canthus, not outer canthus, near the bridge of the nose for 1 or 2 minutes after instilling eyedrops.
3. The nurse should wash hands before and after instilling medications; this is not a sterile procedure.
4. Medication should not be placed directly on the eye but in the lower part of the eyelid.
5. Eyedrops are meant to go in the eye, not on the skin, so the nurse should use a clean tissue to remove excess medication.

**TEST-TAKING HINT:** This is an alternate-type question requiring the test taker to select all the correct options. The test taker should not second-guess the question. The test taker should read each option, and if it is correct, select it.

9. 1. Special eyeglasses are not needed for an enucleation.
2. An enucleation is the removal of the entire eye and part of the optic nerve. An ocular prosthesis will help maintain the shape of the eye socket after the enucleation.
3. The client had the left eye removed but is not blind because the client still has the right eye.
4. The eyeball was totally removed and a pressure dressing was applied; therefore, there will be no need to instill eyedrops.

**TEST-TAKING HINT:** In some questions, the test taker must know the definition of the word ("enucleation") to be able to apply it in a clinical situation.

10. 1. Steroid medication is administered to decrease inflammation.
2. Both systemic and topical medications are used to decrease the intraocular pressure in the eye, which causes glaucoma.
3. Glaucoma does not affect the pupillary reaction.
4. Floaters are a report of clients diagnosed with retinal detachment.

**TEST-TAKING HINT:** To determine the effectiveness of a medication, the nurse must know the findings of the disease process. If the test taker knew glaucoma was the result of an increase in intraocular pressure, then the medication is effective if there was a decrease in intraocular pressure.

11. **Correct answers are 2, 4, and 5.**
    1. The client does not have to wear eye patches after this surgery.
    2. The client should wear sunglasses if outside during the day for the first 24 hours.
    3. The client can read immediately after this surgery but should avoid eye strain for the first 2 to 4 hours.
    4. LASIK surgery is an effective, safe, predictable surgery with minimal postoperative care. Instilling eyedrops can help to lubricate the eye to avoid dryness and discomfort.
    5. The client should avoid swimming pools, hot tubs, lakes, rivers, and the ocean for at least a week after LASIK surgery to help prevent infections.

    **TEST-TAKING HINT: Option "3" has the absolute word "any," so the test taker could eliminate it. LASIK is a corrective surgery with minimal postoperative care.**

12. 1. Movement of the eye should be avoided until the client has received general anesthesia; therefore, this is not the first intervention.
    2. Parenteral broad-spectrum antibiotics are initiated, but not until the eyes are treated first.
    3. Before any further evaluation or treatment, the eyes must be thoroughly flushed with sterile normal saline solution.
    4. Tetanus prophylaxis is recommended for full-thickness ocular wounds.

    **TEST-TAKING HINT: If the test taker is not sure of the answer, the test taker should select the answer directly addressing the client's condition. Options "1" and "3" directly affect the eyes, but when choosing between these two options, the test taker should ask, "How will moving the eyes help treat the eyes?" and then eliminate option "1."**

## Ear Disorders

13. 1. Daily cleaning of the ears does not indicate the client has a hearing loss.
    2. The need to turn up the volume on the television is an early sign of hearing impairment.

3. Pain in the ears is not a clinical manifestation of hearing loss or impairment.
4. This statement may indicate a balance problem secondary to an ear disorder, but it does not indicate a hearing loss.

**TEST-TAKING HINT: If the test taker has no idea of the answer, option "2" is the only answer that has anything to do with sound.**

14. **Correct answers are 1, 2, and 3.**
    1. The tympanic membrane is the eardrum, and if it is punctured, it may lead to hearing loss.
    2. Loud, persistent noise, such as heavy machinery, engines, and artillery, over time may cause noise-induced hearing loss.
    3. Multiple ear infections scar the tympanic membrane, which can lead to hearing loss.
    4. Nephrotoxic means harmful to the kidneys; ototoxic is harmful to the ears.
    5. Multiple pierced earrings do not lead to hearing loss. The auricle (skin attached to the head) is composed mainly of cartilage, except for the fat and subcutaneous tissue in the earlobe.

    **TEST-TAKING HINT: This alternate-type question requires the test taker to select multiple correct answers. Many options can be eliminated as incorrect answers when the test taker knows medical terminology—*nephro*- means kidney-related—and normal anatomy of the body—*auricle* means "skin attached to the head."**

15. 1. Otalgia (ear pain) is experienced by clients diagnosed with otitis media.
    2. Green, foul-smelling drainage supports the diagnosis of external otitis, not of acute otitis media.
    3. A sensation of congestion in the ear supports serous otitis media.
    4. Hearing loss supports a diagnosis of chronic otitis media or serous otitis media.

    **TEST-TAKING HINT: If the test taker were not sure of the answer, the adjective "acute" in the stem should cause the test taker to think "pain," which is included in option "1."**

16. 1. The client should blow the nose with the mouth open to prevent pressure in the eustachian tube.
    2. There may be temporary deafness as a result of postoperative edema, but the hearing will return as the edema subsides.
    3. Ophthalmic drops are used in the eyes, not the ears. Otic drops are used for the ears.

4. Water should be prevented from entering the external auditory canal because it may irritate the surgical incision and is a medium for bacterial growth.

**TEST-TAKING HINT:** The test taker must be aware of adjectives. In option "3," the test taker should know "ophthalmic" refers to the eye, which causes the test taker to eliminate this as a possible answer.

17. 1. Antibiotics will not cure this disease. Surgery is the only cure for Ménière's disease, which may result in permanent deafness as a result of the labyrinth being removed in the surgery.
    2. Ménière's disease does not lead to deafness unless surgery is performed, removing the labyrinth in attempts to eliminate the attacks of vertigo.
    3. Sodium regulates the balance of fluid within the body; therefore, a low-sodium diet is prescribed to help control the symptoms of Ménière's disease.
    4. Sleeping with the head of the bed elevated will not affect Ménière's disease.

**TEST-TAKING HINT:** Sleeping with the HOB elevated is not a medical treatment; therefore, option "4" can be eliminated as a possible answer. The test taker must read the stem carefully.

18. 1. Vertigo is an illusion of movement in which the client reports dizziness.
    2. Otorrhea is drainage of the ear.
    3. Tinnitus is "ringing of the ears." It is a subjective perception of sound with internal origins.
    4. Presbycusis is a progressive hearing loss associated with aging.

**TEST-TAKING HINT:** The test taker familiar with medical terminology can rule out options based on the understanding of medical terms.

19. 1. This is not the rationale for holding the otoscope in this manner.
    2. Holding the otoscope in this manner does not help visualize the membrane any better than holding the otoscope in other ways.
    3. Inserting the speculum of the otoscope into the external ear can cause ear trauma if not done correctly.
    4. If the ear is inflamed, it may be impossible to prevent hurting the client on examination.

**TEST-TAKING HINT:** The scientific rationale is the critical-thinking component of nursing; the test taker must understand the "why" of nursing interventions.

20. 1. This is not the correct way to administer eardrops.
    2. The nurse must straighten the ear canal; therefore, the outside of the ear must be moved.
    3. This will increase pressure in the ear and should not be done before administering eardrops.
    4. This will straighten the ear canal so the eardrops will enter the ear canal and drain toward the tympanic membrane (eardrum).

**TEST-TAKING HINT:** The test taker should notice options "1" and "4" are opposite, which should clue the test taker into either eliminating both or deciding one of these two is the correct answer. Either way, the test taker now has a 50/50 chance of selecting the correct answer.

21. 1. Calcium channel blockers, such as amlodipine, are not going to affect the client's hearing.
    2. Aminoglycoside antibiotics, such as gentamicin, are ototoxic. Overdosage of these medications can cause the client to go deaf, which is why peak and trough serum levels are drawn while the client is taking medication of this type. These antibiotics are also very nephrotoxic.
    3. Steroids, such as methylprednisolone, cause many adverse effects, but damage to the ear is not one of them.
    4. Administering an intravenous push loop diuretic such as furosemide too fast can cause auditory nerve damage, but an oral loop diuretic does not.

**TEST-TAKING HINT:** The test taker must be cautious of adjectives. The designation "po" means "oral" in option "4" and eliminates this option as a possible correct answer.

22. 1. Tight-fitting swim caps or wetsuit hoods should be worn because they prevent water from entering the ear canal.
    2. Silicone earplugs should be worn because they keep water from entering the ear canal without reducing hearing significantly.
    3. A 2% acetic acid solution or 2% boric acid in ethyl alcohol is effective in drying the canal and restoring its normal acidic environment.
    4. A bulb syringe with a Teflon catheter can be used to remove impacted debris from the ear, but it is not used to remove excess water.

**TEST-TAKING HINT:** If the test taker has no idea what the correct answer is, the test taker should evaluate the answer options to see if two are similar. In this question, both options "1" and "2" say not to use ear protectors. Because there cannot be two correct answers, these two could be eliminated as possible correct answers.

23. 1. Mild analgesics such as aspirin or acetaminophen every 4 hours as needed to relieve pain and fever are recommended; aspirin may help decrease inflammation of the ear.
    2. Heat applied to the affected ear is recommended because heat dilates blood vessels, promoting the reabsorption of fluid and reducing edema.
    3. Pain subsiding abruptly may indicate spontaneous perforation of the tympanic membrane within the middle ear and should be reported to the HCP.
    4. Earplugs should not be used in clients diagnosed with otitis media, but cotton balls could be used to keep otic antibiotics in the ear canal.

**TEST-TAKING HINT:** The test taker must use basic principles when answering questions. Cold causes constriction, and heat dilates. Except for aspirin not being administered to children to prevent Reye's syndrome, mild analgesics can be administered for almost any discomfort.

24. 1. Leaving the mouth open when coughing or sneezing will minimize the pressure changes in the middle ear.
    2. Surgery on the ear may disrupt the client's equilibrium, increasing the risk of falling.
    3. Hearing loss secondary to postoperative edema is common after surgery, but the hearing will return after the edema subsides.
    4. **Shampooing, showering, and immersing the head in water are avoided to prevent contamination of the ear canal; therefore, this comment indicates the client does not understand the preoperative teaching.**

**TEST-TAKING HINT:** This is an "except" question. The stem states "needs more teaching"; therefore, three of the options reflect an appropriate understanding of the teaching, and only one indicates a misunderstanding of the teaching.

25. 1. The client is holding the dropper too high. Eyedrops are instilled from 1.5 to 2 cm (0.5–0.8 inch) above the eye.
    2. Eyedrops are instilled from 1.5 to 2 cm (0.5–0.8 inch) above the eye. The client should not hold the dropper too high (Treas et al., 2018).
    3. Eyedrops can be instilled at room temperature or chilled. If a client has trouble recognizing if the drops have been instilled, the nurse can recommend refrigerating the drops so the client can feel when the eyedrops have been administered.
    4. Eyedrops are administered in the lower conjunctival sac.

**TEST-TAKING HINT:** The test taker must remember the basics of medication administration.

26. 1. The pinna should be pulled upward and backward for all clients 3 years of age and older. Before 3 years of age, the pinna is directed upward only.
    2. The pinna should be pulled upward and backward for all clients 3 years of age and older. Before 3 years of age, the pinna is directed upward only.
    3. **The pinna should be pulled upward and backward for all clients 3 years of age and older. Before 3 years of age, the pinna is directed upward only.**
    4. The pinna should be pulled upward and backward for all clients 3 years of age and older. Before 3 years of age, the pinna is directed upward only.

**TEST-TAKING HINT:** The test taker must remember the basics of medication administration.

27. 1. The client should close the eye gently after the ointment is instilled in order for the eyelid to spread the ointment over the eye.
    2. The nurse's nondominant thumb or fingers are placed on the cheekbone to pull the lid down to expose the conjunctival sac.
    3. **The first bead of ointment is considered contaminated and should be discarded. (Callahan, 2015).**
    4. The client should look upward to reduce the amount of blinking during administration.

**TEST-TAKING HINT:** The test taker must remember the basics of medication administration.

28. Correct order is 5, 3, 1, 2, 4.
    5. The client should be offered the opportunity to agree to be tested before any further action is taken.
    3. The nurse should give directions as to what the client is expected to do upon hearing what the nurse says.
    1. The client covers the ear not being tested after the nurse has explained the test.
    2. The nurse should stand to the side but not until talking directly to the client.
    4. One ear at a time is tested.

**TEST-TAKING HINT:** This is a basic assessment tool to determine sensory perception. The test taker should memorize basic tests and normal results.

29. 1. Homonymous hemianopsia (blindness in the same half of each visual field) is a common problem after a stroke. Clients disregard objects in that part of the visual field. The nurse would want to place the client in a room with the bed positioned so that the client will know when someone is entering the room.
    2. Client preference can be taken into consideration but is not a priority.
    3. Requesting dietary to place foods in a certain order will assist the client diagnosed with visual disturbances to know where to find the food on the plate but is not first.
    4. Physical therapy may need to assess the client, but it is not first.

**TEST-TAKING HINT:** The findings of CVA vary, and some of the clinical manifestations may not be immediately observable. The brain impacts the entire body. The test taker must know which symptoms impact the client's daily life.

30. 1. Otic drops go in the ear, not the eye.
    2. Postoperatively the client will be prescribed eyedrops for several weeks; the nurse should teach the client to administer as prescribed.
    3. The light should be brighter for safety.
    4. The client does not need to sleep with the HOB elevated.

**TEST-TAKING HINT:** The test taker must know basic instructions for postoperative clients.

31. 1. Pupil response may be poor, but this is not professionally documented for a clear record of the nurse's observation.
    2. Pinpoint describes the least amount of dilation noted, which is 1 mm. Bilateral means both sides, so equal describes that one side is the same as the other. Nonreactive describes the pupils not constricting. This is clear and concise.
    3. Two to 3 mm is not pinpoint, and nonconstrictive is not describing the response to light.
    4. This is something a layperson might say but is not in professional terms.

**TEST-TAKING HINT:** The findings of eye disorders can be confusing, but the nurse must communicate in professional terminology that all medical personnel can interpret consistently.

32. 1. The nurse should leave the needle where it is but try to make sure the client does not move the eye. The HCP will be the one to remove the obstacle.
    2. The ophthalmologist will need to be notified after the nurse has made sure that the client will not sustain further damage to the eye.
    3. The nurse should try to stabilize the right eye but not do anything that increases the damage to it. The left eye is patched to keep it from moving to see what is going on, and the right eye moves with it.
    4. The nurse should not do anything, including irrigating the eye, that might move the needle and create more damage.

**TEST-TAKING HINT:** The emergency treatment of eye disorders requires the nurse to stabilize the client until the HCP can take care of the situation.

# SENSORY DEFICITS
# COMPREHENSIVE EXAMINATION

1. Which recommendations should the nurse suggest to an older client living alone when discussing normal developmental changes of the olfactory organs? **Select all that apply.**
   1. Suggest installing multiple smoke alarms in the home.
   2. Recommend using a night-light in the hallway and bathroom.
   3. Discuss keeping a high-humidity atmosphere in the bedroom.
   4. Encourage the client to check food expiration dates before eating it.
   5. Have natural gas appliances serviced every year.

2. The older male client tells the nurse, "My spouse says her cooking hasn't changed, but it is bland and tasteless." Which response by the nurse is **most appropriate**?
   1. "Would you like me to talk to your spouse about her cooking?"
   2. "Taste buds change with age, which may be why the food seems bland."
   3. "This happens because the medications sometimes cause a change in taste."
   4. "Why don't you barbecue food on a grill if you don't like your spouse's cooking?"

3. The charge nurse is admitting a 90-year-old client to a long-term care facility. Which intervention should the nurse implement?
   1. Ensure the client's room temperature is cool.
   2. Talk louder to make sure the client hears clearly.
   3. Complete the admission as fast as possible.
   4. Provide extra orientation to the surroundings.

4. Which assessment technique should the nurse implement when assessing the client's cranial nerves for vibration?
   1. Move the big toe up and down and ask in which direction the vibration is felt.
   2. Place a tuning fork on the big toe and ask if the vibrations are felt.
   3. Tap the client's cheek with the finger and determine if vibrations are felt.
   4. Touch the arm with two sharp objects and ask if one vibration or two is felt.

5. Which intervention should the nurse include when conducting an in-service to the ancillary nursing staff on caring for older clients addressing normal developmental sensory changes?
   1. Ensure curtains are open when having the client read written material.
   2. Provide a variety of written material when discussing a procedure.
   3. Assist the client when getting out of the bed and sitting in the chair.
   4. Request a telephone for individuals with hearing impairments for all older clients.

6. Which situation makes the nurse suspect the client has glaucoma?
   1. An automobile accident because the client did not see the car in the next lane.
   2. The cake tasted funny because the client could not read the recipe.
   3. The client has been wearing mismatched clothes and socks.
   4. The client ran a stoplight and hit a pedestrian walking in the crosswalk.

7. The client diagnosed with a retinal detachment has just undergone a pneumatic retinopexy. Which discharge instruction should the nurse include in the teaching?
   1. The client must lie flat with the face down.
   2. The head of the bed must be elevated 45 degrees.
   3. The client should wear sunglasses when outside.
   4. The client should avoid reading for 3 weeks.

8. The nurse is conducting a Weber test on the client suspected of having conductive hearing loss in the left ear. Where should the nurse place the tuning fork when conducting this test?

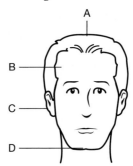

   1. A
   2. B
   3. C
   4. D

9. The student nurse asks the nurse, "Which type of hearing loss involves damage to the cochlea or vestibulocochlear nerve?" Which statement is the **best response** of the RN?
   1. "It is called conductive hearing loss."
   2. "It is called a functional hearing loss."
   3. "It is called a mixed hearing loss."
   4. "It is called sensorineural hearing loss."

10. The client has undergone a bilateral stapedectomy. Which action by the client **warrants immediate** intervention by the nurse?
    1. The client is ambulating without assistance.
    2. The client is sneezing with the mouth open.
    3. There is some slight serosanguineous drainage.
    4. The client reports hearing popping in the affected ear.

11. The female client tells the clinic nurse she is going on a 7-day cruise and is worried about getting motion sickness. Which information should the nurse discuss with the client?
    1. Make an appointment for the client to see the health-care provider.
    2. Recommend getting an over-the-counter scopolamine patch.
    3. Discourage the client to take the trip because she is worried.
    4. Instruct the client to lie down and the motion sickness will go away.

12. The nurse writes the diagnosis "risk for injury related to impaired balance" for the client diagnosed with vertigo. Which nursing intervention should be included in the plan of care?
    1. Provide information about vertigo and its treatment.
    2. Assess for level and type of diversional activity.
    3. Assess for visual acuity and proprioceptive deficits.
    4. Refer the client to a support group and counseling.

13. The nurse is assessing the client's cranial nerves. Which assessment data indicate cranial nerve I is intact?
    1. The client can identify cold and hot on the face.
    2. The client does not have any tongue tremors.
    3. The client has no ptosis of the eyelids.
    4. The client is able to identify a peppermint smell.

14. The older client is reporting abdominal discomfort. Which scientific rationale should the nurse remember when addressing an older client's perception of pain?
    1. Older clients react to pain the same way any other age group does.
    2. The older client usually requires more pain medication.
    3. Reaction to painful stimuli may be decreased with age.
    4. The older client should use the Wong scale to assess pain.

15. Which instruction should the nurse discuss with the client when completing a sensory assessment regarding proprioception?
    1. Instruct the client to lie flat without a pillow during the assessment.
    2. Instruct the client to keep both eyes shut during the assessment.
    3. During the assessment, the client must be in a treatment room.
    4. Keep the lights off during the client's sensory assessment.

16. Which findings should the nurse expect when assessing the client diagnosed with an acoustic neuroma?
    1. Incapacitating vertigo and otorrhea.
    2. Nystagmus and reports of dizziness.
    3. Nausea and vomiting.
    4. Unilateral hearing loss and tinnitus.

17. Which assessment technique should the nurse use to assess the client's optic nerve?
    1. Have the client identify different smells.
    2. Have the client discriminate between sugar and salt.
    3. Have the client read the Snellen chart.
    4. Have the client say "ah" to assess the rise of the uvula.

18. Which referral is **most important** for the nurse to implement for the client diagnosed with permanent hearing loss?
    1. Aural rehabilitation.
    2. Speech therapist.
    3. Social worker.
    4. Vocational rehabilitation.

19. Which instructions should the nurse discuss with the female client diagnosed with viral conjunctivitis? **Select all that apply.**
    1. Contact the HCP if pain occurs.
    2. Do not share towels or linens.
    3. Apply warm compresses to the eyes.
    4. Apply makeup very lightly.
    5. Avoid touching the infected eye.

20. The client is 2 hours postoperative right-ear mastoidectomy. Which assessment data should be reported to the HCP?
    1. Reports of aural fullness.
    2. Hearing loss in the affected ear.

3. No vertigo.

4. Facial drooping.

21. Which behavior by the male client should make the nurse suspect the client has a hearing loss? **Select all that apply.**

    1. The client reports hearing voices in his head.
    2. The client becomes irritable very easily.
    3. The client has difficulty making decisions.
    4. The client's spouse reports he ignores her.
    5. The client does not dominate a conversation.

22. The client diagnosed with cataracts had intraocular lens implants and is being discharged from the day surgery department. Which discharge instructions should the nurse discuss with the client?

    1. Do not push or pull objects heavier than 50 pounds.
    2. Lie on the affected eye with two pillows at night.
    3. Wear glasses or metal eye shields at all times.
    4. Bend and stoop carefully for the rest of your life.

23. The nurse is assessing the client's sensory system. Which assessment data indicate an abnormal stereognosis test?

    1. The client is unable to identify which way the toe is being moved.
    2. The client cannot discriminate between sharp and dull objects.
    3. The toes contract and draw together when the sole of the foot is stroked.
    4. The client is unable to identify a key in hand with both eyes closed.

24. Which statement by the daughter of an 80-year-old female client living alone **warrants immediate** intervention by the nurse?

    1. "I put a night-light in my mother's bedroom."
    2. "I got carbon monoxide detectors for my mother's house."
    3. "I changed my mother's furniture around."
    4. "I got my mother large-print books."

25. The 72-year-old client tells the nurse food does not taste good anymore, and he has lost a little weight. Which information should the nurse discuss with the client?

    1. Suggest using extra seasoning when cooking.
    2. Instruct the client to keep a 7-day food diary.
    3. Refer the client to a dietitian immediately.
    4. Recommend eating three meals a day.

26. The male client diagnosed with type 2 diabetes mellitus tells the nurse he has begun to see yellow spots. Which interventions should the nurse implement? **Rank in order of priority.**

    1. Notify the health-care provider.
    2. Check the client's hemoglobin A1c.
    3. Assess the client's vision using the Amsler grid.
    4. Teach the client about controlling blood glucose levels.
    5. Determine where the spots appear to be in the client's field of vision.

1. Correct answers are 1, 4, and 5.
   1. The decreased sense of smell resulting from atrophy of olfactory organs is a safety hazard, and clients may not be able to smell gas leaks or fire, so the nurse should recommend a carbon monoxide detector and a smoke alarm. This safety equipment is critical for older people.
   2. Night-lights do not address the client's sense of smell.
   3. High humidity may help with breathing, but it does not help the sense of smell.
   4. The client's sense of smell is decreased; therefore, smelling food before eating is not an appropriate intervention. The client should check expiration dates on food and label food with the date when opening.
   5. The client will not be able to smell a natural gas leak; therefore, the client should have any gas appliances serviced yearly and consider a natural gas detector.

2. 1. The nurse needs to discuss possible causes with the client and not talk to the spouse.
   2. The acuity of the taste buds decreases with age, which could cause regular foods to seem bland and tasteless.
   3. Some medications may cause a metallic taste in the mouth, but medication does not cause foods to taste bland.
   4. Telling the client to cook if he doesn't like his spouse's food is an argumentative and judgmental response.

3. 1. Because of altered temperature regulation, the client usually needs a warmer room temperature, not a cooler room temperature.
   2. The nurse should use a low-pitched, normal-volume, clear voice. Talking louder or shouting makes it harder for the client to understand the nurse.
   3. The older client requires adequate time to receive and respond to stimuli, to learn, and to react; therefore, the nurse should take time and not rush the admission.
   4. Sensory isolation resulting from visual and hearing loss can cause confusion, anxiety, disorientation, and misinterpretation of the new environment; therefore, the nurse should provide extra orientation.

4. 1. This assesses proprioception, or position sense; the direction of the toe must be evaluated.
   2. Vibration is assessed by using a low-frequency tuning fork on a bony prominence and asking the client whether the sensation is felt and, if so, when the sensation ceases.
   3. Tapping the cheek assesses for tetany, not cranial nerve involvement.
   4. A two-point discrimination test evaluates the integration of sensation, but it does not assess for vibration.

5. 1. Adequate lighting without a glare should be provided when having the client read written material; therefore, the curtains should be closed, not open.
   2. The nurse should provide short, concise, and concrete material, not a variety of material.
   3. Because fewer tactile cues are received from the bottom of the feet, the client may get confused as to body position and location. Safety is a priority, and assisting the client in getting out of bed and sitting in a chair is appropriate.
   4. This is making a judgment. Not all older clients are hard of hearing, and telephones for people with hearing impairments require special training for the user.

6. 1. Loss of peripheral vision as a result of glaucoma causes the client problems with seeing things on each side, resulting in a "blind spot." This problem can lead to the client having car accidents when switching lanes.
   2. This is indicative of cataracts because clients diagnosed with cataracts have blurred vision and cannot read clearly.
   3. This is indicative of cataracts because there is a color shift to yellow-brown and there is reduced light transmission.
   4. This is indicative of macular degeneration, in which the central vision is affected.

7. 1. If pneumatic retinopexy is utilized to repair retinal detachment, the client will have to be specially positioned to make the gas bubble float into the best position; clients must lie face down or on the side for days.

2. The HOB should not be elevated after this surgery.

3. There is no need for the client to wear sunglasses; this surgery does not cause photophobia.

4. The client does not need to avoid reading.

8. 1. **The tuning fork should be struck to produce vibrations and then placed midline between the ears on top of the head.**

    2. The right temple area is not an appropriate place to assess for conductive hearing loss.

    3. The right occipital area is not the appropriate place to place the tuning fork; this is the area behind the ear where the Rinne test is performed.

    4. The chin area is not the appropriate area to put the tuning fork.

9. 1. Conductive hearing loss results from an external ear disorder, such as impacted cerumen, or a middle ear disorder, such as otitis media or otosclerosis.

    2. Functional (psychogenic) hearing loss is nonorganic and unrelated to detectable structural changes in the hearing mechanisms. It is usually a manifestation of an emotional disturbance.

    3. Mixed hearing loss involves both conductive loss and sensorineural loss. It results from dysfunction of air and bone conduction.

    4. **Sensorineural hearing loss is described in the stem of the question. It involves damage to the cochlea or vestibulocochlear nerve.**

10. 1. **Balance disturbance, or true vertigo, rarely occurs with other middle-ear surgical procedures, but it does occur for a short time after a stapedectomy. Safety is an important issue, and ambulating without assistance requires intervention by the nurse.**

    2. Pressure changes in the middle ear will be minimal if the client sneezes or blows the nose with the mouth open instead of closed.

    3. Slightly bloody or serosanguineous drainage is normal after ear surgery.

    4. Popping and crackling in the operative ear is normal for about 3 to 5 weeks after surgery.

11. 1. This is not a condition requiring an appointment with the health-care provider.

    2. **Anticholinergic medications, such as scopolamine patches, can be**

recommended by the nurse; this is not prescribing. Motion sickness is a disturbance of equilibrium caused by constant motion.

3. Motion sickness can be controlled with medication, and it may not even occur. Therefore, discussing canceling the trip is not providing the client with appropriate information.

4. This is providing the client with false information. Lying down may or may not help motion sickness. To be able to enjoy the cruise, the client needs medication.

12. 1. This is appropriate for a diagnosis of "knowledge deficit."

    2. This is appropriate for a diagnosis of "deficient diversional activity" related to environmental lack of activity.

    3. **Balance depends on visual, vestibular, and proprioceptive systems; therefore, the nurse should assess these systems for findings.**

    4. This is appropriate for a diagnosis of "ineffective coping."

13. 1. Being able to identify cold and hot on the face indicates an intact trigeminal nerve, cranial nerve V.

    2. Not having any tongue tremor indicates an intact hypoglossal nerve, cranial nerve XI.

    3. No ptosis of the eyelids indicates an intact oculomotor nerve (cranial nerve III), trochlear nerve (IV), and abducens nerve (VI). Tests also assess for ocular motion, conjugate movements, nystagmus, and papillary reflexes.

    4. **Cranial nerve I is the olfactory nerve, which involves the sense of smell. With the eyes closed, the client must identify familiar smells to indicate an intact cranial nerve I.**

14. 1. This is an inaccurate statement.

    2. The older client usually requires less pain medication because of the effects of the normal aging process on the liver (metabolism) and renal system (excretion).

    3. **Decreased reaction to painful stimuli is a normal developmental change; therefore, reports of pain may be more serious than the client's perception might indicate, and thus such reports require careful evaluation.**

    4. The Wong scale is used to assess pain for the pediatric client, not the adult client.

15. 1. The client should be in the sitting position during a sensory assessment.
    2. The eyes are closed so tactile, superficial pain, vibration, and position sense (proprioception) can be assessed without the client seeing what the nurse is doing.
    3. The sensory assessment can be conducted at the bedside; there is no reason to take the client to the treatment room.
    4. There is no reason the lights should be off during the sensory assessment; the client's eyes should be closed.

16. 1. Vertigo and otorrhea are not the findings of an acoustic neuroma.
    2. Neither nystagmus, an involuntary rhythmic movement of the eyes, nor dizziness is a sign of an acoustic neuroma.
    3. Nausea and vomiting are not findings of an acoustic neuroma.
    4. **An acoustic neuroma is a slow-growing, benign tumor of cranial nerve VII. It usually arises from the Schwann cells of the vestibular portion of the nerve and results in unilateral hearing loss and tinnitus with or without vertigo.**

17. 1. This assesses cranial nerve I, the olfactory nerve.
    2. This assesses cranial nerve IX, the glossopharyngeal nerve.
    3. **This assesses cranial nerve II, the optic nerve, along with visual field testing and ophthalmoscopic examination.**
    4. This assesses cranial nerve X, the vagus nerve.

18. 1. **The purpose of aural rehabilitation is to maximize the communication skills of clients with hearing impairments. It includes auditory training, speech reading, speech training, and the use of hearing aids and hearing guide dogs.**
    2. A speech therapist may be part of the aural rehabilitation team, but the most important referral is aural rehabilitation.
    3. The client may or may not need financial assistance, but the most important referral is aural rehabilitation.
    4. The client may or may not need assistance with employment because of hearing loss, but the most important referral is aural rehabilitation.

19. **Correct answers are 2 and 5.**
    1. The client should be aware of eye pain (a sandy sensation and sensitivity to light) that will occur with conjunctivitis.

    2. Viral conjunctivitis is a highly contagious eye infection. It is easily spread from one person to another; therefore, the client should not share personal items.
    3. Cold compresses should be placed over the eyes for about 10 minutes four to five times a day to soothe the pain.
    4. The client must not apply any makeup until the disease is over and should discard all old makeup to help prevent reinfection.
    5. **The client should avoid touching their eyes and wash hands thoroughly after touching them.**

20. 1. **Aural fullness or pressure after surgery is caused by residual blood or fluid in the middle ear. This is an expected occurrence after surgery, and the nurse should administer the prescribed analgesic.**
    2. Hearing in the operated ear may be reduced for several weeks because of edema, accumulation of blood and tissue fluid in the middle ear, and dressings or packing, so this does not need to be reported to the HCP.
    3. Vertigo (dizziness) is uncommon after this surgery, but if it occurs, the nurse should administer an antiemetic or antivertigo medication and does not need to report it to the HCP.
    4. The facial nerve, which runs through the middle ear and mastoid, is at risk for injury during mastoid surgery; therefore, a facial paresis should be reported to the HCP.

21. **Correct answers are 2, 3, and 4.**
    1. Voices in the head may indicate schizophrenia, but it is not a symptom of hearing loss.
    2. **Fatigue may be the result of straining to hear, and a client may tire easily when listening to a conversation. Under these circumstances, the client may become irritable very easily.**
    3. **Loss of self-confidence makes it increasingly difficult for a person with a hearing impairment to make a decision.**
    4. **Often it is not the person with the hearing loss but a significant other noticing hearing loss; hearing loss is usually gradual.**
    5. Many clients diagnosed with hearing impairment tend to dominate the conversation because, as long as it is centered on the client, they can control it and are not as likely to be embarrassed by some mistake.

22. 1. The client should not lift, push, or pull objects heavier than 15 pounds; 50 pounds is excessive.
    2. The client should avoid lying on the side of the affected eye at night.
    3. The eyes must be protected by wearing glasses or metal eye shields at all times following surgery. Very few answer options with "all" will be correct, but if the option involves ensuring safety, it may be the correct option.
    4. The client should avoid bending or stooping for an extended period—but not forever.

23. 1. This is an abnormal finding for testing proprioception, or position sense.
    2. This is an abnormal finding for assessing superficial pain perception.
    3. This is a normal Babinski's reflex in an adult client.
    4. Stereognosis is a test evaluating higher cortical sensory ability. The client is instructed to close both eyes and identify a variety of objects (e.g., keys, coins) placed in one hand by the examiner.

24. 1. With normal aging comes decreased peripheral vision, constricted visual field, and tactile alterations. A night-light addresses safety issues and warrants praise, not intervention.
    2. Carbon monoxide detectors help ensure safety in the mother's home, so this comment doesn't warrant intervention.
    3. Decreased peripheral vision, constricted visual fields, and tactile alterations are associated with normal aging. The client needs a familiar arrangement of furniture for safety. Moving the furniture may cause the client to trip or fall. The nurse should intervene in this situation.
    4. As a result of normal aging, vision may become impaired, and the provision of large-print books warrants praise.

25. 1. The acuity of taste buds decreases with age, which may cause a decreased appetite and subsequent weight loss. Spices or other seasonings may help the food taste better to the client.
    2. This may be an appropriate intervention if excessive weight is lost or if seasoning the food does not increase appetite, but it is not necessary at this time.
    3. The client does not need a dietary consult for food not "tasting good." The nurse can address the client's concerns.
    4. This recommendation does not address the client's comment about food not tasting good.

26. Correct order is 5, 3, 2, 1, 4.
    5. The nurse should question the client further to obtain information such as which eye is affected, how long the client has seen the spots, and whether this ever occurred before.
    3. The Amsler grid is helpful in determining losses occurring in the visual fields.
    2. The hemoglobin A1c laboratory test results indicate glucose control over the past 2 to 3 months. Diabetic retinopathy is directly related to poor blood glucose control.
    1. The health-care provider should be notified to plan for laser surgery on the eye.
    4. The client should be instructed about controlling blood glucose levels, but this can wait until the immediate situation is resolved or at least until measures to address the potential loss of eyesight have been taken.

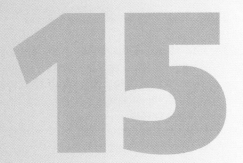

# Emergency Nursing

*The universe is full of magical things, patiently waiting
for our wits to grow sharper.*

—Eden Phillpotts

Nurses in a medical-surgical unit may face emergency situations in the care of their clients.
An important concept is shock. A client diagnosed with shock needs immediate intervention.
Other emergency situations occur because of outside factors—bioterrorism, disasters, physical abuse. Nurses must know what to do immediately, when to notify the rapid response
team (RRT), when to call a code, and what interventions are needed. In addition, because
some emergency situations involve large numbers of people or people posing a threat, there
are specific public health and other governmental agencies that must be notified and rules
must be followed in specific situations.

## KEYWORDS

Corrosive

Epistaxis

Gastric lavage

## PRACTICE QUESTIONS

### Shock

1. The client diagnosed with hypovolemic shock
   has a BP of 100/60. Fifteen minutes later the BP
   is 88/64. How much narrowing of the client's
   pulse pressure has occurred between the two
   readings?

   [                              ]

2. The client is admitted into the emergency department with diaphoresis, pale clammy skin, and BP
   of 90/70. Which intervention should the nurse
   implement **first**?
   1. Start an IV with an 18-gauge catheter.
   2. Administer intravenous dopamine infusion.
   3. Obtain arterial blood gases (ABGs).
   4. Insert an indwelling urinary catheter.

3. The nurse is caring for a client diagnosed with
   septic shock. Which assessment data **warrant
   immediate** intervention by the nurse?
   1. Vital signs T 100.4°F, P 104, R 26, and
      BP 102/60.
   2. A white blood cell count of 18,000/mm³.
   3. Urinary output of 90 mL in the last 4 hours.
   4. The client reports being thirsty.

4. The client diagnosed with septicemia has the following health-care provider (HCP) orders. Which
   HCP order has the **highest priority**?
   1. Provide clear liquid diet.
   2. Initiate IV antibiotic therapy.
   3. Obtain a STAT chest x-ray.
   4. Perform hourly glucometer checks.

5. The client is diagnosed with neurogenic shock. Which clinical manifestations should the nurse assess in this client? **Select all that apply.**
   1. Cool, moist skin.
   2. Bradycardia.
   3. Wheezing.
   4. Decreased bowel sounds.
   5. Hypotension.

6. The nurse in the emergency department administered an intramuscular antibiotic in the left ventrogluteal muscle to the client diagnosed with pneumonia being discharged home. Which intervention should the nurse implement?
   1. Ask the client about drug allergies.
   2. Obtain a sterile sputum specimen.
   3. Have the client wait for 30 minutes.
   4. Place a warm washcloth on the client's left hip.

7. The nurse caring for a client diagnosed with sepsis writes the client diagnosis of "alteration in comfort R/T chills and fever." Which intervention should be included in the plan of care?
   1. Ambulate the client in the hallway every shift.
   2. Monitor urinalysis, creatinine level, and BUN level.
   3. Apply sequential compression devices to the lower extremities.
   4. Administer an antipyretic medication every 4 hours PRN.

8. The registered nurse (RN) and an unlicensed assistive personnel (UAP) are caring for a group of clients on a medical floor. Which action by the UAP **warrants intervention** by the RN?
   1. The UAP places a urine specimen in a biohazard bag in the hallway.
   2. The UAP uses the alcohol foam hand cleanser after removing gloves.
   3. The UAP puts soiled linen in a plastic bag in the client's room.
   4. The UAP obtains a disposable stethoscope for a client in an isolation room.

9. The older female client diagnosed with vertebral fractures and self-medicating with ibuprofen presents to the emergency department (ED) reporting abdominal pain, is pale and clammy, and has a P of 110 and a BP of 92/60. Which **type of shock** should the nurse suspect?
   1. Cardiogenic shock.
   2. Hypovolemic shock.
   3. Neurogenic shock.
   4. Septic shock.

10. The client has recently experienced a myocardial infarction. Which action by the nurse helps **prevent** cardiogenic shock?
    1. Monitor the client's telemetry.
    2. Turn the client every 2 hours.
    3. Administer oxygen via nasal cannula.
    4. Place the client in the Trendelenburg position.

11. The client diagnosed with septicemia is receiving a broad-spectrum antibiotic. Which laboratory data require the nurse to **notify** the HCP?
    1. The client's potassium level is 3.8 mEq/L.
    2. The urine culture indicates high sensitivity to the antibiotic.
    3. The client's pulse oximeter reading is 94%.
    4. The culture and sensitivity is resistant to the client's antibiotic.

12. The nurse is caring for a client diagnosed with shock. The client has hypotension, decreased urine output, and cool, pale skin. Which stage of shock is the client experiencing?
    1. The refractory stage.
    2. The compensatory stage.
    3. The initial stage.
    4. The progressive stage.

## Bioterrorism

13. The nurse in the emergency department has admitted five clients in the last 2 hours with reports of fever and gastrointestinal distress. Which question is **most appropriate** for the nurse to ask each client to determine if there is a bioterrorism threat?
    1. "Do you work or live near any large power lines?"
    2. "Where were you immediately before you got sick?"
    3. "Can you write down everything you ate today?"
    4. "What other health problems do you have?"

14. The health-care facility has been notified an alleged inhalation anthrax exposure has occurred at the local post office. Which category of personal protective equipment (PPE) should the response team wear?
    1. Level A.
    2. Level B.
    3. Level C.
    4. Level D.

15. The nurse is teaching a class on bioterrorism to first responders and is discussing PPE. Which statements are important for the nurse to share with the participants? **Select all that apply.**
    1. Health-care facilities should keep masks at entry doors.
    2. The respondent should be trained in the proper use of PPE.
    3. No single combination of PPE protects against all hazards.
    4. The CDC has divided PPE into levels of protection.
    5. PPE should be properly fitted to each respondent.

16. The nurse is teaching a class on bioterrorism. Which statement is the scientific rationale for designating a specific area for decontamination?
    1. Showers and privacy can be provided to the client in this area.
    2. This area isolates the clients exposed to the agent.
    3. It provides a centralized area for stocking the needed supplies.
    4. It prevents secondary contamination to the health-care providers.

17. The triage nurse in a large trauma center has been notified of an explosion in a major chemical manufacturing plant. Which action should the nurse implement **first** when the clients arrive at the emergency department?
    1. Triage the clients and send them to the appropriate areas.
    2. Thoroughly wash the clients with soap and water and then rinse.
    3. Remove the clients' clothing and have them shower.
    4. Assume the clients have been decontaminated at the plant.

18. The nurse is teaching a class on biological warfare. Which information should the nurse include in the presentation?
    1. Contaminated water is the only source of transmission of biological agents.
    2. Vaccines are available and being prepared to counteract all biological agents.
    3. Biological weapons are less of a threat than chemical agents.
    4. Biological weapons are easily obtained and result in significant mortality.

19. Which clinical manifestations should the nurse assess in the client exposed to the anthrax bacillus via the skin?
    1. A scabby, clear fluid-filled vesicle.
    2. Edema, pruritus, and a 2-mm ulcerated vesicle.
    3. Irregular brownish-pink spots around the hairline.
    4. Tiny purple spots flush with the surface of the skin.

20. The client asks the nurse about the smallpox vaccine. Which information should the nurse provide to the client? **Select all that apply.**
    1. The client should get the vaccine for prevention from the health department.
    2. The client should get the vaccine only after the smallpox rash has developed.
    3. The smallpox vaccine can help if given less than a week after exposure to the virus.
    4. Health officials have enough smallpox vaccine to vaccinate everyone in the United States.
    5. The client should avoid travel to countries with smallpox outbreaks.

21. A chemical exposure has just occurred at an airport. An off-duty nurse, knowledgeable about biochemical agents, is giving directions to the travelers. Which direction should the nurse provide to the travelers?
    1. Hold their breath as much as possible.
    2. Stand up to avoid heavy exposure.
    3. Lie down to stay under the exposure.
    4. Attempt to breathe through their clothing.

22. The nurse is caring for a client diagnosed with the prodromal phase of radiation exposure. Which clinical manifestations should the nurse assess in the client?
    1. Anemia, leukopenia, and thrombocytopenia.
    2. Sudden fever, chills, and enlarged lymph nodes.
    3. Nausea, vomiting, and diarrhea.
    4. Flaccid paralysis, diplopia, and dysphagia.

23. Which cultural issues should the nurse consider when caring for clients during a bioterrorism attack? **Select all that apply.**
    1. Language difficulties.
    2. Religious practices.
    3. Prayer times for the people.
    4. Rituals for handling the dead.
    5. Keeping the family in the designated area.

24. The off-duty nurse hears on the television of a bioterrorism act in the community. Which action should the nurse take **first**?
    1. Immediately report to the hospital emergency department.
    2. Call the American Red Cross to find out where to go.
    3. Pack a bag and prepare to stay at the hospital.
    4. Follow the nurse's hospital policy for responding.

## Codes

25. The nurse finds the client unresponsive on the floor of the bathroom. Which action should the nurse implement **first**?
    1. Check the client for breathing.
    2. Assess the carotid artery for a pulse.
    3. Shake the client and shout.
    4. Notify the rapid response team.

26. The UAP is performing cardiac compressions on an adult client during a code. Which behavior **warrants immediate** intervention by the RN?
    1. The UAP has hand placement on the lower half of the sternum.
    2. The UAP performs cardiac compressions and allows for rescue breathing.
    3. The UAP depresses the sternum 0.5 to 1 inch during compressions.
    4. The UAP asks to be relieved from performing compressions because of exhaustion.

27. Which intervention is **most important** for the nurse to implement when participating in a code?
    1. Elevate the arm after administering medication.
    2. Maintain sterile technique throughout the code.
    3. Treat the client's clinical manifestations; do not treat the monitor.
    4. Provide accurate documentation of what happened during the code.

28. The CPR instructor is discussing an automated external defibrillator (AED) during class. Which statement **best** describes an AED?
    1. It analyzes the rhythm and shocks the client diagnosed with ventricular fibrillation.
    2. The client will be able to have synchronized cardioversion with the AED.
    3. It will keep the health-care provider informed of the client's oxygen level.
    4. The AED will perform cardiac compressions on the client.

29. The nurse is caring for clients on a medical floor. Which client is **most likely** to experience sudden cardiac death?
    1. The 84-year-old client exhibiting uncontrolled atrial fibrillation.
    2. The 60-year-old client exhibiting asymptomatic sinus bradycardia.
    3. The 53-year-old client exhibiting ventricular fibrillation.
    4. The 65-year-old client exhibiting supraventricular tachycardia.

30. Which health-care team member referral should be made by the nurse when a code is being conducted on a client in a community hospital?
    1. The hospital chaplain.
    2. The social worker.
    3. The respiratory therapist.
    4. The director of nurses.

31. Which intervention is the **most important** for the intensive care unit nurse to implement when performing mouth-to-mouth resuscitation on a client diagnosed with pulseless ventricular fibrillation?
    1. Perform the jaw thrust maneuver to open the airway.
    2. Use the mouth to cover the client's mouth and nose.
    3. Insert an oral airway before performing mouth to mouth.
    4. Use a pocket mouth shield to cover the client's mouth.

32. The nurse is teaching CPR to a class. Which statement **best** explains the definition of sudden cardiac death?
    1. Cardiac death occurs after being removed from a mechanical ventilator.
    2. Cardiac death is the time the HCP officially declares the client dead.
    3. Cardiac death occurs within 1 hour of the onset of cardiovascular symptoms.
    4. The death is caused by myocardial ischemia resulting from coronary artery disease.

33. Which statement explains the scientific rationale for having emergency suction equipment available during resuscitation efforts?
    1. Gastric distention can occur as a result of ventilation.
    2. It is needed to assist when intubating the client.
    3. This equipment will ensure a patent airway.
    4. It keeps the vomitus away from the health-care provider.

34. Which equipment must be **immediately** brought to the client's bedside when a code is called for a client diagnosed with a cardiac arrest?
    1. A ventilator.
    2. A crash cart.
    3. A gurney.
    4. Portable oxygen.

35. The nursing administrator responds to a code situation. When assessing the situation, which role must the administrator ensure is performed for legal purposes and continuity of care of the client?
    1. A person is ventilating with an Ambu bag.
    2. A person is performing chest compressions correctly.
    3. A person is administering medications as ordered.
    4. A person is keeping an accurate record of the code.

36. The client in a code is now diagnosed with ventricular bigeminy. The HCP orders a lidocaine drip at 3 mg/min. The lidocaine comes prepackaged with 2 grams of lidocaine in 500 mL of D$_5$W. At which rate will the nurse set the infusion pump?

    [                    ]

## Disasters and Triage

37. Which situation **warrants** the nurse obtaining information from a material safety data sheet (MSDS)?
    1. The custodian spilled a chemical solvent in the hallway.
    2. A visitor slipped and fell on the floor that had just been mopped.
    3. A bottle of antineoplastic agent broke on the client's floor.
    4. The nurse was stuck with a contaminated needle in the client's room.

38. The triage nurse is working in the emergency department. Which client should be assessed **first**?
    1. The 10-year-old child whose dad thinks the child's leg is broken.
    2. The 45-year-old male clutching his chest and diaphoretic.
    3. The 58-year-old female reporting a headache and seeing spots.
    4. The 25-year-old male with a hunting knife wound on the hand.

39. The nurse is teaching a class on disaster preparedness. Which are components of an emergency operations plan (EOP)? **Select all that apply.**
    1. A plan for practice drills.
    2. A deactivation response.
    3. A plan for internal communication only.
    4. A preincident response.
    5. A security plan.

40. According to the North Atlantic Treaty Organization (NATO) triage system, which situation is considered a **level red**?
    1. Injuries are extensive and chances of survival are unlikely.
    2. Injuries are minor and treatment can be delayed hours to days.
    3. Injuries are significant but can wait hours without threat to life or limb.
    4. Injuries are life-threatening but survivable with available interventions.

41. Which statement **best** describes the role of the medical-surgical nurse during a disaster?
    1. The nurse may be assigned to ride in the ambulance.
    2. The nurse may be assigned as a first assistant in the operating room.
    3. The nurse may be assigned to crowd control.
    4. The nurse may be assigned to the emergency department.

42. The nurse in a disaster is triaging the following clients. Which client should be triaged as an Expectant Category and color black?
    1. The alert client diagnosed with a sucking chest wound.
    2. The unresponsive client diagnosed with a head injury.
    3. The client diagnosed with an abdominal wound and stable vital signs.
    4. The client diagnosed with a sprained ankle which may be fractured.

43. Which federal agency is a resource for the nurse volunteering at the American Red Cross on a committee to prepare the community for any type of disaster?
    1. The Joint Commission (JC).
    2. Office of Emergency Management (OEM).
    3. Department of Health and Human Services (HHS).
    4. Metro Medical Response Systems (MMRS).

44. Which situation requires the emergency department manager to schedule and conduct a Critical Incident Stress Management (CISM)?
    1. Caring for a 2-year-old child who died from severe physical abuse.
    2. Performing unsuccessful CPR on a middle-aged male executive.
    3. Responding to a 22-victim bus accident with no apparent fatalities.
    4. Being required to work 16 hours without taking a break.

45. During a disaster, a local news reporter comes to the emergency department requesting information about the victims. Which action is **most appropriate** for the nurse to implement?
    1. Have security escort the reporter off the premises.
    2. Direct the reporter to the disaster command post.
    3. Tell the reporter this is a violation of HIPAA.
    4. Request the reporter to stay out of the way.

46. The triage nurse has placed a disaster tag on the client. Which action **warrants immediate** intervention by the nurse?
    1. The nurse documents the tag number in the disaster log.
    2. The unlicensed assistive personnel documents vital signs on the tag.
    3. The health-care provider removes the tag to examine the limb.
    4. The licensed practical nurse securely attaches the tag to the client's foot.

47. The father of a child brought to the emergency department is yelling at the staff and obviously intoxicated. Which approach should the nurse take with the father?
    1. Talk to the father in a calm and low voice.
    2. Tell the father to wait in the waiting room.
    3. Notify the child's mother to come to the ED.
    4. Call the police department to come and arrest him.

48. A gang war has resulted in 12 young males being brought to the emergency department. Which action by the nurse is a **priority** when a gang member points a gun at a rival gang member in the trauma room?
    1. Attempt to talk to the person with the gun.
    2. Explain to the person the police are coming.
    3. Stand between the client and the man with the gun.
    4. Get out of the line of fire and protect self.

## Poisoning

49. The parents bring their toddler to the ED in a panic. The parents state the child had been playing in the kitchen and got into some cleaning agents and swallowed an unknown quantity of the agents. Which health-care agency should the nurse contact at this time?
    1. Child Protective Services (CPS).
    2. The local police department.
    3. The Department of Health.
    4. The Poison Control Center.

50. Which is the **primary** goal of the ED nurse in caring for a poison ingestion client?
    1. Remove or inactivate the poison before it is absorbed.
    2. Provide long-term supportive care to prevent organ damage.
    3. Administer an antidote to increase the effects of the poison.
    4. Implement treatment prolonging the elimination of the poison.

51. The client has ingested a corrosive solution containing lye. Which intervention should the nurse implement?
    1. Administer syrup of ipecac to induce vomiting.
    2. Insert a nasogastric tube and connect to wall suction.
    3. Assess for airway compromise.
    4. Immediately administer water or milk.

52. The male client was found in a parked car with the motor running. The paramedic brought the client to the ED with reports of a headache, nausea, and dizziness and the client is unable to recall his name or address. On assessment, the nurse notes the buccal mucosa is a cherry red color. Which intervention should the nurse implement **first**?
    1. Check the client's oxygenation level with a pulse oximeter.
    2. Apply oxygen via nasal cannula at 100%.
    3. Obtain a psychiatric consult to determine if this was a suicide attempt.
    4. Prepare the client for transfer to a facility with a hyperbaric chamber.

53. Activated charcoal has been ordered for a client after ingesting a full bottle of acetaminophen. Which statements explain the rationale for using activated charcoal?
    1. Activated charcoal adheres to gastric mucosa to prevent absorption.
    2. Activated charcoal binds with drugs to reduce systemic absorption.
    3. Activated charcoal irritates gastric lining to induce vomiting of drugs.
    4. Activated charcoal irrigates the stomach to be removed by suction.

54. A vat of chemicals spilled onto the client. Which action should the occupational health nurse implement **first**?
    1. Have the client stand under a shower while removing all clothes.
    2. Check the material safety data sheets for the antidote.
    3. Administer oxygen by nasal cannula.
    4. Collect a sample of the chemicals in the vat for analysis.

55. The client presents to the ED with acute vomiting after eating at a fast-food restaurant. There has not been any diarrhea. The nurse suspects botulism poisoning. Which nursing problem is the **highest priority** for this client?
    1. Fluid volume loss.
    2. Risk for respiratory paralysis.
    3. Abdominal pain.
    4. Anxiety.

56. The client has ingested the remaining amount of a bottle of analgesic medication. The medication comes 500 mg per capsule. Two doses of two capsules each have been used by another member of the family. The bottle originally had 250 capsules. How many milligrams of medication did the client take?

    ┌─────────────────────────┐
    │                         │
    └─────────────────────────┘

57. The nurse is providing first aid to a victim of a poisonous snake bite. Which intervention should be the nurse's **first** action?
    1. Apply a tourniquet to the affected limb.
    2. Cut an "X" across the bite and suck out the venom.
    3. Administer a corticosteroid medication.
    4. Have the client lie still and remove constrictive items.

58. The nurse is discharging a client diagnosed with accidental carbon monoxide poisoning. Which statement made by the client indicates the **need for further** teaching?
    1. "I should install carbon monoxide detectors in my home."
    2. "Having a natural bright red color to my lips is good."
    3. "You cannot smell carbon monoxide, so it can be difficult to detect."
    4. "I should have my furnace checked for leaks before turning it on."

59. The RN and a UAP are caring for clients in a medical unit. Which nursing task can be delegated to the UAP? **Select all that apply.**
    1. Obtaining the intake and output of a client diagnosed with food poisoning.
    2. Performing a dressing change on the client diagnosed with a chemical burn.
    3. Assisting a client overdosed on morphine to the bedside commode.
    4. Helping a client diagnosed with carbon monoxide poisoning turn, cough, and deep breathe.
    5. Giving activated charcoal to a client with acetaminophen poisoning.

60. The charge nurse is making assignments. Which client should be assigned to the **most experienced** nurse?
    1. The client diagnosed with a snake bite receiving antivenin.
    2. The client who swallowed a lye preparation and is being discharged.
    3. The angry client following a failed suicide attempt.
    4. The client requiring skin grafting after a chemical spill.

## Violence, Physical Abuse, and Neglect

61. The female client presents to the emergency department with facial lacerations and contusions. The spouse will not leave the room during the assessment interview. Which intervention should be the nurse's **first** action?
    1. Call the security guard to escort the spouse away.
    2. Discuss the injuries while the spouse is in the room.
    3. Tell the spouse the police will want to talk to him.
    4. Escort the client to the bathroom for a urine specimen.

62. The older male client is admitted to the medical unit with a diagnosis of dementia. The client is 74 inches tall and weighs 54.5 kg. The client lives with his son and daughter-in-law, and both work outside the house. Which referral is **most important** for the nurse to implement?
    1. Adult Protective Services.
    2. Social worker.
    3. Medicare ombudsman.
    4. Dietitian.

63. The nurse working in a homeless shelter identifies an adolescent female acting sexually aggressive toward some of the males in the shelter. Which is the **most common** cause for this behavior?
    1. The client is acting in a learned behavior pattern to get attention.
    2. The client had to leave home because of promiscuous behavior.
    3. The client has a psychiatric disorder called nymphomania.
    4. The client is a prostitute and is trying to get customers.

64. The adolescent female comes to the school nurse of an intermediate school and tells the nurse she thinks she is pregnant. During the interview, the client states her father is the baby's father. Which intervention should the nurse implement **first**?
    1. Complete a rape kit.
    2. Notify Child Protective Services.
    3. Call the parents to come to the school.
    4. Arrange for the client to go to a free clinic.

65. The nurse in an outpatient rehabilitation facility is working with convicted child abusers. Which characteristics should the nurse expect to observe in the abusers? **Select all that apply.**
    1. The abuser calls the child a liar.
    2. The abuser has a tendency toward violence.
    3. The abuser exhibits a high self-esteem.
    4. The abuser is unable to admit the need for help.
    5. The abuser was spoiled as a child.

66. The nurse is teaching a class about rape prevention to a group of women at a community center. Which information are common myths about rape? **Select all that apply.**
    1. Raped women asked for it by dressing provocatively.
    2. If a woman says no, it is a come on and she really does not mean it.
    3. Rape is an attempt to exert power and control over the client.
    4. All victims of sexual assault are women; men can't be raped.
    5. A person cannot be raped by their legal spouse.

67. The nurse working in the emergency department is admitting a 34-year-old female client for one of multiple admissions for spousal abuse. The client has refused to leave her spouse or to press charges against him. Which action should the nurse implement?
    1. Insist the woman press charges this time.
    2. Treat the wounds and do nothing else.
    3. Tell the woman her spouse could kill her.
    4. Give the woman the number of a women's shelter.

68. The 84-year-old female client is admitted with multiple burn marks on the torso and under the breasts along with contusions in various stages of healing. When questioned by the nurse, the woman denies any problems have occurred. The woman lives with her son and does the housework.

Which is the **most** probable reason the woman denies being abused?
    1. There has not been any abuse to report.
    2. The client is ashamed to admit to being abused.
    3. The client has Alzheimer's disease and can't remember.
    4. The client fell on a hike.

69. Which question is an appropriate interview question for the nurse to use with clients involved in abuse?
    1. "I know you are being abused. Can you tell me about it?"
    2. "How much does your spouse drink before he hits you?"
    3. "What did you do to cause your spouse to get mad?"
    4. "Do you have a plan if your partner becomes abusive?"

70. The client abused as a child is diagnosed with post-traumatic stress disorder (PTSD). Which intervention should the nurse implement when the client is resting?
    1. Call the client's name to awaken him or her, but don't touch the client.
    2. Touch the client gently to let him or her know you are in the room.
    3. Enter the room as quietly as possible to not disturb the client.
    4. Do not allow the client to be awakened at all when sleeping.

71. The emergency department nurse writes the problem of "ineffective coping" for a client who was raped. Which intervention should the nurse implement?
    1. Encourage the client to take the "morning-after" pill.
    2. Allow the client to admit guilt for causing the rape.
    3. Provide a list of rape crisis counselors.
    4. Discuss reporting the case to the police.

72. The nurse writes a nursing diagnosis of "risk for injury as a result of physical abuse by spouse" for a client. Which is an **appropriate** goal for this client?
    1. The client will learn not to trust anyone.
    2. The client will admit the abuse is happening and get help.
    3. The client will discuss the nurse's suspicions with the spouse.
    4. The client will choose to stay with the spouse.

# CONCEPTS

The concepts covered in this chapter focus on clinical judgment. Exemplars that are covered are shock, disaster and triage, abuse and neglect. The interrelated concepts of the nursing process is covered throughout the questions. The concept of clinical judgment is presented in prioritizing or "first" questions.

73. The nurse is admitting a client with the laboratory results listed. Which **priority** intervention should the nurse implement **first**?

### Date: Today

| Laboratory Test | Client Values | Normal Values |
|---|---|---|
| White blood cell count (WBC) | 25.3 | 4.5–11.1 × 10³/microL |
| Red blood cell count (RBC) | 4.8 | M: 4.21–5.81 × 10⁶/microL<br>F: 3.6–5.11 × 10⁶/microL |
| Hemoglobin (Hgb) | 10 | M: 14–17.3 g/dL<br>F: 11.7–15.5 g/dL |
| Hematocrit (Hct) | 30% | M: 427%–52%<br>F: 36%–48% |
| Platelets | 250 | 140–400 × 10³/microL |

1. Administer the prescribed antibiotic IVPB.
2. Start an intravenous line in the client's left forearm.
3. Perform the admission assessment.
4. Have the laboratory draw blood cultures STAT.

74. The nurse is preparing to administer medications to a newly admitted client with a hemoglobin of 5.3 g/mL. Which medication should the nurse administer **first**?

| Client Name: Mr. J.S. | MR#: 654231 | Diagnosis: GI Bleed | |
|---|---|---|---|
| Age: 68 years | Allergies: NKDA | | |
| Medication | 0701–1900 | 1901–0700 | |
| Normal Saline 1,000 mL<br>150 mL per hour continuous | | | |
| Packed red blood cells 2 units<br>Administer over 2 hours each unit | | | |
| Furosemide 40 mg between units | | | |
| Diphenhydramine 50 mg IVP before<br>   each unit of PRBCs | | | |
| Signature of Nurse: | Day Nurse RN/DN | Night Nurse RN/NN | |

1. Normal saline.
2. Packed red blood cells unit #1.
3. Furosemide.
4. Diphenhydramine.

75. The nurse responded to a cardiac arrest. On which sites should the nurse place the AED pads? **Select all that apply.**

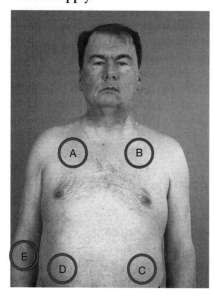

1. Site A.
2. Site B.
3. Site C.
4. Site D.
5. Site E.

76. The nurse is responding to a disaster call from home following a multivehicle motor-vehicle accident. Which action should the nurse take **first**?
    1. Go to the emergency department to triage the clients coming in.
    2. Assist the charge nurse to identify dischargeable clients.
    3. Report to the command center for assignment.
    4. Pack a bag to be able to stay until the emergency is over.

77. The charge nurse of the medical-surgical unit secured the crash cart during the code. Which intervention should the charge nurse implement **first** after transferring the client to the intensive care unit?
    1. Reassign the clients on the floor because one is now gone.
    2. Call the family of the code client and let them know of the transfer.

3. Make sure the crash cart is restocked.
4. Hold a unit meeting to determine if anything could have been done differently during the code.

78. The charge nurse has been notified that a disaster has occurred and that all possible clients should be discharged so the floor can receive the casualties. Which clients can be discharged? **Select all that apply.**
    1. The 13-year-old client scheduled for a tonsillectomy.
    2. The 42-year-old client scheduled for an abdominal aorta aneurysm dissection.
    3. The 76-year-old client diagnosed with a pulmonary embolus with 2.9 INR.
    4. The 80-year-old client refusing to assist in activities of daily living.
    5. The 30-year-old client diagnosed with a small bowel obstruction.

79. The nurse is working at a facility where a client diagnosed with Ebola has been admitted. Which action should the nurse take?
    1. Consult the nurse manager regarding the infection-control standards to follow.
    2. Resign immediately and leave the facility.
    3. Watch the television news reports to identify which station has the client.
    4. Participate in a news report about the quality of care provided at the hospital.

80. The male client presents to the emergency department stating he vomited a "large" amount of bright red blood. Which should the RN implement **first**?
    1. Start an intravenous line with an 18-gauge needle.
    2. Have the UAP take the client's vital signs.
    3. Ask the client to provide a stool specimen for blood.
    4. Send the client to radiology for an abdominal CT scan.

## Shock

1. **16 mmHg pulse pressure.**
   The pulse pressure is the systolic BP minus the diastolic BP.

   > 100 − 60 = 40 mmHg pulse pressure in first BP reading

   > 88 − 64 = 24 mmHg pulse pressure in second reading

   > 40 − 24 = 16 mmHg pulse pressure narrowing.

   A narrowing or decreased pulse pressure is an earlier indicator of shock than a decrease in systolic blood pressure.

   **TEST-TAKING HINT:** If the test taker is not aware of how to obtain a pulse pressure, the only numbers provided in the stem are systolic and diastolic blood pressures. The test taker should do something with the numbers.

2. 1. There are many types of shock, but the one common intervention that should be done first in all types of shock is to establish an intravenous line with a large-bore catheter. The low blood pressure and cold, clammy skin indicate shock.
   2. This blood pressure does not require dopamine; fluid resuscitation is first.
   3. The client may need ABGs monitored, but this is not the first intervention.
   4. An indwelling catheter may need to be inserted for accurate measurement of output, but it is not the first intervention.

   **TEST-TAKING HINT:** This question asks for the first intervention, which means all options may be appropriate interventions for the client, but only one should be implemented first. Remember: When the client *is in* distress, do not assess.

3. 1. These vital signs are expected in a client diagnosed with septic shock.
   2. An elevated WBC count indicates an infection, which is the definition of sepsis.
   3. The client must have a urinary output of at least 30 mL/hr, so 90 mL in the last 4 hours indicates impaired renal perfusion, which is a sign of worsening shock.
   4. The client being thirsty is not an uncommon issue for a client diagnosed with septic shock. This warrants immediate intervention.

**TEST-TAKING HINT:** The words "warrant immediate intervention" mean the nurse must do something, which frequently can be notifying the HCP. Any client diagnosed with shock will have clinical manifestations requiring the nurse to intervene. In this question, the test taker must determine priority and which data require immediate intervention.

4. 1. The client's diet is not a priority when transcribing orders.
   2. An IV antibiotic is the priority medication for the client diagnosed with an infection, which is the definition of sepsis—a systemic bacterial infection of the blood. A new order for an IV antibiotic should be implemented within 1 hour of receiving the order.
   3. Diagnostic tests are important but not priority over intervening in a potentially life-threatening situation such as septic shock.
   4. There is no indication in the stem of the question that this client has diabetes, and glucose levels are not associated with clinical manifestations of septicemia.

**TEST-TAKING HINT:** Remember, if the test taker can rule out two answers—options "1" and "4"—and cannot determine the right answer between options "2" and "3," select the option directly affecting or treating the client, which is antibiotics. Diagnostic tests do not treat the client.

5. Correct answers are 2 and 5.
   1. The client diagnosed with neurogenic shock will have dry, warm skin, rather than cool, moist skin, as seen in hypovolemic shock.
   2. The client will have bradycardia instead of tachycardia, which is seen in other forms of shock.
   3. Wheezing is associated with anaphylactic shock.
   4. Decreased bowel sounds occur in the hyperdynamic phase of septic shock.
   5. Hypotension is a clinical manifestation of most types of shock (Hoffman & Sullivan, 2020).

**TEST-TAKING HINT:** The test taker should identify the body system the question is addressing. In this case, *neuro-* indicates the question relates to the neurological system. With this information only, the test taker could possibly rule out option "4," which refers to the gastrointestinal system, and option "3," which refers to the respiratory system. Although bradycardia is in the cardiac system, the pulse rate is controlled by the brain.

6. 1. It is too late to ask the client about drug allergies because the medication has already been administered.
   2. Obtaining a specimen after the antibiotic has been initiated will skew the culture and sensitivity results. It must be obtained before the antibiotic is started.
   3. Anytime a nurse administers a medication for the first time, the client should be observed for a possible anaphylactic reaction, especially with antibiotics.
   4. The client is being discharged, and the nurse can encourage the client to do this at home, but it is not appropriate to do in the emergency department.

**TEST-TAKING HINT:** The test taker must be observant of information in the stem. The nurse has already administered the medication, and checking for allergies after the fact will not affect the client's outcome. This is a violation of the five rights; this medication cannot be the right medication if the client is allergic to it.

7. 1. Ambulating the client in the hall will not address the etiology of the client's chills and fever; in fact, this could increase the client's discomfort.
   2. Monitoring these laboratory data does not address the etiology of the client's diagnosis.
   3. Sequential compression devices help prevent deep vein thrombosis.
   4. Antipyretic medication will help decrease the client's fever, which directly addresses the etiology of the client's nursing diagnosis.

**TEST-TAKING HINT:** The test taker must know the problem "alteration in comfort" is addressed by the goal and the interventions address the etiology, which is "chills and fever."

8. 1. Specimens should be put into biohazard bags before leaving the client's room.
   2. This is the appropriate way to clean hands and does not warrant intervention.
   3. This is the appropriate way to dispose of soiled linens and does not warrant intervention.
   4. Taking a stethoscope from a client in isolation to another room is a violation of infection-control principles.

**TEST-TAKING HINT:** This is an "except" question. The stem is asking which action warrants intervention; therefore, the test taker must

select the option indicating an inappropriate action by the unlicensed assistive personnel.

9. 1. Cardiogenic shock occurs when the heart's ability to contract and pump blood is impaired and the supply of oxygen to the heart and tissues is inadequate, such as occurs in myocardial infarction or valvular damage.
   2. This client's clinical manifestations make the nurse suspect the client is losing blood, which leads to hypovolemic shock, which is the most common type of shock and is characterized by decreased intravascular volume. The client's taking of ibuprofen, an NSAID, puts her at risk for hemorrhage because NSAIDs inhibit prostaglandin production in the stomach, which increases the risk of developing ulcers, which can erode the stomach lining and lead to hemorrhaging.
   3. In neurogenic shock, vasodilation occurs as a result of a loss of sympathetic tone. It can result from the depressant action of medication or lack of glucose.
   4. Septic shock is a type of circulatory shock caused by widespread infection.

**TEST-TAKING HINT:** The test taker must look at the clinical manifestations and realize this client is in shock. Tachycardia and hypotension with clammy skin indicate shock. The additional information in the stem describes a particular medication, an NSAID, which can cause a peptic ulcer.

10. 1. Monitoring the telemetry will not prevent cardiogenic shock. It might help identify changes in the hemodynamics of the heart, but it does not prevent anything from occurring.
    2. Turning the client every 2 hours will help prevent pressure injuries, but it will do nothing to prevent cardiogenic shock.
    3. Promoting adequate oxygenation of the heart muscle and decreasing the cardiac workload can prevent cardiogenic shock.
    4. Placing the client's head below the heart will not prevent cardiogenic shock. This position can be used when a client is in hypovolemic shock.

**TEST-TAKING HINT:** If the test taker has no idea what the correct answer is, the test taker should apply Maslow's hierarchy of needs, which states oxygenation is most important. The test taker must know positions the client may be put in during different disorders and diseases.

11. 1. This is a normal potassium level (3.5 to 5.5 mEq/L); therefore, the nurse does not need to notify the HCP.
    2. A culture result showing a high sensitivity to an antibiotic indicates this is the antibiotic the client should be receiving.
    3. A pulse oximeter reading of greater than 93% indicates the client is adequately oxygenated.
    4. A sensitivity report indicating resistance to the antibiotic being administered indicates the medication the client is receiving is not appropriate for the treatment of the infectious organism, and the HCP needs to be notified so the antibiotic can be changed.

**TEST-TAKING HINT: The keywords in option "2" are "high sensitivity," and this should make the test taker think this is a good thing. In option "4," the word "resistant" indicates something wrong with the antibiotic and the need for intervention.**

12. 1. The refractory stage is the last and irreversible phase of shock, characterized by multi-system organ failure, coma, and death.
    2. In the compensatory stage of shock, the heart rate and respiratory rate are increased, but the skin may be cold and clammy and urinary output may be decreased. The client exhibits restlessness and confusion (Hoffman & Sullivan, 2020).
    3. In the initial stage of shock the client can have no clinical manifestations or very subtle findings.
    4. The progressive stage of shock is characterized by hypotension, lethargy, weak pulses, and respiratory and metabolic acidosis.

**TEST-TAKING HINT: There are some questions the test taker must know; they are called knowledge-based questions. The stages of shock are important for the nurse to recognize.**

## Bioterrorism

13. 1. Power lines are not typical sources of biological terrorism, which is what these symptoms represent.
    2. The nurse should take note of any unusual illness for the time of year or clusters of clients coming from a single geographical location, all exhibiting clinical manifestations of possible biological terrorism.
    3. This might be appropriate for gastroenteritis secondary to food poisoning but is not the nurse's first thought to determine a biological threat. The nurse must determine if the clients have anything in common.
    4. This is important information to obtain for all clients but is not pertinent to determine a biological threat.

**TEST-TAKING HINT: Option "4" is a question the nurse asks all clients; therefore, the test taker should eliminate it based on the specific question. Power lines are electrical, and most bioterrorism threats involve chemical or biological threats, so option "1" can be eliminated.**

14. 1. Level A protection is worn when the highest level of respiratory, skin, eye, and mucous membrane protection is required. In this situation of possible inhalation of anthrax, such protection is required (National Institute for Occupational Safety and Health, 2014).
    2. Level B protection is similar to Level A protection, but it is used when a lesser level of skin and eye protection is needed.
    3. Level C protection requires an air-purified respirator (APR), which uses filters or absorbent materials to remove harmful substances.
    4. Level D is basically the work uniform.

**TEST-TAKING HINT: If the test taker were totally unaware of the correct answer, then the choice should be either option "1" or option "4" because these are at either end of the spectrum. This gives the test taker a 50/50 chance of selecting the correct answer, instead of a 25% chance.**

15. Correct answers are 2, 3, 4, and 5.
    1. Masks are kept at designated areas, not at every entry door.
    2. This is a true statement, but in an emergency situation, the respondent should use the equipment even if not trained.
    3. The HCPs are not guaranteed absolute protection, even with all the training and protective equipment. This is the most important information individuals wearing protective equipment should know because all other procedures should be followed at all times.
    4. The CDC has divided PPE into different levels based on exposure risk.
    5. Properly fitted PPE increases the protection from exposure to biological agents (NIOSH, 2014).

**TEST-TAKING HINT:** There are very few questions where the test taker should select an option with the word "all." Option "3" is stating this is not an "always" situation. The test taker should not automatically assume it is not a possible answer until understanding the context.

16. 1. This is not a rationale; this is a statement of what is done in the area.
    2. This separates the clients until decontamination occurs, but the question is asking for the scientific rationale.
    3. This is a false statement—the supplies should not be kept in the decontamination area.
    4. Avoiding cross-contamination is a priority for personnel and equipment—the fewer the number of people exposed, the safer the community and area.

**TEST-TAKING HINT:** Options "1" and "2" are not rationales.

17. 1. In most situations, this is the first step, but with a potential chemical or biological exposure, the first step must be the safety of the hospital; therefore, the client must be decontaminated.
    2. This is the second step in the decontamination process.
    3. **This is the first step. Depending on the type of exposure, this step alone can remove a large portion of the exposure.**
    4. This assumption could cost many people in the hospital staff, as well as clients, their lives.

**TEST-TAKING HINT:** If the test taker wants to select option "4" as the correct answer, the test taker should be careful—assumptions are dangerous. The test taker may want to choose option "1" because it involves assessment, but exposure to a chemical agent should be considered distress and an action should be implemented first.

18. 1. Sources of biological agents include inhalation, insects, animals, and people.
    2. Vaccines are not available to counteract all biological agents.
    3. Because of the vast range of agents, biological weapons are more of a threat. A biological agent could be released in one city and affect people in other cities thousands of miles away.

    4. Because of the variety of agents, the means of transmission, and the lethality of the agents, biological weapons, including anthrax, smallpox, and plague, are especially dangerous.

**TEST-TAKING HINT:** Answer option "1" should be eliminated because of the word "only." Even if the test taker has little knowledge of biological warfare, knowledge of the human body suggests a wide range of ways biological agents could be transmitted.

19. 1. Scabby, clear fluid-filled vesicles are characteristic of chickenpox.
    2. **Exposure to anthrax bacilli via the skin results in skin lesions, which cause edema with pruritus and the formation of macules or papules, which ulcerate, forming a 1- to 3-mm vesicle. Then a painless eschar develops, which falls off in 1 to 2 weeks.**
    3. Irregular brownish-pink spots around the hairline are characteristic of rubella.
    4. Tiny purple spots flush with the skin surface are petechiae.

**TEST-TAKING HINT:** This is a knowledge-based question. The test taker should try to determine which disease or condition each answer option describes to rule out the incorrect answers.

20. Correct answers are 3 and 4.
    1. The smallpox vaccine is not available to the general public because smallpox has been eradicated and the virus no longer exists in nature.
    2. Once the smallpox rash has developed, the vaccine does not provide protection from the disease.
    3. If given within 7 days of being exposed to the smallpox virus, the vaccine can provide some protection from the disease.
    4. Health officials have enough smallpox vaccine to vaccinate every person in the United States if an outbreak were to occur (CDC, 2019).
    5. Smallpox is eradicated and the virus no longer exists in nature.

**TEST-TAKING HINT:** This is a knowledge-based question. The test taker should try to determine which answer options to select based on knowledge of immunizations.

21. 1. The absence of breathing is death, and this is neither a viable option nor a sensible recommendation to terrified people.
    2. Standing up will avoid heavy exposure because the chemical will sink toward the floor or ground.

3. Staying below the level of the smoke is the instruction for a fire.
4. Breathing through the clothing, which is probably contaminated with the chemical, will not provide protection from the chemical entering the lung.

**TEST-TAKING HINT: If the test taker does not know the answer, the test taker should realize options "1" and "4" address breathing and options "2" and "3" address positioning, and one set of options should be eliminated, narrowing the choice to one out of two options.**

22. 1. Anemia, leukopenia, and thrombocytopenia, signs of bone marrow depression, are clinical manifestations the client experiences in the manifest illness stage of radiation exposure, which occurs from 72 hours to years after exposure. The client is usually asymptomatic in the prodromal phase of radiation exposure.
2. Sudden fever, chills, and enlarged lymph nodes are clinical manifestations of bubonic plague.
3. The prodromal stage (presenting symptoms) of radiation exposure occurs 48 to 72 hours after exposure, and the clinical manifestations are nausea, vomiting, diarrhea, anorexia, and fatigue. Clinical manifestations of higher exposures of radiation include fever, respiratory distress, and coma (CDC, 2018).
4. These are clinical manifestations of inhalation botulism.

**TEST-TAKING HINT: If the test taker knows the definition of "prodromal," which is an early sign of a developing condition or disease (*prodrom* is Greek for "running before"), then the option with vague and nonspecific clinical manifestations should be selected as the correct answer.**

23. Correct answers are 1, 2, 3, and 4.
1. Language difficulties can increase fear and frustration on the part of the client.
2. Some religions have specific practices related to medical treatments, hygiene, and diet, and these should be honored if at all possible.
3. Prayers in times of grief and disaster are important to an individual and actually can have a calming effect on the situation.
4. Caring for the dead is as important as caring for the living based on religious beliefs.
5. For purposes of organization, this may be needed, but it is not addressing cultural sensitivity and, in some instances, may violate the cultural needs of the client and the family.

**TEST-TAKING HINT: The stem asks the test taker to address cultural needs, and these client needs must be addressed in a bioterrorism attack or with an individual in the hospital. The test taker should select options addressing cultural needs. Dishonoring cultural needs can increase the client's anxiety and increase problems for the health-care team.**

24. 1. Many hospital procedures mandate off-duty nurses should not report immediately to the hospital, so relief is available for initial responders.
2. The nurse's first responsibility is to the facility of employment, not the community.
3. This is a good action to take when the nurse is notified of the next action. For example, if the hospital is quarantined, the nurse may not report for days.
4. The nurse should follow the hospital's policy. Often nurses will stay at home until decisions are made as to where the employees should report.

**TEST-TAKING HINT: After looking at all the options, the test taker should select the option that best assesses the entire situation, which is following policy. There will be a tendency for mass hysteria to occur in the community, but following the terrorist attack on 9/11/2001, all hospitals and communities are now required by Homeland Security to have a disaster preparedness plan in place. The best action the nurse can take is to follow the procedure and remain calm.**

## Codes

25. 1. This is not the first intervention based on the answer options available in this question.
2. This is not the first intervention based on the options available in this question.
3. This is the first intervention the nurse should implement after finding the client unresponsive on the floor.
4. The rapid response team is called if the client is breathing; a code would be called if the client were not breathing.

**TEST-TAKING HINT: Options "1," "2," and "3" are all assessment interventions, which is the first step in the nursing process. Of these three possible options, the test taker should select the intervention easiest and fastest to determine if the client is alert, which is to shake and shout at the client.**

26. 1. This hand position will help prevent positioning the hand over the xiphoid process, which can break the ribs and lacerate the liver during compressions.
    2. This is the correct two-rescuer CPR; therefore, no intervention is needed.
    3. **The sternum should be depressed 1.5 to 2 inches during compressions to ensure adequate circulation of blood to the body; therefore, the nurse needs to correct the UAP.**
    4. The UAP should request another HCP to perform compressions when exhausted.

**TEST-TAKING HINT: The test taker must select which option is an incorrect procedure for cardiac compressions.**

27. 1. This is an appropriate intervention, but it is not the most important.
    2. Sterile technique should be maintained as much as possible, but the nurse can treat a live body with an infection without using sterile technique; however, the nurse cannot treat a dead body without an infection.
    3. **This is the most important intervention. The nurse should always treat the client based on the nurse's assessment and data from the monitors; an intervention should not be based on data from the monitors without the nurse's assessment.**
    4. Documentation is important but not a priority over treating the client.

**TEST-TAKING HINT: The phrase "most important" in the stem is the key to answering this question. All four options are appropriate interventions for the question, but only one is the most important. The test taker should remember to always select the option directly affecting the client, and this may mean not selecting an assessment intervention when the client is in distress.**

28. 1. **This is the correct statement explaining what an AED does when used in a code.**
    2. The defibrillator on the crash cart must be used to perform synchronized cardioversion.
    3. This is the explanation for a pulse oximeter.
    4. This is not the function of the AED.

**TEST-TAKING HINT: The test taker must know the equipment to be able to answer this question. The test taker may be able to eliminate options based on knowledge of what other equipment does.**

29. 1. Atrial fibrillation is not a life-threatening dysrhythmia; it is chronic.
    2. Asymptomatic sinus bradycardia may be normal for the client, especially for athletes or long-distance runners.
    3. **Ventricular fibrillation is the most common dysrhythmia associated with sudden cardiac death (Srinivasan & Schilling, 2018).**
    4. "Supraventricular" means "above the ventricle." The atrium is above the ventricle, and atrial dysrhythmias are not life-threatening.

**TEST-TAKING HINT: The test taker should know the left ventricle is responsible for pumping blood to the body (heart muscle and brain) and could eliminate options "1" and "4" as correct answers. The word "asymptomatic" should cause the test taker to eliminate option "2" as the correct answer.**

30. 1. **The chaplain should be called to help address the client's family or significant others. A small community hospital does not have a 24-hour on-duty pastoral service. A chaplain is part of the code team in large medical center hospitals.**
    2. The social worker does not need to be notified of a code.
    3. The respiratory therapist responds to the code automatically without a referral. The respiratory therapist is part of the code team, and one is on duty 24 hours a day, even in a small community hospital.
    4. The director of nurses does not need to be notified of codes, but possibly the house supervisor should be notified.

**TEST-TAKING HINT: The test taker must know the roles of the multidisciplinary health-care team to make appropriate referrals. The words "community hospital" are an important phrase to help determine the correct answer.**

31. 1. A jaw thrust is used for a possible fractured neck. The nurse should use the head-tilt, chin-lift maneuver to open the airway.
    2. The nurse should cover the client's mouth and nose with the nurse's mouth when giving mouth-to-mouth resuscitation to an infant but not when giving mouth-to-mouth resuscitation to an adult. According to the American Heart Association 2010 Guidelines, mouth to mouth is only performed with a barrier device in place to protect the rescuer.

3. An oral airway is not mandatory to do effective breathing; therefore, it is not the most important intervention.
4. **Nurses should protect themselves against possible communicable diseases, such as HIV and hepatitis, and should be protected if the client vomits during CPR.**

**TEST-TAKING HINT: Unless the stem provides an age for the client, the client is an adult client; therefore, the test taker could eliminate option "2" because it is for an infant.**

32. 1. This is not the definition of sudden cardiac death; this is sometimes known as "pulling the plug" on clients diagnosed as brain dead.
2. This is not the definition of sudden cardiac death.
3. **Unexpected death occurring within 1 hour of the onset of cardiovascular symptoms is the definition of sudden cardiac death (Srinivasan & Schilling, 2018).**
4. This is not the definition of sudden cardiac death.

**TEST-TAKING HINT: If the test taker relates the word "sudden" in the stem with "unexpected," the best answer is option "3." The test taker must be aware of adjectives and adverbs.**

33. 1. **Gastric distention occurs from over ventilating clients. When compressions are performed, the pressure will cause vomiting, which may cause aspiration into the lungs.**
2. The HCP does not require suctioning equipment to intubate.
3. Nothing ensures a patent airway, except a correctly inserted endotracheal tube, and suction is needed to clear the airway.
4. Suction equipment is for the client's needs, not the HCP's needs.

**TEST-TAKING HINT: Option "4" could be eliminated because the equipment is for the client, not for the nurse or HCPs. The word "ensures" in option "3" is an absolute word, so the test taker should be cautious before selecting this option.**

34. 1. A ventilator is not kept on the medical-surgical floors and is not routinely brought to the bedside. The client is manually ventilated until arriving in the intensive care unit.
2. **The crash cart is the mobile unit with the defibrillator and all the medications and supplies needed to conduct a code.**
3. The gurney, a stretcher, may be needed when the client is being transferred to another unit, but it is not an immediate need, and in some hospitals, the client is transferred in the bed.
4. Oxygen is available in the room and portable oxygen is on the crash cart, so it doesn't need to be brought separately.

**TEST-TAKING HINT: This is knowledge the test taker must have. The crash cart is the primary piece of equipment, and in most facilities there is a person assigned to bring the crash cart to the client's bedside.**

35. 1. This is providing immediate direct care to the client and is not performed for legal purposes.
2. The key to answering the question is "legal," and direct care is not performed for legal purposes.
3. This is providing immediate direct care to the client and is not performed for legal purposes. This is an occasion where someone else is allowed to document another nurse's medication administration.
4. **The EHR is a legal document, and the code must be documented in the EHR and provide the information needed in the intensive care unit.**

**TEST-TAKING HINT: Answer options "1," "2," and "3" have the nurse providing direct hands-on care. Option "4" is the only option addressing documentation and should be selected as the correct answer because it is different.**

36. **45 mL/hr.**
The test taker could remember the mnemonic, which is "For 1 mg, 2 mg, 3 mg, 4 mg the rate is 15 mL, 30 mL, 45 mL, 60 mL." If the test taker has not memorized it, it is too late to figure it out in an emergency situation. But for math purposes: First determine the number of milligrams of lidocaine in the 500 mL of $D_5W$:

$$2 \text{ g} \times 1,000 \text{ mg} = 2,000 \text{ mg per } 500 \text{ mL}$$

Then determine how many milligrams per milliliters:

$$2,000 \text{ mg} \div 500 \text{ mL} = 4 \text{ mg/mL}$$

Then find out how many milliliters must be infused per minute to give the ordered dose of 3 mg/min. In algebraic terms:

$$4 \text{ mg} : 1 \text{ mL} = 3 \text{ mg} : x \text{ mL}$$

Cross multiply and divide:

$$x = 3/4 \text{ or } 0.75$$

The number of milliliters to be infused in a minute is 3/4 mL or 0.75.

The infusion pump is set at an hourly rate, so multiply 3/4 by 60 minutes:

$$3/4 \times 60 = 45$$

The pump should be set at 45 mL/hr to infuse 3 mg/min.

**TEST-TAKING HINT: The test taker must be familiar with basic nursing math and become comfortable with the equations the test taker uses to compute dosage calculations.**

## Disasters and Triage

37. 1. The MSDS provides chemical information regarding specific agents, health information, and spill information for a variety of chemicals. It is required for every chemical found in the hospital.
   2. This situation requires an occurrence or accident report.
   3. Any facility administering antineoplastic agents (medications used to treat cancer) is required to have specific chemotherapy spill kits available and a policy and procedure included; in this situation, the nurse already knows the chemical involved.
   4. This requires a hospital variance report and notifying the employee health or infection-control nurse.

**TEST-TAKING HINT: If the test taker were not aware of an MSDS, the name tells the test taker to look for content in the answer options addressing materials; therefore, options "2" and "4" could be eliminated as possible answers.**

38. 1. The child needs an x-ray to confirm the fracture, but the client is stable and does not have a life-threatening problem.
   2. The triage nurse should see this client first because these are symptoms of a myocardial infarction, which is potentially life-threatening.
   3. These are symptoms of a migraine headache and are not life-threatening.
   4. A laceration on the hand is a priority, but not over a client having a myocardial infarction.

**TEST-TAKING HINT: The test taker should evaluate each option on a scale of 1 to 10, with 1 being the least critical client and 10 being life-threatening. Option "2" rates a score of 10.**

39. Correct answers are 1, 2, and 5.
   1. Practice drills allow for troubleshooting any issues before a real-life incident occurs.
   2. A deactivation response is important so resources are not overused, and the facility can then get back to daily activities and routine care.
   3. Communication between the facility and external resources and an internal communication plan are critical.
   4. In a postincident response, it is important to include a critique and debriefing for all parties involved; a preincident response is a plan itself. Be sure to read adjectives closely.
   5. A coordinated security plan involving facility and community agencies is the key to controlling an otherwise chaotic situation (American College of Emergency Physicians, 2019).

**TEST-TAKING HINT: The test taker must notice adjectives such as "only" in option "3" and "preincident" in option "4." These words make these options incorrect. This question requires the test taker to select more than one option as the correct answer.**

40. 1. This describes injuries color-coded black and is called the Expectant Category. It is used for the deceased or those with extensive, unsurvivable injuries
   2. This is a description of injuries color-coded green and is called the Wait Category. These clients are walking wounded.
   3. These injuries are color-coded yellow and are in the Observation Category.
   4. This is called the Immediate Category. Individuals in this group can progress rapidly to Expectant if treatment is delayed (Clarkson & Williams, 2019).

**TEST-TAKING HINT: This is basically a knowledge-based question, but often the color "red" indicates a high priority.**

41. 1. The nurse should not leave the hospital area; the nurse must wait for the casualties to come to the facility.
   2. This is a position requiring knowledge of instruments and procedures not common to the medical-surgical floor.
   3. The people in this area are usually chaplains or social workers, not direct client care personnel. In a disaster, direct care personnel cannot be spared for this duty.
   4. New settings and atypical roles for nurses may be required during

disasters; medical-surgical nurses can provide first aid and may be required to work in unfamiliar settings.

**TEST-TAKING HINT:** The test taker should look at traditional nursing roles requiring nursing expertise and eliminate crowd control or riding in an ambulance.

42. 1. This client should be classified as an Immediate Category and the color red. If not treated STAT, a tension pneumothorax will occur.
    2. This client has a very poor prognosis, and even with treatment, survival is unlikely. This client is classified as a black tag and an Expectant Category (Clarkson & Williams, 2019).
    3. This client should be classified as an Observation Category and the color yellow. This client receives treatment after the casualties requiring immediate treatment are treated.
    4. This client is a Wait Category and the color green. This client can wait for days for treatment.

**TEST-TAKING HINT:** If the test taker did not know the definition of the categories, looking at the word "black," which has a connotation of death, and the word "expectant" might lead the test taker to select the worst-case scenario.

43. 1. This organization mandates all health-care facilities to have an emergency operations plan, but it is a national agency, not a federal agency.
    2. Most cities and all states have an OEM, which coordinates the disaster relief efforts at the state and local levels.
    3. Federal resources include organizations such as the HHS, Federal Emergency Management Agency (FEMA), and the Department of Justice. The American Red Cross provides disaster relief alongside these federal departments.
    4. MMRS teams are local teams located in cities deemed to be possible terrorist targets.

**TEST-TAKING HINT:** The question asks for a federal agency. The word "metro" means "local"; therefore, option "4" could be eliminated. All HCPs should be aware of the role of The Joint Commission in the hospital, so the test taker could eliminate option "1."

44. 1. CISM is an approach to preventing and treating the emotional trauma affecting emergency responders as a consequence of their job. Performing CPR

and treating a young child affects the emergency personnel psychologically, and the death increases the traumatic experience.
    2. Caring for this type of client is an expected part of the job. If the nurse finds this traumatic enough to require a CISM, then the nurse should probably leave the emergency department.
    3. This requires an intense time for triaging and caring for the victims, but without fatalities, this should not be as traumatic for the staff.
    4. This is a dangerous practice because medication errors and other mistakes may occur as a result of fatigue, but this is not a traumatic situation.

**TEST-TAKING HINT:** The test taker should examine the words "critical," "incident," and "stress." Each option should be examined to determine which is the most traumatic. Needless deaths of children are psychologically traumatic.

45. 1. The media have an obligation to report the news and can play a significant positive role in communication, but communication should come from only one source—the disaster command center.
    2. EOPs will have a designated disaster plan coordinator. All public information should be routed through this person.
    3. Client confidentiality must be maintained, but the best action is for the nurse to help the reporter get to the appropriate area for information.
    4. This allows the reporter to stay in the emergency department, which is inappropriate.

**TEST-TAKING HINT:** The nurse should address the situation with the reporter and provide access for the information. Options "1," "3," and "4" do not help the reporter get accurate information.

46. 1. This is the correct procedure when tagging a client and does not warrant intervention.
    2. Vital signs should be documented on the tag. The tag takes the place of the client's EHR, so this does not warrant intervention.
    3. The tag should never be removed from the client until the disaster is over or the client is admitted and the tag becomes a part of the client's record.
    4. The tag can be attached to any part of the client's body.

**TEST-TAKING HINT:** This question is asking the test taker to identify an incorrect option for the situation. Sometimes asking which action is appropriate helps identify the correct answer.

47. 1. This will help diffuse the escalating situation and attempt to keep the father calm.
    2. Sending the father to the waiting room does not help his behavior and could possibly make his behavior worse; loud and obnoxious behavior can become violent.
    3. This will not help the current situation and could make it worse because the nurse doesn't know the home situation.
    4. The nurse should notify hospital security before calling the police department.

**TEST-TAKING HINT:** The rule concerning dealing with anger is to address the client directly and defuse the situation. There is only one option addressing this rule, option "1."

48. 1. This puts the nurse in a dangerous position and might cause the death of the nurse.
    2. This will escalate the situation.
    3. This is a dangerous position for the nurse to be put in.
    4. Self-protection is a priority; the nurse is not required to be injured in the line of duty.

**TEST-TAKING HINT:** Self-protection is a priority. There is no advantage to protecting others if the caregivers are also injured. The only option protecting the nurse is to get out of the line of fire.

## Poisoning

49. 1. CPS should be contacted only if the nurse suspects an intentional administration of the poison, but at this time, determining which poison the child has swallowed and the antidote is the priority.
    2. The local police department is only notified if the nurse suspects child abuse.
    3. The Department of Health does not need to be notified.
    4. The Poison Control Center can assist the nurse in identifying which chemical has been ingested by the child and the antidote.

**TEST-TAKING HINT:** The test taker should analyze each option to determine what information could be obtained. Then the test taker should put this information in order of priority. Even if the nurse suspects child abuse, the priority is to help the child immediately.

50. 1. The primary goal for the ED nurse is to stop the action of the poison and then maintain organ functioning.
    2. ED nurses do not provide long-term care.
    3. Antidotes are administered to neutralize the effects of poisons, not to increase the effects.
    4. Treatment is implemented to hasten the elimination of the poison.

**TEST-TAKING HINT:** The test taker should read each option carefully. ED nurse and "long-term care" don't match. Increasing the effects and prolonging the elimination of the poison is damaging to the client.

51. 1. Vomiting is never induced in clients after ingesting corrosive alkaline substances or petroleum distillates. More damage can occur to the esophagus and pharynx.
    2. Gastric lavage may be done (very rare) but not by inserting an NGT and attaching it to wall suction.
    3. Airway edema or obstruction can occur as a result of the burning action of corrosive substances.
    4. Water or milk may be administered to dilute the substance if the airway is not compromised.

**TEST-TAKING HINT:** This is an emergency situation. If the test taker did not know the answer, Maslow's hierarchy of needs puts the airway first.

52. 1. These are clinical manifestations of carbon monoxide poisoning. Pulse oximetry is not a valid test because the hemoglobin is saturated with the carbon monoxide and a false high reading is being obtained.
    2. These are clinical manifestations of carbon monoxide poisoning. Symptoms include skin color from a cherry red to cyanotic and pale, headache, muscular weakness, palpitations, dizziness, and confusion and can progress rapidly to coma and death. Oxygen should be administered 100% at hyperbaric or atmospheric pressures to reverse hypoxia and accelerate the elimination of the carbon monoxide.
    3. This may be done, but it is not the first action.
    4. This may need to be done, but getting oxygen to the brain is first.

**TEST-TAKING HINT:** Three of the four options concern oxygenation. The test taker must then decide which of the three has the highest priority.

53. 1. Activated charcoal does not adhere to the gastric mucosa; it binds to the drug or toxin.
    2. **Activated charcoal binds to drugs or toxins in the body, reducing systemic absorption. It is the most frequently used method of gastrointestinal decontamination (Juurlink, 2016).**
    3. A client may occasionally vomit when given activated charcoal, but this is not the scientific rationale for the administration. Ipecac can be given to induce vomiting but is not commonly used today.
    4. Gastric lavage can be performed to flush the stomach, and the fluid is removed by suction but not activated charcoal.

**TEST-TAKING HINT: This is a knowledge-based question. The test taker should have knowledge of the actions of medications administered for a drug overdose.**

54. 1. **The skin should be immediately drenched with water from a hose or shower. A constant stream of water is applied. Time should not be lost by removing the clothes first and then proceeding to rinse with water. If a dry powder form of white phosphorus or lye spilled onto the client, it is brushed off and then the client is placed under the shower.**
    2. The first action is to remove the poison from the client's skin and prevent further damage.
    3. If the client becomes dyspneic, the nurse administers oxygen while waiting for the paramedics.
    4. The vat should be labeled as to the chemical contents per Occupational Safety and Health Administration (OSHA) regulations, but if not, the nurse must determine which chemicals are in the vat so the HCP can treat the client appropriately.

**TEST-TAKING HINT: Usually, oxygen is a priority, but in this scenario, the client has dangerous chemicals on the skin. The stem did not tell the test taker the respirations were a problem. It is important not to read into a question.**

55. 1. Fluid volume loss is a concern because of the potential for the client to go into hypovolemic shock, but this is not a priority over the airway.
    2. **Clients diagnosed with botulism are at risk for respiratory paralysis, and this is the priority problem.**
    3. The client will be in pain and pain is a priority, but it does not come before airway and fluid volume.
    4. The client may be anxious, but a psychosocial problem usually can be ranked after a physiological one in priority.

**TEST-TAKING HINT: Maslow's hierarchy of needs lists the airway as the highest priority.**

56. 123,000 mg of analgesic medication were consumed.

    The container originally contained 250 capsules. Two doses of two capsules each were removed.

    $$2 \times 2 = 4.$$

    250 capsules – 4 capsules
    = 246 capsules remaining.

    Each capsule contains 500 mg.

    246 capsules $\times$ 500 mg = 123,000 mg
    of medication consumed.

**TEST-TAKING HINT: The test taker must not overlook a step in the problem. On the NCLEX-RN®, the test taker should check answers with the drop-down calculator.**

57. 1. Although this is seen as the first action in old television westerns, it is not a recommended action for clients been bitten by a snake. This action will cause further damage to the tissue by restricting blood flow to the tissue.
    2. This is an action seen in classic television programs and movies from the 1950s and 1960s, but this is not the current treatment for snakebite. If this is done, the rescuer will suck the venom into the rescuer's mouth and possibly be poisoned.
    3. Corticosteroid medications are contraindicated in the first 6 to 8 hours after the bite because they might interfere with antibody production and hinder the action of the antivenin.
    4. **The client should lie down, all restrictive items such as rings should be removed, the wound should be cleaned and covered with a sterile dressing, the affected body part should be immobilized, and the client should be kept warm.**

**TEST-TAKING HINT: The test taker should not jump to what is depicted in the mass media as the correct answer. Both options "1" and "2" have answers portrayed in the media as the correct method of caring for snake bite. This should give the test taker a clue: If both options cannot be right, then both are probably wrong.**

58. 1. Installing carbon monoxide detectors in the home is a recommended safety measure.
    2. The lips should not be bright red or blue. This indicates saturation of the hemoglobin with carbon monoxide. This client needs more instruction.
    3. Because carbon monoxide is colorless and odorless, it can be dangerous. It is detected with special detectors.
    4. One of the major causes of accidental carbon monoxide poisoning is a faulty furnace.

**TEST-TAKING HINT: Three options, "1," "3," and "4" are about protecting the home and keeping the client from inhaling carbon monoxide. If the test taker did not know the answer, a good choice is the different option.**

59. Correct answers are 1, 3, and 4.
    1. UAPs can obtain intake and outputs, but evaluating the information is the nurse's responsibility.
    2. This is a sterile dressing change and should not be delegated.
    3. A UAP can assist clients in getting up to the bedside commode as long as the UAP is knowledgeable about body mechanics.
    4. The UAP can assist a client in turning and asking the client to cough and deep breathe.
    5. The UAP cannot administer medications to clients. This should not be delegated.

**TEST-TAKING HINT: The task requiring knowledge of sterile technique is the one the nurse should perform. Any task requiring specialized knowledge or nursing judgment cannot be delegated.**

60. 1. Before administering antivenin, the affected body part must be measured. The infusion is begun slowly and increased after 10 minutes. The affected part is measured every 30 to 60 minutes after the infusion and for 48 hours to detect symptoms of compartment syndrome (edema, loss of pulse, increased pain, and paresthesias). Allergic reactions to the antivenin are not uncommon and are usually the result of a too-rapid infusion of the antivenin. The most experienced nurse should be assigned to this client.
    2. This client is beyond critical danger and is being discharged, so a less-experienced nurse could care for this client.
    3. This client has many needs, but anger is not a priority over a physiological need.
    4. A less-experienced nurse could care for this client.

**TEST-TAKING HINT: The test taker can rule out options "2" and "3" because of the discharge information and psychosocial versus physiological problem.**

## Violence, Physical Abuse, and Neglect

61. 1. This action could cause the spouse to become violent. The security personnel should not attempt to remove the spouse unless the client wishes them to do so.
    2. Injuries resulting from spousal abuse should be discussed without the abuser present.
    3. This may or may not be true. The client will have to prosecute, and many times the abused client will not do so. The client may feel responsible for the abuse or may fear for her children's lives or for her own, or there may be a financial hold the spouse has over the client. Battered woman syndrome has many facets.
    4. By escorting the client to a bathroom for any reason, the nurse can get the client to a safe area out of the hearing of the spouse. This is the most innocuous way to get the client alone.

**TEST-TAKING HINT: When dealing with a violent person, the nurse should use discretion to avoid the spouse erupting into violence directed against the nurse, client, or others in the emergency department.**

62. 1. Adult Protective Services should be called only if it is determined willful neglect or abuse of the client is occurring.
    2. The nurse should arrange for the social worker to see the client and family to determine if some arrangements could be made to provide for the client's safety and for the client to be provided with nutritious meals while the adult children are at work. A long-term care facility or adult day care may be needed.
    3. The Medicare ombudsman is a person representing a Medicare client in a long-term care facility.
    4. The dietitian could see this client to determine eating preferences (74 inches = 6 foot 2 inches and 54.5 kg = 120 pounds), but the most appropriate intervention is safety.

**TEST-TAKING HINT: The question asks for the test taker to determine a priority intervention. The client is diagnosed with senile dementia and is being left alone for hours of the day. Safety is a priority.**

**63.** 1. Research suggests at least 67% of runaways or homeless adolescents have been abused in the home. This represents a learned behavior pattern getting the female adolescent attention.
2. One reason adolescents of both sexes run away from home is abuse in the home. Nothing in the stem indicates the client was turned out of the home for any behavior.
3. This has the nurse medically diagnosing the client.
4. This is a judgmental statement.

**TEST-TAKING HINT: The test taker should not read into the question or choose an option allowing the nurse to function outside the scope of practice. Option "2" is assuming facts not in the stem, and option "3" is asking the nurse to make a medical diagnosis.**

**64.** 1. The school nurse is not a Sexual Assault Nurse Examiner (SANE) nurse, and this child thinks she is pregnant, suggesting the abuse has been occurring for a period of time or at least in some months past. The child should be taken to a hospital for examination.
2. Child Protective Services should be notified to protect the child from further abuse and to initiate charges against the father. An intermediate school nurse cares for children in the fourth, fifth, sixth, or seventh grades, depending on the school district.
3. This action brings the abuser to the school.
4. Sending the child to a free clinic does not negate the nurse's responsibility to report suspected child abuse.

**TEST-TAKING HINT: All 50 states require the nurse to report suspected child abuse. CPS is the advocate to notify. Nurses in a school clinic do not have the appropriate facilities to perform rape examinations. Option "4" does not address the abuse.**

**65.** Correct answers are 1, 2, and 4.
1. Frequently child abusers will deny the child's reports of abuse and say the child is a habitual liar.
2. Child abusers believe violence is an acceptable way to reduce tension. They tend to have a low tolerance for frustration and have poor impulse control.
3. Child abusers have a tendency toward feelings of helplessness and hopelessness.
4. Child abusers tend to blame the child for the abuse and not admit the problem is their own.

5. The child abuser may have been abused as a child, but there is no evidence of the child abuser being spoiled as a child.

**TEST-TAKING HINT: This is an alternative-type question. The test taker should examine each option carefully to determine if it could be a correct answer. Option "3" could be eliminated because of the adjective "high," and "5" could be eliminated because of the adjective "spoiled."**

**66.** Correct answers are 1, 2, 4, and 5.
1. This is a myth believed by some people. Many individuals are raped, ranging in age from infants to people in their 90s of all gender identities, and sexual orientations. No one asks to be raped.
2. If a person says I am not interested in any type of sexual activity, it means "no" and therefore, anything else is forced and is rape. "No" means "no." It is considered rape if a prostitute says "no."
3. Rape is an act of violence motivated by the rapist desiring to overpower and control the victim.
4. This is a myth. Men and children can be victims of rape. Sexual arousal and orgasm do not imply consent; it may be a pathological response to stimulation.
5. This is a myth. Sexual assault can occur between spouses and partners.

**TEST-TAKING HINT: This question asks about myths or widely held false beliefs. Only one option is a true statement about rape.**

**67.** 1. The nurse can encourage the client to press charges but has no right to insist.
2. The nurse should treat the wound and may find it frustrating the client will not press charges, but the nurse is obligated to provide the client information to help the client to get to a safe place.
3. The woman is more aware of this fact than the nurse.
4. The nurse should help the client to devise a plan for safety by giving the client the number of a safe house or a women's shelter.

**TEST-TAKING HINT: The test taker could eliminate option "3" based on common sense; the client lives in an abusive situation and realizes the abuser's potential more than the nurse. Option "2" could be eliminated by the phrase "do nothing else." Option "1" could be eliminated because of the principle of nurses empowering their clients, not overpowering them, which is what has been happening to the client already.**

**68.** 1. This client has signs of ongoing abuse such as multiple burns and contusions in different stages of healing.
   2. Often older clients are ashamed to report abuse because they raised the abuser and feel responsible for their child becoming an abuser. The elder parent may feel financially dependent on the child or be afraid of being placed in a long-term care facility. Forty-seven states have Adult Protective Services (APS) created by the states to protect older citizens.
   3. There is no evidence provided in the stem that the client is not mentally competent, and there is evidence in the stem of physical abuse. This client is performing activities of daily living.
   4. The client may have fallen and sustained contusions, but burn marks would not result from a fall.

**TEST-TAKING HINT:** The test taker could eliminate options "1," "3," and "4" by examining the stem and noting the physical abuse occurring and by the fact the client is functioning by performing activities of daily living.

**69.** 1. Unless the nurse is being personally abused in the same manner the client is being abused and has seen the abuse taking place, the nurse cannot "know" the client is being abused.
   2. Alcohol and drugs are implicated in the abuse of many clients, but not all abusers use alcohol or drugs.
   3. This is agreeing with the abuser about the client causing the abuse.
   4. This statement assesses the abused client's safety (or a plan for safety).

**TEST-TAKING HINT:** Option "3" could be eliminated because it blames the victim. Option "1" can be eliminated because the nurse should not tell the client "I know" unless the nurse has proof or has been in the situation.

**70.** 1. Clients diagnosed with PTSD are easily startled and can react violently if awakened from sleep by being touched.
   2. Touching the client can cause the client to become afraid, to feel under attack, and to

react violently. The nurse should not touch a sleeping client diagnosed with PTSD.
   3. If the client awakes with the nurse in the room, the client could become fearful and react to the fear.
   4. There may be times when the nurse must awaken the client to determine if the client is physically stable.

**TEST-TAKING HINT:** Option "4" can be eliminated because of the absolute statement "at all." Options "2" and "3" can be eliminated if the test taker thinks of how it feels to be startled when perceiving another person around him or her when the test taker was not aware of the other person's presence.

**71.** 1. This plan for the client to take RU 486, or the "morning-after" pill, prevents pregnancy from occurring, but it does not directly address coping skills.
   2. The client may talk about "what if I had not done . . .," but the client is not guilty of causing the rape.
   3. The client should be provided the phone number of a rape crisis counseling center or counselor to help the client deal with the psychological effects of having been raped.
   4. This is a legal issue.

**TEST-TAKING HINT:** The test taker should read the stem "ineffective coping" and eliminate the physiological problem in option "1" and the legal problem in option "4."

**72.** 1. The nurse should attempt to develop a relationship in which the client feels they can trust the nurse (people of all gender identities are abused by significant others).
   2. The first step in helping an abused client is to get the client to admit the abuse is happening.
   3. This could cause the abuse to escalate.
   4. This is what the nurse is trying to get the client to avoid.

**TEST-TAKING HINT:** Option "1" could be eliminated because it is the opposite of what the nurse tries to establish in a nurse–client relationship. Option "4" places the client in harm's way.

73. 1. This should be considered a NOW medication but should not be the first intervention because cultures have been ordered.
    2. The IV line must be started before the IVPB can be administered, but it is not first.
    3. The admission assessment must be completed in a timely manner, but it is actually the last intervention of the four listed. Admission assessments involve a thorough head-to-toe assessment and can take time to complete.
    4. The cultures are the priority intervention because the antibiotics should not be administered until the cultures have been drawn.

TEST-TAKING HINT: After looking at all the options, the test taker should select the option that best addresses the abnormal laboratory value, which is the high white blood cell (WBC) count. This client has an infection and must be treated as rapidly as possible, but performing cultures first will give the HCP information about the causative agent without skewing the results.

74. 1. The normal saline can be initiated to maintain the client's circulatory status while the packed red blood cells (PRBCs) are cross-matched.
    2. The PRBCs are the third order to initiate.
    3. Furosemide is not to be administered until after the client has received the first unit of PRBCs.
    4. Diphenhydramine is the second order to initiate because it is to be administered before the PRBCs.

TEST-TAKING HINT: After looking at all the options, the test taker should select the option that best addresses the entire situation. This client has perfusion and hematological regulation issues.

75. Correct answers are 1 and 3.
    1. A is the right upper shoulder. The electrical activity of the client's heart will be read similar to lead II on an electrocardiogram (ECG). Current delivered during defibrillation will be sent from the right shoulder through the heart muscle to the left lower thoracic area.
    2. Site B is the left upper chest area, and current will not be consistent with the normal electrical pattern of the heart.

3. Site C is the left lower thoracic area, and the electrical activity of the client's heart will be read similar to lead II on an ECG. Current delivered during defibrillation will be sent from the right shoulder through the heart muscle to the left lower thoracic area.
4. Site D is the right lower thoracic area, and the electrical current passing from one electrode to the other is opposite the normal electrical pattern of the heart.
5. Site E is the right arm and the electrical activity will not reach the cardiac muscle.

TEST-TAKING HINT: After looking at all the options, the test taker should treat each option like a true or false response. Is the pad placement correct for an ECG?

76. 1. The nurse should wait to be assigned when responding to a disaster; even if the nurse works in the emergency department, the nurse may be assigned to a different area for the disaster.
    2. The nurse should not assume where to be best utilized during a disaster. The command center administrative nurse will determine where the greatest need exists.
    3. The command center administrative nurse will determine where the greatest need exists. The nurse reports there to receive assignments.
    4. The nurse should not delay responding to the hospital to pack a bag.

TEST-TAKING HINT: After looking at all the options, the test taker should think, "How will I know where the greatest need is?" The answer is to ask for instructions, not assume the answer.

77. 1. The charge nurse would not reassign the clients in the middle of the shift. If the nurse caring for the client has time, then the nurse can assist the other staff.
    2. The HCP should notify the family of the client's arrest and current bed assignment.
    3. The charge nurse must maintain a culture of readiness for any emergency. The crash cart must be checked and restocked for a future emergency.
    4. A unit meeting can be held when the crash cart has been restocked and the floor has settled down, but it is not the priority.

**TEST-TAKING HINT:** After looking at all the options, the test taker should select the option that best cares for the remaining clients on the unit.

78. **Correct answers are 1, 3, and 4.**
    1. The 13-year-old is having elective surgery and could be rescheduled.
    2. Abdominal aortic aneurysm surgeries are not scheduled until the aneurysm is at least 7 cm and at risk for rupture. This client should not be discharged.
    3. This client is on oral medication and the INR is in therapeutic range; this client could be discharged.
    4. Not wanting to care for oneself is not a valid reason to remain in the hospital.
    5. A small bowel obstruction can compromise the blood supply to the bowel tissue. This is a life-threatening situation. The client should not be discharged.

**TEST-TAKING HINT:** After looking at all the options, the test taker should select the options that best assess the entire situation. Option "1" describes an elective surgery and could be postponed. The client described in option "3" is on oral medication, warfarin (Coumadin), with an INR that is within the therapeutic range. The client in option "4" has a psychosocial issue, and this does not warrant remaining in the hospital.

79. 1. The nurse should not panic but follow the infection-control procedures as guided by the Centers for Disease Control (CDC).
    2. This is not a professional response to a public health issue. The best action the nurse can take is to follow the procedure and remain calm.
    3. Television news reports are frequently inaccurate and biased.
    4. The nurse should not discuss hospital situations in a public venue; rather, the nurse should refer the news reporter to the Public Relations Officer for the hospital.

**TEST-TAKING HINT:** After looking at all the options, the test taker should select the option that best assesses the entire situation, which is the following of policy. There will be a tendency for mass hysteria to occur in the community, but the CDC has plans for this type of emergency.

80. 1. The nurse should start an intravenous line with a large-bore needle to administer fluids and blood if needed. This client may need a rapid replacement of fluid volume.
    2. The nurse must assess the client to determine if the client is stable or unstable before being able to delegate this task to a UAP.
    3. This will be done, but not first.
    4. The nurse must assess the client to determine if the client is stable or unstable before allowing the client to go to the radiology department.

**TEST-TAKING HINT:** The nurse should initiate an IV because in an emergency, this, followed with rapid fluid replacement, can stabilize an unstable client. Then the nurse must determine if the client is stable before delegating activities or allowing the client to leave the ED.

# EMERGENCY NURSING
# COMPREHENSIVE EXAMINATION

1. The ED nurse is caring for a client diagnosed with multiple rib fractures. Which data should the nurse include in the assessment?
   1. Level of orientation to time and place.
   2. Current use and last dose of medication.
   3. Symmetrical movement of the chest.
   4. Time of last meal the client ate.

2. The nurse is caring for a client in the ED diagnosed with abdominal trauma, and peritoneal lavage was performed. Which intervention should the nurse include in the plan of care?
   1. Assess for the presence of blood, bile, or feces.
   2. Palpate the client for bilateral femoral pulses.
   3. Perform Leopold's maneuver every 8 hours.
   4. Collect information on the client's dietary history.

3. The older client is brought to the ED reporting cramps, headache, and weakness after working outside in the sun. The telemetry shows sinus tachycardia. Which intervention should the nurse implement?
   1. Determine if the client is experiencing any thirst.
   2. Administer $D_5W$ intravenously at 250 mL/hr.
   3. Maintain a cool environment to promote rest.
   4. Withhold the client's oral intake.

4. The ED nurse is caring for a near-drowning victim. Which expected outcome should the nurse include in the plan of care for this client?
   1. Maintain the client's cardiac function.
   2. Promote a continued decrease in lung surfactant.
   3. Warm rapidly to minimize the effects of hypothermia.
   4. Keep the oxygen saturation level above 93%.

5. The nurse is assessing the near-drowning victim. Which data **require immediate** intervention?
   1. The onset of pink, frothy sputum.
   2. An oral temperature of 97°F.
   3. An alcohol level of 100 mg/dL.
   4. A heart rate of 100 beats/min.

6. A nurse is at the lake when a person nearly drowns. The nurse determines the client is breathing spontaneously. Which data should the nurse assess **next**?
   1. Possibility of drug use.
   2. Spinal cord injury.
   3. Level of confusion.
   4. Amount of alcohol.

7. The ED nurse is caring for a male client admitted with carbon monoxide poisoning. Which intervention requires the nurse to notify the rapid response team?
   1. The client has expectorated black sputum.
   2. The client reports trying to kill himself.
   3. The client's pulse oximeter reading is 94%.
   4. The client has stridor and reports dizziness.

8. The ED nurse is working triage. Which client should be triaged **first**?
   1. A client diagnosed with multiple injuries from a motor-vehicle accident.
   2. A client reporting epigastric pain and nausea after eating.
   3. An older client with a fractured left femoral neck from a fall.
   4. The client suffering from a migraine headache and nausea.

9. The nurse is providing discharge teaching for the client with intermaxillary wiring to repair a fractured mandible. Which statement by the client indicates teaching has been **effective**?
   1. Iced alcoholic drinks may be consumed by using a straw.
   2. Only one food item should be consumed at one time.
   3. Carbonated sodas should be limited to two daily.
   4. Teeth can be brushed after tenderness and edema subside.

10. The occupational health nurse is called to the scene of a traumatic amputation of a finger. Which intervention should the nurse implement before sending the client to the ED? **Select all that apply.**
   1. Rinse the amputated finger with sterile normal saline.
   2. Place the amputated finger in a sealed and watertight plastic bag.
   3. Place the amputated finger into an iced saline solution.
   4. Wrap the amputated finger in saline-moistened gauze dressings.
   5. Replace the amputated finger on the hand and wrap it with gauze.

11. The nurse is teaching the client home care instructions for a reimplanted finger after a traumatic amputation. Which information should the nurse include in the teaching?
    1. Perform range-of-motion exercises weekly.
    2. Smoking may be resumed if it does not cause nausea.
    3. Protect the finger and be careful not to reinjure the finger.
    4. An elevated temperature is the only reason to call the HCP.

12. The ED nurse is caring for a client diagnosed with frostbite of the feet. Which intervention should the nurse implement?
    1. Massage the feet vigorously.
    2. Soak the feet in warm water.
    3. Apply a heating pad to feet.
    4. Apply petroleum jelly to feet.

13. A student reports to the school nurse with reports of stinging and burning from a wasp sting. Which intervention should the nurse implement?
    1. Grasp the stinger with tweezers and pull it out.
    2. Apply a warm, moist soak to the area.
    3. Cleanse the site with alcohol.
    4. Apply an ice pack to the site.

14. The ED nurse is caring for a client diagnosed with a severe allergic reaction to a bee sting. Which discharge instructions should the nurse discuss with the client?
    1. Instruct the client to wear a medical identification bracelet.
    2. Apply corticosteroid cream to the site to prevent anaphylaxis.
    3. Administer epinephrine 1:10,000 intravenously every 3 minutes.
    4. Teach the client to avoid attracting insects by wearing bright colors.

15. The ED nurse is caring for a client diagnosed with fractured pelvis and bladder trauma secondary to a motor-vehicle accident. Which data are **most important** for the nurse to assess?
    1. Monitor the creatinine and BUN.
    2. Check urine output hourly.
    3. Note the amount and color of the urine.
    4. Assess for bladder distention.

16. The school nurse is caring for a child with a deep laceration. Which intervention should the nurse implement **first**?
    1. Clean with saline solution.
    2. Apply direct pressure.
    3. Don nonsterile gloves.
    4. Notify the child's parents.

17. The ED receives a client involved in a motor-vehicle accident. The nurse notes a large hematoma on the right flank. Which intervention should the nurse implement **first**?
    1. Insert an indwelling urinary catheter.
    2. Take the vital signs every 15 minutes.
    3. Monitor the skin turgor every hour.
    4. Mark the edges of the bruised area.

18. Which expected outcome is **priority** for the nurse caring for a client diagnosed with chest trauma from a gunshot injury?
    1. The client will have an absence of pain.
    2. The client will maintain a BP of 90/60.
    3. The client will have symmetrical chest expansion.
    4. The client will maintain urine output of 30 mL/hr.

19. Which problem is **most appropriate** for the nurse to identify for the client experiencing renal trauma?
    1. Infection of the renal tract.
    2. Ineffective tissue perfusion.
    3. Alteration in skin integrity.
    4. Alteration in temperature.

20. The nurse is discharging a client from the ED with a sutured laceration on the right knee. Which information is **most important** for the nurse to obtain?
    1. The date of the client's last tetanus injection.
    2. The name of the client's regular health-care provider.
    3. The client's ability to return to the ED for suture removal.
    4. The client's allergies to any drug or food.

21. The nurse working in an outpatient clinic is caring for a client diagnosed with epistaxis. Which intervention should the nurse implement **first**?
    1. Take the client's blood pressure in both arms.
    2. Hold the nose with thumb and finger for 15 minutes.
    3. Have the client sit with the head tilted back and hold a tissue.
    4. Prepare to administer silver nitrate, a cauterizing agent, with a packing applicator.

22. The client with a temperature of 94°F is being treated in the ED. Which intervention should the nurse implement to directly **elevate** the client's temperature?
    1. Remove the client's clothing.
    2. Place a warm air blanket over the client.
    3. Have the client change into a hospital gown.
    4. Raise the temperature in the room.

23. The ED nurse is caring for a client diagnosed with a cocaine overdose. Which intervention should the RN delegate to the UAP?
    1. Evaluate the airway and breathing.
    2. Monitor the rate of intravenous fluids.
    3. Place the cardiac monitor on the client.
    4. Transfer the client to the intensive care unit.

24. The client has been brought to the ED by ambulance following a motor-vehicle accident with a flail chest, an intravenous line, and a Heimlich valve. Which intervention should the nurse implement **first**?
    1. Start a large-bore intravenous access.
    2. Request a portable chest x-ray.
    3. Prepare to insert chest tubes.
    4. Assess the cardiac rhythm on the monitor.

25. The ED nurse is completing the initial assessment on a suddenly unresponsive client. Which intervention should the nurse implement **first**?
    1. Assess the rate and site of the intravenous fluid.
    2. Administer an ampule of sodium bicarbonate.
    3. Assess the cardiac rhythm shown on the monitor.
    4. Prepare to cardiovert the client into sinus rhythm.

26. The ED nurse is caring for a female client diagnosed with a greenstick fracture of the left forearm and multiple contusions on the face, arms, trunk, and legs. The significant other is in the treatment area with the client. Which nursing interventions should the nurse implement? **Rank in order of priority.**
    1. Determine if the client has a plan for safety.
    2. Assess the pulse, temperature, and capillary refill of the left wrist and hand.
    3. Ask the client if she feels safe in her own home.
    4. Request the significant other wait in the waiting room during the examination.
    5. Notify the social worker to consult on the case.

1. 1. Orientation to person, place, and time should be assessed on all clients, but this information will not provide specific information about the chest trauma.
   2. The current use of all medication and the last doses should be assessed for all clients.
   3. **When a client suffers from multiple rib fractures, the client has an increased risk for flail chest. The nurse should assess the client for paradoxical chest wall movement and, if respiratory distress is present, for pallor and cyanosis.**
   4. The time of this last meal is important if the client were to have surgery or intubation planned. A nutritional assessment should be performed on all clients.

2. 1. **A diagnostic peritoneal lavage is performed to assess the presence of blood, bile, and feces from internal bleeding induced by injury. If any of these are present, surgery should be considered to explore the extent of damage and repair of the injury.**
   2. Palpating the client's peripheral pulses indicates blood flow to the extremities. Femoral pulses are not necessarily assessed if all distal pulses are strong.
   3. Leopold's maneuver is performed on pregnant clients to assess the position of the fetus.
   4. A dietary history is information that is assessed but not in an emergency situation. Assessments need to be efficient and direct to eliminate any time-wasting activities.

3. 1. Older clients lose the defense mechanism of increased thirst with dehydration. This does not accurately indicate fluid deficit.
   2. Intravenous fluid should be administered, but the solution should correct fluid and electrolyte imbalances. $D_5W$ does not replace electrolytes lost, and 250 mL/hr could place the client at risk for heart failure if the body cannot adjust rapidly to the fluid replacement.
   3. **The nurse should encourage the client to rest and should maintain a cool environment to assist the client in recovering from heat exhaustion. Older clients are more susceptible to this condition.**
   4. If the client can tolerate oral fluids, the client should be encouraged to drink fluids to replace electrolytes lost in excessive sweating.

4. 1. An expected outcome is a desired occurrence, not a common event. Tachycardia is a common manifestation of a near-drowning event, but it is not desired. A combination of physiological changes, hypothermia, and hypoxia puts the client at risk for life-threatening cardiac rhythms.
   2. Any near-drowning causes a decrease in alveolar surfactant, which results in alveolar collapse. A decrease in surfactant is not the desired outcome.
   3. The client needs to be rewarmed slowly to reduce the influx of metabolites. These metabolites, including lactic acid, remain in the extremities.
   4. **The oxygen level needs to be maintained greater than 93%. The client needs as much support as necessary for this. Mechanical ventilation with peak end-expiratory pressure (PEEP) and high oxygen levels may be needed to achieve this goal.**

5. 1. **The onset of pinky, frothy sputum indicates the client is experiencing pulmonary edema. This needs to be treated to prevent further decline in this client.**
   2. An oral temperature of 97°F is in the lower level of within normal limits.
   3. A blood alcohol of 100 mg/dL is an elevation but should not be considered priority over pulmonary edema. Treatments for elevations in toxicology levels can be considered after the client is stable.
   4. A heart rate of 100 beats/min is tachycardia, but not at a critical level. The nurse needs to remember Maslow's hierarchy of needs, and airway and breathing are physiological needs that take priority.

6. 1. The use of drugs can alter the treatment of and recovery from the near-drowning event. This is information needed, but it is not a priority at this time.
   2. An injury of the spinal cord should be considered and the spine should be assessed, but after the client has been stabilized. The nurse does not complete an assessment of a potential spinal injury before assessing oxygenation status.

3. The nurse should assess the victim for hypoxia. Clinical manifestations of hypoxia include confusion or irritability and alterations in the level of consciousness, such as lethargy.

4. The amount of alcohol ingestion will affect the treatment, but this is not a higher priority than oxygenation.

7. 1. The client diagnosed with carbon monoxide poisoning frequently has black sputum from inhaling soot, so the RRT does not need to be notified.

2. The client admitting to attempting suicide requires the client being placed on one-to-one suicide precautions and psychological counseling.

3. A pulse oximeter reading of 94% indicates the client is being well oxygenated and does not require notifying the RRT.

4. **Stridor or dizziness indicates occlusion of the airway, which is a medical emergency. The RRT is called when the client is experiencing a decline but is still breathing.**

8. 1. **Injuries from a motor-vehicle accident can be life-threatening. This client should be assessed first to rule out respiratory difficulties and hemorrhage.**

2. Epigastric pain with nausea after eating sounds like gallbladder disease. Pain has high priority, but not over breathing and hemorrhage.

3. Older clients have special fluid and electrolyte issues after a fall. The cause of the fall may be cardiac, but the question does not indicate this.

4. Migraine headaches are painful experiences, but they do not have a higher priority than breathing and hemorrhage.

9. 1. Alcoholic beverages should be avoided to prevent nausea and vomiting. The client should be taught where and how to cut wires if vomiting occurs.

2. A combination of foods should be blended into a milkshake and consumed to maintain caloric intake and promote nutrition.

3. Carbonated sodas can cause foam in the back of the throat and may induce vomiting.

4. **Hygiene is helpful in healing. The mouth should be rinsed and an irrigation device should be used frequently. Gentle brushing and rinsing the mouth after each meal and at bedtime can begin after edema and tenderness subside.**

10. Correct answers are 1, 2, and 4.

1. The amputated finger and all tissue should be rinsed with sterile normal saline to remove dirt and sent to the ED with the client.

2. Place the finger and all tissue in a watertight, sealed plastic bag to prevent loss and contamination.

3. The finger or other tissue should not be placed on ice or in saline solution because this will cause severe damage to the tissue cells.

4. The finger should be wrapped in gauze moistened with sterile normal saline.

5. The finger should not be replaced on the hand and wrapped with gauze in the field. The surgeon will determine if reattachment is possible.

11. 1. Exercises should be performed several times each day, not weekly.

2. Smoking causes vasoconstriction, which will compromise the implanted finger's survival.

3. The client should take extra care to protect the finger from injury. The peripheral nerves protecting the finger require months to regenerate.

4. The client needs to report any signs of rejection of the finger, such as infection or impaired circulation, not just an elevated temperature.

12. 1. Massaging or rubbing tissue with frostbite will cause further damage.

2. **Soaking the feet in a warm bath of 107°F causes rapid continuous rewarming.**

3. Heating pads are not used to rewarm tissue with frostbite. Heating pads can cause tissue damage from burns, especially in tissue with impaired sensation.

4. Petroleum jelly does not affect the temperature of the tissue.

13. 1. The stinger should not be grasped because the wasp's venom sac may release more toxin. The stinger should be scraped in the opposite direction.

2. Warmth increases the blood flow, which will increase the edema.

3. The site should be cleaned with soap and water, not alcohol.

4. **The nurse should apply an ice pack to the site. The cold will decrease blood flow and sensation. The ice should be applied intermittently.**

14. 1. Clients with severe reactions to insect stings should wear identifying bracelets to provide information. If the client is unconscious, the bracelet can alert the HCP so treatment can be started.
2. Corticosteroid creams treat local reactions, not systemic ones.
3. Epinephrine 1:10,000 is administered intravenously during a code situation or for a severe anaphylactic reaction to an allergen. This client is being discharged and may need an epinephrine injector (EpiPen) to carry at all times but not IV epinephrine.
4. Bright-colored clothing attracts insects. Clients allergic to insect stings should learn how to avoid them to decrease the risk. Flowery-smelling perfumes and lotions should also be avoided.

15. 1. The creatinine and BUN assess kidney function, but the nurse should assess the bladder function by checking the amount and color of the urine.
2. Checking the urine output hourly is appropriate data to assess but not the most important for a client diagnosed with bladder trauma.
3. **The amount and color of urine assists with diagnosing the extent of the injury. The color of the urine indicates the presence of blood. The amount indicates whether the urine is contained throughout the pathway from bladder to urinary meatus.**
4. The nurse should not palpate a client diagnosed with bladder trauma because it could cause further damage.

16. 1. The laceration should be cleaned well to prevent infection. A sterile saline solution or water should be used. This is done after donning nonsterile gloves and applying pressure.
2. The nurse should apply direct pressure to a deep laceration to stop the bleeding after donning nonsterile gloves.
3. **The nurse must follow standard precautions in the school nurse setting by donning nonsterile gloves before caring for the client.**
4. The school nurse must notify the parents but not before taking care of the client.

17. 1. Inserting an indwelling catheter may cause further injury. Until the extent of the injury is determined, prevention of further damage should have a high priority.
2. **Vital signs should be taken frequently to assess for covert bleeding. The**

hematoma in the flank area may indicate the presence of trauma to the kidney. Because of the large amount of blood flow through the kidney, hemorrhage is a high risk.
3. Assessing skin turgor is important in determining the fluid balance, but it is not a higher priority than monitoring vital signs.
4. The nurse could mark the bruised area to assess if the hematoma is enlarging, but this is not the first intervention.

18. 1. Pain management is a goal for clients. At this time in the care of this client, it is not realistic to expect no pain.
2. Maintaining homeostasis is an appropriate outcome, but the priority is to maintain respiratory status. Remember Maslow's hierarchy of needs.
3. **Symmetrical chest expansion indicates the client's lungs have not collapsed and air is being exchanged. This is the client's priority outcome.**
4. A urine output of 30 mL/hr indicates the tissues are being adequately perfused and is an indicator of kidney functioning. Kidney function is important but is not a priority over respiratory status in a client diagnosed with a gunshot wound.

19. 1. Potential for infection is an appropriate nursing diagnosis, but there is no indication of infection from this question.
2. **Bleeding results in an impairment of tissue perfusion. Because of the large amount of blood flow through the renal system, bleeding is a major problem.**
3. Skin integrity is not necessarily an issue in trauma. There is no indication from the question that the skin is not intact.
4. An alteration in temperature is not a problem for this client unless infection occurs. This intervention is not indicated at this time.

20. 1. **Any client without a tetanus injection within 5 years will need to receive an injection as prophylaxis.**
2. The nurse may need to determine if the usual HCP can remove the sutures or if the client should return to the ED for suture removal, but this is not the most important information.
3. This information is important to teach the client, but preventing tetanus (lockjaw) is a priority.
4. This client has been treated, so it is too late to determine if the client has allergies.

21. 1. The nurse should assess the client's blood pressure but not before stopping the bleeding. The most common cause of spontaneous epistaxis is hypertension.
    2. **Most nosebleeds will stop after applying pressure on the nose between thumb and index finger for 15 minutes.**
    3. The nurse should position the client with the head tilted forward. This position will prevent the client from swallowing the blood. The blood can be aspirated if the head is tilted back.
    4. Most nosebleeds respond to pressure. If pressure for 15 minutes does not stop the bleeding, the HCP may need to use electrocautery or silver nitrate. This is performed by the HCP, not the nurse.

22. 1. Removing clothing causes further chilling.
    2. **The warm air blanket blows warm air over the client and is an active warming method.**
    3. Hospital gowns have openings down the back and can increase chilling.
    4. Raising the temperature of the room will not directly raise the client's temperature.

23. 1. Evaluation of airway and breathing is assessment and cannot be delegated.
    2. Monitoring the rate of intravenous fluid is a part of administering a medication. Medication administration cannot be delegated.
    3. **The UAP can attach leads to the client for the cardiac monitor.**
    4. The nurse cannot delegate an unstable client to the UAP. A client being transferred to the intensive care unit is unstable.

24. 1. The client already has intravenous access; therefore, the nurse would not need to start an intravenous line.
    2. A STAT chest x-ray will be done to evaluate the extent of the chest trauma, but it is not the first intervention.

3. The client will require a chest tube because the Heimlich valve is only temporary; therefore, the nurse should prepare for this first.
    4. Assessing cardiac rhythm is important, but the client is in distress and needs circulatory support, not further assessment.

25. 1. Assessing the site and rate is not the first intervention.
    2. Sodium bicarbonate is not administered unless indicated by ABGs.
    3. **The rhythm on the monitor should be assessed. Many suddenly unresponsive clients have a lethal rhythm requiring defibrillation immediately.**
    4. Cardioversion is not appropriate. Defibrillation may be needed.

26. Correct order is 4, 2, 3, 1, 5.
    4. This is done first before any action is taken to decrease suspicions on the part of the significant other. The nurse needs to ask the client questions regarding the injuries and may not get truthful answers with the significant other in the room.
    2. The nurse should assess the actual physical problems before assessing the potential abuse situation.
    3. This is one of the first questions the nurse should ask to determine if abuse is occurring.
    1. The nurse should determine if the client has a plan to escape the violence. The nurse should provide the client with hotline numbers for safe houses.
    5. The nurse should refer the client to the social worker for further evaluation and referral needs.

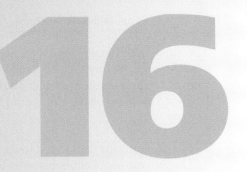

# Perioperative Care

*You don't have to be great to start, but you have to start to be great.*

—Zig Ziglar

Surgery is a serious experience for clients. Before the surgery, in preoperative care, the nurse must prepare clients for the specific surgery, telling them what to expect during the procedure and afterward. During surgery, nurses help monitor the client and maintain the proper condition of the operating room. The postoperative period is also important. The nurse must assess the client frequently during the immediate postoperative period, ensuring that the airway, breathing, and circulation are maintained. The client also must be assessed for any complications, such as hemorrhage, evisceration, or infection. Because acute pain is associated with most surgeries, the nurse also must assess the level and type of pain and dispense pain-relieving medication as ordered by the health-care provider (HCP).

## KEYWORDS

Anesthesia
Anesthesiologist
Circulating nurse

Evisceration
Nurse anesthetist

## PRACTICE QUESTIONS

### Preoperative

1. The nurse requests the client to sign a surgical informed consent form for an emergency appendectomy. Which statement by the client indicates **further teaching** is needed?
   1. "I will be glad when this is over so I can go home today."
   2. "I will not be able to eat or drink anything before my surgery."
   3. "I can practice relaxing by listening to my favorite music."
   4. "I will need to get up and walk as soon as possible."

2. The nurse in the holding area of the surgery department is interviewing a client requesting to keep his religious medal on during surgery. Which intervention should the nurse implement?
   1. Notify the surgeon about the client's request to wear the medal.
   2. Tape the medal to the client and allow the client to wear the medal.
   3. Request the family member to take the medal before surgery.
   4. Explain taking the medal to surgery is against the policy.

3. The nurse must obtain surgical consent forms for the scheduled surgery. Which clients are able to consent legally to surgery? **Select all that apply.**
   1. The 65-year-old client who cannot read or write.
   2. The 30-year-old non-English speaking client.
   3. The 16-year-old client with a fractured ankle.
   4. The 80-year-old client not oriented to the day.
   5. The 45-year-old client who is blind and cannot read Braille.

4. The nurse is preparing a client for surgery. Which intervention should the nurse implement **first**?
   1. Check the permit for the spouse's signature.
   2. Take and document intake and output.
   3. Administer the "on call" sedative.
   4. Complete the preoperative checklist.

5. The nurse is interviewing a surgical client in the holding area. Which information should the nurse report to the anesthesiologist? **Select all that apply.**
   1. The client has loose, decayed teeth.
   2. The client is experiencing anxiety.
   3. The client smokes two packs of cigarettes a day.
   4. The client has a chest x-ray that shows no infiltrates.
   5. The client reports using herbs.

6. Which task would be **most appropriate** for the RN to delegate to the unlicensed assistive personnel (UAP)?
   1. Complete the preoperative checklist.
   2. Assess the client's preoperative vital signs.
   3. Teach the client about coughing and deep breathing.
   4. Assist the client in removing clothing and jewelry.

7. The nurse is assessing a client in the day-surgery unit stating, "I am really afraid of having this surgery. I'm afraid of what they will find." Which statement would be the **most therapeutic** response by the nurse?
   1. "Don't worry about your surgery. It is safe."
   2. "Tell me why you're worried about your surgery."
   3. "Tell me about your fears of having this surgery."
   4. "I understand how you feel. Surgery is frightening."

8. The 68-year-old client scheduled for intestinal surgery does not have clear fecal contents after three tap water enemas. Which intervention should the nurse implement **first**?
   1. Notify the surgeon of the client's status.
   2. Continue giving enemas until clear.
   3. Increase the client's IV fluid rate.
   4. Obtain STAT serum electrolytes.

9. The nurse is caring for a male client scheduled for abdominal surgery. Which interventions should the nurse include in the plan of care? **Select all that apply.**
   1. Perform passive range-of-motion exercises.
   2. Discuss how to cough and deep breathe effectively.
   3. Tell the client he can have a meal in the post-anesthesia care unit.
   4. Teach ways to manage postoperative pain.
   5. Discuss events that occur in the postanesthesia care unit.

10. The nurse is caring for a client scheduled for total hip replacement. Which behavior indicates the **need for further** preoperative teaching?
    1. The client uses the diaphragm and abdominal muscles to inhale through the nose and exhale through the mouth.
    2. The client demonstrates dorsiflexion of the feet, flexing of the toes, and moves the feet in a circular motion.
    3. The client uses the incentive spirometer and inhales slowly and deeply, so the piston rises to the preset volume.
    4. The client gets out of bed by lifting straight upright from the waist and then swings both legs along the side of the bed.

11. The nurse is completing a preoperative assessment on a male client who states, "I am allergic to codeine." Which intervention should the nurse implement **first**?
    1. Apply an allergy bracelet on the client's wrist.
    2. Label the client's allergies on the front page of the EHR.
    3. Ask the client what happens when he takes the codeine.
    4. Document the allergy on the medication administration record.

12. Which laboratory result would require **immediate intervention** by the nurse for the client scheduled for surgery?

| Laboratory Test | Client Results | Normal Values |
|---|---|---|
| Prothrombin time (PT) | 12 | 10–13 seconds |
| Hemoglobin (Hgb) | 15 | Male: 14–17.3 g/dL Female: 11.7–15.5 g/dL |
| Calcium | 9.2 | 8.2–10.2 mg/dL |
| Potassium (K⁺) | 2.4 | 3.5–5.3 mEq/L or mmol/L |

1. Calcium.
2. Prothrombin time (PT).
3. Hemoglobin (Hgb).
4. Potassium ($K^+$).

## Intraoperative

13. Which activities are the circulating nurse's responsibilities in the operating room?
    1. Monitor the position of the client, prepare the surgical site, and ensure the client's safety.
    2. Give preoperative medication in the holding area and monitor the client's response to anesthesia.
    3. Prepare sutures; set up the sterile field; and count all needles, sponges, and instruments.
    4. Prepare the medications to be administered by the anesthesiologist and change the tubing for the anesthesia machine.

14. The circulating nurse observes the surgical scrub technician remove a sponge from the edge of the sterile field with a clamp and place the sponge and clamp in a designated area. Which action should the RN implement?
    1. Place the sponge back where it was.
    2. Tell the technician not to waste supplies.
    3. Do nothing because this is the correct procedure.
    4. Take the sponge out of the room immediately.

15. The circulating nurse and the scrub technician find a discrepancy in the sponge count. Which action should the RN take **first**?
    1. Notify the client's surgeon.
    2. Complete an occurrence report.
    3. Contact the surgical manager.
    4. Recount all sponges.

16. Which violation of surgical asepsis would require **immediate intervention** by the circulating nurse?
    1. Surgical supplies were cleaned and sterilized before the case.
    2. The circulating nurse is wearing a long-sleeved sterile gown.
    3. Masks covering the mouth and nose are being worn by the surgical team.
    4. The scrub nurse setting up the sterile field is wearing artificial nails.

17. The nurse identifies the nursing diagnosis "risk for injury related to positioning" for the client in the operating room. Which nursing intervention should the nurse implement?
    1. Avoid using the cautery unit that does not have a biomedical tag on it.
    2. Carefully pad the client's elbows before covering the client with a blanket.
    3. Apply a warming pad on the OR table before placing the client on the table.
    4. Check the EHR for any prescription or over-the-counter medication use.

18. The circulating nurse is positioning clients for surgery. Which client has the **greatest potential** for nerve damage?
    1. The 16-year-old client in the dorsal recumbent position having an appendectomy.
    2. The 68-year-old client in the Trendelenburg position having a cholecystectomy.
    3. The 45-year-old client in the reverse Trendelenburg position having a biopsy.
    4. The 22-year-old client in the lateral position having a nephrectomy.

19. Which situation demonstrates the circulating nurse acting as the client's advocate?
    1. Plays the client's favorite audiobook during surgery.
    2. Keeps the family informed of the findings of the surgery.
    3. Keeps the operating room door closed at all times.
    4. Calls the client by the first name when the client is recovering.

20. The circulating nurse is planning the care for an intraoperative client. Which statement is the **expected** outcome?
    1. The client has no injuries from the OR equipment.
    2. The client has no postoperative infection.
    3. The client has stable vital signs during surgery.
    4. The client recovers from anesthesia.

21. Which nursing intervention has the **highest priority** when preparing the client for a surgical procedure?
    1. Pad the client's elbows and knees.
    2. Apply soft restraint straps to the extremities.
    3. Prepare the client's incision site.
    4. Document the temperature of the room.

22. The nursing manager is making assignments for the OR. Which case should the manager assign to the **inexperienced** nurse?
    1. The client having open-heart surgery.
    2. The client having a biopsy of the breast.
    3. The client having laser eye surgery.
    4. The client having a laparoscopic knee repair.

23. The circulating nurse assesses tachycardia and hypotension in the client. Which interventions should the nurse implement?
    1. Prepare cooling blankets and dantrolene sodium.
    2. Request the defibrillator be brought into the OR.
    3. Draw a PTT and prepare a heparin drip.
    4. Obtain finger stick blood glucose immediately.

24. The nurse is planning the care of the surgical client having procedural sedation. Which intervention has the **highest priority**?
    1. Assess the client's respiratory status.
    2. Monitor the client's urinary output.
    3. Take a 12-lead ECG before injection.
    4. Attempt to keep the client focused.

## Postoperative

25. The PACU nurse is receiving the client from the OR. Which intervention should the nurse implement **first**?
    1. Assess the client's breath sounds.
    2. Apply oxygen via nasal cannula.
    3. Take the client's blood pressure.
    4. Monitor the pulse oximeter reading.

26. Which assessment data indicate the postoperative client after spinal anesthesia is suffering a **complication** of the anesthesia?
    1. Loss of sensation at the lumbar (L5) dermatome.
    2. Absence of the client's posterior tibial pulse.
    3. The client has a respiratory rate of eight.
    4. The blood pressure is within 20% of the client's baseline.

27. The surgical client's vital signs are populated in the vital sign flowsheet below. The client is awake and oriented times three, and the skin is pale and damp. Which intervention should the nurse implement **first**?

    | Vital Sign Flowsheet | Client Results | Normal Values |
    |---|---|---|
    | Blood pressure | 88/40 | 100–119 mmHg systolic 60–80 mmHg diastolic |
    | Temperature | 98°F | Oral: 98°F (36.7°C) |
    | Pulse | 106 | 60–100 beats/min |
    | Respirations | 24 | 12–20 breaths/min |

    1. Call the surgeon and report the vital signs.
    2. Start an IV of $D_5RL$ with 20 mEq KCl at 125 mL/hr.
    3. Elevate the feet and lower the head.
    4. Monitor the vital signs every 15 minutes.

28. The PACU nurse administers naloxone to a postoperative client. Which client problem should the nurse include in the plan of care based on this medication?
    1. Alteration in comfort.
    2. Risk for depressed respiratory pattern.
    3. Potential for infection.
    4. Fluid and electrolyte imbalance.

29. The 26-year-old male client in the PACU has a heart rate of 110 and a rising temperature and reports muscle stiffness. Which interventions should the nurse implement? **Select all that apply**.
    1. Give a back rub to the client to relieve stiffness.
    2. Apply ice packs to the axillary and groin areas.
    3. Prepare an ice slush for the client to drink.
    4. Prepare to administer dantrolene.
    5. Reposition the client on a warming blanket.

30. Which data indicate to the nurse that the client 1 day postoperative right total hip replacement is progressing as **expected**?
    1. Urine output was 160 mL in the past 8 hours.
    2. Paralysis and paresthesia of the right leg.
    3. T 99.0°F, P 98, R 20, and BP 100/60.
    4. Lungs are clear bilaterally in all lobes.

31. The nurse and the UAP are working on the surgical unit. Which tasks can the RN delegate to the UAP? **Select all that apply**.
    1. Take routine vital signs on clients.
    2. Check the Jackson Pratt insertion site.
    3. Hang the client's next IV bag.
    4. Ensure the client obtains pain relief.
    5. Reposition the client every 2 hours.

32. The charge nurse is making shift assignments. Which postoperative client should be assigned to the **most experienced** nurse?
    1. The 4-year-old client after tonsillectomy and able to swallow fluids.
    2. The 74-year-old client after repair of the left hip and unable to ambulate.
    3. The 24-year-old client after an uncomplicated appendectomy the previous day.
    4. The 80-year-old client diagnosed with small bowel obstruction and congestive heart failure.

33. Which statement would be an expected outcome for the postoperative client with general anesthesia?
    1. The client will be able to sit in the chair for 30 minutes.
    2. The client will have a pulse oximetry reading of 97% on room air.

3. The client will have a urine output of 30 mL per hour.
4. The client will be able to distinguish sharp from dull sensations.

34. The postoperative client is transferred from the PACU to the surgical floor. Which action should the nurse implement **first**?
    1. Apply antiembolism hose to the client.
    2. Attach the drain to 20 cm suction.
    3. Assess the client's vital signs.
    4. Listen to the report from the anesthesiologist.

35. Which problem should the nurse identify as a **priority** for the client 1 day postoperative?
    1. Potential for hemorrhaging.
    2. Potential for injury.
    3. Potential for fluid volume excess.
    4. Potential for infection.

36. The UAP reports the vital signs for a first-day postoperative client populated in the vital sign flowsheet below. Which intervention would be **most appropriate** for the RN to implement?

| Vital Sign Flowsheet | Client Results | Normal Values |
|---|---|---|
| Blood pressure | 148/80 | 100–119 mmHg systolic 60–80 mmHg diastolic |
| Temperature | 100.8°F | Oral: 98°F (36.7°C) |
| Pulse | 80 | 60–100 beats/min |
| Respirations | 24 | 12–20 breaths/min |

1. Administer the antibiotic earlier than scheduled.
2. Change the dressing over the wound.
3. Have the client turn, cough, and deep breathe every 2 hours.
4. Encourage the client to ambulate in the hall.

## Acute Pain

37. The client is reporting left shoulder pain. Which intervention should the nurse implement **first**?
    1. Assess the neurovascular status of the left hand.
    2. Check the medication administration record.
    3. Ask if the client wants pain medication.
    4. Administer the client's pain medication.

38. The nurse is caring for a client in acute pain as a result of surgery. Which intervention should the nurse implement?
    1. Administer pain medication as soon as the time frame allows.
    2. Use nonpharmacological methods to replace medications.

3. Use cryotherapy after heat therapy because it works faster.
4. Instruct family members to administer medication with the PCA.

39. Which situation is an example of the nurse fulfilling the role of client advocate?
    1. The nurse brings the client pain medication when it is due.
    2. The nurse collaborates with other disciplines during the care conference.
    3. The nurse contacts the health-care provider when pain relief is not obtained.
    4. The nurse teaches the client to ask for medication before the pain gets to a "5."

40. Which statement should the nurse identify as the expected outcome for a client experiencing acute pain?
    1. The client will have decreased use of medication.
    2. The client will participate in self-care activities.
    3. The client will use relaxation techniques.
    4. The client will repeat instructions about medications.

41. Which nursing intervention is the **highest priority** when administering pain medication to a client experiencing acute pain?
    1. Monitor the client's vital signs.
    2. Verify the time of the last dose.
    3. Check for the client's allergies.
    4. Discuss the pain with the client.

42. Which intervention is **appropriate** for the RN to delegate to UAP when caring for the female client experiencing acute pain?
    1. Take the pain medication to the room.
    2. Apply an ice pack to the site of pain.
    3. Check on the client 30 minutes after she takes the pain medication.
    4. Observe the client's ability to use the PCA.

43. The nurse is administering an opioid narcotic to the client. Which interventions should the nurse implement for client safety? **Select all that apply.**
    1. Compare the hospital number on the MAR to the client's bracelet.
    2. Have a witness verify the wasted portion of the narcotic.
    3. Assess the client's vital signs before administration.
    4. Determine if the client has any allergies to medications.
    5. Clarify all pain medication orders with the health-care provider.

44. Which technique would be **most appropriate** for the nurse to implement when assessing a 4-year-old client in acute pain?
    1. Use words a 4-year-old child can remember.
    2. Explain the 0-to-10 pain scale to the child's parent.
    3. Have the child point to the face which describes the pain.
    4. Administer the medication every 4 hours.

45. Which nursing intervention is a **priority** for the client experiencing acute pain?
    1. Assess the client's verbal and nonverbal behavior.
    2. Wait for the client to request pain medication.
    3. Administer the pain medication on a scheduled basis.
    4. Teach the client to use only imagery every hour for the pain.

46. The nurse is conducting an interview with a 75-year-old client admitted with acute pain. Which question would have **priority** when assisting with pain management?
    1. "Have you ever had difficulty getting your pain controlled?"
    2. "What types of surgery have you had in the last 10 years?"
    3. "Have you ever been addicted to narcotics?"
    4. "Do you have a list of your prescription medications?"

47. The nurse clears the PCA pump and discovers the client has used only a small amount of medication during the shift. Which intervention should the nurse implement?
    1. Determine why the client is not using the PCA pump.
    2. Document the amount and take no action.
    3. Document the client is not having pain in the EHR.
    4. Contact the HCP and request oral medication.

48. Which problem would be **most appropriate** for the nurse to identify for the client experiencing acute pain?
    1. Ineffective coping.
    2. Potential for injury.
    3. Alteration in comfort.
    4. Altered sensory input.

## CONCEPTS

The concepts covered in this chapter focus on comfort. Exemplars that are covered are acute pain, infection, and perioperative care. Interrelated concepts of the nursing process and clinical judgment are covered throughout the questions. The concept of clinical judgment is presented in prioritizing or "**first**" questions.

49. The nurse is preparing a client for surgery with general anesthesia. Which medication should the nurse **question** administering?

| Client Name: Mr. S.A. Operation | MR#: 654231 | Diagnosis: Right Inguinal Hernia |
|---|---|---|
| DOB: 7/15/1955 | Allergies: PCN | |
| Medication | 0701–1900 | 1901–0700 |
| Metoprolol 50 mg PO daily | | 0700 |
| Cefazolin sodium 1,000 mg IVPB on call to OR | | |
| EMLA cream topical before IV start | | 0700 |
| Dabigatran etexilate 100 mg PO daily | 0900 | |
| Signature of Nurse: | Day Nurse RN/DN | Night Nurse RN/NN |

1. Metoprolol PO.
2. Cefazolin sodium IVPB.
3. EMLA cream topical.
4. Dabigatran etexilate.

50. The client has undergone an abdominal perineal resection of the colon for colon cancer with a left lower quadrant colostomy. Which interventions should the nurse implement? **Select all that apply.**
    1. Assess the stoma for color every 4 hours and prn.
    2. Encourage the client to turn, cough, and deep breathe every 2 hours.
    3. Maintain the head of the bed 30 to 40 degrees elevated at all times.
    4. Auscultate for bowel sounds every 4 hours.
    5. Administer pain medications sparingly to prevent addiction.

51. The nurse is reviewing the pathology report of a client post-cervical neck node dissection. The HCP has explained the results of the biopsy to the client. Which should the nurse implement?

| Specimen and Site | Pathological Finding |
|---|---|
| Excisional biopsy of cervical neck lymph nodes | **Lymph Node #1**<br>9 × 5 cm; multi-nodularity noted; positive for Reed-Sternberg cells<br><br>**Lymph Node #2**<br>4 × 4 cm<br>Consistent with finding in node #1<br><br>**Lymph Node #3**<br>3 × 2 cm<br>Consistent with finding in node #1<br><br>**Lymph Node #4**<br>Findings consistent with Hodgkin's lymphoma Stage 3 |

    1. Allow the client the opportunity to discuss feelings about the results.
    2. Assess the client's neck dissection dressing for bleeding.
    3. Monitor the client's white blood cell count for elevation.
    4. Call the pathology department to verify the report is correct.

52. The client returned to the medical surgical unit at 1800 following a 2-hour surgery and 1 hour in the post-anesthesia care unit (PACU). The nurse is reviewing the client's intake and output at midnight. Which intervention should the nurse implement based on the recorded data?

**Intake and Output Record**

| Day 1 | Oral (mL) | Intravenous (mL) | Urine (mL) | Nasogastric Tube (mL) | Other (Specify) (mL) |
|---|---|---|---|---|---|
| 0701–1500 | 0 | In OR | | | |
| 1501–2300 | 250 | 750 | 120 | | 120 |
| 2301–0700 | | | | | |
| Total | | | | | |

    1. Immediately place an indwelling catheter in the client.
    2. Assess the client's skin turgor in the abdominal area.
    3. Recheck the client's urinary output in 2 hours.
    4. Encourage the client to drink 500 mL of clear liquids.

53. The nurse is completing the preoperative checklist for the client scheduled for a laparoscopic cholecystectomy. The preoperative complete blood count (CBC) results are in the EHR. Which action should the nurse implement **first**?

| Laboratory Test | Client Values | Normal Values |
|---|---|---|
| White blood cell count (WBC) | 12.3 | 4.5–11.1 × 10³ cells/microL |
| Red blood cell count (RBC) | 6.8 | Male: 4.21 to 5.81 (10⁶ cells/microL)<br>Female: 3.61–5.1 (10⁶ cells/microL) |
| Hemoglobin (Hgb) | 14.4 | Male: 14–17.3 g/dL<br>Female: 11.7–15.5 g/dL |
| Hematocrit (Hct) | 41.8 | Male: 42%–52%<br>Female: 36%–48% |
| Platelets | 168 | 140–400 × 10³/microL |

1. Check off that the CBC report is in the EHR.
2. Notify the surgeon of the WBC.
3. Assess the client for dyspnea.
4. Teach the client to turn, cough, and deep breathe.

54. The nurse is receiving a client from the post-anesthesia care unit (PACU). Which interventions should the nurse implement? **Select all that apply.**
   1. Ambulate the client to the bathroom to void.
   2. Take the client's vital signs to compare with PACU data.
   3. Monitor all lines into and out of the client's body.
   4. Assess the client's surgical site.
   5. Push the client's PCA button to treat for pain during movement.

55. The 3-day postoperative client is reporting unrelieved pain at the incision site 1 hour after the administration of narcotic pain medication. Which action should the nurse implement **first**?
   1. Check the MAR for another medication to administer.
   2. Teach the client to use guided imagery to relieve the pain.
   3. Assess the client for complications.
   4. Elevate the head of the client's bed.

## Preoperative

**1.** 1. The client will be in the hospital for a few days. This is not a day-surgery procedure. The client needs more teaching.
   2. Clients are NPO (nothing by mouth) before surgery to prevent aspiration during and after anesthesia. The client understands the teaching.
   3. Listening to music and other relaxing techniques can be used to alleviate anxiety and pain. This statement indicates the client understands the teaching.
   4. Clients are encouraged to get out of bed as soon as possible and progress until a return to daily activity is achieved. The client understands the teaching.

**TEST-TAKING HINT:** This question is asking the test taker to identify the answer option that is incorrect. Three options will be appropriate statements that indicate the client understands the teaching.

**2.** 1. The surgeon does not need to be notified of the client's request; this can be addressed by the nursing staff.
   2. The medal should be taped, and the client should be allowed to wear the medal because meeting spiritual needs is essential to this client's care.
   3. The client should be allowed to bring the medal to surgery if the medal is taped to the client.
   4. Hospital policies should be established for the well-being of clients, and spiritual needs should be addressed.

**TEST-TAKING HINT:** Because options "3" and "4" do not allow the client to wear the medal to surgery, these can be eliminated as possible answers because they are both saying the same thing.

**3.** Correct answers are 1, 2, 4, and 5.
   1. The 65-year-old client unable to read can mark an "X" on the form and is legally able to sign a surgical permit as long as the client understands the benefits, alternatives, and all potential complications of the surgery.
   2. The non-English-speaking client can and should have information given and questions answered in the client's native language.

3. A 16-year-old client is not legally able to give permission for surgery unless the adolescent has been given an emancipated status by a judge. This information was not given in the stem.
   4. A client is able to give permission unless determined incompetent. Not knowing the day of the week is not significant.
   5. The client who is blind can consent to surgery. The validity of the consent does not depend on if the form is verbal or written. It depends on voluntary consent and a complete understanding of the surgery by the client (Saleh, 2004).

**TEST-TAKING HINT:** Age in a stem or option gives the test taker a clue as to the correct answer. The nurse must be aware of legal issues when caring for the client.

**4.** 1. The client's signature, not the spouse's, should be on the surgical permit.
   2. This would be important information if abnormal, but it is not the first intervention.
   3. "On call" sedatives should be administered after the surgical checklist is completed.
   4. Completing the preoperative checklist has the highest priority to ensure all details are completed without omissions.

**TEST-TAKING HINT:** A client should never be sedated until the permit has been verified and all legal issues are settled. The test taker should not read into a question by inserting facts not in the stem. For example, the test taker may think option "1" could be a correct answer if the client is confused, but the stem does not include this information.

**5.** Correct answers are 1, 3, and 5.
   1. Loose teeth or caries need to be reported to the anesthesiologist so provisions can be made to prevent breaking the teeth and causing the client to aspirate pieces possibly.
   2. The nurse should report any extremely anxious client, but the nurse can address the needs of a client experiencing expected surgical anxiety.
   3. Smokers are at a higher risk of complications from anesthesia.
   4. No infiltrates on a chest x-ray is a normal finding and does not have to be reported.

5. Herbs—for example, St. John's wort, licorice, and ginkgo—have serious interactions with anesthesia and with bodily functions such as coagulation.

**TEST-TAKING HINT:** This question is an alternate-type question requiring the test taker to select more than one option as the correct answer. Safety is a priority for a client undergoing surgery.

6. 1. The nurse should complete this form because it requires analysis, which cannot be delegated to the UAP.
   2. Nurses cannot delegate assessment.
   3. The nurse cannot delegate teaching to a UAP.
   4. The UAP can remove clothing and jewelry.

**TEST-TAKING HINT:** The nurse should consider the knowledge and training of the person receiving the assignments. The nurse should never delegate assessment, teaching, administering medications, evaluation, or care of an unstable client to a UAP.

7. 1. This statement is giving false reassurance.
   2. "Why" is never therapeutic. The client does not owe the nurse an explanation.
   3. This statement focuses on the emotion that the client identified and is therapeutic.
   4. This statement belittles the client's fear, and no person understands how another person feels.

**TEST-TAKING HINT:** There are rules the test taker should implement when answering these types of questions. The test taker should not select an option that asks the client "why," such as option "2," or an option that states, "I understand," such as option "4."

8. 1. The nurse should contact the surgeon because the client is at risk for fluid and electrolyte imbalance after three enemas. NPO clients, older clients, and pediatric clients are more likely to have these imbalances.
   2. Administering more enemas will put the client at further risk for fluid volume deficit and electrolyte imbalance.
   3. The IV may need to be increased, but the nurse would need to fully assess the fluid status of the client before initiating this intervention. Intravenous fluids would not directly affect the peristalsis of the gastrointestinal tract so that the bowels would move more rapidly.

4. The electrolyte status may need to be assessed, but the nurse would need an order for this intervention.

**TEST-TAKING HINT:** Very few questions will require the nurse to notify the HCP, but there will be some; the test taker must know when a potential complication may occur. The nurse cannot prescribe or order laboratory tests without an HCP's order.

9. Correct answers are 2, 4, and 5.
   1. Passive means the nurse performs the range-of-motion exercises. The client in the PACU should do active range-of-motion exercises.
   2. Effective coughing aids in the removal of pooled secretions, which can cause pneumonia. Deep-breathing exercises keep the alveoli inflated and prevent atelectasis.
   3. The client having abdominal surgery will be NPO until bowel sounds return, which will not occur in the PACU; therefore, the client is not given a meal.
   4. The client's postoperative pain should be kept within a tolerable range.
   5. These interventions help decrease the client's anxiety.

**TEST-TAKING HINT:** This is an alternate-type question, which requires the test taker to select more than one option as the correct answer. The nurse's priority after surgery is to prevent postoperative complications.

10. 1. This is the correct way to perform deep-breathing exercises; therefore, no further teaching is needed.
    2. This is the correct way to perform range-of-motion exercises; therefore, no further teaching is needed.
    3. This is the way to use a volume incentive spirometer; therefore, no further teaching is needed.
    4. The correct way to get out of bed postoperatively is to roll onto the side, grasp the side rail to maneuver to the side, and then push up with one hand while swinging the legs over the side. The client needs further teaching.

**TEST-TAKING HINT:** This is an "except" question. Therefore, the test taker must select an option that shows the client does not understand the teaching. Sometimes flipping the question and asking which behavior indicates the client understands the teaching will help in answering this type of question.

11. 1. This is an important step for the nurse to implement, but it is not the first intervention.
   2. This must be done, but it is not the first intervention.
   3. The nurse should first assess the events that occurred when the client took this medication because many clients think a side effect, such as nausea, is an allergic reaction.
   4. This information must be put on the MAR, but it is not the first intervention.

**TEST-TAKING HINT: The stem is asking the test taker to identify the first intervention. Therefore, all four options could be interventions that should be implemented, but assessment is the first part of the nursing process, so option "3" is the correct answer.**

12. 1. This laboratory value is within normal limits. The normal calcium is 8.2 to 10.2 mg/dL.
   2. This laboratory value is within normal limits. The normal prothrombin time (PT) is 10 to 13 seconds.
   3. This laboratory value is within normal limits. The normal hemoglobin is 17 to 17.3 g/dL in males and 11.7 to 15.5 g/dL in females.
   4. This potassium level is low (normal potassium is 3.5 to 5.3 mEq/L) and should be reported to the HCP because potassium is important for muscle function, including the cardiac muscle (Van Leeuwen & Bladh, 2017).

**TEST-TAKING HINT: There are some items, such as normal laboratory values, the test taker must memorize. Laboratory values may differ slightly between laboratories, but the test taker must know them.**

## Intraoperative

13. 1. The circulating nurse has many responsibilities in the OR, including coordinating the activities in the OR; keeping the OR clean; ensuring the safety of the client; and maintaining the humidity, lighting, and safety of the equipment.
   2. This is the role of the nurse anesthetist or anesthesiologist.
   3. This is the role of the scrub nurse or technologist.
   4. If there is an anesthesia technologist, this would be the anesthesia technologist's role, or the nurse anesthetist and the anesthesiologist would assume the role.

**TEST-TAKING HINT: Options "2" and "4" discuss anesthesia and an anesthesiologist, which may lead the test taker to eliminate these as possible correct answers. Some questions are knowledge-based questions that require the test taker to know the information; this is an example of this type of question.**

14. 1. Items that are on the edge of the sterile field are considered contaminated and should be removed from the field.
   2. The technician is not wasting supplies; the technician is following principles of asepsis.
   3. The technician followed the correct procedure. Sponges are counted to maintain client safety, so all sponges must be kept together to repeat the count before the incision site is sutured. The sponge must be removed, not used, and placed in a designated area to be counted later.
   4. Taking the contaminated sponge out of the room would cause a discrepancy in the sponge count.

**TEST-TAKING HINT: When answering this question, the test taker must consider safety, which is always of the utmost importance during surgery. Sponge count is a basic concept in operating room nursing theory.**

15. 1. When discrepancies occur in the count, it is usually a simple mistake discovered with a recount. The surgeon will be notified if the count is wrong after a recount.
   2. If an error is found to have been made, an occurrence report will be completed, but it is not the first intervention.
   3. This would be done if a correct count is not maintained, but it is not the first intervention.
   4. A recount of sponges may lead to the discovery of the cause of the presumed error. Usually, it is just a miscount or a result of a sponge being placed in a location other than the sterile field, such as the floor or a lower shelf.

**TEST-TAKING HINT: When the test taker has no idea of the correct answer, the test taker should apply the nursing process and choose the option that addresses assessment because it is the first step in the nursing process.**

16. 1. These are appropriate activities in a surgery department; therefore, no intervention is required.
   2. This is required to maintain surgical asepsis.

3. This follows the principles of surgical asepsis.
4. According to the Centers for Disease Control and Prevention (CDC), the Association of Operating Room Nurses (AORN) (2016), and the Association for Practitioners in Infection Control, artificial nails harbor microorganisms, which increase the risk for infection.

**TEST-TAKING HINT: The adjective "artificial" in option "4" and the word "violation" in the stem should cause the test taker to select option "4" as the correct answer if the test taker had no idea which distracter to select.**

17. 1. This would prevent an electrical injury, but the interventions must address positioning, which is the etiology of the nursing diagnosis.
2. Padding the elbows decreases pressure, so nerve damage and pressure ulcers are prevented. This addresses the etiology of the nursing diagnosis.
3. This would help to decrease hypothermia, but it does not address the etiology of the nursing diagnosis.
4. Checking the EHR for medication use would help prevent interactions between anesthesia and routine medications, but it does not address the etiology of the nursing diagnosis.

**TEST-TAKING HINT: The test taker must be knowledgeable of nursing diagnosis and the nursing process. The assessment data support the response "risk for injury" and the interventions address the etiology "positioning."**

18. 1. The young client is not a high risk for nerve damage secondary to positioning.
2. The client's age, along with the Trendelenburg position, places increased weight and pressure on the shoulders, putting this client at higher risk.
3. This client is sitting in an upright position, which would not put this client at risk for nerve damage.
4. A younger client would not be at high risk of nerve damage when lying on the side.

**TEST-TAKING HINT: Clients at the highest risk for nerve damage are older, obese or emaciated, and clients placed in positions that increase pressure on bony prominences.**

19. 1. The client is not awake during surgery, so playing a favorite audiobook would not be an example of client advocacy.
2. This would be a nice action to take, but it is not an example of client advocacy.

3. This would keep the client's dignity by maintaining privacy. With this action, the nurse is speaking for the client while the client cannot speak as a result of anesthesia; this is an example of client advocacy.
4. Clients should be referred to by their last names rather than first names unless a client requests the staff to use the first name. This is not an example of client advocacy.

**TEST-TAKING HINT: The definition of a client advocate is a person designated to speak up for the client's rights when the client cannot.**

20. 1. This expected outcome addresses the safety of the client while in the OR.
2. This would be an expected outcome in the postoperative period.
3. The anesthesiologist or nurse anesthetist would monitor the client's vital signs during surgery.
4. This would be an expected outcome for the anesthesiologist or nurse anesthetist.

**TEST-TAKING HINT: The adjectives "intraoperative" and "circulating" are the keywords for answering this question. Safety is priority in the operating room.**

21. 1. This intervention prevents nerve damage from positioning, but it is not a higher priority than preventing the client from falling off the OR table.
2. This action would prevent the client from falling off the table, which is the highest priority.
3. Preparing the incision site is not a higher priority than preventing the client from falling off the OR table.
4. The temperature of the room does not have a higher priority than safety.

**TEST-TAKING HINT: Client safety should always be a high priority. In order, the priorities would be preventing a fall, preventing nerve damage, preventing infection, and then documenting.**

22. 1. Open-heart surgery is complex, and the care of the client should be assigned to an experienced nurse with special training.
2. The case of a client having a biopsy of the breast would be a good case for an inexperienced nurse because it is simple.
3. Laser eye surgery requires the nurse in the OR to have additional training to operate the equipment.
4. Additional training to be in the OR would be required for this case because special care to prevent infection is needed in orthopedic cases.

**TEST-TAKING HINT:** The test taker should select the option that requires the least amount of additional training because the nurse is new to the operating room. The technology required for specific surgeries requires additional training.

23. 1. Unexplained tachycardia, hypotension, and elevated temperature are signs of malignant hyperthermia, which is treated with cooling blankets and dantrolene sodium (Harvard Health Publishing, 2018).
    2. A defibrillator would be needed if the client were in ventricular tachycardia or ventricular fibrillation.
    3. These interventions would not be appropriate for malignant hyperthermia.
    4. This would be important if the client had diabetes, but it does not address malignant hyperthermia.

**TEST-TAKING HINT:** The test taker could eliminate options based on basic concepts. Option "2" could be eliminated because the client is not coding. Option "3" would increase bleeding, which would not be appropriate for a client having surgery.

24. 1. Assessing the respiratory rate, rhythm, and depth is the most important action.
    2. The nurse needs to monitor all systems, but monitoring the urine output would not be a priority over monitoring breathing.
    3. Monitoring the client's ECG is appropriate, but it is not a priority.
    4. The client needs to be relaxed, not focused, but this is not a priority over respiratory status.

**TEST-TAKING HINT:** When the test taker must prioritize nursing care, assessment is usually first. Using Maslow's hierarchy of needs to prioritize, assessment of respiration is always first. All sedation agents can depress respiration.

## Postoperative

25. 1. The airway should be assessed first. When caring for a client, the nurse should follow the ABCs: airway, breathing, and circulation.
    2. After assessing the client's airway and breathing, the nurse can apply oxygen via a nasal cannula if it is necessary.
    3. The blood pressure is taken automatically by the monitor, but this is not a priority over airway.

    4. The pulse oximeter is applied to the client's finger to obtain the peripheral oxygenation status, but the nurse should assess the client's breathing first.

**TEST-TAKING HINT:** When the stem of the question asks the test taker to implement a nursing intervention first, the test taker should think of assessment and then apply Maslow's hierarchy of needs.

26. 1. Loss of sensation in the L5 dermatome is expected from spinal anesthesia.
    2. The absence of a posterior tibial pulse is indicative of a block in the blood supply, but it is not a complication of spinal anesthesia.
    3. If the effects of the spinal anesthesia move up rather than down the spinal cord, respirations can be depressed and even blocked.
    4. This is an expected outcome and does not indicate a complication.

**TEST-TAKING HINT:** The test taker must know normal rates for vital signs, and a respiratory rate of eight would be significantly low for any client and indicate a possible complication.

27. 1. The surgeon should be notified, but this is not the first action; the client must be cared for.
    2. The postoperative client had lactated Ringer's infused during surgery. The rate should be increased during hemorrhage—which the vital signs indicate is occurring—but potassium should not be added.
    3. By lowering the head of the bed and raising the feet, the blood is shunted to the brain until volume-expanding fluids can be administered, which is the first intervention for a hemorrhaging client.
    4. When findings of shock are observed, the nurse will monitor the vital signs more frequently than every 15 minutes.

**TEST-TAKING HINT:** These are the signs of hypovolemic shock. The test taker should select the intervention that will directly affect the client's problem and can be implemented the fastest to ensure the client's safety.

28. 1. Naloxone (Narcan), an opioid antagonist, does not cause pain for the client.
    2. A client diagnosed with respiratory depression treated with Naloxone (Narcan), an opioid antagonist, can have another episode within 15 minutes after receiving the drug as a result of the short half-life of the medication.

3. Infection would not be a concern immediately after surgery.
4. Although the client may experience an imbalance in fluid or electrolytes, this problem would not be of concern as a result of the administration of Narcan.

**TEST-TAKING HINT: The test taker should be knowledgeable about medications commonly used in the postoperative period. If the test taker had no idea of the answer, selecting an option addressing the airway is an appropriate action.**

29. Correct answers are 2 and 4.
    1. A back rub is a therapeutic intervention, but it is not appropriate for a life-threatening complication of surgery.
    2. **Ice packs should be applied to the axillary and groin areas for a client experiencing malignant hyperthermia.**
    3. The client would be NPO to prepare for intubation, but an ice slush would be used to irrigate the bladder and stomach per nasogastric tube.
    4. **Dantrolene, a smooth-muscle relaxant, is the drug of choice for treatment.**
    5. Cooling blankets, not a warming blanket, are used to decrease the fast-rising temperature.

**TEST-TAKING HINT: This is an alternate-type question, which requires the test taker to select more than one option as the correct answer. Malignant hyperthermia is a medical emergency requiring immediate treatment.**

30. 1. Adequate urine output should be 30 mL/hr or at least 240 mL in an 8-hour period.
    2. Paralysis (inability to move) and paresthesia (numbness and tingling) indicate neurovascular compromise to the right leg, which indicates a complication and is not an expected outcome.
    3. The client's temperature and pulse are slightly elevated and the BP is low, which does not indicate effective nursing care.
    4. **Lung sounds, which are clear bilaterally in all lobes, indicate the client has adequate gas exchange, which prevents postoperative complications and indicates effective nursing care.**

**TEST-TAKING HINT: If the test taker does not know the answer, then applying the testing rule that the airway is priority would cause the test taker to select option "4" as the correct answer.**

31. Correct answers are 1 and 5.
    1. **Taking the vital signs of the stable client may be delegated to the UAP.**
    2. Assessments cannot be delegated; "check" is a word which means "to assess."
    3. IVs cannot be hung by the UAP; this is considered administering a medication.
    4. Evaluating the client's pain relief is the responsibility of the RN.
    5. **Repositioning a stable client every 2 hours may be delegated to the UAP.**

**TEST-TAKING HINT: The test taker cannot delegate assessment, teaching, or evaluating the care of the client.**

32. 1. The client appears stable; pediatric clients can become unstable quickly, but the most experienced nurse would not need to care for this client.
    2. A client diagnosed with a fractured hip will be ambulated by the physical therapist and this client is stable, so the most experienced nurse does not need to care for this client.
    3. A young client after an appendectomy would require routine postoperative care.
    4. **An older client diagnosed with a chronic disease would be a complicated case, requiring the care of a more experienced nurse.**

**TEST-TAKING HINT: When questions ask for assignments for the most experienced nurse, the test taker should realize clients whose condition can change quickly, such as older clients with complications, should be assigned to the most experienced nurse.**

33. 1. The postoperative client is expected to be out of bed as soon as possible, but this goal is not specific to having general anesthesia.
    2. **The anesthesia machine takes over the function of the lungs during surgery, so the expected outcome should directly reflect the client's respiratory status; the alveoli can collapse, causing atelectasis.**
    3. Urine output should be 30 mL/hr, but the expected outcome is not specific to general anesthesia.
    4. Sensation would be an outcome assessed after the use of spinal anesthesia or block, but it is not specific to general anesthesia.

**TEST-TAKING HINT: If the test taker has no idea what the answer is, the test taker should apply Maslow's hierarchy of needs and select the option addressing the airway. This will not always result in the correct answer, but the rule can be followed if the test taker has no idea of the correct answer.**

34. 1. Applying antiembolism hose may be appropriate, but it is not the first intervention.
    2. Attaching a drain would be appropriate but not before assessing the client.
    3. Assessing the client's status after transfer from the PACU should be the nurse's first intervention.
    4. Receiving reports is not the nurse's first intervention.

**TEST-TAKING HINT:** The test taker should apply the nursing process when answering questions that require identifying the first intervention. Assessment is the first step of the nursing process.

35. 1. All clients undergoing surgery are at risk for hemorrhaging, which is the priority problem.
    2. The client is at risk for injury, but the priority problem the first-day postoperative is hemorrhaging.
    3. A potential fluid imbalance would be for less fluid as a result of blood loss and decreased oral intake; it would not be for fluid volume excess.
    4. Infection would be a potential problem but not a priority over hemorrhaging on the first postoperative day.

**TEST-TAKING HINT:** Remember to apply the ABCs of care: airway, breathing, and circulation. The test taker must apply testing rules when answering questions that require identifying priority problems.

36. 1. Antibiotics need to be administered at the scheduled time.
    2. These data would not support the need to change the dressing, and surgeons usually want to change the surgical dressing for the first time.
    3. Having the client turn, cough, and deep breathe is the best intervention for the nurse to implement because, if a client has a fever within the first day, it is usually caused by a respiratory problem.
    4. The client is first-day postoperative, and ambulating in the hall would not be appropriate.

**TEST-TAKING HINT:** For clients after surgery, the priority problems are respiration and hemorrhaging. The test taker should select an option that addresses one of these two areas.

## Acute Pain

37. 1. The nurse should first assess the client for potential complications to determine if this is expected pain or pain requiring notifying the HCP.
    2. The nurse must check the MAR to determine when the last pain medication was administered, but it is not the first intervention.
    3. The nurse must rule out complications that require medical intervention before medicating the client.
    4. The nurse should not administer any pain medication before ruling out complications and checking the MAR.

**TEST-TAKING HINT:** The test taker should apply the nursing process when answering the question and select an option that addresses assessment.

38. 1. Pain medications should be administered at the frequency ordered by the HCP, not just when the client requests them, especially for acute pain.
    2. Nonpharmacological methods should never replace medications, but they should be used in combination to help keep the client comfortable.
    3. Cryotherapy (cold) is used immediately postoperative or postinjury. Heat applications are applied at a later time.
    4. Only clients should activate the PCA to prevent overdosing.

**TEST-TAKING HINT:** Option "4" should be eliminated because a basic concept is the client should be the person in control of the pain, not a family member; pain is subjective.

39. 1. This exemplifies the role of provider of care, and it does not address client advocacy.
    2. This action is addressing the role of collaborator.
    3. When the nurse contacts the HCP about unrelieved pain, the nurse is speaking when the client cannot, which is the definition of a client advocate.
    4. This action is providing care to the client and does not address client advocacy.

**TEST-TAKING HINT:** One of the most important roles of the nurse is to be a client advocate. The nurse must always identify problems and follow through to their resolution.

**40.** 1. A decrease in the use of pain medication does not mean the client's pain is managed; the client may be concerned about possible addiction to pain medication.
2. Clients experiencing acute pain will not be involved in self-care because of their reluctance to move, which increases the pain; therefore, participation indicates the client's pain is tolerable.
3. Using relaxation techniques does not indicate the client's pain is under control.
4. This would be an expected outcome of a knowledge-deficit problem.

**TEST-TAKING HINT:** The test taker must first determine what is the expected outcome, which should be "relief of pain," and then determine which option addresses the client's relief of pain.

**41.** 1. It is important to monitor vital signs, but it is not a priority intervention before administering the medication.
2. The nurse should verify the time the last dose was administered to determine the time the next dose could be administered, but this is not the priority intervention.
3. Before giving any medication, the nurse should assess any allergies, but it is not the priority intervention.
4. The nurse should question the client to rule out complications and to determine which medication and amount would be most appropriate for the client. This is assessment.

**TEST-TAKING HINT:** When questions require a priority answer, the test taker should look for an option that addresses assessment, but the test taker should remember there are many words that reflect assessment, such as "discuss," "determine," "monitor," or "obtain," to name a few.

**42.** 1. Medication administration cannot be delegated to a UAP.
2. This task does not require teaching, evaluating, or nursing judgment and therefore can be delegated.
3. Assessment cannot be delegated to a UAP.
4. Evaluation of teaching cannot be delegated to a UAP.

**TEST-TAKING HINT:** The terms "observe" and "check" in options "3" and "4" are different from the term "evaluate," but reading the options, the tasks are clearly addressing the evaluation step of the nursing process. Evaluation cannot be delegated to the UAP.

**43.** Correct answers are 1, 3, and 4.
1. This procedure ensures client safety by preventing the medication from being given to the wrong client.
2. This is a legal requirement, not a safety issue.
3. This intervention would prevent giving a narcotic to an unstable or compromised client.
4. Determining allergies addresses client safety.
5. It would not be realistic to recheck all orders.

**TEST-TAKING HINT:** This question specifically asks the test taker to identify interventions for safely administering medication to the client. Therefore, options "2" and "5" could be eliminated because they do not address the client's safety. This is an alternate-type question requiring the test taker to select more than one option as the correct answer.

**44.** 1. The nurse should use words a 4-year-old child understands and remembers, but this is not the best way to assess pain.
2. A 4-year-old child cannot be expected to use the numeric pain scale because of a lack of cognitive abilities, and explaining it to the parents does not address the child's pain.
3. The Faces Scale is the best way to assess pain in a 4-year-old child (Wong-Baker FACES® Foundation, 2019).

**Wong-Baker FACES® Pain Rating Scale**

| 0 | 2 | 4 | 6 | 8 | 10 |
|---|---|---|---|---|---|
| No Hurt | Hurts Little Bit | Hurts Little More | Hurts Even More | Hurts Whole Lot | Hurts Worst |

4. This does not assess the child's pain, and administering the pain medication every four (4) hours may compromise the child's safety.

**TEST-TAKING HINT:** When age is listed, it is an indication the question is asking for age-specific information. The test taker should consider developmental levels for that particular age.

45. 1. Assessing verbal and nonverbal cues is the priority intervention because pain is subjective.
    2. Some clients are hesitant to ask for medication or believe it is a sign of weakness to ask.
    3. There are times when pain medications are given on a routine basis, but it is not the best answer because assessment takes priority.
    4. Alternative therapies, such as imagery, are used in combination with medications, but they never replace medications.

**TEST-TAKING HINT:** Options such as option "4," which have absolute words such as "only," usually can be eliminated as a correct answer. The test taker should remember to apply the nursing process, and the first step is assessment.

46. 1. The answer to this request would indicate if the client has had a negative experience that may influence the client's pain management.
    2. Previous surgeries would be pertinent information but not for pain management.
    3. Before asking this question, the nurse should have specific information to suspect drug use.
    4. Discussing the client's prescription medications is necessary, but asking for a list of medications will not address the client's pain management.

**TEST-TAKING HINT:** Assessment, the first step of the nursing process, of pain perception is indicated when caring for a client diagnosed with acute pain.

47. 1. Assessing why the client is not using the medication is a priority, and then, based on the client's response, a plan of care can be determined.
    2. The fact a client is not using pain medication warrants the nurse to determine the cause so appropriate action can be taken.
    3. This may or may not be why the client is not using the PCA pump. The nurse must first determine why the client is not using pain medication.
    4. This may or may not be indicated, but until the nurse determines why the client is not taking the medication, this action should not be implemented.

**TEST-TAKING HINT:** Assessment is a priority when caring for a client. It is the first step of the nursing process, and if the test taker is unsure of the correct answer, it is the best choice to select.

48. 1. This is a psychosocial problem, which is not appropriate for an acute physiological problem.
    2. A potential problem is not a priority for a client in acute pain.
    3. Alteration in comfort is addressing the client's acute pain.
    4. Altered sensory input does not address the client's acute physical pain.

**TEST-TAKING HINT:** The test taker should be familiar with NANDA's list of client problems and nursing diagnoses, which includes alteration in comfort for pain. Potential problems do not have priority over actual problems.

**49.** 1. Even though metoprolol (Lopressor) is an oral medication and the client is NPO, beta blocker medications are not held for surgery. They are administered with a sip of water. Beta blockers can cause rebound cardiac dysrhythmias if not administered as routinely taken. Beta blocker medications should be tapered off to avoid cardiac issues. The nurse would not question this medication.

2. Cefazolin sodium (Ancef), an antibiotic medication, would be expected to be administered prophylactically to prevent infections postoperatively. This is a cephalosporin, not penicillin. The nurse would not question this medication.

3. Some facilities apply EMLA topical cream before initiating the IV to decrease pain during the procedure. The nurse would not question this medication.

4. Dabigatran etexilate (Pradaxa) is an anticoagulant; the nurse would question this medication. The medication should have stopped 5 to 7 days preoperatively. The nurse would question this medication, and the surgery may have to be postponed because the client is receiving an anticoagulant.

**TEST-TAKING HINT: Because options "1" and "4" are oral medications and clients receiving general anesthesia are NPO, the test taker would choose from these options. The nurse must know which medications have specific requirements, such as steroids and beta blockers are tapered off.**

**50.** Correct answers are 1, 2, and 4.
1. The colostomy stoma should be assessed to determine circulation to the stoma at least every 4 hours. A purple or bluish purple indicates that the circulation to the stoma is impaired and is a medical emergency.

2. This is an extensive surgery requiring the client to be under general anesthesia for several hours. Turning, coughing, and deep-breathing exercises done at least every 2 hours helps to prevent pneumonia.

3. The client is not allowed to sit on the perineal area for several days and should be maintained in a side-lying position when possible.

4. The nurse should assess for bowel activity at regularly scheduled intervals.

5. Pain medication is administered to control the client's pain; the nurse is concerned with client comfort, not addiction. Poorly controlled pain is more likely to result in drug-seeking behavior than adequately treated pain.

**TEST-TAKING HINT: "Select all that apply" questions must be answered with each option considered a true or false freestanding question. The test taker cannot use one option to rule out another.**

**51.** 1. The client will have been told about the cancer diagnosis. The nurse should allow the client to verbalize feelings.

2. The nurse should routinely monitor any dressing, but assessing the dressing does not address the pathology report and its implications for the client.

3. The report indicates a diagnosis of cancer, not infection.

4. The pathology report is performed on the actual cells removed from the tissues. The report does not need to be verified.

**TEST-TAKING HINT: The test taker could reason out the correct answer from some keywords in the report. Reed-Sternberg cells are only associated with Hodgkin's lymphoma, but if the test taker did not know this then "Stage 3" is usually used to designate the severity of the cancer being diagnosed.**

**52.** 1. This client has been without food or water for several hours before the surgery, so the client needs fluid intake to urinate. Indwelling catheters carry with them the risk of a urinary tract infection. The nurse should continue to monitor the client's output before taking this action.

2. Skin turgor should not be assessed for indicating a fluid volume deficit yet. The client received fluids during surgery and would have had an indwelling catheter to prevent incontinence during surgery.

3. The nurse should wait and monitor the client before taking another action. The client has an IV running at 150 mL/hr. The client should be given a chance to produce urine before rushing to take another action.

4. The client should be allowed to rest. It has been a long day of waiting for the surgery to take place and then having the surgery. Pushing liquids at midnight is not advised, considering the need for rest.

**TEST-TAKING HINT: Timing is important to consider when answering this question—midnight, return from surgery, and PACU at 1800. Basic knowledge of surgical procedure is the client is NPO for at least 8 hours before general anesthesia.**

53. 1. The nurse should recognize the WBC count is high, possibly indicating a current infection. The HCP should be notified immediately, and surgery may be canceled because a laparoscopic cholecystectomy is an elective procedure.
    2. **The nurse should notify the surgeon. Surgery may be canceled because a laparoscopic cholecystectomy is an elective procedure.**
    3. The client may have any of a number of infections. The high WBC could indicate pneumonia, but it could indicate another type of infection.
    4. The client may have any of a number of infections. The high WBC could indicate pneumonia, but it could indicate another type of infection.

**TEST-TAKING HINT: The test taker should find the abnormal data in the EHR before deciding what action to take. If all the data presented are within normal limits, then option "1" would be the answer.**

54. Correct answers are 2, 3, and 4.
    1. The client should not be ambulated until the nurse has a chance to assess for the client's ability to ambulate safely.
    2. **The nurse should assess the vital signs from PACU with the current vital signs to be sure that the client is stable.**

3. **The nurse should assess the intravenous lines, indwelling catheters, and tubes upon receiving the client.**
4. **The nurse must assess the surgical site for bleeding to know if the client is stable or not.**
5. Only the client should push the PCA pump's button; otherwise, the client may receive an overdose of medication.

**TEST-TAKING HINT: The client is "returning" from PACU. This client may still be groggy from anesthesia and should not be ambulating until the nurse has assessed the client and is aware the client is awake enough to ambulate safely.**

55. 1. This may be an appropriate intervention, but unrelieved pain 3 days after the surgery may indicate a problem. The nurse should assess the client first.
    2. A client in pain is not ready to learn. If narcotic medication is not successful, something else may be occurring.
    3. **The first step of the nursing process is to assess. Pain unrelieved 3 days postoperative needs to be investigated.**
    4. Repositioning the client may or may not help, but the nurse should assess the client.

**TEST-TAKING HINT: The first step of the nursing process is to ASSESS. The test taker must have some systematic method of problem solving. The test taker must also remember "if in stress—do not assess." In other words, the test taker has been given enough information to implement an intervention immediately.**

# PERIOPERATIVE CARE
# COMPREHENSIVE EXAMINATION

1. Which client would the nurse identify as having the **highest risk** for developing postoperative complications?
   1. The 67-year-old client who is obese, has diabetes, and takes insulin.
   2. The 50-year-old client diagnosed with arthritis and taking nonsteroidal anti-inflammatory drugs.
   3. The 45-year-old client having abdominal surgery to remove the gallbladder.
   4. The 60-year-old client diagnosed with anemia who smokes one pack of cigarettes per day.

2. The nurse is completing the preoperative checklist on a client going to surgery. Which information should the nurse **report** to the surgeon?
   1. The client understands the purpose of the surgery.
   2. The client stopped taking aspirin 3 weeks ago.
   3. The client uses the oral supplements licorice and garlic.
   4. The client has mild levels of preoperative anxiety.

3. Which statement explains the **nurse's responsibility** when obtaining informed consent for the client undergoing a surgical procedure?
   1. The nurse should provide detailed information about the procedure.
   2. The nurse should inform the client of any legal consultation needed.
   3. The nurse should write a list of the risks for postoperative complications.
   4. The nurse should ensure the client is voluntarily giving consent.

4. Which client outcome would the nurse identify for the preoperative client?
   1. The client's abnormal laboratory data will be reported to the anesthesiologist.
   2. The client will not have any postoperative complications for the first 24 hours.
   3. The client will demonstrate the use of a pillow to splint during deep breathing.
   4. The client will complete an advance directive before having the surgery.

5. Which problem would be **appropriate** for the nurse to identify for the preoperative client having an open reduction and internal fixation of the right ankle?
   1. Alteration in skin integrity.
   2. Knowledge deficit of postoperative care.
   3. Alteration in gas exchange and pattern.
   4. Alteration in urinary elimination.

6. The nurse and a UAP are caring for clients in a surgery unit. Which task would be **most appropriate** for the RN to delegate to the UAP?
   1. Explain to the client how to cough and deep breathe.
   2. Discuss preoperative plans with the client and family.
   3. Determine the ability of the caregivers to provide postoperative care.
   4. Assist the client to take a povidone-iodine shower.

7. Which action by the client indicates that the nurse's preoperative teaching has been **effective**?
   1. The client demonstrates how to use the incentive spirometer device.
   2. The client demonstrates the use of the patient-controlled analgesia pump.
   3. The client can name two anesthesia agents used during surgery.
   4. The client ambulates down the hall to the nurse's station each hour.

8. Which intervention has **priority** for the nurse in the surgical holding area?
   1. Verify the surgical checklist.
   2. Prepare the client's surgical site.
   3. Assist the client to the bathroom.
   4. Restrain the client on the surgery table.

9. The client in the surgical holding area tells the nurse "I am so scared. I have never had surgery before." Which statement would be the nurse's **most appropriate** response?
   1. "Why are you afraid of the surgery?"
   2. "This is the best hospital in the city."
   3. "Does having surgery make you afraid?"
   4. "There is no reason to be afraid."

10. The UAP can be overheard talking loudly to the scrub technologist discussing a problem that occurred during one of the surgeries. Which intervention should the RN in the surgical holding area with a female client implement?
    1. Close the curtains around the client's stretcher.
    2. Instruct the UAP and scrub tech to stop the discussion.
    3. Tell the surgeon on the case what the nurse overheard.
    4. Inform the client the discussion was not about her surgeon.

11. The nurse is completing the preoperative checklist. Which laboratory value should be reported to the HCP **immediately**?

| Laboratory Test | Client Results | Normal Values |
|---|---|---|
| Glucose | 60 | Fasting < 100 mg/dL Random < 200 mg/dL |
| Hemoglobin (Hgb) | 14.1 | Male: 14–17.3 g/dL Female: 11.7–15.5 g/dL |
| White blood cells (WBC) | 6 | 4.5–11.1 × (10³/cells/ microL) |
| Potassium (K⁺) | 3.8 | 3.5–5.3 mEq/L or mmol/L |

1. Hemoglobin (Hgb).
2. Glucose.
3. White blood cells (WBCs).
4. Potassium (K⁺).

12. Which problem is appropriate for the nurse to identify for a client in the intraoperative phase of surgery?
1. Alteration in comfort.
2. Disuse syndrome.
3. Risk for injury.
4. Altered gas exchange.

13. The client is in the lithotomy position during surgery. Which nursing intervention should be implemented to **decrease** a complication from the positioning?
1. Increase the intravenous fluids.
2. Lower one leg at a time.
3. Raise the foot of the stretcher.
4. Administer epinephrine.

14. The circulating nurse observes the surgeon tossing a bloody gauze sponge onto the sterile field. Which action should the circulating nurse implement **first**?
1. Include the sponge in the sponge count.
2. Obtain a new sterile instrument pack.
3. Tell the surgical technologist about the sponge.
4. Throw the sponge in the sterile trashcan.

15. The circulating nurse notes a discrepancy in the needle count. What intervention should the nurse implement **first**?
1. Inform the other members of the surgical team about the problem.
2. Assume the original count was wrong and change the record.
3. Call the radiology department to perform a portable x-ray.
4. Complete an occurrence report and notify the risk manager.

16. The client in the surgery holding area identifies the left arm as the correct surgical site, but the operative permit designates surgery to be performed on the right arm. Which interventions should the nurse implement? **Select all that apply.**
1. Review the client's EHR.
2. Notify the surgeon.
3. Immediately call a "time-out."
4. Correct the surgical permit.
5. Request the client mark the left arm.

17. The nurse received a male client from the post-anesthesia care unit (PACU). Which assessment data would **warrant immediate** intervention?
1. The client's vital signs are T 97°F, P 108, R 24, and BP 80/40.
2. The client is sleepy but opens the eyes to his name.
3. The client is reporting pain at a "5" on a 1-to-10 pain scale.
4. The client has 20 mL of urine in the urinary drainage bag.

18. The client received naloxone in the post-anesthesia care unit (PACU). Which nursing intervention should the nurse include in the care plan?
1. Measure the client's intake and output hourly.
2. Administer sleep medications at night.
3. Encourage the client to verbalize feelings.
4. Monitor respirations every 15 to 30 minutes.

19. Which nursing task would be **most appropriate** to delegate to the UAP on a postoperative unit?
1. Change the dressing over the surgical site.
2. Teach the client how to perform incentive spirometry.
3. Empty and record the amount of drainage in the JP drain.
4. Auscultate the bowel sounds in all four quadrants.

20. Which client assessment data are a **priority** for the postanesthesia care nurse?
1. Bowel sounds.
2. Vital signs.
3. IV fluid rate.
4. Surgical site.

21. The male client in the day-surgery unit reports difficulty urinating postoperatively. Which intervention should the nurse implement?
1. Insert an indwelling catheter.
2. Increase the intravenous fluid rate.
3. Assist the client to stand to void.
4. Encourage the client to increase fluids.

22. The postoperative client reports hearing a "popping sound" and feeling "something opening" when ambulating in the room. Which intervention should the nurse implement **first**?
    1. Notify the surgeon the client has had an evisceration.
    2. Contact the surgery department to prepare for emergency surgery.
    3. Assess the operative site and cover the site with a moistened dressing.
    4. Explain this is a common feeling and tell the client to continue with the activity.

23. The nurse received a report the older postoperative client became confused during the previous shift. Which client problem would the nurse include in the plan of care?
    1. Risk for injury.
    2. Altered comfort level.
    3. Impaired circulation.
    4. Impaired skin integrity.

24. The client 1 day postoperative develops an elevated temperature. Which intervention would have **priority** for the client?
    1. Encourage the client to deep breathe and cough every hour.
    2. Encourage the client to drink 200 mL of water every shift.
    3. Monitor the client's wound for drainage every 8 hours.
    4. Assess the urine output for color and clarity every 4 hours.

25. Which statement made by the postoperative abdominal surgery client indicates the discharge teaching has been **effective**?
    1. "I will take my temperature each week and report any elevation."
    2. "I will not need any pain medication when I go home."
    3. "I will take all of my antibiotics until they are gone."
    4. "I will not take a shower until my 3-month checkup."

26. The client diagnosed with appendicitis has undergone an appendectomy. At 2 hours postoperative, the nurse takes the vital signs populated in the vital sign flowsheet below. Which interventions should the nurse implement? **Rank in order of priority**.

| Vital Sign Flowsheet | Client Results | Normal Values |
|---|---|---|
| Blood pressure | 92/46 | 100–119 mmHg systolic 60–80 mmHg diastolic |
| Temperature | 102.6°F | Oral: 98°F (36.7°C) |
| Pulse | 132 | 60–100 beats/min |
| Respirations | 26 | 12–20 breaths/min |

   1. Increase the IV rate.
   2. Notify the health-care provider.
   3. Elevate the foot of the bed.
   4. Check the abdominal dressing.
   5. Determine if the IV antibiotics have been administered.

1. 1. This client has comorbid conditions—advanced age, obesity, and diabetes—which put this client at a higher risk for postoperative complications.
   2. This client's risk factor of arthritis can make positioning in surgery and movement in the postoperative period more difficult, but this does not put the client at greater risk for postoperative complications. The NSAIDs can be held a few days before surgery to decrease the problems associated with NSAIDs.
   3. The client after abdominal surgery may have respiratory complications, but the client is not at as high risk as the older client diagnosed with diabetes and obesity.
   4. The client's smoking increases the risk of pulmonary complications and increases the blood level of carboxyhemoglobin, but this client does not have the problems of delayed healing and age the 67-year-old client diagnosed with diabetes has.

2. 1. The surgeon should be notified if the client does not understand the surgical procedure, not if the client understands.
   2. Aspirin should be stopped before surgery to help prevent bleeding.
   3. Licorice and garlic can interfere with coagulation; therefore, the surgeon should be notified.
   4. Mild levels of anxiety and apprehension before surgery are normal.

3. 1. The nurse is not responsible for explaining the details of the surgery. This is the surgeon's responsibility.
   2. The nurse is not responsible for informing the client of any need for legal representation.
   3. The surgeon is responsible for informing the client of the risks and hazards of the surgery.
   4. The nurse is responsible for ensuring the client voluntarily signs the surgical consent form giving permission for the surgery without coercion.

4. 1. This would be an outcome for the health-care team, not the client.
   2. This would be an appropriate postoperative, not preoperative, outcome.
   3. This would be the expected outcome for the client during the preoperative phase. After the teaching has been completed, the client should be able to demonstrate how to splint with the pillow during deep breathing and coughing.
   4. This would not be an expected outcome for the preoperative client. All clients should be encouraged to complete an advance directive, but it is not required by law.

5. 1. This client problem would not be written until after the surgery.
   2. This would be an appropriate client problem for the preoperative client scheduled for ankle repair. Teaching is a priority.
   3. This would not be a problem for a client scheduled for surgery.
   4. This would not be a problem for a client scheduled for surgery.

6. 1. Teaching cannot be delegated.
   2. Discussing the preoperative plans is part of the planning process and cannot be delegated.
   3. Evaluation cannot be delegated to the UAP.
   4. The UAP can assist a stable client in taking a shower whether or not it is with povidone-iodine (Betadine).

7. 1. The teaching is effective if the client is able to demonstrate the use of the spirometer before surgery.
   2. The patient-controlled analgesia pump would not be available before surgery because the pumps are charged to the client on a daily basis and the client would not be able to demonstrate how to use it.
   3. Determining allergies to anesthesia medications is important before surgery, but the nurse would not teach specific medication names.
   4. This would demonstrate increased mobility and would be encouraged after surgery, but it would not determine if teaching was effective.

8. 1. The surgical checklist is assessed when the client arrives in the surgery department holding area where clients wait for a short time before entering the operating room.
   2. Preparing the surgical site is completed in the surgery suite, but not until the client and surgery have been verified.
   3. The client should have voided just before being transported to the surgery department.
   4. Securing the client onto the surgical table would be important in the operating room, not in the holding area.

9. 1. The nurse should never ask the client, "why." The client does not owe the nurse an explanation.
   2. This response defends the hospital and does not address the client's feelings.
   3. This response is therapeutic and promotes communication of feelings.
   4. This statement is closed-ended and will not encourage the continued discussion of "fear."

10. 1. Closing curtains will not keep loud conversations from being overheard.
    2. The UAP and scrub tech are violating HIPAA and should be told to stop the conversation immediately.
    3. This is a nursing problem, and the nurse should handle the situation. The surgeon is not in the chain of command of the UAP or the scrub tech.
    4. Telling the client the situation does not involve her surgeon involves the client even more in the overheard conversation.

11. 1. This hemoglobin is within normal limits (Male: 14 to 17.3 g/dL, Female 11.7 to 15.5 g/dL) and would not warrant immediate action.
    2. This glucose level indicates hypoglycemia, which requires medical intervention.
    3. This white blood cell value (4.5 to 11.1 × 10³/microL) is within the normal range and would not be reported.
    4. This potassium level (3.5 to 5.3 mEq/L) is within normal limits and would not require intervention.

12. 1. This client problem would be appropriate for a postoperative client or, in some circumstances, a preoperative client, but not for a client in surgery.
    2. This is a problem of long-term immobility and would not apply during surgery.

3. This problem would be appropriate for the intraoperative phase. The circulating nurse would strap and carefully pad areas to prevent damage to tissues and nerves.
4. The client is receiving oxygen or breathing by the ventilator. The client should not have an alteration in gas exchange.

13. 1. The anesthesiologist, not the nurse in the operating room, manages the intravenous fluids.
    2. The lithotomy position has both legs elevated and placed in stirrups. The legs should be lowered one leg at a time to prevent hypotension from the shift of the blood.
    3. Raising the foot of the bed would be a treatment of hypotension, but not hypotension resulting from the lithotomy position.
    4. Epinephrine, a vasopressor, is used during codes to shunt blood from the periphery to the central circulation.

14. 1. All sponges must be included in the sponge count, but it is not the first intervention.
    2. The circulating nurse should obtain another sterile pack for the operation to continue, but it is not the first intervention.
    3. The circulating nurse should inform the surgical technologist of any break in sterile technique or field. This is the first intervention because the field is now contaminated (Association of Operating Room Nurses, 2016).
    4. This action is below the standards of the Association of Operating Room Nurses and violates the principles of sterility. The sponge is included in the count and will not be discarded until the end of the case and all sponges have been accounted for.

15. 1. If the needle count does not correlate, the surgical technologist and the other surgical team members should be informed. After repeating the count, a search for the missing needle should be conducted.
    2. Assuming the original count was wrong is illegal and dangerous for the client.
    3. If the needle is not located, an x-ray will be done, but this is not the first intervention.
    4. If the missing needle is not located, an occurrence report should be completed and sent to the risk manager, but this is not the first intervention.

16. Correct answers are 1, 2, 3, and 5.
    1. When the client in the holding area states that the surgery site differs from the scheduled surgery, the nurse should identify the client and review the client's EHR.
    2. If there is a discrepancy, the nurse should notify the surgeon to explain the situation and resolve the issue.
    3. The Joint Commission surgical standards state a "time-out" period is called and everything stops until the discrepancy is resolved.
    4. The nurse should not change a permit. If an error is discovered, the nurse should correct the situation within legal and ethical guidelines.
    5. Clients are encouraged to mark the correct side or site with indelible ink.

17. 1. These are symptoms of hypovolemic shock and require immediate intervention.
    2. This is a common response to anesthesia. Clients are sleepy until the anesthesia wears off.
    3. Pain management is required, but this does not indicate a life-threatening complication.
    4. Urine outputs should be monitored in the postoperative period, but indwelling catheter bags are emptied in the PACU before transferring the client to the floor, so 20 mL would not warrant immediate intervention.

18. 1. Naloxone (Narcan), an opioid antagonist, does not alter the urinary elimination; therefore, this is not an appropriate intervention for this client.
    2. Anesthesia may alter sleep patterns, but this nursing intervention does not take into account the need for Narcan to be administered to the client.
    3. This nursing intervention does not address the use of Narcan.
    4. Naloxone (Narcan), an opioid antagonist, is given to reverse respiratory depression from opioid analgesic medications and has a short half-life. The client may experience a rebound respiratory depression in 15 to 20 minutes, so this nursing intervention of monitoring respirations every 15 to 30 minutes is appropriate.

19. 1. The surgeon usually removes the first surgical dressing. The nurse performs surgical dressing changes so asepsis is maintained and the incision can be assessed.
    2. Nurses cannot delegate teaching and assessment.
    3. Emptying the drainage devices and recording the amounts on the bedside intake and output forms can be delegated.
    4. Listening to bowel sounds is assessing and cannot be delegated.

20. 1. Bowel sounds should be assessed, but it is not a priority for the surgical client in the PACU.
    2. The post-anesthesia (PACU) care unit nurse should follow the standards for post anesthesia care monitoring oxygenation, ventilation, circulation, level of consciousness, and temperature (Kaplow, 2010). Vital signs assess for hemodynamic stability; this is a priority in the PACU.
    3. Intravenous fluids should be assessed after breathing and circulation have been assessed.
    4. The surgical site should be assessed after the intravenous fluid rate is assessed.

21. 1. This intervention is invasive, increases the client's risk for infection, and should be the last resort.
    2. Increasing the IV fluids might increase the amount of urine in the bladder and cause further discomfort.
    3. Helping the male client to stand can offer the assistance needed to void. The safety of the client should be ensured.
    4. Drinking more fluids helps to increase urinary output but will not assist the client in emptying the bladder.

22. 1. The nurse should assess the client before notifying the surgeon the client felt or heard a "pop" and "something opening."
    2. The surgery department may or may not need to be notified. The incision should be assessed.
    3. The nurse should assess the surgical site and, if the site has eviscerated, cover the opening with a sterile dressing moistened with sterile 0.9% saline. This will prevent the tissues from becoming dry and infected.
    4. The nurse should not dismiss any report from a client without further assessment.

23. 1. Any time the nurse has a disoriented client, the nurse must initiate fall and safety precautions.
    2. Confusion would not indicate a change in comfort level.
    3. Sudden confusion is usually not a circulation problem.
    4. Impaired skin integrity would not cause confusion.

24. 1. When a postoperative client develops a fever within the first 24 hours, the cause is usually in the respiratory system. The client should increase deep breathing and coughing to assist the client in expanding the lungs and decrease pulmonary complications.
    2. Drinking fluid can bring down the temperature, but 200 mL would not be a sufficient amount to accomplish this. Unless contraindicated, the client should drink from 1 to 2 L/day.
    3. Wound infections may cause a fever later in the recovery but will usually not elevate within the first 24 hours after surgery.
    4. A urinary tract infection may occur later but would probably not be the cause of elevated temperature within 24 hours after surgery.

25. 1. The client should check the temperature twice a day.
    2. It is not realistic to expect the client to experience no pain after surgery.
    3. This statement about taking all the antibiotics ordered indicates the teaching is effective.
    4. Clients may shower after surgery, but not taking a tub bath for 3 months after surgery is too long a time.

26. Correct order is 1, 3, 4, 5, 2.
    1. The nurse should increase the IV rate to maintain the circulatory system function until further orders can be obtained.
    3. The foot of the bed should be elevated to help treat shock, the symptoms of which include elevated pulse and decreased blood pressure. Those findings and an elevated temperature indicate an infection may be present and the client could be developing septicemia.
    4. The dressing should be assessed to determine if bleeding is occurring.
    5. The nurse should administer any IV antibiotics ordered after addressing hypovolemia. The nurse will need this information when reporting to the HCP.
    2. The HCP should be notified when the nurse has the needed information.

# Cultural and Spiritual Nursing and Alternative Health Care

**17**

*Remember that our nation's first great leaders were also great scholars.*

—John F. Kennedy

The use of alternative therapies to treat specific disorders and to promote health and well-being has increased in recent years. Many people use herbs, massage therapy, aromatherapy, Rolfing, guided imagery, yoga, and numerous other techniques either alone or in addition to the techniques and drugs used by conventional medicine. The nurse should be aware of these practices and of the various health-related beliefs and traditions that people of different cultures have.

## KEYWORDS

Ayurveda

Curandero

Mezuzah

Nattuvidhyar

Rolfing

Tallis

Yom Kippur

## PRACTICE QUESTIONS

1. The nurse is admitting the client to a medical unit. Which questions should the nurse specifically ask the client about the current use of medications? **Select all that apply**.
   1. "Have you used or do you currently use any type of herb?"
   2. "What over-the-counter medications do you take?"
   3. "Are you allergic to any medications or foods?"
   4. "When is the last time you took any medication?"
   5. "Do you take any prescription medications?"

2. The client with a cold for the last week is reporting congestion and a stuffy nose. The client has been using medicated nasal spray several times a day. Which information should the nurse teach the client about the frequent use of nasal spray?
   1. Nasal sprays are safe because they are available over the counter.
   2. Nasal sprays cause rebound congestion when used frequently.
   3. Nasal sprays have no adverse reactions, unlike over-the-counter oral decongestants.
   4. Nasal sprays must be alternated to help prevent developing a tolerance to the spray.

3. The client using contraceptive foam for birth control has not had her menses for the last 2 months. Which intervention should the nurse implement **first**?
   1. Perform a vaginal examination.
   2. Check the urine for glucose and protein.
   3. Obtain vital signs to determine a baseline.
   4. Request a pregnancy test for this client.

4. The female client diagnosed with a cold is prescribed warfarin for chronic atrial fibrillation. The client calls the clinic and tells the nurse she is bleeding and bruising more than normal. Which information indicates a need for **further** teaching?
   1. The client reports taking echinacea.
   2. The client had blood drawn for an INR last month.
   3. The client uses acetaminophen for pain.
   4. The client reads labels on packaged foods.

5. Which intervention should the nurse implement when discussing health promotion activities for a client with German heritage leading a sedentary lifestyle?
   1. Refer the client to a support group for weight loss.
   2. Teach the client never to drink alcoholic beverages.
   3. Help the client to identify a routine exercise program.
   4. Assist the client in making a list of foods that must be avoided.

6. The older female client is upset and tells the nurse that the unlicensed assistive personnel (UAP), a member of a different culture from the client, complimented her grandchild's hair. Which intervention should the RN implement?
   1. Ask the client why she is upset about the UAP saying the child's hair is pretty.
   2. Take no action because the UAP was being friendly.
   3. Notify the psychologist of the client's response to the UAP's compliment.
   4. Explain to the UAP the importance of being aware of client's cultural beliefs.

7. The home health-care nurse is visiting an older female client talking loudly. The client weighs 102 kg, is 5′4″ tall, and has a BP of 154/98. The client lives with her daughter, son-in-law, and two grandchildren. Which intervention should the nurse implement?
   1. Maintain extended direct eye contact during the interview.
   2. Address what is assumed to be the client's anger because she is talking loudly.
   3. Discuss the client's care with the daughter and son-in-law.
   4. Discuss a weight-loss program for the client.

8. The home health nurse is making the initial visit to a client diagnosed with terminal cancer. The client is of a different culture and ethnicity from that of the nurse. Which questions would **best promote** a therapeutic nurse-client relationship? **Select all that apply**.
   1. "How would you prefer for me to address you?"
   2. "Who do you want to be involved in decisions about your care?"
   3. "What language do you prefer to communicate in?"
   4. "Why did you come to this country?"
   5. "Do you have any values or beliefs I need to know about to provide you optimal care?"

9. When interviewing the client who practices the Hindu religion and also does not speak English, which information should the nurse obtain to plan culturally sensitive care?
   1. Determine if the client has an advance directive.
   2. Assess if or to what extent the client uses Ayurveda.
   3. Request an interpreter to obtain the client's chief concerns.
   4. Inquire if the client has allergies to any foods or medications.

10. The UAP notices an amulet pinned to the client's gown and offers to remove it. The client does not want it removed. Which rationale should the RN give the UAP for allowing the client to continue to wear the amulet?
    1. The client is superstitious and may become distressed if it is removed.
    2. The amulet is a silly trinket that won't hurt the client in any way.
    3. The client brought the amulet because it gives the client emotional support.
    4. The amulet is worthless and no one would try to steal it if it stays on the gown.

11. After evaluating the meal tray of a Jewish client, the nurse notices the client did not eat any of the meal. Which intervention should the nurse implement **first**?
    1. Request the client's family to bring meals the client can eat.
    2. Contact the dietary department and request a kosher meal.
    3. Notify the local rabbi to request meals be provided for the client.
    4. Determine why the client did not eat any of the meal.

12. The client approaches the nurse about a weight-loss program. Which complementary therapies should the nurse suggest to assist the client's plan? **Select all that apply.**
    1. Music therapy.
    2. Hypnotherapy.
    3. Hatha yoga.
    4. Alexander technique.
    5. Acupuncture.

13. The nurse is incorporating complementary therapies in the routines of residents of a long-term care facility. Which information should the nurse consider when matching the clients with the therapy? **Select all that apply.**
    1. The client's preferences.
    2. The client's likes and dislikes.
    3. The benefits obtained from the therapy.
    4. The significant other's concerns.
    5. The client's ability to perform therapies.

14. Which form of complementary therapy should the nurse encourage as a relaxation technique for the anxious older client admitted for surgery?
    1. Meditation.
    2. Deep breathing.
    3. Rolfing.
    4. Scented candle.

15. The nurse is preparing the plan of care for the client diagnosed with migraine headaches. Which information regarding complementary therapies should the nurse include in this plan?
    1. Encourage the use of therapeutic touch.
    2. Purchase a textbook on autogenic therapy.
    3. Explain how to perform massage therapy.
    4. Discuss the need to avoid aromatic oils.

16. The rehabilitation nurse is caring for an older client after the surgical repair of a fractured hip. The client states she misses her dog. Which intervention should the nurse implement?
    1. Put the television on a show with animal performers.
    2. Arrange for the family to bring the client's dog for a visit.
    3. Arrange for the client to have a visit from the pet therapy dog.
    4. Share that the client's feelings are completely understood by the nurse.

17. In the rehabilitation unit, the nurse is caring for an anxious client with a hearing impairment and elevated blood pressure. The client enjoys pet therapy but is allergic to dogs and cats. Which intervention should the nurse implement?
    1. Administer antihistamine medication before pet therapy.
    2. Spend extra time visiting at the client's bedside.
    3. Arrange for a volunteer to bring the client a radio.
    4. Provide a colorful fish in a small bowl for the client.

18. The nurse arranges for a dance movement therapist to lead a group session for clients diagnosed with osteoarthritis. Which statement **best** describes the rationale for this intervention?
    1. Participants in dance movements form a unique bond while moving in unison.
    2. Dancing will help increase the amount of synovial fluid in the affected joints.
    3. Dance therapy helps decrease the client's pain in inflamed joints.
    4. Dancing causes the release of endorphins and helps the clients deal with pain.

19. The nurse is providing preoperative teaching about pain management techniques for the client having surgery. The client has a history of drug abuse. What should the nurse include in this client's plan of care?
    1. The nurse should know these clients always require too much nursing care.
    2. The client should select two alternate therapies to replace medications.
    3. The client should receive complementary therapies in addition to medications.
    4. The nurse should plan to administer a double dose of medication to this client.

20. Which intervention should the circulating nurse implement for the preoperative older client who is anxious and diaphoretic?
    1. Play soft, slow-beat music in the operating room.
    2. Encourage the client to take rapid, shallow breaths.
    3. Continue to talk to the client to promote relaxation.
    4. Open the door to the operating suite to increase the airflow.

21. The UAP is bathing a comatose client with the radio playing current rock music. The client has tachycardia and elevated blood pressure. Which intervention should the RN implement?
    1. No action by the nurse is indicated in this situation.
    2. Instruct the UAP to select baroque music to play for the client.
    3. Administer medication to decrease the client's heart rate and blood pressure.
    4. Assist the UAP to turn the client into the lateral position.

22. The nurse is caring for the surgical client experiencing pain at a "4" on a 1-to-10 pain scale and receiving pain medication via patient-controlled analgesia (PCA). Which intervention should the nurse implement **first** to assist the client's pain management?
    1. Notify the health-care provider (HCP) to increase the dosage of medication.
    2. Inform the client to relax and the medication will relieve the pain soon.
    3. Assist the client to perform guided imagery to increase relaxation.
    4. Instruct the family member to continue to push the button for the medication.

23. Which expected outcome should be included in the plan of care for a postoperative client practicing guided imagery?
    1. The client will have a decreased white blood cell count.
    2. The client will report a decrease in pain using the pain scale.
    3. The client will have a urine output of 360 mL each shift.
    4. The client will have no drainage on the surgical dressing.

24. The nurse is teaching the client how to use guided imagery. Which information would indicate the teaching has been **effective**?
    1. The client closes both eyes and makes a one-syllable-sounding chant.
    2. The client rubs the right arm in firm stroking motions.
    3. The client selects meaningful music that has 50 beats per minute.
    4. The client visualizes a scene from a favorite place.

25. The client is reporting nonspecific body aches, congestion, and coughing. The client's blood pressure is elevated. Which intervention should the nurse implement **first**?
    1. Instruct the client to decrease salt in the diet.
    2. Notify the HCP to request an antihypertensive medication.
    3. Determine if the client takes any over-the-counter medication.
    4. Discuss the long-term effects of atherosclerosis and hypertension.

# CONCEPTS

The concepts covered in this chapter focus on cultural diversity and safety as well as alternative medicine. Exemplars that are covered are cultures, values, health beliefs, religion, spiritual distress, and alternative therapies to Western medicine. Interrelated concepts of the nursing process and clinical judgment are covered throughout the questions. The concept of clinical judgment is presented in the prioritizing or "**first**" questions.

26. The nurse is caring for a client who recently immigrated to the United States and doesn't speak English. The family is present in the room, and one member of the family speaks English. Which action should the nurse implement to complete the admission assessment?
    1. Ask the family to interpret the questions for the client and provide the information.
    2. Use hand gestures with the client to get and receive the needed information.
    3. Notify the HCP that only limited information can be obtained about the client.
    4. Use the medical interpretation phone to ask the admission questions.

27. The male client is wearing a silver amulet to protect from evil spirits. Which action should the nurse take when sending the client to surgery?
    1. Tell the client that the amulet will be placed near him during surgery but cannot be allowed to stay on him.
    2. Inform the client to send the amulet home with the family because it is an infection control risk in the hospital.
    3. Ask the client why he thinks the amulet will protect him during the hospital stay and then respond accordingly.
    4. Tape the amulet to the client's skin so that it will not become separated from him during surgery.

28. The nurse is admitting a female client to the medical-surgical unit when the client tells the nurse she takes many vitamins to keep her healthy. Which statement is the nurse's **most appropriate** response to the information provided by the client?
    1. "Vitamins are just a way that the manufacturers bilk people out of money."
    2. "You need to make sure that your health-care provider knows which ones you take."

3. "If you take vitamins, then be careful when taking too many water-soluble vitamins."

4. "Most people are deficient in getting enough vitamins. It is good you take supplements."

29. The nurse is preparing to administer morning medications. Which order would the nurse **question**?

| Client Name: I.M. Client | MR# 654231 | Diagnosis: Atrial Fibrillation |
|---|---|---|
| DOB: 7/15/1950 | Allergies: NKDA | |
| Medication | 0701–1900 | 1901–0700 |
| Vitamin C 500 mg PO daily | 0900 | |
| Tamsulosin 0.4 mg PO twice a day | 0900 1800 | |
| St. John's wort 1 tablet daily | 0900 | |
| Warfarin 5 mg PO daily | 0900 | |
| Signature of Nurse: | Day Nurse RN/DN | Night Nurse RN/NN |

1. Vitamin C.
2. Tamsulosin.
3. St. John's wort.
4. Warfarin.

30. The male client tells the nurse that he has been using acupuncture to control his chronic back pain. Which is the nurse's **best** response?
   1. "Insurance and Medicare will not pay for acupuncture treatments."
   2. "Can you describe the pain before and after the acupuncture treatments?"
   3. "Make sure you sterilize the needles before using them to relieve the pain."
   4. "You should try to use guided imagery to control your pain."

31. The client expresses anxiety before an upcoming procedure. Which should the nurse implement **first** to assist the client?
   1. Call the HCP for a sedative order.
   2. Notify the family the client is nervous about the procedure.
   3. Encourage the client to take slow deep breaths.
   4. Tell the client not to think about the procedure and soon it will be over.

32. The nurse is preparing a female client for surgery. The client tells the nurse that she is a Jehovah's Witness and is afraid that the staff will administer blood to her during the procedure while she is under anesthesia. Which is the nurse's **best** response to the client?
   1. "I will place a notice in your EHR and report to the surgical team that you will not allow blood or blood products to be given."
   2. "If you go into surgery, then all interventions there have to be administered in order for you to have the desired results."

3. "You do not want a blood transfusion? Tell me why you would not want something that could save your life."
   4. "Your HCP must write an order that you do not want blood or blood products to be given."

33. The nurse educator is preparing to teach a class on cultural diversity to new graduate nurses. Which information should the nurse include in the teaching? **Select all that apply**.
   1. Be aware of your own biases and preconceptions.
   2. Avoid making assumptions and stereotypes about people from other cultures.
   3. Use everyday language to explain procedures.
   4. Use assertive body language to obtain respect.
   5. Explain to clients the importance of interpreters in providing safe care.

34. The new graduate nurse is performing a cultural assessment on a client using the LEARN method of cross-cultural communication. Which steps are included in the LEARN method? **Select all that apply**.
   1. Listen to the client's perception of the problem.
   2. Explain your perception of the problem
   3. Acknowledge and discuss differences and similarities
   4. Require treatment decisions from the client.
   5. Notify HCPs of the client's decisions

**1** Correct answers are 1, 2, 3, 4, and 5.
1. The nurse should ask specifically about herbs because many clients do not consider them drugs and will not volunteer the information.
2. The nurse should ask about the use of over-the-counter medications because many clients believe HCPs are only concerned about prescribed medications.
3. The nurse should assess the client for any previous reaction to medications.
4. The nurse should be aware of when the last medication was taken to determine the effectiveness of the medication and to ensure any further medication will not have an untoward effect.
5. The health-care team must be aware of all prescriptions so the medications may be continued during hospitalization or discontinued if necessary.

**TEST-TAKING HINT:** This is an example of an alternative-type question. There could be more than one correct answer. The test taker should key into the descriptive words, such as "specifically," in the stem of the question.

**2.** 1. All medications have side effects, even the drugs that are available over the counter.
2. Medicated nasal sprays, such as Afrin nasal spray, cause the arterioles to constrict, resulting in increased congestion after several days of use.
3. Medicated nasal sprays, as well as oral decongestants, have adverse effects.
4. Alternating several nasal sprays will not prevent the client from developing a tolerance to the sprays.

**TEST-TAKING HINT:** If the test taker has no idea of the correct answer, option "2" has the word "congestion" in the answer, and the word "congestion" is in the stem of the question. This would be an appropriate option to select as the correct answer.

**3.** 1. A vaginal examination would be performed after the pregnancy test result has been obtained.
2. The first intervention is to determine if the client is pregnant.
3. Baseline vital signs would be needed if the client were pregnant.

4. The first intervention should be determining if the client is pregnant. The results of a pregnancy test will determine which interventions should be implemented next.

**TEST-TAKING HINT:** The test taker must key in on the word "first," which indicates all four interventions are appropriate, but only one should be implemented first.

**4.** 1. Echinacea, an herb, combines with warfarin (Coumadin), an anticoagulant, to increase bleeding time. It does not, however, alter the INR.
2. Clients taking warfarin (Coumadin) should have their INR tested routinely.
3. Clients taking anticoagulants should use acetaminophen (Tylenol), a nonopioid analgesic, for pain rather than aspirin or NSAIDs because these can cause bleeding.
4. Prepared foods can interact with medications and medical treatments, but not many foods cause bleeding and bruising.

**TEST-TAKING HINT:** Herbs often interfere with over-the-counter medications and prescription medications. Therefore, option "1" would be an appropriate choice for the correct answer if the test taker had no idea of the correct answer to this question.

**5.** 1. Nothing in the stem indicates the client is overweight.
2. Unless contraindicated, a more realistic goal would be to restrict the number of alcoholic beverages to two per day.
3. All clients would benefit from a routine daily exercise program, which promotes health, especially for those with a sedentary lifestyle.
4. There is nothing in the stem indicating the client has a specific disease process that warrants restricting foods.

**TEST-TAKING HINT:** The adjective "sedentary" is the key to answering this question correctly. The test taker should not become distracted by excess verbiage in the stem. In option "2," the word "never" is an absolute term and makes this option incorrect.

**6.** 1. The nurse should not ask the client "why"; the client has a right to her feelings.
2. An action should be implemented because the client is upset, and the client's emotional state should be addressed.

3. There is no reason for the nurse to refer the client to a psychologist.
4. The UAP should be informed about how certain actions can be perceived differently in clients from a different cultural background. The UAP should be encouraged to learn about different cultures to avoid actions that are culturally insensitive.

**TEST-TAKING HINT: The phrase "of a different culture" informs the test taker the question is focused on cultural differences and insensitivities. Option "4" is good advice for all health-care professionals.**

7. 1. The nurse should realize maintaining direct eye contact with members of some cultures can be interpreted as aggressive behavior.
   2. Loud expression of needs does not mean the client is angry.
   3. The nurse should discuss the care with the client. Discussing her care with family members is a violation of HIPAA, and just because the client lives in their home does not mean the family members are the client's guardians.
   4. The nurse should discuss the importance of the management of ideal body weight because the client is overweight and hypertensive.

**TEST-TAKING HINT: The test taker must realize 102 kg is 224 pounds, which is overweight for a 5′4″ woman. The test taker should not automatically select option "2" because the word "loudly" is in both the stem and the answer option. Speaking loudly could indicate a hearing impairment or her normal speech.**

8. Correct answers are 1, 2, 3, and 5.
   1. The nurse should always ask clients how they would like to be addressed. Some clients may prefer use of their first name, others may prefer a more formal title.
   2. The nurse should ask the client if any family should be involved in decisions about the client's care.
   3. The client may speak or read a different language. The nurse should assess the language the client prefers to communicate with and provide translation services if needed.
   4. The nurse should not ask a "why" question.
   5. The nurse should ask the client for values or beliefs the client practices and attempt to incorporate those beliefs in the plan of care for the client if they are not detrimental to the client's health.

**TEST-TAKING HINT: The question is asking for interventions that will help establish a rapport with the client, and cultural influences must be addressed, especially in the home. Option "4" can be eliminated because a "why" question is not appropriate for building a therapeutic relationship.**

9. 1. An advance directive would not be information that would help provide culturally sensitive nursing care.
   2. Ayurveda is the traditional health care of India, and the nurse should determine if the client practices Ayurveda or uses a faith healer. Many clients self-medicate with medications brought from home.
   3. An interpreter would not help the nurse provide culturally sensitive care but would help the nurse understand what the client is saying.
   4. Allergies to medications and environmental elements are assessed in the initial interviews of all clients and would not reflect the cultural aspects of care.

**TEST-TAKING HINT: This question is requesting specific information about the culture of the client who practices Hinduism. Options "1" and "4" are information the nurse would require of any client and, therefore, could be eliminated because the stem is asking about culturally sensitive care.**

10. 1. The nurse should not refer to the client's beliefs in a negative manner.
    2. This statement is belittling to the client's beliefs and would interfere with the nurse-client relationship.
    3. Good luck charms, amulets, or medals provide clients with emotional support. Folk remedies that are not harmful should be allowed while caring for the client.
    4. Personal belongings are usually sent home to prevent the loss of the items, but this statement would be false because the client values the amulet.

**TEST-TAKING HINT: A basic concept in nursing is that the nurse should always try to support the client's cultural beliefs if they do not harm the client or interfere with the medical treatment.**

11. 1. The nurse could request the family bring meals, but this is not the first intervention.
    2. The nurse should notify the dietary department once it is determined why the client is not eating the meals provided.

3. Many local Jewish communities will provide kosher meals for clients in the hospital if the dietary department is unable to provide them, but this is not the first intervention.
4. The nurse should first assess and determine why the client is not eating. It could be because of illness, medication, or cultural beliefs.

**TEST-TAKING HINT: Religious practices should be considered when clients are in the hospital. However, the nurse must first assess the situation to determine why the client is not eating. Remember, the first step of the nursing process is assessment.**

12. Correct answers are 2 and 5.
    1. Music therapy has been used in pain management and relaxation, but it is not used for weight loss.
    2. Hypnotherapy, or self-hypnosis, has been used successfully in weight-loss programs.
    3. There are several types of yoga exercises that increase relaxation and promote health, but they do not assist with weight loss.
    4. The Alexander technique focuses on assisting clients become aware of movements and the relationship with health and performance, but it has not been used for weight loss.
    5. Acupuncture has been regarded as an alternative treatment for obesity (Esteghamati et al., 2015).

**TEST-TAKING HINT: The test taker should be familiar with current treatments. Current treatment options being advertised for weight loss are hypnosis and self-hypnosis.**

13. Correct answers are 1, 2, 3, and 5.
    1. The selection of various therapies offers the client the ability to have some control over care and may help maintain personal independence.
    2. Clients can select treatments that are pleasurable, in addition to being effective.
    3. Many therapies decrease heart rate and blood pressure. Therefore, the nurse should be knowledgeable, so referrals can be effective.
    4. The nurse should explain the benefits of the therapy to the significant other to alleviate concerns, but this would not be considered when the nurse is planning the therapy.

5. Many therapies require movement or specific cognitive abilities to perform. If the client cannot perform the therapy, the client can become frustrated.

**TEST-TAKING HINT: This is an example of an alternative-type question. The test taker may have to select more than one correct answer.**

14. 1. Meditation takes practice and the ability to focus. It is not the best way to help an anxious older client manage stress.
    2. Deep breathing begins to relax the muscles in the body, and this would be a method for an older client to learn and use to relax.
    3. Rolfing is a holistic method of structural integration. The client would not be able to perform this therapy independently because a therapist is needed to perform it.
    4. Scented candles would be unsafe in a hospital setting. Aromatherapy using essential oils can be used, but the client is admitted for surgery and any scent postoperatively can initiate nausea.

**TEST-TAKING HINT: The adjective "older" should cause the test taker to select the easiest and simplest way to help the client relax. The test taker must pay close attention to adjectives such as "older."**

15. 1. Therapeutic touch is used in the treatment of migraine headaches by some clients. The practitioner uses the hands to direct energy to correct imbalances, which cause the migraine headache.
    2. Autogenic training is a method using mental relaxation to lead the body to healing. Because it may require several sessions by a certified trainer, the client would find it difficult to learn this technique from a book.
    3. Massage is the manual manipulation of the client's tissue, which affects the entire body and produces generalized relaxation and a feeling of well-being, but the client cannot perform massage therapy alone.
    4. Aromatherapy has been linked to the relief of the symptoms of migraine headaches by using certain essential oils such as rosemary, chamomile, and lavender.

**TEST-TAKING HINT: The test taker should be aware that the client will be unable to perform therapies alone. The test taker should be cautious when selecting an answer option that encourages the client to purchase a book explaining the therapy.**

16. 1. The nurse should not ignore the client's feelings of sadness and loneliness by turning on the television.
    2. The client is in a rehabilitation setting, which often allows for pet visits. Therefore, the nurse should investigate having the family bring the dog to the facility. This is being a client advocate.
    3. Pet therapy is being used to promote relaxation and a sense of well-being, but the client wants to see her own dog.
    4. The nurse should never claim to have a complete understanding of the client's feelings. This would belittle the client's feelings.

**TEST-TAKING HINT:** The test taker must be aware of adjectives, and "rehabilitation" in the stem indicates the client is not in an acute care setting. Many rehabilitation units allow family pets to visit.

17. 1. The nurse should not administer medication so the client can visit with animals. The nurse cannot control all of the client's symptoms and this could present a danger to the client.
    2. The nurse cannot realistically spend extra time visiting with the client when the nurse has many clients to care for and duties to complete.
    3. Arranging for the volunteer to bring a radio for the client with a hearing impairment would not be helpful because it would need to be played loudly for the client to hear and would interfere with other clients and staff.
    4. For clients with allergies to pet dander, the nurse can provide fish therapy. Studies indicate watching fish swim can decrease blood pressure and promote a calming effect.

**TEST-TAKING HINT:** The descriptive terms should guide the test taker to the correct answer. The test taker should eliminate option "3" because of the words "hearing impairment" in the stem of the question.

18. 1. Dance movement therapy incorporates synchronized movement and creates an experience shared by all the participants, which, in turn, contributes to the establishment of a bond between the participants. The sharing of emotions and experiences strengthens support-group relationships.
    2. Dance movements do not help increase the amount of synovial fluid in joints.
    3. Dance movements don't help decrease pain; in fact, they may increase pain in some clients.
    4. Endorphins are released by laughing, not dancing, and their release does not necessarily help with the pain.

**TEST-TAKING HINT:** The test taker should apply knowledge of anatomy and physiology to help answer this question. Synovial fluid does not increase for any reason; therefore, option "2" should be eliminated as a correct answer. Inflamed joints respond to cold or heat; therefore, option "3" should be eliminated as a correct answer.

19. 1. The nurse is responsible for ensuring the client receives quality care regardless of the client's history or the amount of care required.
    2. The client should be encouraged to use alternative therapies for pain management to supplement medication, not replace medication.
    3. The nurse should assist the client's pain management by using complementary therapies as well as medication but never in place of pain medication.
    4. A double dose of medication requires an HCP's order, and, if administered, careful monitoring is required.

**TEST-TAKING HINT:** The descriptive term "preoperative teaching" can assist the test taker in eliminating options. Option "1" is judgmental and should be eliminated. Options "2" and "3" are opposites. Most of the time one of these options is correct.

20. 1. Studies show music can calm the anxious client when the music has a slow beat. Faster beats or irregular rhythms tend to irritate older clients.
    2. Taking deep breaths may help decrease anxiety. Rapid shallow breathing could cause the client to hyperventilate and lead to dizziness.
    3. Talking makes some clients more anxious; a quiet environment would assist this client in relaxing.
    4. The increased airflow could increase the risk of client infection and will not help the client's diaphoresis.

**TEST-TAKING HINT:** The test taker should understand basic concepts in operating room nursing, and, often, music is played to help decrease the anxiety of the client as well as the staff. Music can have a calming effect on people.

**21.** 1. This situation indicates the nurse should take some type of action. The client has an elevated heart rate and blood pressure.
2. Baroque music has a slower pace, and studies have shown that client's bodies attempt to synchronize with the beat and rhythm of the sounds in the room. The client's elevated vital signs could be a result of rock music in the room.
3. Medications should be used if other methods are not effective.
4. Changing the client's position should be done routinely and may decrease discomfort, but it will not affect the client's pulse and blood pressure.

**TEST-TAKING HINT:** The test taker should recognize words in the questions that can aid in the selection of the correct answer. The description of "rock" music in the stem of the question and answer option "2" to change the music should assist in selecting the correct answer.

**22.** 1. The pain and evaluation of the medication should be assessed before contacting the HCP.
2. Telling the client to relax does not help when the client is uncomfortable.
3. Guided imagery can be used to increase relaxation and decrease the sensation of pain.
4. When clients are using a PCA pump, family members should be discouraged from administering the medication for the client. The client can become oversedated and develop respiratory depression.

**TEST-TAKING HINT:** If the test taker wants to select the answer option that says "notify the health-care provider," the test taker must evaluate the other options to make sure another option does not include assessment data or an independent nursing intervention.

**23.** 1. Guided imagery is not used to prevent or treat infection; therefore, assessing the white blood cell count would not be appropriate.
2. The postoperative client uses guided imagery to increase relaxation, which helps decrease the perception of pain.
3. This is a goal for a postoperative client, but it is not based on the use of guided imagery.
4. The expected outcome for the postoperative client would be to have a clean, dry dressing, but guided imagery would not affect the dressing.

**TEST-TAKING HINT:** The expected outcome must reflect the goal of guided imagery. Therefore, the test taker must have knowledge of why guided imagery is used to be able to answer this question.

**24.** 1. This would be done during meditation.
2. Rubbing the arm in firm stroking motions is performing self-massage.
3. Music therapy is purposefully using music that has 50 to 60 beats per minute.
4. The client using guided imagery should use as many senses as possible to create an image of a scene that has meaning for the client.

**TEST-TAKING HINT:** Each answer option describes a type of complementary therapy. The test taker should pay attention to the words "imagery" and "visualizes." To visualize is to use the imagination.

**25.** 1. Instructing on a low-salt diet may be needed, but assessment should be the first intervention implemented.
2. Antihypertensive medications may be needed, but an assessment should be the first intervention implemented.
3. The nurse should first assess the client to determine if the client is taking any over-the-counter medication that may increase the blood pressure. Decongestants that contain ephedrine or pseudoephedrine elevate blood pressure and should be used with caution.
4. Teaching about the complications of hypertension would be important but not done before assessing the client.

**TEST-TAKING HINT:** The test taker should use the nursing process when answering questions that ask the test taker to select the first intervention. Assessment is the first intervention of the nursing process.

26. 1. The family may or may not understand the medical questions. The client may not wish to have a family member be involved in knowing the personal information required on the admission assessment.
 2. Hand gestures are inadequate for determining the information required on an admission assessment.
 3. The nurse is responsible for obtaining accurate information. Not speaking a language is not a relevant excuse for not attempting to perform a thorough assessment.
 4. Hospitals are required by the Joint Commission to have a method of communicating with non-English-speaking clients from other cultures. Most facilities pay a fee to have medical interpreters available 24 hours a day.

**TEST-TAKING HINT: This is an example of a nurse being required to know rules and regulations that govern the practice of nursing. In this question, the test taker could rule out options "2" and "3" because these options violate the basic rules of nursing practice.**

27. 1. The amulet is metal and cannot stay on the client during surgery because the cautery machine could create an electrical burn for the client. It should be allowed near the client and replaced on the client as soon as it is safe to do so.
 2. The amulet can stay with the client and in the room. Requesting the client to send it home is not sensitive to his beliefs.
 3. The client believes it helps him; he does not owe the nurse an explanation of his beliefs.
 4. Taping the amulet to the client's skin could result in an electrical burn during surgery.

**TEST-TAKING HINT: The test taker must understand the equipment used in a hospital and make adjustments to be culturally sensitive but maintain safety for the client.**

28. 1. This may be somewhat true in this country but many people do benefit from taking a multivitamin daily. "Many" indicates the client may be overdoing it, but challenging the client without determining what is being taken can result in the client continuing to take the vitamins but next time not telling the health-care personnel.
 2. The HCP should be aware of all medications, both prescribed and over the counter, the client takes because they can interact with one another and be inappropriate for some diagnoses.
 3. Water-soluble vitamins, when taken to excess, are eliminated from the body in the urine. Fat-soluble vitamins can build up in the body and create a problem.
 4. Most people could get sufficient vitamins daily if they eat a balanced diet. This statement would be misleading to the client.

**TEST-TAKING HINT: The test taker must read all words in the question and in the options carefully. Would a nurse tell a client that manufacturers "bilk" people? Basic guidelines for discharge instructions encourage clients to make all HCPs aware of medications being taken.**

29. 1. Vitamin C 500 mg is not an excessive dose, and the medication administration record (MAR) does not indicate a problem that the client might expect in taking the vitamin.
 2. Tamsulosin (Flomax) is a medication prescribed for a client diagnosed with benign prostatic hypertrophy (BPH). A 70+-year-old man could be expected to have mild to moderate BPH.
 3. St. John's wort is commonly taken by clients for depression. It has significant interactions with various prescription medications, including warfarin (Coumadin). It will decrease the effectiveness of Coumadin. The nurse would question this medication while the client is on Coumadin.
 4. Warfarin (Coumadin) is prescribed to prevent clot formation in clients diagnosed with atrial fibrillation.

**TEST-TAKING HINT: This is an example of an alternative-type question. The test taker must read all of the MAR to determine if the medications are appropriate. Next, the nurse must realize that even though St. John's wort is an over-the-counter preparation, it can still impact other medications. There could be more than one correct answer. The test taker should key into the descriptive words, such as "specifically," in the stem of the question.**

30. 1. The client has been using the treatments and will know how to pay for the treatments.
    2. This is an assessment question to determine the success of the treatment.
    3. The client would not sterilize the needles; this is the responsibility of the acupuncturist.
    4. The client is not asking for a different method to control the pain.

**TEST-TAKING HINT:** The test taker could use the nursing process to answer this question; assessment is the first step in the nursing process.

31. 1. The HCP may need to be notified of the anxiety but not for a sedative order. This is not assisting the client, but the first action is to allow the client to cope with the situation. The nurse should allow the client to verbalize the anxious feelings and assist the client in coping with the situation.
    2. The client may ask the nurse to notify the family, but the nurse should not automatically assume the client has a relationship with the family that would decrease the anxiety.
    3. During anxiety situations, a client's breathing increases in a "fight or flight" reaction. The nurse can assist the client in remaining calm and coping with the anxiety by coaching the client in deep-breathing exercises.
    4. The client cannot automatically turn off anxious thoughts just by not thinking about something.

**TEST-TAKING HINT:** This is an example of an alternative-therapy question. The nurse should be open to nonpharmacological interventions to assist the client in coping. This is a temporary situation at this point, worrying over a procedure.

32. 1. The nurse should assure the client that her wishes will be respected and then proceed to make sure that the information is provided to all other health-care personnel.
    2. An adult client has the legal right to make decisions of this nature, and the health-care team is required to abide by those decisions.
    3. This is a poor attempt at a therapeutic conversation; the client has given factual information. "Why" is never therapeutic. A therapeutic conversation is not required in this question. The nurse can address the issue.
    4. The HCP would have to write an order to administer blood and blood products. An order to refuse the blood does not have to be written.

**TEST-TAKING HINT:** This is an example of knowing differences in cultures and religions.

33. Correct answers are 1, 2, 3, and 5.
    1. The nurse should be aware of their own biases and preconceptions about other cultures to provide culturally competent care.
    2. Cultural stereotypes should be avoided. The client should be assessed for their own beliefs and approaches to health care.
    3. Everyday language, in lay terms, will facilitate the client's understanding of procedures or disease processes.
    4. Open, approachable body language should be used to facilitate communication. The nurse should avoid crossing their arms when speaking and should try to be at the same eye level as the client.
    5. Clients have the right to refuse an interpreter, but the nurse should reinforce to the client that an interpreter can enhance the quality and safety of the client's care.

**TEST-TAKING HINT:** This is an example of an alternative-type question. There will be more than one correct answer. The test taker should read each option as a true or false question.

34. Correct answers are 1, 2, and 3.
    1. The nurse should always listen to the client's perception of the health-care problem.
    2. The nurse should present the perception of the problem to the client based on knowledge and evidence-based practice.
    3. Acknowledgment and discussing differences and similarities can resolve conflicts in client care (Berlin & Fowkes, 1983).
    4. The nurse should not require treatment decisions from the client. This step is to recommend and explain treatment options.
    5. The final step is to negotiate, involving the client in the decision-making process.

**TEST-TAKING HINT:** This is an example of a priority question. A physiological need is a priority over psychosocial needs. If every other option is within normal limits or expected for the disease process and not life-threatening, the psychosocial need can be addressed first.

# CULTURAL NURSING AND ALTERNATIVE HEALTH CARE COMPREHENSIVE EXAMINATION

1. The client diagnosed with rheumatoid arthritis asks the nurse, "Is it all right for me to wear this copper bracelet to help cure my arthritis?" Which statement by the nurse would be **most appropriate**?
   1. "How do you know the copper bracelet will help cure your arthritis?"
   2. "The bracelet will not cure your arthritis, but if it helps the pain, wear it."
   3. "You should talk to your health-care provider before wearing the copper bracelet."
   4. "I recommend not wearing the bracelet and taking your prescribed medications."

2. The client asks the nurse about using herbs and special teas to decrease blood pressure. Which question is **most important** for the nurse to consider before addressing the client's concerns?
   1. "How expensive is this treatment?"
   2. "Is this practice safe for the client?"
   3. "Do I have the knowledge to answer this question?"
   4. "Is this within the scope of the state's Nurse Practice Act?"

3. The client is using acupuncture to help relieve severe back pain. Which client problem would the home health nurse identify in the plan of care?
   1. The likelihood of paralysis.
   2. The potential for infection.
   3. The possibility of contracting AIDS.
   4. No resolution of the pain.

4. The male Navajo client comes to the clinic reporting chest pain and has a pouch filled with objects around his neck. Which statement **best** supports the nurse allowing the client to wear the pouch?
   1. This is a cultural practice shared by many Navajo clients, and the nurse should not remove it unless it interferes with the client's care.
   2. The client may get very upset and angry with the nurse if the pouch is removed and lose faith in the health-care system.
   3. The nurse should never ask any client to remove any type of cultural objects from the body.
   4. This is a preventive measure prescribed by the medicine man to ward off evil.

5. The Mexican client requests a curandero to come to the hospital to visit. Which statement explains the role of the curandero in the Mexican culture?
   1. He treats muscle and joint problems using massage and manipulation.
   2. He uses herbs, teas, and roots to prevent or treat illnesses.
   3. He is a spiritualist and treats conditions caused by witchcraft.
   4. He receives gifts from God and treats traditional illnesses.

6. The home health nurse is visiting a Jewish client who has a small container on the doorpost of the house. Which term **best** describes this container?
   1. A tallis.
   2. A mezuzah.
   3. A synagogue.
   4. Yom Kippur.

7. The home health nurse is assessing a client diagnosed with congestive heart failure. The client has a slice of raw potato on an abdominal carbuncle. Which action should the nurse implement **first**?
   1. Explain the client should not put raw potatoes on the boil.
   2. Ask the client to explain why there is a raw potato on the boil.
   3. Cleanse the wound and determine if there is an infection.
   4. Leave the raw potato on the boil and take no further action.

8. The female client is reporting dyspepsia, insomnia, and upper respiratory infection symptoms and has an elevated blood pressure. The client tells the nurse she recently moved to the area to care for an ill parent. Which statement **best** explains the client's clinical manifestations?
   1. The client has a psychosomatic illness.
   2. The client's immune system is altered by stress.
   3. The client's symptoms are caused by gastric reflux.
   4. The client has essential hypertension.

9. The nurse assessing an older client diagnosed with chronic obstructive pulmonary disease notes purple, round, nontender areas on the client's back. Which question should the nurse ask the client?
   1. "Have you had cupping performed?"
   2. "Do you always bruise this easily?"
   3. "Did someone living with you hurt you?"
   4. "What have you done to cause these?"

10. The nurse is preparing a teaching plan for a client diagnosed with chronic stress. Which information should the nurse include in the teaching care plan? **Select all that apply**.
    1. Discuss the relationship between stress and illness with the client.
    2. Define the terms "stress" and "relaxation" in words the client understands.
    3. Explain methods used to decrease stress that the nurse has used.
    4. Refer the client to a practitioner of traditional Chinese medicine.
    5. Provide Web site addresses for the client to investigate.

11. The nurse is assisting the client diagnosed with chronic pain to identify methods of complementary and alternative medicine (CAM). Which would indicate an **expected** outcome was achieved?
    1. The client will spend 18 out of 24 hours in bed.
    2. The client will have an enhanced sensation of pain.
    3. The client will take medication on a routine basis.
    4. The client will be able to perform three ADLs without pain.

12. The nurse and the UAP are performing postmortem care on a client. Two of the family members are seen laughing about a memory they shared with the client. What explanation of this behavior would be **best** for the RN to give the UAP?
    1. The two family members probably did not love the client.
    2. The behavior is inappropriate for the situation and inexcusable.
    3. The family members are using laughter to cope with the pain.
    4. This behavior is demonstrated only by uneducated individuals.

13. The UAP asked the wound care nurse why a client has cabbage leaves on the wound. Which statement would be the **best** response by the nurse?
    1. "Cabbage leaves have antibacterial and anti-inflammatory properties."
    2. "Some people are ignorant and will believe or try anything to get better."
    3. "This is the placebo effect. If people believe something will work, it will."
    4. "The cabbage leaves will keep the wound moist and clean until it heals."

14. The nurse at the Family Planning Clinic is preparing a discussion about contraception and methods to prevent pregnancy for students attending a community college. What information should

the nurse include in the presentation? **Select all that apply**.
    1. Condoms should be used to prevent sexually transmitted diseases.
    2. Sexually active females should have vaginal examinations yearly.
    3. Hormonal therapy can be used orally, subcutaneously, or topically.
    4. All methods of contraception need prescriptions from the HCP.
    5. Sterilization is the only way to avoid unintended pregnancy.

15. The occupational health nurse is caring for the client diagnosed with a superficial burn on the arm. The client states a preference for using holistic natural medication. Which medicinal plant should the nurse recommend to the client?
    1. Black cohosh.
    2. Fennel.
    3. Witch hazel.
    4. Aloe vera.

16. The client has been diagnosed with bronchitis. The client asks the nurse, "Can I use eucalyptus oil in steam and breathe it in deeply?" Which response by the nurse would be **most appropriate**?
    1. "I would not recommend using any type of folk medicine."
    2. "The steam and the oil may help open up your airway."
    3. "This type of treatment could interfere with your other medications."
    4. "Inhaled eucalyptus oil is not as effective as rubbing it on the chest."

17. The client diagnosed with a deficiency of the immune system questions the nurse about the use of ginseng. Which information should the nurse teach the client?
    1. Take the ginseng daily to achieve a therapeutic level.
    2. Take ginseng with caffeine drinks to enhance its effects.
    3. Do not take ginseng continuously for more than 2 months.
    4. There are no contraindications for any client taking ginseng.

18. The client diagnosed with severe itching from an insect bite calls the clinic and asks the nurse, "What do I need to do for the itching?" Which intervention should the nurse implement for the client problem of alteration in comfort?
    1. Alternate acetaminophen with acetylsalicylic acid every 2 hours.
    2. Cover the area with diphenhydramine topical every 6 hours as needed for itching.

3. Wash the area with soap and hot water and cover with gauze pads.

4. Apply 1% hydrocortisone cream every 2 hours.

19. The client diagnosed with anemia has been taking iron supplements. Which data would indicate to the nurse the treatment has been **effective**?
    1. The client is able to prepare a menu high in iron.
    2. The client is able to perform ADLs.
    3. The client has an increase in black tarry stools.
    4. The client has an increase in dystrophy of nails.

20. The nurse is teaching the older client about taking oral iron supplements. Which intervention should the nurse include in the teaching?
    1. Take the iron with an antacid to prevent a bleeding ulcer.
    2. If a dose is missed, take the dose with the next dose.
    3. The client should take the medication between meals.
    4. The client should recline for 30 minutes after the dosage.

21. The nurse is teaching a 28-year-old client about recently prescribed birth control pills. Which statement by the client indicates teaching has been **effective**?
    1. "I will use another birth control method if I have to take antibiotics."
    2. "If I miss a pill, I will take it at the end of the prescription."
    3. "I will use the contraceptive patch because it has fewer side effects."
    4. "If the contraceptive ring comes out, I will have to get a new one."

22. Which method of birth control would the nurse recommend for the homeless client with two unplanned pregnancies?
    1. Cavity-rim cervical cap device.
    2. Subdermal levonorgestrel implants.
    3. Combination oral contraceptives.
    4. Medroxyprogesterone acetate injections intramuscularly.

23. Which information would be **most important** for the public health department nurse to obtain before giving the client condoms?
    1. The frequency of sexual activity.
    2. Type of condom the client prefers.
    3. If the client is allergic to latex.
    4. The client's sexual history.

24. The nurse and the UAP are caring for an anxious client. Which task should the RN delegate to the UAP?
    1. Teach the client how to breathe deep.
    2. Give the client a back rub.
    3. Listen to the client's concerns.
    4. Instruct the client on how to perform guided imagery.

25. The nurse is teaching the client about relaxation techniques. Which interventions should be included in the teaching? **Select all that apply.**
    1. Instruct the client to contract and relax the muscles.
    2. Explain the importance of playing soothing music.
    3. Use all five senses when using guided imagery.
    4. Discuss the need to eliminate all stress in the client's life.
    5. Insist the client write about personal feelings in a journal.

26. The client is reporting acute abdominal pain, and the next pain medication is not due for 2 hours. Which interventions should the nurse implement? **Rank in order of priority.**
    1. Notify the HCP to increase pain medication.
    2. Auscultate for bowel sounds and palpate the abdomen.
    3. Instruct the client to visualize a pleasant memory.
    4. Turn on the radio to soft, easy-listening music.
    5. Offer the client a therapeutic back massage.

1. 1. This is challenging the client's question and will not help establish a therapeutic relationship with the client.
   2. The nurse should present facts and support the client's alternative health belief unless it hurts the client or makes the disease process worse.
   3. The nurse does not need to pass the buck to the HCP to answer this question.
   4. Alternative medicine is often helpful to the client, and the nurse should support a client's beliefs as much as possible if it does not hurt the client.

2. 1. The nurse can be concerned about the cost of the herbs and teas, but it is not the most important question to consider.
   2. The client's safety is a priority, but if the nurse does not have the knowledge, then the nurse cannot answer the question.
   3. Teaching about herbs and alternative therapies is not a priority in nursing programs. Therefore, the nurse must determine sufficient personal knowledge or expertise to answer the client's question. The nurse should find a reputable resource before answering this question.
   4. The nurse must always practice within the scope of nursing, but providing correct and factual information is within the scope of the nurse's practice.

3. 1. Acupuncture does not usually cause paralysis because of the size of the needles and wires used.
   2. Acupuncture is a method of producing analgesia or altering the function of a system of the body by inserting fine, wire-thin needles into the skin at specific sites on the body. Infection does occur if a sterile procedure is not used when inserting the needles.
   3. AIDS is not a great concern because the health department regulates the centers that perform acupuncture and there is no sharing of the needles.
   4. The pain not being resolved is a concern, but the potential for infection is a priority.

4. 1. Some Navajo people wear medicine bags, and the nurse should support the client's culture if it does not interfere with the medical regimen.
   2. Most clients will not get upset and angry and lose faith if the nurse explains the importance of removing an object.
   3. "Never" is an absolute word, and sometimes objects must be removed, such as when going to surgery.
   4. This may be the reason the object is worn, but it is not the best statement to explain why the nurse should not remove the pouch. Even if the nurse does not understand the reason for the object, the nurse should respect and honor the practice if possible.

5. 1. This is a Mexican folk practitioner known as a *sobadore*.
   2. This is a Mexican folk practitioner known as a *yerbera* or *jerbera*.
   3. This is a Mexican folk practitioner known as an *espiritista*.
   4. Curanderos receive their gift from God or serve an apprenticeship. Some even prescribe over-the-counter medications. They treat mental, physical, and spiritual illnesses.

6. 1. A tallis (or tallith) is a rectangular prayer shawl with fringes used during prayer.
   2. A mezuzah is a small container with scripture inside that is placed on the doorpost of the home; some wear the mezuzah as a necklace.
   3. A synagogue is a Jewish house of prayer; Jews may pray alone, or they may pray as a group.
   4. Yom Kippur is a high holy day celebrated in September or early October. On Yom Kippur, one fasts for a day to cleanse and purify oneself.

7. 1. The nurse should be sensitive to folk medicine, and if it does not hurt the client, the nurse should be respectful and honor the practice.
   2. The nurse should not make the client explain personal folk medicine beliefs.

3. The nurse should first assess the carbuncle to determine if the raw potato is making the carbuncle worse; if it is not, the nurse should support the client's folk medicine.
4. The nurse should assess the carbuncle before deciding not to take any further action.

8. 1. These are not typical findings of a psychosomatic disorder.
2. This would be the best explanation because the client has experienced major life changes—moving to another area and assuming the role of caregiver to a parent. Chronic unrelieved stress has been shown to decrease immunity, resulting in frequent upper respiratory tract infections and increased blood pressure.
3. Gastric reflux has been linked to asthma-type symptoms but not upper respiratory infections.
4. These clinical manifestations do not support the diagnosis of essential hypertension.

9. 1. Cupping is an alternative treatment modality in which heated cups are applied to the body. They produce round, red, or purple circles that may remain for as long as 1 week. It may be used for clients diagnosed with respiratory difficulty.
2. This response assumes the areas are bruises resulting from injury or illness.
3. This response assumes the areas are bruises resulting from abuse, which could lead to false accusations and legal issues.
4. This response sounds judgmental and blaming, and the nurse should avoid responses that damage the client-nurse relationship.

10. Correct answers are 1, 2, 3, and 5.
1. The client should understand the relationship between stress and illness.
2. For effective teaching, the nurse should use terms the client understands.
3. Methods the nurse has experienced personally or has observed to be successful with other clients can aid the client's selection.
4. The nurse should not refer the client to alternative HCPs. This is imposing the nurse's cultural beliefs onto the client.
5. The nurse should provide a variety of referrals and resources to use to help reduce and control stressful situations.

11. 1. If the client spends more than three-fourths of the time in bed, then this would be a low quality of life and would not be the expected outcome.
2. An expected outcome would be relief of pain or enhanced pain management. An enhanced sensation of pain would be unrelieved pain.
3. CAM would not include prescription medication, and taking medication is an intervention, not an expected outcome.
4. A client performing ADLs without pain represents an appropriate expected outcome.

12. 1. This behavior does not indicate a lack of love; it is a coping mechanism.
2. Family members' coping mechanisms should not be criticized by staff.
3. Laughter during times of stress aids in coping with pain and increases relaxation.
4. Laughter is used by many individuals as stress relief, regardless of educational levels.

13. 1. Cabbage leaves have been shown to have some antibacterial and anti-inflammatory properties. Softened leaves are applied to wounds, ulcers, and arthritic joints.
2. This response is belittling the client's beliefs and actions.
3. Studies support the placebo effect, but this response does not answer the UAP's question about the use of cabbage leaves.
4. The leaves would not be the best way to keep the wound moist and clean.

14. Correct answers are 1 and 3.
1. Condoms are helpful in preventing sexually transmitted diseases and in preventing pregnancy.
2. Sexually active females do need vaginal examinations, but this statement does not address preventing pregnancy.
3. Routes of hormonal therapy include birth control pills, creams, patches, and injections. All address ways to help prevent conception.
4. All methods of birth control do not require a prescription. Condoms and contraceptive creams and ointments are sold over the counter.
5. Sterilization does not guarantee unintended pregnancies. This information is incorrect.

15. 1. Black cohosh is used for gynecological disorders.
2. Fennel is used as an expectorant or diuretic.
3. Witch hazel has anti-inflammatory properties, but it is prepared with an alcohol base, which would cause pain to the client when applying it to the burned area.
4. **Aloe vera has been used to promote wound healing. It has some antifungal properties and helps soothe the pain from a superficial burn.**

16. 1. The nurse should support the use of folk and home remedies as long as they are not contraindicated by medical treatment.
2. **Eucalyptus has been used by clients diagnosed with congestion and as an expectorant, steam helps open the airway and liquefies secretions.**
3. This is an inhaled treatment that will provide the medication directly to the lungs and will limit systemic effects.
4. The steam provides moisture to the lungs to liquefy secretions, and the efficacy of rubbing on the chest is provided by inhalation.

17. 1. Continuous, daily doses will not increase the effectiveness of the herb and could cause harm to the client.
2. Ginseng is a stimulant; therefore, additional stimulants such as caffeine should be avoided.
3. **Clients should take ginseng intermittently and short-term for safety. Infants, children, and women who are pregnant or breastfeeding should not use ginseng. Some evidence suggests ginseng can affect blood sugar and blood pressure (National Center for Complementary and Integrative Health, 2016).**
4. There are contraindications to all medications. Ginseng elevates the blood pressure, so clients diagnosed with hypertension should avoid ginseng.

18. 1. Alternating acetaminophen (Tylenol), an analgesic, with acetylsalicylic acid (aspirin), an antiplatelet, is recommended for clients diagnosed with fevers unresponsive to Tylenol alone.
2. **Diphenhydramine topical (Benadryl gel) can be applied to the area three to four times a day. The medication is absorbed topically. If the medication is applied more often, the client can develop systemic effects.**
3. Washing the area with soap and hot water will increase the itching.
4. Hydrocortisone cream, a steroid, is applied three to four times daily, not every 2 hours.

19. 1. This outcome would be for a knowledge-deficit problem.
2. **Clients diagnosed with anemia have decreased energy and are unable to complete ADLs. The ability to complete ADLs indicates the treatment has been effective.**
3. Green-black stools are an expected side effect of taking iron supplements and can be confused with tarry stools, which indicate blood in the stool.
4. Dystrophy of fingernails is an indication the treatment is ineffective.

20. 1. Antacids should be taken 1 hour before or 2 hours after taking iron.
2. Clients should not double up on doses because that may lead to gastrointestinal upset.
3. **Food interferes with the absorption of oral supplements, so it is recommended clients take iron between meals to minimize gastrointestinal upset and maximize iron absorption.**
4. The client needs to remain in an upright position for 30 minutes after taking oral iron supplements to reduce esophageal irritation or corrosion.

21. 1. **Antibiotics such as ampicillin and tetracycline increase the elimination of the oral contraceptive by killing the flora in the gastrointestinal tract. Clients should use another method of birth control while taking an antibiotic.**
2. The pills should be taken at the same time each day. If the client misses one, that pill should be taken as soon as the client remembers. If the client misses taking the pill 2 days in a row, then two pills should be taken each day for the next 2 days.
3. The transdermal patch has the same side effects as oral birth control pills. The advantage of the patch is it does not have to be taken every day.
4. If the contraceptive ring comes out, it should be washed with warm water and replaced. One ring can be used for 3 weeks.

22. 1. The cavity-rim cervical cap (Prentif) has a 40% failure rate for multiparous women.
2. **Subdermal levonorgestrel implants (Norplant) are an effective method of birth control for up to 5 years.**

3. When taken as directed, oral contraceptives can be effective, but because this client has had two unplanned pregnancies, compliance should be questioned.
4. Medroxyprogesterone acetate (Depo-Provera) is one of the most effective methods of birth control but lasts for only 3 months; therefore, it should not be recommended for this client.

23. 1. The frequency of sexual activity would indicate the number of condoms to be distributed, but it would not be the most important information.
2. The public health department provides free condoms and is not concerned with the client's style preference.
3. The most effective condoms are made of latex, but they should not be used if the client is allergic to latex. The client should be instructed to ask the partner about latex allergies.
4. Sexual history should be discussed only if the client has a sexually transmitted disease because the public health department must notify all partners.

24. 1. Deep breathing would aid the client to relax, but teaching cannot be delegated.
2. This relaxing intervention can be delegated to the UAP.
3. Listening to why the client is anxious is part of the assessment, which cannot be delegated.
4. Guided imagery is a method that assists clients to relax, but teaching it cannot be delegated.

25. Correct answers are 1, 2, and 3.
1. Progressive muscle relaxation is the systematic contracting and relaxing of muscles. It helps aid in relaxation when the client feels anxious.
2. Soothing music with a rate of 50 to 60 beats per minute can slow the client's heart rate and relax the client.
3. Guided imagery is helpful in decreasing anxiety. The more senses involved, the better the results of the guided imagery.
4. Stress is not always harmful, and the absence of all stress is death.
5. Journaling is useful for some individuals, but the nurse cannot insist or demand that the client do anything.

26. Correct order is 2, 4, 5, 1, 3.
2. Any pain not relieved with prescribed pain medication warrants assessment by the nurse to rule out any complications.
4. Soft music is a method of distraction that can be implemented quickly and may have a calming effect on the client.
5. According to the gate control theory of pain, flooding the brain with pleasurable sensations will block the transmission of pain.
1. The nurse should notify the HCP and discuss other possible medication regimens that can be provided for the client.
3. Clients in acute pain are not receptive to being taught; therefore, this intervention should be implemented as soon as the pain is tolerable and may be used by the client for future pain episodes.

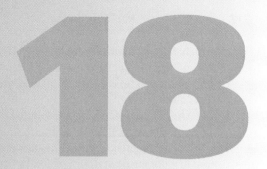

# End-of-Life Issues

*In the end, it is not the years in your life that count.*
*It is the life in your years.*

—Edward J. Stieglitz

End-of-life issues include some of the most sensitive issues a nurse must handle. Many times a nurse will need to confront personal feelings and fears about death to be able to help clients. This chapter deals with advance directives, death and dying, chronic pain, ethical and legal issues, and organ and tissue transplants.

## KEYWORDS

Advance directive
Brain death
Do not resuscitate (DNR)
Durable power of attorney

Kübler-Ross stages of grief
Nonmaleficence
Organ donation
Persistent vegetative state

## PRACTICE QUESTIONS

### Advance Directives (AD)

1. The client tells the nurse, "Every time I come to the hospital you hand me one of these advance directives (ADs). Why should I fill one of these out?" Which statement by the nurse is **most** appropriate?
   1. "You must fill out this form because Medicare laws require it."
   2. "An AD lets you participate in decisions about your health care."
   3. "This paper will ensure no one can override your decisions."
   4. "It is part of the hospital admission packet, and I have to give it to you."

2. The nurse is presenting an in-service discussing do not resuscitate (DNR) orders and ADs. Which statements should the nurse discuss with the class? **Select all that apply.**
   1. ADs must be notarized by a notary public.
   2. The client must use an attorney to complete the AD.
   3. Once the AD is written, it can be used for every hospital admission.
   4. The HCP must write the DNR order in the client's EHR.
   5. A DNR order must be included in the AD.

3. In which client situation would the AD be consulted and used in decision making?
   1. The client diagnosed with Guillain-Barré on a ventilator.
   2. The client diagnosed with a C6 spinal cord injury in the rehabilitation unit.
   3. The client diagnosed with end-stage renal disease in a comatose state.
   4. The client with Down syndrome and diagnosed with cancer.

4. The nurse is moving to another state, which is part of the multistate licensure compact. Which information regarding ADs should the nurse be aware of when practicing nursing in other states?
   1. The laws regarding ADs are the same in all the states.
   2. ADs can be transferred from state to state.
   3. A significant other can sign a loved one's AD.
   4. ADs are state regulated, not federally regulated.

5. Which client would be **most** likely to complete an AD?
   1. A 65-year-old female who visits her provider yearly.
   2. A 34-year-old male licensed practical nurse.
   3. A 22-year-old female attending college.
   4. A 55-year-old male without a high school diploma.

6. The client with an AD tells the nurse, "I have changed my mind about my AD. I really want everything possible done if I am near death since I have a grandchild." Which action should the nurse implement?
   1. Notify the health information systems department to talk to the client.
   2. Remove the AD from the client's EHR and shred any paper documents.
   3. Inform the client of the right to revoke the AD at any time.
   4. Explain this document cannot be changed once it is signed.

7. The client has just signed an AD at the bedside. Which intervention should the nurse implement **first**?
   1. Notify the client's HCP about the AD.
   2. Instruct the client to discuss the AD with significant others.
   3. Scan a copy of the advance directive into the client's EHR.
   4. Give the original AD to the client.

8. The HCP has notified the family of a client diagnosed with being in a persistent vegetative state on a ventilator of the need to "pull the plug." The client does not have an AD or a durable power of attorney for health care, and the family does not want their loved one removed from the ventilator. Which action should the nurse implement?

   1. Refer the case to the hospital ethics committee.
   2. Tell the family they must do what the HCP orders.
   3. Follow the HCP's order and "pull the plug."
   4. Determine why the client did not complete an AD.

9. The client asks the nurse, "When will the durable power of attorney for health care take effect?" On which scientific rationale would the nurse base the response?
   1. It goes into effect when the client needs someone to make financial decisions.
   2. It will be effective when the client is under general anesthesia during surgery.
   3. The client must say it is all right for it to become effective and enforced.
   4. It becomes valid only when the clients cannot make their own decisions.

10. The male client requested a DNR per the AD, and the HCP wrote the order. The client's death is imminent, and the client's spouse tells the nurse, "Help him, please. Do something. I am not ready to let him go." Which action should the nurse take?
    1. Ask the spouse if she would like to revoke her husband's AD.
    2. Leave the spouse at the bedside and notify the hospital chaplain.
    3. Sit with the spouse at the bedside and encourage her to say good-bye.
    4. Request the client to tell the spouse he is ready to die, and don't do anything.

11. Which situation would cause the nurse to **question** the validity of an AD when caring for the older client?
    1. The client's child insists the client make decisions.
    2. The nurse observes the wife making the spouse sign the AD.
    3. A nurse encouraged the client to think about end-of-life decisions.
    4. A friend witnesses the client's signature on the AD form.

12. The nurse is aware of the Patient Self-Determination Act (PSDA) of 1991 requires the health-care facility to implement which action? **Select all that apply**.
    1. Make available an AD on admission to the facility.
    2. Assist the client with legally completing a will.
    3. Provide ethically and morally competent care to the client.
    4. Educate the facility staff about ADs.
    5. Discuss the importance of understanding consent forms.

## Death and Dying

13. The spouse of a client dying from lung cancer states, "I don't understand this death rattle. She has not had anything to drink in days. Where is the fluid coming from?" Which is the hospice care nurse's **best** response?
    1. "The body produces about 2 teaspoons of fluid every minute on its own."
    2. "Are you sure someone is not putting ice chips in her mouth?"
    3. "There is no reason for this, but it does happen from time to time."
    4. "I can administer a patch to her skin to dry up the secretions if you wish."

14. The nurse is discussing placing the client diagnosed with chronic obstructive pulmonary disease in hospice care. Which prognosis must be determined to place the client in hospice care?
    1. The client is doing well but could benefit from the added care by hospice.
    2. The client has a life expectancy of 6 months or less.
    3. The client will live for about 1 to 2 more years.
    4. The client has about 8 weeks to live and needs pain control.

15. The client diagnosed with end-stage congestive heart failure and type 2 diabetes is receiving hospice care. Which action by the nurse demonstrates an understanding of the client's condition? **Select all that apply.**
    1. The nurse monitors the blood glucose four times a day.
    2. The nurse keeps the client on a strict fluid restriction.
    3. The nurse limits the visitors the client can receive.
    4. The nurse brings the client a small piece of cake.
    5. The nurse reports uncontrolled pain to the HCP.

16. The hospice care nurse is conducting a spiritual care assessment. Which statement is the scientific rationale for this intervention?
    1. The client will ask spiritual questions and get answers.
    2. The nurse is able to explain to the client how death will affect the spirit.
    3. Spirituality provides a sense of meaning and purpose for many clients.
    4. The nurse is an expert when assisting the client with spiritual matters.

17. The nurse is caring for a dying client and the family. The male client is a practicing Muslim. Which intervention should the female nurse implement at the time of death?
    1. Delay notification of the Islamic funeral home to allow for bedside death rituals.
    2. Call the client's imam to perform last rites when the client dies.
    3. Place incense around the bed, but do not allow anyone to light it.
    4. Do not touch the body, and have family members perform care.

18. The nurse writes a client problem of "spiritual distress" for the dying client. Which statement is an appropriate goal?
    1. The client will reconcile himself and the higher power of personal beliefs.
    2. The client will be able to express anger at the terminal diagnosis.
    3. The client will reconcile himself to estranged members of the family.
    4. The client will have a dignified and pain-free death.

19. The hospice care nurse is planning the care of an older client diagnosed with end-stage renal disease. Which interventions should be included in the plan of care? **Select all that apply.**
    1. Discuss financial concerns.
    2. Assess any comorbid conditions.
    3. Monitor increased visual or auditory abilities.
    4. Note any spiritual distress.
    5. Encourage euphoria at the time of death.

20. The nurse is orienting to a hospice organization. Which statements describe the rights of the terminal client? **Select all that apply.**
    1. Be treated with respect and dignity.
    2. Have particulars of the death withheld.
    3. Receive optimal and effective pain management.
    4. Receive holistic and compassionate care.
    5. Choose the attending physician.

21. The client is on the ventilator and has been declared brain dead. The spouse refuses to allow the ventilator to be discontinued. Which collaborative action by the nurse is **most** appropriate?
    1. Discuss the referral of the case to the ethics committee.
    2. Pull the plug when the spouse is not in the room.
    3. Ask the HCP to discuss the futile situation with the spouse.
    4. Inform the spouse what is happening is cruel.

22. The client has been in a persistent vegetative state for several years. The family, having decided to withhold tube feedings because there is no hope of recovery, asks the nurse, "Will the death be painful?" Which intervention should the nurse implement?
    1. Tell the family that death will be painful, but the HCP can order medications.
    2. Inform the family dehydration provides a type of natural euphoria.
    3. Relate other cases where the clients have died in excruciating pain.
    4. Ask the family why they are concerned because they want the client to die anyway.

23. The family is dealing with the imminent death of the client. Which information is **most important** for the nurse to discuss when planning interventions for the grieving process?
    1. How angry are the family members about the death?
    2. Which family member will be making decisions?
    3. What previous coping skills have been used?
    4. What type of funeral service has been planned?

24. The nurse is caring for five clients in different stages of the grieving process. **Rank each client in order of the Kübler-Ross stages from first to last**.
    1. The hospice client who called his family to the room and said good-bye, then dismissed them and now lies quietly and refuses to eat.
    2. The male client diagnosed with lung cancer tells the nurse, "If I can live long enough to walk my daughter down the aisle at her wedding, then I can deal with this cancer."
    3. The 20-year-old female client after being told she has breast cancer tells the HCP, "I can't have breast cancer. I am too young."
    4. The female client is refusing to get out of bed to go to chemotherapy treatments for cancer because she feels the treatment is hopeless.
    5. The young man is punching the wall when told his father has just died.

## Chronic Pain

25. The nurse is assessing a client diagnosed with chronic pain. Which clinical manifestations should the nurse observe?
    1. The client's blood pressure is elevated.
    2. The client has rapid shallow respirations.
    3. The client has facial grimacing.
    4. The client is lying quietly in bed.

26. The client had a mastectomy and lymph node dissection 3 years ago and has experienced post-mastectomy pain syndrome (PMPS) since. Which intervention should the nurse implement?
    1. Have the client see a psychologist because the pain is not real.
    2. Tell the client that the pain is cancer coming back.
    3. Refer the client to a physical therapist to prevent a frozen shoulder.
    4. Discuss changing the client to a more potent narcotic medication.

27. The male client diagnosed with chronic pain since a construction accident that broke several vertebrae tells the nurse he has been referred to a pain clinic and asks, "What good will it do? I will never be free of this pain." Which statement is the nurse's **best** response?
    1. "Are you afraid of the pain never going away?"
    2. "The pain clinic will give you medication to cure the pain."
    3. "Pain clinics work to help you achieve relief from pain."
    4. "I am not sure. You should discuss this with your HCP."

28. The client diagnosed with cancer is experiencing severe pain. Which regimen would the nurse teach the client about to control the pain?
    1. NSAIDs around the clock with narcotics used for severe pain.
    2. Morphine, sustained release, routinely with a liquid morphine preparation for breakthrough pain.
    3. Extra-strength acetaminophen plus therapy to learn alternative methods of pain control.
    4. Meperidine every 6 hours orally with a suppository when the pain is not controlled.

29. The client is being discharged from the hospital for intractable pain secondary to cancer and is prescribed morphine. Which statements indicate the client **understands** the discharge instructions? **Select all that apply**.
    1. "I will be sure to have my prescriptions filled before any holiday."
    2. "There should not be a problem having the prescriptions filled anytime."
    3. "If I run out of medications, I can call the HCP to phone in a prescription."
    4. "There are no side effects to morphine I should be concerned about."
    5. "I can get only a 30-day supply of the prescription morphine."

30. The client diagnosed with intractable pain is receiving an IV constant infusion of morphine. The concentration is 50 mg of morphine in 250 mL of normal saline. The IV is infusing at 10 mL/hr. The client has required bolus administration of 2 mg IV push (IVP) × 2 during the 12-hour shift. How much morphine has the client received during the shift?

    ```
    _____ mg
    ```

31. The male client has a DNR order in the EHR and is in pain. The client's vital signs are populated in the vital sign flowsheet below. Which intervention should be the nurse's **priority** action?

    | Vital Sign Flowsheet | Client Results | Normal Values |
    |---|---|---|
    | Blood Pressure | 108/70 | 100 to 119 mmHg systolic 60 to 80 mmHg diastolic |
    | Pulse | 88 | 60 to 100 beats/min |
    | Respirations | 8 | 12 to 20 breaths/min |

    1. Refuse to give the medication because it could kill the client.
    2. Administer the medication as ordered and assess for relief from pain.
    3. Wait until the client's respirations improve and then administer the medication.
    4. Notify the HCP the client is unstable, and pain medication is being held.

32. The charge nurse is making assignments on an oncology floor. Which client should be assigned to the **most** experienced nurse?
    1. The client diagnosed with leukemia and has a hemoglobin of 6 g/dL.
    2. The client diagnosed with lung cancer with a pulse oximeter reading of 89%.
    3. The client diagnosed with colon cancer who needs the colostomy irrigated.
    4. The client diagnosed with Kaposi's sarcoma and is yelling at the staff.

33. The nurse and an unlicensed assistive personnel (UAP) are caring for a group of clients in a pain clinic. Which intervention would be inappropriate for the RN to delegate to the UAP?
    1. Assist the client diagnosed with intractable pain to the bathroom.
    2. Elevate the head of the bed for a client diagnosed with back pain.
    3. Perform passive range of motion for a bedfast client.
    4. Monitor the potassium levels on a client about to receive medication.

34. The client diagnosed with chronic back pain is being placed on a transcutaneous electrical nerve stimulation (TENS) unit. Which information should the nurse teach? **Select all that apply**.
    1. The TENS unit can be controlled by the client adjusting the intensity.
    2. The TENS unit will deaden the nerve endings, and the client will not feel pain.
    3. The TENS unit could cause paralysis if the client gets the unit wet.
    4. The TENS unit stimulates the nerves in the area, blocking the pain sensation.
    5. The TENS unit should be left on for an hour and then taken off for an hour.

35. The nurse is caring for clients on the medical floor. Which client should the nurse assess **first** after the shift report?
    1. The client with arterial blood gases of pH 7.36, $PaCO_2$ 40, $HCO_3$ 26, $PaO_2$ 90.
    2. The client with vital signs of T 99°F, P 101, R 28, and BP 120/80.
    3. The client reporting pain at a "10" on a 1-to-10 scale but can't localize it.
    4. The postappendectomy client with pain at a "3" on a 1-to-10 scale.

36. The client in the oncology clinic tells the nurse she has a great deal of pain but does not like to take pain medication. Which action should the nurse implement **first**?
    1. Tell the client it is important to take the medication.
    2. Find out how the client has been dealing with the pain.
    3. Have the HCP tell the client to take the pain medications.
    4. Instruct the client not to worry—the pain will resolve itself.

## Ethical and Legal Issues

37. The nurse is teaching an in-service on legal issues in nursing. Which situations are examples of battery, an intentional tort? **Select all that apply**.
    1. The nurse threatens the client refusing to take a hypnotic medication.
    2. The nurse forcibly inserts a Foley catheter in a client refusing it.
    3. The nurse tells the client a nasogastric tube insertion is not painful.
    4. The nurse gives confidential information over the telephone.
    5. The nurse pushes the client out of the bed after the client says "no."

38. Which act protects the nurse against a malpractice claim when the nurse stops at a motor vehicle accident and renders emergency care?
    1. The Health Insurance Portability and Accountability Act.
    2. The State Nurse Practice Act.
    3. The Emergency Rendering Aid Act.
    4. The Good Samaritan Act.

39. The family has requested a client diagnosed with terminal cancer not be told of the diagnosis. The client tells the nurse, "I think something is really wrong with me, but the doctor says everything is all right. Do you know if there is something wrong with me?" Which response by the nurse would support the ethical principle of veracity?
    1. "I think you should talk to your doctor about your concerns."
    2. "What makes you think something is really wrong?"
    3. "Your family has requested you not be told your diagnosis."
    4. "The doctor would never tell you incorrect information."

40. The nurse is obtaining the client's signature on a surgical permit form. The nurse determines the client does not understand the surgical procedure and possible risks. Which action should the nurse take **first**?
    1. Notify the client's surgeon.
    2. Document the information in the EHR.
    3. Contact the operating room staff.
    4. Explain the procedure to the client.

41. The client is in the psychiatric unit in a medical center. Which actions by the psychiatric nurse are violations of the client's legal and civil rights? **Select all that apply**.
    1. The nurse tells the client to wear a hospital gown in the unit.
    2. The nurse allows the client to have family visits during visiting hours.
    3. The nurse permits the client to eat food family members brought from home.
    4. The nurse delivers unopened mail and packages to the client.
    5. The nurse listens to the client talking on the telephone to a friend.

42. The client receiving dialysis for end-stage renal disease wants to quit dialysis and die. Which ethical principle supports the client's right to die?
    1. Autonomy.
    2. Self-determination.
    3. Beneficence.
    4. Justice.

43. Which document is the **best** professional source to provide direction for a nurse when addressing ethical issues and behavior?
    1. The Hippocratic Oath.
    2. The Nuremberg Code.
    3. Home Health Care Bill of Rights.
    4. ANA Code of Ethics.

44. Which elements are necessary to prove nursing malpractice? **Select all that apply**.
    1. Duty to the client.
    2. Identification of an ethical issue.
    3. Failure to follow the standard of care.
    4. Injury to the client.
    5. Proximate cause.

45. The nurse is caring for a client who is confused and fell, trying to get out of bed. There is no family at the client's bedside. Which action should the nurse implement **first**?
    1. Contact a family member to come and stay with the client.
    2. Administer a sedative medication to the client.
    3. Place the client in a chair with a sheet tied around him or her.
    4. Notify the HCP to obtain a restraint order.

46. Which entity mandates the registered nurse's behavior when practicing professional nursing?
    1. The state's Nurse Practice Act.
    2. Client's Bill of Rights.
    3. The U.S. legislature.
    4. American Nurses Association.

47. The nurse must be knowledgeable regarding ethical principles. Which is an example of the ethical principle of justice?
    1. The nurse administers a placebo, and the client asks if it will help the pain.
    2. The nurse accepts a work assignment in an area of inexperience.
    3. The nurse refuses to tell a family member the client has a positive HIV test.
    4. The nurse provides an indigent client with safe and appropriate nursing care.

48. The nurse is discussing malpractice issues in an in-service class. Which situation is an example of malpractice?
    1. The nurse fails to report a neighbor abusing his two children.
    2. The nurse does not intervene in a client with a BP of 80/50 and an apical pulse of 122.
    3. The nurse is suspected of taking narcotics prescribed for a client.
    4. The nurse falsifies vital signs in the client's medical records.

## Organ and Tissue Donation

49. The mother of a 20-year-old male client receiving dialysis asks the nurse, "My son has been on the transplant list longer than that woman. Why did she get the kidney?" Which statement is the nurse's **best** response?
    1. "The woman was famous, and so more people will donate organs now."
    2. "I understand you are upset your son is ill. Would you like to talk?"
    3. "No one knows who gets an organ. You just have to wait and pray."
    4. "The tissues must match or the body will reject the kidney and it will be wasted."

50. The nurse is discussing the HCP's recommendation for removal of life support with the client's family. Which information concerning brain death should the RN teach the family?
    1. Positive waves on the electroencephalogram (EEG) mean the brain is dead and any further treatment is futile.
    2. When putting cold water in the ear, if the client reacts by pulling away, this demonstrates brain death.
    3. Tests will be done to determine if any brain activity exists before the machines are turned off.
    4. Although the blood flow studies don't indicate activity, the client can still come out of the coma.

51. The client diagnosed with septicemia has died. The family tells the nurse the client is an organ donor. Which intervention should the nurse implement?
    1. Notify the organ and tissue organizations to make the retrieval.
    2. Explain a systemic infection prevents the client from being a donor.
    3. Call and notify the HCP of the family's request.
    4. Take the body to the morgue until the organ bank makes a decision.

52. The client has received a kidney transplant. Which assessment would **warrant immediate** intervention by the nurse?
    1. Fever and decreased urine output.
    2. Decreased creatinine and BUN levels.
    3. Decreased serum potassium and calcium.
    4. Bradycardia and hypotension.

53. The client received a liver transplant and is preparing for discharge. Which discharge instructions should the nurse teach? **Select all that apply.**
    1. The immune-suppressant drugs must be tapered off when discontinuing them.
    2. There may be slight foul-smelling drainage on the dressing for a few days.
    3. Notify the HCP immediately if a cough or fever develops.
    4. The skin will turn yellow from the antirejection drugs.
    5. Immunizations are recommended, but avoid live virus vaccinations.

54. The pregnant client asks the nurse about banking the cord blood. Which information should the nurse teach the client?
    1. The procedure involves a lot of pain with a very poor result.
    2. The client must deliver at a large public hospital to do this.
    3. The client will be charged a yearly storage fee on the cells.
    4. The stem cells can be stored for about 4 years before they ruin.

55. The nurse is caring for a client who received a kidney transplant from an unrelated cadaver donor. Which interventions should be included in the plan of care? **Select all that apply.**
    1. Collect a urine culture every other day.
    2. Prepare the client for dialysis three times a week.
    3. Monitor urine osmolality studies.
    4. Monitor intake and output every shift.
    5. Check abdominal dressing every 4 hours.

56. The client is 3 hours post–heart transplantation. Which data would **support** a complication of this procedure?
    1. The client has nausea after taking oral antirejection medication.
    2. The client has difficulty coming off the heart-lung bypass machine.
    3. The client has saturated three abdominal dressing pads in 1 hour.
    4. The client reports pain at a "6" on a 1-to-10 scale.

57. The nurse and a UAP are caring for clients on a postoperative transplant unit. Which task should the RN delegate to the UAP?
    1. Assess the hourly outputs of the post–kidney transplantation client.
    2. Raise the head of the bed for a post–liver transplantation client.
    3. Monitor the serum blood studies of a rejected organ transplant client.
    4. Irrigate the nasogastric tube of a pancreas transplant client.

58. The experienced medical-surgical nurse is being oriented to the transplant unit. Which client should the charge nurse assign to this nurse?
    1. The client who donated a kidney to a relative 3 days ago and will be discharged in the morning.
    2. The client who had a liver transplantation 3 days ago and was transferred from the intensive care unit 2 hours ago.
    3. The client who received a corneal transplant 4 hours ago and has developed a cough and is vomiting.
    4. The client who had pancreas transplantation and who has a fever, chills, and a blood glucose monitor reading of 342.

59. The 6-year-old client diagnosed with cystic fibrosis (CF) needs a lung transplant. Which individual would be the **best** donor for the client?
    1. The 20-year-old brother without CF.
    2. The 45-year-old father who carries the CF gene.
    3. The 18-year-old fatality victim of an MVA matching on 4 points.
    4. The 5-year-old drowning victim with a 3-point match.

60. Which tissue or organ can be repeatedly donated to clients needing a transplant?
    1. Skin.
    2. Bones.
    3. Kidneys.
    4. Bone marrow.

# CONCEPTS

The concepts covered in this chapter focus on end-of-life issues, including grief and loss, ethics, spirituality, diversity, regulations, and nursing. Exemplars that are covered are chronic pain, advanced directives, end-of-life care, legal decisions, patient rights, and death and dying. Interrelated concepts of the nursing process, assessment, and critical thinking are covered throughout the questions.

61. The nurse is admitting a client to the medical-surgical unit. Which is required to be offered to the client if the hospital accepts Medicare reimbursement?
    1. The opportunity to make an AD.
    2. The client must be referred to a case manager.
    3. The client must apply for Medicare supplement insurance.
    4. The opportunity to discuss end-of-life issues.

62. The nurse pronounced Dr. Smith's client to be **clinically dead**. Which should the RN document in the client's EHR?
    1. Brain scan indicates no brain wave activity; the client pronounced deceased. The family refuses to talk with the organ bank.
    2. Cardiac arrest noted, CPR initiated but unsuccessful. Pronounced dead.
    3. Pulse, respirations, and blood pressure absent at 0900, pronounced dead. Dr. Smith to sign death certificate.
    4. Client found without a pulse, body cold to touch. Pronounced deceased at 0900.

63. The nurse is caring for an 82-year-old female client crying and asking for her mother to come to see her. Which statement represents the ethical principle of **nonmaleficence**?
    1. "You must miss your mother very much. Can you tell me about her?"
    2. "You are 82 years old. Your mother is dead and can't come to see you."
    3. "Why do you need your mother? Can I get something for you?"
    4. "Your mother would not want you to worry. I will tell her you want to see her."

64. The hospice nurse is admitting a client. Which question concerning end-of-life care is **most important** for the nurse to discuss with the client and family?
    1. Encourage the client and family to make funeral arrangements.
    2. Assess the client's pain medication regimen for effectiveness.
    3. Determine if the client has made an AD or living will.
    4. Ask what durable medical equipment is in place in the home.

65. The client is dying and wants to talk to the nurse about heaven. Which is the nurse's **best** nursing action?
    1. Make a referral to the chaplain to come to see the client.
    2. Tell the client that nurses are not allowed to discuss spiritual matters.
    3. Ask the client to describe heaven and hell.
    4. Allow the client to discuss the beliefs about heaven.

66. The male client in the long-term care facility has been told that he will not live for many more months. The client has been estranged from his son for years. He tells the nurse that he could die a happy man if he could talk to his son just one more time. Which statement is the nurse's **best** response?
    1. "You should not feel bad. Things will work out for the best before your death."
    2. "What did you do to make your son not talk to you all this time?"
    3. "If you would like, I can try to contact your son and ask him to come see you."
    4. "Tell me more about being unhappy that you don't have a relationship with your son."

67. The nurse is caring for the family of the deceased client. Which is the nurse's **priority** action?
    1. Be with the family.
    2. Call the funeral home.
    3. Notify the minister.
    4. Fill out the death certificate.

## Advance Directives (AD)

1. 1. ADs are not legally required. It is a standard of the Joint Commission, and any facility that accepts federal funds must ask and offer the AD.
   2. ADs allow the client to make personal health-care decisions about end-of-life issues, including cardiopulmonary resuscitation (CPR), ventilators, feeding tubes, and other issues concerning the client's death (National Institute on Aging, n.d.).
   3. This is not a legal document guaranteed to stand up in a court of law; therefore, the client should make sure all family members know the client's wishes.
   4. It is part of the hospital admission requirements, but it is not the reason why the client should complete an AD.

   **TEST-TAKING HINT:** The test taker could eliminate option "1" because the nurse cannot make the client do anything. The client has a right to say no. Option "3" is an absolute, and unless the test taker knows for sure this is correct information, the test taker should not select this option.

2. Correct answers are 3 and 4.
   1. This is not true; someone who is not family or directly involved in the client's care must witness the AD, but the document does not always have to be notarized. The notary requirements vary by state.
   2. This form can be filled out without the use of an attorney; copies of an AD can be obtained at hospitals or online from various sources.
   3. The AD does not expire; therefore, it does not need to be updated with each hospital readmission. However, the client can change or cancel the AD at any time. In contrast, a DNR order must be written on each admission.
   4. The HCP writes the DNR order in the client's EHR.
   5. A DNR order does not have to be included in an AD. The client may use the AD form or may tell the HCP they do not want to be resuscitated.

   **TEST-TAKING HINT:** Options "1" and "2" are absolute, and unless the test taker knows for sure this is correct information, the test taker should eliminate them.

3. 1. A client diagnosed with Guillain-Barré syndrome is mentally competent, and being on a ventilator does not indicate the client has lost decision-making capacity.
   2. A client in the rehabilitation unit would be alert, and spinal cord injuries do not cause the client to lose decision-making capacity.
   3. The client must have lost decision-making capacity as a result of a condition that is not reversible or must be in a condition specified under state law, such as a terminal, persistent vegetative state; an irreversible coma; or as specified in the AD.
   4. A client diagnosed with Down syndrome may have some intellectual challenges, but unless the client has been declared legally incompetent in a court of law, the client can complete an AD and participate in care.

   **TEST-TAKING HINT:** If the test taker knows what an AD is, then the words "end-stage" and "comatose" would lead the test taker to select option "3" as a correct answer. Remember, clients with congenital or genetic disorders are not incompetent, even if they are mentally challenged.

4. 1. Individual states are responsible for specific legal requirements for ADs.
   2. Moving from one state to another does not nullify or honor the AD; the nurse must be aware of the individual state's requirements.
   3. Only the individual can complete and sign an AD. The significant other may be asked to implement the AD.
   4. The state determines the definition of terms and requirements for an AD; individual states are responsible for specific legal requirements for ADs.

   **TEST-TAKING HINT:** The test taker should know the RN must obtain a copy of the Nurse Practice Act of the state being practiced in. The test taker should realize every state has different regulations regarding ADs and other health-care issues. Option "4" is the only option that reflects this thought.

5. 1. ADs are most frequently completed by women, whites, married individuals, individuals with a college degree, those individuals in the middle- to upper-socioeconomic class, and those with a chronic disease and regular access to care. This client has the most characteristics of this listed (Rao et al., 2014).

2. Many nurses do not have ADs, although they discuss them with clients daily.
3. Although this client is female, she does not have the most characteristics assigned to clients who complete ADs.
4. ADs are most frequently completed by women, whites, married individuals, individuals with a college degree, middle- to upper-class socioeconomic status, and those with a chronic disease and regular access to care. This client does not have a college degree.

**TEST-TAKING HINT: If the test taker were not aware of the research, the test taker could examine the characteristics of the clients and ask themselves, "Which client would want to direct care and make decisions?" Nurses may want this, but many do not have ADs.**

6. 1. This department has nothing to do with the AD.
2. The most appropriate action would be for the nurse to have the client write on the AD that the document is revoked; the nurse cannot shred legal documents from the client's EHR.
3. The client must be informed the AD can be rescinded or revoked at any time for any reason verbally, in writing, or by destroying the AD. The nurse cannot destroy the client's AD, but the client can.
4. This is an incorrect answer because the client always has the right to a change of mind.

**TEST-TAKING HINT: Option "4" can be eliminated by remembering statements with absolutes should not be selected as correct answers unless the test taker knows for sure the answer is correct. The nurse should record in the EHR that the client has rescinded or revoked the document. Any paper copies of the AD should be returned to the client to destroy.**

7. 1. The HCP should be made aware of the AD, but this is not the first intervention.
2. This is the most important intervention because the legality of the document is sometimes not honored if the family members disagree and demand other actions. If the client's family is aware of the client's wishes, then the health-care team can support and honor the client's final wishes.
3. Copies of the AD should be placed in the EHR and given to significant others, the client's attorney, and all HCPs.
4. The original should be given to the client, and a copy should be placed in the EHR, but this is not the first intervention.

**TEST-TAKING HINT: This is a priority-setting question, and the test taker should read all the answer options and try to rank them in order of priority.**

8. 1. The ethics committee is composed of health-care workers and laypeople from the community to objectively review the situation and make a recommendation that is fair to both the client and the health-care system. The family has the right to be present and discuss their feelings.
2. The nurse is legally obligated to be a client advocate.
3. This action could create a multitude of ramifications, including a lawsuit and possible criminal charges.
4. It really doesn't matter at this point why the client didn't complete an AD; the client cannot do it now.

**TEST-TAKING HINT: The test taker must be aware of the ethics committee and its role in helping resolve ethical dilemmas. Any answer option that has the word "why" should be evaluated closely before selecting it as the correct answer. Removing the endotracheal tube or turning off the ventilator ("pulling the plug") is a medical responsibility; therefore, option "3" could be eliminated as the correct answer.**

9. 1. It is a power of attorney executed by a lawyer that allows a delegated other person to make financial decisions. That document has nothing to do with a durable power of attorney for health care.
2. The client has not lost the capacity to make decisions; therefore, a durable power of attorney cannot be used by the assigned person to make decisions.
3. The client must not be able to make decisions before this document can be used.
4. The client must have lost decision-making capacity as a result of a condition that is not reversible or must be in a condition that is specified under state law, such as a terminal, persistent vegetative state; an irreversible coma; or as specified in the AD.

**TEST-TAKING HINT: The test taker should not confuse a power of attorney and a durable power of attorney for health care. These are two separate, yet very important, documents with similar names.**

10. 1. Only the client can revoke the AD.
    2. The spouse should not be left alone, and the hospital chaplain may not be available for the client and his spouse.
    3. At the time of death, loved ones become scared and find it difficult to say good-bye. The nurse should support the client's decision and acknowledge the spouse's psychological state. Research states hearing is the last sense to go, and talking to the dying client is therapeutic for the client and the family.
    4. The client is dying and should not be asked to exert himself for his wishes to be carried out.

**TEST-TAKING HINT:** Logic would suggest option "4" is not a viable answer. Leaving a grieving spouse would not be appropriate in any situation; therefore, the test taker should eliminate option "2." Option "1" denies the client's autonomy and is not an ethical or a legal choice.

11. 1. This is appropriate for completing an AD and would not make the nurse question the validity of the AD.
    2. This is coercion and is illegal when signing an AD. The AD must be signed by the client's own free will; an AD signed under duress may not be valid.
    3. The nurse encouraging the client to think about ADs is an excellent intervention and would not make the AD invalid.
    4. A friend can sign the AD as a witness; this would not cause the nurse to question its validity.

**TEST-TAKING HINT:** This is an "except" question. The test taker could ask, "Which situation is valid for an AD?" Remember, three answers are valid information for the AD and only one is not. The test taker should read all answer options and not jump to conclusions.

12. Correct answers are 1 and 4.
    1. The PSDA of 1991 requires health-care facilities that receive Medicare or Medicaid funding to make ADs available to clients on admission into the facility (American Bar Association, 2013).
    2. This act is not concerned with completing a legal will.
    3. Client care is not based on this act.
    4. The PSDA requires that health-care facilities educate their staff about ADs (American Bar Association, 2013).
    5. Consent forms are legal documents, which are not discussed in this act.

**TEST-TAKING HINT:** The test taker should examine the word "self-determination" in the stem of the question, which matches the AD in option "1." Also, the facility should ensure the staff is familiar with all federal laws impacting the care of a client. The words "legally," "ethically," and "morally" in options "2" and "3" apply to the nurse in the health-care setting, not the client.

## Death and Dying

13. 1. The respiratory tract cells produce liquid as a defense mechanism against bacteria and other invaders. About 9 mL a minute are produced. The "death rattle" can be disturbing to family members; the nurse should intervene, but not with suctioning, which will increase secretions and the need to suction more.
    2. This is a natural physical phenomenon and should be addressed.
    3. There is an explanation.
    4. The scopolamine patch applied to the skin helps to limit the secretions, but this does not answer the question.

**TEST-TAKING HINT:** The test taker could eliminate option "3" because it states there is no reason, option "4" because it does not answer the question, and option "2" because it is attempting to fix blame.

14. 1. Hospice care does not assume care of a client with a prognosis of more than 6 months and who is doing well.
    2. The HCP must think that, without life-prolonging treatment, the client has a life expectancy of 6 months or less. The client may continue receiving hospice care if the client lives longer.
    3. The client may live this long, but the HCP must think life expectancy is much shorter.
    4. Hospice will attempt to manage symptoms of pain, nausea, and any other discomfort the client is experiencing, but the life expectancy is 6 months.

**TEST-TAKING HINT:** This is a knowledge-based question requiring an understanding of hospice.

15. Correct answers are 4 and 5.
    1. This would be basic care, but it does not indicate the nurse is aware of the client's terminal prognosis.
    2. This does not indicate an understanding of the client's terminal status.

3. The nurse should encourage visitors. There is not much time left for making memories, which will assist those left behind in dealing with the loss and allow the client time to say good-bye.

4. The client may have diabetes, but the client is also terminal, and allowing some food for pleasure is an understanding of the client's life expectancy.

5. The nurse should inform the HCP of a client who has pain that is not controlled. There is no basis for fear of this client becoming addicted to pain medications with an understanding of the client's life expectancy.

**TEST-TAKING HINT: This question requires the test taker to look not only at the disease processes but also at the descriptive words "end-stage" and "hospice" and ask, "What do these descriptors mean to the disease process?" Not limiting the client in small ways indicates the nurse is aware the client has a limited time to live. Pain control is a priority for hospice clients. Federal guidelines require hospice to make every reasonable effort to control a client's pain.**

16. 1. The nurse is not able to provide all spiritual answers to the client.

2. The nurse can explain the physical aspects of death, but no one is able to tell the client with absolute knowledge what will happen to the soul or spirit at death. The beliefs of the client may differ greatly from those of the nurse.

3. Clients facing death may wish to find meaning and purpose in life through a higher power. This gives the clients hope, even if life on earth will be temporary.

4. The nurse is not an expert but should be comfortable in private beliefs to be able to allow the client to discuss personal beliefs and hopes. The experts would be chaplains and spiritual advisers from the client's faith.

**TEST-TAKING HINT: The test taker should recognize the nurse's expertise is not in the spiritual realm, although the nurse is frequently the one called on to perform the assessment and refer to the appropriate person.**

17. 1. Muslim burials are often performed quickly after death, sometimes on the same day. The nurse should not delay notification of the Islamic funeral home.

2. Last rites are performed by a Catholic priest, not a Muslim imam.

3. Many Hindus use incense to pray, but Muslims typically do not.

4. If possible, the male client should not be handled or washed by a female nurse for cultural sensitivity. Often, members of the Muslim community wish to make arrangements for the washing, shrouding, and burial of the client according to Islamic requirements (Attum et al., 2019).

**TEST-TAKING HINT: The question requires culturally sensitive knowledge. The test taker must be aware of the different beliefs of the clients being cared for.**

18. 1. The primary goal of spiritual care is to allow the client to be able to reconcile with a higher being, maybe God. This goal is based on the belief that life comes from God, and to some degree, for many people the process of living includes some separation from God.

2. This could be a goal for a diagnosis of anger, but it does not recognize the spiritual aspect of the client.

3. This would be a goal for altered family functioning.

4. This is the physiological goal for any client who is dying, but it is not a goal for spiritual distress.

**TEST-TAKING HINT: The identified problem is "spiritual distress," and the goal must have information that addresses the spiritual. This would eliminate option "4." Personal relationships with family members (option "3") could also be eliminated.**

19. Correct answers are 1, 2, and 4.

1. Older clients are frequently on fixed incomes, and financial concerns are important for the nurse to address. A social services referral may be needed.

2. Older clients may have many comorbid conditions, which affect the type and amount of medications the client can tolerate and the client's quality of life.

3. Visual and auditory senses decrease with age; they do not increase.

4. The client may feel some spiritual distress at the terminal diagnosis. Even if the client possesses a strong faith, the unknown can be frightening.

5. A type of euphoria may accompany dehydration before death. This is a natural physiological occurrence the nurse should recognize, but it is not an intervention the nurse can implement.

**TEST-TAKING HINT:** The test taker can decide on three of the answer options based on the descriptive word "elderly." Option "5" is not a nursing intervention.

20. Correct answers are 1, 3, 4, and 5.
    1. The client has the right to be cared for with respect and dignity.
    2. The client has the right to discuss feelings and direct care. Withholding information would be lying to the client.
    3. The client has the right to the best care available and to have pain treated, regardless of the potential for hastening death.
    4. All clients, even if they are not dying, have the right to holistic and compassionate care.
    5. Clients have a right to choose their attending physician or HCP without undue influence from the hospice organization.

**TEST-TAKING HINT:** This is an alternative format question. The test taker should select more than one option as correct and must select all appropriate options to receive credit for a correct answer. There are no partially correct answers.

21. 1. The nurse should discuss using the ethics committee with the HCP to assist the family in making the decision to terminate life support. Many families feel there may be a racial or financial reason the HCP wants to discontinue life support.
    2. This would be an illegal act on the part of the nurse and would destroy the nurse-client relationship with the family.
    3. The stem already indicates the spouse is aware of the situation.
    4. This is expressing a personal bias on the part of the nurse.

**TEST-TAKING HINT:** The test taker could eliminate option "2" based on the legal and ethical issues. Option "3" is asking the HCP to do something that has already been done.

22. 1. Death from dehydration occurs when the client is unable to take in fluids, but dehydration is not painful.
    2. Death from dehydration occurs when the client is unable to take in fluids. A natural euphoria occurs with dehydration. This is the body's way of allowing comfort at the time of death.
    3. This is needless.

4. Families who make this decision tend to do so from a deep sense of love and commitment. It is an extremely difficult decision to make, and the nurse should not condemn the family decision.

**TEST-TAKING HINT:** The test taker could examine options "3" and "4" and eliminate them based on the needless information or the nurse stepping outside of professional boundaries.

23. 1. The family may or may not be angry, and this would need to be addressed, but it is not the most important.
    2. Who makes the decisions is not as important as discovering which coping skills the family uses when under stress.
    3. The nurse should assess previous coping skills used by the family and build on those to assist the family in dealing with their loss. Coping mechanisms are learned behaviors and should be supported if they are healthy behaviors. If the client and family use unhealthy coping behaviors, then the nurse should attempt to guide the family to a counselor or support group.
    4. The type of funeral service may help the family to grieve, but it is not the most important intervention.

**TEST-TAKING HINT:** The test taker must prioritize the interventions listed. All of the interventions could be addressed in option "3."

24. Correct order is 3, 5, 2, 4, and 1.
    3. This client is experiencing the first stage of Kübler-Ross' stages of grief. She is in denial and experiencing avoidance and shock.
    5. This client is experiencing the second stage of grief known as anger.
    2. This client is trying to negotiate with his grief by trying to change the circumstances. This is the third stage of Kübler-Ross' stages of grief called bargaining.
    4. This client is in the fourth stage of Kübler-Ross' stages of grief, which is depression, and experiencing hopelessness and withdrawal from others.
    1. This client has accepted his imminent death and is withdrawing from his family. Acceptance is the last stage of Kübler-Ross' stages of grief.

**TEST-TAKING HINT:** There are five stages to Dr. Elisabeth Kübler-Ross's grieving process, and some authorities list several more. The test taker should be familiar with the five stages of grief.

## Chronic Pain

25. 1. Blood pressure elevates in acute pain. Chronic pain, by definition, lasts more than 6 months, lasts far beyond the expected time for the pain to resolve, and may have an unclear onset. Changes in vital signs result from the fight-or-flight response by the body. The body cannot maintain this response and must adjust.
    2. Rapid shallow respirations might be attributed to acute pain if it was painful to breathe. The client diagnosed with a chest injury or pain will splint the area and slow the respirations or attempt to breathe shallowly and rapidly.
    3. Facial grimacing will occur in acute pain and is an objective sign the nurse can identify. Clients with chronic pain may be laughing and still be in pain. Remember, pain is whatever the client says it is and occurs whenever the client says it does.
    4. The client diagnosed with chronic pain will have adapted to living with the pain, and lying quietly may be the best way for the client to limit the feeling of pain.

**TEST-TAKING HINT:** The test taker must be able to differentiate between acute and chronic pain. Options "1," "2," and "3" are objective symptoms of acute pain. If the test taker were aware of this, then choosing the only option left would be a good choice.

26. 1. Pain is whatever the client says it is and occurs whenever the client says it does. The nurse should never deny the client's pain exists.
    2. This has been occurring for the past 3 years and does not mean cancer has come back. Many clients will fear cancer has recurred and delay treatment; denial is a potent coping mechanism.
    3. PMPS is characterized as a constriction accompanied by a burning sensation or prickling in the chest wall, axilla, or posterior arm resulting from movement of the arm. The pain can cause the client to limit movement of the arm and the shoulder, resulting in a frozen shoulder, also known as adhesive capsulitis of the shoulder.
    4. There are many problems associated with long-term narcotic use. Other strategies should be attempted before resigning the client to a lifetime of taking narcotic medications.

**TEST-TAKING HINT:** The test taker could eliminate option "1" because it violates all principles of pain management. Option "2" is not in the realm of the nurse's responsibility.

27. 1. This is a therapeutic response and the client is requesting information.
    2. Pain clinics do not cure pain; they do help identify measures to relieve pain.
    3. Pain clinics use a variety of methods to help the client to achieve relief from pain. Some measures include guided imagery, transcutaneous electrical nerve stimulation (TENS) units, nerve block surgery or injections, or medications.
    4. This is not an appropriate answer, even if the nurse is not sure. The nurse should attempt to discover the information for the client and then give factual information.

**TEST-TAKING HINT:** The test taker should answer a question with factual information. If the stem asks for a therapeutic response, then the test taker should choose one that addresses feelings.

28. 1. NSAIDs around the clock are dangerous because of the potential for gastrointestinal ulceration. NSAIDs are not the drug of choice for cancer pain.
    2. Opioids, such as morphine, are the drug of choice for cancer pain. There is no ceiling effect, it metabolizes without harmful by-products, and it is relatively inexpensive. A sustained-release formulation, such as MS Contin, can be administered every 6 to 8 hours, and a liquid fast-acting form is administered sublingually for any pain that is not controlled.
    3. Extra-strength acetaminophen (Tylenol), a nonnarcotic analgesic, is not strong enough for this client's pain. The maximum adult dose within a 24-hour period is 4 g. Extra-strength Tylenol is toxic to the liver in higher amounts.
    4. Meperidine (Demerol), an opioid narcotic, metabolizes into normeperidine and is not cleared by the body rapidly. A buildup of normeperidine can cause the client to seize.

**TEST-TAKING HINT:** The test taker must be aware of medications and their uses.

29. Correct answers are 1 and 5.
    1. Narcotic medications require a prescription handwritten in ink or typewritten and manually signed by the practitioner (Drug Enforcement

Administration, n.d.). Many local pharmacies will not have the medication available or may not have it in the quantities needed. The client should anticipate the needs before any time when the HCP may not be available or the pharmacy may be closed.

2. There can be several reasons a legitimate prescription is not filled.

3. In most cases, morphine, an opioid, needs a handwritten or typewritten prescription that is manually signed by the practitioner. Telephone orders are only permitted in emergency situations.

4. All medications have side effects; most notably, narcotics slow peristalsis and cause constipation.

5. Although federal regulations do not limit quantities of drugs dispensed with a prescription, many states and insurance carriers limit the quantity of a controlled substance to a 30-day supply.

**TEST-TAKING HINT:** The test taker could eliminate options "1" and "2" because they are opposites. Option "4" is untrue of all medications. The test taker should be familiar with prescription requirements for opioids.

30. 28 mg of morphine.
First, determine how many milligrams of morphine, a narcotic opioid, are in each milliliter of saline:

$50 \div 250$ mL $= 0.2$ mg/mL

Then determine how many milliliters are given in a shift:

10 mL/hr $\times$ 12 hour $= 120$ mL infused
1 shift $= 120$ mL infused

If each milliliter contains 0.2 mg of morphine, then

0.2 mg $\times$ 120 mL $= 24$ mg by constant infusion

Then determine the amount given IVP:

$2 \times 2 = 4$ mg given IVP

Finally, add the bolus amount to the amount constantly infused:

$24 + 4 = 28$ mg

**TEST-TAKING HINTS:** The nurse is responsible for being knowledgeable regarding all medications and the amount the client is receiving. The test taker can use the drop-down calculator on the NCLEX-RN® examination or ask the examiner for scratch paper.

31. 1. The client is in pain and has the right to have pain-control measures taken.

2. The client is in pain. The American Nurses Association Code of Ethics (2015) states clients have the right to die as comfortably as possible even if the measures used to control the pain indirectly hasten the impending death. The Dying Client's Bill of Rights reiterates this position. The client should be allowed to die with dignity and with as much comfort as the nurse can provide.

3. The client may be splinting to prevent the pain from being too severe. The client's respirations actually may improve when the nurse administers the pain medication.

4. The HCP is aware the client is unstable because the HCP must write the DNR order on the EHR. There is no reason to withhold the needed medication.

**TEST-TAKING HINT:** The position of administering medication that could hasten a client's death is a difficult one and requires the nurse to be aware of ethical position statements. Nurses never administer medications for the purpose of hastening death but sometimes must administer medications to provide the best comfort.

32. 1. This hemoglobin is low but would be expected for a client diagnosed with leukemia. A less-experienced nurse could care for this client. Leukemia affects the production of all cells produced by the bone marrow—either there is too much production of immature cells overpowering the ability of the bone marrow to use the pluripotent cells to produce other needed blood cells or because the bone marrow is not producing enough cells as needed. It effectively produces pancytopenia.

2. This represents an arterial blood gas of less than 60%; this client should be assigned to the most experienced nurse.

3. A client who needs a colostomy irrigated could be assigned to a less-experienced nurse.

4. Psychological problems come second to physiological ones.

**TEST-TAKING HINT:** This is a priority question. The test taker should realize option "1" is expected and may even be good for this client; option "3" is expected and not life-threatening; and option "4," although not expected, is not life-threatening. By doing this, the test taker could then look at what was determined for each option and realize option "2" needs the most experienced nurse.

**33.** 1. The UAP could perform this function.
   2. The UAP could perform this function.
   3. The UAP could perform this function.
   4. The nurse should monitor any laboratory work needed to administer medication safely.

**TEST-TAKING HINT: The rules for delegation state assessment, teaching, evaluating, or anything requiring nursing judgment cannot be delegated.**

**34.** Correct answers are 1 and 4.
   1. The TENS unit has a dial allowing the client to adjust the intensity of the electrical stimulation.
   2. The TENS unit does not deaden nerve endings; this would be accomplished through local anesthesia.
   3. The unit could stop functioning if it got wet, but this would not cause paralysis.
   4. The TENS unit works on the gate control theory of pain control and works by flooding the area with stimulation and blocking the pain impulses from reaching the brain.
   5. The TENS unit should be applied and left in place unless the client is showering.

**TEST-TAKING HINT: A medical device that causes paralysis so easily would not be approved for use by the general population, so option "2" could be eliminated. The test taker would need to be aware of the gate control theory of pain control to select option "4." The test taker should be familiar with how a TENS unit operates.**

**35.** 1. These are normal arterial blood gases.
   2. These temperature, pulse, and respiration rates are only slightly elevated, and the blood pressure is normal.
   3. This is typical of clients with chronic pain. They cannot localize the pain and frequently describe the pain as always being there, as disturbing rest, and as demoralizing. This client should be seen, and appropriate pain-control measures should be taken.
   4. This is considered mild pain, and this client can be seen after the client diagnosed with chronic pain.

**TEST-TAKING HINT: Options "1" and "2" could be eliminated because the values are within normal limits or only slightly above normal. Option "4" could be eliminated because 3 is low on the 1-to-10 pain scale.**

**36.** 1. This could be appropriate once the nurse assesses the situation further.
   2. The nurse should assess the situation fully. The client may be afraid of becoming addicted or may have been using alternative forms of treatment, such as music therapy, distraction techniques, acupuncture, or guided imagery.
   3. This is not appropriate. It is in the nurse's realm of responsibility to investigate the client's reasons for not wanting to take pain medication.
   4. Chronic cancer pain does not resolve on its own.

**TEST-TAKING HINT: Option "1" is advising without assessing. Assessment is the first step of the nursing process and should be implemented first in most situations unless a direct intervention treats the client in an emergency.**

## Ethical and Legal Issues

**37.** Correct answers are 2 and 5.
   1. This is an example of assault, which is a mental or physical threat without touching the client.
   2. When a mentally competent adult is forced to have a treatment that has been refused, battery occurs.
   3. This is fraud, a willful and purposeful misrepresentation that could cause harm to a client.
   4. This is called "defamation," a divulgence of privileged information or communication. This is a violation of the Health Insurance Portability and Accountability Act (HIPAA).
   5. When a mentally competent adult is forced to perform an action the client has refused, this is battery, even if it did not result in physical harm to the client.

**TEST-TAKING HINT: If the test taker knows battery is "bad," it may lead to selecting option "2" and option "5" because both indicate the patient has refused the treatment or action. The test taker could attempt to eliminate options based on knowledge. For example, breaking confidentiality is a violation of HIPAA; thus option "4" can be eliminated.**

**38.** 1. HIPAA is a federal act protecting the client's privacy while receiving health care.
   2. The state Nurse Practice Acts provide the laws that control the practice of nursing in each state.

3. There is no such law as this act.
4. The Good Samaritan Act protects HCPs against malpractice claims for care provided in emergency situations.

**TEST-TAKING HINT:** The test taker should be knowledgeable regarding the Good Samaritan Act and its implications in the nurse's professional career. The NCLEX-RN® often asks questions on this act.

39. 1. This response does not support veracity.
2. This response does not support veracity.
3. The principle of veracity is the duty to tell the truth. This response is telling the client the truth.
4. This response does not support veracity.

**TEST-TAKING HINT:** The test taker must know certain ethical principles, such as veracity, beneficence, nonmaleficence, fidelity, autonomy, and justice, to name a few. Without knowing the definition of veracity, the test taker would not be able to answer this question correctly.

40. 1. The surgeon is responsible for explaining the surgical procedure to the client; therefore, the nurse should first notify the surgeon.
2. This information should be documented in the EHR, but it is not the first intervention.
3. The operating room staff may or may not need to be notified based on when or if the permit is being signed, but it is not the first intervention.
4. The nurse is not responsible for explaining the surgical procedure. The nurse is responsible for making sure the client understands and for obtaining the consent.

**TEST-TAKING HINT:** The nurse is responsible for getting the permit signed and in the EHR before going to surgery, but the nurse is not responsible for explaining the procedure to the client.

41. Correct answers are 1 and 5.
1. This is a violation of the client's rights. The civil rights of clients include the right to wear their own clothes, keep personal items, and have a small amount of money in a psychiatric unit.
2. Seeing visitors is the civil right of the client.
3. Clients are allowed to eat food brought from home by family members.
4. Receiving and sending unopened mail is a civil right of the client, but any packages must be inspected when the client is opening them to check for sharp items, weapons, or any type of medication.
5. This is a violation of the client's rights. The client has a right to have reasonable access to a telephone and the opportunity to have private conversations by telephone.

**TEST-TAKING HINT:** The test taker must be aware of the client's legal and civil rights. The client in the psychiatric unit has the same rights as the client in the medical unit. Clients in a psychiatric hospital do not have to wear hospital gowns; they can wear their own clothes.

42. 1. Autonomy implies the client has the right to make choices and decisions about care, even if it may result in death or is not in agreement with the healthcare team.
2. Self-determination is not an ethical principle.
3. Beneficence is the duty to actively do good for clients.
4. Justice is the duty to treat all clients fairly.

**TEST-TAKING HINT:** The test taker should be aware of ethical principles that mandate a nurse's behavior. Clients have rights, and autonomy is an important principle that the nurse must ensure every client has.

43. 1. The Hippocratic Oath is the oath taken by medical doctors.
2. The Nuremberg Code identifies the need for voluntary informed consent when medical experiments are conducted on human beings. This source does not provide direction for the nurse addressing ethical issues.
3. This document informs clients and families receiving home health care of the ethical conduct they can expect from home care agencies and their employees when they are in the home. This source is not the best professional source for all nurses.
4. The American Nurses Association (ANA) Code of Ethics outlines to society the values, concerns, and goals of the nursing profession. The code provides direction for ethical decisions and behavior by emphasizing the obligations and responsibilities that are entailed in the nurse-client relationship.

**TEST-TAKING HINT:** The test taker must be aware of the word "best" to be able to answer this question. All four answer options may or may not be potential answers, but the test taker must select the option that addresses all nurses. Option "3" should be eliminated as a possible answer because it addresses only home health care.

44. Correct answers are 1, 3, 4, and 5.
 1. The duty to the client must be established. The nurse assumes a legal duty by accepting to care for the client. Establishing duty to the client is one of the four elements necessary to prove nursing malpractice. It is a failure to perform according to the established standard of conduct.
 2. This is one of the four steps in ethical decision making. It is not an element necessary to prove nursing malpractice.
 3. Failure to perform according to the established standards of care is necessary to prove nursing malpractice.
 4. Breach of duty resulting in an actual injury or damage to the client is required to prove nursing malpractice.
 5. A connection must exist between conduct and the resulting injury to prove nursing malpractice.

**TEST-TAKING HINT:** This is a knowledge-based question, but the test taker should realize that ethical issues and legal issues are two different concerns and that malpractice is a legal concern. The test taker should also know the four elements necessary to prove nursing malpractice: (1) The nurse has a duty to the client. (2) The duty has been breached. The nurse failed to uphold a standard of care. (3) There is some harm to the client. (4) The breach of duty caused the harm.

45. 1. This action should be taken, but this is not the first action to keep the client safe.
 2. This is a form of chemical restraint, and the nurse must have an HCP's order.
 3. This is a form of restraint and is against the law unless the nurse has an HCP's order.
 4. The nurse must notify the HCP before putting the client in restraints. Restraints are used in an emergency situation and for a limited time and must be for the protection of the client.

**TEST-TAKING HINT:** The test taker must realize that when the stem asks which action is first, more than one option may be appropriate for the situation, but only one is implemented first. Restraining a client is considered battery and is against the law unless the client is a danger to self and there is an HCP's order.

46. 1. Nurse Practice Acts provide the laws that control the practice of nursing in each state. All states have Nurse Practice Acts.
 2. The Client's Bill of Rights, also known as "Your Rights as a Hospital Patient," is a document that explains the client's rights to participate in health care; it does not address the nurse's behavior.
 3. Each state, not the U.S. Congress, is responsible for writing and implementing the state's Nurse Practice Act.
 4. The American Nurses Association is a voluntary organization that provides standards of care and a code of ethics. It addresses issues in nursing, but it does not mandate the registered nurse's behavior.

**TEST-TAKING HINT:** This is a knowledge-based question that the test taker must know.

47. 1. This addresses the ethical principle of veracity. Should the nurse tell the client truthfully a placebo will not help the pain?
 2. This is an example of nonmaleficence, the duty to prevent or avoid doing harm, whether intentional or unintentional. Is it harmful for the nurse to work in an area of inexperience?
 3. This is an example of the ethical principle of fidelity, the duty to be faithful to commitments. It involves keeping promises and information confidential and maintaining privacy.
 4. Justice involves the duty to treat all clients fairly, without regard to age, socioeconomic status, or any other variables. Providing safe and appropriate nursing care to all clients is an example of justice.

**TEST-TAKING HINT:** The test taker must be knowledgeable regarding ethical principles; they are part of the NCLEX-RN®. The word "justice" should make the test taker think about fairness, which might lead the test taker to select option "4" as the correct answer. The test taker should not automatically think, "I don't know the answer." Think about the words before selecting the correct answer.

48. 1. The law states child abuse or suspected child abuse must be reported. The nurse is legally responsible for reporting child abuse or suspected child abuse. This is a legal issue, not malpractice.
 2. Malpractice is a failure to meet the standards of care that results in harm to or death of a client. Failing to heed warnings of shock is an example of malpractice.

3. Stealing narcotics is a legal situation, not a malpractice issue. The nursing license could be revoked for this illegal behavior.
4. Falsifying documents is against the law. It is not a malpractice issue.

**TEST-TAKING HINT: The test taker must be knowledgeable regarding malpractice. Legal issues are dealt with by the laws of the state and federal government, and malpractice issues are dealt with in the state Nurse Practice Acts.**

## Organ and Tissue Donation

49. 1. There is a feeling during times of stress that organs may be distributed unfairly. Tissue and organ banks use the United Network of Organ Sharing (UNOS) to be as fair as possible in the allocation of organs and tissues. Organs will be given to the best match for the organ in the community where the donor dies. If no match is found in that area, then the search for a human leukocyte antigen (HLA) match will be expanded to other areas of the country. The recipient is chosen based on the HLA match, not fame or fortune.
    2. The client is asking for information, which the nurse should provide.
    3. There is a definitive method of allocation of organs.
    4. HLAs are the principal histocompatibility system used to match donors and recipients. The greater the number of matches, the less likely the client will reject the organ. Different races have different HLAs (Organ Procurement and Transplantation Network, 2019).

**TEST-TAKING HINT: Option "2" can be eliminated because the client asked for information. Option "1" can be eliminated because the statement supports an unethical situation.**

50. 1. Positive brain waves on the EEG indicate brain activity, and the client is not brain dead.
    2. This is called the oculovestibular test. If the client reacts, then it indicates brain activity and the client is not brain dead.
    3. The Uniform Determination of Brain Death Act states brain death is determined by accepted medical standards, which indicate irreversible loss of all brain function. Cerebral blood flow studies, EEG, and oculovestibular and oculocephalic tests may be done.

4. If the cerebral blood flow studies do not show acceptable blood flow to the brain, the client will not come out of the vegetative state.

**TEST-TAKING HINT: If the test taker examined all answer options and did not understand options "1," "2," and "4," then reading option "3" again would prove it to be the best choice because it simply states the machine won't be turned off until brain death has been proved.**

51. 1. Many states require tissue and organ banks to be notified of all deaths, but the systemic infection eliminates this client from becoming a donor.
    2. **Septicemia is a systemic infection and will prevent the client from donating tissues or organs.**
    3. There is no reason to notify the HCP.
    4. If the client were to be an organ donor, then the client's body would remain in the intensive care unit on the ventilator and with IV medication support until the organ bank team arrives and takes the client to the operating room.

**TEST-TAKING HINT: Option "3" could be eliminated from consideration because the nurse should be able to handle this situation. Option "4" could be eliminated because the client would have to stay on life support if the organ bank were to retrieve viable organs.**

52. 1. Oliguria, fever, increasing edema, hypertension, and weight gain are signs of organ rejection.
    2. A decrease in serum creatinine and BUN would indicate the transplanted kidney is functioning well.
    3. Potassium and calcium are not monitored for rejection.
    4. The client diagnosed with a fever might have tachycardia. Hypertension is a sign of rejection.

**TEST-TAKING HINT: Option "2" could be eliminated because of the word "decreased." If the test taker were aware of the role the kidneys play in controlling blood pressure, then option "4" could be eliminated. Decreased urine output in option "1" would make the most sense to choose because the kidneys produce urine.**

53. Correct answers are 3 and 5.
    1. The client must take an immune-suppressant medication forever unless a rejection occurs, and then the client would die without another transplant.

2. Foul-smelling drainage would indicate infection and is not expected. This would be an emergency situation.

3. Clients should be taught to notify the HCP immediately of any signs of an infection. The immune-suppressant drugs will mask the sign of an infection and superinfections can develop.

4. The skin turns yellow in liver failure; the antirejection drugs do not cause jaundice.

5. Clients should be instructed to get routine immunizations, such as the flu vaccine. Live attenuated vaccines are contraindicated, but some are currently under investigation by the U.S. Food and Drug Administration.

**TEST-TAKING HINT: Standard postoperative instructions include teaching the client to watch for any sign of an infection. Foul-smelling drainage is never normal.**

54. 1. There is no pain associated with storing cord blood. The blood is taken from the separated placenta at birth. From 40 to 150 mL of stem cells can be retrieved from the umbilical vein.

2. All hospitals that have an obstetrics department should be able to assist with the collection of stem cells. The client should notify the HCP to be prepared with the kit to obtain the specimens and to be able to send the stem cells to the Cord Blood Registry for processing and storage.

3. In private cord blood banks, there is an initial fee to process the stem cells and a yearly fee to maintain the stored stem cells until needed. Stem cells may be used by the infant in case of a devastating illness or can be donated at the discretion of the owner. In a public cord blood bank, there is no fee to store the cord blood, but the stem cells would be donated to anyone who matches.

4. This is true of stem cells that have been stored for more than 20 years.

**TEST-TAKING HINT: The test taker should recognize pain could not be associated with tissue that is no longer a part of the body.**

55. Correct answers are 1 and 2.
1. Urine cultures are performed frequently because of the bacteriuria present in the early stages of transplantation.
2. A cadaver kidney may have undergone acute tubular necrosis and may not function for 2 to 3 weeks, during which time the client may experience anuria, oliguria, or polyuria and require dialysis.

3. Serum creatinine and BUN levels are monitored, but there is no need to monitor the urine osmolality.

4. Hourly outputs are monitored and compared with the intake of fluids.

5. The dressing is a flank dressing.

**TEST-TAKING HINT: The test taker should notice time frames. Anytime a specific time reference is provided, the test taker must determine if the time frame is the appropriate interval for performing the activity. In option "4," "every shift" is not appropriate.**

56. 1. The client would be NPO at this time and would be receiving parenteral antirejection medications.
2. The client would have been taken off the heart-lung bypass machine in the operating room.
3. Saturating three dressing pads in 1 hour would indicate hemorrhage.
4. Pain is expected and is not a complication of the procedure.

**TEST-TAKING HINT: The test taker should notice the time frame provided in the stem—in this case, 3 hours after surgery. This could eliminate options "1" and "2."**

57. 1. Assessment is always the nurse's responsibility and cannot be delegated. Hourly outputs are monitored to determine kidney function.
2. The UAP can perform this function. There is no nursing judgment required.
3. This requires nursing judgment and is outside the UAP's expertise.
4. Irrigating a nasogastric tube for a client who has undergone a pancreas transplant should be done by the nurse; this is a high-level nursing task.

**TEST-TAKING HINT: When asked to choose a task that can be delegated, the test taker should determine which task requires the least amount of judgment and choose that option.**

58. 1. This client is ready for discharge and is presumably stable. The client donated the kidney and still has one functioning kidney. An experienced medical-surgical nurse could care for this client.
2. This client must be observed closely for rejection of the organ and is newly transferred from the intensive care unit; therefore, a more experienced nurse in transplant care should care for this client.
3. This client has developed symptoms of a problem unrelated to the corneal transplant, but these symptoms will increase

intracranial pressure, resulting in indirect pressure to the cornea. Therefore, a more experienced transplant nurse should care for this client.

4. This client is showing symptoms of organ rejection, which is a medical emergency and requires a more experienced transplant nurse.

**TEST-TAKING HINT: The test taker should choose the client with the fewest potential problems. The nurse is experienced as a medical-surgical nurse, but transplant recipients require more specialized knowledge.**

59. 1. Living donors are able to donate some organs. The kidneys, a portion of the liver, and a lung may be donated, and the donor will still have functioning organs. An identical twin is the best possible match. However, in the situation in this question, the identical twin would also have CF because the genes would be identical. The next best chance for a compatible match comes from a sibling with both parents in common.

2. The father would have only half of the genetic makeup of the child.

3. There are at least 27 HLA types. A match requires at least 7, and preferably 10 to 11, points.

4. This is not an acceptable match; the client would reject the organ.

**TEST-TAKING HINT: If the test taker did not know the rationale, then a choice between options "1" and "2" would be the best option because of the direct familial relationships.**

60. 1. Skin is taken from cadaver donors, so it is given once.

2. Bones are taken from cadaver donors, so it is given once.

3. A kidney can be donated while the donor is living or both can be donated as cadaver organs, but either way, the donation is only once.

4. The human body reproduces bone marrow daily. There is a bone marrow registry for participants willing to undergo the procedure to donate to clients when a match is found.

**TEST-TAKING HINT: The test taker could eliminate option "3" because the stem asks for repeated times and the client cannot live without kidney function. The client would have to be placed on dialysis or die.**

61. 1. In the 1990s, Congress added the requirement for health-care facilities to offer clients the opportunity to receive an AD form and to be able to complete it to provide the health-care team with knowledge of the clients' wishes. It was added to a Medicare funding bill.
    2. The client has to refuse or accept or alert the facility of an intact document about advanced decisions made by the client, but referral to a case manager is not attached to Medicare funding.
    3. The client does not have to apply for supplemental insurance.
    4. The opportunity may include end-of-life issues, but it is not limited to end of life; it does include issues of irreversible situations and surrogate decision makers.

**TEST-TAKING HINT:** The test taker could eliminate option "3" because the nurse cannot make the client do anything. The client has a right to say no.

62. 1. Clinical death is the absence of pulse, respirations, and blood pressure. It does not include radiology or other diagnostic tests.
    2. If CPR is unsuccessful, the nurse cannot pronounce death. A physician must determine the reason for the death.
    3. For it to be legal for a nurse to pronounce death, the client must have a disease process that could lead to death. The physician must write a clear order that the nurse can pronounce and be willing to document the cause of death on the death certificate. The observed clinical signs must be documented and the time pronounced.
    4. This is an incomplete entry.

**TEST-TAKING HINT:** The test taker could eliminate option "1" because clinical death is the absence of clinical signs of life. Option "3" is complete documentation; the nurse states the facts without embellishment in the documentation.

63. 1. The nurse is caring for a client who is at best disoriented; challenging this cognitive deficiency will only create frustration and anxiety in the client. Nonmaleficence is the duty to prevent or do no harm. This is a therapeutic response that validates the client's

concern but does not include lying to the client.
    2. This is veracity, to tell the truth.
    3. The client does not owe the nurse an explanation of why she wishes to see her mother. "Why" is not appropriate in this situation.
    4. This is the opposite of veracity; it is lying to the client. If the nurse believes the client's mother to be dead, then how will the nurse contact her?

**TEST-TAKING HINT:** The test taker could eliminate option "2" because it is veracity and "4" because it is lying.

64. 1. The nurse could possibly help the family to guide them about the need for eventual arrangements, but it is not appropriate during the admission process.
    2. The client may or may not have pain; nothing indicates pain is an issue in the stem of the question.
    3. ADs provide guidance for end-of-life care; the nurse needs this information in order to plan the care per the client's wishes.
    4. This could be determined, but the priority is knowing the client's wishes.

**TEST-TAKING HINT:** The test taker should recognize timing when reading a stem or option in a question. "On admission," "every day," "every 2 hours" will help to determine a correct answer.

65. 1. Chaplains work with all faiths and are spiritual advisers. If the nurse feels comfortable with discussing heaven, and if the client wishes to talk with the nurse, it is appropriate.
    2. Nurses are not prohibited from discussing spiritual issues with a client; the nurse should not challenge the client's personal beliefs.
    3. Hell is not what the client wants to talk about.
    4. The nurse should allow the client to verbalize feelings regarding what to expect when death occurs.

**TEST-TAKING HINT:** The nurse student is taught in first-level courses to allow the client to verbalize feelings; the test taker should recognize this as basic nursing skills.

66. 1. This is false reassurance.
    2. The blame for the lack of communication may not be the client's; it could be all on the son. This is an accusatory statement.
    3. The nurse is asking permission to divulge the client's location and health status to the son; this is appropriate for complying with HIPAA and is addressing the voiced concerns of the client.
    4. The nurse can perform an intervention that directly affects the client's situation. A therapeutic conversation might be used if the client's son is not willing to reconcile with the client.

    **TEST-TAKING HINT:** The test taker could eliminate option "1" because it is advising the client about how he should feel. Option "2" asks why and blames the client. Option "4" does not address the client's needs.

67. 1. When a death occurs, the need is for the nurse's presence; just being there with the family is what will help the family grieve.
    2. The nurse may need to notify the funeral home, but the family is the priority need.
    3. If the family wants the minister to be called, the nurse could do this, but frequently, the family has a relationship with the minister and will need to speak directly with the minister to arrange the services.
    4. The death certificate is completed by the physician signing it, not the nurse.

    **TEST-TAKING HINT:** The test taker could eliminate all options besides "1" because none of these will assist the grieving process.

# END-OF-LIFE ISSUES
# COMPREHENSIVE EXAMINATION

1. The 38-year-old client was brought to the emergency department with CPR in progress and died 15 minutes after arrival. Which intervention should the nurse implement for postmortem care?
   1. Do not allow significant others to see the body.
   2. Do not remove any tubes from the body.
   3. Prepare the body for the funeral home.
   4. Send the client's clothing to the hospital laundry.

2. The primary nurse caring for the deceased client is crying with the family at the bedside. Which action should the charge nurse implement?
   1. Request the primary nurse to come out in the hall.
   2. Refer the nurse to the employee assistance program.
   3. Allow the nurse and family this time to grieve.
   4. Ask the chaplain to relieve the nurse at the bedside.

3. The nurse is discussing ADs with the client. The client asks the nurse, "Why is this so important to do?" Which statement would be the nurse's **best** response?
   1. "The federal government mandates this form must be completed by you."
   2. "This will make sure your family does what you want them to do."
   3. "Don't you think it is important to let everyone know your final wishes?"
   4. "Because of technology, there are many options for end-of-life care."

4. The client of the Jewish faith died during the night. The nurse notified the family, and the family prefers not to come to the hospital. Which intervention should the nurse implement to address the family's behavior?
   1. Take no further action because this is an accepted cultural practice.
   2. Notify the hospital supervisor and report the situation immediately.
   3. Call the local synagogue and request the rabbi go to the family's home.
   4. Assume the family does not care about the client and follow hospital protocol.

5. The hospice nurse is making the final visit to the wife, whose spouse died a little more than a year ago. The nurse realizes the spouse's clothes are still in the closet. Which action should the nurse implement **first**?

   1. Discuss what the wife is going to do with the clothes.
   2. Refer the wife to a grief recovery support group.
   3. Do not take any action because this is a normal grieving.
   4. Remove the clothes from the house and dispose of them.

6. The nurse is giving an in-service to nurses on end-of-life issues. Which activity should the nurse encourage the participants to perform?
   1. Discuss with another participant the death of a client.
   2. Review the hospital postmortem care policy.
   3. Justify not putting the client in a shroud after dying.
   4. Write down their own beliefs about death and dying.

7. The 78-year-old Catholic client is in end-stage congestive heart failure and has a DNR order. The client has vital signs populated in the vital sign flowsheet below and Cheyne-Stokes respirations. Which action should the nurse implement?

   | Vital Sign Flowsheet | Client Results | Normal Values |
   | --- | --- | --- |
   | Blood Pressure | 80/50 | 100 to 119 mmHg systolic 60 to 80 mmHg diastolic |
   | Pulse | 50 | 60 to 100 beats/min |
   | Respirations | 10 | 12 to 20 breaths/min |

   1. Bring the crash cart to the bedside.
   2. Apply oxygen via nasal cannula.
   3. Notify a priest for last rites.
   4. Turn the bed to face the sunset.

8. The Hispanic client diagnosed with terminal cancer is requesting a curandero to come to the bedside. Which intervention should the nurse implement?
   1. Tell the client it is against policy to allow faith healers.
   2. Assist with planning the visit from the curandero.
   3. Refer the client to the pastoral care department.
   4. Determine the reason the client needs the curandero.

9. Which interventions should the nurse implement at the time of a client's death? **Select all that apply**.
   1. Allow gaps in the conversation at the client's bedside.
   2. Avoid giving the family advice about how to grieve.
   3. Tell the family the nurse understands their feelings.
   4. Explain this is God's will to prevent further suffering.
   5. Allow the family time with the body in private.

10. The male client asks the nurse, "Should I designate my spouse as a durable power of attorney for health care?" Which statement would be the nurse's **best** response?
    1. "Yes, because your spouse is your next of kin."
    2. "Most people don't allow their spouse to do this."
    3. "Will your spouse be able to support your wishes?"
    4. "Your children are probably the best ones for the job."

11. The client has been declared brain dead and is an organ donor. The nurse is preparing the spouse of the client to enter the room to say good-bye. Which information is **most important** for the nurse to discuss with the spouse?
    1. Inform the spouse the client will still be on the ventilator.
    2. Instruct the spouse to only stay a few minutes at the bedside.
    3. Tell the spouse it is all right to talk to the client.
    4. Allow another family member to go in with the spouse.

12. Which clients would the nurse consider as potential organ and tissue donors? **Select all that apply**.
    1. The 60-year-old female client diagnosed with an inoperable primary brain tumor.
    2. The 45-year-old female client diagnosed with a subarachnoid hemorrhage.
    3. The 22-year-old male client involved in a motor vehicle accident.
    4. The 36-year-male client diagnosed as HIV positive and recently released from prison.
    5. The 51-year-old male client diagnosed with sepsis from a perforated bowel.

13. The intensive care nurse is caring for a deceased organ donor client, and the organ donation team is en route to the hospital. Which statement would be an appropriate goal of treatment for the client?
    1. The urinary output is 20 mL/hr via a Foley catheter.
    2. The systolic blood pressure is greater than 90 mmHg.
    3. The pulse oximeter reading remains between 88% and 90%.
    4. The telemetry shows the client in sinus tachycardia.

14. The nurse is teaching a class on ethical principles in nursing. Which statement **supports** the definition of beneficence?
    1. The duty to prevent or avoid doing harm.
    2. The duty to actively do good for clients.
    3. The duty to be faithful to commitments.
    4. The duty to tell the truth to the clients.

15. Which action by the UAP would **warrant immediate** intervention by the RN?
    1. The UAP is holding the phone to the ear of a quadriplegic client.
    2. The UAP refuses to discuss the client's condition with the visitor in the room.
    3. The UAP put a vest restraint on an older client found wandering in the hall.
    4. The UAP is assisting the client diagnosed with arthritis to open up personal mail.

16. The nurse is teaching a class on chronic pain to new graduates. Which information is **most important** for the RN to discuss?
    1. The nurse must believe the client's report of pain.
    2. Clients in chronic pain may not show objective signs.
    3. Alternative pain-control therapies are used for chronic pain.
    4. Referral to a pain clinic may be necessary.

17. The client diagnosed with chronic low back pain is having trouble sleeping at night. Which nonpharmacological therapy should the nurse teach the client? **Select all that apply**.
    1. Proper sleep hygiene.
    2. Acupuncture.
    3. Massage therapy.
    4. Herbal remedies.
    5. Progressive relaxation techniques.

18. The client diagnosed with cancer is unable to attain pain relief despite receiving large amounts of narcotic medications. Which intervention should be included in the plan of care?
    1. Ask the HCP to increase the medication.
    2. Assess for any spiritual distress.
    3. Change the client's position every 2 hours.
    4. Turn on the radio to soothing music.

19. The client diagnosed with chronic pain is laughing and joking with visitors. When the nurse asks the client to rate the pain on a 1-to-10 scale, the client rates the pain as 10. According to the FACES® pain scale, how would the nurse chart the client's pain (see figure below)?

**Wong-Baker FACES® Pain Rating Scale**

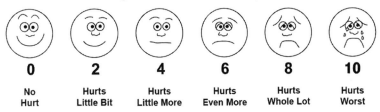

| 0 | 2 | 4 | 6 | 8 | 10 |
|---|---|---|---|---|---|
| No Hurt | Hurts Little Bit | Hurts Little More | Hurts Even More | Hurts Whole Lot | Hurts Worst |

   1. The client's pain is between 0 and 2 on the FACES® scale.
   2. The client's pain is a "10" on a 1-to-10 pain scale.
   3. The client is unable to rate the pain on a scale accurately.
   4. The client's pain is moderate on the pain scale.

20. The client diagnosed with diabetes mellitus type 2 wants to be an organ donor and asks the nurse, "Which organs can I donate?" Which statement is the nurse's **best** response?
   1. "It is wonderful you want to be an organ donor. Let's discuss this."
   2. "You can donate any organ in your body if the organ is usable when you die."
   3. "You have to donate your body to science to be an organ donor."
   4. "You cannot donate any organs, but you can donate some tissues."

21. The client diagnosed with multiple sclerosis becoming very debilitated tells the home health nurse the Final Exit Network sent information on Physician Aid in Dying (PAD) laws. Which question should the nurse ask the client?
   1. "Why did you get in touch with the Final Exit Network?"
   2. "Did you know this is an illegal organization?"
   3. "Did you know someone who committed suicide?"
   4. "What religious beliefs do you practice?"

22. Which intervention should the nurse implement to provide culturally sensitive health care to the white older client diagnosed as terminal?
   1. Discuss health-care issues with the oldest male child.
   2. Determine if the client will be cremated or have an earth burial.
   3. Do not talk about death and dying in front of the client.
   4. Encourage the client's autonomy and answer questions truthfully.

23. Which action by the primary nurse would require the unit manager to intervene?
   1. The nurse overwrites an erroneous EHR entry, so it is erased.
   2. The nurse is shredding the paper worksheet at the end of the shift.
   3. The nurse documents a medication not given on the MAR.
   4. The nurse documents narcotic wastage with another nurse.

24. Which action should the nurse implement for the client's family requesting to light incense around the dying client?
   1. Suggest the family bring potpourri instead of incense.
   2. Tell the client the door must be shut at all times.
   3. Inform the family the scent will make the client nauseated.
   4. Explain the fire code does not allow any burning in a hospital.

25. The nurse is caring for the client diagnosed with active tuberculosis of the lungs. The client does not have a DNR order. The client experiences a cardiac arrest, and there is no resuscitation mask at the bedside. The nurse waits for the crash cart before beginning resuscitation. According to the ANA Code of Ethics for Nurses (see Table 18-1), which disciplinary action should be taken against the nurse?
   1. Report the action to the State Board of Nurse Examiners.
   2. The nurse should be terminated for failure to perform duties.
   3. No disciplinary action should be taken against the nurse.
   4. Refer the nurse to the American Nurses Association.

## Table 18–1 The American Nurses Association Code of Ethics for Nurses

- The nurse practices with compassion and respect for the inherent dignity, worth, and unique attributes of every person.
- The nurse's primary commitment is to the patient, whether an individual, family, group, community, or population.
- The nurse promotes, advocates for, and protects the rights, health, and safety of the patient.
- The nurse has authority, accountability, and responsibility for nursing practice; makes decisions; and takes action consistent with the obligation to promote health and to provide optimal care.
- The nurse owes the same duties to self as to others, including the responsibility to promote health and safety, preserve wholeness of character and integrity, maintain competence, and continue person and professional growth.
- The nurse, through individual and collective effort, establishes, maintains, and improves the ethical environment of the work setting and conditions of employment that are conducive to safe, quality health care.
- The nurse, in all roles and settings, advances the profession through research and scholarly inquiry, professional standards development, and the generation of both nursing and health policy.
- The nurse collaborates with other health professionals and the public to protect human rights, promote health diplomacy, and reduce health disparities.
- The profession of nursing collectively through its professional organizations, must articulate nursing values, maintain the integrity of the profession, and integrate principles of social justice into nursing and health policy.

The American Nurses Association Code of Ethics for Nurses with Interpretative Statements. Copyright 2015, American Nurses Publishing, American Nurses Foundation/American Nurses Association, Washington, DC. Reprinted with permission.

26. The spouse of a client receiving hospice care being cared for at home calls the nurse to report the client is restless and agitated. Which interventions should the nurse implement? **Rank in order of priority.**
    1. Request an order from the HCP for antianxiety medications.
    2. Call the medical equipment company and request oxygen for the client.
    3. Go to the home and assess the client and address the spouse's concerns.
    4. Reassure and calm the spouse over the telephone.
    5. Notify the chaplain about the client's change in status.

1. 1. There is no reason the family members should not be able to see the client; this is important to allow closure for the significant others.
   2. This death should be reported to the medical examiner because the death occurred less than 24 hours after hospital admission and an autopsy may be required. Therefore, the nurse must leave all tubes in place; the medical examiner will remove the tubes.
   3. This is a medical examiner's case, and the nurse should not prepare the body by removing tubes or washing the body before taking the client to a funeral home.
   4. The client's clothing should be given to the family or to the police if foul play is suspected.

2. 1. The nurse is providing care for the family and should not have to leave the bedside.
   2. An employee assistance program is available at many facilities for counseling employees who are having psychosocial issues, but this nurse is humane.
   3. Crying was once considered unprofessional, but today it is recognized as simply an expression of empathy and caring.
   4. The chaplain may come to the client's room and offer support but should not relieve the nurse who has developed a therapeutic nurse-client relationship with the client.

3. 1. ADs are not mandated by the federal government. The nurse must discuss this with the client, but the client does not have to complete it.
   2. ADs can be overridden by the family because the HCP is worried about being sued by family survivors.
   3. This response is not answering the client's question and it is argumentative.
   4. Technology now allows for the body to maintain life functions indefinitely in some futile situations. ADs allow clients to make decisions, which hopefully will be honored at the time of their death.

4. 1. The nurse should not be judgmental of the family's decision. In the Jewish faith, the body may be sent to the funeral home for burial within 24 hours, and a closed casket may be preferred (Jewish Virtual Library, n.d.).
   2. The hospital supervisor does not need to be notified the family did not want to come to the hospital.
   3. The nurse needs to take care of the client, not the family, and should not call to request a rabbi to go visit the family.
   4. The nurse must be aware of cultural differences and not be judgmental.

5. 1. The nurse must first confront the wife about moving on through the grieving process. After 1 year, the wife should be seriously thinking about what to do with her spouse's belongings.
   2. This is an appropriate intervention, but the nurse must first talk directly to the client.
   3. After 1 year, the wife should be progressing through the grieving process and needs encouragement to remove her spouse's belongings.
   4. This will need to be done at some point, but it is not the nurse's responsibility. This action is crossing professional boundaries unless the wife asks the nurse to do this.

6. 1. This activity will not help the nurse address a personal fear of death.
   2. This activity will not help the nurse address a personal fear of death.
   3. This activity will not help the nurse address a personal fear of death.
   4. Many nurses are reluctant to discuss death openly with their clients because of their own anxieties about death. Therefore, coming face to face with the nurse's own mortality will address the fear of death.

7. 1. The client has a DNR; therefore, there is no need to bring the crash cart to the bedside.
   2. The client has a DNR, and the nurse needs to help the client die peacefully.
   3. The Catholic religion requires last rites to be performed immediately before or after death.
   4. The client is Catholic, and there is no specific way for the bed to be placed.

8. 1. The hospital should not prevent the client from practicing personal culture rituals or beliefs, and denying faith healers would be denying the client's spiritual guidance.
   2. The nurse should support the client's culture as long as it is not contraindicated in the client's care. This client is terminal; therefore, allowing the curandero, a folk healer and religious person in the Hispanic culture, would be appropriate.
   3. There is no reason to refer this client to the pastoral care department; the nurse can assist the client.
   4. The nurse does not need to know why the client wants the curandero; the nurse should support the client's request without prejudice.

9. Correct answers are 1, 2, and 5.
   1. The nurse needs to be sensitive to the family, and simply being present to support the family emotionally is important; the nurse does not have to talk.
   2. The nurse should avoid the impulse to give advice; each person grieves in an individual way.
   3. The nurse should not tell the family she understands; even if the test taker has lost a loved one, the test taker should never select an option that says the nurse understands another person's feelings.
   4. This is projecting the nurse's personal religious beliefs on the family and could cause more anger at God when the family needs to be able to draw on their own spiritual beliefs.
   5. The family needs time for closure, and allowing the family to stay at the bedside is meeting the family's need to say good-bye.

10. 1. The client can designate anyone he wishes to be the durable power of attorney.
    2. This is not true; many spouses are designated as the durable power of attorney for health care.
    3. No matter who the client selects as a power of attorney, the most important aspect is to make sure the person, whether it be the spouse, child, or friend, will honor the client's wishes no matter what happens.
    4. The children must be at least 18 years old and willing to honor the client's wishes.

11. 1. This is the most important action because, when the spouse walks into the room, the client's chest will be rising and falling, the monitor will show a heartbeat, and the client will be warm. Many family members do not realize this and think the client is still alive. The organs must be perfused until retrieved for organ donation.
    2. The spouse should be encouraged to stay a short time and leave the facility before the client is taken to the operating room, but it is not the most important intervention.
    3. It is all right for the spouse to talk to the client, but because the client is brain dead and cannot hear her, it is not the most important intervention.
    4. It is all right for another family member to go into the room, but it is not the most important intervention.

12. Correct answers are 1, 2, 3, and 4.
    1. Primary brain tumors rarely metastasize outside the skull, and this client can be a donor; cancers other than primary brain tumors can prevent organ and tissue donation.
    2. This is an excellent potential donor because all other organs are probably healthy.
    3. This is an excellent candidate because this is a young person with a traumatic death, not a chronic illness.
    4. According to the HIV Organ Policy Equity (HOPE) Act, the client diagnosed with HIV could be an organ donor to an HIV-positive recipient. Therefore, the nurse should consider this client a potential organ donor (Organ Procurement and Transplantation Network, 2019).
    5. The client diagnosed with sepsis from a perforated bowel is not a candidate for organ donation due to systemic infection.

13. 1. The urinary output should be at least 30 mL/hr.
    2. The systolic blood pressure must be maintained at this rate to keep the client's organs perfused until removal.
    3. The pulse oximeter should be greater than 93%.
    4. The client's heart must be beating, but it can be a normal sinus rhythm or even sinus bradycardia.

14. 1. This is the ethical principle of nonmaleficence.
2. **This is the ethical principle of beneficence.**
3. This is the ethical principle of fidelity.
4. This is the ethical principle of veracity.

15. 1. The client has a right to private phone conversations but, because the client is a quadriplegic, holding the phone to the ear does not require immediate intervention.
2. This is the appropriate action for the UAP and should be praised.
3. **Restraints are not allowed unless there is an HCP's order with documentation by the nurse of the client being a danger to himself or others. The UAP putting the client in restraints warrants immediate intervention because it is battery.**
4. The client has a right to send and receive mail, and the UAP is helping the client open the mail; therefore, this does not require immediate intervention.

16. 1. **The most important information for a nurse caring for a client diagnosed with acute or chronic pain is to believe the client. Pain is subjective, and the nurse should not be judgmental.**
2. This is a true statement because the client's sympathetic nervous system cannot remain in a continual state of readiness. This results in no objective data to support the pain and a normal pulse and blood pressure. However, it is not the most important information a new graduate should know.
3. TENS, distraction, imagery, acupuncture, and acupressure are all alternate pain therapies that may be used for chronic pain, but it is not the most important information the new graduate should know.
4. Pain clinics treat clients with chronic pain, but it is not the most important information a new graduate should know.

17. Correct answers are 1 and 5.
1. **The nurse should teach proper sleep hygiene including limiting daytime naps, avoiding caffeine and alcohol, regular exercise, and establishing a regular bedtime routine.**
2. Acupuncture is an alternative therapy, but a nurse cannot teach it and the client cannot perform it.
3. A client cannot perform self-massage therapy.
4. The nurse should not prescribe herbal remedies.

5. **Progressive relaxation techniques involve visualizing a specific muscle group and mentally relaxing each muscle; this can be taught to the client, and it will allow the client to relax, which will foster sleep.**

18. 1. The client is already receiving large amounts of medication. The nurse should assess for other causes of pain.
2. **Pain has many components, and spiritual distress or psychosocial needs will affect the client's perception of pain; remember, assessment is the first step of the nursing process.**
3. Usually, clients will naturally assume the most comfortable position, and forcing them to move may increase their pain.
4. The client may or may not like this type of music, but it would not be the first intervention.

19. 1. The FACES pain scale was devised to help children identify pain when they are unable to understand the concept of numbers. The nurse can use this pain scale when caring for adults unable to use the 1-to-10 numerical scale. This client rated the pain at a 10.
2. **Pain is whatever the client says it is and occurs whenever the client says it does. Pain is a wholly subjective symptom, and the nurse should not question the client's perception of pain. The client's pain is a 10.**
3. The client did rate the pain on the pain scale. Laughing and talking with visitors may occur with excruciating chronic pain. The client diagnosed with chronic pain must learn to adapt to pain and try to live as normal a life as possible.
4. The client rated the pain at a 10.

20. 1. This is not answering the client's question.
2. **The usable condition of the organs at death is the main consideration of donation. The client diagnosed with type 2 diabetes can have organ damage as a result of the high glucose over time, but the quality of the organ at death is the consideration. Everyone is eligible to sign up as an organ donor.**
3. This is a false statement. The client does not have to will the body to science to be a tissue and organ donor.
4. The client can donate corneas, skin, and some joints. Organs can be donated if the organ is deemed usable at the time of the client's death.

21. 1. The nurse should not ask "why" the client does something; this is judgmental.
    2. This answer option is giving erroneous information because it is not illegal. The Final Exit Network, originally called the Hemlock Society, is an organization that supports members in states with death with dignity or Physician Aid in Dying (PAD) laws and support and education in all states.
    3. This question is not relevant to the situation.
    4. **This question must be asked because some religious belief supports the view that suicide is a violation of natural law and the laws of God. The tenets of the Final Exit Network, originally named the Hemlock Society, are in direct opposition to these beliefs.**

22. 1. Many Middle Eastern cultures practice this, but the Caucasian culture does not.
    2. Caucasians, as a culture, do not necessarily have a preference, but this does not affect culturally sensitive health care.
    3. Frequently, Caucasians do not like to talk about death and dying, but this is an individual preference of the client and the nurse should allow the discussion.
    4. **The Western Caucasian society values autonomy and truth telling in individual decision making.**

23. 1. **The client's EHR is a legal document, and if a mistake occurs, it should be acknowledged by flagging the erroneous entry per facility protocol and documenting the correct information. Both the original error and the correction should be documented for future reference. Overwriting of the entry could be considered the improper alteration of the medical record.**
    2. This is the correct method for disposing of any paper that has client information on it that is not a part of the client's permanent medical record.
    3. This is the correct method to document a medication not administered to the client. The nurse should include a comment in the MAR explaining why the medication was not administered (i.e., digoxin not given due to bradycardia).
    4. All narcotics not administered to the client must be verified when being wasted and then documented.

24. 1. **The nurse must support the client's culture. Potpourri provides the scent without having the burning incense, which is against fire code, and this is a compromise that supports the client's culture.**
    2. Having the door shut does not matter; open flames are not allowed in any health-care facility.
    3. This is not necessarily true, and if it is part of the cultural beliefs about dying, then the nurse should medicate the client if nauseated.
    4. This is a fact, but the nurse should attempt to compromise and support the client and family's cultural needs, especially at the time of death.

25. 1. There is no need to report this action to the state board; this is not malpractice.
    2. This action does not warrant the nurse being terminated.
    3. **The Code states, "The nurse owes the same duty to self as to others, including the responsibility to preserve integrity and safety." Therefore, if the nurse realizes TB could be contracted if unprotected mouth-to-mouth resuscitation is performed, then not doing this action does not violate the Code of Ethics.**
    4. The ANA cannot discipline nurses; it is a voluntary nurse's organization.

26. **Correct order is 4, 3, 2, 1, 5.**
    4. The nurse should calm and reassure the spouse over the telephone.
    3. The nurse should then visit the client immediately to assess the change in condition.
    2. Restlessness and agitation are symptoms of a lack of oxygen. Therefore, calling the medical equipment company to send oxygen would be the next intervention.
    1. Terminal restlessness is difficult for the family to watch and the client to experience, so antianxiety medications would be the next logical intervention.
    5. Referral to the chaplain is needed because the death may be imminent.

# Pharmacology

19

*Learning is a weightless treasure you can always carry easily.*

—Chinese Proverb

This chapter contains test-taking hints specific to pharmacology-related questions. The general hints in Chapter 1 and answer rationales throughout this book are also immensely beneficial. Remember, however, test-taking hints are useful for discriminating information and choosing among answer options, but they cannot substitute for knowledge. Nurses must be familiar with medications—their specific uses, modes of administration, side effects, possible adverse reactions, and ways to gauge their effectiveness in treating specific disorders and diseases.

## KEYWORDS

| | |
|---|---|
| Agranulocytosis | Echinacea |
| Ataxia | Mydriasis |
| Doll's eye test | Tetany |

## TEST-TAKING HINTS FOR PHARMACOLOGY QUESTIONS

The test taker must know medications and memorize specific facts, including their actions, uses, dosages, adverse reactions, side effects, and methods of administration (for example, oral, intravenous, intramuscular). This knowledge is part of administering medications safely. There are some specific tips to assist the test taker in learning about medications, and they will apply to the questions in this chapter.

The NCLEX-RN® examination provides the generic name, not the brand or trade name, of medications. Some questions may have the general classifications of the medications. The student nurse should focus on learning the medications primarily by their generic name. The suffix of the word can give the test taker a hint as to the drug classification, such as "ol," atenolol or propranolol—Tenormin and Inderal—respectively, are both beta blockers and as such have similar administration guidelines. Other suffixes include "il" for ACE inhibitors, "pam" for benzodiazepines, "toin" for hydantoins, and "parin" for low molecular weight heparins.

It is helpful to learn the different classifications of drugs—for example, diuretics, antibiotics, nonsteroidal anti-inflammatory drugs (NSAIDs). The test taker should learn the actions, uses, side effects, adverse effects, possible interactions, and methods of administration (for example, oral, intravenous, intramuscular) of these drugs. Generally speaking, the various drugs in each classification will be similar in these characteristics.

Avoid overgeneralizing drug classifications. For example, do not combine all medications administered for hypertension in the same category. Angiotensin-converting enzyme (ACE) inhibitors, beta blockers, and calcium channel blockers, for example, are all used to treat hypertension, but they are different categories of medications, acting differently in the body and producing different effects. Diuretics and oral medications for diabetes mellitus fall into different specific classifications and must be learned by the specific classification. Each classification has effects on the body, side effects, and adverse effects, and each has steps the nurse must take before administering the medication.

When administering medications for a group of clients, the test taker must realize time is a real problem. The nurse will be unable to look up 50 to 60 medications and administer them all within the dosing time frame, so it is imperative that nurses learn the most common medications.

One tip for learning the medications is for the test taker to complete drug memory cards or flashcards. Making the drug cards by hand is helpful because, in making the card, the test taker must read about the drug, decide which information is pertinent, and finally write the pertinent information on the card. The multifaceted redundancy will assist the test taker in memorizing the information. If preprinted drug cards are used, be sure to highlight the important information for ease of use and retention.

## Drug Cards

When the test taker is deciding which information is the most important to include or highlight on a drug card, there are five questions that can be used as a guide.

1. **What is the scientific rationale for administering the medication?**
   - Why is this intervention being implemented?
   - What classification of medication is the nurse administering to the client?
   - Why is this client receiving this medication?
   - What action does the medication have in the body?

The answers to these questions provide the scientific rationale for administering the medication. It is also important to remember that in many cases medication may be in a particular classification, but the client is receiving the medication for a different reason—for example, the anticonvulsant divalproex sodium (Depakote) is also administered as an antimania medication.

### EXAMPLE 1

Digoxin (Lanoxin) 0.25 mg PO

- The classification of this medication is a cardiac glycoside.
- The medication is administered to clients diagnosed with congestive heart failure or rapid atrial fibrillation.
- Cardiac glycosides increase the contractility of the heart and decrease the heart rate.

### EXAMPLE 2

Furosemide (Lasix) 40 mg an intravenous push (IVP).

- The classification of this medication is a loop diuretic.
- The medication is administered to clients diagnosed with essential hypertension.
- This medication helps remove excess fluid from the body.
- Loop diuretics remove water from the kidneys along with potassium.

**2. When should the administration of medication be questioned?**
- Does the medication have a therapeutic serum level?
- Which vital signs must be monitored?
- Which physiological parameters should be monitored when the medication is being administered?

The answers to these questions will provide the nurse with information on which to base a decision regarding which medication orders should be questioned.

## EXAMPLE 1

Digoxin (Lanoxin)

- Is the apical pulse less than 60 bpm?
- Is the digoxin level within the therapeutic range?
- Is the potassium level within normal range?

## EXAMPLE 2

Furosemide (Lasix)

- Is the potassium level within normal range?
- Does the client have clinical manifestations of dehydration?
- Is the client's blood pressure below 90/60?

**3. How can the nurse ensure the safety of the administration of medications?**
- What interventions must the client be taught to ensure the medication is administered safely in the hospital?
- What interventions must the client be taught to ensure medication is taken safely at home?

## EXAMPLE 1

Digoxin (Lanoxin)

- Explain to the client the importance of getting serum levels regularly.
- Teach the client to take the radial pulse and take the medication only if the pulse is greater than 60.
- Tell the client to take the medication as ordered and to notify the health-care provider (HCP) of any failure to comply.

## EXAMPLE 2

Furosemide (Lasix)

- Teach the client about orthostatic hypotension.
- Instruct the client to drink water to replace insensible fluid loss.
- Because the medication is an IVP, for how many minutes should the medication be pushed? What primary IV is hanging? Is it compatible with Lasix?

**4. What are the possible side effects and possible adverse reactions associated with a specific medication?**
- What are the side effects of this medication?
- What are the possible adverse reactions to this medication?

Side effects are not expected but are not unusual. Adverse reactions are any events that require notifying the HCP or discontinuing the medication.

### EXAMPLE 1

Digoxin (Lanoxin)

- Inform the client of the clinical manifestations of toxicity, which are nausea, vomiting, anorexia, and yellow haze.

### EXAMPLE 2

Furosemide (Lasix)

- Side effects include dizziness and light-headedness.
- Adverse effects include hypokalemia and tinnitus (if Lasix is administered too quickly).

**5. How can the effectiveness of medications be monitored?**

### EXAMPLE 1

Digoxin (Lanoxin)

- Have the clinical manifestations of congestive heart failure improved?
- Is the client able to breathe easier?
- How many pillows does the client need to sleep when lying down?
- Is the client able to perform activities of daily living without shortness of breath?

### EXAMPLE 2

Furosemide (Lasix)

- Is the client's urinary output greater than the intake?
- Has the client lost any weight?
- Does the client have sacral or peripheral edema?
- Does the client have jugular vein distention?
- Is the client's blood pressure decreased?

## Sample Drug Cards

| Classification of Drug: | Route: |
|---|---|
| Action of Drug: | |
| Uses: | |
| Nursing Implications (When would I question giving the medication?) | |
| How will I monitor to see if it is working? | |
| Side Effects: | |
| Teaching Needs: | |
| Drug Names: | |

It is suggested the test taker complete these cards using a pharmacology textbook rather than a drug handbook because most test questions come from a pharmacology textbook.

## EXAMPLE 1: DIGOXIN

| Classification of Drug: **Cardiac Glycosides**   Route: **PO/IV** | |
|---|---|
| Action: | Positive inotropic action; increases the force of ventricular contraction and thereby increases cardiac output; slows the heart, allowing for increased filling time. |
| Uses: | Congestive heart failure and rapid atrial cardiac dysrhythmias. |
| Nursing Implications: | Check apical pulse for 1 full minute, hold if less than 60. Check digoxin level (0.5–2 normal; greater than 2 is toxic). Check K$^+$ level (3.5–5.5 mEq/L is normal). Hypokalemia is the most common cause of dysrhythmias in clients receiving digoxin. Monitor for clinical manifestations of CHF, crackles in lungs, I & O, edema. Question if the AP is less than 60 or abnormal laboratory values. |
| | IVP more than **5 minutes**: maintenance dose 0.125–0.25 mg q day. |
| Effective: | Breathing improves, activity tolerance improves, atrial rate decreases. |
| Side Effects: | TOXIC = YELLOW HAZE OR NAUSEA AND VOMITING, VENTRICULAR RATE DECREASES. IF A DIURETIC IS GIVEN SIMULTANEOUSLY, IT MIGHT INCREASE THE LIKELIHOOD OF HYPOKALEMIA. |
| Teaching Needs: | Take pulse and hold digoxin if the pulse is less than 60 and notify HCP. |
| K$^+$ replacement: | Eat food high in K$^+$ or may need supplemental K$^+$. |
| | Report weight gain of 3 lb or more. |
| Brand or Trade names: | Lanoxin, Lanoxicaps, Toloxin |

## EXAMPLE 2: FUROSEMIDE

| Classification of Drug: **Loop Diuretic**   Route: **PO/IVP** | |
|---|---|
| Actions: | Blocks reabsorption of sodium and chloride in the loop of Henle, which prevents the passive reabsorption of water and leads to diuresis. |
| Uses: | CHF, fluid volume overload, pulmonary edema, HTN. |
| Nursing Implications: | I & O, monitor K$^+$ level, check skin turgor, monitor for leg cramps, provide K$^+$-rich foods or supplements, give early in the day to prevent nocturia. If giving IVP: Give at the prescribed rate, ototoxic if given faster. |
| Effective: | Decrease in weight, output greater than intake, less edema, lungs sound clear. |
| Side Effects: | Hypokalemia, muscle cramps, hyponatremia, dehydration. |
| Teaching Needs: | Take early in the day. |
| | Eat foods high in K$^+$. |
| Brand or Trade Names: | Lasix |

# MEDICATIONS ADMINISTRATION IN A MEDICAL-SURGICAL SETTING COMPREHENSIVE EXAMINATION

The test taker is encouraged to use the clinical judgment guide previously provided when taking the following medication test. The test is comprehensive for medications administered in a medical-surgical setting.

1. The client asks the clinic nurse about taking 2,000 mg of ascorbic acid (vitamin C) a day to prevent getting a cold. On which scientific rationale should the nurse base the response?
   1. Vitamin C in this dosage will help cure a common cold.
   2. This vitamin must be taken with echinacea to be effective.
   3. This dose of vitamin C is not high enough to help prevent colds.
   4. Megadoses of vitamin C may cause crystals to form in the urine.

2. The client recently has had a myocardial infarction (MI). Which medication should the nurse anticipate the health-care provider (HCP) recommending to **prevent** another heart attack?
   1. Nonsteroidal anti-inflammatory drug.
   2. Low-dose acetylsalicylic acid.
   3. An anticoagulant medication.
   4. An iron supplement.

3. The client diagnosed with essential hypertension calls the clinic and tells the nurse she needs something for the flu. Which information should the nurse tell the client?
   1. OTC medications for the flu should not be taken because of your hypertension.
   2. If OTC medications do not relieve symptoms within 3 days, contact the HCP.
   3. Tell the client to ask the pharmacist to recommend an OTC medication for the flu.
   4. Make an appointment for the client to receive the influenza vaccine.

4. Which laboratory test should the nurse monitor for the client receiving an intravenous steroid?
   1. Potassium level.
   2. Sputum culture and sensitivity.
   3. Glucose level.
   4. Arterial blood gases.

5. The client diagnosed with asthma is prescribed cromolyn. Which statement by the client indicates the need for **further** teaching?
   1. "I will take two puffs of my inhaler before I exercise."
   2. "I will rinse my mouth with water after taking the medication."

3. "After inhaling the medication, I will hold my breath for 10 seconds."
   4. "When I start to wheeze, I will use my inhaler immediately."

6. The client diagnosed with methicillin-resistant *Staphylococcus aureus* (MRSA) is receiving vancomycin. Peak and trough levels are ordered for the dose the nurse is administering. Which **priority** intervention should the nurse implement?
   1. Ask if the client has had any diarrhea.
   2. Monitor the aminoglycoside peak level.
   3. Determine if the trough level has been drawn.
   4. Check the client's culture and sensitivity report.

7. The nurse is caring for an older client 8 hours postoperative hip replacement who is reporting incisional pain. Which intervention is a **priority** for this client?
   1. Assist the client in sitting in the bedside chair.
   2. Initiate pain medication at the lowest dose.
   3. Assess the client's pupil size and accommodation.
   4. Monitor the client's urinary output hourly.

8. The client is diagnosed with pernicious anemia. Which HCP order should the nurse anticipate in treating this condition?
   1. Subcutaneous iron dextran.
   2. Intramuscular vitamin $B_{12}$.
   3. Intravenous folic acid.
   4. Oral thiamine medication.

9. The client diagnosed with type 2 diabetes mellitus is prescribed glyburide. Which statement indicates the client **understands** the medication teaching?
   1. "I should carry some hard candy when I go walking."
   2. "I must take my insulin injection every morning."
   3. "There are no side effects I need to worry about."
   4. "This medication will make my muscles absorb insulin."

10. The unlicensed assistive personnel (UAP) reports the client's glucometer reading is 380 mg/dL. The client is on regular sliding-scale insulin which reads:

| Glucometer Reading | Units of Insulin |
|---|---|
| Less than 150 | 0 |
| 151–250 | 5 |
| 251–350 | 8 |
| 351–450 | 10 |
| 451+ | Notify the HCP |

How much insulin should the RN administer to the client?

| units |
|---|

11. The nurse administers 18 units of insulin isophane at 1630. Which **priority** intervention should the nurse implement?
    1. Monitor the client's hemoglobin $A_{1c}$.
    2. Make sure the client eats the evening meal.
    3. Check the a.c. blood glucometer reading.
    4. Ensure the client eats a snack.

12. The nurse is administering the following 1800 medications. Which medication should the nurse **question** before administering?
    1. The sliding-scale insulin to the client just released to have the evening meal.
    2. The antibiotic to the client 1 day postoperative exploratory abdominal surgery.
    3. Metformin to the client having a CT scan with contrast dye in the morning.
    4. Pantoprazole to the client diagnosed with peptic ulcer disease.

13. The nurse is administering insulin glargine to the client at 2200. The nurse asks the charge nurse to check the dosage. Which action should the charge nurse implement?
    1. Ask the nurse why the insulin is being given late.
    2. Check the MAR versus the dosage in the syringe.
    3. Instruct the nurse to complete a medication error form.
    4. Have the nurse notify the health-care provider.

14. The nurse is preparing to administer levothyroxine to the client diagnosed with hypothyroidism. Which assessment data would indicate the client is receiving **too much** medication?
    1. Bradypnea and weight gain.
    2. Lethargy and hypotension.
    3. Irritability and tachycardia.
    4. Normothermia and constipation.

15. The client is receiving a continuous intravenous infusion of heparin. Based on the most recent laboratory data:

| Laboratory Test | Client Results | Normal Values |
|---|---|---|
| Prothrombin time (PT) | 13.2 (Control: 12.1) | 10–13 seconds |
| Partial thromboplastin time (PTT) | 72 (Control: 39) | 25–35 seconds |
| International normalized ratio (INR) | 1.3 | 0.9–1.1 w/o anticoagulation therapy 2–3 with therapy 2.5–3.5 if the client has a mechanical heart valve |

Which action should the nurse implement?
    1. Continue to monitor the infusion.
    2. Prepare to administer protamine sulfate.
    3. Have the laboratory reconfirm the results.
    4. Assess the client for bleeding.

16. The older client is admitted to the emergency department from a long-term care facility. The client has multiple ecchymotic areas on the body. The client is receiving digoxin, furosemide, warfarin, and alprazolam. Which order should the nurse request from the HCP?
    1. A STAT serum potassium level.
    2. An order to admit to the hospital for observation.
    3. An order to administer diazepam intravenous push.
    4. A STAT international normalized ratio (INR).

17. The client diagnosed with postmenopausal osteoporosis is prescribed alendronate sodium. Which discharge instruction should the nurse discuss with the client? **Select all that apply.**
    1. The medication must be taken with the breakfast meal only.
    2. Remain upright for at least 30 minutes after taking medication.
    3. The tablet should be chewed thoroughly before swallowing.
    4. Stress the importance of having monthly hormone levels.
    5. Notify the health-care provider for new or worsening heartburn.

18. The nurse is administering morning medications. Which medication should the nurse administer **first**?
    1. The daily digoxin to the client diagnosed with congestive heart failure.
    2. The loop diuretic to the client with a serum potassium level of 3.1 mEq/L.
    3. Sucralfate to the client diagnosed with peptic ulcer disease.
    4. Methylprednisolone IVP to a client diagnosed with chronic lung disease.

19. The HCP ordered an angiotensin-converting enzyme (ACE) inhibitor for the client diagnosed with MI. Which statement **best** explains the rationale for administering this medication to this client?
    1. It will help prevent the development of congestive heart failure.
    2. This medication will help decrease the client's blood pressure.
    3. ACE inhibitors increase the contractility of the heart muscle.
    4. They will help decrease the development of atherosclerosis.

20. The client is receiving enalapril. When would the nurse **question** administering this medication?
    1. The client is not receiving potassium supplements.
    2. The client reports a persistent irritating cough.
    3. The blood pressure for two consecutive readings is 110/70.
    4. The client's urinary output is 400 mL for the last 8 hours.

21. The nurse is preparing to administer the morning dose of digoxin to a client diagnosed with congestive heart failure. Which data would indicate the medication is **effective**?
    1. The apical heart rate is 72 beats per minute.
    2. The client denies having any anorexia or nausea.
    3. The client's blood pressure is 120/80 mm Hg.
    4. The client's lungs sounds are clear bilaterally.

22. The client diagnosed with multiple sclerosis (MS) is receiving baclofen. Which information should the nurse teach the client and family?
    1. The importance of tapering off when discontinuing the medication.
    2. Baclofen may cause diarrhea, so the client should take antidiarrheal medication.
    3. The client should not be allowed to drive alone while taking this medication.
    4. The client should have follow-up visits to obtain a monthly white blood cell count.

23. The nurse is administering digoxin to the client diagnosed with congestive heart failure. Which interventions should the nurse implement? **Select all that apply**.
    1. Check the apical heart rate for 1 full minute.
    2. Monitor the client's serum sodium level.
    3. Teach the client how to take a radial pulse.
    4. Evaluate the client's serum digoxin level.
    5. Assess the client for buffalo hump and moon face.

24. The client's vital signs are populated in the vital sign flowsheet below. Which medication would the nurse **question** administering?

| Vital Sign Flowsheet | Client Results | Normal Values |
|---|---|---|
| Blood pressure | 108/72 | 100–119 mmHg systolic 60–80 mmHg diastolic |
| Temperature | 99.2°F | Oral: 98°F (36.7°C) |
| Pulse | 59 | 60–100 beats/min |
| Respirations | 20 | 12–20 breaths/min |

    1. Theophylline.
    2. Propranolol.
    3. Ampicillin.
    4. Diltiazem.

25. The client diagnosed with end-stage renal disease is a Jehovah's Witness. The HCP orders erythropoietin subcutaneously for anemia. Which action should the nurse take?
    1. Question this order because of the client's religion.
    2. Encourage the client to talk to the minister.
    3. Administer the medication subcutaneously as ordered.
    4. Obtain the informed consent before administering.

26. The older male client is admitted for severe acute diverticulitis. He has been taking alprazolam for nervousness three to four times a day prn for 6 years. Which intervention should the nurse implement **first**?
    1. Prepare to administer an intravenous antianxiety medication.
    2. Notify the HCP to obtain an order for the client's alprazolam prn.
    3. Explain alprazolam causes addiction and he should quit taking it.
    4. Assess for clinical manifestations of medication withdrawal.

27. The nurse is administering an ophthalmic drop to the right eye. Which anatomical location would be **correct** when administering eyedrops?

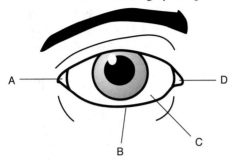

   1. A
   2. B
   3. C
   4. D

28. The nurse is administering furosemide to the client diagnosed with essential hypertension. Which assessment data would warrant the nurse to **question** administering the medication?
   1. The client's potassium level is 4.2 mEq/L.
   2. The client's urinary output is greater than the intake.
   3. The client has tented skin turgor and dry mucous membranes.
   4. The client has lost 2 pounds in the last 24 hours.

29. The client had a kidney transplant and told the nurse about taking St. John's wort for depression. Which action should the nurse take **first**?
   1. Praise the client for taking the initiative to treat the depression.
   2. Remain nonjudgmental about the client's alternative treatments.
   3. Refer the client to a psychologist for counseling for depression.
   4. Instruct the client to quit taking the medication immediately.

30. The nurse is administering an antacid to a client diagnosed with gastroesophageal reflux disease (GERD). Which statement **best** describes the scientific rationale for administering this medication?
   1. This medication will suppress gastric acid secretion.
   2. This medication will decrease the gastric pH.
   3. This medication will coat the stomach lining.
   4. This medication interferes with prostaglandin production.

31. The client is diagnosed with essential hypertension and is receiving a calcium channel blocker. Which assessment data would **warrant** the nurse **holding** the client's medication?

   1. The client's oral temperature is 102°F.
   2. The client reports a dry, nonproductive cough.
   3. The client's blood pressure reading is 106/76.
   4. The client reports being dizzy when getting out of bed.

32. The nurse has received the morning report and has the following medications due or being requested. In which order should the nurse administer the medications? **Rank in order of priority**.
   1. Administer furosemide IVP daily to a client diagnosed with heart failure and is dyspneic on exertion.
   2. Administer morphine IVP prn to a client diagnosed with lower back pain reporting pain at a "10" on a 1-to-10 scale.
   3. Administer neostigmine PO to a client diagnosed with myasthenia gravis.
   4. Administer lidocaine IVP prn to a client in normal sinus rhythm with multifocal premature ventricular contractions.
   5. Administer vancomycin to a client diagnosed with a *Staphylococcus* infection and a trough level of 14 mg/dL.

33. The nurse is preparing to administer the initial dose of an antibiotic in the emergency department. Which interventions should the nurse implement? **Select all that apply**.
   1. Assess for drug allergies.
   2. Collect needed specimens for culture.
   3. Check the client's armband.
   4. Ask the client for a birth date.
   5. Draw peak and trough levels.

34. For which client should the nurse **question** administering oxybutynin?
   1. The client diagnosed with an overactive bladder.
   2. The client diagnosed with type 2 diabetes.
   3. The client diagnosed with glaucoma.
   4. The client diagnosed with peripheral vascular disease.

35. The nurse is administering a topical ointment to the client's rash on the right leg. Which interventions should the nurse implement? **Rank in order of performance**.
   1. Perform hand hygiene and don nonsterile gloves.
   2. Cleanse the skin site and dry thoroughly.
   3. Check the client's ID band and have the client state name and date of birth.
   4. Explain the procedure and purpose to the client.
   5. Apply the medication to the rash.

36. The client is exhibiting multifocal premature ventricular contractions. Which antidysrhythmic medication should the nurse anticipate the HCP ordering for this dysrhythmia?
    1. Adenosine.
    2. Epinephrine.
    3. Atropine.
    4. Amiodarone.

37. The client in the intensive care department is receiving 2 mcg/kg/min of dopamine. Which interventions should the nurse include in the plan of care? **Select all that apply**.
    1. Monitor the client's blood pressure every 2 hours.
    2. Palpate the client's peripheral pulses often.
    3. Use a urometer to assess hourly output.
    4. Ensure the IV tubing is not exposed to the light.
    5. Assess IV site for extravasation every hour.

38. The client is receiving fibrinolytic therapy (thrombolytic therapy) for a diagnosed MI. Which assessment data indicate the therapy is **successful**?
    1. The client's ST segment is becoming more depressed.
    2. The client is exhibiting reperfusion dysrhythmias.
    3. The client's cardiac isoenzyme CK-MB is not elevated.
    4. The client's platelet count is increased 2 hours post-MI.

39. The client diagnosed with arthritis is self-medicating with acetylsalicylic acid. Which complication should the nurse discuss with the client?
    1. Tinnitus.
    2. Diarrhea.
    3. Tetany.
    4. Paresthesia.

40. The client is receiving a loop diuretic for congestive heart failure. Which medication would the nurse expect the client to be receiving while taking this medication?
    1. A potassium supplement.
    2. A cardiac glycoside.
    3. An ACE inhibitor.
    4. A potassium cation.

41. The nurse is reviewing laboratory values for the female client diagnosed with cancer. Based on the laboratory report, which biologic response modifier would the nurse anticipate administering to the client?

| Laboratory Test | Client Values | Normal Values |
|---|---|---|
| Red blood cells | 4.11 | M: $4.21–5.81 \times 10^6$/microL<br>F: $3.61–5.11 \times 10^6$/microL |
| Hemoglobin | 12.2 | M: 14.5–17.5 g/dL<br>F: 11.7–15.5 g/dL |
| Hematocrit | 37 | M: 42%–52%<br>F: 34%–48% |
| White blood cells | 2 | $4.5–11.1 \times 10^3$/microL |
| Platelets | 160 | $140–400 \times 10^3$/microL |

1. Interferon.
2. Filgrastim.
3. Oprelvekin.
4. Epoetin alfa.

42. The client admitted with pneumonia is taking azathioprine. Which question should the nurse ask the client regarding this medication?
    1. "Do you know this medication has to be tapered off when discontinued?"
    2. "Have you been exposed to viral hepatitis B or C recently?"
    3. "Why are you taking this medication, and how long have you taken it?"
    4. "Do you have a lot of allergies or sensitivities to different medications?"

43. The older male client is in a long-term care facility. If the client does not have a daily bowel movement in the morning he requests a cathartic, bisacodyl. Which action is **most important** for the nurse to take?
    1. Ensure the client gets a cathartic daily.
    2. Discuss the complications of a daily cathartic.
    3. Encourage the client to increase fiber in the diet.
    4. Refuse to administer the medication to the client.

44. The client received naloxone following a procedure. Which action by the nurse has the **highest priority**?
    1. Document the occurrence in the nurse's notes.
    2. Prepare to administer narcotic medication IV.
    3. Administer oxygen via nasal cannula.
    4. Assess the client every 15 to 30 minutes.

45. The client diagnosed with chronic obstructive pulmonary disease is being discharged and is prescribed prednisone. Which scientific rationale supports why the nurse instructs the client to taper off the medication?
    1. The pituitary gland must adjust to the decreasing dose.
    2. The beta cells of the pancreas have to start secreting insulin.
    3. This will allow the adrenal gland time to start functioning.
    4. The thyroid gland will have to start producing cortisol.

46. The client is diagnosed with tuberculosis and prescribed rifampin and isoniazid (INH). Which instruction is **most important** for the public health nurse to discuss with the client?
    1. The client will have to take the medications for 6 to 12 months.
    2. The client will have to stay in isolation as long as medications are taken.
    3. Explain the client cannot eat any type of pork products while taking the medication.
    4. The urine may turn turquoise in color, but this is an expected occurrence and harmless.

47. The employee health RN is observing a student nurse administer a Mantoux tuberculin skin test with purified protein derivative (PPD) to a new employee. Which behavior would **warrant immediate** intervention by the employee health nurse?
    1. The student nurse inserts the needle at a 45-degree angle.
    2. The student nurse cleanses the forearm with alcohol.
    3. The student nurse circles the injection site with ink.
    4. The student nurse instructs the employee to return in 3 days.

48. The female client diagnosed with herpes simplex 2 is prescribed valacyclovir. Which information should the nurse discuss with the client? **Select all that apply**.
    1. Do not take this medication while pregnant; it will harm the fetus.
    2. The medication does not prevent the transmission of the disease.
    3. There are no side effects when taking this medication by mouth.
    4. The client should get monthly liver function study tests.
    5. Drink plenty of fluids while taking this medication.

49. The client diagnosed with coronary artery disease is prescribed an HMG-CoA reductase inhibitor to help reduce the cholesterol level. Which assessment data should be reported to the HCP?
    1. Reports of flatulence.
    2. Weight loss of 2 pounds.
    3. Reports of muscle pain.
    4. No bowel movement for 2 days.

50. The client diagnosed with coronary artery disease is prescribed one low-dose acetylsalicylic acid (ASA) a day. Which instructions should the nurse provide the client concerning this medication? **Select all that apply**.
    1. Take the medication on an empty stomach.
    2. Do not crush or chew enteric-coated tablets.
    3. Do not take acetaminophen while taking this drug.
    4. If experiencing joint pain, notify the HCP.
    5. Notify the HCP if stools become dark and tarry.

51. The nurse is preparing to administer phenytoin, 100 mg intravenous push, to the client diagnosed with a head injury with an IV of $D_5W$ at 50 mL/hr. Which intervention should the nurse implement?
    1. Flush the IV tubing before and after with normal saline.
    2. Administer the medication if the phenytoin level is 22 mcg/mL.
    3. Push the phenytoin intravenously rapidly over 1 minute.
    4. Expect the intravenous tubing to turn cloudy when infusing the medication.

52. The client diagnosed with epilepsy is being discharged from the hospital with a prescription for phenytoin by mouth. Which discharge instructions should the nurse discuss with the client? **Select all that apply**.
    1. The client should purchase a self-monitoring phenytoin machine.
    2. The client should see the dentist at least every 6 months.
    3. The client should never drive when taking this medication.
    4. The client should not take phenytoin within 3 hours of taking an antacid.
    5. The client should drink no more than one glass of wine a day.

53. The female client diagnosed with *Trichomonas vaginalis* is prescribed metronidazole. Which statement indicates the client **understands** the discharge teaching? **Select all that apply**.
    1. "I will not be able to drink any alcohol while taking this drug."
    2. "My boyfriend will need to take this same medication."

3. "I cannot transmit the disease through oral sex."
4. "I must make sure I take all the pills no matter how I feel."
5. "I should call my doctor if I get a rash."

54. The client diagnosed with angina must receive a 2-inch nitroglycerin paste application. Which interventions should the nurse implement? **Select all that apply**.
    1. Wear gloves when administering.
    2. Remove the old nitroglycerin paste paper.
    3. Apply the paper on a hairy spot.
    4. Put medication only on the legs.
    5. Report any headache to the HCP.

55. The nurse is hanging 1,000 mL of IV fluids to run for 8 hours. The intravenous tubing is a microdrip. How many drops per minute (gtt/min) should the IV rate be set?

    > _____ gtt/min

56. The client diagnosed with osteoarthritis is prescribed an NSAID. Which intervention should the nurse implement?
    1. Time the medication to be given with meals.
    2. Notify the HCP if abdominal striae develop.
    3. Do not administer if the oral temperature is greater than 102°F.
    4. Monitor liver function tests and renal studies.

57. The client in the intensive care department has a nasogastric tube for continuous feedings. The nurse is preparing to administer nifedipine extended release (XL) via the NG tube. Which procedure should the nurse follow?
    1. Crush the medication and dissolve it in water.
    2. Administer and flush the NG tube with cranberry juice.
    3. Give the medication orally with pudding.
    4. Do not administer the medication and notify the HCP.

58. The employee health nurse is discussing hepatitis B vaccines with new employees. Which statement **best** describes the proper administration of the hepatitis B vaccine?
    1. The vaccine must be administered once a year.
    2. Two milliliters of vaccine should be given in each hip.
    3. The vaccine is given in three doses over a 6-month time period.
    4. The vaccine is administered intradermally into the deltoid muscle.

59. The UAP reported an intake of 1,000 mL and urinary output of 1,500 mL for a client receiving a thiazide diuretic. Which nursing task could the RN delegate to the nursing assistant?
    1. Instruct the UAP to restrict the client's fluid intake.
    2. Request the UAP to insert a Foley catheter with a urometer.
    3. Tell the UAP urinary outputs are no longer needed.
    4. Ask the UAP to document fluids on the I & O record at the bedside.

60. The charge nurse is observing the new graduate administering a fentanyl patch to a client diagnosed with cancer. Which action by the new graduate **requires intervention** by the RN charge nurse?
    1. The new graduate documents the date and time on the patch.
    2. The new graduate removes the patch 24 hours after it is placed on the client.
    3. The new graduate rotates the application site on the client's body.
    4. The new graduate checks the client's name band and date of birth.

61. The 68-year-old client is admitted to the emergency department with reports of slurred speech, right-sided weakness, and ataxia. The emergency department physician ordered thrombolytic therapy for the client. Which action should the nurse implement **first**?
    1. Administer thrombolytic therapy via the protocol.
    2. Send the client for a STAT CT of the head.
    3. Arrange for admission to the intensive care unit (ICU).
    4. Check to determine if the client is cross-sensitive to the thrombolytic.

62. The client is admitted to the burn unit and prescribed pantoprazole. Which statement **best** supports the scientific rationale for administering this medication to a client diagnosed with a severe burn?
    1. This medication will help prevent a stress ulcer.
    2. This medication will help prevent systemic infections.
    3. This medication will provide continuous vasoconstriction.
    4. This medication will stimulate new skin growth.

63. The nurse administered an IV broad-spectrum antibiotic scheduled every 6 hours to the client diagnosed with a systemic infection at 0800. At 1000, the culture and sensitivity prompted the HCP to change the IV antibiotic. When transcribing the new antibiotic order, when would the **initial dose** be administered?
    1. Schedule the dose for 1400.
    2. Schedule the dose for the next day.
    3. Check with the HCP to determine when to start.
    4. Administer the dose within 1 hour of the order.

64. The client is receiving a continuous heparin drip, 20,000 units/500 mL D$_5$W, at 23 mL/min. How many units of heparin is the client receiving an hour?

    | units/hr |
    |---|

65. The client diagnosed with epilepsy is prescribed carbamazepine. Which discharge instruction should the nurse include in the teaching? **Select all that apply.**
    1. Wear SPF 30 sunscreen when outside.
    2. Obtain regular serum drug levels.
    3. Be sure to floss teeth daily.
    4. Instruct the client to take tub baths only.
    5. Avoid grapefruit and grapefruit juice.

66. The client diagnosed with bipolar disorder has been taking valproic acid for 4 months. Which assessment data would **warrant** the medication being **discontinued**?
    1. The client's eyes are yellow.
    2. The client has mood swings.
    3. The client's BP is 164/94.
    4. The client's serum level is 75 mcg/mL.

67. The client is reporting nausea, and the nurse administers promethazine, IM. Which intervention has **priority** for this client after administering this medication?
    1. Instruct the client to call the nurse before getting out of bed.
    2. Evaluate the effectiveness of the medication.
    3. Assess the client's abdomen and bowel sounds.
    4. Tell the client not to eat or drink for at least 1 hour.

68. The client on bedrest is receiving enoxaparin. Which anatomical site is recommended for administering this medication?
    1. The abdominal wall 1 inch away from the umbilicus.
    2. The vastus lateralis with a 23-gauge needle.
    3. In the deltoid area, subcutaneously.
    4. In the anterolateral abdomen.

69. The male client comes to the emergency department and reports he stepped on a rusty nail at home about 2 hours ago. Which question would be **most important** for the nurse to ask during the admission assessment?
    1. "What have you used to clean the puncture site?"
    2. "Did you bring the nail with you so we can culture it?"
    3. "Do you remember when you had your last tetanus shot?"
    4. "Are you able to put any weight on your foot?"

70. The nurse is administering carbidopa and levodopa to the client. Which assessment should the nurse perform to determine if the medication is **effective**?
    1. Assess the client's muscle strength.
    2. Assess for cogwheel rigidity.
    3. Assess the carbidopa serum level.
    4. Assess the client's blood pressure.

71. The client diagnosed with coronary artery disease is prescribed atorvastatin to help decrease the client's cholesterol level. Which interventions should the nurse discuss with the client? **Select all that apply.**
    1. The client should eat a low-cholesterol, low-fat diet.
    2. The client should take this medication with each meal.
    3. The client should take this medication in the evening.
    4. The client should monitor daily cholesterol levels.
    5. The client should take this medication at the same time each day.

72. The client is in end-stage renal disease and is receiving sodium polystyrene sulfonate via an enema. Which data indicate the medication is **effective**?
    1. The client has 30 mL/hr of urine output.
    2. The serum phosphorus level has decreased.
    3. The client is in normal sinus rhythm.
    4. The client's serum potassium level is 5 mEq/L.

73. The client has arterial blood gases populated in the ABG chart below. Which medication would the nurse prepare to administer based on the results?

| Arterial Blood Gas | Client Results | Normal Values |
|---|---|---|
| pH | 7.19 | 7.35–7.45 |
| PCO$_2$ | 33 | 35–45 mmHg |
| HCO$_3$ | 19 | 22–26 mEq/L |
| PaO$_2$ | 95 | 80–95 mmHg |

1. Intravenous sodium bicarbonate.
2. Oxygen via nasal cannula.
3. Epinephrine intravenous push.
4. Magnesium hydroxide orally.

74. The client diagnosed with migraine headaches is prescribed propranolol for prophylaxis. Which information should the nurse teach the client?
1. Instruct client to take the medication at the first sign of a headache.
2. Teach the client to take a radial pulse for 1 minute.
3. Explain this drug may make the client thirsty and have a dry mouth.
4. Discuss the need to increase artificial light in the home.

75. The client is experiencing supraventricular tachycardia (SVT). Which antidysrhythmic medication should the nurse prepare to administer?
1. Atropine.
2. Amiodarone.
3. Adenosine.
4. Dobutamine.

76. The client diagnosed with Parkinson's disease is taking levodopa and is experiencing an "on-off" phenomenon. Which action should the nurse take regarding this medication?
1. Document the occurrence and take no action.
2. Request the HCP to increase the dose of medication.
3. Discuss the client's imminent death as a result of this complication.
4. Explain this is a desired effect of the medication.

77. The client in the emergency department requires sutures for a laceration on the left leg. Which information is **most pertinent before** suturing the wound?
1. The client tells the nurse she has never had sutures.
2. The spouse refuses to leave the room during suturing.

3. The client shares she is scared of needles.
4. The client reports hives after having dental surgery.

78. The client diagnosed with diabetes insipidus is receiving vasopressin intranasally. Which assessment data indicate the medication is **effective**?
1. The client reports being able to breathe through the nose.
2. The client reports being thirsty all the time.
3. The client has a blood glucose of 99 mg/dL.
4. The client is urinating every 3 to 4 hours.

79. The nurse is administering an otic drop to the 45-year-old client. Which procedure should the nurse implement when administering the drops?
1. Place the drops when pulling the ear down and back.
2. Place the drops when pulling the ear up and back.
3. Place the drops in the lower conjunctival sac.
4. Place the drops in the inner canthus and apply pressure.

80. The male client diagnosed with a chronic urinary tract infection is prescribed trimethoprim-sulfamethoxazole. Which statement indicates the client **needs more** teaching?
1. "I will drink six to eight glasses of water a day."
2. "I am going to have to take this medication forever."
3. "I can stop taking this medication if there is no more burning."
4. "I may get diarrhea with this medication, but I can take loperamide hydrochloride."

81. The 54-year-old female client diagnosed with severe menopausal clinical manifestations is prescribed hormone replacement therapy (HRT). Which **secondary** health screening activity should the nurse recommend for HRT?
1. A Pap smear every 6 months.
2. A yearly mammogram.
3. A bone density test every 3 months.
4. A serum calcium level monthly.

82. The LPN is administering 0800 medications to clients on a medical floor. Which action by the LPN would **warrant immediate** intervention by the RN?
1. The LPN scores the medication to give the correct dose.
2. The LPN checks the client's armband and birth date.
3. The LPN administers sliding-scale insulin intramuscularly.
4. The LPN is 30 minutes late hanging the IV antibiotic.

83. The client diagnosed with end-stage renal disease is receiving aluminum hydroxide. Which assessment data indicate the medication is **effective**?
    1. The client denies reports of indigestion.
    2. The client is not experiencing burning on urination.
    3. The client has had a normal, soft bowel movement.
    4. The client's phosphate level has decreased.

84. The client diagnosed with diabetes mellitus type 2 is scheduled for bowel resection in the morning. Which medication should the nurse **question** administering to the client?
    1. Ticlopidine.
    2. Ticarcillin.
    3. Pioglitazone.
    4. Bisacodyl.

85. The client diagnosed with type 2 diabetes is diagnosed with gout and prescribed allopurinol. Which instructions should the nurse discuss when teaching about this medication? **Select all that apply**.
    1. The client will probably develop a red rash on the body.
    2. The client should drink 2 to 3 liters of water a day.
    3. The client should take this medication on an empty stomach.
    4. The client will need to decrease oral diabetic medications.
    5. The client should discontinue medication during an acute attack of gout.

86. The nurse realizes he did not administer a medication on time to the client diagnosed with an MI. Which action should the nurse implement?
    1. Administer the medication and take no further action.
    2. Notify the director of nurses of the medication error.
    3. Complete a medication error report form.
    4. Report the error to the Peer Review Committee.

87. The client is showing ventricular ectopy, and the HCP orders amiodarone intravenously. Which interventions should the nurse implement? **Select all that apply**.
    1. Monitor telemetry continuously.
    2. Assess the client's respiratory status.
    3. Evaluate the client's liver function studies.
    4. Confirm the original order with another nurse.
    5. Prepare to defibrillate the client at 200 joules.

88. The HCP has ordered an intramuscular antibiotic. After reconstituting the medication, the clinic nurse must administer 5.5 mL of the medication. Which action should the nurse implement **first** when administering this medication?
    1. Inform the HCP the amount of medication is too large.
    2. Administer the medication in the dorsogluteal muscle.
    3. Discard the medication in the sharps container.
    4. Divide the medication and give 2.75 mL in each hip.

89. The client diagnosed with status asthmaticus is prescribed intravenous aminophylline. Which assessment data would **warrant immediate** intervention?
    1. The theophylline level is 12 mcg/mL.
    2. The client has expiratory wheezing.
    3. The client reports muscle twitching.
    4. The client is refusing to eat the meal.

90. For which client would the nurse **question** administering mannitol?
    1. The client diagnosed with 4+ pitting pedal edema.
    2. The client diagnosed with decorticate posturing.
    3. The client diagnosed with widening pulse pressure.
    4. The client diagnosed with a positive doll's eye test.

91. The male client is self-medicating with cimetidine. Which side effects can occur while taking this medication? **Select all that apply**.
    1. Melena.
    2. Gynecomastia.
    3. Pyrosis.
    4. Eructation.
    5. Myalgia.

92. The client is reporting low back pain and is prescribed carisoprodol. Which teaching intervention has **priority**?
    1. Explain this medication causes GI distress.
    2. Discuss the need to taper off this medication.
    3. Warn this medication will cause drowsiness.
    4. Instruct the client to limit alcohol intake.

93. The client diagnosed with adult-onset asthma is being discharged. Which medication would the nurse expect the HCP to prescribe?
    1. A nonsteroidal anti-inflammatory medication.
    2. An antihistamine medication.
    3. An angiotensin-converting enzyme inhibitor.
    4. A proton pump inhibitor.

94. The client is reporting incisional pain. Which intervention should the nurse implement **first**?
    1. Administer the pain medication STAT.
    2. Determine when the last pain medication was given.
    3. Assess the client's pulse and blood pressure.
    4. Teach the client distraction techniques to address pain.

95. The nurse is evaluating the client's home medications and notes the client diagnosed with angina is taking an antidepressant. Which intervention should the nurse implement because the client is taking this medication?
    1. Ask the client if there is a plan for suicide.
    2. Assess the client's depression on a 1-to-10 scale.
    3. Explain this medication cannot be taken because of angina.
    4. Request a referral to the hospital psychologist.

96. The nurse is assessing the older client first thing in the morning. The client is confused and sleepy. Which intervention should the nurse implement **first**?
    1. Determine if the client received a sedative last night.
    2. Allow the client to continue to sleep and do not disturb.
    3. Encourage the client to ambulate in the room with assistance.
    4. Notify the health-care provider about the client's status.

97. The nurse is preparing to administer 37.5 mg of meperidine IM to a client reporting pain. The medication comes in a 50-mg/mL vial. Which action should the nurse implement?
    1. Notify the pharmacist to bring the correct vial.
    2. Have another nurse verify the wastage of medication.
    3. Administer 1 mL of medication to the client.
    4. Request the HCP to increase the client's dose.

98. The client is to receive 3,000 mg of medication daily in a divided dose every 8 hours. The medication comes 500 mg per tablet. How many tablets will the nurse administer at each dose?

    [                    ]

99. The 38-year-old client diagnosed with chronic asthma is prescribed a leukotriene receptor antagonist. Which is the scientific rationale for administering this medication?
    1. This medication is used prophylactically to control asthma.
    2. This medication will cure the client's chronic asthma.
    3. It will stabilize mast cell activities and reduce asthma attacks.
    4. It will cause the bronchioles to dilate and increase the airway.

100. The client diagnosed with chronic alcoholism is prescribed intravenous multivitamins. The solution turns yellow after injecting the multivitamins. Which action should the nurse implement?
    1. Notify the pharmacist about the yellow discoloration of the IV.
    2. Cover the IV bag and tubing with light-resistant material.
    3. Administer the medication as prescribed.
    4. Discard the IV bag and obtain another vial of multivitamins.

1. 1. The normal recommended daily dose of vitamin C is 60 to 90 mg for healthy adults, but nothing cures the virus that causes the common cold.
   2. Echinacea is an herbal preparation thought to limit the severity of a cold and is sold in OTC preparations, but it does not have to be taken with vitamin C.
   3. This dose is already too high, and water-soluble vitamins in excess of the body's needs are excreted in the urine.
   4. **Megadoses can lead to crystals in the urine, and crystals can lead to the formation of renal calculi (stones) in the kidneys (Knight et al., 2016).**

2. 1. NSAIDs are recommended for inflammatory disorders and to relieve mild to moderate pain.
   2. **A daily, low dose of acetylsalicylic acid (aspirin) is an antiplatelet that prevents platelet aggregation.**
   3. Anticoagulants are prescribed for clients diagnosed with a high risk for clot formation.
   4. Iron supplements are recommended for clients diagnosed with iron-deficiency anemia.

3. 1. **OTC decongestant medications used for the flu cause vasoconstriction of the blood vessels, which would increase the client's hypertension and therefore should be avoided. The client should let the flu run its course.**
   2. OTC medications should not be taken by the client diagnosed with essential hypertension.
   3. The nurse should provide the information to the client about what medications to take and should not refer the client to the pharmacist.
   4. It is too late for the flu vaccine because the client is already ill with the flu.

4. 1. The potassium level is not affected by the administration of the intravenous steroid (Solu-Medrol).
   2. Culture and sensitivity reports should be monitored to determine if the proper antibiotic is being administered.
   3. Steroids, including the intravenous steroid (Solu-Medrol), are excreted as glucocorticoids from the adrenal gland and are responsible for insulin resistance by the cells, which may cause hyperglycemia.
   4. There is no reason why the nurse would question administering a steroid based on an arterial blood gas result.

5. 1. Cromolyn, a mast cell inhibitor, is used prophylactically to prevent exercise-induced asthma attacks. It is administered in routine daily doses to prevent asthma attacks.
   2. Rinsing the mouth will help prevent the growth of bacteria secondary to medication left in the mouth.
   3. Holding the breath for 10 seconds keeps the medication in the lungs.
   4. **The mast cell inhibitor, cromolyn, is used to stabilize the mast cells in the lungs. During an asthma attack, the mast cells are already unstable; therefore, this medication will not be effective in treating the acute asthma attack. This statement would require the nurse to reteach about the medication.**

6. 1. Diarrhea may indicate the client may have a superinfection, but it is not the priority intervention at this time because the aminoglycoside antibiotic, vancomycin, would still be administered.
   2. The peak level is not drawn until 1 hour after the medication has been infused.
   3. **The trough level must be drawn before administering the aminoglycoside antibiotic vancomycin; therefore, it is the priority intervention.**
   4. The culture and sensitivity (C&S) has already been done because it is known the client has MRSA.

7. 1. At 8 hours postoperative, the client should be on bedrest, and moving the client to a chair will not help the incisional pain and could cause hip dislocation.
   2. **Normal developmental changes in the organs of older clients, especially the kidneys and liver, result in lower doses of pain medication needed to achieve therapeutic levels.**

3. This is a neurological assessment, which is not pertinent to the extremity assessment.

4. The urinary output would not affect the administration of pain medication.

8. 1. Iron dextran is administered for iron-deficiency anemia intravenously or intra-muscularly, not subcutaneously.

2. **Vitamin B$_{12}$ is administered for pernicious anemia because there is insufficient intrinsic factor produced by the rugae in the stomach to be able to absorb and use vitamin B$_{12}$ from food sources.**

3. Folic acid is administered orally or intravenously for folic acid deficiency, which is usually associated with chronic alcoholism.

4. Thiamine is administered intravenously in high doses to clients detoxifying from chronic alcoholism to prevent rebound nervous system dysfunction.

9. 1. **Glyburide (Diabeta), a sulfonylurea, stimulates the pancreas to secrete insulin. Therefore, the client is at risk for developing hypoglycemic reactions, especially during exercise.**

2. This is an oral hypoglycemic medication.

3. There are side effects to every medication; glyburide (Diabeta), a sulfonylurea, can cause hypoglycemia.

4. The medication stimulates the pancreas to produce more insulin, but it does not affect the muscles' absorption of glucose.

10. **10 units.**
The nurse should administer the dosage for the appropriate parameters.

11. 1. This test monitors the client's average blood glucose level over the previous 3 months.

2. The evening meal would prevent hypoglycemia for regular insulin administered at 1630.

3. The before-meal (a.c.) blood glucose level done at 1630 would not be affected by the insulin administered after that time.

4. **Insulin isophane (Humulin N), an intermediate-acting insulin, peaks 6 to 8 hours after being administered; therefore, the nighttime snack (h.s.) will prevent late-night hypoglycemia.**

12. 1. The nurse would not question administering insulin to a client about to eat.

2. The client 1 day postoperative would be receiving a prophylactic antibiotic.

3. **Metformin (Glucophage), a biguanide, must be held 24 to 48 hours before receiving contrast media (dye) because Glucophage, along with the contrast dye, can damage kidney function.**

4. The client diagnosed with peptic ulcer disease would be ordered a proton pump inhibitor to help decrease gastric acid production.

13. 1. The long-acting insulin glargine (Lantus) is scheduled for bedtime.

2. **The charge nurse should double-check the dosage against the MAR to make sure the client is receiving the correct dose; the long-acting insulin glargine (Lantus) does not peak and works for 24 hours.**

3. There is not a medication error at this time.

4. The HCP would only need to be notified if a serious medication error has occurred.

14. 1. These are clinical manifestations of hypothyroidism, which indicates not enough levothyroxine (Synthroid), a thyroid hormone replacement.

2. These indicate not enough medication is being administered.

3. **Irritability and tachycardia are clinical manifestations of hyperthyroidism, which indicates the client is receiving too much levothyroxine (Synthroid), a thyroid hormone replacement.**

4. Normothermia indicates a normal temperature, which does not indicate hypothyroidism or hyperthyroidism, and constipation is a sign of hypothyroidism.

15. 1. **The therapeutic heparin, an anticoagulant, level is 1.5 to 2 times the control, which is 58 to 78; therefore, a PTT of 72 is within therapeutic range so the nurse should continue to monitor the infusion. PT and INR are used to monitor the oral anticoagulant warfarin (Coumadin).**

2. Protamine sulfate is the antidote for heparin toxicity, but the client is in the therapeutic range.

3. There is no need for the laboratory to reconfirm the results.

4. The nurse would not need to assess for bleeding because the results are within the therapeutic range.

**16.** 1. A STAT potassium level would be needed for problems with digoxin, a cardiac glycoside, or furosemide (Lasix), a loop diuretic, but not for bleeding.
2. The nurse needs more information before requesting an admission to the hospital.
3. Diazepam (Valium) IVP does not help bleeding.
4. **Ecchymotic areas are secondary to bleeding. The nurse should order an INR to rule out warfarin (Coumadin) toxicity.**

**17.** **Correct answers are 2 and 5.**
1. The bisphosphonate, alendronate sodium (Fosamax), must be taken first thing in the morning before breakfast on an empty stomach; no food, juice, or coffee should be consumed for at least 30 minutes.
2. **Remaining in the upright position minimizes the risk of esophagitis; the bisphosphonate, alendronate sodium (Fosamax), should be taken with 8 ounces of water.**
3. The tablet should be swallowed, not chewed, and should not be allowed to dissolve until it is in the stomach.
4. There is no monthly hormone level to determine the effectiveness of the bisphosphonate, alendronate sodium (Fosamax); it is determined by a bone density test.
5. **The client should notify the HCP if pain or difficulty swallowing or new or worsening heartburn occurs.**

**18.** 1. A daily digoxin dose is not a priority medication.
2. This potassium level is very low, and the nurse should not administer the loop diuretic.
3. **The mucosal barrier, sucralfate (Carafate), must be administered on an empty stomach; therefore, it should be administered first.**
4. Methylprednisolone (Solu-Medrol), an IVP medication, is not a priority over administering a medication that must be given on an empty stomach.

**19.** 1. **Attempting to prevent CHF is the rationale for administering ACE inhibitors to clients diagnosed with MIs. This medication is administered for a variety of medical diagnoses, such as heart failure and stroke, and to help prevent diabetic nephropathy.**

2. ACE inhibitors are prescribed to help decrease blood pressure, but the stem states the client has had an MI, not essential hypertension.
3. Cardiac glycosides such as digoxin, not ACE inhibitors, increase the contractility of the heart.
4. Antilipidemics, not ACE inhibitors, help decrease the development of atherosclerosis.

**20.** 1. ACE inhibitors may increase potassium levels. The client should avoid potassium salt substitutes and supplements; therefore, the nurse would not question the fact the client is not receiving potassium supplements.
2. **An adverse effect of ACE inhibitors, including enalapril (Vasotec), is the possibility of a persistent irritating cough, which might precipitate the HCP's changing the client's medication.**
3. This blood pressure indicates the ACE inhibitor enalapril (Vasotec), is effective.
4. The urinary output of 30 mL/hr indicates the kidneys are functioning properly.

**21.** 1. The apical heart rate is assessed before administering the digoxin, a cardiac glycoside, but it does not indicate the medication is effective.
2. Anorexia and nausea are clinical manifestations of digoxin toxicity and do not indicate if the medication is effective.
3. Digoxin has no effect on the client's blood pressure.
4. **Digoxin, a cardiac glycoside, is administered for heart failure and dysrhythmias. Clear lung sounds indicate the heart failure is being controlled by the medication.**

**22.** 1. **Abrupt discontinuation of baclofen (Lioresal), a muscle relaxant, is associated with hallucinations, paranoia, and seizures.**
2. This medication causes constipation and urinary retention.
3. The client should not be allowed to drive at all when taking this medication because it causes drowsiness, and the spasticity of MS makes driving dangerous for the client.
4. White blood cell levels do not need to be monitored because the baclofen (Lioresal), a muscle relaxant, does not cause bone marrow suppression.

23. Correct answers are 1, 3, and 4.
    1. If the apical heart rate is less than 60, the nurse should question administering digoxin, a cardiac glycoside.
    2. The client's potassium level, not the sodium level, should be monitored.
    3. The client should be taught to monitor the radial pulse at home and not to take the medication if the pulse is less than 60 because digoxin, a cardiac glycoside, will further decrease the heart rate.
    4. The digoxin level should be between 0.5 and 2 ng/mL to be therapeutic.
    5. The client diagnosed with digoxin toxicity would complain of anorexia, nausea, and yellow haze; buffalo hump and moon face would be assessed for the client taking prednisone, a glucocorticoid.

24. 1. The respiratory rate and pulse rate would not affect the administration of theophylline (Theo-Dur), a bronchodilator.
    2. The apical heart rate (AP) of 59 would cause the nurse to question administering propranolol (Inderal) because beta blockers decrease the sympathetic stimulation to the heart, thereby decreasing the heart rate.
    3. These vital signs would not warrant the nurse questioning administering ampicillin, an antibiotic.
    4. The blood pressure is higher than 90/60; therefore, the nurse would not question administering diltiazem (Cardizem), a calcium channel blocker.

25. 1. Erythropoietin (Epogen), a biologic response modifier, stimulates the client's own bone marrow to produce red blood cells; therefore, this is not a violation of the client's religious beliefs about blood products.
    2. There is no reason for the client to have problems receiving this medication because of religious beliefs, so the client does not need to talk to the minister.
    3. This medication does not violate the client's Jehovah's Witness beliefs concerning receiving blood products; therefore, the nurse should administer the erythropoietin (Epogen), a biologic response modifier, via the correct route.
    4. This is not an invasive procedure or investigational medication, and thus, informed consent is not needed.

26. 1. Because the client is NPO as a result of the admitting diagnosis, the client needs alternative antianxiety medication to prevent clinical withdrawal manifestations, but this is not the first intervention.
    2. The client will be NPO as a result of the diverticulitis, and alprazolam (Xanax), a benzodiazepine, is administered orally; therefore, another route of medication administration is needed, but this is not the first intervention.
    3. This is correct information, but it is not the priority intervention.
    4. Alprazolam (Xanax) has a greater dependence problem than all the other benzodiazepines; therefore, the nurse must assess for clinical withdrawal manifestations first. Then the nurse can implement the other interventions. The client needs to be withdrawn slowly from the benzodiazepines, but an assessment is a priority.

27. 1. This is the outer canthus, and medications are not administered to this area.
    2. The correct placement of ophthalmic drops is to administer the medication in the lower conjunctival sac.
    3. This is the sclera, and the correct placement of eyedrops is in the lower conjunctival sac.
    4. This is the inner canthus, where pressure can be applied gently after instilling eyedrops to help prevent the systemic absorption of ophthalmic medications.

28. 1. This potassium level is within normal limits; therefore, the nurse would administer the loop diuretic furosemide (Lasix).
    2. This indicates the medication is effective and the nurse should not question administering the medication.
    3. This indicates the client is dehydrated and the nurse should discuss this with the HCP before administering another dose of the loop diuretic furosemide (Lasix), which could increase the dehydration and could cause renal failure.
    4. This indicates the medication is effective. Daily weight changes reflect fluid gain and loss.

29. 1. The nurse should investigate any herbs, such as St. John's wort, a client is taking, especially if the client has a condition that requires long-term medication, such as antirejection medication.

2. The nurse should remain nonjudgmental but must intervene if the alternative treatment, St. John's wort, poses a risk to the client.

3. The client may need to be referred for psychological counseling, but it is not the first action the nurse should take.

4. St. John's wort, an herb, decreases the effects of many medications, including oral contraceptives, antiretrovirals, and transplant immunosuppressant drugs. Rejection of the client's kidney could occur if the client continues to use St. John's wort.

30. 1. This is the rationale for H-2 antagonists and proton pump inhibitors.
2. Antacids neutralize gastric acidity.
3. This is the rationale for mucosal barrier agents.
4. Prostaglandin is responsible for the production of gastric acid. Antacids do not interfere with prostaglandin production.

31. 1. The client's temperature would not affect the administration of this medication.
2. ACE inhibitors sometimes cause the client to develop a cough, which requires discontinuing the medication, but this is a calcium channel blocker.
3. This blood pressure reading indicates the client's medication is effective.
4. **This indicates orthostatic hypotension, and the nurse should assess the client's BP before administering the medication.**

32. Correct order is 4, 3, 2, 1, 5.
4. Although the lidocaine, an antidysrhythmic, is a prn order, this client is exhibiting a life-threatening dysrhythmia, multifocal premature ventricular contractions.
3. The client diagnosed with myasthenia gravis must have this medication as close to the specific time as possible. Neostigmine (Prostigmin), a cholinesterase inhibitor, allows skeletal muscle to function; if this medication is delayed, the client may experience respiratory distress.
2. Pain is a priority, and morphine, a narcotic analgesic, should be administered after administering medications to clients diagnosed with life-threatening situations.

1. This client is symptomatic, and the furosemide (Lasix), a loop diuretic, should relieve some of the clinical manifestations of dyspnea.
5. Intravenous antibiotics are a priority, but this client has received several doses of vancomycin, an aminoglycoside antibiotic, or there would not be a trough level, so this client's medication could wait until the other medications have been administered.

33. Correct answers are 1, 2, 3, and 4.
1. The nurse should always assess for allergies, but especially when administering antibiotics, which are notorious for allergic reactions.
2. If specimens are not obtained for C&S before administering the first dose of antibiotic, the results will be skewed.
3. One of the five rights is to administer the medication to the "right client." Checking the armband on the client with the MAR and medication is a way to ensure this.
4. The 2005 Joint Commission standards require two forms of identification before administering medications. The client's armband and medical record number provide one form of identifying information, and the client's birthday is the second form of identification in most health-care facilities. This is a nationwide emphasis to help prevent medication errors.
5. The stem does not state it is an aminoglycoside antibiotic, and it is the initial dose, which means there is no medication in the system even if it were an aminoglycoside antibiotic.

34. 1. The muscarinic cholinergic agonist oxybutynin (Ditropan) is prescribed for clients diagnosed with an overactive bladder.
2. There is no contraindication for a client diagnosed with type 2 diabetes receiving this medication.
3. These drugs cause mydriasis. The muscarinic cholinergic agonist oxybutynin (Ditropan) increases intraocular pressure, which could lead to blindness. Glaucoma is caused by increased intraocular pressure.
4. There is no contraindication for a client diagnosed with peripheral vascular disease receiving this medication.

35. Correct order is 3, 4, 1, 2, and 5.

    3. The nurse should always check the ID band of the client and ask the client to state name and date of birth before beginning any procedure.
    4. The nurse should explain the procedure and the purpose of the procedure to the client before beginning but after the identification of the client.
    1. The nurse should perform hand hygiene when entering and exiting a client's room and before administering a topical ointment. Nonsterile gloves should be used for this procedure.
    2. The client's leg should be cleansed before administering a new application of ointment and dried thoroughly.
    5. The topical medication should be applied smoothly and evenly over the rash with a gloved hand (Treas et al., 2018).

36. 1. Adenosine is ordered for supraventricular tachycardia.
    2. Epinephrine is administered during a code to vasoconstrict the periphery and shunt the blood to the central circulating system.
    3. Atropine is used for symptomatic sinus bradycardia.
    4. Amiodarone is the suggested drug of choice for ventricular irritability according to the ACLS (AHA, 2016) algorithm to suppress ventricular ectopy.

37. Correct answers are 2, 3, and 5.
    1. The blood pressure must be continuously monitored more often, at least every 10 to 15 minutes.
    2. The peripheral pulses should be palpated frequently and the appearance of extremities should be evaluated for evidence of vasoconstriction such as cold or mottled skin.
    3. The client's urine output should be monitored because low-dose dopamine, an inotropic vasopressor, is administered to maintain renal perfusion; higher doses can cause vasoconstriction of the renal arteries.
    4. Dopamine is not inactivated when exposed to light.
    5. Dopamine should be infused in a large vein and the administration site should be evaluated frequently for extravasation. Extravasation can cause necrosis and sloughing of surrounding tissue (Vallerand & Sanoski, 2019).

38. 1. The ST segment becoming more depressed indicates a worsening of the oxygenation of the myocardial tissue.
    2. Reperfusion dysrhythmias indicate the ischemic heart tissue is receiving oxygen and is viable heart tissue.
    3. The creatine kinase CK-MB isoenzyme elevates when there is necrotic heart tissue and does not indicate if thrombolytic therapy is successful.
    4. The platelet count can decrease with administration of fibrinolytic therapy for an MI.

39. 1. Tinnitus, ringing in the ears, is a sign of ASA (aspirin) toxicity and needs to be reported to the HCP; the aspirin should be stopped immediately.
    2. Diarrhea is a complication of many medications but not with aspirin.
    3. Tetany is muscle twitching secondary to hypocalcemia.
    4. ASA (aspirin) does not cause paresthesia, which is numbness or tingling.

40. 1. Loop diuretics cause loss of potassium in the urine output; therefore, the client should be receiving potassium supplements. Hypokalemia can lead to life-threatening cardiac dysrhythmias.
    2. A cardiac glycoside, digoxin, is administered for congestive heart failure, but it is not necessary when administering a loop diuretic.
    3. An ACE inhibitor is not prescribed along with a loop diuretic. It may be ordered for congestive heart failure.
    4. A potassium cation, Kayexalate, is ordered to remove potassium through the bowel for clients diagnosed with hyperkalemia.

41. 1. Interferon is administered to treat hepatitis and some cancers, but it does not stimulate the bone marrow.
    2. Filgrastim (Neupogen) is a granulocyte-stimulating factor that stimulates the bone marrow to produce white blood cells (WBCs), which this client needs because the normal WBC count is 4.5 to $11.1 \times 10^3$/microL.
    3. Oprelvekin (Neumega) stimulates the production of platelets, but the client's platelet count of 160 is normal (100 to $400 \times 10^3$/microL).
    4. Epoetin alfa (Procrit) stimulates the production of red blood cells and hemoglobin, but a hemoglobin of 12.2 is normal for a woman (11.7 to 15.5 g/dL).

42. 1. Azathioprine (Imuran), an immunosuppressive agent, must be taken for life because the client has to have received some type of transplant or have severe rheumatoid arthritis for it to be prescribed.
   2. Exposure to hepatitis does not have anything to do with receiving this medication.
   3. **Azathioprine (Imuran), an immunosuppressive agent, is not a drug of choice for treating pneumonia; therefore, the nurse must find out why the client is taking it (either for a renal transplant or for severe rheumatoid arthritis).**
   4. Azathioprine (Imuran) does not affect the antigen–antibody reaction.

43. 1. A daily cathartic is a colonic stimulant, which results in dependency and a narrowing of the lumen of the colon, which increases constipation.
   2. **Although the client may think a medication for bowel movements is necessary, the nurse should teach the client that bisacodyl (Dulcolax) can cause serious complications, such as dependency and narrowing of the colon.**
   3. Fiber will help increase the roughage, which may help prevent constipation, but the most important action is to empower the client to make informed decisions about medications.
   4. The nurse should not refuse to administer the medication; the nurse should talk to the client and, if needed, the HCP before administering the bisacodyl (Dulcolax).

44. 1. This should be documented in the client's nurse's notes because this is a prn medication, but it is not the priority action.
   2. The nurse would not administer another narcotic, which is what caused the need for naloxone (Narcan), a narcotic antagonist, in the first place.
   3. Oxygen will not help reverse respiratory depression secondary to a narcotic overdose.
   4. **Naloxone (Narcan), a narcotic antagonist, is administered when the client has received too much of a narcotic. Narcan has a short half-life of about 30 minutes, and the client will be at risk for respiratory depression for several hours; therefore, the nurse should assess the client frequently.**

45. 1. The pituitary gland is not directly affected by the steroid prednisone and is not why the medication must be gradually tapered.

2. Steroids do not affect the pancreas's production of insulin.
   3. **When the client is receiving exogenous steroids, the adrenal glands stop producing cortisol, and if the steroid prednisone is not tapered, the client can have a severe hypotensive crisis, known as adrenal gland insufficiency or Addisonian crisis.**
   4. The adrenal gland, not the thyroid gland, produces cortisol.

46. 1. **Rifampin and isoniazid (INH), both antituberculosis medications, are taken for 6 months to 1 year and often in combination with two other medications. Directly observed therapy (DOT) is recommended to ensure medication compliance because TB is a public health issue and the most common cause of infectious disease-related mortality worldwide (Herchline, 2019).**
   2. The client is in isolation until three consecutive early-morning sputum cultures are negative, which is usually in about 2 to 4 weeks.
   3. Pork products do not interact with rifampin and isoniazid (INH), both antituberculosis medications.
   4. The client's urine and all body fluids may turn orange from the rifampin.

47. 1. **This medication should be administered intradermally with the needle barely inserted under the skin so a wheal (bubble) forms after the injection.**
   2. Cleansing the forearm with an alcohol swab is standard procedure and would not warrant immediate intervention.
   3. Circling the site is an appropriate intervention so, when the skin test is read and no reaction is occurring, the nurse will be able to document a negative skin test reading.
   4. The skin test is read in 3 days to determine the results.

48. **Correct answers are 2 and 5.**
   1. Valacyclovir (Valtrex), an antiviral, is used to prevent transmission of this virus to the fetus during pregnancy and is FDA pregnancy category B. Therefore, when taken as prescribed, the client may be pregnant while taking the medication (Prescribers' Digital Reference, 2019).
   2. **Condoms reduce the risk of or abstinence prevents transmission of the herpes virus.**

3. There are side effects to every drug; vala-cyclovir (Valtrex), an antiviral, causes head-ache, dizziness, nausea, and anorexia.

4. This medication does not directly affect the liver, and liver function tests (LFTs) are not required monthly.

5. **The client should be instructed to main-tain adequate hydration during the course of therapy to avoid renal side effects.**

49. 1. Flatulence ("gas") is an expected side effect that is not life-threatening and does not need to be reported to the HCP.

2. A weight loss of 2 pounds would not need to be reported to the HCP because this medication does not affect the client's weight.

3. **Muscle pain may indicate arthralgias, myositis, or rhabdomyolysis, which are complications that would cause the HCP to discontinue the medication because its continued use may lead to liver failure.**

4. Not having a bowel movement may be important to the client, but clients do not have to have daily bowel movements.

50. Correct answers are 2 and 5.
1. ASA (aspirin) causes GI distress and should be taken with food.

2. **Enteric-coated tablets should be swal-lowed whole to avoid GI distress.**

3. Acetaminophen (Tylenol) is recommended for pain and can be safely taken with a daily low-dose aspirin.

4. ASA (aspirin) does not cause joint pain; in fact, it may provide some relief because of its anti-inflammatory action, but when aspirin is taken daily, it is an antiplatelet medication.

5. **ASA is known to cause gastric upset, which can lead to gastric bleeding, and dark, tarry stools may indicate upper GI bleeding.**

51. 1. **Phenytoin (Dilantin) will crystallize in the tubing and is not compatible with any IV fluid except normal saline. The IV tubing must be flushed before the medication is administered.**

2. The therapeutic phenytoin (Dilantin) level is 10 to 20 mcg/mL; therefore, this is a toxic level.

3. The medication is administered undiluted at a rate not to exceed 50 mg/min.

4. If the tubing turns cloudy, it means it is not compatible, and the nurse must stop the IVP immediately and discontinue the IV.

52. Correct answers are 2 and 4.
1. There is no machine for home use that monitors phenytoin (Dilantin) levels. Levels are usually checked every 6 months to 1 year by venipuncture and laboratory tests.

2. **Phenytoin (Dilantin) causes gingival hyperplasia, and mouth care and dental care are a priority to help prevent rot-ting of the teeth.**

3. Some states allow seizure-free clients diagnosed with epilepsy to drive, but some states don't. The word "never" in this distracter should eliminate it as a possible correct answer.

4. **Clients should be instructed to avoid taking phenytoin (Dilantin) within 2 to 3 hours of antacids.**

5. Alcohol should be strictly prohibited when taking anticonvulsant medications.

53. Correct answers are 1, 2, 4, and 5.
1. **Alcohol creates a disulfiram-like reac-tion to the metronidazole (Flagyl), an antibiotic and antiprotozoal agent, which causes severe nausea, vomiting, and extreme hypertension.**

2. *Trichomonas vaginalis* **is an asymptom-atic sexually transmitted disease in males. If the male partner is not simul-taneously treated, then he can reinfect the female.**

3. This sexually transmitted infection can be transmitted via oral routes.

4. **This is a concept that must be taught to all clients taking antibiotics: Take all the medications as prescribed.**

5. **Metronidazole can, in rare cases, cause Stevens-Johnson syndrome. The client should notify the HCP for the appear-ance of a rash.**

54. Correct answers are 1 and 2.
1. **If the nurse does not wear gloves, the nurse can absorb the nitroglycerin paste (Nitro-Bid) and get a headache.**

2. **The old nitroglycerin paste must be removed because it could cause an over-dose of the medication.**

3. The paper should be applied to a clean, dry, hairless area.

4. The nitroglycerin paste (Nitro-Bid) can be placed on the chest, arms, back, or legs.

5. A headache is a common side effect and should not be reported to HCP.

55. 125 gtt/min.
A microdrip is 60 gtt/mL. The formula for this dosage problem is as follows:

$$\frac{1000 \text{ mL} \times 60}{480 \text{ min}} = \frac{60,000}{480} = 125 \text{ gtt/min}$$

56. 1. This medication is harsh on the lining of the stomach and should be taken with meals.
2. Abdominal striae occur with steroids, not NSAIDs.
3. The temperature does not affect the administration of this medication. NSAIDs would be prescribed for fever.
4. The liver and kidneys are responsible for metabolizing and excreting all medications, but the tests are not routinely monitored for NSAIDs.

57. 1. The XL means the nifedipine (Procardia XL) is extended release and cannot be crushed.
2. Whole capsules or tablets cannot be administered through a feeding tube.
3. The client has a feeding tube and is not able to swallow; therefore, the nurse should not administer the nifedipine (Procardia XL) orally.
4. Tablets that are enteric coated or extended release cannot be crushed and administered via the NG tube. This would allow 24 hours' worth of medication into the client's system at one time. The nurse should ask the HCP to change the nifedipine (Procardia XL) medication to a form that is not enteric coated and not extended release. Then it can be crushed and administered through the feeding tube.

58. 1. The vaccine is administered in a series of three injections and is reported to be effective for life, but boosters may be given every 5 years.
2. This is the incorrect administration for the hepatitis B vaccine.
3. Hepatitis B (Engerix-B or Recombivax HB) is given in three doses—initially, then at 1 month, and then again at 6 months. An alternative administration is a two-dose hepatitis series (Heplisav-B)—two doses at least 4 weeks apart (Centers for Disease Control and Prevention, 2019).
4. Hepatitis B vaccine is given intramuscularly in the deltoid muscle.

59. 1. Output greater than intake indicates the medication is effective, and there is no need to restrict fluid intake.
2. There is no reason to insert a Foley catheter in the client urinating without difficulties.
3. As long as the client is receiving diuretics, the client should be on intake and output monitoring.
4. The UAP can document the client's fluid intake and output numbers on the bedside record; this is one of the UAP's duties.

60. 1. This is a correct intervention when applying a fentanyl (Duragesic) patch; therefore, the charge nurse would not have to intervene.
2. The fentanyl (Duragesic) patch takes about 24 hours to develop a full analgesic effect; the patch should be replaced every 72 hours.
3. The sites should be rotated to prevent irritation to the skin.
4. This is the correct way to administer all medications.

61. 1. The nurse should prepare to administer the medication, but it is not the first intervention.
2. A CT scan must be done to rule out a hemorrhagic CVA because, if it is a hemorrhagic stroke, thrombolytic therapy will increase bleeding in the head.
3. The client receiving thrombolytic therapy will be in the ICU because the client needs constant surveillance during therapy. Heparin will be started, but this is not the first intervention.
4. The nurse should check to determine if the client is allergic to medications, but in this situation, the client must have a CT before any other action is taken. Cross sensitivity usually occurs with antibiotics, not thrombolytic therapy.

62. 1. Pantoprazole (Protonix), a proton pump inhibitor (PPI), decreases gastric secretion and is prescribed for clients to prevent Curling's stress ulcer. PPIs are ordered for most clients in the intensive care department, not just clients diagnosed with burns.
2. PPIs do not treat infections; antibiotics treat infections.

3. Pantoprazole (Protonix), a PPI, does not cause continuous constriction. Dopamine might do this.

4. A positive nitrogen balance accomplished through nutritional interventions will help promote tissue regeneration.

63. 1. The new antibiotic must be started as soon as the medication arrives from the pharmacy.

2. Waiting until the next day could cause serious harm, with the client possibly going into septic shock.

3. The HCP does not determine when the medications are administered; this is a nursing intervention.

4. **A new IV antibiotic must be initiated as soon as possible, at least within 1 hour. A broad-spectrum antibiotic is ordered until C&S results are determined. Then, an antibiotic that will specifically target the infectious organism must be started immediately.**

64. 920 units/hr.

20000 units ÷ 500 mL = 40 units/mL
40 units/mL × 23 mL/hr = 920 units/hr

65. Correct answers are 1, 2, and 5.

1. **Carbamazepine (Tegretol), an anticonvulsant, is photosensitive, and the client must wear SPF of at least 30 to be protected.**

2. **Carbamazepine (Tegretol), an anticonvulsant medication, has a therapeutic level that must be maintained to help prevent seizures. The therapeutic range is from 4 to 12 mcg/mL (Vallerand & Sanoski, 2017).**

3. Dilantin, another anticonvulsant, causes hyperplastic gingivitis, but carbamazepine does not.

4. The client diagnosed with a seizure disorder should only take showers because, if a seizure occurs in the bathtub, the client could drown.

5. **Grapefruit and grapefruit juice can increase the amount of carbamazepine absorbed by the body, increasing side effects.**

66. 1. **Yellow eyes would indicate the client is experiencing some type of hepatic toxicity, which would warrant the valproic acid (Depakote), an anticonvulsant, being discontinued immediately. During the first few months of treatment, the client is closely monitored for hepatic toxicity because deaths have occurred.**

2. The medication dose may need to be increased, but valproic acid (Depakote), an anticonvulsant, is administered to prevent the mood swings.

3. The BP is slightly elevated, but it is not related to the medication.

4. The therapeutic serum valproic acid level is 50 to 125 mcg/mL; therefore, the client is within the therapeutic range (Vallerand & Sanoski, 2017).

67. 1. **Safety is a priority when administering the antiemetic promethazine (Phenergan) because it causes sedative-like effects.**

2. Evaluation is not a priority over safety.

3. The nurse should have assessed the client's GI system before administering the antiemetic, not after.

4. Withholding fluids and food is an appropriate intervention to help prevent emesis, but it is not a priority over safety after administering promethazine (Phenergan).

68. 1. This is the correct area to administer subcutaneous heparin, but not enoxaparin (Lovenox), a low molecular weight heparin.

2. This is in the client's anterior thigh, which may be used for insulin administration but not for Lovenox, and a 25-gauge 1/2-inch needle is used to administer Lovenox.

3. This is the upper arm area, which is used for subcutaneous insulin, but not enoxaparin (Lovenox), a low molecular weight heparin.

4. **Enoxaparin (Lovenox), a low molecular weight heparin, is administered in the "love handles," which is in the anterolateral or posterolateral abdomen to enhance absorption. Sites should be rotated frequently (Vallerand & Sanoski, 2017).**

69. 1. This may be a question the nurse asks, but it doesn't matter because the nurse will clean the site again.

2. The nail does not matter and it will not be cultured; it is assumed the nail is contaminated.

3. **The tetanus shot must be received every 10 years to prevent tetany, also known as "lockjaw."**

4. Being able to walk on the foot is not a priority question. Determining the status of the tetanus shot is the priority.

70. 1. Carbidopa and levodopa (Sinemet) does not affect the client's muscle strength; it affects the smoothness of muscle movement.
   2. **Cogwheel rigidity (jerky, uneven movements when moving a limb) is a symptom of Parkinson's disease, and if the client is not experiencing this rigidity, then the carbidopa and levodopa (Sinemet) is effective.**
   3. There is no such thing as a carbidopa therapeutic level. The client's clinical manifestations determine the effectiveness of the medication.
   4. The client's blood pressure should be assessed to determine if the client is having hypotension, which is a side effect of carbidopa and levodopa (Sinemet), but this does not determine the effectiveness of the medication.

71. **Correct answers are 1 and 5.**
   1. **This diet is recommended for clients diagnosed with coronary artery disease.**
   2. This medication is taken once a day in the evening.
   3. Atorvastatin (Lipitor) can be taken at any time of day. Other HMG-CoA reductase inhibitors such as fluvastatin (Lescol), pravastatin (Pravachol), and simvastatin (Zocor) must be taken at night to enhance the enzymes that metabolize cholesterol (Vallerand & Sanoski, 2017).
   4. There is no machine to test daily cholesterol levels. The cholesterol level is checked every 3 to 6 months.
   5. **Atorvastatin (Lipitor) can be taken at any time of the day, but the client should be instructed to take the medication at the same time each day.**

72. 1. The client diagnosed with end-stage renal disease does not normally urinate, and urine output does not determine if this medication is effective.
   2. Sodium polystyrene sulfonate (Kayexalate) does not affect phosphorus levels.
   3. The client being in normal sinus rhythm is good, but it does not determine if the medication is effective.
   4. **Sodium polystyrene sulfonate (Kayexalate) is a cation and exchanges sodium ions for potassium ions in the intestines, thereby lowering the serum potassium level. Therefore, a serum potassium level within normal limits would indicate the medication is effective. Normal potassium levels are 3.5 to 5.3 mEq/L.**

73. 1. **The ABG results indicate metabolic acidosis, and the treatment of choice is sodium bicarbonate.**
   2. Oxygen is the treatment of choice for respiratory acidosis.
   3. Epinephrine is administered in a code situation.
   4. This is milk of magnesia, which is an antacid and laxative, but it is not the treatment for metabolic acidosis.

74. 1. Propranolol is taken prophylactically, which means the client should take the medication routinely whether the client has a headache or not.
   2. **Beta blockers decrease the heart rate. If the radial pulse is less than 60 bpm, the client should hold the propranolol (Inderal), a beta blocker, and notify the HCP.**
   3. Propranolol (Inderal), a beta blocker, will mask tachycardia in clients diagnosed with diabetes, an early symptom of hypoglycemia. Thirst and dry mouth are clinical manifestations of hyperglycemia, but this client does not have diabetes.
   4. Beta blockers do not affect the client's visual acuity; therefore, a change in light is not necessary.

75. 1. Atropine is used in clients diagnosed with asystole or symptomatic sinus bradycardia.
   2. Amiodarone is a Class C medication used for ventricular dysfunction.
   3. **Adenosine is the drug of choice for clients diagnosed with SVT.**
   4. Dobutamine is used for clients diagnosed with heart failure.

76. 1. **The loss of effect of the medication occurs near the end of a dosing interval and indicates the plasma drug level has declined to subtherapeutic value. This is an expected occurrence with levodopa (L-dopa) and the chronic nature of the disease.**
   2. Increasing the dose increases the peripheral action of levodopa (L-dopa) on the heart and vessels. Because 75% of the drug never crosses the blood-brain barrier, the dose may not be increased.
   3. This effect does not mean the client is dying. It means the levodopa (L-dopa) is wearing off.
   4. This is not the desired effect of the medication.

**77.** 1. This information really doesn't have a bearing on the current situation.
2. The spouse can stay in the room if able to stay calm and not upset the client.
3. The nurse should address the client's fear, but it is not the most pertinent information.
4. **A local anesthetic will be administered to numb the area before suturing. The same classification of drugs is used to numb the mouth before dental procedures, and this client may be allergic to the numbing medication.**

**78.** 1. The medication is administered through the nose, but it has no effect on the client's ability to breathe.
2. Being thirsty all the time would indicate the vasopressin is not effective.
3. Neither the medication nor the disease process has anything to do with the glucose level. A disease that affects the glucose level is diabetes mellitus, not diabetes insipidus.
4. **Diabetes insipidus is characterized by the client not being able to concentrate urine and excreting large amounts of dilute urine. If the client is able to delay voiding for 3 to 4 hours, it indicates the vasopressin medication is effective.**

**79.** 1. This is the correct procedure for instilling eardrops for children.
2. **"Otic" refers to the ear. Instilling eardrops in the adult must be done by pulling the ear up and back to straighten the eustachian tube.**
3. This is the correct procedure for placing ophthalmic drops in the eye.
4. Pressure is applied to the inner canthus to prevent eye medication from entering the systemic circulation.

**80.** 1. The client should increase fluid intake to help flush the bacteria through the kidneys and bladder.
2. The client has a chronic UTI, which will require an antibiotic such as trimethoprim-sulfamethoxazole (Bactrim) on a daily basis to keep the bacteria count under control.
3. **The key to answering this question is the word "chronic," which indicates a continuing problem; this statement would be appropriate for an acute UTI.**
4. Diarrhea is a sign of superinfection, which occurs when the antibiotic trimethoprim-sulfamethoxazole (Bactrim) kills the good flora in the bowel. However, the client must keep taking the antibiotic, and loperamide hydrochloride (Imodium) is an OTC antidiarrheal.

**81.** 1. A Pap smear is usually done yearly and is used to detect cervical cancer; HRT does not increase the risk.
2. **The risk of developing breast cancer increases when the client is receiving HRT.**
3. A bone density test is used to detect osteoporosis, and HRT improves bone density.
4. Calcium levels are not affected by HRT.

**82.** 1. One of the rights of medication administration is the correct dose, and some medications must be divided before administering.
2. One of the rights of medication administration is the correct client, and this is making sure it is the correct client.
3. **One of the rights of medication administration is the correct route. Insulin cannot be administered intramuscularly. It must be administered subcutaneously or intravenously; therefore, this action warrants immediate intervention.**
4. One of the rights of medication administration is the right time, and the LPN has 30 minutes to 1 hour to administer medications depending on hospital policy; therefore, this would not require intervention by the RN.

**83.** 1. Aluminum hydroxide (Amphojel) is an antacid, but it is not being administered to this client for that reason.
2. The client is in end-stage renal disease (ESRD), but burning on urination is not a sign of ESRD; it is a sign of urinary tract infection.
3. A side effect of this medication is constipation, but having a normal bowel movement does not indicate the aluminum hydroxide (Amphojel) is effective.
4. **Aluminum hydroxide (Amphojel) decreases the absorption of phosphates in the intestines, thereby decreasing serum phosphate levels. The normal phosphate level is 2.5 to 4.5 mg/dL.**

**84.** 1. **Any medication that will prolong bleeding as a platelet aggregate inhibitor does, including ticlopidine (Ticlid), should not be administered to the client for at least 2 to 3 days before surgery.**
2. The nurse should not question administering Ticarcillin (Timentin), an extended-spectrum antibiotic before surgery, especially not before gastrointestinal surgery.

3. Pioglitazone (Actos), a thiazolidinedione, is a medication for type 2 diabetes and should be administered the day before the surgery.
4. The client will be receiving medications to evacuate the bowel. Bisacodyl (Dulcolax) is a cathartic laxative.

85. Correct answers are 2 and 4.
    1. This rash indicates a sensitivity reaction, and the allopurinol (Zyloprim) medication may need to be discontinued permanently or the dose should be decreased.
    2. **Increased fluid intake minimizes the risk of renal calculi formation.**
    3. The medication should be taken with food or milk to minimize gastric irritation.
    4. **Allopurinol (Zyloprim) increases the effects of oral diabetic medications; therefore, the dose should be decreased.**
    5. Allopurinol (Zyloprim) helps prevent acute gout attacks but does not relieve them. The client should continue the medication during an acute attack.

86. 1. Although many nurses will do this, the correct and ethical action is to take responsibility for the error and just be thankful the client did not have a problem.
    2. There is a chain of command to report medication errors, which includes the charge nurse and the HCP, not the director of nurses.
    3. **The ethical and correct action is to report and document the medication error; remember always to assess the client.**
    4. The Peer Review Committee will not be involved in one medication error unless the client died or a life-threatening complication occurred, or if the nurse has a pattern of behavior with multiple medication errors.

87. Correct answers are 1, 2, 3, and 4.
    1. **Telemetry should be monitored during amiodarone (Cordarone) therapy to ensure the client does not develop worsening of dysrhythmias.**
    2. **The client taking amiodarone (Cordarone) is at risk for pulmonary toxicity and developing adult respiratory distress syndrome (ARDS); therefore, the nurse should monitor the client's respiratory status.**
    3. **When the client is receiving medications intravenously, monitoring the liver and renal function is appropriate; amiodarone (Cordarone) causes hepatomegaly.**
    4. **Intravenous vasoactive medications are inherently dangerous; fatalities have occurred from amiodarone (Cordarone), so the nurse confirming the order with another nurse is appropriate.**
    5. The nurse should never defibrillate a client with a heartbeat, and nothing in the stem states the client is in ventricular fibrillation.

88. 1. This medication amount is too much and must be divided into two injections to be given safely, but the nurse can do this independently and does not need to notify the HCP.
    2. The nurse should not administer 5.5 mL in one injection. No more than 3 to 5 mL should be administered in an intramuscular injection (Treas et al., 2018).
    3. There is no reason for the nurse to discard this medication. Divide the medication and give two injections.
    4. **The nurse should never administer more than 3 to 5 mL in an intramuscular injection because a larger amount could cause damage to the muscle. The nurse should divide the dose and administer two injections (Treas et al., 2018).**

89. 1. The client's aminophylline drug level is within the therapeutic range of 10 to 20 mcg/mL.
    2. Expiratory wheezing would be expected in the client diagnosed with status asthmaticus and, therefore, would not warrant intervention.
    3. **Muscle twitching indicates the client is receiving too much aminophylline, a bronchodilator, and may experience a seizure.**
    4. The client is having trouble breathing, and eating requires energy. Therefore, the client may not want to eat a meal or the client may not like the hospital food, which would not warrant immediate intervention.

90. 1. The client diagnosed with pitting pedal edema is in fluid volume overload, which should make the nurse question administering an osmotic diuretic because the osmotic diuretic mannitol (Osmitrol) will pull more fluid from the tissues into the circulatory system, causing further fluid volume overload.
    2. An osmotic diuretic is administered for increased intracranial pressure; therefore, a client exhibiting decorticate posturing would need this medication.

3. A widening pulse pressure indicates increased intracranial pressure; therefore, the client needs the osmotic diuretic mannitol (Osmitrol).

4. The doll's eye test indicates increased intracranial pressure, which is why the HCP would prescribe the osmotic diuretic mannitol (Osmitrol).

91. Correct answers are 1, 2, and 5.
    1. **Melena is a black, tarry stool, which could indicate an adverse reaction to this medication.**
    2. **Gynecomastia, or breast development in men, is a complication of the H-2 antagonist cimetidine (Tagamet).**
    3. Pyrosis, or heartburn, is why the client would be taking this medication and not a side effect.
    4. Eructation, or belching, is not a side effect or complication of the H-2 antagonist cimetidine (Tagamet).
    5. **Myalgia is mild to severe muscle aches and pain and can be a side effect of the H-2 antagonist cimetidine (Tagamet).**

92. 1. Muscle relaxants do not cause GI distress.
    2. Muscle relaxants, with the exception of baclofen, do not need to be tapered off.
    3. **Initially, muscle relaxants cause drowsiness, so safety is an important issue.**
    4. As a safety precaution, the client should avoid drinking alcohol while taking the muscle relaxant carisoprodol (Soma).

93. 1. The client may be given a steroid, such as prednisone, but not an NSAID.
    2. An antihistamine is prescribed to decrease clinical manifestations of a cold or the flu, but it is not prescribed for asthma.
    3. An ACE inhibitor prevents deterioration of heart muscle and kidneys, but it is not a drug of choice for the respiratory system.
    4. **Adult-onset asthma can be caused or aggravated by gastroesophageal reflux disease; therefore, a proton pump inhibitor would be prescribed to decrease acid reflux into the esophagus and subsequent aspiration (American Academy of Allergy, Asthma, & Immunology, 2019).**

94. 1. The pain medication should be administered as soon as possible but not before assessing for complications that might be causing pain.
    2. The nurse must not administer the medication too close to the last dose, but this is not the first intervention the nurse would implement.

3. **The first step of the nursing process is to assess, and the nurse must determine if this is routine postoperative pain the client should have or if this is a complication that requires immediate intervention. Decreased blood pressure and increased pulse indicate hemorrhaging.**

4. Teaching distraction techniques is an appropriate intervention, but the nurse should medicate the client.

95. 1. Just because a client is taking an antidepressant does not mean the client is suicidal.
    2. **The nurse should determine if the client is in a depressed state or if the medication is effective, so the nurse should ask the client to rate the depression on a 1-to-10 scale, with 1 being no depression and 10 being the most depressed.**
    3. Antidepressants must be tapered off because of rebound depression.
    4. The client taking an antidepressant medication does not automatically need a referral to a psychologist.

96. 1. **Many times, especially with older clients, sedatives extend the desired effects longer than expected; therefore, the nurse should check to see if the client received any sleeping medication.**
    2. The nurse should assess why the client is sleepy and then allow the client to sleep if the sleepiness is a result of receiving a sedative the previous night.
    3. If an older client is confused and drowsy, the client should not be allowed to ambulate, even if assistance is being provided, because of safety issues.
    4. The nurse must determine if this is an expected occurrence or a decrease in neurological function before notifying the HCP.

97. 1. Medication does not always come in the exact amount of the HCP's order.
    2. **Because meperidine (Demerol) is a narcotic, the nurse preparing the medication must have someone to verify and document the wastage of 12.5 mg of the Demerol.**
    3. This would be a medication error because the order is for 37.5 mg, not 50 mg.
    4. This would not be an appropriate intervention. The nurse can safely and accurately administer the prescribed meperidine (Demerol) dose to the client. If the pain is not controlled with the amount, then the HCP should be notified.

**98.** 2 tablets.

The nurse needs to determine how many doses are to be given in 1 day (24 hours) if doses are to be 8 hours apart.

$$24 \div 8 = 3 \text{ doses}$$

If 3,000 mg is to be given in three doses, then determine how much is given in each dose:

$$3000 \div 3 = 1,000 \text{ mg per dose}$$

If the medication comes in 500-mg tablets, then to give 1,000 mg, the nurse must give:

$$1000 \div 500 = 2 \text{ tablets}$$

**99.** 1. This medication decreases inflammation by stabilizing the leukotrienes in the lung, which initiate an asthma attack.

2. Children may outgrow asthma attacks, whereas adult asthmatics can control their disease, but there is no cure for asthma at this time.

3. This is the scientific rationale for mast cell inhibitors.

4. This is the scientific rationale for bronchodilators.

**100.** 1. The multivitamins in the IV solution cause the IV solution to be yellow. There is no reason to notify the HCP.

2. The IV does not need to be protected from light.

3. **Multivitamins cause the IV solution to turn a yellow color and is commonly called a "banana bag." The nurse should administer the medication as prescribed.**

4. The yellow color is normal for this medication.

# Comprehensive Final Examination

*The great thing in this world is not so much where we stand as in what direction we are moving.*

—Oliver Wendell Holmes

This book is designed to assist the test taker with recognizing elements of test construction, thinking critically, and arriving at the correct answer. Many hints appear in previous chapters. Some are general hints applying to class preparations and taking examinations (Chapter 1), some are specific tips for varied question types about disorders and diseases of body systems (Chapters 2–18), and some are specific to pharmacology (Chapter 19). The test taker should apply these hints, use all the knowledge gained in class, study, and take the comprehensive examination.

## COMPREHENSIVE FINAL EXAMINATION

1. The 44-year-old female client calls the clinic and tells the nurse she felt a lump while performing breast self-examination (BSE). Which question should the nurse ask the client?
   1. "Are you taking birth control pills?"
   2. "Do you eat a lot of chocolate?"
   3. "When was your last period?"
   4. "Are you sexually active?"

2. Which problem is a **priority** for the 24-year-old client admitted to the gynecological unit diagnosed with endometriosis?
   1. Hemorrhage.
   2. Pain.
   3. Constipation.
   4. Dyspareunia.

3. The 28-year-old client diagnosed with testicular cancer is scheduled for a unilateral orchiectomy. Which intervention should have **priority** in the client's plan of care?
   1. Encourage the client to bank his sperm.
   2. Discuss completing an advance directive.
   3. Explain follow-up chemotherapy and radiation.
   4. Allow the client to express his feelings regarding having cancer.

4. The nurse is teaching a class on sexually transmitted infections (STIs) to high school sophomores. Which information should be included in the discussion? **Select all that apply.**
   1. Oral sex decreases the chance of transmitting a sexual disease.
   2. Sexual activity during menses decreases the transmission of diseases.
   3. Frequent sexual activity is necessary to transmit a sexual disease.
   4. Unprotected sex puts the individual at risk for many diseases.
   5. Get vaccinated to prevent the most common STI.

5. The nurse has taught Kegel exercises to the client, who is para 5, gravida 5. Which information indicates the exercises have been **effective**?
   1. The client reports no SOB when walking upstairs.
   2. The client has no reports of stress incontinence.
   3. The client denies being pregnant at this time.
   4. The client has lost 10 lbs. in the last 2 months.

6. Which diagnostic procedure does the nurse anticipate being ordered for the 27-year-old female client reporting irregular menses and lower left abdominal pain during menses?
   1. Pelvic sonogram.
   2. Complete blood count (CBC).
   3. Kidney, ureter, bladder (KUB) x-ray.
   4. Computed tomography (CT) of the abdomen.

7. The client diagnosed with stage IV prostate cancer is receiving chemotherapy. Which laboratory value should the nurse assess **before** administering the chemotherapy?
   1. Prostate-specific antigen (PSA).
   2. Serum calcium level.
   3. Complete blood count (CBC).
   4. Alpha-fetoprotein (AFP).

8. Which client should the registered nurse (RN) charge nurse of the day surgery unit, assign to a **new graduate** nurse in orientation?
   1. The client after an arthroscopy with an AP of 110 and BP of 94/60.
   2. The client with open reduction of the ankle who is confused.
   3. The client with a total hip replacement being transferred to the ICU.
   4. The client diagnosed with low back pain after a myelogram.

9. The client diagnosed with severe osteoarthritis is in the long-term care facility. Which nursing task should the RN delegate to the unlicensed assistive personnel (UAP)?
   1. Feed the client the breakfast meal.
   2. Give the client an OTC antacid.
   3. Monitor the client's INR results.
   4. Assist the client to the shower room.

10. The primary nurse is applying antiembolism hose to the client postoperative total hip replacement. Which situation **warrants immediate** intervention by the charge nurse?
    1. Two fingers can be placed under the top of the band.
    2. The peripheral capillary refill time is less than 3 seconds.
    3. There are wrinkles in the hose behind the knees.
    4. The nurse does not place a hose on the foot with a venous pressure injury.

11. The 54-year-old female client is diagnosed with osteoporosis. Which interventions should the nurse discuss with the client? **Select all that apply.**
    1. Instruct the client to swim 30 minutes every day.
    2. Encourage drinking milk with added vitamin D.
    3. Determine if the client smokes cigarettes.
    4. Recommend the client not go outside.
    5. Teach about safety and fall precautions.

12. The 33-year-old client had a traumatic amputation of the right forearm as a result of a work-related injury. Which referral by the RN rehabilitation nurse is **most appropriate**?
    1. Physical therapist.
    2. Occupational therapist.
    3. Workers' compensation.
    4. State rehabilitation commission.

13. The client has a fractured right tibia. Which assessment data **warrant immediate** intervention?
    1. The client reports right calf pain.
    2. The nurse cannot palpate the radial pulse.
    3. The client's right foot is cold to touch.
    4. The nurse notes ecchymosis on the right leg.

14. The nurse identifies the problem "high risk for complications" for the client with a right total hip replacement being discharged from the hospital. Which problem would have the **highest priority**?
    1. Self-care deficit.
    2. Impaired skin integrity.
    3. Abnormal bleeding.
    4. Prosthetic infection.

15. The client has sustained severe burns on both the anterior right and left leg and the anterior chest and abdomen. According to the rule of nines, what **percentage** of the body has been burned?

   [            %            ]

   **Rule of Nines for Establishing Extent of Body Surface Burned**

   | Anatomic Surface | Total Body Surface (%) |
   |---|---|
   | Head and neck | 9% |
   | Anterior trunk | 18% |
   | Posterior trunk | 18% |
   | Arms, including hands | 9% each |
   | Legs, including feet | 18% each |
   | Genitalia | 1% |

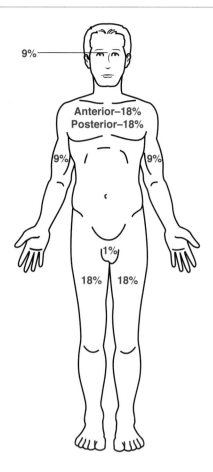

9%

Anterior–18%
Posterior–18%

9% 9%

1%

18% 18%

16. The nurse is planning the care for the client diagnosed with multiple stage IV pressure injuries. Which **complication** results from these pressure injuries?
    1. Wasting syndrome.
    2. Osteomyelitis.
    3. Renal calculi.
    4. Cellulitis.

17. The client comes to the clinic, reporting itching on the left wrist near a wristwatch. The nurse notes an erythematous area along with pruritic vesicles around the left wrist. Which condition should the nurse suspect?
    1. Contact dermatitis.
    2. Herpes simplex 1.
    3. Impetigo.
    4. Seborrheic dermatitis.

18. Which diagnostic test should the nurse expect to be ordered for the client diagnosed with a nevus, which is purple and brown with irregular borders?
    1. Bone scan.
    2. Skin biopsy.
    3. Carcinoembryonic antigen (CEA).
    4. Sonogram.

19. The client diagnosed with a closed head injury is admitted to the neuro-intensive care department following a motor vehicle accident. Which goal is an appropriate short-term goal for the client?

1. The client will maintain an optimal level of functioning.
2. The client will not develop extremity contractures.
3. The client's intracranial pressure will not be greater than 15 mmHg.
4. The client will be able to verbalize feelings of anger.

20. The 25-year-old client diagnosed with a C6 spinal cord injury is crying and asks the nurse, "Why did I have to survive? I wish I was dead." Which statement is the nurse's **best response**?
    1. "Don't talk like that. At least you are alive and able to talk."
    2. "God must have something planned for your life. Pray about it."
    3. "You survived because the people at the accident saved your life."
    4. "This must be difficult to cope with. Would you like to talk?"

21. The client is newly diagnosed with epilepsy. Which statement indicates the client **needs clarification** of the discharge teaching?
    1. "I can drive as soon as I see my HCP for my follow-up visit."
    2. "I should get at least 8 hours of sleep at night."
    3. "I should take my medication every day even if I am sick."
    4. "I will take showers instead of taking tub baths."

22. The RN observes the UAP taking vital signs on an unconscious client. Which action by the UAP **warrants intervention** by the nurse?
    1. The UAP uses a vital sign machine to check the BP.
    2. The UAP takes the client's temperature orally.
    3. The UAP verifies the blood pressure manually.
    4. The UAP counts the respirations for 30 seconds.

23. The client diagnosed with a brain tumor having radiation treatment is developing alopecia. The client and asks, "When will my hair grow back?" Which statement is the nurse's **best response?**
    1. "Your hair should start growing back within 3 weeks."
    2. "Are you concerned your hair will not grow back?"
    3. "It may take months if your hair grows back at all."
    4. "It may take a couple of years for the hair to grow back."

24. Which assessment data indicate the treatment for the client diagnosed with bacterial meningitis is **effective?**
    1. There is a positive Brudzinski's sign and photophobia.
    2. The client tolerates meals without nausea.

3. There is a positive Kernig's sign and elevated temperature.

4. The client is able to flex the neck without pain.

25. The client is being evaluated to rule out Parkinson's disease. Which diagnostic test **confirms** this diagnosis?
    1. A positive magnetic resonance imaging (MRI) scan.
    2. A biopsy of the substantia nigra.
    3. A stereotactic pallidotomy.
    4. There is no test that confirms this diagnosis.

26. The client diagnosed with a transient ischemic attack (TIA) is being discharged from the hospital. Which medication should the nurse expect the HCP to prescribe?
    1. Warfarin.
    2. Low-dose acetylsalicylic acid.
    3. Propranolol.
    4. Valproic acid.

27. The nurse has just received the shift assessment. Which client should the nurse assess **first**?
    1. The client diagnosed with encephalitis reporting myalgia.
    2. The client reporting chest pain.
    3. The client refusing to eat hospital food.
    4. The client scheduled to go to the whirlpool.

28. Which client should the RN charge nurse on the substance abuse unit assign to the licensed practical nurse (LPN)?
    1. The client diagnosed with chronic alcoholism in the unit now 3 days.
    2. The client reporting palpitations and has a history of cocaine abuse.
    3. The client diagnosed with amphetamine abuse and has tried to commit suicide.
    4. The client diagnosed with cannabinoid abuse threatening to leave AMA.

29. The telemetry nurse is monitoring the following clients. Which client should the telemetry nurse instruct the primary nurse to assess **first**?
    1. The client diagnosed with occasional premature ventricular contractions (PVCs).
    2. The client post-cardiac surgery with three unifocal PVCs in a minute.
    3. The client diagnosed with myocardial infarction has two multifocal PVCs.
    4. The client diagnosed with atrial fibrillation has an AP of 116 and no P wave.

30. The nurse is teaching the client in a cardiac rehabilitation unit. Which dietary information should the nurse discuss with the client?
    1. No more than 30% of daily food intake should be fats.
    2. Eighty percent of calories should come from carbohydrates.

3. Red meat should comprise at least 50% of daily intake.

4. Monounsaturated fat in the daily diet should be increased.

31. The client diagnosed with end-stage heart failure is being cared for by the home health nurse. Which intervention should the nurse teach the caregiver?
    1. Report any time the client starts having difficulty breathing.
    2. Notify the HCP if the client gains more than 3 lbs. in a week.
    3. Teach how to take the client's apical pulse for 1 full minute.
    4. Encourage the client to participate in 30 minutes of exercise a day.

32. The client is diagnosed with aortic stenosis. Which assessment data indicate a **complication** is occurring?
    1. Barrel chest and clubbing of the fingers.
    2. Intermittent claudication and rest pain.
    3. Pink, frothy sputum and dyspnea on exertion.
    4. Bilateral wheezing and friction rub.

33. The client, after receiving a permanent pacemaker, is admitted to the telemetry floor. The nurse writes the problem "knowledge deficit." Which interventions should be included in the plan of care? **Select all that apply.**
    1. Take tub baths instead of showers from now on.
    2. Avoid holding electrical devices near the pacemaker.
    3. Carry the pacemaker identification card at all times.
    4. Count the radial pulse 1 full minute every morning.
    5. Notify the HCP if the pulse is 12 beats slower than the preset rate.

34. Which question should the nurse ask the client being admitted to rule out infective endocarditis?
    1. "Do you have a history of a heart attack?"
    2. "Have you had a cardiac valve replacement?"
    3. "Is there a family history of rheumatic heart disease?"
    4. "Do you take nonsteroidal anti-inflammatory medications?"

35. The client diagnosed with peripheral arterial disease is prescribed clopidogrel. Which assessment data indicate the medication is **effective?**
    1. The client's pedal pulse is bounding.
    2. The client's blood pressure has decreased.
    3. The client does not exhibit clinical manifestations of a stroke.
    4. The client has decreased pain when ambulating.

36. The client is diagnosed with atherosclerosis and coronary artery disease. The client experiences sudden chest pain when walking to the nurse's station. Which intervention should the nurse implement **first?**
    1. Administer sublingual nitroglycerin.
    2. Apply oxygen via nasal cannula.
    3. Obtain a STAT electrocardiogram.
    4. Have the client sit in a chair.

37. The RN and the UAP are caring for clients on a medical floor. Which nursing task could be delegated to the UAP? **Select all that apply.**
    1. Retake the BP on a client having received a STAT nitroglycerin sublingual.
    2. Notify the health-care provider of the client's elevated blood pressure.
    3. Obtain and document the routine vital signs on all the clients on the floor.
    4. Call the laboratory technician and discuss a hemolyzed blood specimen.
    5. Pass breakfast trays to the clients on the medical floor with diets ordered.

38. The client diagnosed with venous insufficiency tells the nurse, "The doctor just told me about my disease and walked out of the room. What am I supposed to do?" Which statement is the nurse's **best response?**
    1. "I will have your HCP come back and discuss this with you."
    2. "One thing you can do is elevate your legs above your heart while watching TV."
    3. "You will probably need to have surgery within a few months."
    4. "This will go away after you lose about 20 pounds and start walking."

39. The client is admitted with rule-out leukemia. Which assessment data **support** the diagnosis of leukemia?
    1. Cervical lymph node enlargement.
    2. An asymmetrical dark-purple nevus.
    3. Petechiae covering the trunk and legs.
    4. Brownish-purple nodules on the face.

40. The client diagnosed with non-Hodgkin's lymphoma tells the nurse, "I am so tired. I just wish I could die." Which stage of the grieving process does this statement represent?
    1. Anger.
    2. Denial.
    3. Bargaining.
    4. Acceptance.

41. The nurse writes the goal "the client will list three food sources of cobalamin vitamin $B_{12}$" for the client diagnosed with pernicious anemia. Which foods listed by the client indicate the goal has been **met?**
    1. Brown rice, dried fruits, and oatmeal.
    2. Beef, chicken, and pork.
    3. Broccoli, asparagus, and kidney beans.
    4. Liver, cheese, and eggs.

42. The client diagnosed with stomach cancer has developed disseminated intravascular coagulopathy (DIC). Which **collaborative** intervention should the nurse expect to implement?
    1. Prepare to administer intravenous heparin.
    2. Assess for frank hemorrhage from venipuncture sites.
    3. Monitor for a decreased level of consciousness.
    4. Prepare to administer total parenteral nutrition.

43. The nurse is administering 250 mL of packed red blood cells with 50 mL of preservative. The client has no jugular vein distention and has clear breath sounds. After the first 15 minutes, at **what rate** should the nurse set the IV infusion pump?

    [                    ]

44. The 24-year-old African American female client tells the nurse she has a brother with sickle cell disease. She is engaged to be married and is concerned about passing this disease to her future children. Which information is **most important** to provide to the client?
    1. Tell the client that she won't pass this on if she has never had symptoms.
    2. Encourage the client to discuss this concern with her fiancé.
    3. Recommend that she and her fiancé see a genetic counselor.
    4. Discuss the possibility of adopting children after she gets married.

45. The nurse is at home preparing for the 7 a.m. to 7 p.m. shift and has the flu with a temperature of 100.4°F. Which action should the nurse take?
    1. Notify the hospital that the nurse will not be coming into work.
    2. Go to work and wear an isolation mask when caring for the clients.
    3. Request an alternative assignment, not involving direct client care.
    4. Take over-the-counter cold medication and report to work on time.

46. The client is being admitted into the hospital with a diagnosis of pneumonia. Which HCP order should the nurse implement **first?**
    1. Initiate intravenous antibiotics.
    2. Collect a sputum specimen for culture.
    3. Obtain a clean voided midstream urinalysis.
    4. Request a chest x-ray to confirm the diagnosis.

47. Which medical client problem should the nurse include in the plan of care for a client diagnosed with cardiomyopathy?
    1. Heart failure.
    2. Activity intolerance.
    3. Paralytic ileus.
    4. Atelectasis.

48. The client comes to the emergency department reporting pain in the right forearm. The nurse notes a large area of redness and edema over the forearm, and the client has an elevated temperature. Which condition should the nurse suspect?
    1. Cellulitis.
    2. Intravenous drug abuse.
    3. Raynaud's phenomenon.
    4. Thromboangiitis obliterans.

49. The client is performing breast self-examination (BSE) by the American Cancer Society's recommended steps and has completed palpating the breast. Which **step is next** when completing the BSE?
    1. Stand before the mirror and examine the breast.
    2. Lean forward and look for dimpling or retractions.
    3. Examine the breast using a circular motion.
    4. Pinch the nipple to see if any fluid can be expressed.

50. Which assessment information is the **most critical indicator** of a neurological deficit?
    1. Changes in pupil size.
    2. Level of consciousness.
    3. A decrease in motor function.
    4. Numbness of the extremities.

51. The nurse is initiating a blood transfusion. Which interventions should the nurse implement? **Select all that apply.**
    1. Assess the client's lung fields.
    2. Have the client sign a consent form.
    3. Start an IV with a 22-gauge IV catheter.
    4. Hang 250 mL of D$_5$W at a keep-open rate.
    5. Check the EHR for the HCP's order.

52. The nurse is assessing the client diagnosed with psoriasis. Which data support this diagnosis?
    1. Appearance of red, elevated plaques with silvery-white scales.
    2. A burning, prickling row of vesicles located along the torso.
    3. Raised, flesh-colored papules with a rough surface area.
    4. An overgrowth of tissue with an excessive amount of collagen.

53. Which comment by the client, diagnosed with rule-out Guillain-Barré (GB) syndrome, is **most significant** when completing the admission interview?
    1. "I had a bad case of gastroenteritis a few weeks ago."
    2. "I never use sunblock, and I use a tanning bed often."
    3. "I started smoking cigarettes about 20 years ago."
    4. "I was out of the United States for the last 2 months."

54. Which laboratory result **warrants immediate** intervention by the nurse for the female client diagnosed with systemic lupus erythematosus (SLE)?

| Laboratory Test | Client Values | Normal Values |
|---|---|---|
| Serum albumin | 4.5 | 3.4–5 g/dL |
| Hemoglobin (Hgb) | 13 | Male: 14–17.3 g/dL<br>Female: 11.7–15.5 g/dL |
| Hematocrit (Hct) | 40 | Male: 42%–52%<br>Female: 36%–48% |
| White blood cells (WBC) | 15 | 4.5–11.1 × (10³/cells/microL) |
| Erythrocyte sedimentation rate (ESR) | 9 | Adult < 50 yr:<br>  Male: 0–15 mm/hr<br>  Female: 0–25 mm/hr<br>Adult ≥ 50 yr:<br>  Male: 0–20 mm/hr<br>  Female: 0–30 mm/hr |

1. The hemoglobin and hematocrit (Hgb, Hct).
2. The erythrocyte sedimentation rate (ESR).
3. The serum albumin level.
4. The white blood cell count (WBC).

55. The client diagnosed with gastroesophageal reflux disease (GERD) has undergone surgery for a hiatal hernia repair. The client has a nasogastric tube in place. Intravenous fluid replacement is to be at 125 mL/hr plus the amount of drainage. The drainage from 0800 to 0900 is 45 mL. At which **rate** should the IV pump be set for the next hour?

56. Which assessment data indicate to the nurse the client has a conductive hearing loss?
    1. The Rinne test results in air-conducted sound being louder than bone-conducted sound.
    2. The client is unable to hear accurately when conducting the whisper test.
    3. The Weber test results in the sound being heard better in the affected ear.
    4. The tympanogram results in the ticking watch heard better in the unaffected ear.

57. The client reports a painful twisting motion injury of the knee during a basketball game. The client is scheduled for arthroscopic surgery to repair the injury. Which information should the nurse teach the client about postoperative care? **Select all that apply.**
    1. The client should begin strengthening the postsurgical leg.
    2. The client should take pain medication routinely.
    3. The client should remain on bedrest for 2 weeks.
    4. The client should return to the doctor in 6 months.
    5. The client should keep the dressing on the knee dry.

58. The nurse is preparing the client newly diagnosed with asthma for discharge. Which data indicate the teaching about the peak flowmeter has been **effective?**
    1. "I can continue my usual activities without medication if I am in the yellow zone."
    2. "It takes 1 to 2 days to establish my personal best."
    3. "When I can't talk while walking, I need to take my quick-relief medicine."
    4. "When I am in the red zone, I must take my quick-relief medication and not exercise."

59. Which assessment data indicate the client has developed a deep vein thrombosis (DVT) in the left leg?
    1. A negative Homans' sign of the left leg.
    2. Increased left leg calf circumference.
    3. Elephantiasis of the left lower leg.
    4. Brownish pigmentation of the left lower leg.

60. The 85-year-old client diagnosed with severe, end-stage chronic obstructive pulmonary disease has a chest x-ray incidentally revealing an 8-cm abdominal aortic aneurysm (AAA). Which intervention should the nurse implement?
    1. Discuss possible end-of-life care issues.
    2. Prepare the client for abdominal surgery.

    3. Teach the client how to do pursed-lip breathing.
    4. Talk with the family about the client's condition.

61. The UAP notifies the RN that the client diagnosed with chronic obstructive pulmonary disease is reporting shortness of breath and would like his oxygen level increased. Which intervention should the nurse implement?
    1. Notify the respiratory therapist (RT).
    2. Ask the UAP to increase the oxygen.
    3. Obtain a STAT pulse oximeter reading.
    4. Tell the UAP to leave the oxygen alone.

62. Which psychosocial client problem should the nurse write for the client diagnosed with cancer of the lung and metastasis to the brain?
    1. Altered role performance.
    2. Grieving.
    3. Body image disturbance.
    4. Anger.

63. The client diagnosed with cancer of the larynx had a partial laryngectomy. Which client problem has the **highest priority?**
    1. Impaired communication.
    2. Ineffective coping.
    3. Risk for aspiration.
    4. Social isolation.

64. The client receiving a continuous heparin drip reports sudden chest pain on inspiration and tells the nurse, "Something is really wrong with me." Which intervention should the nurse implement **first?**
    1. Increase the heparin drip rate.
    2. Notify the health-care provider.
    3. Assess the client's lung sounds.
    4. Apply oxygen via nasal cannula.

65. The nurse is assessing the client diagnosed with a pneumothorax who has a closed-chest drainage system. Which data indicate the client's condition is **stable?**
    1. There is fluctuation in the water-seal compartment.
    2. There is blood in the drainage compartment.
    3. The trachea deviates slightly to the left.
    4. There is bubbling in the suction compartment.

66. The client is admitted to the intensive care unit diagnosed with rule-out adult respiratory distress syndrome (ARDS). The client is receiving 10 L/min of oxygen via nasal cannula. Which arterial blood gases indicate the client does **not** have ARDS?

    1.

    | Arterial Blood Gas | Client Results | Normal Values |
    |---|---|---|
    | pH | 7.38 | 7.35–7.45 |
    | PCO2 | 45 | 35–45 mmHg |
    | HCO3 | 26 | 22–26 mEq/L |
    | PaO2 | 82 | 80–95 mmHg |

    2.

    | Arterial Blood Gas | Client Results | Normal Values |
    |---|---|---|
    | pH | 7.35 | 7.35–7.45 |
    | PCO2 | 43 | 35–45 mmHg |
    | HCO3 | 24 | 22–26 mEq/L |
    | PaO2 | 74 | 80–95 mmHg |

    3.

    | Arterial Blood Gas | Client Results | Normal Values |
    |---|---|---|
    | pH | 7.45 | 7.35–7.45 |
    | PCO2 | 45 | 35–45 mmHg |
    | HCO3 | 28 | 22–26 mEq/L |
    | PaO2 | 60 | 80–95 mmHg |

    4.

    | Arterial Blood Gas | Client Results | Normal Values |
    |---|---|---|
    | pH | 7.32 | 7.35–7.45 |
    | PCO2 | 55 | 35–45 mmHg |
    | HCO3 | 28 | 22–26 mEq/L |
    | PaO2 | 50 | 80–95 mmHg |

67. The client has gastroesophageal reflux disease. Which HCP order should the nurse **question?**
    1. Elevate the head of the client's bed with blocks.
    2. Administer pantoprazole four times a day.
    3. A regular diet with no citrus or spicy foods.
    4. Activity as tolerated and sit up in a chair for all meals.

68. The client is diagnosed with an acute exacerbation of Crohn's disease. Which laboratory assessment data **warrant immediate** attention?

    | Laboratory Test | Client Results | Normal Values |
    |---|---|---|
    | Glucose | 148 | Fasting <100 mg/dL Random <200 mg/dL |
    | Serum amylase | 100 | 100–300 units/L |
    | White blood cells (WBC) | 10 | 4.5–11.1 × (10³/cells/ microL) |
    | Potassium (K+) | 3.3 | 3.5–5.3 mEq/L or mmol/L |

    1. The client's WBC count.
    2. The client's serum amylase.
    3. The client's potassium level.
    4. The client's blood glucose.

69. Which information should the nurse discuss with the client to prevent an acute exacerbation of diverticulitis? **Select all that apply.**
    1. Increase the fiber in the diet.
    2. Drink at least 1,000 mL of water a day.
    3. Encourage sedentary activities.
    4. Take cathartic laxatives daily.
    5. Avoid heavy lifting.

70. The client diagnosed with peptic ulcer disease is being discharged. Which nursing task can be delegated to a trained UAP?
    1. Complete the discharge instructions sheet.
    2. Remove the client's saline lock.
    3. Clean the client's room after discharge.
    4. Check the client's hemoglobin and hematocrit.

71. The client diagnosed with colon cancer tells the nurse, "All I do is sit and watch TV all day. I can barely go to the bathroom." According to the Oncology Nursing Society's cancer fatigue scale, how would the nurse document the fatigue objectively?

**FATIGUE SCALE**
Select the number that best describes how you feel today

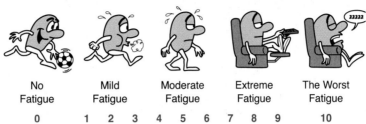

| No Fatigue | Mild Fatigue | Moderate Fatigue | Extreme Fatigue | The Worst Fatigue |
|---|---|---|---|---|
| 0 | 1  2  3 | 4  5  6 | 7  8  9 | 10 |

   1. Mild fatigue.
   2. Moderate fatigue.
   3. Extreme fatigue.
   4. Worst fatigue.

72. The home health nurse must see the following clients. Which client should the nurse assess **first**?
   1. The client postoperative from an open cholecystectomy with green drainage coming from the T-tube.
   2. The client diagnosed with heart failure reporting shortness of breath while fixing meals.
   3. The client diagnosed with AIDS dementia whose family called and reported that the client is vomiting "coffee grounds stuff."
   4. The client diagnosed with end-stage liver disease gaining 3 pounds and unable to wear house shoes.

73. Which data indicate to the nurse the client diagnosed with end-stage liver disease is **improving?**
   1. The client has a tympanic wave.
   2. The client is able to perform asterixis.
   3. The client is confused and lethargic.
   4. The client's abdominal girth has decreased.

74. The nurse is discussing funeral arrangements with the family of a deceased client having organs and tissues donated today. Which information should the nurse discuss with the family?
   1. The family can request an open casket funeral.
   2. Your loved one must wear a long-sleeved shirt.
   3. You might want to have a private viewing only.
   4. This will not delay the timing of the funeral.

75. The public health nurse is discussing hepatitis with a client traveling to a developing country in 1 month. Which recommendations should the nurse discuss with the client? **Select all that apply.**
   1. A gamma globulin injection.
   2. A hepatitis A vaccination.
   3. A PPD skin test on the left arm.
   4. A hepatitis B vaccination.
   5. No additional vaccinations are required.

76. The client diagnosed with chronic pancreatitis is admitted with an acute exacerbation of the disease. Which laboratory result **warrants immediate** intervention by the nurse?
   1. The client's amylase is elevated.
   2. The client's WBC count is WNL.
   3. The client's blood glucose is elevated.
   4. The client's lipase is within normal limits.

77. The client had abdominal surgery and is receiving bag #5 of total parenteral nutrition (TPN) via a subclavian line infusing at 126 mL/hr. The nurse realizes bag #6 is not on the unit and TPN bag #5 has 50 mL left to infuse. Which intervention should the nurse implement?
   1. Decrease the rate of bag #5 to a keep-open rate.
   2. Prepare to hang a 1,000-mL bag of normal saline.
   3. When bag #5 is empty, convert to a heparin lock.
   4. Infuse $D_{10}W$ at 126 mL/hr via the subclavian line.

78. Which **priority** problem should the clinic nurse identify for the client exceeding ideal body weight at 87 kg?
    1. Risk for complications.
    2. Altered nutrition.
    3. Body image disturbance.
    4. Activity intolerance.

79. Which assessment data indicate to the nurse the client diagnosed with diarrhea is experiencing a complication?
    1. Moist buccal mucosa.
    2. A 3.6-mEq/L potassium level.
    3. Tented tissue turgor.
    4. Hyperactive bowel sounds.

80. The client diagnosed with type 2 diabetes mellitus asks the nurse, "What does it matter if my glucose level is high? I don't feel bad." Which statement by the nurse is **most appropriate?**
    1. "The high glucose level can damage your eyes and kidneys over time."
    2. "The glucose level causes microvascular and macrovascular problems."
    3. "As long as you don't feel bad, everything will probably be all right."
    4. "A high blood glucose level will cause you to get metabolic acidosis."

81. The client diagnosed with type 1 diabetes asks the nurse, "What causes me to get dehydrated when my glucose level is elevated?" Which statement would be the nurse's **best response?**
    1. "The kidneys are damaged and cannot filter out the urine."
    2. "The glucose causes fluid to be pulled from the tissues."
    3. "The sweating as a result of the high glucose level causes dehydration."
    4. "You get dehydrated with high glucose because you are so thirsty."

82. The client calls the clinic first thing in the morning and tells the nurse, "I have been vomiting and having diarrhea since last night." Which response is appropriate for the nurse to make?
    1. Encourage the client to eat dairy products.
    2. Have the client go to the emergency department.
    3. Request the client to obtain a stool specimen.
    4. Tell the client to stay on a clear liquid diet.

83. Which clinical manifestations should the nurse expect to assess in the client diagnosed with Addison's disease? **Select all that apply.**
    1. Hypotension and bronze skin pigmentation.
    2. Water retention and osteoporosis.
    3. Hirsutism and abdominal striae.
    4. Truncal obesity and thin, wasted extremities.
    5. Hypotension and hypoglycemia.

84. The client diagnosed with neurogenic diabetes insipidus (DI) asks the nurse, "What is wrong with me? Why do I urinate so much?" Which statement by the nurse is **most appropriate?**
    1. "The islet cells in your pancreas are not functioning properly."
    2. "Your pituitary gland is not secreting a necessary hormone."
    3. "Your kidneys are in failure and you are overproducing urine."
    4. "The thyroid gland is speeding up all your metabolism."

85. The client is admitted into the medical unit diagnosed with heart failure and is prescribed levothyroxine orally. Which intervention should the nurse implement?
    1. Call the pharmacist to clarify the order.
    2. Administer the medication as ordered.
    3. Ask why the client takes levothyroxine.
    4. Request serum thyroid function levels.

86. Which client should the nurse consider **at risk** for developing acute renal failure?
    1. The client diagnosed with essential hypertension.
    2. The client diagnosed with type 2 diabetes.
    3. The client diagnosed with an anaphylactic reaction.
    4. The client after having an autologous blood transfusion.

87. The client diagnosed with chronic renal failure is receiving peritoneal dialysis. Which assessment by the nurse **warrants immediate** intervention?
    1. The dialysate return is cloudy.
    2. There is a greater dialysate return than input.
    3. The client reports abdominal fullness.
    4. The client voided 50 mL during the day.

88. Which action by the UAP requires intervention by the RN?
    1. The UAP used two washcloths when washing the perineal area.
    2. The UAP emptied the indwelling catheter and documented the amount.
    3. The UAP applied moisture barrier cream to the anal area.
    4. The UAP is wiping the client's perineal area from back to front.

89. The UAP empties the indwelling urinary catheter for a client 4 hours postoperative transurethral resection of the prostate then informs the RN the urine is red with some clots. Which intervention should the nurse implement **first?**
    1. Assess the client's urine output immediately.
    2. Notify the HCP that the client has gross hematuria.
    3. Explain this is expected with this surgery.
    4. Medicate for bladder spasms to decrease bleeding.

90. The client with a history of substance abuse presents to the emergency department reporting right flank pain, and the urinalysis indicates microscopic blood. Which intervention should the nurse implement?
    1. Determine the last illegal drug use.
    2. Insert a #22 French indwelling catheter.
    3. Give the client a back massage.
    4. Medicate the client for pain.

91. Which assessment data would make the nurse suspect the client has cancer of the bladder?
    1. Gross painless hematuria.
    2. Burning on urination.
    3. Terminal dribbling.
    4. Difficulty initiating the stream.

92. The client asks the nurse, "What are the risk factors for developing multiple sclerosis?" Which statement is a risk factor for MS?
    1. A close relative with MS may indicate a risk for MS.
    2. Living in the southern United States predisposes a person to MS.
    3. Use of tobacco product is the number-one risk for developing MS.
    4. A sedentary lifestyle can cause a person to develop MS.

93. The older client from the long-term care facility is admitted into the hospital diagnosed with septicemia. Which area of the body is the **most appropriate** place for the nurse to assess the hydration status of the client?

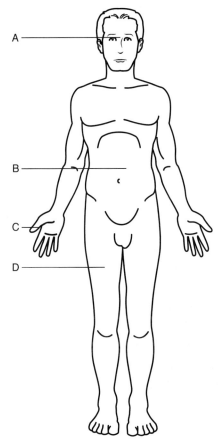

    1. A
    2. B
    3. C
    4. D

94. The student nurse accidentally punctured her finger with a contaminated needle. Which action should the student nurse take **first?**
    1. Notify the infection control nurse.
    2. Allow the puncture site to bleed.
    3. Report to the emergency department.
    4. Cleanse the site with povidone-iodine.

95. The client is admitted to the medical unit reporting severe abdominal pain. Which intervention should the nurse implement **first?**
    1. Assess for complications.
    2. Medicate for pain.
    3. Turn the television on.
    4. Teach relaxation techniques.

96. The female client is admitted to the orthopedic floor diagnosed with a spiral fracture of the arm and multiple contusions and abrasions covering the trunk of the body. Her husband accompanies her. During the admission interview, which intervention is a **priority?**
    1. Notify the local police department of the client's admission.
    2. Provide privacy to discuss how the injuries occurred to the client.
    3. Refer the client to the social worker for names of women's shelters.
    4. Ask the client if she prefers the husband to stay in the room.

97. Which interventions should the emergency department nurse implement for a client with an AP of 122 and a BP of 80/50? **Select all that apply.**
    1. Put the client in reverse Trendelenburg position.
    2. Start an intravenous line with an 18-gauge catheter.
    3. Have the client complete the admission process.
    4. Cover the client with blankets and keep warm.
    5. Request the laboratory to draw a type and crossmatch.

98. The client is 8 hours postoperative for small bowel resection. Which data indicate the client has a complication from the surgery?
    1. A hard, rigid, boardlike abdomen.
    2. High-pitched tinkling bowel sounds.
    3. Absent bowel sounds.
    4. Reports of pain at "6" on the pain scale.

99. Which intervention will help prevent the nurse from being sued for malpractice throughout professional practice?
    1. Keep accurate and legible documentation of client care.
    2. A kind, caring, and compassionate bedside manner at all times.
    3. Maintain knowledge of medications for disease processes.
    4. Follow all health-care provider orders explicitly.

100. According to the nursing process, which interventions should the nurse implement when caring for the client diagnosed with a right-sided cerebrovascular accident (stroke) having difficulty swallowing? **Rank in order of performance.**
    1. Write the client problem of "altered tissue perfusion."
    2. Assess the client's level of consciousness and speech.
    3. Request dietary send a full liquid tray with beverage thickener.
    4. Instruct the UAP to elevate the head of the bed 30 degrees.
    5. Note the amount of food consumed on the dinner tray.

1. 1. Birth control pills regulate the hormones in the body but will not cause changes in the breast tissue.
   2. There is a theory that chocolate increases breast discomfort in women with fibrocystic breast changes.
   3. **During the menstrual cycle, pregnancy, and menopause, variations in breast tissue occur and must be distinguished from the pathological disease. BSE is best performed on days 5 to 7 after menses, counting the first day of menses as day 1. Although BSE is no longer recommended by the American Cancer Society, some women might still be comfortable doing regular self-exams and the nurse should be prepared to provide information (American Cancer Society, 2020).**
   4. Sexual manipulation of the breast does not cause malignant changes in breast tissue.

2. 1. Anemia caused by endometriosis occurs over time and is not an acute complication, such as hemorrhaging.
   2. **Pain is the primary concern of the client; the pain occurs as a result of ectopic tissue bleeding into the abdominal cavity during menses.**
   3. Endometriosis does not cause constipation, and this would not be a priority problem. The client may experience pain during a bowel movement.
   4. Dyspareunia is pain during intercourse, and this client is in the hospital (and unlikely to be having sex there).

3. 1. With a remaining testicle, the client will be able to maintain sexual potency, but radiation and chemotherapy may cause the client to become sterile. Therefore, banking his sperm will allow him to father a child later in life.
   2. Testicular cancer has a 90% cure rate with standard therapy; therefore, completing an advance directive is not a priority.
   3. The client will not be undergoing chemotherapy for at least 6 weeks to allow the client to heal; therefore, this is not a priority intervention.
   4. This is important, but when preparing the client for surgery, the priority intervention is to accomplish presurgical interventions.

4. Correct answers are 4 and 5.
   1. Oral sex still involves mucous membrane–to–mucous membrane contact, and disease transmission is possible; herpes simplex 2 is simply herpes simplex 1 transferred to the genitalia.
   2. This is a myth.
   3. The more often the person engages in sexual contact and the more sexual partners, the more likely the person will contract an STI; however, one time is enough to contract a deadly STI, such as AIDS.
   4. **According to developmental theories, adolescents think they are invincible, and nothing will happen to them. This attitude leads adolescents to participate in high-risk behaviors without regard to consequences.**
   5. **Teenagers and preteens should get vaccinated for HPV, the most common STI prevented by a vaccine (Centers for Disease Control and Prevention, 2016).**

5. 1. Kegel exercises do not have anything to do with activity endurance.
   2. **Kegel exercises are exercises that strengthen the perineal muscles. Multiple pregnancies weaken the pelvic muscles, resulting in bladder incontinence; a report of no stress incontinence indicates the Kegel exercises are effective.**
   3. Kegel exercises do not affect pregnancy.
   4. Kegel exercises do not have anything to do with weight loss.

6. 1. **The pelvic sonogram, which visualizes the ovary using sound waves, is a diagnostic test for an ovarian cyst, which would be suspected with the client's clinical manifestations.**
   2. A CBC may be ordered to rule out appendicitis, but this client does not have right lower abdominal pain.
   3. A KUB x-ray is ordered for a client diagnosed with possible kidney stones.
   4. A CT of the abdomen would not visualize contents in the pelvis.

7. 1. PSA is a tumor marker monitored to determine the progress of the disease and treatment, but it is not monitored before chemotherapy.
2. Serum calcium levels may be monitored to determine metastasis to the bone, but it would not be done before chemotherapy.
3. **The CBC is monitored to determine if the client is at risk for developing an infection or bleeding as a result of the side effects of the chemotherapy medications. The chemotherapy could be held or decreased based on these results.**
4. AFP is a tumor marker monitored to determine the progress of the disease and treatment, but it is not monitored before chemotherapy.

8. 1. This client is showing clinical manifestations of hypovolemic shock and should not be assigned to an inexperienced nurse.
2. Confusion could be a clinical manifestation of many complications after surgery, so this client should not be assigned to an inexperienced nurse.
3. This client is being transferred to the ICU, which indicates the client is not stable; therefore, this client should not be assigned to an inexperienced nurse.
4. **A myelogram is a routine diagnostic test. With minimal instruction, an inexperienced nurse could care for this client.**

9. 1. The RN should encourage the client to maintain independent functioning, and delegating the UAP to feed the client would be encouraging dependence.
2. Although the antacid aluminum hydroxide, magnesium hydroxide, simethicone (Maalox) is an over-the-counter (OTC) medication, a UAP cannot administer any medication to a client.
3. The UAP cannot assess or evaluate any of the client's diagnostic information.
4. **The UAP could assist the client in ambulating to the shower room and assist with morning care.**

10. 1. This would not warrant intervention because this indicates the hose are not too tight.
2. This indicates the hose are not too tight.
3. **There should be no wrinkles in the hose after application. Wrinkles could cause constriction in the area, resulting in clot formation or skin breakdown;** therefore, this would warrant immediate intervention by the charge nurse.
4. Antiembolism hose should not be put over a wound; they would restrict the circulation to the wound and cause a decrease in wound healing.

11. **Correct answers are 2, 3, and 5.**
1. The nurse should suggest a daily walk because bones need stress to maintain strength.
2. **Vitamin D helps the body absorb calcium.**
3. **Smoking interferes with estrogen's protective effects on bones, promoting bone loss.**
4. Lack of exposure to sunlight results in decreased vitamin D, which is necessary for calcium absorption and normal bone mineralization. The client should go outside.
5. **The client is at risk for fractures; therefore, a fall could result in serious complications.**

12. 1. The physical therapist focuses on evaluating, diagnosing movement dysfunctions (injured tissues and structures), and treating these issues. The PT helps restore movement and mobility.
2. **The occupational therapist focuses on evaluating and improving functional abilities to optimize independence and address activities of daily living, which would be an appropriate referral.**
3. Workers' compensation is an insurance provider for the employer and employee to cover medical expenses and loss of wages. This is not an appropriate referral by the rehabilitation nurse.
4. The client may need this referral, but after the occupational therapist has worked with the client and determined the ability to perform skills.

13. 1. The nurse would expect the client diagnosed with a fractured right leg to have pain, but it would not warrant immediate intervention.
2. The nurse would assess the client's pedal or posterior tibial pulse for a client diagnosed with a fractured right tibia.
3. **Any abnormal neurovascular assessment data, such as coldness, paralysis, or paresthesia, warrant immediate intervention by the nurse.**
4. Ecchymosis is bruising and would be expected in the client diagnosed with a fractured tibia.

14. 1. The client is being discharged, so a self-care deficit would not be a potential complication.
    2. The client is being discharged and is ambulating; therefore, impaired skin integrity should not be a problem.
    3. The client would have been taking a prophylactic anticoagulant but would not be at risk for abnormal bleeding.
    4. **The client must inform all HCPs, especially the dentist, of the hip prosthesis, because the client should be taking prophylactic antibiotics before any invasive procedure. Any bacteria invading the body may cause an infection in the joint, and this may result in the client having the prosthesis removed (American Dental Association, 2019).**

15. 36%.
    Each leg is 18%, with the anterior surface (front) being 9%. Because the anterior of both legs are burned (9% each), that would be 18%. That 18% plus the anterior surface of the trunk, which is 18%, totals 36% of the total body surface burned.

16. 1. Wasting syndrome occurs in clients diagnosed with protein-calorie malnutrition. This syndrome leads to pressure injuries not healing, but it is not a complication of the pressure injury.
    2. **Stage IV pressure injuries frequently extend to the bone tissue, predisposing the client to develop a bone infection—osteomyelitis—which can rarely be treated effectively.**
    3. Renal calculi may be a result of immobility, but they are not a complication of pressure injuries.
    4. Cellulitis is an inflammation of the skin, which is not a complication of pressure injuries.

17. 1. **Contact dermatitis is a type of dermatitis caused by a hypersensitivity response. In this case, it is a hypersensitivity reaction to metal salts in the watch the client is wearing. Any time the nurse assesses redness or irritation in areas where jewelry (such as rings, watches, necklaces) or clothing (such as socks, shoes, or gloves) are worn, the nurse should suspect contact dermatitis.**
    2. Herpes simplex 1 virus occurs in oral or nasal mucous membranes.
    3. Impetigo is a superficial infection of the skin caused by a staph or strep infection and occurs on the body, face, hands, or neck.

    4. Seborrheic dermatitis is a chronic inflammation of the skin involving the scalp, eyebrows, eyelids, ear canals, nasolabial folds, axillae, and trunk.

18. 1. A bone scan would not be ordered unless a biopsy proves malignant melanoma.
    2. **This is an abnormal-appearing mole on the skin, and the HCP would order a biopsy to confirm skin cancer.**
    3. A CEA is a test used to mark the presence or prognosis of several cancers but not skin cancer.
    4. A sonogram would not be ordered to diagnose skin cancer.

19. 1. This could be an appropriate long-term goal for the client based on the extent of the injury, but it is not an appropriate short-term goal.
    2. This is an appropriate long-term goal to prevent immobility complications, but it is not an appropriate short-term goal.
    3. **The worst-case scenario with a closed head injury is increased intracranial pressure resulting in death. An appropriate short-term goal would be the intracranial pressure remaining within normal limits, which is 7 to 15 mmHg.**
    4. This is a psychosocial goal, which would not be a short-term goal, and the client may not be angry. The stem did not indicate the client is angry.

20. 1. This is negating the client's feelings and will abruptly end any conversation the client may want or need to have.
    2. This is imposing the nurse's religious beliefs on the client, and these are clichés, which do not address the client's feelings.
    3. This is explaining why the client survived, but the client isn't really asking for information. The client is expressing and showing emotions that must be addressed by the nurse.
    4. **This is a therapeutic response that allows the client to verbalize feelings.**

21. 1. This statement indicates the client does not understand the discharge teaching. The client will not be able to drive until the client is seizure-free for a certain period of time. The laws in each state differ.
    2. Lack of sleep is a risk factor for having seizures.
    3. Noncompliance with medication is a risk factor for having a seizure.
    4. If the client has a seizure in the bathtub, the client could drown.

22. 1. Using the vital sign machine to take the client's BP is an appropriate intervention.
   2. **The body temperature of an unconscious client should never be taken by mouth because the client is unable to hold the thermometer safely.**
   3. Manually verifying the blood pressure is an appropriate intervention if the UAP questions the automatic blood pressure reading. This action should be praised.
   4. Counting the respiration for 30 seconds and multiplying by 2 is appropriate.

23. 1. This is incorrect information for radiation therapy. It is correct for chemotherapy.
   2. This is a therapeutic response, which does not answer the client's question.
   3. **Radiation therapy can cause permanent damage to the hair follicles, and the hair may not grow back at all; the nurse should answer the client's question honestly.**
   4. This is not a true statement.

24. 1. A positive Brudzinski's sign—flexion of the knees and hip when the neck is flexed—indicates the presence of meningitis. Therefore, the treatment is not effective. Sensitivity to light is a common clinical manifestation of meningitis.
   2. This does not indicate whether the meningitis is resolving.
   3. Kernig's sign—the leg cannot be extended when the client is lying with the thigh flexed on the abdomen—is a clinical manifestation of meningitis. An elevated temperature indicates the client still has meningitis.
   4. **The client does not have nuchal rigidity, which indicates the client's treatment is effective.**

25. 1. An MRI is not able to confirm the diagnosis of Parkinson's disease.
   2. This is the portion of the brain where Parkinson's disease originates, but this area lies deep in the brain and cannot be biopsied.
   3. This is a surgery that relieves some of the clinical manifestations of Parkinson's disease. To be eligible for this procedure, the client must have failed to achieve an adequate response with medical treatment.
   4. **Many diagnostic tests are completed to rule out other diagnoses, but Parkinson's disease is diagnosed based on the clinical presentation of the client and the presence of two of the three cardinal manifestations: tremor, muscle rigidity, and bradykinesia.**

26. 1. An oral coagulant such as warfarin (Coumadin) is ordered if the TIA was caused by atrial fibrillation, and that information is not presented in the stem.
   2. **Atherosclerosis is the most common cause of a TIA or stroke, and taking a low-dose acetylsalicylic acid (aspirin) [ASA], antiplatelet medication, every day helps prevent clot formation around plaques.**
   3. If the client had hypertension, then the beta blocker propranolol (Inderal) may be prescribed, but this information is not in the stem.
   4. Anticonvulsant medications, such as valproic acid (Depakote), are not prescribed to help prevent TIAs.

27. 1. Myalgia is muscle pain, which is expected in a client diagnosed with encephalitis.
   2. **The client reporting chest pain is the priority. Remember Maslow's hierarchy of needs.**
   3. Refusing to eat hospital food is not a priority.
   4. The client going to the whirlpool is stable and is not a priority over chest pain.

28. 1. The client should be assessed for delirium tremens and should be assigned to an RN.
   2. Palpitations indicate cardiac involvement, and because the client has a history of cocaine abuse, this client should be assigned to an RN.
   3. This client is at high risk for injury to self and should be assigned to an RN and be on one-to-one precautions.
   4. **The client has a right to leave against medical advice (AMA), and marijuana abuse is not life-threatening to him or to others. Therefore, the LPN could be assigned to this client.**

29. 1. An occasional PVC does not warrant intervention; it is normal for most clients.
   2. Less than six unifocal PVCs in 1 minute is not life-threatening.
   3. **Multifocal PVCs indicate the ventricle is irritable, and this client is at risk for a cardiac event such as ventricular fibrillation.**
   4. Atrial fibrillation is not life-threatening, and the nurse would expect the client not to have a P wave when exhibiting this dysrhythmia.

30. 1. This is a correct statement. The recommended proportions of food are 50% carbohydrates, 30% or less from fat, and 20% protein.
    2. Only 50% of the calories should come from carbohydrates.
    3. Red meat is an excellent source of protein but should only comprise 20% of the diet, and red meat is very high in fat.
    4. Polyunsaturated fats, not the monounsaturated fats, are the better fats.

31. 1. The client diagnosed with heart failure will be short of breath on exertion and with activity. The significant other should report difficulty breathing not subsiding with rest or stopping the activity.
    2. Weight gain of 2 to 3 pounds reflects fluid retention as a result of heart failure, which warrants notifying the HCP.
    3. The caregiver must not administer the digoxin if the radial pulse is less than 60 bpm. The apical pulse is more difficult to assess in a client than the radial pulse.
    4. The client diagnosed with end-stage heart failure is dying and should not exercise daily; activity intolerance as a result of decreased cardiac output is the number-one life-limiting problem.

32. 1. Barrel chest and clubbing of the fingers are clinical manifestations of chronic lung disease.
    2. Intermittent claudication and rest pain are clinical manifestations of peripheral arterial disease.
    3. Pink, frothy sputum and dyspnea on exertion are clinical manifestations of heart failure, which occurs when the heart can no longer compensate for the strain of an incompetent valve.
    4. Friction rub occurs with pericarditis, and bilateral wheezing occurs with asthma.

33. Correct answers are 2, 3, and 4.
    1. Once the chest incision heals, the client can shower or bathe, whichever the client prefers.
    2. Electrical devices may interfere with the functioning of the pacemaker.
    3. This alerts any HCP as to the presence of a pacemaker.
    4. The client should be taught to take the radial pulse for 1 full minute before getting out of bed. If the count is more than 5 bpm less than the preset rate, the HCP should be notified immediately because this may indicate the pacemaker is malfunctioning.

    5. The client should notify the HCP if the pulse is 5 bpm less than the preset rate. This may indicate a pacemaker malfunction.

34. 1. Having a history of myocardial infarction is not a risk factor for developing infective endocarditis.
    2. This is why clients must receive prophylactic antibiotic treatment before dental work and invasive procedures.
    3. A personal history of rheumatic fever, not a family history, increases the risk of developing infective endocarditis.
    4. NSAIDs have no effect on the development of infective endocarditis.

35. 1. The client's pedal pulse does not evaluate the effectiveness of this medication.
    2. Clopidogrel (Plavix), an antiplatelet medication, is not administered to help decrease blood pressure.
    3. Clopidogrel (Plavix), an antiplatelet medication, inhibits platelet aggregation and is considered effective when there is a decrease in atherosclerotic events, an example of which is a stroke.
    4. This medication will not help the pain associated with peripheral arterial disease.

36. 1. Sublingual nitroglycerin is the medication of choice for angina, but it is not the first intervention.
    2. Applying oxygen is appropriate, but it is not the first intervention.
    3. A STAT ECG should be ordered, but it is not the first intervention.
    4. Stopping the client from whatever activity the client is doing is the first intervention because this decreases the oxygen demands of the heart muscle and may decrease or eliminate the chest pain.

37. Correct answers are 3 and 5.
    1. This client is unstable and received medication for chest pain. The RN cannot delegate any task for an unstable client.
    2. The UAP cannot notify the HCP because UAPs are not allowed to take verbal or telephone orders.
    3. The UAP can take routine vital signs. The RN must evaluate the vital signs and take action if needed. The nurse should not delegate teaching, assessing, evaluating, or any unstable client.
    4. This is outside the level of a UAP's expertise.
    5. The UAP can pass food trays on the floor to the clients who have diets ordered.

38. 1. This might be what the nurse wants to do, but the nurse should teach the client about the disease process.
2. **Elevating the legs above the heart as much as possible will help decrease edema.**
3. There are no surgical procedures to correct venous insufficiency.
4. Losing weight and walking are excellent lifestyle modifications, but there is no guarantee the venous insufficiency will resolve.

39. 1. Cervical lymph node enlargement would indicate Hodgkin's lymphoma.
2. An asymmetrical dark-purple nevus would indicate malignant melanoma.
3. **Petechiae covering the trunk and legs is one of the indicators of bone marrow problems, which could be leukemia.**
4. Brownish-purple nodules on the face indicate Kaposi's sarcoma, a complication of AIDS.

40. 1. This statement does not represent the anger stage of grieving.
2. This statement does not represent the denial stage of grieving.
3. This statement does not represent the bargaining stage of grieving.
4. **This statement indicates the client is ready to die and is in the acceptance stage of the grieving process.**

41. 1. Brown rice, dried fruit, and oatmeal are sources of nonheme iron. Nonheme iron comes from vegetable sources.
2. Beef, chicken, and pork are sources of heme iron or animal sources of iron.
3. Broccoli, asparagus, and kidney beans are sources of folic acid.
4. Liver, cheese, and eggs are sources of vitamin $B_{12}$.

42. 1. **Heparin interferes with the clotting cascade and may prevent further clotting factor consumption resulting from uncontrolled thromboses formation.**
2. Assessment is an independent intervention; it is not collaborative and does not require an HCP's order.
3. Assessment is an independent intervention; it is not collaborative and does not require an HCP's order.
4. TPN is not a treatment for a client diagnosed with DIC.

43. **150 mL/hr.**
The nurse should infuse the blood in 2 hours because the client does not have clinical manifestations of fluid volume overload.

44. 1. This is a false statement. The client could have the sickle cell trait.
2. This should be discussed with her fiancé, but it is not the most important information.
3. **Referral to a genetic counselor is the most important information to give the client. If she and her fiancé both have the sickle cell trait, there is a 25% chance of a child having sickle cell disease with each pregnancy.**
4. Adoption may be a choice, but at this time, the most important information is to refer the couple to a genetic counselor.

45. 1. **The nurse should stay at home because the nurse will expose all other personnel and clients to the illness. Flu, especially with a fever, places the nurse at risk for secondary pneumonia.**
2. The nurse is ill, and many errors are made when the nurse is not functioning at 100%.
3. Even if the nurse doesn't have direct client care, the nurse will expose other employees to the virus.
4. OTC medications will not prevent the transmission of flu to others, nor will they prevent the nurse from developing secondary pneumonia.

46. 1. The nurse should not administer antibiotics until the culture specimen is obtained.
2. **The sputum must be collected first to identify the infectious organism so appropriate antibiotics can be prescribed. Administering broad-spectrum antibiotics before collecting sputum could alter the culture and sensitivity (C&S) results.**
3. This is not a priority over sputum culture, and getting the antibiotic started.
4. Always treat the client first.

47. 1. **Medical client problems indicate the nurse and the HCP must collaborate to care for the client; the client must have medications for heart failure.**
2. Without an HCP's order, the nurse can instruct the client to pace activities and teach about rest versus activity.
3. Paralytic ileus is a medical problem but would not be expected in a client diagnosed with cardiomyopathy.
4. Atelectasis occurs when airways collapse, which would not occur in a client diagnosed with cardiomyopathy.

48. 1. Cellulitis is the most common infectious cause of limb edema as a result of bacterial invasion of the subcutaneous tissue. This assessment would make the nurse suspect this condition.
    2. Intravenous drug use can cause cellulitis, but the assessment did not include track marks or needle insertion sites.
    3. Raynaud's phenomenon is a form of intermittent arteriolar vasoconstriction resulting in coldness, pain, and pallor of fingertips or toes. The client should keep warm to prevent vasoconstriction of extremities.
    4. Buerger's disease (thromboangiitis obliterans) is a relatively uncommon occlusive disease limited to medium and small arteries and veins. The cause is unknown, but there is a strong association with tobacco use.

49. 1. This step is the first step in BSE.
    2. This is step three in the BSE process.
    3. This is included in steps four and five and is described as using a systematic process of examining the breast. Using circular motions and dividing the breast into wedges or vertical strips to palpate the entire breast is encouraged. This step was described in the stem as having been completed.
    4. **The American Cancer Society no longer recommends breast self-exam as a screening tool for women with an average risk of breast cancer. A woman at high risk may need to be instructed on the process. The last step of BSE after palpation is to express the nipple by gently squeezing the nipple. Any discharge should be brought to the attention of an HCP. Nipple discharge can be caused by many factors such as carcinoma, papilloma, pituitary adenoma, cystic breasts, and some medications.**

50. 1. Changes in pupil size are a late clinical manifestation of a neurological deficit.
    2. A change in the level of consciousness is the first and most critical indicator of any neurological deficit.
    3. A decrease in motor function occurs with a neurological deficit, but it is not the most critical indicator.
    4. Numbness of the extremities occurs with a neurological deficit, but it is not the most critical indicator.

51. Correct answers are 1, 2, and 5.
    1. The nurse must make a decision on the amount of blood to infuse per hour. If the client is showing any clinical manifestation of heart or lung compromise, the nurse will infuse the blood at the slowest possible rate.
    2. Blood products require the client to give specific consent to receive blood.
    3. The IV should be started with an 18-gauge catheter if possible; the smallest possible catheter is a 20-gauge. Smaller gauge catheters break down the blood cells.
    4. Blood is not compatible with $D_5W$; the nurse should hang 0.9% normal saline to keep open.
    5. The nurse should verify the HCP's order before having the client sign the consent form.

52. 1. Most clients diagnosed with psoriasis have red, raised plaques with silvery-white scales.
    2. A burning, prickling row of vesicles located along the torso is the description of herpes zoster.
    3. A raised, flesh-colored papule with a rough surface area is a description of a wart.
    4. An overgrowth of tissue with an excessive amount of collagen is the definition of keloids.

53. 1. The cause of GB syndrome is unknown, but a precipitating event usually occurs 1 to 3 weeks before the onset. The precipitating event may be a respiratory or gastrointestinal viral or bacterial infection.
    2. These are not precipitating events or risk factors for developing GB syndrome.
    3. Smoking is not a risk factor for developing GB syndrome.
    4. GB syndrome is not more prominent in foreign countries than in the United States.

54. 1. A normal hemoglobin is 12 to 15 g/dL, and normal hematocrit is 36% to 45%.
    2. A normal ESR is between 1 and 20 mm/hr for a female client.
    3. A normal albumin level is between 3.5 and 5 g/dL.
    4. The client diagnosed with SLE is at an increased risk for infection, and this WBC count indicates an infection requiring medical intervention.

55. 170 mL/hr.

    125 mL + 45 mL = 170 mL

    The IV pump should be set at this rate.

56. 1. The Rinne test result indicates normal hearing; in conductive hearing loss, the bone-conducted sound is heard as long as or longer than air-conducted sound.
    2. The whisper test is used to make a general estimation of hearing, but it is not used to diagnose for conductive hearing loss specifically.
    3. **The Weber test uses bone conduction to test lateralization of sound by placing a tuning fork in the middle of the skull or forehead. A normal test results in the client hearing the sound equally in both ears.**
    4. The tympanogram (impedance audiometry) measures middle-ear muscle reflex to sound stimulation and compliance of the tympanic membrane by changing air pressure in a sealed ear canal. It does not specifically support the diagnosis of conductive hearing loss.

57. Correct answers are 1 and 5.
    1. **The client should begin exercises that will strengthen the surgical leg as soon as the surgery is completed.**
    2. Pain medication should be taken as needed, not routinely.
    3. The client may ambulate with the restrictions ordered by the surgeon.
    4. The client will return to see the surgeon before 6 months. The surgeon will need to monitor for healing and complications.
    5. **The client will have a dressing on the surgical site that should remain dry. The dressing will stay on for 3 days after surgery and is then covered with adhesive bandages.**

58. 1. Yellow means caution. The client should follow some, but not all, usual activities.
    2. The client's personal best takes 2 to 3 weeks to establish.
    3. When a client can't talk while walking, there is shortness of breath, which indicates the client does not have tight control, but this has nothing to do with the peak flow meter.
    4. **When the client is in the red zone, the client should take the quick-relief medication and should not exercise or follow regular routines.**

59. 1. A positive Homans' sign would indicate a DVT.
    2. **The calf with DVT becomes edematous, so there is an increase in the size of the calf when compared to the other leg.**
    3. Elephantiasis is characterized by tremendous edema, usually of the external genitalia and legs and is not associated with DVT. Elephantiasis is a lymphatic problem, not a venous problem.
    4. The brownish discoloration is a clinical manifestation of chronic venous insufficiency.

60. 1. **The client diagnosed with end-stage COPD would not be a candidate for an AAA repair, although the size of the aneurysm places the client at risk for rupture. Although many nurses do not like to address end-of-life issues, this would be an important and timely intervention.**
    2. The client is not a surgical candidate because of the comorbid condition and age.
    3. The client should know how to pursed-lip breathe at this point in the disease process.
    4. Although the client is 85 years old, the nurse should discuss all health-care issues with the client and not the family. This is a violation of HIPAA.

61. 1. The RN can take care of this situation and does not need to notify the RT.
    2. The UAP cannot increase oxygen. The RN should treat oxygen as a medication. Also, increasing the oxygen level could cause the client to stop breathing as a result of carbon dioxide narcosis.
    3. The pulse oximeter reading will be low because the client has COPD.
    4. **The oxygen level for a client diagnosed with COPD must remain between 2 and 3 L/min because the client's stimulus for breathing is low blood oxygen levels. If the client receives increased oxygen, the stimulus for breathing will be removed, and the client will stop breathing.**

62. 1. Metastasis indicates advanced disease; therefore, altered role performance would not be an appropriate client problem.
    2. **Metastasis indicates advanced disease, and the client should be allowed to express feelings of loss and grieving; the client is dying.**

3. Body image is a psychosocial problem but would not be applicable in this scenario.
4. Anger is part of the grieving process.

63. 1. The client has a partial laryngectomy, and the voice quality may change, but the client can still speak.
2. This is a psychosocial problem, but it is not a priority over a potential physiological problem.
3. **As a result of the injury to the musculature of the throat area, this client is at high risk for aspirating.**
4. This is a psychosocial problem, but it is not a priority over a potential physiological problem.

64. 1. The heparin drip may be increased because the client has now thrown a pulmonary embolus (PE), but this needs an HCP's order.
2. The HCP will be notified because the client has a suspected embolus, but it is not the first intervention.
3. The client has probably thrown a PE, and assessing the lungs will not do anything for a client in imminent risk of death. PEs are life-threatening, and assessing the client is not a priority in a life-threatening situation.
4. **The client probably has a PE, and the priority is to provide additional oxygen, so oxygenation of tissues can be maintained.**

65. 1. **Fluctuation in the water-seal compartment with respirations indicates the system is working properly, and the client is stable.**
2. Blood in the drainage compartment indicates there is a problem because the client is diagnosed with a pneumothorax, and there should not be any bleeding.
3. Any deviation of the trachea indicates a tension pneumothorax, a potentially life-threatening complication.
4. Bubbling in the suction compartment does not indicate a stable or unstable client.

66. 1. **These are normal ABGs, which would not be expected if the client has ARDS.**
2. This client has an oxygen level below 80 to 100; therefore, this client may be developing early ARDS.
3. This is respiratory acidosis, which would be expected in a client diagnosed with ARDS.
4. These are the expected ABGs of a client diagnosed with ARDS. There is a low oxygen level despite high oxygen administration.

67. 1. The HOB is elevated to prevent the reflux of stomach contents into the esophagus.
2. **Proton pump inhibitors are only administered once or twice a day; they should not be given four times a day because the pantoprazole (Protonix) decreases gastric acidity, and the stomach needs some gastric acid to digest foods. The nurse would question this order.**
3. The client is not prescribed any special diet; limiting spicy and citrus foods decrease acid in the stomach.
4. Sitting upright after all meals decreases the reflux of stomach contents into the esophagus.

68. 1. This white blood cell (WBC) level is WNL and would not warrant immediate intervention.
2. This amylase level is within normal limits (100 to 300 units/L).
3. **This potassium level is low as a result of excessive diarrhea and puts the client at risk for cardiac dysrhythmias. Therefore, these assessment data warrant immediate intervention.**
4. The client's blood glucose level is elevated, but it would not warrant immediate intervention for a client diagnosed with Crohn's disease and hypokalemia.

69. Correct answers are 1 and 5.
1. **Increasing fiber will help prevent constipation, the best way to prevent an acute diverticulitis exacerbation.**
2. The client should increase fluid intake to at least 2,000 to 2,500 mL/day to prevent constipation.
3. The client should exercise daily to prevent constipation.
4. The client should take bulk-forming laxatives, which help prevent constipation by adding bulk to the stool. Cathartic laxatives are harsh colonic stimulants and should not be taken on a daily basis.
5. **The client should avoid activities that increase intra-abdominal pressure because it could cause an exacerbation.**

70. 1. The discharge instruction sheet is teaching, which cannot be delegated to a UAP.
2. **The trained UAP can remove a saline lock from a stable client.**
3. The UAP does not clean hospital rooms; this is the housekeeping department's responsibility.
4. The RN cannot delegate evaluation, which is checking the client's laboratory data before discharge; this is out of the UAP's area of expertise.

71. 1. Mild fatigue represents fatigue that the client has only occasionally.
    2. Moderate fatigue would be fatigue occurring about 40% to 60% of the time.
    3. **Extreme fatigue occurs 70% to 90% of the time, which is indicated by the client still being able to watch TV and get to the bathroom.**
    4. The worst fatigue occurs all the time and the client spends most of the day sleeping and is not able to stay awake to watch television.

72. 1. The T-tube is inserted into the common bile duct to drain bile until healing occurs, and bile is green, so this is expected.
    2. The client diagnosed with congestive heart failure would be expected to experience dyspnea on exertion.
    3. **Coffee-ground emesis indicates gastrointestinal bleeding, and this client should be seen first.**
    4. The client diagnosed with end-stage liver disease is unable to assimilate protein from the diet, which leads to fluid volume retention and resulting weight gain. This is expected for this client.

73. 1. The tympanic wave indicates ascites, which is not an indicator of improving health.
    2. Asterixis is a flapping of the hands, which indicates an elevated ammonia level.
    3. Confusion and lethargy indicate increased ammonia levels.
    4. **A decrease in the abdominal girth indicates an improvement in the ascitic fluid.**

74. 1. **The procurement of organs and tissues from the client will not be noticeable if there is an open casket funeral.**
    2. There is no reason for the client to wear a long-sleeved shirt because the skin is not removed from the arms.
    3. There is no reason for a private viewing as a result of the organ and tissue donation.
    4. The funeral may or may not have to be delayed depending on when the procurement team can make arrangements; the nurse should not give false information to the family.

75. **Correct answers are 2 and 4.**
    1. A gamma globulin injection is administered to provide passive immunity to clients exposed to hepatitis.
    2. **Hepatitis A is contracted through the fecal-oral route of transmission; poor sanitary practices in developing countries place the client at risk for hepatitis A.**
    3. This is a test to determine exposure to tuberculosis and does not have anything to do with hepatitis.
    4. **The hepatitis B vaccination is administered for exposure to blood and body fluids and recommended for individuals traveling to a developing country.**
    5. The CDC recommends routine vaccinations for individuals traveling outside the United States. Additionally, the CDC provided travel health notices, updated frequently on their Web site, with recommendations for enhanced precautions and vaccinations (Centers for Disease Control and Prevention, 2020).

76. 1. The client's amylase would be elevated in acute exacerbation of pancreatitis.
    2. The WBC count is not elevated in this disease process.
    3. **In clients diagnosed with chronic pancreatitis, the beta cells of the pancreas are affected, and therefore, insulin production is affected. An elevated glucose level would warrant the nurse assessing the client.**
    4. Lipase is an enzyme that is excreted by the pancreas. Normal lipase levels indicate a normally functioning pancreas.

77. 1. The client could experience hypoglycemia if the rate of infusion is decreased. TPN must be tapered when discontinuing.
    2. Normal saline does not have glucose, so the client would be at risk for hypoglycemia.
    3. The client must be tapered off TPN to prevent hypoglycemia; therefore, the line cannot be converted to a heparin lock.
    4. **Dextrose 10% has enough glucose to prevent hypoglycemia and should be administered until bag #6 arrives at the unit.**

78. 1. This client is overweight but not morbidly obese, which would place the client at risk for complications.
    2. **"Altered nutrition: more than body requirements" is an appropriate client problem for a client weighing 175 pounds.**

3. This is a psychosocial problem, which is not a priority over a physiological problem.

4. The client may or may not be active, but altered nutrition is a priority.

79. 1. A moist mouth indicates the client is not dehydrated.

2. This is within normal limits for potassium—3.5 to 5.5 mEq/L.

3. **Tented tissue turgor indicates dehydration, which is a complication of diarrhea.**

4. Hyperactive bowel sounds would be expected in a client with diarrhea.

80. 1. **The long-term complications of increased blood glucose levels to organs are the primary reasons for keeping the blood glucose level controlled.**

2. This is the medical explanation for keeping the glucose under control, but this answer is not appropriate for laypeople.

3. The client diagnosed with type 2 diabetes often doesn't feel bad, but the organs are still being damaged as a result of increased blood glucose levels.

4. Metabolic acidosis occurs in clients diagnosed with type 1 diabetes, not type 2. Clients diagnosed with type 2 diabetes have hyperosmolar hyperglycemic nonketotic syndrome (HHNS).

81. 1. This is not the rationale as to why the client becomes dehydrated.

2. **The glucose in the bloodstream is hyperosmolar, which causes water from the extracellular space to be pulled into the vessels, resulting in dehydration.**

3. The client has diaphoresis in hypoglycemia, not hyperglycemia.

4. The dehydration causes the client to be thirsty; the thirst does not cause dehydration.

82. 1. Dairy products contain milk and increase flatus and peristalsis. These products should be discouraged.

2. Symptoms lasting less than 24 hours would not warrant the client going to the emergency department; if anything, an appointment at a clinic would be appropriate.

3. A stool specimen may be needed at some point, but not this early in the disease process.

4. **A clear liquid diet is recommended because it maintains hydration without stimulating the gastrointestinal tract; diarrhea and vomiting lasting longer than 24 hours, along with dehydration and weakness, would warrant the client being evaluated.**

83. Correct answers are 1 and 5.

1. **These are clinical manifestations of Addison's disease, which is adrenal cortex insufficiency.**

2. These are clinical manifestations of Cushing's syndrome, which is adrenal cortex hyperfunction.

3. These are clinical manifestations of Cushing's syndrome, which is adrenal cortex hyperfunction.

4. These are clinical manifestations of Cushing's syndrome, which is adrenal cortex hyperfunction.

5. **These are clinical manifestations of Addison's disease.**

84. 1. This would cause the client to have diabetes mellitus.

2. **The pituitary gland secretes vasopressin, the antidiuretic hormone (ADH) causing the body to conserve water, and if the pituitary is not secreting ADH, the body will produce large volumes of dilute urine.**

3. There are two types of diabetes insipidus: neurogenic DI and nephrogenic DI. In neurogenic DI, the pituitary gland fails to produce ADH; in nephrogenic DI, the kidneys fail to respond to ADH.

4. The thyroid gland has nothing to do with DI.

85. 1. There is no reason to question or clarify this order; the nurse is responsible for clarifying the order with the HCP, not the pharmacist.

2. **The thyroid hormone levothyroxine (Synthroid) is prescribed for hypothyroidism. Many older clients have comorbid conditions requiring daily medications, which are not the primary reason for admission into the hospital.**

3. The nurse should know why the client is taking this medication; the thyroid hormone levothyroxine (Synthroid) is prescribed for only one reason, hypothyroidism.

4. The serum thyroid function levels are monitored by the HCP, usually yearly after maintenance doses have been established.

86. 1. The client diagnosed with essential hypertension is at risk for chronic renal failure.
    2. The client diagnosed with diabetes type 2 is at risk for chronic renal failure.
    3. **Anaphylaxis leads to circulatory collapse, which decreases perfusion of the kidneys and can lead to acute renal failure.**
    4. This is a transfusion of the client's own blood, which should not cause a reaction.

87. 1. **A cloudy dialysate indicates an infection and must be reported immediately to prevent peritonitis.**
    2. The dialysate should be greater than the intake, so fluid is being removed from the body.
    3. After infusing 1,000 mL of dialysate, abdominal fullness is not unexpected.
    4. The client voiding any amount does not warrant immediate intervention.

88. 1. Using two washcloths to clean the client's perineal area is an appropriate action to prevent a urinary tract infection.
    2. This action does not require intervention.
    3. Moisture barrier cream is not considered a medication and can be applied by the UAP after the perineum is cleaned.
    4. **The UAP should wipe the area from front to back to prevent fecal contamination of the urinary meatus, which could result in a urinary tract infection.**

89. 1. This is a normal postoperative expectation with this procedure.
    2. This is gross hematuria, but it is expected with this type of surgery, and the nurse should not call the surgeon.
    3. **The client has a three-way indwelling 30-mL catheter inserted in surgery. This type of catheter instills an irrigant into the bladder to flush the clots and blood from the bladder; bloody urine is expected after this surgery.**
    4. The stem does not indicate the client is having bladder spasms and bladder spasms are not causing the bleeding. Clots left in the bladder and not flushed out can cause bladder spasms.

90. 1. This is not pertinent to the client's current situation.
    2. The nurse should strain all the client's urine, but a large indwelling catheter does not need to be inserted into this client; this isn't a bladder stone, it is a ureteral stone.
    3. A back massage is a nice thing to do, but it will not help renal colic caused by ureteral calculi.

    4. **The client should be medicated for pain, which is excruciating, and the client's history of substance abuse should not be an issue.**

91. 1. **This is the most common presenting clinical manifestation of bladder cancer.**
    2. Burning on urination is a clinical manifestation of a urinary tract infection.
    3. Terminal dribbling is a clinical manifestation of benign prostatic hypertrophy.
    4. Difficulty initiating a urine stream is a clinical manifestation of benign prostatic hypertrophy or neurogenic bladder.

92. 1. **A close relation (parent or sibling) diagnosed with MS may indicate a risk for the client also to develop MS. Other common risk factors are age, race, gender, environment, immune factors, and smoking.**
    2. There is a higher incidence of MS in people living in the northeastern United States and Canada, but there is no known reason for this occurrence.
    3. Tobacco use is a risk factor but not the primary risk factor for MS.
    4. A sedentary lifestyle does not predispose a person to develop MS.

93. 1. The eyeball will lose its elasticity secondary to dehydration, but most people do not like the eyes being touched.
    2. **The tissue on the chest is protected from sun exposure and has adequate subcutaneous tissue to provide a more accurate assessment of hydration status.**
    3. The client's hand has decreased subcutaneous tissue and has been exposed to the sun, which results in decreased tissue elasticity, so this is not the best place to assess for skin turgor.
    4. The client's thigh area is not the best place to assess skin turgor.

94. 1. The infection control nurse must be notified, but it is not the first action.
    2. **Allowing the site to bleed allows any pathogen to bleed out; the student nurse should not apply pressure or attempt to stop the flow of blood.**
    3. This would be done to document the occurrence and start early prophylaxis if necessary, but it is not the first intervention.
    4. Cleaning the site with povidone-iodine (Betadine) is an appropriate intervention once the wound is allowed to bleed; this is a needle stick, so the nursing student will not bleed to death.

95. 1. The nurse must rule out any complication requiring immediate intervention before masking the pain with medication. Pain indicates a problem in some instances; pain is expected after surgery, but complications should always be ruled out.
    2. The nurse should not medicate for pain until ruling out complications.
    3. The television provides a distraction, but it is not the first intervention. Assessment is the first intervention.
    4. Teaching relaxation techniques will help the client's pain, but the first intervention must be an assessment to rule out any complication.

96. 1. The police can be notified if the woman requests this course of action; otherwise, this cannot be done. It is not a priority at this time.
    2. The nurse must ensure the husband cannot hear the client discussing how she was injured. The client needs to feel safe when answering these questions because a spiral fracture indicates a twisting motion, and the bruises are on areas covered with clothing. The nurse should suspect abuse with these types of injuries.
    3. The nurse should refer to the social worker if it is determined the client has been abused, but the nurse should not refer during the admission interview.
    4. The nurse should make every attempt to interview the client without the possible abuser present; the client will probably be afraid to tell the nurse she wants the husband to leave the room if he is the abuser.

97. Correct answers are 2, 4, and 5.
    1. The client would be placed in the Trendelenburg position, which is with the head lower than the feet.
    2. The client is in shock and may need blood transfusions; therefore, a large-bore catheter should be started to infuse fluids, plasma expanders, and possible blood.
    3. The admission process cannot be completed by the client because the condition is life-threatening.
    4. The client will be cold as a result of vasoconstriction of the periphery resulting from a low pulse and blood pressure.

    5. The client will more than likely need blood transfusions that require a type and crossmatch.

98. 1. A hard, rigid, boardlike abdomen is the hallmark clinical manifestation of peritonitis, which is a life-threatening complication of abdominal surgery.
    2. This occurs when the client has a nasogastric tube connected to suction and has minimal peristalsis, and it is not a complication of the surgery.
    3. The client has had general anesthesia for this surgery, and absent bowel sounds at 8 hours postoperative does not indicate a complication.
    4. The client with this type of surgery is expected to have pain at a "6" or higher on a 1-to-10 scale; this is not considered a complication.

99. 1. Documentation can help the nurse defend nursing actions if a lawsuit occurs, but it will not help prevent a lawsuit.
    2. Research indicates nurses forming a trusting nurse-client relationship are less likely to be sued; if the nurse were to make an error, the client and family are often more forgiving.
    3. Knowledge of medications will prevent medication errors but will not keep the nurse from being sued. Nurses are human and can make mistakes with medications even if they are knowledgeable.
    4. The nurse is a client advocate and is legally, morally, and ethically required to question the HCP's orders when caring for assigned clients.

100. Correct order is 2, 1, 3, 4, 5.
    2. This is the assessment step, the first step of the nursing process.
    1. Diagnosis is the second step in the nursing process. In this case, it is "altered tissue perfusion."
    3. Planning is the third step of the nursing process.
    4. Implementation is the fourth step in the nursing process.
    5. Evaluation is the last step of the nursing process.

# Glossary of English Words Commonly Encountered on Nursing Examinations

**Abnormality** — defect, irregularity, anomaly, oddity

**Absence** — nonappearance, lack, nonattendance

**Abundant** — plentiful, rich, profuse

**Accelerate** — go faster, speed up, increase, hasten

**Accumulate** — build up, collect, gather

**Accurate** — precise, correct, exact

**Achievement** — accomplishment, success, reaching, attainment

**Acknowledge** — admit, recognize, accept, reply

**Activate** — start, turn on, stimulate

**Adequate** — sufficient, ample, plenty, enough

**Angle** — slant, approach, direction, point of view

**Application** — use, treatment, request, claim

**Approximately** — about, around, in the region of, more or less, roughly speaking

**Arrange** — position, place, organize, display

**Associated** — linked, related

**Attention** — notice, concentration, awareness, thought

**Authority** — power, right, influence, clout, expert

**Avoid** — keep away from, evade, let alone

**Balanced** — stable, neutral, steady, fair, impartial

**Barrier** — barricade, blockage, obstruction, obstacle

**Best** — most excellent, most important, greatest

**Capable** — able, competent, accomplished

**Capacity** — ability, capability, aptitude, role, power, size

**Central** — middle, mid, innermost, vital

**Challenge** — confront, dare, dispute, test, defy, face up to

**Characteristic** — trait, feature, attribute, quality, typical

**Circular** — round, spherical, globular

**Collect** — gather, assemble, amass, accumulate, bring together

**Commitment** — promise, vow, dedication, obligation, pledge, assurance

**Commonly** — usually, normally, frequently, generally, universally

**Compare** — contrast, evaluate, match up to, weigh or judge against

**Compartment** — section, part, cubicle, booth, stall

**Complex** — difficult, multifaceted, compound, multipart, intricate

**Complexity** — difficulty, intricacy, complication

**Component** — part, element, factor, section, constituent

**Comprehensive** — complete, inclusive, broad, thorough

**Conceal** — hide, cover up, obscure, mask, suppress, secrete

**Conceptualize** — form an idea

**Concern** — worry, anxiety, fear, alarm, distress, unease, trepidation

**Concisely** — briefly, in a few words, succinctly

**Conclude** — make a judgment based on reason, finish

**Confidence** — self-assurance, certainty, poise, self-reliance

**Congruent** — matching, fitting, going together well

**Consequence** — result, effect, outcome, end result

**Constituents** — elements, components, parts that make up a whole

**Contain** — hold, enclose, surround, include, control, limit

**Continual** — repeated, constant, persistent, recurrent, frequent

**Continuous** — constant, incessant, nonstop, unremitting, permanent

**Contribute** — be a factor, add, give

**Convene** — assemble, call together, summon, organize, arrange

**Convenience** — expediency, handiness, ease

**Coordinate** — organize, direct, manage, bring together

**Create** — make, invent, establish, generate, produce, fashion, build, construct

**Creative** — imaginative, original, inspired, inventive, resourceful, productive, innovative

**Critical** — serious, grave, significant, dangerous, life threatening

**Cue** — signal, reminder, prompt, sign, indication

**Curiosity** — inquisitiveness, interest

**Damage** — injure, harm, hurt, break, wound

**Deduct** — subtract, take away, remove, withhold

**Deficient** — lacking, wanting, underprovided, scarce, faulty

**Defining** — important, crucial, major, essential, significant, central

**Defuse** — resolve, calm, soothe, neutralize, rescue, mollify

**Delay** — hold up, wait, hinder, postpone, slow down, hesitate, linger

**Demand** — insist, claim, require, command, stipulate, ask

**Describe** — explain, tell, express, illustrate, depict, portray

**Design** — plan, invent, intend, aim, propose, devise

**Desirable** — wanted, pleasing, enviable, popular, sought after, attractive, advantageous

**Detail** — feature, aspect, element, factor, facet

**Deteriorate** — worsen, decline, weaken

**Determine** — decide, conclude, resolve, agree on

**Dexterity** — skillfulness, handiness, agility, deftness

**Dignity** — self-respect, self-esteem, decorum, formality, poise

**Dimension** — aspect, measurement

**Diminish** — reduce, lessen, weaken, detract, moderate

**Discharge** — release, dismiss, set free

**Discontinue** — stop, cease, halt, suspend, terminate, withdraw

**Disorder** — concern, issue, problem, confusion, chaos

**Display** — show, exhibit, demonstrate, present, put on view

**Dispose** — get rid of, arrange, order, set out

**Dissatisfaction** — displeasure, discontent, unhappiness, disappointment

**Distinguish** — separate and classify, recognize

**Distract** — divert, sidetrack, entertain

**Distress** — suffering, trouble, anguish, misery, agony, concern, sorrow

**Distribute** — deliver, spread out, hand out, issue, dispense

**Disturbed** — troubled, unstable, concerned, worried, distressed, anxious, uneasy

**Diversional** — serving to distract

**Don** — put on, dress oneself in

**Dramatic** — spectacular

**Drape** — cover, wrap, dress, swathe

**Dysfunction** — abnormality, impairment

**Edge** — perimeter, boundary, periphery, brink, border, rim

**Effective** — successful, useful, helpful, valuable

**Efficient** — not wasteful, effective, competent, resourceful, capable

**Elasticity** — stretch, spring, suppleness, flexibility

**Eliminate** — get rid of, eradicate, abolish, remove, purge

**Embarrass** — make uncomfortable, make self-conscious, humiliate, mortify

**Emerge** — appear, come, materialize, become known

**Emphasize** — call attention to, accentuate, stress, highlight

**Ensure** — make certain, guarantee

**Environment** — setting, surroundings, location, atmosphere, milieu, situation

**Episode** — event, incident, occurrence, experience

**Essential** — necessary, fundamental, vital, important, crucial, critical, indispensable

**Etiology** — assigned cause, origin

**Exaggerate** — overstate, inflate

**Excel** — stand out, shine, surpass

**Excessive** — extreme, too much, unwarranted

**Exhibit** — show signs of, reveal, display

**Expand** — get bigger, enlarge, spread out, increase, swell, inflate

**Expect** — wait for, anticipate, imagine

**Expectation** — hope, anticipation, belief, prospect, probability

**Experience** — knowledge, skill, occurrence, know-how

**Expose** — lay open, leave unprotected, allow to be seen, reveal, disclose, exhibit

**External** — outside, exterior, outer

**Facilitate** — make easy, make possible, help, assist

**Factor** — part, feature, reason, cause, think, issue

**Focus** — center, focal point, hub

**Fragment** — piece, portion, section, part, splinter, chip

**Function** — purpose, role, job, task

**Furnish** — supply, provide, give, deliver, equip

**Further** — additional, more, extra, added, supplementary

**Generalize** — take a broad view, simplify, make inferences from particulars

**Generate** — make, produce, create

**Gentle** — mild, calm, tender

**Girth** — circumference, bulk, weight

**Highest** — uppermost, maximum, peak, main

**Hinder** — hold back, delay, hamper, obstruct, impede

**Humane** — caring, kind, gentle, compassionate, benevolent, civilized

**Ignore** — pay no attention to, disregard, overlook, discount

**Imbalance** — unevenness, inequality, disparity

**Immediate** — insistent, urgent, direct

**Impair** — damage, harm, weaken

**Implant** — insert, embed, inseminate, graft, prosthesis, fixture

**Impotent** — powerless, weak, incapable, ineffective, unable

**Inadvertent** — unintentional, chance, unplanned, accidental

**Include** — comprise, take in, contain

**Indicate** — point out, be a sign of, designate, specify, show

**Ineffective** — unproductive, unsuccessful, useless, futile

**Inevitable** — predictable, expected, unavoidable, foreseeable

**Influence** — power, pressure, sway, manipulate, affect, effect

**Initiate** — start, begin, open, commence, instigate

**Insert** — put in, add, supplement, introduce

**Inspect** — look over, check, examine

**Inspire** — motivate, energize, encourage, enthuse

**Institutionalize** — place in a facility for treatment

**Integrate** — put together, mix, add, combine, assimilate

**Integrity** — honesty

**Interfere** — get in the way, hinder, obstruct, impede, hamper

**Interpret** — explain the meaning of, make understandable

**Intervention** — action, activity

**Intolerance** — bigotry, prejudice, narrow-mindedness

**Involuntary** — instinctive, reflex, unintentional, automatic, uncontrolled

**Irreversible** — permanent, irrevocable, irreparable, unalterable

**Irritability** — sensitivity to stimuli, fretfulness, quick excitability

**Justify** — explain in accordance with reason

**Likely** — probable, possible, expected

**Logical** — using reason

**Longevity** — long life

**Lowest** — inferior in rank

**Maintain** — continue, uphold, preserve, sustain, retain

**Majority** — the greater part of

**Mention** — talk about, refer to, state, cite, declare, point out

**Minimal** — least, smallest, nominal, negligible, token, minimum

**Minimize** — reduce, diminish, lessen, curtail, decrease to smallest possible

**Mobilize** — activate, organize, assemble, gather together, rally

**Modify** — change, adapt, adjust, revise, alter

**Moist** — slightly wet, damp

**Multiple** — many, numerous, several, various

**Natural** — normal, ordinary, unaffected

**Negative** — not positive, not abnormal, no, harmful, pessimistic

**Negotiate** — bargain, talk, discuss, consult, cooperate, settle

**Notice** — become aware of, see, observe, discern, detect

**Notify** — inform, tell, alert, advise, warn, report

**Nurture** — care for, raise, rear, foster

**Obsess** — preoccupy, consume

**Occupy** — live in, inhabit, reside in, engage

**Occurrence** — event, incident, happening

**Odorous** — scented, stinking, aromatic

**Offensive** — unpleasant, distasteful, nasty, disgusting

**Opportunity** — chance, prospect, break

**Organize** — put in order, arrange, sort out, categorize, classify

**Origin** — source, starting point, cause, beginning, derivation

**Pace** — speed, rate, stride, tempo

**Parameter** — limit, factor, limitation, issue

**Participant** — member, contributor, partaker, applicant

**Perspective** — viewpoint, view, perception

**Position** — place, location, point, spot, situation

**Practice** — do, carry out, perform, apply, follow

**Precipitate** — cause to happen, bring on, hasten, abrupt, sudden

**Predetermine** — fix or set beforehand

**Predictable** — expected, knowable

**Preference** — favorite, liking, first choice

**Prepare** — get ready, plan, make, train, arrange, organize

**Prescribe** — set down, stipulate, order, recommend, impose

**Previous** — earlier, prior, before, preceding

**Primarily** — first, above all, mainly, mostly, largely, principally, predominantly

**Primary** — first, main, basic, chief, most important, key, prime, major, crucial

**Priority** — main concern, given first attention to, order of importance

**Production** — making, creation, construction, assembly

**Profuse** — a lot of, plentiful, copious, abundant, generous, prolific, bountiful

**Prolong** — extend, delay, put off, lengthen, draw out

**Promote** — encourage, support, endorse, sponsor

**Proportion** — ratio, amount, quantity, part of, percentage, section of

**Provide** — give, offer, supply, make available

**Rationalize** — explain, reason

**Realistic** — practical, sensible, reasonable

**Receive** — get, accept, take delivery of, obtain

**Recognize** — acknowledge, appreciate, identify, be aware of

**Recovery** — healing, mending, improvement, recuperation, renewal

**Reduce** — decrease, lessen, ease, moderate, diminish

**Reestablish** — reinstate, restore, return, bring back

**Regard** — consider, look upon, relate to, respect

**Regular** — usual, normal, ordinary, standard, expected, conventional

**Relative** — comparative, family member

**Relevance** — importance of, germane, pertinent, apropos

**Reluctant** — unwilling, hesitant, disinclined, indisposed, averse

**Remove** — take away, get rid of, eliminate, eradicate

**Reposition** — move, relocate, change position

**Require** — need, want, necessitate

**Resist** — oppose, defend against, keep from, refuse to go along with, defy

**Resolution** — decree, solution, decision, ruling, promise

**Resolve** — make up your mind, solve, determine, decide

**Response** — reply, answer, reaction, retort

**Restore** — reinstate, reestablish, bring back, return to, refurbish

**Restrict** — limit, confine, curb, control, contain, hold back, hamper

**Retract** — take back, draw in, withdraw, apologize

**Reveal** — make known, disclose, divulge, expose, tell, make public

**Review** — appraisal, reconsider, evaluation, assessment, examination, analysis

**Ritual** — custom, ceremony, formal procedure

**Rotate** — turn, go around, spin, swivel

**Routine** — usual, habit, custom, practice

**Satisfaction** — approval, fulfillment, pleasure, happiness

**Satisfy** — please, convince, fulfill, make happy, gratify

**Secure** — safe, protected, fixed firmly, sheltered, confident, obtain

**Sequential** — chronological, in order of occurrence

**Significant** — important, major, considerable, noteworthy, momentous

**Slight** — small, slim, minor, unimportant, insignificant, insult

**Source** — basis, foundation, starting place, cause

**Specific** — exact, particular, detail, explicit, definite

**Stable** — steady, even, constant

**Statistics** — figures, data, information

**Subtract** — take away, deduct

**Success** — achievement, victory, accomplishment

**Surround** — enclose, encircle, contain

**Suspect** — think, believe, suppose, guess, deduce, infer, distrust, doubtful

**Sustain** — maintain, carry on, prolong, continue, nourish, suffer

**Synonymous** — same as, identical, equal, tantamount

**Thorough** — careful, detailed, methodical, systematic, meticulous, comprehensive, exhaustive

**Tilt** — tip, slant, slope, lean, angle, incline

**Translucent** — see-through, transparent, clear

**Unique** — one and only, sole, exclusive, distinctive

**Universal** — general, widespread, common, worldwide

**Unoccupied** — vacant, not busy, empty

**Unrelated** — unconnected, unlinked, distinct, dissimilar, irrelevant

**Unresolved** — unsettled, uncertain, unsolved, unclear, in doubt

**Various** — numerous, variety, range of, mixture of, assortment of

**Verbalize** — express, voice, speak, articulate

**Verify** — confirm, make sure, prove, attest to, validate, substantiate, corroborate, authenticate

**Vigorous** — forceful, strong, brisk, energetic

**Volume** — quantity, amount, size

**Withdraw** — remove, pull out, take out, extract

# Abbreviations

| | |
|---|---|
| **A&P repair** | Anterior and posterior repair |
| **AAA** | Abdominal aortic aneurysm |
| **ABG** | Arterial blood gas |
| **ABGs** | Arterial blood gases |
| **a.c.** | Before meals |
| **ACE** | Angiotensin-converting enzyme |
| **ACS** | American Cancer Society |
| **ACTH** | Adrenocorticotropic hormone |
| **AD** | Advance directive |
| **ADH** | Antidiuretic hormone |
| **ADL** | Activities of daily living |
| **AED** | Automated external defibrillator |
| **AIDS** | Acquired immunodeficiency syndrome |
| **AKA** | Above-the-knee amputation |
| **AKI** | Acute kidney injury |
| **ALS** | Amyotrophic lateral sclerosis |
| **ANA** | American Nurses Association |
| **ANC** | Absolute neutrophil count |
| **AORN** | Association of Operating Room Nurses |
| **AP** | Apical pulse |
| **aPTT** | Activated partial thromboplastin time |
| **ARDS** | Acute respiratory distress syndrome |
| **BKA** | Below-the-knee amputation |
| **BMI** | Body mass index |
| **BMP** | Basal metabolic panel |
| **BNP** | B-type natriuretic peptide |
| **BP** | Blood pressure |
| **BPH** | Benign prostatic hypertrophy |
| **BPM** | Beats per minute |
| **BSE** | Breast self-examination |
| **BUN** | Blood urea nitrogen |
| **CAD** | Coronary artery disease |
| **CAM** | Complementary and alternative medicine |
| **CAUTI** | Catheter-associated urinary tract infection |
| **CBC** | Complete blood count |
| **CDC** | Centers for Disease Control and Prevention |
| **CHF** | Congestive heart failure |
| **CKD** | Chronic kidney disease |
| **CLL** | Chronic lymphocytic leukemia |
| **COPD** | Chronic obstructive pulmonary disease |

| | |
|---|---|
| CPAP | Continuous positive airway pressure |
| CPM | Continuous passive motion |
| CPR | Cardiopulmonary resuscitation |
| CRT | Capillary refill time |
| CT | Computed tomography |
| CVA | Cerebrovascular accident |
| CXR | Chest x-ray |
| DI | Diabetes insipidus |
| DIC | Disseminated intravascular coagulation |
| DKA | Diabetic ketoacidosis |
| DM | Diabetes mellitus |
| DNA | Deoxyribonucleic acid |
| DNR | Do not resuscitate |
| DOE | Dyspnea on exertion |
| DOT | Directly observed treatment |
| DRE | Digital rectal examination |
| DVT | Deep vein thrombosis |
| ECG | Electrocardiogram |
| ED | Emergency department |
| EEG | Electroencephalogram |
| EGD | Esophagogastroduodenoscopy |
| EHR | Electronic health record |
| EIA | Exercise-induced asthma |
| ELISA | Enzyme-linked immunosorbent assay |
| EMG | Electromyogram |
| EPA | U.S. Environmental Protection Agency |
| ERCP | Endoscopic retrograde cholangiopancreatography |
| ESR | Erythrocyte sedimentation rate |
| ESRD | End-stage renal disease |
| ET | Endotracheal |
| ET | Endotracheal tube |
| FVD | Fluid volume deficit |
| GB | Guillain-Barré syndrome |
| GERD | Gastroesophageal reflux disease |
| GFR | Glomerular filtration rate |
| GI | Gastrointestinal |
| GI | Gastrointestinal tract |
| H&H | Hemoglobin and hematocrit |
| hCG | Human chorionic gonadotropin |
| $HCO_3$ | Bicarbonate |
| HCP | Health-care provider |
| Hct | Hematocrit |
| HDL | High-density lipoprotein |
| Hgb | Hemoglobin |
| HHNS | Hyperosmolar hyperglycemic nonketotic syndrome |
| HIPAA | Health Insurance Portability and Accountability Act |
| HIT | Heparin-induced thrombocytopenia |
| HIV | Human immunodeficiency virus |
| HLA | Human leukocyte antigen |

| | |
|---|---|
| **HOB** | Head of bed |
| **HPV** | Human papillomavirus |
| **HRT** | Hormone replacement therapy |
| **h.s.** | Hour of sleep (at bedtime) |
| **I&D** | Incision and drainage |
| **I&O** | Intake & output |
| **IBD** | Inflammatory bowel disease |
| **ICD** | Implantable cardioverter defibrillator |
| **ICP** | Intracranial pressure |
| **ICU** | Intensive care unit |
| **IM** | Intramuscular |
| **INR** | International normalized ratio |
| **ITP** | Idiopathic thrombocytopenic purpura |
| **IV** | Intravenous |
| **IVP** | Intravenous push |
| **IVP** | Intravenous pyelogram |
| **IVPB** | Intravenous piggyback |
| **JVD** | Jugular vein distention |
| **LDL** | Low-density lipoprotein |
| **LHRH** | Luteinizing hormone–releasing hormone |
| **LMP** | Low malignancy potential |
| **LMWH** | Low molecular weight heparin |
| **LPM** | Liters per minute |
| **LPN** | Licensed practical nurse |
| **MAR** | Medication administration record |
| **MG** | Myasthenia gravis |
| **MI** | Myocardial infarction |
| **MRI** | Magnetic resonance imaging |
| **MS** | Multiple sclerosis |
| **MSDS** | Material safety data sheet |
| **NCCAM** | National Center for Complementary and Alternative Medicine |
| **NG** | Nasogastric |
| **NG** | Nasogastric tube |
| **NGT** | Nasogastric tube |
| **NP** | Nurse practitioner |
| **NPO** | Nothing by mouth |
| **NS** | Normal saline |
| **NSAID** | Nonsteroidal anti-inflammatory drug |
| **OA** | Osteoarthritis |
| **OR** | Operating room |
| **OTC** | Over-the-counter |
| **P** | Pulse |
| **PACU** | Post-anesthesia care unit |
| **Pao$_2$** | Arterial partial pressure of oxygen |
| **PCA** | Patient-controlled analgesia |
| **Pco$_2$** | Partial pressure of carbon dioxide |
| **PCP** | *Pneumocystis* pneumonia |
| **PD** | Parkinson's disease |
| **PE** | Pulmonary embolus |

| | |
|---|---|
| PEG | Percutaneous endoscopic gastrostomy |
| PEG | Percutaneous endoscopic gastrostomy tube |
| PID | Pelvic inflammatory disease |
| po | By mouth (per os) |
| PRBCs | Packed red blood cells |
| prn | When required (as needed) |
| PSA | Prostate-specific antigen |
| PT | Physical therapy |
| PT | Prothrombin time |
| PTCA | Percutaneous transluminal coronary angioplasty |
| PTSD | Post-traumatic stress disorder |
| PTT | Partial thromboplastin time |
| PVC | Premature ventricular contraction |
| PVD | Peripheral vascular disease |
| R | Respirations |
| R/O | Rule out |
| R/T | Related to |
| RBC | Red blood cell |
| RBCs | Red blood cells |
| ROM | Range of motion |
| RR | Respiratory rate |
| RRT | Rapid response team |
| SARS | Severe acute respiratory syndrome |
| SCA | Sickle cell anemia |
| SCI | Spinal cord injury |
| SIADH | Syndrome of inappropriate antidiuretic hormone |
| SLE | Systemic lupus erythematosus |
| SOB | Shortness of breath |
| SPF | Sun protection factor |
| SQ | Subcutaneous |
| STAT | Immediately |
| STI | Sexually transmitted infection |
| SVT | Supraventricular tachycardia |
| T | Temperature |
| TBI | Traumatic brain injury |
| TENS | Transcutaneous electrical nerve stimulation |
| THR | Total hip replacement |
| TIA | Transient ischemic attack |
| t.i.d. | Three times a day |
| TKR | Total knee replacement |
| TPN | Total parenteral nutrition |
| TURP | Transurethral resection of the prostate |
| UAP | Unlicensed assistive personnel |
| URI | Upper respiratory infection |
| UTI | Urinary tract infection |
| UV | Ultraviolet light |
| V/Q | Ventilation/perfusion |
| WBC | White blood cell |
| WBCs | White blood cells |
| WNL | Within normal limits |

# Appendix A

**Table A.1 The Joint Commission's "Do Not Use" Abbreviation List***

| Do Not Use | Potential Problem | Use Instead |
|---|---|---|
| U (Unit) | Mistaken for "0" (zero), the number "4" (four), or "cc" | Write "unit." |
| IU (International Unit) | Mistaken for "IV" (intravenous) Or the number "10" (ten) | Write "International Unit." |
| Q.D., QD, q.d., qd (daily) Q.O.D., QOD, q.o.d., qod (every other day) | Mistaken for each other; period after the "Q" mistaken for "I," and the "O" mistaken for "I" | Write "daily." Write "every other day." |
| Trailing zero (X.0 mg)† Lack of leading zero (.X mg) | Decimal point is missed. | Write "X mg." Write "0.X mg." |
| MS MSO4 and MgSO4 | Can mean morphine sulfate or magnesium sulfate; confused for one another | Write "morphine sulfate." Write "magnesium sulfate." |

*Applies to all orders and all medication-related documentation that is handwritten (including free-text computer entry) or on preprinted forms.
† Exception: A "trailing zero" may be used only where required to demonstrate the level of prevision of the value being reported, such as for laboratory results, imaging studies that report size of lesions, or catheter/tube sizes. It may not be used in medication orders or other medication-related documentation.

## NORMAL LABORATORY VALUES

These values are obtained from *Davis's Comprehensive Handbook of Laboratory and Diagnostic Tests with Nursing Implications (7th edition)*. Laboratory results may differ slightly depending on the resource manual or the laboratory normal values.

| Arterial Blood Gas | Adult |
|---|---|
| pH | 7.35–7.45 |
| $Pco_2$ | 35–45 mmHg |
| $Hco_3$ | 22–26 mmol/L |
| $Po_2$ | 80–95 mmHg |
| $O_2$ saturation | 95%–99% |

| Chemistry | Adult |
|---|---|
| Cholesterol<br>HDL<br>LDL | Less than 200 mg/dL<br>40–60 mg/dL<br>Less than 100 mg/dL |
| Creatinine | Male: 0.61–1.21 mg/dL<br>Female: 0.51–1.11 mg/dL |
| Glucose | Fasting: Less than 100 mg/dL<br>Random: Less than 200 mg/dL |
| Potassium | 3.5–5.3 mEq/L or mmol/L |
| Sodium | 135–145 mEq/L or mmol/L |
| Calcium | 8.2–10.2 mg/dL |
| Triglycerides | Less than 150 mg/dL |
| Blood urea nitrogen | 8–21 mg/dL<br>Adult over 90 years: 10–31 mg/dL |

| Blood Count | Adult |
|---|---|
| Hematocrit (Hct) | Male: 42%–52%<br>Female: 36%–48% |
| Hemoglobin (Hgb) | Male: 14–17.3 g/dL<br>Female: 11.7–15.5 g/dL |
| Activated partial thromboplastin time (aPTT) | 25–35 seconds |
| Prothrombin time (PT) | 10–13 seconds |
| Red blood cell count (RBC) | Male: 4.21–5.81 ($10^6$ cells/microL)<br>Female: 3.61–5.11 ($10^6$ cells/microL) |
| White blood cell count (WBC) | 4.5–11.1 $\times$ $10^3$/microL |
| Platelets | 140–400 $\times$ $10^3$/microL |
| Erythrocyte sedimentation rate (ESR) | Adult less than 50 years: 0–15 mm/hr<br>Adult 50 years and older: 0–20 mm/hr |

| Drug Levels | Adult |
|---|---|
| Digoxin (Lanoxin) | 0.5–2.0 ng/mL |
| International normalized ratio (INR) | 0.9–1.1 without anticoagulation therapy<br>2–3 with therapy<br>2.5–3.5 if the client has a mechanical<br>  heart valve |
| Lithium | 0.6–1.2 mEq/L |
| Phenytoin (Dilantin) | 10–20 mcg/mL |
| Theophylline (Aminophylline) | 10–20 mcg/mL |
| Valproic acid (Depakote) | 50–125 mcg/mL |
| Vancomycin (trough level) | 5–15 mcg/mL |

| Urinalysis | |
|---|---|
| pH | 4.5–8 |
| Specific gravity | 1.005–1.03 |
| Glucose<br>Ketones<br>Hemoglobin<br>Bilirubin<br>Nitrite<br>Leukocyte esterase | Negative |
| Urobilinogen | Up–1 mg/dL |
| Protein | Less than 20 mg/dL |
| *MICROSCOPIC* | |
| RBC | Less than 5/hpf (high power field) |
| WBC | Less than 5/hpf |
| Bacteria | None seen |

# Appendix B

# SAMPLE NURSING CONCEPT CARE MAP

**CONDITION:** Seizure Disorders

**PHYSIOLOGY:** Seizure disorders are characterized by convulsions or other clinically detectable events caused by a sudden discharge of electrical activity that temporarily interrupts brain activity. In idiopathic seizures, which encompass 75% of all seizures, no cause is identified. In acquired seizure disorder, the causes include acidosis, electrolyte imbalances, hypoglycemia, hypoxia, hyperthermia, alcohol and drug withdrawal, septicemia, brain tumors, head trauma.

### Classification
The source of the seizure within the brain can be localized, called partial, or distributed, called generalized.
1. *Partial seizures* can be simple (consciousness is unaffected) or complex (consciousness is affected).
2. *Generalized seizure* involves loss of consciousness and is further classified by the effect on the body: absence (brief periods of impaired consciousness without convulsions), myoclonic (brief jerky motor movements), clonic (rhythmic jerky movements involving upper and lower extremities), tonic (sudden tonic extension or flexion of neck, head, trunk, extremities), tonic-clonic or grand mal (rhythmic clonic movements with prolonged postictal phase), atonic (brief loss of postural tone resulting in falls and injury).

## HANDOFF COMMUNICATION

| | | | |
|---|---|---|---|
| **S** Situation | Assess what is currently happening in a short statement. | Client presents as _____ | |
| **B** Background | Summarize important past assessment data for your client here. Place lab results and medications on the concept map. | **Age:** <br> **Allergies:** <br> **Isolation:** | **Sex:** <br> **Fall Risk:** |
| **A** Assessment | Use the assessment data to complete your concept map. | **Nursing Diagnosis:** Place the Nursing Diagnoses in prioritized order on the concept map and add any needed for your specific client. <br> **Plan:** Place any further Nursing Interventions Classifications (NIC) needed on the map. | |

## Implement Your Plan of Care

| | | **EVALUATE YOUR CARE** | | |
|---|---|---|---|---|
| **R** Recommendation | Evaluate your nursing care and make recommendations related to the achievement of your desired outcomes. Were they met, or do new goals need to be established? | **Diag** | **Nursing Outcomes Classification (NOC)** | **Outcome met** |
| | | 1 | Client demonstrates behaviors and lifestyle changes to reduce risk factors and protects self from future seizure events and injury. | ☐ Yes <br> ☐ No |
| | | 2 | Client maintains effective respiratory pattern with patent airway and prevention of aspiration. | ☐ Yes <br> ☐ No |
| | | 3 | Client verbalizes increased sense of self-esteem in relation to diagnosis. | ☐ Yes <br> ☐ No |
| | | 4 | Client verbalizes a positive attitude toward life changes. | ☐ Yes <br> ☐ No |
| | | 5 | Client verbalizes identification of options and use of resources. | ☐ Yes <br> ☐ No |

## Nursing Diagnosis1

Risk for injury related to loss of muscle coordination, emotional difficulties.

**NIC:**
**1)** Explore with client the various stimuli such as alcohol, drugs, flashing lights that may precipitate seizure activity; **2)** Maintain bedrest when prodromal signs or aura is present; **3)** Stay with client before and after seizure; **4)** Keep padded side rails up or in accordance with facility protocol. Keep bed in lowest position. Utilize a floor mat if side rails are not available; **5)** If client is out of bed when a seizure begins, assist client to the floor and place head on a soft surface; **6)** Discuss safety measures regarding activities such as climbing ladders, swimming, use of mechanical equipment, driving; **7)** Perform neurological and VS checks after seizure. Reorient client; and **8)** Document preseizure activity, presence of aura, type of seizure, type and duration of motor activity, incontinence, eye activity, vocalizations, respiratory impairment.

## Nursing Diagnosis2

Risk for ineffective airway clearance/breathing pattern related to neuromuscular impairment.

**NIC:**
**1)** Encourage client to empty mouth of dentures or food if aura occurs. Avoid chewing gum or sucking lozenges if seizure can occur without warning; **2)** Place client in a lying position on a flat surface during seizure. Turn head to the side; **3)** Loosen clothing around the neck, chest, and abdominal area; **4)** Turn head to side and suction airway as needed; **5)** Administer supplemental oxygen as needed postictally; and **6)** Use bag-valve mask and prepare for intubation if needed.

## Nursing Diagnosis3

Self-esteem (situational or chronic low) related to stigma associated with condition evidenced by fear of rejection; negative feelings about body.

**NIC:**
**1)** Discuss feelings about diagnosis and perception of threat to self. Encourage expression of feelings; **2)** Identify possible public reaction to condition. Encourage client to refrain from concealing problem; **3)** Avoid overprotecting client, encourage participation in activities; **4)** Stress importance of family remaining calm during seizure activity; and **5)** Refer client to a support group such as Epilepsy Foundation to gain information and ideas for dealing with problems.

## Nursing Diagnosis4

Deficient knowledge regarding condition, prognosis, treatment regimen, self-care, and discharge needs related to information misinterpretation evidenced by increased frequency and lack of control of seizure activity.

**NIC:**
**1)** Review pathology and prognosis of condition and lifelong need for treatment as indicated; **2)** Discuss trigger factors such as loud noises, video games, blinking lights, TV viewing; **3)** Discuss importance of maintaining general health such as adequate rest, moderate exercise, avoidance of alcohol, caffeine, and stimulant drugs; **4)** Evaluate the need for head gear if frequent severe seizures are common; **5)** Discuss local laws pertaining to persons with a seizure disorder; **6)** Recommend taking medications with meals when possible; **7)** Review prescribed drugs and discuss the need to continue therapy; and **8)** Discuss the adverse effects of drugs such as drowsiness, hyperactivity, visual disturbances, rashes, syncope.

## Condition:
### Seizure Disorders
Age:

_ _ _ _ _ _ _ _ _ _ _ _ _ _
Link & Explain
• Nursing Interventions Classification (NIC)
• Laboratory and Diagnostic Procedures
• Medications

## Nursing Diagnosis5

Ineffective coping related to threat of physical and social well-being evidenced by lack of correct information about frequency of seizures.

**NIC:**
**1)** Encourage the client to express feelings, including hostility and anger, denial, depression, and sense of disconnectedness; **2)** Identify previous methods of dealing with life problems; **3)** Determine presence and quality of support systems; **4)** Support behaviors such as increased interest and participation in care; and **5)** Monitor for sleep disturbance, increased difficulty concentrating, statements of lethargy, withdrawal.

## Medications
**a.** Carbamazepine (Tegretol), divalproex (Depakote), gabapentin (Neurontin), topiramate (Topamax)
**b.** Valproic acid (Depakene), clonazepam (Klonopin), phenobarbital, phenytoin (Dilantin)
**c.**
**d.**

## Laboratory & Diagnostic Procedures
**a.** Electrolytes, glucose, BUN, liver function tests, CBC
**b.** Serum drug levels, toxicology screen
**c.** Electroencephalogram (EEG), CT scan, MRI
**d.**

# Bibliography

## All Chapters

Hoffman, J. J., & Sullivan, N. J. (2020). *Medical-surgical nursing* (2nd ed.). F.A. Davis.

Treas, L. S., Wilkinson, J. M., Barnett, K. L., & Smith, M. H. (2018). *Basic nursing: Thinking, doing, and caring* (2nd ed.). F.A. Davis.

Vallerand, A. H., & Sanoski, C. A. (2019). *Davis's drug guide for nurses* (16th ed.). F.A. Davis.

Van Leeuwen, A. M., & Bladh, M. L. (2017). *Davis's comprehensive handbook of laboratory & diagnostic tests with nursing implications* (7th ed.). F.A. Davis.

## Chapter 2

American Stroke Association. (2020). *Stroke symptoms*. https://www.stroke.org/en/about-stroke/stroke-symptoms

Centers for Disease Control and Prevention. (2019). *Epilepsy and seizures in older adults*. https://www.cdc.gov/epilepsy/communications/features/olderadults.htm

Centers for Disease Control and Prevention. (2018). *West Nile virus*. https://cdc.gov/westnile/index.html

Chen, P. H., Tsai, S. Y., Pan, C. H., Chang, C. K., Su, S. S., & Kuo, C. J. (2019). Mood stabilisers and risk of stroke in bipolar disorder. *British Journal of Psychiatry, 15*(1), 409–414. https://doi.org/10.1192/bjp.2018.203

National Center for Advancing Translational Sciences. (2016). *Waterhouse-Friderichsen syndrome*. https://www.rarediseases.info.nih.gov/diseases/9449/waterhouse-friderichsen-syndrome

National Institutes of Health. (2016). *How many people are affected by/at risk for stroke?* https://www.nichd.nih.gov/health/topics/stroke

National Institute of Neurological Disorders and Stroke. (2019). *Amyotrophic lateral sclerosis (ALS) fact sheet*. https://www.ninds.nih.gov/Disorders/Patient-Caregiver-Education/Fact-Sheets/Amyotrophic-Lateral-Sclerosis-ALS-Fact-Sheet

National Institute of Neurological Disorders and Stroke. (2019). *Trigeminal neuralgia fact sheet*. https://www.ninds.nih.gov/Disorders/Patient-Caregiver-Education/Fact-Sheets/Trigeminal-Neuralgia-Fact-Sheet

Snarska, K. K., Bachorzewska-Gajewska, H., Kapica-Topczewska, K., Drozdowski, W., Chorazy, M., Kulakowska, A., & Malyszko, J. (2017) Hyperglycemia and diabetes have different impacts on outcome of ischemic and hemorrhagic stroke. *Archives of Medical Science, 13*(1), 100–108. https://www.ncbi.nlm.nih.gov/pmc/articles/PMC5206364/

Stoker, T. B., Torsney, K. M., & Barker, R. A. (2018). Emerging treatment approaches for Parkinson's disease. *Frontiers in Neuroscience, 12*. http://doi.org/10.3389/frins.2018.00693

West, B., & Varacallo, M. (2019). *Good Samaritan laws*. https://www.ncbi.nlm.nih.gov/books/NBK542176/

## Chapter 3

American Heart Association. (2016). *Devices that may interfere with ICDS and pacemakers.* https://www.heart.org/en/health-topics/arrhythmia/prevention–treatment-of-arrhythmia/devices-that-may-interfere-with-icds-and-pacemakers

American Heart Association. (2020). *Life's simple 7®.* https://www.heart.org/en/professional/workplace-health/lifes-simple-7

Centers for Disease Control and Prevention. (2017). *Leading causes of death.* https://www.cdc.gov/nchs/fastats/leading-causes-of-death.htm

Myocarditis Foundation. (2018). *Cause of myocarditis.* https://www.myocarditisfoundation.org/research-and-grants/faqs/causes-of-myocarditis/

## Chapter 4

American Heart Association. (2018). *Diagnosing and managing hypertension in adults.* https://www.heart.org/-/media/files/health-topics/high-blood-pressure

National Heart, Lung, and Blood Institute. (n.d.). *DASH eating plan.* https://nhlbi.nih.gov/health-topics/dash-eating-plan

National Organization for Rare Disorders. (2019). *Elephantiasis.* https://rarediseases.org/rare-diseases/elephantiasis/

Shaikh, A., O'Leary, B., & Bajwa, T. (2015). Subclavian steal syndrome treated with endovascular repair. *Journal of the American College of Cardiology, 65*(10). https://doi.org/10.1026/S0735-1097(15)60695-7

Teasdale, E. J., Lalonde, A., Muller, I., Chalmers, J., Smart, P., Hooper, J., El-Gohary, M., Thomas, K. S., & Santer, M. (2019). Patients' understanding of cellulitis and views about how best to prevent recurrent episodes: Mixed methods study in primary and secondary care. *British Journal of Dermatology, 180*(4), 810–820. https://doi.org/10/111/bjd.17445

Vallabhaneni, R. (n.d.). Aortoiliac occlusive disease. *Society for Vascular Surgery.* https://vascular.org/patient-resources/vascular-conditions/aortoiliac-occlusive-disease

## Chapter 5

American Red Cross. (2020). *Frequently asked questions.* https://www.redcrossblood.org/faq.html#eligibility.\

American Society of Hematology. (2019). *Hydroxyurea for sickle cell disease.* https://www.hematology.org/education/patients

National Cancer Institute. (2019). *Adult Hodgkin lymphoma treatment.* https://www.cancer.gov/types/lymphoma/patient/adult-hodgkin-treatment-pdq

National Hemophilia Foundation. (2020). *Von Willebrand disease.* https://www.hemophilia.org/Bleeding-Disorders/Types-of-Bleeding-Disorders/Von-Willebrand-Disease

National Organization for Rare Disorders. (2019). *Hereditary spherocytosis.* https://rarediseases.org/rare-diseases/anemia-hereditary-spherocytic-hemolytic/

## Chapter 6

American Cancer Society. (2017). *Radiation therapy for laryngeal and hypopharyngeal cancers.* https://www.cancer.org/cancer/laryngeal-and-hypopharyngeal-cancer/treating/radiation.html

American Cancer Society. (2020). *Cancer facts & figures 2020.* https://www.cancer.org/content/dam/cancer-org/research/cancer-facts-and-statistics/annual-cancer-facts-and-figures/2020/cancer-facts-and-figures-2020.pdf

American Lung Association. (2019). *Asbestosis.* https://www.lung.org/lung-health-diseases/lung-disease-lookup/asbestosis/learn-about-asbestosis

Centers for Disease Control and Prevention. (2018). *Allocating and targeting pandemic influenza vaccine during an influenza pandemic.* cdc.gov/flu/pandemic-resources/pdf/2018-Influenza-Guidance.pdf

Centers for Disease Control and Prevention. (2019). *Mantoux tuberculin skin test.* cdc.gov/tb/publications/posters/images/Mantoux_wallchart.pdf

Centers for Disease Control and Prevention. (2020). *Coronavirus disease 2019 (COVID-19). Infection control guidance for healthcare professionals about coronavirus (COVID-19).* https://cdc.gov/coronavirus/2019-nCoV/hcp/infection-control.html

National Center for Advancing Translational Sciences. (n.d.). *Bronchiolitis obliterans.* https://rarediseases.info.nih.gov/diseases/9551/bronchiolitis-obliterans

Thyroid, Head & Neck Cancer Foundation (THANC). (n.d.). https://headandneckcancerguide.org/adults/cancer-diagnosis-treatments/surgery-and-rehabilitation/cancer-removal-surgeries/neck-dissection/

## Chapter 7

American Cancer Society. (2018). *American Cancer Society guideline for colorectal cancer screening.* https://www.cancer.org/cancer/colon-rectal-cancer/detection-diagnosis-staging/acs-recommendations.html

American Diabetes Association. (2019). *Understanding Carbs. Find your balance. Get smart on carbs.* https://www.diabetes.org/nutrition/understanding-carbs

Banki, F. (2020). *Reflux related adult onset asthma.* Memorial Herman. http://www.memorialhermann.org/digestive/reflux-related-adult-onset-asthma/

Centers for Disease Control and Prevention. (2019). *Handwashing: Clean hands save lives. When and how to wash your hands.* cdc.gov/handwashing/when-how-handwashing.html

Centers for Disease Control and Prevention. (2019). *Salmonella.* cdc.gov/salmonella/index.html

Denis, E. A., Dengo, A. L., Comber, D. L., Flack, K. D., Savia, J., Davy, K. P., & Davy, B. M. (2010). Water consumption increases weight loss during a hypocaloric diet intervention in middle-aged and older adults. *Obesity, 18*(2), 300–307. https://doi.org/10.1038/oby.2009.235

Foodsafety.gov. (2019). *Food poisoning: Bacteria and viruses.* foodsafety.gov/food-poisoning/bacteria-and-viruses#salmonella.

Hepatitis B Foundation. (2019). *What is silymarin (milk thistle), and is it helpful for managing my hepatitis B and D?* https://www.hepb.org/blog/tag/milk-thistle/

National Heart, Lung, and Blood Institute. (2020). *Calculate your body mass index.* https://www.nhlbi.nih.gov/health/educational/lose_wt/BMI/bmicalc.htm

National Institute of Diabetes and Digestive and Kidney Diseases. (2017). *Irritable bowel syndrome (IBS).* https://www.niddk.nih.gov/health-information/digestive-diseases/irritable-bowel-syndrome

Nguyen, D. L., & Morgan, T. (2014). Protein restriction in hepatic encephalopathy is appropriate for selected patients: A point of view. *Hepatology International, 8*(2), 447–451. https://www.ncbi.nlm.nih.gov/pmc/articles/PMC4267851/

Waldum, H. L., Kleveland, P. M., and Sordal, O. F. (2016). *Helicobacter pylori* and gastric acid: An intimate and reciprocal relationship. *Therapeutic Advances in Gastroenterology, 9*(6), 836–844.

## Chapter 8

American College of Gastroenterology. (n.d.). *ERCP: A patient's guide.* https://gi.org/topics /ercp-a-patients-guide/

American Diabetes Association. (2020). *Understanding A1c. A1C does it all.* https://www .diabetes.org/a1c

Lipska, K., Flory, J., Hennessy, S., & Inzucchi, S. (2016). Modifying prescribing guidelines by petitioning the FDA: The metformin experience. *Circulation, 134*(18), 1405–1408. https://doi.org/10.1161/CIRCULATIONAHA.116.023041

Matsusue, E., Fujihara, Y., Maeda, K., Okamoto, M., Yanagitani, A., et. al. (2016). Three cases of mediastinal pancreatic pseudocysts. *Acta Radiologica Open, 5*(6), https: //doi.org/10.1177/2058460116647213

Milas, K. (2020). *Endocrineweb. Radioactive iodine for hyperthyroidism.* https://www .endocrineweb.com/conditions/hyperthyroidism/radioactive-iodine-hyperthyroidism

Ramsey, M. L., Conwell, D. L., & Hart, P. A. (2017). Complications of chronic pancreatitis. *Digestive Diseases and Sciences, 62*(7), 1745–1750. https://www.ncbi.nlm.nih.gov /pubmed/28281169

Salazar, J. J., Ennis, W. J., & Koh, T. J. (2016). Diabetes medications: Impact on inflammation and wound healing. *The Journal of Diabetes Complications, 30*(4), 746–752. https://doi.org/10.1016/j.jdiacomp.2015.12.017

U.S. National Library of Medicine. (2019). *Von Hippel-Lindau syndrome.* https://ghr.nlm .nih.gov/condition/von-hippel-lindau-syndrome

## Chapter 9

American Urological Association. (2019). *Intravesical administration of therapeutic medication.* https://www.auanet.org/guidelines/intravesical-administration-of-therapeutic-medication

Berns, J. S. (2019) *Patient education: Hemodialysis (beyond the basics).* https://www.uptodate .com/contents/hemodialysis-beyond-the-basics

Davis, N. G., & Silberman, M. (2019). *Bacterial acute prostatitis.* https://ncbi.nlm.gov/books /NBK459257/

Federal Drug Administration (2012). *Medication guide.* https://www.accessdata.fda.gov /drugsatfda_docs/nda/2012/202799Orig1s000PharmR.pdf

Lohr, J. W. (2019). *Chronic pyelonephritis.* emedicine.medscape.com/article/245464

National Institute of Diabetes and Digestive and Kidney Diseases. (n.d.). *Hemodialysis.* niddk.nih,gov/health-information/kidney-disease/kidney-failure/hemodialysis.

Saardi, K. M., & Schwartz, R. A. (2016) Uremic frost: A harbinger of impending renal failure. *International Journal of Dermatology, 55*(1), 17–20. https://doi.org/10.1111/ijd.12963.

Society of Urologic Nurses and Associates. (2013). *Prostatitis.* https://www.suna.org /download/members/prostatitisFactSheet.pdf

Thornburg, B., & Gray-Vickrey, P. (2016). Acute kidney injury. *Nursing 2016, 46*(6), 24–34.

U.S. National Library of Medicine. (2019*). Kidney removal-discharge.* medlineplus.gov/ency /patientinstructions/000295.htm.

Vagefi, P. (2018). *Xenotransplantation: How pigs could one day save kidney patients' lives.* utswmed.org/medblog/xenotransplantation-kidney/

## Chapter 10

American Cancer Society. (2015). *New breast cancer guidelines.* cancer.org/latest-news /American-cancer-society-releases-new-breast-cancer- guidelines.html.

American Cancer Society. (2019). *Hormone therapy for prostate cancer.* cancer.org/cancer /prostate-cancer/treating/hormone-therapy.html

American Society of Colon and Rectal Surgeons. (n.d.). *Rectocele expanded information.* fascrs.org/patients/disease-condition/rectocele-expanded-information.

Centers for Disease Control and Prevention. (2013). *Condom fact sheet in brief.* cdc.gov /condomeffectiveness/brief.html.

Komen.org. (2011). *Komen perspectives: Lumpectomy versus mastectomy for early invasive breast cancer.* ww5.komen.org/KomenPerspectives/Komen-Perspectives-Lumpectomy-versus -mastectomy-for-early-invasive-breast-cancer-(February-20110).html.

National Cancer Institute. (2019). *Sentinel lymph node biopsy.* https://www.cancer.gov /about-cancer/diagnosis-staging/staging/sentinel-node-biopsy-fact-sheet

National Cancer Institute. (2018). *Ovarian low malignant potential tumors treatment.* https: //www.cancer.gov/types/ovarian/patient/ovarian-low-malignant-treatment-pdq

Zuckerman, D., & Shapiro, D. (2019). *National Center for Health Research. Talcum powder and ovarian cancer.* center4research.org/talcum-powder-ovarian-cancer/

## Chapter 11

Franchini, M., Marano, G., Mengoli, C., Pupella, S., Vaglio, S., Munoz, M., & Liumbruno, G. (2017). Red blood cell transfusion policy: A critical literature review. *Blood Transfusion, 15*(4), 307–317. https://www.ncbi.nlm.nih.gov/pmc/articles/PMC5490725

National Center for Complementary and Integrative Health. (2017). *Glucosamine and chondroitin for osteoarthritis.* https://www.nccih.nih.gov/health/glucosamine -and-chrondroitin-for-osteoarthritis

National Institute of Arthritis and Musculoskeletal and Skin Diseases. (n.d.). *Bone mass measurement: What the numbers mean.* https://bones.nih.gov/health-info/bone /bone-health/bone-mass-measure

National Institutes of Health. (2019). *Calcium.* ods.od.nih.gov/factsheets/Calcium -HealthProfessional/

Shiva.com. (2019). *Tattoos, piercings, amputation, cremation, and suicide.* shiva.com /learning-center/death-and-mourning/burial/tattoos-amputation-cremation

Topfer, L. (2016). *Portable compression to prevent venous thromboembolism after hip and knee surgery: The ActiveCare system.* Canadian Agency for Drugs and Technology in Health (2016-14). http://ncbi.nlm.nih.gov/books/NBK378970/

## Chapter 12

American Cancer Society. (2019). *How do I protect myself from ultraviolet (UV) rays?* https://www.cancer.org/healthy/be-safe-in-sun.html

Celakovska, J., & Bukac, J. (2017). Severity of atopic dermatitis in relation to food and inhalant allergy in adults and adolescents. *Food and Agricultural Immunology, 28*(1), 121–133. https://doi.org/10.1080/09540105.2016.1228838

Centers for Disease Control and Prevention. (2019). *Lyme disease.* https://www.cdc.gov /lyme/transmission/index.html

Centers for Disease Control and Prevention. (2019). *Parasites.* https://www.cdc.gov /parasites/lice/head/treatment.html

Centers for Disease Control and Prevention. (2019). *Skin cancer.* https://www.cdc.gov/skin /basic_info/symptoms.htm

Clark, A., Imran, J., Madni, T., & Wolf, S. E. (2017). Nutrition and metabolism in burn patients. *Burns & Trauma, 5*(11). http://doi.org/burnstrauma.biomedcentral.com /articles/10.1186/s41038-017-0076-x

The Joint Commission. (2019). *CLABSI Toolkit.* https://www.jointcommission.org/resources /patient-safety-topics/infection-prevention-and-control/central-line-associated -bloodstream-infections-toolkit-and-monograph/clabsi-toolkit—chapter-3/

National Center for Biotechnology Information. (2018). *What helps to get rid of athlete's foot.* https://www.ncbi.nlm.nih.gov/books/NBK279548/

U.S. Department of Health and Human Services. (2019). *Chemical hazard and emergency management. Burn triage and treatment – thermal injury.* https://www.chemm.nlm.nih.gov/burns.htm

Vig, K., Chaudhari, A., Tripathi, S., Dixit, S., Sahu, R., Pillai, S., Dennis, V., & Singh, S. (2017). Advances in skin regeneration using tissue engineering. *International Journal of Molecular Sciences, 18,*789. https://doi.org/10.3390/ijms18040789.

## Chapter 13

American Academy of Dermatology. (2019). *Poison ivy, oak, and sumac: How to treat the rash.* https://www.aad.org/public/everyday-care/itchy-skin/poison-ivy/treat-rash.

American Academy of Ophthalmology. (2019). *Diagnosis.* https://www.aao.org/bcscsnippetdetail.aspx?id=d036a1a0-4cac-4281-837a-4bb2af32171e

Kolaczek, A., Skorupa, D., Antczak-Marczak, M., Kuna, P., & Kupcyzk, M. (2017). Safety and efficacy of venom immunotherapy: A real life study. *Postępy Dermatologii i Alergologii, 34*(2), 159–167. https://doi.org/10.5114/ada.2017.67082

Muscular Dystrophy Association. (2019). *Polymyositis (PM).* https://www.mda.org/disease/polymyositis/medical-management

Myasthenia Gravis Foundation of America. (2019). *For a world without myasthenia gravis.* myasthenia.org.

National Institute of Biomedical Imaging and Bioengineering. (n.d.). *Magnetic resonance imaging (MRI).* https://www.nibib.nih.gov/science-education/science-topics/magnetic-resonance-imaging-mri

National Institute of Neurological Disorders and Stroke. (2019). *Guillain-Barre syndrome.* https://www.ninds.nih.gov/Disorders/Patient-Caregiver-Education/Fact-Sheets/Guillain-Barr%C3%A9-Syndrome-Fact-Sheet

National Institute of Neurological Disorders and Stroke. (2019). *Multiple sclerosis: Hope through research.* https://www.ninds.nih.gov/disorders/all-disorders/multiple-sclerosis-information-page

U.S. Department of Health and Human Services. (2019). What is a preventive HIV vaccine. https://www.aidsinfo.nih.gov/understanding-hiv-aids/fact-sheets/19/96/what-is-a-preventive-hiv-vaccine-

## Chapter 14

Callahan, B. (Ed.). (2015). *Clinical nursing skills: A concept-based approach to learning* (2nd ed.). Pearson.

National Eye Institute (2018*). Facts about age-related macular degeneration.* National Institute of Health. https://www.nei.nih.gov/learn-about-eye-health/eye-conditions-and-diseases/age-related-macular-degeneration

Stewart, S., & Chan, W. (2018). Pneumatic retinopexy: Patient selection and specific factors. *Clinical Ophthalmology, 12,* 493–502. https://doi.org/10.2147/OPTH.S137607

## Chapter 15

American College of Emergency Physicians. (2019). *Hospital emergency management program checklist.* California Hospital Association. https://www.calhospitalprepare.org/post/cha-hospital-activation-emergency-operations-plan-eop-checklist

Centers for Disease Control and Prevention. (2019). *Smallpox.* https://www.cdc.gov/smallpox/prevention-treatment/index.html

Centers for Disease Control and Prevention. (2018). *Radiation and your health*. https://www
.cdc.gov/nceh/radiation/emergencies/arsphysicianfactsheet.htm

Clarkson, L. & Williams, M. (2019). *EMS, mass casualty triage*. https://pubmed.ncbi.nlm
.nih.gov/29083791.

Juurlink, D. N. (2016). Activated charcoal for acute overdose: A reappraisal. *British Journal
of Clinical Pharmacology, 81*(3), 482–487.

National Institute for Occupational Safety and Health (NIOSH). (2014). *Recommendations
for the selection and use of respirators and protective clothing for protection against biological
agents.* DHHS (NIOSH) Publication Number 2009-132. https://www.cdc.gov/niosh
/docs/2009-132/default.html

Srinivasan, N. T., & Schilling, R. (2018). Sudden cardiac death and arrhythmias.
*Arrhythmia & Electrophysiology Review 2018, 7*(2), 111–117. http://doi.org/aerjournal
.com/articles/sudden-cardiac-death-arrhythmias

## Chapter 16

Association of Operating Room Nurses (AORN). (2016). *Guidelines for perioperative practice.*
AORN, Inc.

Harvard Health Publishing. (2018). *Malignant hypertension*. https://www.health.harvard
.edu/a_to_z/malignant-hyperthermia-a-to-z

Kaplow, R. (2010). Care of postanesthesia patients. *Crit Care Nurse, 30*(1), 60–62. https:
//doi.org/10.4037/ccr2010386

Saleh, G. M. (2004). Consent of the blind and visually impaired: A time to change practice.
*British Journal of Ophthalmology, 88*(2), 310–311. https://doi.org/10/1136
/bjo.2003.025239

## Chapter 17

Esteghamati, A., Mazaheri, T., Rad, M. V., & Noshad, S. (2015). Complementary and
alternative medicine for the treatment of obesity: A critical review. *International Journal
of Endocrinology and Metabolic Disorders, 13*(2):e19678.

National Center for Complementary and Integrative Health. (2016). *Asian ginseng.*
National Institutes of Health. https://www.nccih.nih.gov/health/asian-ginseng

## Chapter 18

American Bar Association (March). *Law for older Americans*. https://www.americanbar
.org/groups/public_education/resources/law_issues_for_consumers/patient_self
_determination_act/

American Nurses Association. (2015). *Code of ethics for nurses with interpretive statements.*
American Nurses Association.

Attum, B., Waheed, A., & Shamoon, Z. (2019). *Cultural competence in the care of Muslim
patients and their families.* StatPearls. https://www.ncbi.nlm.nih.gov/books/NBK499933/

Centers for Medicaid and Medicare Services (2008). Medicare and Medicaid programs:
Hospice conditions of participation. *Federal Registry*. https://www.federalregister
.gov/documents/2008/06/05/08-1305/medicare-and-medicaid-programs
-hospice-conditions-of-participation

Chong, P. P., & Avery, R. K. (2017). A comprehensive review of immunization practices
in solid organ transplant and hematopoietic stem cell transplant recipients. *Journal of
Clinical Therapeutics, 39*(8), 1581–1598. https://www.clinicaltherapeutics.com/article
/S0149-2918(17)30774-9/pdf

Drug Enforcement Administration. (n.d.) *Practitioner's manual*, section V–Valid prescription requirements. https://www.deadiversion.usdoj.gov/21cfr/cfr/1306/1306_11.htm

Habkirk, S., & Chang, H. (2017) Scents, community, and incense in traditional Chinese religion. *Material Religion, 13*(2), 156–174.

Jewish Virtual Library. (n.d.). *Death & bereavement in Judaism: Death and mourning.* jewishvirtuallibrary.org/death-and-mourning-in-judaism

National Institute on Aging. (n.d.). *Advanced care planning: Healthcare directives.* https://www.nia.nih.gov/health/advance-care-planning-healthcare-directives

Organ Procurement and Transplantation Network (OPTN). (2019). *Policies.* https://optn.transplant.hrsa.gov/media/1200/optn_policies.pdf#nameddest=Policy_15

Rao, J. K., Anderson, L. A., Lin, F., & Laux, J. P. (2014). Completion of advance directives among U.S. consumers. *American Journal of Preventive Medicine, 46*(1), 65–70.

## Chapter 19

American Academy of Allergy, Asthma, & Immunology. (2019). *Gastroesophageal reflux disease.* https://www.aaaai.org/conditions-and-treatments/related-conditions/gastroesophageal-reflux-disease

American Heart Association. (2016) *Advanced cardiovascular life support: Provider manual.* (16th ed.). American Heart Association.

Centers for Disease Control and Prevention (CDC). (2019). *Adult immunization schedules.* https://www.cdc.gov/vaccines/schedules/hcp/imz/adult.html

Herchline, T. E. (2019). Tuberculosis (TB). *Drugs & diseases.* Medscape. emedicine.medscape.com/article/230802

Knight, J., Madduma-Liyanage, K., Mobley, J. A., Assimos, D. G., & Holmes, R. P. (2016). Ascorbic acid intake and oxalate synthesis. *Urolithiasis, 44*(4), 289–297. https://doi.org/10.1007/s00240-016-0868-7

Prescribers' Digital Reference. (2019). *Valacyclovir hydrochloride–drug summary.* https://www.pdr.net/drug-summary/Valtrex-valacyclovir-hydrochloride-233

## Chapter 20

American Cancer Society. (2020). *American Cancer Society recommendations for the early detection of breast cancer.* https://www.cancer.org/cancer/breast-cancer/screening-tests-and-early-detection/american-cancer-society-recommendations-for-the-early-detection-of-breast-cancer.html

American Dental Association. (2019). *Oral health topics.* https://www/ada.org/en/member-center/oral-health-topics/antibiotic-prophylaxis

Centers for Disease Control and Prevention. (2016). *The lowdown on how to prevent STDs.* https://www.cdc.gov/std/prevention/lowdown/lowdown-text-only.htm

Centers for Disease Control and Prevention (2020). *Traveler's health.* https://wwwnc.cdc.gov/travel/notices

# Illustration Credits

## Chapter 2

Page 56 From Teasdale, G., & Jennett B. Assessment of coma and impaired consciousness. A practical scale. Lancet 1974;2:81–84. Reprinted with permission.

## Chapter 3

Page 75 From Jones: ECG Notes, 2e (2010). Philadelphia: F.A. Davis, with permission.
Page 76 From Geiter: E-Z ECG Rhythm Interpretation (2007). Philadelphia: F.A. Davis, with permission.

## Chapter 11

Page 419 From Wise: Orthopaedic Manual Therapy (2015). Philadelphia: F.A. Davis, with permission.
Page 440 From Williams, L. S., & Hopper, P. D. (2015). Understanding Medical Surgical Nursing, 5e. Philadelphia: F.A. Davis, with permission.

## Chapter 14

Page 520 Image used under license from Shutterstock.com.
Page 521 From Wilkinson, J. M., & Treas, L. S. (2015). Fundamentals of Nursing, 3e. Philadelphia: F.A. Davis Company.
Page 521 From Myers: LPN Notes, 4e (2016). Philadelphia: F.A. Davis, with permission.

## Chapter 18

Page 643 © 1983 Wong-Baker FACES ® Foundation, www.WongBakerFACES.org. Used with permission. Originally published in Whaley & Wong's Nursing Care of Infants and Children. © Elsevier Inc.
Page 644, Table 18-1 The American Nurses Association Code of Ethics for Nurses with Interpretative Statements. Copyright 2001, American Nurses Publishing, American Nurses Foundation/American Nurses Association, Washington, DC. Reprinted with permission.

## Chapter 20

Page 689 Reprinted with permission from the Oncology Nursing Society.

# Index

## A

## Q

## R